The
Washington
Manual® of
Surgery
Fourth Edition

The Washington Manual of Surgery

Fourth Edition

Department of Surgery
Washington University
School of Medicine
St. Louis, Missouri

Mary E. Klingensmith, MD
Keith D. Amos, MD
Douglas W. Green, MD
Valerie J. Halpin, MD
Steven R. Hunt, MD

Foreword by
Timothy J. Eberlein, MD
Bixby Professor and
Chair of Surgery
Director, Siteman Cancer Center
Washington University
School of Medicine
St. Louis, Missouri

LIPPINCOTT WILLIAMS & WILKINS
A **Wolters Kluwer** Company
Philadelphia • Baltimore • New York • London
Buenos Aires • Hong Kong • Sydney • Tokyo

Acquisitions Editor: Brian Brown
Developmental Editor: Jenny Kim
Project Manager: Nicole Walz
Senior Manufacturing Manager: Ben Rivera
Senior Marketing Manager: Adam Glazer
Design Coordinator: Holly McLaughlin
Cover Designer: Marie Clifton
Compositor: TechBooks
Printer: R.R. Donnelley, Crawfordsville

Library of Congress Cataloging-in-Publication Data

The Washington manual of surgery / Department of Surgery, Washington University School of Medicine, St. Louis, Missouri; Mary E. Klingensmith . . . [et al.]; foreword by Timothy J. Eberlein.— 4th ed.
    p. ; cm.
  Includes index.
  ISBN 0-7817-5048-2 (alk. paper)
    1. Surgery, Operative—Handbooks, manuals, etc. I. Title: Manual of surgery. II. Klingensmith, Mary E. III. Washington University (Saint Louis, Mo.). Dept. of Surgery.
  [DNLM: 1. Surgical Procedures, Operative–methods. WO 500 W317 2005]
  RD37.W37 2005
  617′.91—dc22

                                        2005001037

10 9 8 7 6 5 4 3 2 1

Contents

Foreword

This is the fourth edition of *The Washington Manual® of Surgery*. This effort reflects the ongoing commitment by the Department of Surgery at Washington University to the medical education of medical students, residents, and practicing surgeons. The commitment to resident and medical student education began with the first full-time head of the Department of Surgery at Washington University, Dr. Evarts A. Graham (1919–1951). Dr. Graham was a superb educator. He was a founding member of the American Board of Surgery and made seminal contributions to the management of surgical patients. His work in the development of oral cholecystography helped establish the Mallinckrodt Institute of Radiology. His work in identifying the epidemiological link of cigarette smoking to lung cancer was the beginning of our current public health consciousness about the health effects of smoking.

Dr. Carl Moyer (1951–1965) was also a superb educator. Dr. Moyer was particularly well known for his bedside teaching, linking pathophysiology to patient outcome. Dr. Walter Ballinger (1967–1978) incorporated the Halsted traditions of resident education and emphasized the importance of laboratory research in fostering the development of the surgeon/scientist. Dr. Samuel A. Wells (1978–1997) assembled a world-class faculty and increased the focus on research within the Department of Surgery. Dr. Wells also placed a great emphasis on educating academic leaders of surgery. He is currently the group chair and principal investigator of the American College of Surgeons Oncology Group (ACOSOG), where he is helping to translate basic science concepts into improvements in patient care.

The current residents have authored this fourth edition of *The Washington Manual® of Surgery*, ably assisted by faculty coauthor and senior editor Dr. Mary Klingensmith. The combination of resident and faculty authorship has helped to focus the chapters on issues that will be particularly helpful to the reader. This edition of the manual is intended to be a complete reference that provides medical students, residents, and practicing surgeons with brief and logical approaches to the management of patients with various surgical problems. This manual does not attempt to extensively cover pathophysiology or history, but it does provide the most up-to-date and important diagnostic and management information for a given topic. Each chapter has selected references that the reader may use to further his or her education about the topic. The manual is also standardized so that the reader will be able to easily obtain information regardless of the subject matter.

The fourth edition offers several new sections, including an expanded section on endovascular surgical techniques. In the section on breast cancer and breast diseases, there are updates on treatment and new diagnostic techniques, such as ductoscopy and the utilization of MRI. The section on bariatric surgery has been expanded to reflect the increased variety of surgical options and the unique issues associated with the management of these patients. Additionally, the pediatric section has been expanded to include the utilization of minimally invasive surgery in that patient population. Finally, all of the sections have been updated and rewritten to reflect the current standards of practice. The updates have been carefully integrated so that the number of pages remains approximately the same. The goal is to make this edition the most up-to-date and user-friendly edition that we have published.

I am indebted to Dr. Klingensmith for her devotion to this project. Additionally, I feel that the residents and faculty have done an outstanding job in this fourth edition. I hope that you will find *The Washington Manual* ® *of Surgery* a useful tool as you take care of patients with surgical disease.

Timothy J. Eberlein, M.D.
St. Louis, Missouri

Preface

As with the previous three editions, this fourth edition of *The Washington Manual* ® *of Surgery* is designed to complement *The Washington Manual* ® *of Medical Therapeutics.* Written by resident and faculty members of the Department of Surgery, it presents a brief, rational approach to the management of patients with surgical problems. The text is directed to the reader at the level of the second- or third-year surgical house officer, although surgical and nonsurgical attendings, medical students, physician assistants, and others who provide care for patients with surgical problems will find it of interest and assistance. The book provides a succinct discussion of surgical diseases, with algorithms for addressing problems based on the opinions of the physician authors. Although multiple approaches may be reasonable for some clinical situations, this manual attempts to present a single, effective approach for each. We have limited coverage of diagnosis and therapy; this is not an exhaustive surgical reference. Coverage of pathophysiology, the history of surgery, and extensive reference lists have been excluded from most areas. This fourth edition of the manual, whose first edition was published in 1997, followed by editions in 1999 and 2002, includes updates on each topic as well as substantial new material.

This is a resident-prepared manual. Each chapter was updated and revised by a resident with assistance from a faculty coauthor. The project was separated into four subsections; editorial oversight was performed for each section by one of the four chief resident coeditors (Valerie J. Halpin, MD, Chapters 1–9; Steven Hunt, MD, Chapters 10–20; Douglas W. Green, MD, Chapters 21–31; and Keith D. Amos, MD, Chapters 32–42 and the Appendix). The tremendous effort of all involved—residents and faculty members and particularly the chief resident coeditors—is reflected in the quality and consistency of the chapters.

I am indebted to the former senior editor of this work, Gerard M. Doherty, MD, who developed and oversaw the first three editions, then handed over to me an exceptionally well-organized project. I am grateful for the continued outstanding support from Lippincott Williams & Wilkins, who have been supportive of the effort and have supplied dedicated assistance. Lisa McAllister and Brian Brown were tremendously helpful early on, overseeing the transition between senior editors, and Jenny Kim has been a terrific developmental editor, keeping me in line and on schedule.

Finally, I am grateful to have an outstanding mentor and friend in my department chair, Timothy J. Eberlein, MD A faculty contributor, Dr. Eberlein has a very full professional life, overseeing both a productive department and cancer center, yet he continues to appreciate the individuals with whom he interacts. He is an inspiration for his friendship, leadership, hard work, and dedication.

M.E.K.

Contributing Authors

Mary E. Abusief, MD
Resident in Obstetrics and Gynecology
Washington University School of Medicine
Saint Louis, Missouri

Keith D. Amos, MD
Fellow in Surgical Oncology
MD Anderson Cancer Center
Houston, Texas

Richard J. Battafarano, MD
Assistant Professor of Surgery
Washington University School of Medicine
Saint Louis, Missouri

Jay S. Belani, MD
Instructor in Urologic Surgery
Washington University School of Medicine
Saint Louis, Missouri

Morey A. Blinder, MD
Associate Professor of Medicine
Washington University School of Medicine
Saint Louis, Missouri

Joseph Borrelli, Jr., MD
Associate Professor of Orthopaedic Surgery
Washington University School of Medicine
Saint Louis, Missouri

Daniel C. Brennan, MD
Associate Professor of Medicine
Washington University School of Medicine
Saint Louis, Missouri

L. Michael Brunt, MD
Associate Professor of Surgery
Washington University School of Medicine
Saint Louis, Missouri

Timothy G. Buchman, MD, PhD
Professor of Surgery
Washington University School of Medicine
Saint Louis, Missouri

Celine Buckley, MD
Resident in Surgery
Washington University School of Medicine
Saint Louis, Missouri

Arnold D. Bullock, MD
Assistant Professor of Urologic Surgery
Washington University School of Medicine
Saint Louis, Missouri

Barbara M. Buttin, MD
Resident in Obstetrics and Gynecology
Washington University School of Medicine
Saint Louis, Missouri

William Chapman, MD	Professor of Surgery Washington University School of Medicine Saint Louis, Missouri
Michael R. Chicoine, MD	Assistant Professor of Neurological Surgery Washington University School of Medicine Saint Louis, Missouri
T. Philip Chung, MD	Resident in Surgery Washington University School of Medicine Saint Louis, Missouri
J. Perren Cobb, MD	Associate Professor of Surgery Washington University School of Medicine Saint Louis, Missouri
Mark S. Cohen, MD	Resident in Surgery Washington University School of Medicine Saint Louis, Missouri
David E. Cohn, MD	Fellow in Gynecological Oncology Washington University School of Medicine Saint Louis, Missouri
Craig M. Coopersmith, MD	Associate Professor of Surgery Washington University School of Medicine Saint Louis, Missouri
John A. Curci, MD	Assistant Professor of Surgery Washington University School of Medicine Saint Louis, Missouri
Ralph J. Damiano, Jr. MD	Professor of Surgery Washington University School of Medicine Saint Louis, Missouri
Ketan M. Desai, MD	Resident in Surgery Washington University School of Medicine Saint Louis, Missouri
Sekhar Dharmarajan, MD	Resident in Surgery Washington University School of Medicine Saint Louis, Missouri
David W. Dietz, MD	Assistant Professor of Surgery Washington University School of Medicine Saint Louis, Missouri
Jill R. Dietz, MD	Assistant Professor of Surgery Washington University School of Medicine Saint Louis, Missouri
Patrick A. Dillon, MD	Assistant Professor of Surgery Washington University School of Medicine Saint Louis, Missouri

Toby J. Dunn, MD	Fellow in Vascular Surgery Washington University School of Medicine Saint Louis, Missouri
J. Christopher Eagon, MD	Assistant Professor of Surgery Washington University School of Medicine Saint Louis, Missouri
Timothy J. Eberlein, MD	Professor of Surgery Washington University School of Medicine Saint Louis, Missouri
Felix G. Fernandez, MD	Resident in Surgery Washington University School of Medicine Saint Louis, Missouri
James W. Fleshman, MD	Professor of Surgery Washington University School of Medicine Saint Louis, Missouri
Bradley D. Freeman, MD	Assistant Professor of Surgery Washington University School of Medicine Saint Louis, Missouri
Sean C. Glasgow, MD	Resident in Surgery Washington University School of Medicine Saint Louis, Missouri
Jeremy Goodman, MD	Resident in Surgery Washington University School of Medicine Saint Louis, Missouri
Douglas W. Green, MD	Fellow in Vascular Surgery Washington University School of Medicine Saint Louis, Missouri
Bruce L. Hall, MD, PhD	Assistant Professor of Surgery Washington University School of Medicine Saint Louis, Missouri
Valerie J. Halpin, MD	Assistant Professor of Surgery Washington University School of Medicine Saint Louis, Missouri
Bruce Haughey, MD	Professor of Otolaryngology Washington University School of Medicine Saint Louis, Missouri
Virginia M. Herrmann, MD	Professor of Surgery Washington University School of Medicine Saint Louis, Missouri
Thomas J. Herzog, MD	Associate Professor of Gynecological Oncology Washington University School of Medicine Saint Louis, Missouri

Richard S. Hotchkiss, MD, PhD	Professor of Surgery and Anesthesia Washington University School of Medicine Saint Louis, Missouri
David M. Hovsepian, MD	Associate Professor of Surgery Washington University School of Medicine Saint Louis, Missouri
Steven R. Hunt, MD	Fellow in Colon and Rectal Surgery Washington University School of Medicine Saint Louis, Missouri
Christopher J. Hussussian, MD	Plastic Surgery Associates Waukesha, Wisconsin
Abraham Jacob, MD	Resident in Otolaryngology Washington University School of Medicine Saint Louis, Missouri
Cassandra M. Kelleher, MD	Resident in Surgery Brigham & Women's Hospital Boston, Massachusetts
Mary E. Klingensmith, MD	Assistant Professor of Surgery Washington University School of Medicine Saint Louis, Missouri
Elbert Y. Kuo, MD	Resident in Surgery Washington University School of Medicine Saint Louis, Missouri
Jason Lee, MD	Fellow in Vascular Surgery SUNY-Downstate Brooklyn, New York
David Linehan, MD	Associate Professor of Surgery Washington University School of Medicine Saint Louis, Missouri
Udaya Liyanage, MD	Resident in Surgery Washington University School of Medicine Saint Louis, Missouri
Jeffrey A. Lowell, MD	Professor of Surgery Washington University School of Medicine Saint Louis, Missouri
Kim C. Lu, MD	Fellow in Colon and Rectal Surgery Washington University School of Medicine Saint Louis, Missouri
Susan E. Mackinnon, MD	Professor of Surgery Washington University School of Medicine Saint Louis, Missouri

Julie A. Margenthaler, MD
Resident in Surgery
Washington University School of Medicine
Saint Louis, Missouri

Sean E. McLean, MD
Resident in Surgery
Washington University School of Medicine
Saint Louis, Missouri

Bryan F. Meyers, MD
Associate Professor of Surgery
Washington University School of Medicine
Saint Louis, Missouri

Nader Moazami, MD
Assistant Professor of Surgery
Washington University School of Medicine
Saint Louis, Missouri

Nahush A. Mokadam, MD
Resident in Surgery
Washington University School of Medicine
Saint Louis, Missouri

Jeffrey F. Moley, MD
Professor of Surgery
Washington University School of Medicine
Saint Louis, Missouri

Matthew Mutch, MD
Assistant Professor of Surgery
Washington University School of Medicine
Saint Louis, Missouri

Jack Oak, MD
Resident in Surgery
Washington University School of Medicine
Saint Louis, Missouri

Sunil M. Prasad, MD
Resident in Surgery
Washington University School of Medicine
Saint Louis, Missouri

F. Jay Quayle, MD
Resident in Surgery
Washington University School of Medicine
Saint Louis, Missouri

Dennis J. Rivet, MD
Resident in Neurosurgery
Washington University School of Medicine
Saint Louis, Missouri

Emily B. Rivet, MD
Resident in Surgery
Washington University School of Medicine
Saint Louis, Missouri

Brian Rubin, MD
Associate Professor of Surgery
Washington University School of Medicine
Saint Louis, Missouri

J.R. Rudzki, MD
Resident in Orthopedic Surgery
Washington University School of Medicine
Saint Louis, Missouri

Aalok Sahai, MD

Resident in Surgery
Washington University School of Medicine
Saint Louis, Missouri

Luis A. Sanchez, MD

Associate Professor of Surgery
Washington University School of Medicine
Saint Louis, Missouri

Rodney E. Schmelzer, MD

Fellow in Craniofacial Surgery
Medical City Hospital
Dallas, Texas

Douglas Schuerer, MD

Assistant Professor of Surgery
Washington University School of Medicine
Saint Louis, Missouri

Surendra Shenoy, MD, PhD

Associate Professor of Surgery
Washington University School of Medicine
Saint Louis, Missouri

Gregario A. Sicard, MD

Professor of Surgery
Washington University School of Medicine
Saint Louis, Missouri

Steven M. Strasberg, MD

Professor of Surgery
Washington University School of Medicine
Saint Louis, Missouri

Robert W. Thompson, MD

Professor of Surgery
Washington University School of Medicine
Saint Louis, Missouri

Thomas Tung, MD

Assistant Professor of Plastic Surgery
Washington University School of Medicine
Saint Louis, Missouri

Nirmal K. Veeramachaneni, MD

Resident in Surgery
Washington University School of Medicine
Saint Louis, Missouri

Ravi K. Veeraswamy, MD

Resident in Surgery
Washington University School of Medicine
Saint Louis, Missouri

Benjamin Verdine, MD

Fellow in Orthopedic Hand Surgery
University of Pittsburgh
Pittsburgh, Pennsylania

Robb R. Whinney, MD

Assistant Professor of Surgery
Washington University School of Medicine
Saint Louis, Missouri

Alliric I. Willis, MD

Fellow in Surgical Oncology
Fox Chase Cancer Center
Philadelphia, Pennsylvania

Emily R. Winslow, MD

Resident in Surgery
Washington University School of Medicine
Saint Louis, Missouri

Joseph J. Wizorek, MD

Resident in Surgery
Washington University School of Medicine
Saint Louis, Missouri

Yolanda Y. L. Yang, MD, PhD

Fellow in Hepatobilcony Surgery
Cleveland Clinic
Cleveland, Ohio

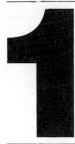

General and Perioperative Care of the Surgical Patient

Emily B. Rivet and
Bruce L. Hall

I. **Preoperative evaluation and management**
  A. **General evaluation of the surgical patient.** The goals of preoperative evaluation are to (1) identify the patient's medical problems, (2) determine if further information is needed to characterize the patient's medical status, (3) establish if the patient is medically optimized, and (4) confirm the appropriateness of the planned procedure.
    1. **History.** Key elements of the history should include preexisting medical conditions known to increase operative risk, such as ischemic heart disease, congestive heart failure (CHF), renal insufficiency, prior cerebrovascular accident (CVA), and diabetes mellitus. Prior operations and any operative complications should be noted. Patients should be questioned carefully about their use of tobacco, alcohol, drugs, or other personal habits that increase operative risk. Pertinent family history and a description of functional status should be elicited. Review of systems should screen for disease by system—cardiac, pulmonary, neurologic, endocrine, peripheral vascular, infectious, and renal—and include deep venous thrombosis (DVT), pulmonary embolism (PE), and occult bleeding disorders.
    2. **Physical examination.** Physical examination includes assessment of vital signs as well as head and neck, lung, cardiac, abdominal, neurologic, and a peripheral vascular examination.
    3. **Routine diagnostic testing.** Minor surgical procedures and procedures on young, healthy patients often require minimal or no diagnostic testing. Table 1-1 lists routine preoperative diagnostic tests and reasons for their use. Inclusion or exclusion of these tests should be selected on a case-by-case basis with consideration of the probability that results will alter management. (See also Chapter 6, Section I.A.)
    4. **Preoperative medications.** In general, patients should continue their medications in the immediate preoperative period. Exceptions to this rule include diabetic medications (see Section I.B.6), anticoagulants (see Section I.B.9.a), and antiplatelet agents. The use of some medications such as statins and ace-inhibitors should be individualized. It is important to query patients regarding their use of over-the-counter and herbal medications.
  B. **Specific considerations in preoperative management**
    1. **Cerebrovascular disease.** Perioperative stroke is an uncommon surgical complication, occurring in fewer than 1% of general patients and in 2% to 5% of cardiac surgical patients. The majority (>80%) of these events are postoperative, and they most often are caused by hypotension or cardiogenic emboli during atrial fibrillation. Acute surgical stress might cause focal signs from a previous stroke to recur, mimicking acute ischemia.
      a. **Risk factors** for perioperative stroke include previous CVA, age, hypertension, coronary artery disease (CAD), diabetes, and tobacco use. Known or suspected cerebrovascular disease requires special consideration.
        (1) **The asymptomatic carotid bruit** is relatively common, occurring in approximately 14% of surgical patients older than 55. However, fewer than 50% of bruits reflect hemodynamically significant

1

Table 1-1. Routine preoperative testing

Test	Comment
Complete blood cell count	Possibility of substantial blood loss, patients with chronic illnesses or symptoms of anemia
Urinalysis	Urologic symptoms, instrumentation of the urinary tract, possibility of surgical placement of prosthetic materials
Serum electrolytes, creatinine, and blood urea nitrogen	Age >50, chronic diarrhea, renal disease, liver disease, diabetes, CHF or other cardiac disease, hypertension (HTN), major procedure, diuretic use, digoxin use, ace inhibitor use
Coagulation studies	Family history of bleeding disorder, patient history of abnormal bleeding, anticoagulant usage, liver disease, malnutrition, chronic antibiotics
Biochemical profiles (including liver enzymes)	History of liver or biliary disease. (Albumin strong predictor of perioperative morbidity and mortality, should be considered for major procedures.)
Pregnancy testing	Any woman of childbearing age (except posthysterectomy patients)
Chest x-ray	Acute cardiac or pulmonary symptoms
Electrocardiogram	Men >40, women >50, history of cardiovascular disease or arrhythmia, diabetes, HTN
Type and cross/type and screen	None if very low risk of blood loss. Type and screen if risk of substantial blood loss is low to moderate; type and cross if moderate to high risk of substantial blood loss

disease. Although no increase in risk of stroke has been demonstrated during noncardiac surgery in the presence of an asymptomatic bruit, it is reasonable to evaluate such patients with carotid duplex before major general surgical procedures.

   (2) **Patients with recent transient ischemic attacks** are at increased risk for perioperative stroke and should have preoperative neurologic evaluation [e.g., computed tomography (CT) of head, echocardiography, carotid Doppler]. Patients with symptomatic carotid artery stenosis should have an endarterectomy before elective general surgery. The timing of carotid endarterectomy in the setting of cardiac surgery remains controversial.

   (3) **Elective surgery for patients with recent cerebrovascular accident** should be delayed for a minimum of 2 weeks, ideally for 6 weeks, depending on the severity of the event.

2. **Cardiovascular disease.** Cardiovascular disease is one of the leading causes of death after noncardiac surgery; therefore, risk stratification by the operating surgeon, anesthesiologist, and consulting internist is important. An important recent paradigm shift entails minimizing risk via perioperative pharmacologic therapy, rather than further stratification of intermediate-risk patients with noninvasive testing.

   a. **Risk factors.** The following risk factors have been associated with perioperative cardiac morbidity:

   (1) The **patient's age** (>70 years) has been identified as an independent multivariate risk factor for cardiac morbidity in many studies.

   (2) **Unstable angina** is defined as chest pain that does not correlate with the level of physical activity and, therefore, occurs at

rest or with minimal physical exertion. It typically implies a more serious degree of CAD. Elective operation in patients with unstable angina is contraindicated and should be postponed pending further evaluation. *Stable angina* has not been consistently identified as a risk factor for adverse cardiac outcome.

(3) A **recent myocardial infarction (MI)** is a well-defined risk factor for cardiac morbidity. The risk of reinfarction is significant if an operation is performed within 6 months of an MI (11% to 16% at 3 to 6 months). This risk still is increased substantially after 6 months, in contrast to patients without a history of MI (4% to 5% versus 0.13%).

(4) **Untreated congestive heart failure is** a predictor of perioperative cardiac morbidity. Consequently, these patients should be optimized before any operative procedures are performed.

(5) **Diabetes mellitus,** especially if insulin requiring, is thought to confer additional independent risk for an adverse cardiac outcome.

(6) **Valvular heart disease.** Aortic stenosis is a significant risk factor and may confer a 14-fold increase in relative risk independent of the manifestations of CHF. Consequently, any uncharacterized systolic ejection murmur deserves further evaluation with echocardiography. Other valvular heart diseases have not been evaluated systematically as risk factors for adverse cardiac outcome. However, patients with unexplained symptoms of dyspnea on exertion, shortness of breath, chest pain, or syncope should undergo further diagnostic evaluation before elective operation. All patients with valvular heart disease, even hemodynamically insignificant disease (excluding patients with mitral valve prolapse alone without a murmur), should receive prophylactic antibiotics before any operation that can introduce bacteria into the bloodstream or any dental procedure to reduce the risk of infectious endocarditis (Table 1-2).

(7) **Arrhythmias and conduction defects.** Both supraventricular and ventricular arrythmias have been identified as independent risk factors for perioperative coronary events. The existence of a preoperative arrhythmia should prompt a search for underlying cardiac or pulmonary disease. Although frequent premature ventricular contractions and nonsustained ventricular tachycardia are associated with increased long-term risk for arrhythmias, these findings are not associated with perioperative MI or cardiac death and therefore aggressive management may not be necessary. High-grade conduction abnormalities can also increase operative risk.

(8) **Peripheral vascular disease.** Because of the high coexistence of CAD with peripheral vascular disease, a lower threshold for obtaining diagnostic testing is warranted.

(9) **Type of procedure.** Patients who are undergoing thoracic surgery, vascular surgery, or upper abdominal surgery are at a higher risk of adverse cardiac outcome. Other procedures considered high risk include emergent major operations, especially in the elderly, and prolonged procedures associated with large fluid shifts or blood loss.

(10) **Functional Impairment.** Patients with a poor functional capacity have a significantly higher risk of experiencing a postoperative cardiac event. Poor function is an indication for more aggressive preoperative evaluation, whereas patients who exercise regularly generally have sufficient cardiac reserve to withstand even stressful operations.

Table 1-2. Antibiotic prophylaxis of bacterial endocarditis for adult patients

Procedure	Situation	Regimen
Dental, oral, respiratory, esophageal	Standard	**Amoxicillin** 2 g PO 1 hr before procedure
	Unable to take PO	**Ampicillin** 2 g IM or IV 30 min before procedure
	Penicillin allergic	**Clindamycin** 600 mg PO 1 hr before procedure; or **cephalexin**[a] or **cefadroxil**[a] 2 g PO 1 hr before procedure; or **clarithromycin** or **azithromycin** 500 mg PO 1 hr before procedure
	Penicillin-allergic and unable to take PO	**Clindamycin** 600 mg IV within 30 min before procedure or **cefazolin**[a] 1 g IV within 30 min before procedure
Gastro intestinal and genitourinary	High-risk patients	**Ampicillin** 2 g IM or IV, plus **gentamicin** 1.5 mg/kg (max 120 mg) within 30 min before procedure. 6 hrs later **ampicillin** 1 g IV/IM or **amoxicillin** 1 g PO.
	High-risk, penicillin-allergic patients	**Vancomycin** 1g IV plus **gentamicin** 1.5 mg/kg (max 120 mg) timed to finish within 30 min of starting procedure
	Moderate-risk patients	**Amoxicillin** 2 g PO 1 hr before procedure or **ampicillin** 2 g IM or IV 30 min before procedure
	Moderate-risk, penicillin allergic patients	**Vancomycin** 1 g IV timed to finish within 30 min of starting procedure

[a]Cephalosporins should not be used in patients with anaphylactic or urticarial reactions to penicillin.

  b. Revised cardiac risk index. See Table 1-3.
  c. Preoperative testing. Patients at intermediate risk for a perioperative myocardial event may require additional studies to determine if
  further therapy is needed to optimize their status.
    (1) A **preoperative electrocardiogram (ECG)** is warranted in inter-
    mediate or high-risk patients with a history of recent chest pain
    or ischemic equivalent scheduled for an intermediate or high-risk
    procedure, as well as for patients with diabetes mellitus. ECG is
    also recommended for patients with prior coronary revasculariza-
    tion, men older than 45 and women older than 55 with risk factors,
    and patients with a prior hospitalization for cardiac reasons.
    (2) Noninvasive testing. Patients who are identified to be at risk of
    a perioperative cardiovascular event by the revised cardiac risk
    index or who have other risk factors (e.g., peripheral vascular dis-
    ease, unexplained chest pain, diabetes, ECG abnormalities) should
    undergo further evaluation.
      (a) Exercise stress testing provides useful information for risk
      stratification. An inability to achieve even modest levels of ex-
      ercise or the presence of ECG changes with exercise identifies
      patients at significant risk of adverse outcome.
      (b) Dipyridamole thallium imaging has a very high negative pre-
      dictive value of approximately 99%, but a moderate positive
      predictive value ranging from 4% to 20%.

Table 1-3. Revised cardiac risk index[a]

Risk factor	Comment
High-risk type of surgery	Intrathoracic, intraperitoneal, major vascular
Ischemic heart disease	History of myocardial infarction, positive exercise test, angina, nitrate therapy, electrocardiogram with abnormal Q waves
History of CHF	History of CHF, pulmonary edema, or paroxysmal nocturnal dyspnea, bilateral rales, S_3 gallop, chest x-ray showing pulmonary vascular redistribution
History of cerebrovascular disease	History of transient ischemic attack or stroke
Preoperative insulin therapy for diabetes	—
Preoperative serum creatinine >2.0 mg/dL	

[a]Rates of major cardiac complication with 0, 1, 2, or 3 of these factors were 0.4%, 0.9%, 7.0%, and 11.0%, respectively.
CHF, congestive heart failure.
Adapted with permission from Lee TH, Marcantonio ER, Mangione CM, et al. Derivation and prospective validation of a simple index for prediction of cardiac risk of major noncardiac surgery. *Circulation* 1999;100:1043.

       (c) Dobutamine stress echocardiography is believed to provide similar adrenergic stimulus to perioperative stress. Positive and negative predictive values are similar to those for dipyridamole thallium imaging.
    (3) Invasive testing. Patients with evidence of high risk identified on noninvasive testing can be further evaluated with angiography. Angiography may also be indicated to characterize equivocal noninvasive testing results in high-risk patients undergoing high-risk procedures. Patients with significant cardiac lesions should have definitive treatment (angioplasty or coronary artery bypass grafting) before any elective general surgical procedures are performed.
  d. Preoperative management
    (1) Patients with pacemakers should have their pacemakers turned to the uninhibited mode (e.g., DOO) before surgery. In addition, a bipolar cautery should be used when possible in these patients. If it is necessary to use a unipolar cautery, the grounding pad should be placed away from the heart.
    (2) Patients with internal defibrillators should have these devices turned off during surgery.
    (3) Perioperative beta-blockade can be used for intermediate risk patients with good functional status to obviate the need for noninvasive testing.
 3. Pulmonary disease. Preexisting lung disease confers a dramatically increased risk of perioperative pulmonary complications.
  a. Preoperative evaluation and screening
    (1) Risk factors
      (a) Chronic obstructive pulmonary disease (COPD) is by far the most important risk factor, increasing pulmonary complications threefold to fourfold.
      (b) Smoking is also a significant risk factor. Operative risk reduction has only been documented after 8 weeks of smoking cessation; however, there are physiologic benefits to stopping as little as 48 hours before surgery.

        (c) **Increased age** >60 years

        (d) **Obesity [Body mass index (BMI)** >27 kg/m², **in some studies]**

        (e) **Type of surgery.** Pulmonary complications occur at a much higher rate for thoracic and upper abdominal procedures than for other procedures.

        (f) **Acute respiratory infections.** Postoperative pulmonary complications occur at a much higher rate for patients with acute respiratory infections; therefore, elective operations should be postponed in these individuals.

        (g) **Functional status.** In the patient with pulmonary disease or a history of smoking, a detailed evaluation of the patient's ability to climb stairs, walk, and perform daily duties is vital to stratify risk. Clinical judgment has been shown to be of equal or greater value as pulmonary function testing for most patients.

    (2) Physical examination should be performed carefully, with attention paid to signs of lung disease (e.g., wheezing, prolonged expiratory–inspiratory ratio, clubbing, or use of accessory muscles of respiration).

    (3) Diagnostic evaluation

        (a) **Chest x-ray (CXR)** for acute symptoms related to pulmonary disease.

        (b) An **arterial blood gas (ABG)** is useful in patients with a history of lung disease or smoking to provide a baseline for comparison with postoperative studies. This test is not useful for routine screening.

        (c) **Preoperative pulmonary function testing** is controversial and probably unnecessary in stable patients with previously characterized pulmonary disease undergoing non-thoracic procedures.

  b. Preoperative prophylaxis and management

    (1) Pulmonary toilet. Increasing lung volume by the use of preoperative incentive spirometry is potentially effective in reducing pulmonary complications.

    (2) Antibiotics do not reduce pulmonary infectious complications in the absence of preoperative infection. Elective operations should be postponed in patients with respiratory infections. If emergent surgery is required, patients with acute pulmonary infections should receive intravenous antibiotic therapy.

    (3) Cessation of smoking. All patients should be encouraged and assisted to stop smoking before surgery

    (4) Bronchodilators. In the patient with obstructive airway disease and evidence of a significant reactive component, bronchodilators may be required in the perioperative period. When possible, elective operation should be postponed in the patient who is wheezing actively.

4. Renal disease

  a. Preoperative evaluation of patients with existing renal insufficiency

    (1) Risk factors

        (a) **Underlying medical disease.** A substantial percentage of patients who require chronic hemodialysis for chronic renal insufficiency (CRI) have diabetes or hypertension. Furthermore, the incidence of CAD is substantially higher in these patients. Much of the perioperative morbidity and mortality arises from these coexisting illnesses.

        (b) **Metabolic and physiologic derangements of chronic renal insufficiency.** A variety of abnormalities in normal physiology that occur as a result of CRI can affect operative outcome adversely; these include alterations in electrolytes, acid-base balance, platelet function, the cardiovascular system, and the immune system. Specifically, the most common abnormalities in the perioperative period include hyperkalemia, intravascular volume overload, and infectious complications.

   (c) **Type of operative procedure.** Minor procedures under local or regional anesthesia are usually well tolerated in patients with CRI; however, major procedures are associated with an increased morbidity and mortality.

(2) Evaluation

   (a) **History.** It is important to ascertain the specific etiology of CRI because patients with hypertension or diabetes and CRI are at a substantially increased risk of perioperative morbidity and mortality. The timing of last dialysis, the amount of fluid removed, and the preoperative weight provide important information about the patient's expected volume status.

   (b) **Physical examination** should be performed carefully to assess the volume status. Elevated jugular venous pulsations or crackles on lung examination can indicate intravascular volume overload.

   (c) **Diagnostic testing**

      (i) **Laboratory data.** Serum sodium, potassium, calcium, phosphorus, magnesium, and bicarbonate levels should be measured, as well as blood urea nitrogen (BUN) and creatinine levels. A complete blood cell (CBC) count should be obtained to evaluate for significant anemia or a low platelet level. Normal platelet numbers can mask platelet dysfunction in patients with chronic uremia.

      (ii) **Supplemental tests** such as noninvasive cardiac evaluation may be warranted in patients with CRI and other risk factors.

(3) Management

   (a) **Timing of dialysis.** Dialysis should be performed within 24 hours of the planned operative procedure.

   (b) **Intravascular volume status.** CAD is the most common cause of death in patients with CRI. Consequently, because of the high incidence of coexisting CAD, patients with CRI undergoing major operations may require invasive monitoring in the intraoperative and postoperative period. Hypovolemia and volume overload are both tolerated poorly.

b. Patients at risk for perioperative renal dysfunction. The reported incidence of acute renal failure (ARF) after operations in patients without preexisting CRI ranges from 1.5 to 2.5% for cardiac surgical procedures to more than 10% for patients who are undergoing repair of supraceliac abdominal aortic aneurysms.

(1) Risk factors for the development of ARF include elevated preoperative BUN or creatinine, CHF, advanced age, intraoperative hypotension, sepsis, aortic cross-clamping, and intravascular volume contraction. Additional risk factors include administration of nephrotoxic drugs, such as aminoglycosides, and the administration of radiocontrast agents.

(2) Prevention

   (a) **Intravascular volume expansion.** Adequate hydration is the single most important preventive measure for reducing the incidence of ARF, because all mechanisms of renal failure are exacerbated by renal hypoperfusion caused by intravascular volume contraction.

   (b) **Radiocontrast dye administration.** Patients undergoing radiocontrast dye studies have an increased incidence of postoperative renal failure. Fluid administration (1 to 2 L isotonic saline) alone appears to confer protection against ARF. Additional measures to reduce the incidence of contrast dye-mediated ARF include the use of low-osmolality contrast agents and oral n-acetylcysteine (600 mg orally 2 times a day on the day of and day after contrast agent administration).

   (c) **Other nephrotoxins**, including aminoglycoside antibiotics, nonsteroidal antiinflammatory drugs, and various anesthetic drugs, can predispose to renal failure and should be used judiciously in patients with other risk factors for the development of ARF.

5. **Infectious complications.** Infectious complications may arise in the surgical wound itself or in other organ systems. They may be initiated by changes in the physiologic state of the respiratory, genitourinary, or immune systems associated with surgery. It is impossible to overemphasize the importance of frequent hand washing or antiseptic foam use by all health care workers to prevent the spread of infection.

   a. **Assessment of risk.** Risk factors for infectious complications after surgery can be grouped into risk factors arising from the type of procedure or patient-specific risk factors.

   (1) **Surgical risk factors** include the type of procedure and degree of wound contamination (Table 1-4), the duration of operation, and the urgency of operation.

Table 1-4. Classification of surgical wounds

Wound class	Definition	Examples of typical procedures	Wound infection rate (%)	Usual organisms
Clean	Nontraumatic, elective surgery; No entry of GI, biliary, tracheo bronchial, respiratory, or GU tracts	Wide local excision of breast mass	2	*Staphylococcus aureus*
Clean-contaminated	Respiratory, genitourinary, gastrointestinal tract entered but minimal contamination	Gastrectomy, hysterectomy	<10	Related to the viscus entered
Contaminated	Open, fresh, traumatic wounds; uncontrolled spillage from an unprepared hollow viscus; minor break in sterile technique	Ruptured appendix; resection of unprepared bowel	20	Depends on underlying disease
Dirty	Open, traumatic, dirty wounds; traumatic perforated viscus; pus in the operative field	Intestinal fistula resection	28–70	Depends on underlying disease

(2) Patient-specific risk factors include age, diabetes, obesity, immunosuppression, malnutrition, preexisting infection, and chronic illness.

b. **Prophylaxis**

(1) Nonantimicrobial strategies documented to decrease the risk of postoperative infection include strict sterile technique, maintaining normal body temperature, maintaining normal blood glucose levels, and hyperoxygenation.

(2) Surgical wound infection. Antibiotic prophylaxis has contributed to a reduction in superficial wound infection rates (see Table 1-5 for specific recommendations). Coverage should be initiated not more than 1 hour (oral administration) or 1/2 hour (intramuscularly or intravenously) before the skin incision is made and, in the absence of gross contamination or overt infection, should not be administered beyond 24 to 48 hours after surgery. Repeat doses should be administered according to the usual dosing protocol during prolonged procedures.

(3) Respiratory infections. Risk factors and measures to prevent pulmonary complications are discussed in Section I.B.3.

(4) Genitourinary infections may be caused by instrumentation of the urinary tract or an indwelling urinary catheter. Preventive measures include sterile insertion of the catheter and removal of the catheter as soon as possible postoperatively. A prophylactic dose of antibiotics should be given after a difficult catheter insertion or excessive manipulation of the urinary tract.

6. **Diabetes mellitus.** Diabetic patients experience significant stress during the perioperative period and are at an estimated 50% increased risk of morbidity and mortality over nondiabetic patients. Diabetic patients experience more infectious complications and have impaired wound healing. Most important, vascular disease is common in diabetics, and silent CAD must always be considered. MI, often with an atypical presentation, is the leading cause of perioperative death among diabetic patients.

a. **Preoperative evaluation** of diabetic patients must include an assessment of the chronic complications of diabetes and an estimation of recent glycemic control. Diabetic patients should be evaluated to exclude the existence of common comorbid conditions such as cardiovascular and renal disease. In general, diabetic patients should be well controlled before elective surgery, with procedures scheduled early in the day. All diabetic patients should have their blood glucose checked on call to the operating room and during general anesthesia to prevent unrecognized hyperglycemia or hypoglycemia. Recent evidence demonstrates improved outcomes in critically ill patients with intensive insulin therapy to maintain blood sugars between 80 and 110 mg/dL.

(1) Patients with **diet-controlled diabetes mellitus** can be maintained safely without food or glucose infusion before surgery.

(2) Patients who are **taking oral hypoglycemic agents** should discontinue these medications the evening before scheduled surgery. Patients who take such long-acting agents as chlorpropamide or glyburide should discontinue these medications 2 to 3 days before surgery.

(3) Patients who normally **take insulin** require insulin and glucose preoperatively to prevent ketosis and catabolism. Patients undergoing major surgery should receive one half of their morning insulin dose and 5% dextrose intravenously at 100 to 125 mL/hour. Subsequent insulin administration by either subcutaneous sliding-scale or insulin infusion is guided by frequent (every 4 to 6 hours) blood glucose determinations. Subcutaneous insulin pumps should be inactivated the morning of surgery.

Table 1-5. Recommendations for antibiotic prophylaxis

Nature of operation	Likely pathogens	Recommended antibiotics	Adult dosage before surgery[a]
Cardiac: prosthetic valve and other procedures	Staphylococci, corynebacteria, enteric gram-negative bacilli	Cefazolin Vancomycin Cefuroxime	1–2 g IV 1 g IV 1.5 g IV
Vascular: peripheral bypass or aortic surgery with prosthetic graft	Staphylococci, Streptococci, enteric gram-negative bacilli, clostridia	Cefazolin Vancomycin Cefoxitin	1–2 g IV 1–2 g IV 1–2 g IV
Orthopedic: total joint replacement or internal fixation of fractures	Staphylococci	Cefazolin Vancomycin	1–2 g IV 1 g IV
Ophthalmic	Staphylococci, streptococci, enteric gram-negative bacilli, Pseudomonas spp.	Gentamicin Tobramycin Ciprofloxacin Ofloxacin Neomycin–gramicidin–polymyxin B	Multiple drops topically over 2–24 hr
Head and neck, entering oral cavity or pharynx	Oral anaerobes, enteric gram-negative bacilli, staphylococci	Cefazolin Ampicillin–sulbactam Clindamycin Gentamycin	1–2 g IV 1.5–3 g IV 600–900 mg IV 1.5 mg/kg IV
Gastroduodenal (high-risk pt)	Enteric gram-negative bacilli, gram-positive cocci	Cefazolin	1–2 g IV
Biliary	Enteric gram-negative bacilli, enterococci, clostridia	Cefazolin Cefoxitin Cefotetan	1–2 g IV 1–2 g IV 1–2 g IV

Procedure	Organisms	Antibiotic	Dose
Colorectal	Enteric gram-negative bacilli, anaerobes, enterococci	Oral: neomycin + erythromycin base	1 g of each at 1 PM., 2 PM., and 11 PM. the day before an 8 AM operation
		IV:	
		Cefoxitin	1–2 g IV
		Cefotetan	1–2 g IV
		Cefazolin plus flagyl	1–2 g IV
		Parenteral: cefoxitin	500 mg IV
			1 g i.v.
Appendectomy (no perforation)	Enteric gram-negative bacilli, anaerobes, enterococci	Cefoxitin	1–2 g IV
		Cefotetan	1–2 g IV
Vaginal or abdominal hysterectomy	Enteric gram-negative bacilli, anaerobes, group B streptococci, enterococci	Cefazolin	1–2 g IV
		Cefoxitin	1–2 g IV
		Cefotetan	1–2 g IV
Cesarean section (high-risk patient)	Same as for hysterectomy	Cefazolin	1 g IV after cord clamped
Traumatic wound	Staphylococci, group A streptococci, clostridia	Cefazolin or	1 g IV q8h
		Ampicillin-sulbactam	1.5–3.0 g IV q6h

[a]Parenteral antibiotics for clean and clean-contaminated surgery can be given as a single intravenous dose completed 30 min before incision. For prolonged procedures, additional doses should be administered at usual dosing intervals. In general, antibiotics should not be continued postoperatively except in dirty wounds.

(4) For **poorly controlled diabetic patients with diabetic ketoacidosis (DKA)** who require emergency surgery, every attempt should be made to correct acidosis, electrolyte imbalance, hypokalemia, and volume depletion before operation. Control of blood glucose in these critically ill patients is best managed with insulin infusion (see Section III.G.1.e).

7. **Thyroid disorders**
    a. **Preoperative evaluation.** Patients with known thyroid disorders should be evaluated for symptoms of thyroid hyperfunction or hypofunction. TSH suffices to screen asymptomatic patients. TSH, T4, and possibly T3 should be obtained in symptomatic patients.
    b. **Hyperthyroidism.** Thyroid storm, cardiac arrhythmias, and cardiac ischemia are the prinicipal risks of surgery in the hyperthyroid patient, although nonthyroid surgery in the treated hyperthyroid patient is well tolerated.
        (1) **Clinically euthyroid patients** who are treated medically with either propylthiouracil (PTU) or methimazole should take their medication the day of surgery, and these drugs should be resumed either orally or per nasogastric tube within 72 hours of surgery. Patients on beta-blockers should also be maintained on these medications, with short-acting intravenous agents used during the perioperative period, if necessary.
        (2) **Untreated hyperthyroid patients** should have elective procedures postponed until euthyroid. Thyrotoxic patients who require emergency surgery should be premedicated with beta-blockers, antithyroid agents, and possibly corticosteroids.
    c. **Hypothyroidism:** In general, the presence of medically controlled thyroid disease or even mild to moderate untreated disease does not adversely affect the outcome of nonthyroid surgery. Fluid and electrolyte disorders, intraoperative hypotension, prolonged ileus, impaired febrile response to infection, and neuropsychiatric problems may be encountered with increased frequency.
        (1) **Clinically euthyroid** patients may have their thyroid hormone withheld the day of surgery. Postoperatively, patients may resume thyroid replacement when tolerating oral intake. Intravenous thyroid replacement is seldom necessary because the half-life of T_4 exceeds 7 days.
        (2) **Profoundly hypothyroid patients** tolerate surgical stress poorly. These individuals should receive 300 to 500 mg of T_4 intravenously and stress steroids if they are subjected to trauma or emergent surgery. Intraoperative hypotension should be anticipated.

8. **Adrenal insufficiency and steroid dependence**
    a. **Exogenous steroids** are used to treat a variety of diseases that are encountered in surgical patients. Perioperative management of these individuals requires knowledge of the dose and type of steroid (long acting versus short acting), schedule, and length of treatment with exogenous steroids.
    b. **Perioperative stress-dose steroids** are indicated for patients who have received chronic steroid replacement or immunosuppressive steroid therapy within the past year.
    c. **Dosage recommendations** for perioperative steroids reflect estimates of normal adrenal responses to major surgical stress. The normal adrenal gland produces 250 to 300 mg cortisol per day under maximal stress, peaking at 6 hours after surgery and returning to baseline after 24 hours unless stress continues. A regimen of hydrocortisone sodium succinate, 100 mg intravenously, on the evening before major surgery, at the beginning of surgery, and every 8 hours on the day of surgery, approximates the normal adrenal stress response. Tapering is not necessary in uncomplicated cases. Patients who are undergoing

Table 1-6. Recommendations for preoperative and postoperative anticoagulation in patients taking oral anticoagulants[a]

Indication	Preoperative	Postoperative
Acute venous thromboembolism		
Within 1 mo of surgery	i.v. heparin[b]	i.v. heparin[b]
Within 3 mo of surgery	No therapy[d]	i.v. heparin
Recurrent venous thromboembolism[c]	No therapy[d]	s.c. heparin
Acute arterial embolism (within 30 days)	i.v. heparin	i.v. heparin[e]
Mechanical heart valve	No therapy[d]	s.c. heparin
Nonvalvular atrial fibrillation	No therapy[d]	s.c. heparin

[a]*i.v. heparin* denotes intravenous heparin at therapeutic doses, and *s.c. heparin* denotes subcutaneous unfractionated and lowmolecular-weight heparin at doses recommended for prophylaxis against venous thromboembolism.
[b]A vena caval filter should be considered if acute venous thromboembolism has occurred within 2 weeks or if the risk of bleeding during i.v. heparin therapy is high.
[c]*Recurrent venous thromboembolism* refers to patients whose last episode of venous thromboembolism occurred more than 3 months before evaluation but who require long-term anticoagulation because of a high risk of recurrence.
[d]If patients are hospitalized, s.c. heparin can be administered, but hospitalization is not necessary solely for this purpose.
[e]i.v. heparin should be used after surgery only if the risk of bleeding is low.
Adapted with permission from Kearon C, Hirsh J. Management of anticoagulation before and after elective surgery. *N Engl J Med* 336:1506, 1997. Copyright ©1997, Massachusetts Medical Society. All rights reserved.

minor surgery or diagnostic procedures usually do not require stress-dose steroids.

9. **Anticoagulation.** The most common indications for warfarin therapy are atrial fibrillation, venous thromboembolism, and mechanical heart valves. Mitigation of warfarin's anticoagulant effect occurs only after several days of cessation from the drug, and it requires several days to reestablish the effect after warfarin is resumed. Recommendations for the management of anticoagulation (summarized in Table 1-6) in the perioperative period require weighing the risk of subtherapeutic anticoagulation (thromboembolic events) against the benefits (reduced incidence of perioperative bleeding).

   a. **Preoperative anticoagulation.** It is generally considered safe to perform surgery when the international normalized ratio (INR) value is below 1.5. Patients whose INR is maintained between 2.0 and 3.0 normally require withholding of the medication for 4 days preoperatively. For patients whose INR is maintained at a value greater than 3.0, withholding for a longer period of time is necessary. The INR should be measured the day before surgery, if possible, to confirm that the anticoagulation is reversed. Alternate prophylaxis should be considered for the preoperative period when the INR is less than 2.0 (Table 1-6).

   b. **Postoperative anticoagulation.** The anticoagulant effects of warfarin require several doses before therapeutic levels are reached. For this reason, in patients who can tolerate oral or nasogastric medications, warfarin therapy can be resumed on postoperative days 1 or 2. If indicated (Table 1-6), intravenous heparin should generally not be restarted until 12 hours after surgery and should be delayed even longer if there is any evidence of bleeding.

   c. **Emergent procedures.** In urgent or emergent situations in which there is no time to reverse anticoagulation before surgery, plasma products must be administered. To provide sufficient functional coagulation factors, several units of fresh frozen plasma are necessary. Vitamin K may have observable effects within 8 hours and should often be given with other products.

Table 1-7. Prophylaxis for deep venous thrombosis and pulmonary embolus

Patient group[a]	Surgery type	Prophylaxis
Low risk	Minor	None
Low or moderate risk	Major	GCS, SQH-12, or IPC
High risk	Major	SQH-8 or LMWH[b]
Highest risk	Major	SQH-8/12 or LMWH + IPC

[a]Low risk, age less than 40 years, no risk factors; moderate risk, major surgery & age less than 40 years or minor procedure with risk factors or between 40 and 60 years of age; high risk, major procedure over age 40 or with risk factors, or minor procedure over age 60 or with risk factors; highest risk, age greater than 40 years, multiple risk factors present, major procedure.
[b]Can use IPC if risk of hematoma or infection is high.
GCS, graded compression stockings; IPC, intermittent pneumatic compression; LMWH, low molecular-weight heparin; SQH-8, subcutaneous heparin every 8 hours; SQH-12, subcutaneous heparin every 12 hours.

II. **Postoperative care of the patient.** This section summarizes general considerations in all postoperative patients and then addresses specific concerns in patients with significant comorbid disease.
   A. **Routine postoperative care**
      1. **Intravenous fluids.** The intravascular volume of surgical patients is depleted by both insensible fluid losses and redistribution into the third space. As a general rule, patients should be maintained on intravenous fluids until they are tolerating oral intake. Extensive abdominal procedures require aggressive fluid resuscitation (see Chapter 4). Insensible fluid losses associated with an open abdomen can reach 500 to 1000 mL/hour.
      2. **Deep venous thrombosis prophylaxis.** Many postoperative patients are not immediately ambulatory. In these individuals, it is important to provide prophylactic therapy to reduce the risk of DVT and PE (see Table 1-7). Prophylaxis should be started preoperatively in patients undergoing major procedures because venous stasis and relative hypercoagulability occur during the operation. Management of patients with a history of DVT or PE is discussed in Section **I.B.9a.**
         a. **Mechanical prophylaxis** includes graded compression stockings and intermittent pneumatic compression devices, either of which are nearly as effective as unfractionated heparin in reducing DVT in most low-risk to moderate-risk patients who are undergoing general surgical procedures. These devices alone are inadequate prophylaxis for high-risk (especially cancer) patients and should be avoided in individuals with peripheral vascular disease.
         b. **Unfractionated heparin,** 5,000 units subcutaneously, starting 2 hours before surgery and continuing every 8 to 12 hours postoperatively, markedly decreases the incidence of DVT after general surgery. No increase in major hemorrhagic complications is observed with this regimen, although the rate of wound hematoma is higher. This increase may be detrimental in operations that involve prosthetic materials (i.e., hernia repair with mesh), in which case intermittent pneumatic compression devices can be substituted.
         c. **Low–molecular-weight heparins,** such as enoxaparin (1 mg/kg subcutaneously every 12 to 24 hours), are derivatives of unfractionated heparin and have become an important class of agents in the prevention and treatment of thromboembolic disease. These agents have a clinical efficacy that is nearly equivalent to that of intravenous heparin and they do not require frequent measurement of coagulation times. Prophylactic efficacy has been demonstrated in patients who have undergone total hip replacement and in those who are undergoing elective abdominal or pelvic operation for malignancy, as well as after major trauma.

    d. Warfarin is indicated in some lower extremity orthopaedic procedures and in certain high-risk patients (i.e., antithrombin III deficiency). Dosing is usually targeted to an INR of 2.0 to 3.0. This method of prophylaxis carries a significantly higher rate of major postoperative bleeding (5% to 10%) than low-dose heparin and is usually not indicated in general surgery patients.

3. Pulmonary toilet. Pain and immobilization in the postoperative patient decrease clearance of pulmonary secretions and alveolar recruitment. Patients with inadequate pulmonary toilet can develop fevers, hypoxemia, and pneumonia. Early mobilization, incentive spirometry, and cough and deep breathing exercises are indispensable to avoiding these complications. Patients must be educated and have adequate pain control prior to the initiation of these modalities.

4. Medications

    a. Antiemetics. Postoperative nausea is common in patients after general anesthesia and in patients receiving narcotics.

    b. Ulcer prophylaxis. Patients with a history of peptic ulcer disease should have some form of ulcer prophylaxis in the perioperative period, either with acid-reducing agents or with cytoprotective agents, such as sucralfate. Routine ulcer prophylaxis in patients without a history of peptic ulcer disease has only been of proven benefit in those with a coagulopathy or prolonged ventilator dependence; however, it is a common practice to use antiulcer agents in all patients who are nil per os (n.p.o.) for a prolonged period of time.

    c. Pain control. Inadequate pain control can slow the recovery or contribute to complications in postoperative patients. Individuals whose pain is poorly controlled are less likely to ambulate and may take shallow breaths, contributing to atelectasis and interfering with the clearance of pulmonary secretions. Pain can also contribute to tachycardia and relative hypertension, increasing myocardial work and possibly increasing the risk of cardiac complications.

    d. Antibiotics. Surgeon preferences often dictate the use of postoperative antibiotics in particular cases. Recommendations for specific procedures can be found in Table 1-5. Antibiotic therapy for specific infectious etiologies is discussed in Section III.E.2.

5. Laboratory tests. Postoperative laboratory tests should be individualized; however, the following considerations are important when planning laboratory evaluations:

    a. A **complete blood count** should be obtained in the immediate postoperative period and on subsequent postoperative days in any procedure in which significant blood loss occurred. This test is also useful on subsequent postoperative days if concern of infection arises. Serial hematocrits should be ordered in any patient in whom there is concern for ongoing blood loss.

    b. Serum electrolytes, blood urea nitrogen, and creatinine are important postoperatively in patients who are n.p.o. or are receiving large volumes of intravenous fluids, total parenteral nutrition, or transfusions. In patients with large transfusion requirements, it is important to obtain frequent calcium and magnesium measurements.

    c. Coagulation studies are important in patients who have had insults to the liver or large transfusion requirements.

    d. Chest x-rays are a necessity after any procedure in which the thoracic cavity is entered or when central venous access is attempted. CXRs on subsequent postoperative days should be considered on an individual basis if significant pulmonary or cardiovascular disease is present.

B. Specific considerations in postoperative care

1. Seizure disorders. Perioperative management of patients with known seizure disorders should be directed toward an understanding of the type (i.e., partial versus generalized, simple partial versus complex partial), frequency, and degree of control of the disorder. Well-controlled seizure disorders pose little additional risk if proper attention is paid to perioperative management of anticonvulsants. Standard seizure precautions should be included in the postoperative nursing orders.

a. **Phenytoin and phenobarbital** are available in parenteral form. If patients are expected to resume oral intake within 24 hours of operation, these oral anticonvulsants can be withheld. If oral intake is withheld for more than 24 hours, the equivalent parenteral dose can be given, using a divided schedule.

b. **Carbamazepine, ethosuximide, and valproic acid** are not available parenterally; decisions to withhold these medications or to substitute parenteral phenytoin must take into account type, frequency, and severity of seizures. Patients with frequent generalized tonic-clonic seizures likely require parenteral anticonvulsant substitution. Phenytoin can be given intravenously as a loading dose of 18 to 20 mg/kg over 30 minutes (<50 mg/minute) followed by 5 mg/kg per day as maintenance, divided into three daily doses.

2. **Cardiovascular disease**
   a. **Coronary artery disease**
      (1) **Control of precipitants.** A basic tenet in the postoperative management of patients with known or suspected CAD is the avoidance of stressors that may exacerbate ischemia through increased myocardial oxygen consumption.
         (a) **Acute hypertension** increases oxygen demand by increasing ventricular wall stress. The management of acute hypertension is described in Section III.H.2.
         (b) **Pain control** is critical in CAD patients, as pain can precipitate tachycardia and hypertension.
         (c) **Oxygen** should be administered in the early postoperative period to maximize the oxygen content of the blood.
         (d) **Anemia** should be avoided in patients with known CAD, as it decreases the oxygen-carrying capacity. Transfusions should be considered when the hemoglobin falls below 9.0.
      (2) **Monitoring.** Patients at high risk for perioperative myocardial morbidity should have telemetry monitoring in the early postoperative period. Invasive monitoring of arterial, venous, and intracardiac pressures should be considered in patients undergoing urgent or emergent surgery with a history of CAD or poorly compensated CHF, those with unstable or severe angina, and those with a recent MI for whom operation cannot be delayed.
      (3) **Rule out myocardial infarction protocol.** No consensus has been reached regarding the appropriate protocol to rule out MI or the indications for this protocol. Daily ECGs and a series of three troponin-I levels 12 hours apart are appropriate in patients with significant risk factors who have had a major surgical procedure.
      (4) **Medications**
         (a) Patients who are receiving **beta-adrenergic receptor antagonists** (beta-blockers) should have this medication continued through the perioperative period. Additionally, beta-blockers should be considered in all intermediate or high-risk patients undergoing noncardiac major surgery. Perioperative beta-blockers can be administered in either the oral or parenteral form (metoprolol, 25 to 50 mg orally 2 times a day or 2.5 to 5.0 mg intravenously every 6 hours).
         (b) Patients who are receiving **nitrate therapy** should be given these medications during the perioperative period. Those who are receiving oral nitrate therapy can be switched to topical therapy.

(c) **Calcium channel blockers** should also be continued in the perioperative period if they were taken preoperatively.
b. **Congestive heart failure.** The etiology of CHF should be determined, recognizing the strong association with ischemic cardiac disease. Patients with poor preoperative cardiac function should be monitored in an intensive care setting for careful titration of volume replacement. Invasive monitoring and daily CXRs assist in evaluating volume status. Patients who are given digoxin therapy for CHF should continue receiving this drug in the postoperative period, either in the oral or parenteral form. The management of florid failure in the postoperative period is discussed in Section III.B.2.
3. **Renal disease**
   a. **Fluids and electrolytes.** Patients with chronic renal insufficiency require replacement of operative fluid losses in the same manner as normal patients; however, care should be taken to avoid excessive fluid replacement. Maintenance fluids should not contain potassium. Frequent measurement of serum electrolytes is required and early dialysis may be necessary because of hyperkalemia or intravascular volume overload.
   b. **Drug therapy in renal insufficiency.** Many drugs and their metabolites are cleared by the kidneys. In patients with reduced creatinine clearance, it is important to adjust the dose or the dosing interval of many drugs, including antibiotics. Some medications, such as meperidine, are contraindicated in patients with renal insufficiency.
4. **Diabetes.** Postoperative management of diabetic surgical patients centers on maintenance of euglycemia and management of chronic complications. All diabetic patients should have blood glucose checked on arrival to the postanesthesia recovery room. There is recent evidence suggesting decreased morbidity and mortality in critically ill patients admitted to the intensive care unit (ICU) with maintenance of blood sugars <110 mg/dl.
   a. **Diet-controlled diabetics** infrequently need glucose infusion or insulin therapy after minor surgery. After major surgery, these patients require dextrose infusion while fasting, blood glucose monitoring every 6 hours, and sliding-scale insulin coverage as needed.
   b. **Diabetic patients who are receiving oral hypoglycemic agents** frequently need insulin postoperatively. These patients require dextrose infusion while fasting, blood glucose monitoring 4 times a day (performed before meals and at bedtime), and subcutaneous regular insulin coverage as needed. When oral intake is tolerated, the preoperative oral hypoglycemic regimen should be resumed.
   c. **Patients who are taking insulin preoperatively** usually require insulin postoperatively to achieve adequate control of the serum glucose level. Brittle diabetics must receive their basal insulin requirements or they are at risk for development of DKA. DKA may develop in the fasting or metabolically stressed patient with a serum glucose level of only 100 to 200 mg/dL. Patients generally require at least their total daily dose given in divided doses postoperatively. Stress related to anesthesia, the operative procedure, and concurrent illness increases this requirement, especially during the first 24 to 48 hours after surgery. Regularly scheduled insulin dosing based on basal requirements plus anticipated patient needs is much more physiologic and thus preferable to the more common sliding-scale method. Parenteral glucose (100 to 150 g/day), given as 5% dextrose in intravenous fluids, should be given to all fasting diabetic patients to promote anabolism and to prevent ketosis and inadvertent hypoglycemia.
   d. **Intermittent dosing of subcutaneous insulin** can be given as intermediate-acting [neutral protamine Hagedorn (NPH)] insulin

twice a day, with hyperglycemia managed by supplemental dosing of regular insulin based on blood glucose determinations performed every 4 to 6 hours. Alternatively, regular insulin can be given in four divided doses before meals and at midnight if the patient is eating or simply every 6 hours if the patient is receiving intravenous glucose.

e. **Continuous intravenous insulin infusion in a monitored setting** is indicated in patients with hyperglycemia that is not controlled by intermittent subcutaneous dosing. The infusion should be started at 1 to 2 units per hour and titrated to effect. Initial blood glucose determinations should be done hourly. Conversion to a scheduled dose of regular or intermediate-acting subcutaneous insulin is based on clinical stability and should begin before discontinuation of the intravenous insulin infusion.

III. Complications
A. Neurologic complications
1. **Perioperative stroke**
   a. **Presentation.** Transient ischemic attacks (neurologic deficits that resolve in 24 hours) and stroke cannot be differentiated at the onset of symptoms. The patient usually describes rapid onset of focal loss of neurologic function (unilateral weakness or clumsiness, sensory loss, speech disorder, diplopia, or vertigo). Massive strokes can also present with altered mental status.
   b. **Examination.** A thorough neurologic examination, in addition to vital signs, finger-stick glucose, and pulse oxymetry, should be assessed.
   c. **Evaluation**
      (1) **Laboratory evaluation** should include a CBC, electrolytes, BUN, creatinine, and coagulation studies. An ECG should be done to rule out cardiac arrhythmia.
      (2) A **CT scan of the head** should be obtained urgently to rule out a hemorrhagic stroke.
      (3) **Further studies**, including echocardiography, carotid and transcranial ultrasound, and MR scan should only be ordered in consultation with a neurologist.
   d. **Treatment**
      (1) **General supportive measures** include supplemental oxygen and intravenous fluid.
      (2) **Aspirin** (325 mg orally) should be given immediately in ischemic stroke.
      (3) **Thrombolysis** has been proven effective in improving outcomes from ischemic strokes; however, it is usually contraindicated in postoperative patients and should only be initiated in close consultation with a neurologist.
2. **Seizures.** Evaluation and treatment of postoperative seizures involve the same principles as those encountered in other settings. Most seizures in surgical patients without a history of seizure can be attributed to metabolic derangements, including electrolyte abnormalities (e.g., hyponatremia, hypocalcemia), hypoglycemia, sepsis, fever, and drugs (e.g., imipenem).
   a. **Determine from patient history whether a true seizure was witnessed**; if so, note its type, characteristics (i.e., general versus focal onset), and similarity to any previous seizures. New-onset seizures are worrisome, and iatrogenic causes (e.g., medications) and cerebrovascular accident must be considered. A history of preoperative alcohol use should prompt an evaluation for withdrawal.
   b. **Complete physical and neurologic examination** should focus on airway, oxygenation, and hemodynamics and then on any sequelae of seizure, including trauma, aspiration, or rhabdomyolysis. A focally abnormal neurologic examination, especially in the setting of a new-onset focal seizure, suggests a possible cerebrovascular event.

c. **Laboratory and diagnostic studies.** Begin with rapid blood glucose determination, CBC, and serum chemistries, including calcium and magnesium as well as an oxygen saturation. Serum levels of anticonvulsants should be measured in patients receiving these medications. Patients with new-onset seizures who do not have identifiable metabolic or systemic causes warrant further evaluation with a head CT scan followed by a lumbar puncture.

d. **Treatment** of new-onset, single, nonrecurring seizures or recurrent generalized seizures with identifiable metabolic or systemic causes usually requires only correction of the underlying abnormality.

   (1) **Recurrent generalized tonic-clonic seizures** require anticonvulsant therapy. A 15- to 20-mg/kg load of phenytoin, given parenterally in three divided doses followed by maintenance dosing of 5 mg/kg per day in three divided doses, controls most seizures. Therapeutic serum levels are 10 to 20 mg/mL.

   (2) **Status epilepticus** is a medical emergency.

      (a) **Monitor cardiopulmonary parameters and stabilize the patient's airway with a soft oral or nasal airway.** Endotracheal intubation might be required to protect the airway, especially in the setting of status epilepticus when significant doses of antiepileptic agents may be required to terminate the seizure. It should be noted that phenobarbital and benzodiazepines in combination severely depress respiratory drive. Intravenous access should be established peripherally.

      (b) **Administer parenteral anticonvulsants promptly.**

         (i) **Diazepam** (5 to 10 mg intravenously every 5 to 10 minutes) or **lorazepam** (1 to 2 mg intravenously every 5 to 10 minutes) should be administered to patients with generalized convulsions of greater than 5 minutes' duration. Results usually are obtained within 10 minutes. These agents are relatively short acting, however, and a second parenteral anticonvulsant should be started concurrently.

         (ii) **Phenytoin** administered parenterally is the first choice to supplement the benzodiazepines in this setting, with dosing as noted previously.

         (III) **Phenobarbital** is a second-line agent and should be used when phenytoin is contraindicated (e.g., heart block) or ineffective. A loading dose of 10 mg/kg can be given at 100 mg/minute. Maintenance doses of 1 to 5 mg/kg per day intravenously or orally are required to achieve therapeutic plasma levels. Institution of a phenobarbital coma should be considered if status epilepticus continues.

3. **Delirium.** Delirium is common in patients (especially the elderly) who undergo the stress of operation. An underlying cause usually can be identified and in most cases involves medications or infection. Other causes include hypoxemia, electrolyte abnormalities, cardiac arrhythmias, MI, and stroke. Alcohol withdrawal, discussed in Section III.A.4, is another common cause of postoperative delirium.

   a. **Symptoms** include impaired memory, altered perception, and paranoia. Altered sleep patterns result in drowsiness during the day and wakefulness and agitation at night (sundowning). Combativeness is common.

   b. **Management** begins with eliminating the possibility of an underlying physiologic or metabolic derangement. Pulse, blood pressure (BP), temperature, and pulse oximetry should be assessed and a thorough physical exam performed with attention to the possibility of infection. CBC and electrolytes should be obtained. Other testing, including ECG, arterial blood gas (ABG), urinalysis (UA), and CXR, is dictated by clinical suspicion. Medications should be reviewed carefully, with consideration directed toward anticholinergic agents, opiate analgesics, and antihistamines. If no underlying organic cause is identified, alteration in sleep patterns or sensory deprivation can be invoked, and haloperidol (1 to 5 mg orally or intramuscularly) can be prescribed. Often, family reassurance or transfer to a naturally lighted room is curative. Physical restraints might be necessary to prevent self-harm.

4. **Alcohol withdrawal.** Alcohol withdrawal carries a significant risk of morbidity and mortality and a high level of vigilance is required to prevent this complication.

   a. **Symptoms.** Minor withdrawal can begin 6 to 8 hours after cessation of alcohol intake and is characterized by anxiety, tremulousness, anorexia, and nausea. Signs include tachycardia, hypertension, and hyperreflexia. These signs and symptoms generally resolve within 24 to 48 hours. Delirium tremens typically occurs 72 to 96 hours or longer after cessation of alcohol intake and is characterized by disorientation, hallucinations, and autonomic lability that includes tachycardia, hypertension, fever, and profuse diaphoresis.

   b. **Treatment**

   (1) **Benzodiazepines**, such as chlordiazepoxide, 25 to 100 mg orally every 6 hours; oxazepam, 5 to 15 mg orally every 6 hours; or diazepam, 5 to 20 mg orally or intravenously every 6 hours, can be used as prophylaxis in alcoholics who have a history of withdrawal or to alleviate symptoms of minor withdrawal. Patients with delirium tremens should be given diazepam, 5 to 10 mg intravenously every 10 to 15 minutes, to control symptoms. Oversedation must be avoided through close monitoring. The dosage of benzodiazepines should be reduced in patients with liver impairment. Moderate alcohol intake with meals can be a simple way to prevent and treat alcohol withdrawal.

   (2) **Clonidine**, 0.1 mg orally 4 times a day, or atenolol, 50 to 100 mg orally, every day, can be used to treat tachycardia or hypertension resulting from autonomic hyperactivity. These patients require close hemodynamic monitoring during therapy.

   (3) **General medical care.** Fluid and electrolyte abnormalities should be corrected, and fever should be treated with acetaminophen or cooling blankets as needed. Thiamine, 100 mg intramuscularly for 3 days, followed by 100 mg orally every day, should be given to all suspected alcoholic patients to prevent development of Wernicke's encephalopathy. Many chronic alcoholics have hypomagnesemia, and, if it is present, magnesium sulfate should be administered to patients with normal renal function. Folate should be given 1 mg intramuscularly or orally every day.

   (4) **Restraints** should be used only when necessary to protect the patient from self-harm.

   (5) **Alcohol withdrawal seizures** occur 12 to 48 hours after cessation of alcohol and are most often generalized tonic-clonic. They are usually brief and self-limited, although status epilepticus occurs in approximately 3% of cases. Benzodiazepines are most helpful in preventing recurrent seizures.

B. **Cardiovascular complications**

1. **Myocardial ischemia and infarction**

   a. The **presentation** of myocardial ischemia in the postoperative patient is often subtle, as incisional pain may be difficult to differentiate from chest pain. Frequently, perioperative MI is silent or presents with dyspnea, hypotension, or atypical pain.

   b. In postoperative patients who present with chest pain, the **differential diagnosis** includes myocardial ischemia or infarction, PE, pneumonia, and, less commonly, pericarditis, aortic dissection, and pneumothorax.

c. Evaluation

(1) Physical examination should be performed carefully to assess BP, heart rate, and general organ and tissue perfusion. The lungs should be auscultated for signs of pulmonary edema (with myocardial ischemia or infarction and CHF) and diminished or absent breath sounds unilaterally (pneumothorax). Auscultation of the heart can reveal a new murmur suggestive of ischemic mitral regurgitation or a pericardial friction rub suggestive of pericarditis. All peripheral pulses should be palpated, and BP should be measured in both arms.

(2) Diagnostic testing

(a) An **electrocardiogram** is warranted in virtually all cases of postoperative chest pain, with comparison to prior tracings. Of note, sinus tachycardia is one of the most common rhythms associated with myocardial ischemia.

(b) Laboratory data

(i) Cardiac enzymes. An elevated troponin-I level is diagnostic of MI. A series of three samplings of troponin-I 12 hours apart has a sensitivity and specificity of more than 90% for detecting myocardial injury.

(ii) Routine chemistries and hemoglobin should be determined.

(iii) Oxygen saturation should be determined via pulse oximetry, and supplemental oxygen should be administered. Patients with chest pain should have arterial oxygen saturation determined with a noninvasive oxygen saturation monitor. Patients with oxygen saturations of less than 93% on room air or with symptoms of dyspnea or other signs of respiratory compromise should have ABG determined. Significant hypoxia can be seen with MI, CHF, pneumonia, and PE.

(c) Chest x-rays should be obtained and evaluated for pneumothorax, infiltrate, or evidence of pulmonary edema.

(d) Further diagnostic evaluation (e.g., echocardiography, coronary catheterization, ventilation-perfusion scintigraphy, or CT scan) should be pursued as indicated by the diagnostic workup.

(3) Treatment

(a) Telemetry should be used in all patients with suspected myocardial ischemia.

(b) Oxygen therapy. The arterial oxygen saturation should be kept at greater than 90% with supplemental oxygen. Endotracheal intubation and mechanical ventilation are indicated for patients with hypoxia that is refractory to supplemental oxygen therapy, progressive hypercapnia, or respiratory fatigue.

(c) Pharmacologic therapy

(i) Nitrates. In the absence of hypotension (systemic BP <90 mm Hg), initial management of patients with chest pain of presumed cardiac origin includes the use of sublingual nitroglycerin (0.4 mg), which can be repeated every 5 minutes. Additionally, topical nitrate therapy (0.5 to 2.0 in. every 6 hours) can be instituted. Ongoing myocardial ischemia or infarction should be treated with intravenous nitroglycerin, starting with an infusion rate of 5 μg/minute and increased at 5-μg/minute increments until the chest pain is relieved or significant hypotension develops (systemic BP <90 mm Hg).

(ii) Beta-adrenergic receptor antagonists. In the absence of significant contraindications (e.g., heart failure, bradycardia, heart block, or significant COPD), patients should be treated with intravenous beta-adrenergic receptor antagonists (e.g., metoprolol, 15 mg intravenously, in 5- mg doses every 5 minutes, followed by a 50- to 100-mg oral dose every 12 hours).

(iii) **Intravenous morphine sulfate** (1 to 4 mg intravenously every hour) is also useful in the acute management of chest pain to decrease the sympathetic drive of an anxious patient.

(iv) **Antiplatelet therapy** in the form of a non–enteric-coated aspirin (325 mg) can also be given, if the patient is at low risk of perioperative bleeding.

(d) **Other therapeutic measures.** Thrombolytic therapy, anticoagulation, or coronary catheterization should be considered on an individual basis in consultation with a cardiologist.

2. **Congestive heart failure**

a. **Differential diagnosis** of shortness of breath or hypoxia in the perioperative period includes CHF, pneumonia, atelectasis, PE, reactive airway disease (asthma, COPD exacerbation), and pneumothorax. These conditions are discussed in Section III.C.

b. **Evaluation**

(1) **History.** CHF typically occurs immediately postoperatively as a result of excessive intraoperative administration of fluids, or 24 to 48 hours postoperatively, related to mobilization of fluids that are sequestered in the extracellular space. Myocardial ischemia or infarct can also lead to CHF.

(2) **Physical examination** should be directed toward signs and symptoms of fluid overload and myocardial ischemia. Net fluid balance and weight for the preceding days should be assessed.

(3) **Diagnostic testing**

(a) **Laboratory data.** Troponin-I, ABG, CBC, electrolytes, and renal function tests may be of value. B-type natriuretic peptide (BNP), a cardiac neurohormone, has shown promise in the diagnosis of CHF. A level of <100 pg/mL generally excludes acutely decompensated CHF.

(b) **Pulse oximetry**

(c) **Electrocardiogram**

(d) **Chest x-ray**

(e) An **echocardiogram** is frequently indicated in patients with new CHF to evaluate the valves, assess the dimensions of each cardiac chamber, and rule out tamponade.

(f) Invasive measurement of cardiac output with a **pulmonary artery catheter** may be of use in assessing volume status.

c. **Management of congestive heart failure**

(1) **Supplemental oxygen** should be administered. Mechanical ventilation (either noninvasive or via endotracheal intubation) is indicated in patients with refractory hypoxemia.

(2) **Diuretics.** Treatment should be initiated with furosemide (20 to 40 mg intravenously push), with doses up to 200 mg every 6 hours as necessary to achieve adequate diuresis. Furosemide drips can be effective in promoting diuresis. Fluid intake should be limited and serum potassium should be monitored closely.

(3) **Morphine** (1 to 4 mg intravenously push every 1 hour)

(4) **Arterial vasodilators.** To reduce afterload and help the failing heart in the acute setting, sodium nitroprusside or angiotensin-converting enzyme inhibitors can be administered to lower the systolic BP to 90 to 100 mm Hg.

(5) **Inotropic agents.** Digoxin increases myocardial contractility and can be used to treat patients with mild failure. Patients with florid failure may need invasive monitoring and titration of drips if they

Table 1-8. Doses of commonly used vasopressors

Vasopressor	Preparation	Infusion	Comments
Dobutamine	250 mg/250 mL NS or D5W	Start at 3 μg/kg/min and titrate up to 20 μg/kg/min based on clinical response	Beta agonist
Dopamine	800 mg in 500 mL NS or D5W	Start at 3 μg/kg per min and titrate to systolic BP	Beta-adrenergic effects dominate at lower infusion rates
Epinephrine	5 mg/ 500 mL NS or D5W	1–4 μg/min, titrate to effect	Alpha and beta
Norepinephrine	8 mg in 500 mL D5W	Start at 2 μg per min and titrate to systolic BP	Strong alpha-adrenergic agonist
Phenylephrine (NeoSynephrine)	10 mg in 250 mL D5W or NS	Start at 10 μg per min and titrate to systolic BP	May be ineffective in severe distributive shock

BP, blood pressure; D5W, 5% dextrose in water; NS, normal saline.

do not respond to these measures. If there is a low cardiac index (<2.5 L/minute per m^2) with elevated filling pressures, inotropic agents are indicated. Therapy can be initiated with dobutamine (3 to 20 μg/kg per minute) to increase the cardiac index to a value near 3 L/minute per m^2. Milrinone is also a useful agent for refractory CHF. (A loading dose of 50 μg/kg is administered over 10 minutes, followed by a continuous infusion of 0.375 to 0.750 μg/kg per minute titrated for clinical response.) If hypotension is accompanied by low systemic vascular resistance, vasopressors may be useful (Table 1-8).

   (6) Recombinant human BNP (**nesiritide**) is now available for the treatment of decompensated CHF, but the optimal role of this agent versus other therapies has not yet been defined.
C. **Pulmonary complications**
   1. The **differential diagnosis** of dyspnea includes atelectasis, pneumonia, CHF, COPD or asthma exacerbation, pneumothorax, PE, and aspiration.
   2. **Evaluation**
      a. **History.** Additional factors that help to differentiate disease entities include the presence of a fever, chest pain, and the time since surgery.
      b. **Physical examination** with attention to jugular venous distention, breath sounds (wheezing, crackles), symmetry, and respiratory effort.
      c. **Diagnostic testing**
         (1) **Laboratory.** CBC, chemistry profile, and pulse oximetry or ABG
         (2) **Electrocardiograms** should be obtained for any patient older than 30 years with significant dyspnea or tachypnea to exclude myocardial ischemia and in any patient who is dyspneic in the setting of tachycardia.
         (3) **Chest x-rays** are mandatory in all dyspneic patients.
         (4) **V/Q scan, pulmonary embolism protocol chest computed tomography scan,** or pulmonary angiogram may be helpful.
   3. **Management** of specific diagnoses
      a. **Atelectasis** commonly occurs in the first 36 hours after operation and typically presents with dyspnea and hypoxia. Therapy is aimed at reexpanding the collapsed alveoli. For most patients, deep breathing

and coughing along with the use of incentive spirometry is adequate. Postoperative pain should be sufficiently controlled so that pulmonary mechanics are not significantly impaired. In patients with significant atelectasis or lobar collapse, chest physical therapy and nasotracheal suctioning might be required. In rare cases, bronchoscopy can aid in clearing mucus plugs that cannot be cleared using less invasive measures.

b. **Pneumonia** is discussed in Section III.E.2.b.

c. **Pulmonary embolism** is discussed in Section III.F.

d. **Gastric aspiration** usually presents with acute dyspnea and fever. CXR might be normal initially, but subsequently can demonstrate a pattern of diffuse interstitial infiltrates. Therapy is supportive, and antibiotics are typically not given empirically.

e. **Pneumothorax** is treated with tube thoracostomy. If tension pneumothorax is suspected, immediate needle decompression through the second intercostal space in the midclavicular line using a 14-gauge needle should precede controlled placement of a thoracostomy tube.

f. **Chronic obstructive pulmonary disease and asthma** exacerbations present with dyspnea or tachypnea, wheezing, hypoxemia, and possibly hypercapnia. Acute therapy includes administration of supplemental oxygen and inhaled beta-adrenergic agonists [albuterol, 3.0 mL (2.5 mg) in 2 mL normal saline every 4 to 6 hours of nebulization]. Beta-adrenergic agonists are indicated primarily for acute exacerbations rather than for long-term use. Anticholinergics such as ipratropium bromide metered-dose inhaler (Atrovent, 2 puffs every 4 to 6 hours) can also be used in the perioperative period, especially if the patient has significant pulmonary secretions. Patients with severe asthma or COPD may benefit from parenteral steroid therapy (methylprednisolone, 50 to 250 mg intravenously every 4 to 6 hours) as well as inhaled steroids (beclomethasone metered-dose inhaler, 2 puffs 4 times a day), but steroids require 6 to 12 hours to take effect.

D. **Renal complications**

1. **Acute renal failure**

a. **Causes.** The etiologies of postoperative renal insufficiency can be divided into prerenal, intrinsic renal, and postrenal classes (Table 1-9).

(1) **Prerenal azotemia** results from decreased renal perfusion that might be secondary to hypotension, intravascular volume contraction, or decreased effective renal perfusion (CHF, hepatorenal syndrome).

(2) **Renal.** Intrinsic renal causes of ARF include drug-induced acute tubular necrosis, pigment-induced renal injury, radiocontrast dye administration, acute interstitial nephritis, and prolonged ischemia from suprarenal aortic cross-clamping.

(3) **Postrenal causes** of ARF can result from obstruction of the ureters or bladder. Operations that involve dissection near the ureters, such as colectomy, colostomy closure, or total abdominal hysterectomy, have a higher incidence of ureteral injuries. In addition to

Table 1-9. Laboratory evaluation of oliguria and acute renal failure

Category	FE_{Na}	U_{Osm}	RFI	U_{Cr}/P_{Cr}	U_{Na}
Prerenal	<1	>500	<1	>40	<20
Renal (acute tubular necrosis)	>1	<350	>1	<20	>40
Postrenal	>1	<50	>1	<20	>40

FE_{Na}, fractional excretion of sodium; RFI, renal failure index; U_{Cr}/P_{Cr}, urine-plasma creatinine ratio; U_{Na}, urine sodium; U_{Osm}, urine osmolality.

ureteral injuries or obstruction, obstruction of the bladder from an enlarged prostate, postoperative pain and medication administration, or obstructed urinary catheter can occur.

b. **General evaluation**
   (1) History and physical examination
   (2) Laboratory evaluation
   (a) **Urinalysis** can help to differentiate between etiologies of renal failure.
   (b) **Serum chemistries**
   (c) **Urinary indices** help to classify ARF into prerenal, postrenal, or intrinsic renal categories (Table 1-9). Fractional excretion of sodium (Fe_{Na}) can be calculated from this formula:

$$Fe_{Na} = (U_{Na}/P_{Na})/(U_{Cr}/P_{Cr}).$$

   The renal failure index (RFI) is $(U_{Na})(P_{Cr})/U_{Cr}$. These measurements must be obtained before diuretic administration.
   (3) Other diagnostic testing
   (a) **Renal ultrasonography** can be used to exclude the diagnosis of obstructive uropathy, evaluate the chronicity of renal disease, and evaluate the renal vasculature with Doppler.
   (b) **Radiologic studies** using intravenous contrast are contraindicated in patients with suspected ARF due to the potential to exacerbate renal injury.
c. **Management of specific problems**
   (1) Oliguria (<500 mL per day) in the postoperative period
   (a) **Evaluation.** Laboratory evaluation should include serum chemistries, BUN, and creatinine and the urinary indices, such as Fe_{Na}, U_{Na}, and U_{Osm}. Because management of the causes of oliguria differs substantially, the goal of this evaluation is to determine the patient's intravascular volume status and to differentiate the causes of oliguria. Cardiac echocardiography, or invasive monitoring of central venous pressures, or pulmonary artery pressures can assist with evaluation of volume status.
   (b) **Management**
      (I) Prerenal. In most surgical patients, oliguria is caused by hypovolemia. Initial management includes fluid challenges (normal saline, 500 mL). Patients with adequate fluid resuscitation and CHF may benefit from invasive monitoring and optimization of cardiac function.
      (ii) Intrinsic renal. Treat underlying cause, if possible, and manage volume status.
      (iii) Postrenal. Ureteral injuries or obstruction can be treated with percutaneous nephrostomy tubes and generally are managed in consultation with a urologist. Urinary retention and urethral obstruction can be managed by placement of a Foley catheter or, if necessary, a suprapubic catheter.
   (2) Elevated creatinine and acute renal failure
   (a) **Evaluation.** The laboratory and diagnostic evaluation for patients with a rising creatinine is similar to the evaluation for patients with oliguria and is discussed above.
   (b) **Management** includes careful attention to the intravascular volume status. The patient should be weighed daily, and intakes and outputs should be recorded carefully. Serum electrolytes should be monitored closely. The patient should be maintained in a euvolemic state. Hyperkalemia, metabolic acidosis, and hyperphosphatemia are common problems in patients with ARF and should be managed as discussed in

Chapter 4. Medication doses should be adjusted appropriately and potassium removed from maintenance intravenous fluids (IVF).

   (i) Dialysis. Indications for dialysis include intravascular volume overload, hyperkalemia, severe metabolic acidosis, and complications of uremia (encephalopathy, pericarditis).

E. Infectious complications

   1. Management of infection and fever

   a. Evaluation of fever should take into context the time after operation in which the fever occurs.

   (1) Intraoperative fever may be secondary to malignant hyperthermia, a transfusion reaction, or a preexisting infection.

   (a) Diagnosis and management of a transfusion reaction are discussed in Chapter 5.

   (b) Malignant hyperthermia is discussed in Chapter 6.

   (c) Preexisting infections should be treated with empiric intravenous antibiotics.

   (2) High fever (>39°C) in the first 24 hours is commonly the result of a streptococcal or clostridial wound infection, aspiration pneumonitis, or a preexisting infection.

   (a) Streptococcal wound infections present with severe local erythema and incisional pain. Penicillin G (2 million units intravenously every 6 hours) or ampicillin (1 to 2 g intravenously every 6 hours) is effective therapy. Rarely, patients with a **severe necrotizing clostridial infection** present with systemic toxemia, pain, and crepitus near the incision. Treatment includes emergent operative débridement and metronidazole (500 mg intravenously every 6 hours) or clindamycin (600 to 900 mg intravenously every 8 hours).

   (3) Fever that occurs more than 72 hours after surgery has a broad differential diagnosis, including pneumonia, urinary tract infection, thrombophlebitis, wound infection, intraabdominal abscess, and drug allergy.

   b. Diagnostic evaluation. The new onset of fever or leukocytosis without an obvious source of infection requires a thorough history and physical examination (including inspection of all wounds, tubes, and catheter sites) and selected laboratory tests.

   c. Specific laboratory tests

   (1) Complete blood count

   (2) Urinalysis

   (3) Chest x-ray

   (4) Gram stain/culture. Cultures of the blood, sputum, urine, or wound should be dictated by the clinical situation.

   d. Antibiotics. Empiric antibiotics can be initiated, with therapy directed by clinical suspicion.

   e. Imaging studies such as ultrasound or CT should be chosen based on clinical context.

   2. Management of specific infectious etiologies

   a. Wound infection is diagnosed by local erythema, swelling, pain and tenderness, and wound drainage. Fever and leukocytosis are usually present but may be absent in superficial wound infections. The primary treatment is to open and pack the wound at the site of erythema and to allow drainage. The wound should be cultured at this time. If the infection is contained in the superficial tissue layers, antibiotics are not required. In the case of a clean procedure that did not enter the bowel, the usual pathogens are staphylococcal and streptococcal species. If surrounding erythema is extensive, parenteral antibiotics should be initiated. Wound infections in the perineum or after bowel surgery are more likely to be caused by enteric pathogens and anaerobes. More aggressive infections with involvement of underlying fascia require emergent operative débridement and broad-spectrum intravenous antibiotics.

b. **Respiratory infections.** Pneumonia is diagnosed by the presence of fever, leukocytosis, purulent sputum production, and an infiltrate on CXR. After Gram stain and culture of the sputum and blood is performed, empiric antibiotics can be started. Pneumonias that occur in postoperative patients should be treated as nosocomial infections. Patients requiring mechanical ventilation for longer than 48 hours are at risk for ventilator-associated pneumonia (VAP), which may require bronchoscopy for diagnosis.

c. **Gastrointestinal infections** may present with fever, leukocytosis, and diarrhea. *Clostridium difficile* is a common cause of diarrhea in hospitalized patients and assay for the *C. difficile* organism or toxin should be performed. Initial therapy includes fluid resuscitation and metronidazole (500 mg orally every 6 to 8 hours) or vancomycin (250–500 mg orally every 6 hours).

d. **Intraabdominal abscess or peritonitis** presents with fever, leukocytosis, abdominal pain, and tenderness. If the patient has generalized peritonitis, emergency laparotomy is indicated. If the inflammation appears to be localized, a CT scan of the patient's abdomen and pelvis should be obtained. The primary management of an intraabdominal abscess is drainage. In some circumstances, this can be performed percutaneously with radiologic guidance. In other situations, operative débridement and drainage are required. Empiric antibiotic therapy should cover enteric pathogens and anaerobes.

e. **Genitourinary infections.** After the urine is cultured, simple lower-tract infections can be managed with oral antibiotics. Ill patients or those with pyelonephritis require more aggressive therapy.

f. **Prosthetic device–related infections** may present with fever, leukocytosis, and systemic bacteremia. Infection of prosthetic valves may present with a new murmur. Management may require removal of the infected device and the use of long-term antibiotics.

g. **Catheter-related infections** also are diagnosed by the presence of fever, leukocytosis, and systemic bacteremia. Local erythema and purulence may be present around central venous catheter insertion sites. Erythema, purulence, a tender thrombosed vein, or lymphangitis may be present near an infected peripheral intravenous line. Management includes removal of the catheter and intravenous antibiotic coverage.

h. **Fascial or muscle infections** may result from gross contamination of a surgical wound or from a previously infected wound. Fasciitis and deep-muscle infections present with hemorrhagic bullae over the infected area, rapidly progressive edema, erythema, pain, and crepitus. Fever, tachycardia, and ultimately cardiovascular collapse occur in rapid succession. Therapy includes emergent operative débridement, management of shock, and broad-spectrum antibiotics (including anaerobic coverage). Necrotizing fasciitis is a surgical emergency; death may result within a few hours of the development of symptoms.

i. **Viral infections** complicating operations are uncommon in immunocompetent patients.

j. **Fungal infections** (primarily with *Candida* species) occur most commonly after long-term antibiotic administration. In these patients, evaluation of persistent fever without an identified bacterial source should include several sets of routine and fungal blood cultures, removal of all intravenous catheters, and examination of the retina for *Candida endophthalmitis*. Therapy includes either amphotericin B or fluconazole.

F. Deep venous thrombosis and pulmonary embolism
   1. Diagnosis and treatment of deep venous thrombosis
      a. Diagnosis
         (1) Symptoms of DVT vary greatly, although classically they include pain and swelling of the affected extremity distal to the site of venous obstruction. Signs of DVT on physical examination may include edema, erythema, warmth, a palpable cord, or calf tenderness with dorsiflexion of the foot (Homans' sign). Physical examination alone is notoriously inaccurate (<50%) in the diagnosis of DVT, and a high index of suspicion is often required to pursue further diagnostic measures.
         (2) Noninvasive studies of the venous system, most notably B-mode ultrasonography plus color Doppler (duplex scanning), have revolutionized the diagnosis and management of suspected DVT. Reported sensitivity and specificity of this test for the detection of proximal DVT are greater than 90%, with nearly 100% positive predictive value. This modality is less reliable in the detection of infrapopliteal thrombi, and a negative study in symptomatic patients should be followed by repeat examination in 48 to 72 hours to evaluate for propagation of clot proximally. Patients in whom a negative study contrasts with a strong clinical suspicion may require contrast venography, the gold standard for diagnosis of DVT.
      b. Treatment (see also Chapter 5, Section V)
         (1) Superficial thrombophlebitis is treated effectively by local measures and poses little risk of PE. Elevation of the affected extremity, range-of-motion exercises, and elastic stockings enhance venous outflow, whereas heat improves arterial microcirculation, promoting clot lysis. Anti-inflammatory agents (aspirin, nonsteroidal antiinflammatory drugs) also can be administered. Antibiotics are not indicated in this setting unless there is evidence of cellulitis.
         (2) Deep venous thrombosis of the proximal veins requires aggressive treatment to avoid potentially lethal PE and to decrease the incidence of postphlebitic venous insufficiency. Although not all isolated calf DVTs require treatment, they must be taken seriously, because up to 30% extend proximally and are at risk for embolization. If anticoagulation is withheld in these cases, serial noninvasive examinations are indicated.
            (a) Heparin is the traditional acute treatment for proximal DVT. It usually is administered intravenously at approximately 100 units/kg bolus (5,000 to 10,000 units) followed by a constant infusion (600 to 1,000 units/hour) targeted to an activated partial thromboplastin time (PTT) of 50 to 80 seconds. Patients who receive heparin should have platelet determinations performed at least every 3 days to detect heparin-induced thrombocytopenia.
            (b) Anticoagulation with warfarin typically requires 1 to 3 days, during which time concurrent anticoagulation with heparin is necessary. Although the dosing regimen should be individualized, in most patients, 5 mg warfarin can be given the first day that heparin is started, with a subsequent 5 mg/day for 1 to 2 days. Dosage thereafter should be directed toward obtaining an INR of 2.0 to 3.0. Duration of therapy for uncomplicated DVT in a patient with no other risk factors (i.e., immobility) is 6 months.
   2. Diagnosis and treatment of pulmonary embolism
      a. Diagnosis
         (1) Symptoms of PE are neither sensitive nor specific. Mental status changes, dyspnea, pleuritic chest pain, and cough can occur

and hemoptysis is encountered occasionally. Signs of PE most commonly include tachypnea and tachycardia. Patients with massive PE may experience syncope or cardiovascular collapse. PE should be considered in any postoperative patient with unexplained dyspnea, hypoxia, tachycardia, or dysrhythmia.

(2) Laboratory studies. Initial evaluation of patients with suspected PE must include noninvasive arterial oxygen saturation, ECG, and CXR. Findings that are suggestive of PE include arterial oxygen desaturation, nonspecific ST-wave or T-wave changes on ECG, and atelectasis, parenchymal abnormalities, or pleural effusion on CXR. Such classic signs as $S_1Q_3T_3$ on ECG or a prominent central pulmonary artery with decreased pulmonary vascularity (Westermark's sign) on CXR are uncommon. ABG determination is a helpful adjunctive test; a decreased PaO_2 (<80 mm Hg), an elevated alveolar-arterial oxygen gradient, or a respiratory alkalosis may support clinical suspicion. Data that are obtained from these initial studies collectively may corroborate clinical suspicion but alone are neither sensitive nor specific for PE. **D-Dimer** assays have a high negative predictive value; however, positive values, particularly in the setting of recent surgery, are less helpful as the postoperative period is one of many conditions that can cause an elevation of this test.

(3) Imaging studies

   (a) Spiral computed tomography scan is becoming the primary diagnostic modality for PE. The advantages of CT scans for PE include increased sensitivity, the ability to simultaneously evaluate other pulmonary and mediastinal abnormalities, greater after-hours availability, and the ability to obtain a CT venogram with the same dye load. This study subjects the patient to a contrast dye load and requires a large (18g) IV in the antecubital vein, but is not invasive. There are still wide variations in technology and institutional expertise with this modality, with reported sensitivities ranging from 57 to 100% and specificity ranging from 78 to 100%.

   (b) A **V/Q scan** that demonstrates one or more perfusion defects in the absence of matched ventilation defects is abnormal and may be interpreted as high, intermediate, or low probability for PE, depending on the type and degree of abnormality. V/Q scans alone are neither sensitive nor specific for PE, however, and their interpretation may be difficult in patients with pre-existing lung disease, especially COPD. Nevertheless, high-probability scans are 90% predictive and suffice for diagnosis of PE. In the appropriate clinical setting, a high probability V/Q scan should prompt treatment. Likewise, a normal scan virtually excludes PE (96%). Scans of intermediate probability require additional confirmatory tests.

   (c) Pulmonary angiography is the reference standard for the diagnosis of PE, but is an invasive test with some element of risk. This test is rapidly being supplanted by spiral CT for most circumstances. Its use should be reserved for (1) resolution of conflicting or inconclusive clinical and noninvasive data; (2) patients with high clinical suspicion for PE and extensive preexisting pulmonary disease, in whom interpretation of V/Q scans is difficult, without access to spiral CT; and (3) confirmation of clinical and noninvasive data in patients who are at high risk for anticoagulation or in unstable patients being considered for thrombolytic therapy, pulmonary embolectomy, or vena caval interruption.

b. Treatment

(1) Supportive measures include administration of oxygen to correct hypoxemia and use of intravenous fluids to maintain BP. Hypotensive patients with high clinical suspicion of PE (i.e., high-risk patient, acute right heart failure, right ventricular ischemia on ECG) require immediate transfer to an ICU, where hemodynamic monitoring and vasoactive medications may be required.

(2) Anticoagulation with intravenous heparin should be started immediately with a target-activated PTT of 50 to 80 seconds. Oral warfarin can be started concurrently while heparin is continued until a therapeutic prothrombin time is achieved. Anticoagulation should continue for 6 months unless risk factors persist or DVT recurs. Some studies have shown that low-molecular-weight heparin administered subcutaneously (1 mg/kg every 12 hours) may be as effective as intravenous heparin.

(3) Thrombolytic therapy is not indicated in the routine treatment of PE in surgical patients because the risk of hemorrhage in individuals with recent (<10 days) surgery outweighs the uncertain long-term benefits of this therapy. Surgical patients with shock secondary to angiographically proved massive PE that is refractory to anticoagulation should be considered for either transvenous embolectomy or open pulmonary embolectomy. These aggressive measures rarely are successful.

(4) Inferior vena caval filter placement is indicated when a contraindication to anticoagulation exists (i.e., active peptic ulcer disease, bleeding tendency, patients prone to falling), when a bleeding complication occurs while receiving anticoagulation, or when a DVT or PE recurs during anticoagulation therapy.

G. Complications of diabetes

1. Diabetic ketoacidosis may occur in any diabetic patient who is sufficiently stressed by illness or surgery. DKA patients who require surgery should be provided every attempt at correction of metabolic abnormalities before operation, although in cases such as gangrene, surgery may be essential for treatment of the underlying cause of DKA. DKA may occur without excessive elevation of the blood glucose. Management of this disorder should emphasize volume repletion, correction of acidosis and electrolyte abnormalities, and regulation of blood glucose with insulin infusion.

a. Laboratory evaluation

(a) Blood glucose

(b) Complete blood count

(c) Serum electrolytes

(d) Serum osmolarity

(e) Arterial blood gas

b. Restoration of intravascular volume should be initiated with isotonic (0.9%) saline or lactated Ringer's solution without glucose. Patients without cardiac disease should receive 1 L or more of fluid per hour until objective evidence of normalization of intravascular volume is demonstrated by a urine output greater than 30 mL/hour and stabilization of hemodynamics. Invasive hemodynamic monitoring may be required to guide fluid replacement in some circumstances (i.e., CHF, suspected MI, and renal failure). Maintenance fluids of 0.45% NaCl with potassium (20 to 40 mEq/L) can be instituted when intravascular volume has been restored. Dextrose can be added to fluids when the blood glucose is less than 400 mg/dL.

c. Correction of acidosis with bicarbonate therapy is controversial but should be considered if the blood pH is less than 7.1 or shock is present. Two ampules (88 mEq $NaHCO_3$) of bicarbonate can be added to 0.45% NaCl and given during the initial resuscitation.

    d. Potassium replacement should be instituted immediately unless hyperkalemia with ECG changes exists. In nonoliguric patients, replacement should begin with 30 to 40 mEq/hour KCl for serum potassium of less than 3.0; 20 to 30 mEq/hour KCl for serum potassium of 3.0 to 4.0; and 10 to 20 mEq/hour KCl for potassium of more than 4.0 mEq/L.

    e. Blood glucose can be controlled with 10 units insulin as an intravenous bolus followed by insulin infusion at 2 to 10 units per hour to a target range of 200 to 300 mg/dL. When the blood glucose falls to 300 to 400 mg/dL, 5% dextrose must be added to the intravenous fluids. Therapy is guided by hourly blood glucose determinations.

  2. Nonketotic hyperosmolar syndrome is characterized by severe hyperglycemia and dehydration without ketoacidosis. This occurs most often in elderly non–insulin-dependent diabetes mellitus patients with renal impairment and may be precipitated by surgical illness or stress. Laboratory findings include blood glucose that exceeds 600 mg/dL and serum osmolarity of more than 350 mOsm/L. Therapy is similar to that for DKA but with two notable exceptions: (1) Fluid requirements are often higher and replacement should be with 0.45% saline, and (2) total insulin requirements are less.

H. Hypertension

  1. Definition. Postoperative hypertension should be defined by the patient's preoperative blood pressure. Patients with chronic hypertension have a shift in their cerebral autoregulatory system that may not allow for adequate cerebral perfusion at normotensive blood pressures. A reasonable goal of therapy for acute postoperative hypertension is within 10% of the patient's normal blood pressure.

  2. Treatment. Before using antihypertensive drugs in the treatment of postoperative hypertension, it is essential to diagnose and treat underlying causes, such as pain, hypoxemia, hypothermia, and acidosis. Acute hypertension can be managed with clonidine (0.1 mg orally every 6 hours), hydralazine (10 to 20 mg intravenously every 6 hours), labetalol (10 to 20 mg intravenously every 10 minutes, to a total dose of 300 mg), or a nitroprusside drip (0.25 to 8.00 μg/kg per minute intravenously). In situations in which the patient is unable to take oral medications and intravenous medications are not appropriate, nitroglycerin paste (0.5 to 2.0 in. every 6 hours) can be used.

IV. Documentation

Optimal patient care requires not only appropriate management but also effective communication and documentation. Documentation is essential for risk management, reimbursement, and communication between members of the health care team. All documentation should include a date, time, legible signature, and contact information (such as phone or pager number) in case clarification is necessary.

A. Hospital orders

  1. Admission orders should detail every aspect of a patient's care. **ADC-VAANDIML** is a simple mnemonic to organize admission, postoperative, and transfer orders.

    a. Admit. Include nursing division, surgical service, attending physician, and admission status (in-patient versus 23-hour observation).

    b. Diagnosis. The principal diagnosis, and, if relevant, care path. Include the operation or procedure performed.

    c. Condition. Distinguish between good, satisfactory, serious, and critical.

    d. Vitals. Include the frequency that vital signs should be obtained and special instructions such as pulse oximetry and neurologic and vascular checks.

    e. Allergies. Include specific reactions if known.

    f. Activity. Include necessary supervision and weightbearing status, if applicable. If mobilizing the patient, include specific instructions for ambulation. Patients on bedrest should be considered for DVT prophylaxis.

g. Nursing orders. Dressing care, drain care, urine output monitoring, and antiembolic stockings. Include specific parameters for physician notification for abnormal results (such as low urine output or low blood pressure). Daily weights, "ins and outs," pulmonary toilet (such as incentive spirometry), and regimens for turning patients should be addressed here. Also, **ventilator settings** (if applicable). Include mode, tidal volume, rate, pressure support, positive end-expiratory pressure, and oxygen percentage.

h. Diet. Include diet type (regular, American Diabetes Association, renal, etc.) and consistency (clear liquids, full liquids, pureed, etc.) as well as supervision instructions, if applicable. Patients are n.p.o. after midnight if a procedure requiring sedation is planned for the following day.

i. Intravenous fluids. Include fluid type, rate, and time interval.

j. Medications. Include home medicines if appropriate. Reference to patient-controlled anesthesia forms should be made here. Indications for new medications should be provided.

k. Laboratories. All necessary laboratory and radiographic investigations should be listed here, as well as electrocardiograms, cardiac diagnostic laboratory testing, pulmonary function tests, and other special procedures.

2. **Review orders with nursing staff.** All orders should be reviewed with the nursing staff, particularly any unusual orders or orders that must be expedited.

3. **STAT orders** should be designated as such on the order form and brought to the attention of the nursing staff. This is especially true for orders for new medicines because the pharmacy must be notified and the medicine brought to the floor.

4. **Discharge orders**

   a. Discharge should include location and condition. If a transfer to another institution is planned, copies of all medical records and a copy of current orders should be included.

   b. Activity limitations, if applicable, should be included. Workplace or school documentation may also be necessary.

   c. Medicines. Prescriptions for new medicines as well as detailed instructions are required.

   d. Follow-up. Follow-up plans with the appropriate physicians should be clearly indicated with contact information for their offices.

   e. Special. Wound care, catheter care, physical therapy, home health care needs, or special studies should be described before discharge.

B. **Hospital notes**

1. **History and physical examination.** The admission history and physical examination should be a complete record of the patient's history. Include past medical and surgical history, social history and family history, allergies, and home medicines with dosage and schedule. A complete review of systems should be documented. Outpatient records are often helpful and should be obtained if possible.

2. **Preoperative notes** summarize the pertinent laboratory and other investigations before one proceeds to the operating room (Table 1-10).

3. **Operative notes.** A brief operative note should be placed in the written medical record immediately following the operation, including the operative findings and patient's condition at the conclusion of the procedure (Table 1-11). The surgeon should also complete a dictated operative note immediately after the operation. In addition, a dictated note should include specific operative indications, preparation and drape position, sponge and instrument count, and copy distribution.

Table 1-10. Preoperative note

Preoperative diagnosis
Procedure planned
Attending physician
Laboratory investigations
Electrocardiogram (if applicable)
Chest x-ray and other radiology (if applicable)
Informed consent
n.p.o. past midnight
Type and screen/cross (if applicable)

    4. **Postoperative check.** Several hours after an operation, a patient should be examined and vital signs and urine output reviewed. Documentation in the medical record in the form of a SOA/P (subjective-objective-assessment/plan) note should be included.

    5. **Discharge summary.** A detailed account of a patient's hospitalization should be dictated at the time of discharge (Table 1-12). If a dictation confirmation number is provided, it should be recorded in the written medical record as the final note of the hospitalization. A dictated discharge summary must accompany any patients who are being transferred to other institutions.

V. Informed consent

    A. **Obtaining informed consent.** Recognition of patient autonomy dictates that physicians provide adequate information so that patients can make informed decisions regarding their medical care. Patients should understand the disease process, the natural course of the disease, the risks and benefits of the procedure under consideration, and potential alternative therapies. The most common and serious risks of the procedure and the patient's condition that might affect the outcome of a planned procedure or might place the patient at increased risk should be discussed. Recovery time, including amount and expected duration of postoperative pain, hospitalization, and future functional status should also be reviewed. The use of invasive monitoring devices, including arterial and pulmonary artery catheters, should

Table 1-11. Brief operative note

Preoperative diagnosis
Postoperative diagnosis
Procedure performed
Attending surgeon
Assistant/resident surgeons
Type of anesthesia
Operative findings and complications
Specimens removed
Packs, drains, and catheters
Estimated blood loss
Urine output
Fluids administered
   Blood products administered
   Antibiotics administered
Documentation that "time-out" to verify correct patient, procedure, and site was
   performed
Patient disposition and condition

Table 1-12. Discharge summary (dictated)

Your name, date, and time of dictation
Patient name
Patient registration number
Attending physician
Date of admission
Date of discharge
Principal diagnosis
Secondary diagnosis
Brief history and physical examination
Laboratory/radiographic findings
Hospital course
List of procedures performed with dates
Discharge instructions
Discharge condition
Copy distribution

be explained. These discussions should use terms that are readily understood by the patient. This is also an important opportunity for physicians to learn about the patient's wishes for aggressive treatment and acceptance of limitations to functional status.

B. **Documentation of informed consent.** An informed consent form is completed and signed by the patient before any elective operative procedure. In addition to the generic consent form, informed consent discussions should be documented in the progress notes section of the medical record. These notes should document the salient features of the informed consent discussion and specifically document that the potential complications and outcomes were explained to the patient. The patient's refusal to undergo a procedure that has been recommended by the physician should be documented clearly in the chart. In certain situations, such as a medical emergency, it is impossible to obtain informed consent. Inability to obtain consent should be documented carefully in the medical record. Local medical bylaws generally have provisions for these types of situations and should be consulted on a case-by-case basis.

VI. **Advance directives.** These are legal documents that allow patients to provide specific instructions for health care treatment in the event that the patient is unable to make or communicate these decisions personally. Advance directives commonly include standard living wills and durable powers of attorney for health care. With the growing realization that medical technology can prolong life considerably and sometimes even indefinitely beyond the point of significant or meaningful recovery, the importance of these issues is clear. Patients should be offered the opportunity to execute an advance directive on admission to the hospital.

A. **Living wills** provide specific instructions for the withdrawal of medical treatment in the event that a patient is unable to make treatment decisions and is terminally ill. Living wills do not include withdrawal or withholding of any procedure to provide nutrition or hydration.

B. **Durable powers of attorney for health care.** These directives allow a patient to legally designate a surrogate or proxy to make health care decisions if the patient is unable to do so. Because of the difficulty of predicting the complexities of aggressive medical management, powers of attorney are often more helpful than living wills in making difficult treatment decisions.

C. **Implementation.** Advance directives are personal documents and therefore differ from patient to patient. These documents should be reviewed carefully before implementation. Advanced directives are legal documents, and they should be displayed prominently in the medical record. To be legally binding,

the documents must be executed properly. If there is any question of validity, the risk management or legal staff of the hospital should be consulted. The most effective advance directives include specific instructions for health care decisions. Important issues to be addressed include the following:
1. Intravenous fluids
2. Enteral and parenteral nutrition
3. Medicines
4. Inotropic support
5. Renal dialysis
6. Mechanical ventilation
7. Cardiopulmonary resuscitation
D. **Conflicts.** Although advance directives can be helpful in the management of critically ill patients, their implementation often is difficult. Advance directives, by their nature, cannot provide for every medical situation. For this reason, it is important to communicate with the patient and family before the execution of an advance directive and with the family in the event that a patient becomes incapacitated. If no advance directive is available, the physician and family must consider carefully when life-prolonging medical treatments are no longer beneficial to the patient. In such a case, the state's interest in preserving life might conflict with the desires of the family and physician. If the family and physician do not agree, the hospital ethics committee or risk management staff should be consulted.

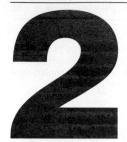

Nutrition

Sean C. Glasgow and
Virginia M. Herrmann

Nutrition plays a vital and often overlooked role in the care of patients on a surgical service. Between 30% and 50% of hospitalized patients are malnourished, and malnutrition is clearly associated with increased morbidity and mortality in select subsets of general surgical patients. Although most healthy patients can tolerate 7 days of starvation (with adequate glucose and fluid replacement), those who have been subject to major trauma, a prolonged operative course, sepsis, cancer-related cachexia, or other physiologic stressors require nutritional intervention much sooner. However, the prudent use of nutritional support is important, as misuse is not only cost-inefficient but can also adversely impact patient recovery. The only patient populations that have been identified as clearly benefiting from perioperative nutrition support are severely malnourished patients (*JPEN J Parenter Enteral Nutr* 2002;26:S63).

METABOLISM

I. **Metabolism of proteins, carbohydrates, and fats**
   A. **Proteins** are important for the biosynthesis of enzymes, structural molecules, and immunoglobulins. Accordingly, the balance between protein synthesis and degradation is critical.
      1. **Digestion of proteins** yields dipeptides and single amino acids, which are actively absorbed. Gastric pepsin initiates the process of digestion. Pancreatic proteases, activated on exposure to enterokinase found throughout the duodenal mucosa, are the principal effectors of protein degradation. Once digested, almost 50% of protein absorption occurs in the duodenum, and complete protein absorption is achieved by the midjejunal level. Protein absorption can effectively occur at every level of the small intestine; therefore, clinically significant protein malabsorption is relatively infrequent, even after extensive intestinal resection. The 20 amino acids are divided into essential and nonessential groups, depending on whether they can be synthesized de novo in the body. Only the L-isotype is utilized in human protein.
      2. **Major roles of amino acids** include the following:
         a. **Synthesis and recycling** of proteins
         b. **Catabolic reactions**, resulting in energy generation and the production of CO_2
         c. **Incorporation of nitrogen** into nonessential amino acids and nucleotides
         d. **Transport and storage** of small molecules and ions
      3. **Metabolism of absorbed amino acids**, primarily by the liver, regulates accumulation of plasma amino acids. Administration of parenteral nutrition initially bypasses the liver by delivering amino acids directly into the systemic circulation. A baseline nitrogen loss of 10 to 15 g per day occurs through urinary excretion.
      4. **Total body protein** in a 70-kg person is approximately 10 to 11 kg, concentrated mostly in skeletal muscle. Daily protein turnover is 250 to 300 g, or approximately 3% of total body protein. The primary site of protein turnover is the gastrointestinal (GI) tract, where shed enterocytes and secreted digestive enzymes are regularly lost. Excessive GI tract losses from

a fistula, ileostomy, or draining gastrostomy, as well as partial- or full-thickness skin burns or seeping wounds, provide other potential sources of significant protein loss in surgical patients. Protein turnover decreases with age, from 25 g/kg per day in the neonate to 3 g/kg per day in the adult.

5. **Protein requirements** in the average healthy adult without excessive losses are approximately 0.8 g/kg body weight. In the United States, the typical daily intake averages twice this amount. Requirements for patients with acute illness increase to 1.2 g/kg per day, and up to 2.5 g/kg per day is necessary for severely physiologically stressed patients in the intensive care unit. Generally, protein intake of 6.25 g is equivalent to 1 g of nitrogen. Amino acids contribute only 15% of the normal energy expenditure, with the remainder supplied by carbohydrates and fat. Each gram of protein can be converted into **4 kcal** energy.

B. **Carbohydrates** are the body's primary energy source, providing 30% to 40% of calories in a typical diet.
1. **Carbohydrate digestion** is initiated by the action of salivary amylase, and absorption is generally completed within the first 1.0- to 1.5 m of the small intestine. Salivary and pancreatic amylases cleave starches into oligosaccharides on contact. Surface oligosaccharidases then hydrolyze and transport these molecules across the GI tract mucosa. Deficiencies in carbohydrate digestion and absorption are rare in surgical patients. Since pancreatic amylase is abundant, even in patients with limited pancreatic function, maldigestion of starch does not usually occur. Diseases that result in generalized mucosal flattening (e.g., celiac sprue, Whipple's disease, and hypogammaglobulinemia) may cause diminished uptake of carbohydrate byproducts because of resultant deficiencies in oligosaccharidases.
2. **Glucose stores.** More than 75% of ingested carbohydrate is broken down and absorbed as glucose. Hyperglycemia leads to insulin secretion, which in turn influences protein synthesis. A minium intake of 400 calories of carbohydrate per day minimizes protein breakdown, particularly after adaptation to starvation. Cellular uptake of glucose (stimulated by insulin) also inhibits lipolysis and promotes glycogen formation. Conversely, glucagon is released in response to starvation or stress; it promotes proteolysis, glycogenolysis, lipolysis, and increased serum glucose. Glucose is essential for wound repair, but excessive amounts can have adverse effects, including hepatic steatosis and neutrophil dysfunction. Each gram of enteral carbohydrate provides **4 kcal** energy, similar to protein. Parenteral carbohydrate (e.g., dextrose) provides **3.4 kcal** per gram.
C. **Lipids** comprise the remaining 25% to 45% of calories in the typical diet. During starvation, lipids provide the majority of energy in the form of ketone bodies converted by the liver from long-chain fatty acids (see section II.A).
1. **Digestion and absorption of lipids** is complex and requires coordination between **biliary and pancreatic secretions**, as well as a functional jejunum and ileum. The introduction of fat to the duodenum produces secretion of cholecystokinin and secretin, which lead to gallbladder contraction and pancreatic enzyme release, respectively. **Pancreatic secretions** contain a combination of lipase, cholesterol esterase, and phospholipase A_2. In the alkaline environment of the duodenum, lipase hydrolyzes triglycerides to one monoglyceride and two fatty acids. Bile salts lead to emulsification. **Micelle formation** is the most important step in lipid absorption, facilitating absorption of fats across the mucosal barrier. Reabsorption of bile salts is necessary to maintain the bile salt pool (i.e., the enterohepatic circulation). The liver is able to compensate for moderate intestinal bile salt losses by increased synthesis from cholesterol. Major ileal resection may lead to depletion of the bile salt pool and subsequent fat malabsorption. Lipolysis is stimulated by steroids, catecholamines, and

glucagon but is inhibited by insulin. **Stress causes dramatic lipolysis.** Each gram of lipid provides **9 kcal** energy.

2. The **essential fatty acids**, linoleic and linolenic acid, are required for cell membrane integrity. Dietary fats are the sole precursors to eicosanoid production and as such are potent immunomodulators. Arachidonic acid, a vital component in prostaglandin synthesis, can be manufactured from linoleic acid. Clinical deficiency results in a generalized scaling rash, poor wound healing, hepatic steatosis, and bone changes. This condition is usually a consequence of long-term fat-free parenteral nutrition, in which high glucose levels stimulate relative hyperinsulinemia, thus inhibiting lipolysis and preventing peripheral essential fatty acid liberation. This can be avoided by providing at least 3% of caloric intake as parenteral lipid.

II. Stress metabolism

A. **Starvation.** After an overnight fast, liver glycogen is rapidly depleted due to decreased plasma insulin and a rise in glucagon levels. Carbohydrate stores are exhausted after a 24-hour fast. Liver glycogen is used first, followed soon thereafter by muscle glycogen. In the first few days of starvation, caloric needs are supplied by fat and protein degradation. Most of the available protein is from the breakdown of skeletal and visceral muscle. Protein is converted to glucose via hepatic gluconeogenesis. The brain preferentially uses this endogenously produced glucose, with the remainder consumed by red blood cells and leukocytes. Within approximately 10 days of starvation, the brain adapts to use fat as its fuel source. Because the brain cannot use free fatty acids in the same manner as other tissues do, it relies on ketoacids produced by the liver. This adaptation to ketone usage has a protein-sparing effect. In summary, the adaptive changes to starvation are a decrease in basal energy expenditure (up to 30%), a change in the type of fuel consumed (which maximizes the caloric potential), and relative preservation of protein.

B. **Physiologic stress.** The interaction of metabolic and endocrine responses that result from major operation, trauma, or sepsis can be divided into three phases.

1. **Catabolic phase.** After major injury, the metabolic demand is dramatically increased, as reflected in a significant rise in the urinary excretion of nitrogen (beyond that seen in simple starvation). Following a major surgical procedure, protein depletion inevitably occurs because patients are commonly prevented from eating in addition to having an elevated basal metabolic rate. The hormonal response of physiologic stress includes elevation in the serum levels of glucagon, glucocorticoids, and catecholamines and reduction in insulin.

2. The **early anabolic phase** is also called the *corticoid-withdrawal phase*, as the body shifts from catabolism to anabolism. The timing of this event is variable, depending on the severity of stress, and ranges from several days to several weeks. The period of anabolism can last from a few weeks to a few months, depending on many factors, including the ability of the patient to obtain and use nutrients and the extent to which protein stores have been depleted. This phase is marked by a positive nitrogen balance, and there is a rapid and progressive gain in weight and muscular strength. The total amount of nitrogen gained is equivalent to the amount lost in the catabolic phase; however, the rate of repletion is much slower than the rapid rate of protein depletion after the original insult.

3. The **late anabolic phase** is the final period of recovery and may last from several weeks to months. Adipose stores are replenished gradually, and nitrogen balance equilibrates. Weight gain is much slower during this period than in the early anabolic phase due to the high caloric content of fat—the primary energy stores deposited during the early anabolic phase—as compared to protein.

NUTRITIONAL ASSESSMENT AND ADMINISTRATION

I. **Nutritional assessment** is essential for identifying patients who are at risk of developing complications related to significant malnutrition. Preoperative nutritional support can significantly reduce perioperative morbidity and mortality in patients with severe malnutrition (*N Engl J Med* 1991;325:525). In addition, the incidence of postoperative morbidities, such as intra-abdominal abscess, anastomotic leakage, and ileus, may be decreased by the use of preoperative enteral or parenteral hyperalimentation in malnourished patients. Preoperative nutritional support for patients with only mild or moderate malnutrition is not routinely indicated. Table 2-1 presents several nutritional and biologic indices developed to predict the risk of perioperative complications and mortality.

   A. **Types of malnutrition.** Originally identified in children, two forms of malnutrition can be generalized to adults.

   1. **Marasmus** is characterized by inadequate protein *and* caloric intake, typically caused by illness-induced anorexia. It is a chronic nutritional deficiency marked by losses in weight, body fat, and skeletal muscle mass (as identified by anthropometric measurements). Visceral protein stores remain normal, as do most lab nutritional indices. Patients with marasmus may lose substantial body weight but are able to resist infection and respond appropriately to minor or moderate stress.

   2. **Kwashiorkor** is characterized by catabolic protein loss, resulting in **hypoalbuminemia** and generalized **edema**. This form of malnutrition develops when the period of starvation is prolonged or if the stress is severe. Even in a well-nourished patient, a severe stress (e.g., major burn or prolonged sepsis) may rapidly lead to the depletion of visceral protein stores and impairment in immune function. Conventional anthropometric measurements may not identify these patients as being significantly malnourished.

   B. **Evaluation of preexisting deficits.** A dietary history, physical examination (including anthropometric measurements), and relevant laboratory data are the appropriate tools needed to make an accurate evaluation of a patient's preoperative nutritional status.

Table 2-1. Nutritional indices

Body mass index (BMI)

BMI = weight (kg)/[height (m)]^2 = 703 $\times$ weight (lbs)/[height (in)]^2
BMI: normal 18.5–24.9, overweight 25–29.9, obese 30–40, morbid obesity >40

Prognostic nutritional index (PNI)

PNI = 158 − 16.6 (Alb) − 0.78 (TSF) − 0.2 (TFN) − 5.8 (DH)
DH: >5 mm induration = 2; 1–5 mm induration = 1; anergy = 0
PNI: >50% = high risk for complications; 40–49% = intermediate risk; <40% = low risk

Nutrition risk index

NRI = 15.19 (Alb) + 41.7 [weight (kg)/ideal weight (kg)]
NRI: <100 = malnourished

Catabolic index (CI)

CI = UUN − [0.5 (dietary nitrogen intake in g)]
CI: 0 = no significant stress; 0–5 = mild stress; >5 = moderate to severe stress

Alb, albumin (g/dL); DH, delayed cutaneous hypersensitivity; TFN, transferrin (mg/dL); TSF, triceps skinfold thickness (mm); UUN, 24-hr urine urea nitrogen excretion (g).
Adapted from Charney PJ. Nutrition screening and assessment. In: Skipper A, ed. *Dietitian's handbook of enteral and parenteral nutrition*, 2nd ed. Gaithersburg, MD: Aspen Publishers, Inc., 1998:324.

1. A **history** of weight fluctuation or a change in dietary habits is particularly relevant. In most cases, the possibility of malnutrition is suggested by the underlying disease or by a history of recent weight loss. Anorexia, nausea, vomiting, dysphagia, odynophagia, gastroesophageal reflux, or a history of generalized muscle weakness should prompt further evaluation. Recent weight loss (5% in the last month or 10% over 6 months) or a current body weight of 80% to 85% (or less) of ideal body weight suggests significant malnutrition. A complete history of current medications is essential to alert caretakers to potential underlying deficiencies as well as drug-nutrient interactions.

2. **Physical examination** may identify muscle wasting (especially thenar and temporal muscles), loose or flabby skin, and peripheral edema (as a result of hypoproteinemia). More subtle findings of nutritional deficiency include skin rash, pallor, glossitis, gingival lesions, hair changes, hepatomegaly, neuropathy, and dementia (*Aspen nutrition support practice manual*, 2nd ed. Gaithersburg, MD: Aspen, 1998).

3. **Anthropometric measurements** such as triceps skinfold thickness and midarm muscle circumference reflect body-fat stores and skeletal muscle mass, respectively. These values are standardized for gender and height, and they should be reported as a percentage of the predicted value. Along with body mass index, these values allow the clinician to assess the patient's visceral and somatic protein mass and fat reserve.

4. **Laboratory tests** that suggest malnutrition correlate with perioperative morbidity (*N Engl J Med* 1991;325:525) and mortality (*Arch Surg* 1999;134:36).

   a. **Serum albumin** of less than 3.5 g/dL (35 g/L) in a stable, hydrated patient; half-life of 14 to 20 days.

   b. **Serum prealbumin** may be a more useful indicator of acute changes in nutritional status: 10 to 17 mg/dL equals mild depletion, 5 to 10 mg/dL equals moderate depletion, and less than 5 mg/dL equals severe depletion; half-life of 2 to 3 days.

   c. **Serum transferrin** of less than 200 mg/dL; half-life of 8 to 10 days.

5. **Immune function** is frequently altered by malnutrition. The degree of derangement may be determined by assessing:

   a. **Delayed-type hypersensitivity** (anergy to common skin antigens).

   b. **Total lymphocyte count (TLC)** is calculated by the following formula:

   $$TLC = \frac{\% \text{ lymphocytes} \times WBC}{100}$$

   where 1,500 to 1,800 mm^3 equals mild depletion, 900 to 1,500 mm^3 equals moderate depletion, and less than 900 mm^3 equals severe depletion.

C. **Estimation of caloric requirements** is necessary to provide adequate substrates for healing and tissue repair. Failure to provide adequate amounts of both calories and protein leads to further depletion of lean body mass.

   1. **Basal energy expenditure (BEE)** can be predicted using the Harris-Benedict equation:

      a. BEE in kilocalaries per day for men equals 66.4 + [13.7 × weight (kg)] + [5.0 × height (cm)] − [6.8 × age (years)]

      b. BEE in kilocalories per day for women equals 655 + [9.6 × weight (kg)] + [1.7 × height (cm)] − [4.7 × age (years)]

   2. These equations provide a reliable estimate of the energy requirements in approximately 80% of hospitalized patients. The actual caloric need is obtained by multiplying BEE by specific stress factors (Table 2-2). Most stressed patients require 25 to 35 kcal/kg per day.

D. **Estimates of protein requirements.** The appropriate calorie:nitrogen ratio is approximately 150:1 (for a calorie:protein ratio of 24:1). This ratio increases to 300-400:1 in uremic patients. In the absence of severe renal or hepatic

Table 2-2. Disease stress factors used in calculation of total energy expenditure

Clinical condition	Stress factor
Starvation	0.80–1.00
Elective operation	1.00–1.10
Peritonitis or other infections	1.05–1.25
Adult respiratory distress syndrome or sepsis	1.30–1.35
Bone marrow transplant	1.20–1.30
Cardiopulmonary disease (noncomplicated)	0.80–1.00
Cardiopulmonary disease with dialysis or sepsis	1.20–1.30
Cardiopulmonary disease with major surgery	1.30–1.55
Acute renal failure	1.30
Liver failure	1.30–1.55
Liver transplant	1.20–1.50
Pancreatitis	1.30–1.80

Adapted from Shoppell JM, Hopkins B, Shronts EP. Nutrition screening and assessment. In: Gottschlich M, ed. *The science and practice of nutrition support: a case based core curriculum*. Dubuque, IA: Kendall/Hunt Publishing, 2001:107–140.

dysfunction, approximately 1.5 g protein per kilogram body weight should be provided daily (Table 2-3).

1. **Twenty-four–hour nitrogen balance** is calculated by subtracting nitrogen loss from nitrogen intake. Nitrogen intake is the sum of nitrogen delivered from enteral and parenteral feedings. Nitrogen is lost through excretion in urine, fistula drainage, diarrhea, and so forth. The usual approach is to measure the urine urea nitrogen (UUN) concentration of an aliquot of a 24-hour urine collection and multiply by urine volume to estimate 24-hour urinary loss. Nitrogen loss then equals 1.2 × [24-hour UUN (grams per day)] + 2 g per day as a correction factor to account for nitrogen losses in the stool and from skin exfoliation.

2. **Creatinine-height index (CHI)** can be used to determine the degree of malnutrition. A 24-hour urinary creatinine excretion is measured and compared to normal standards. The creatinine height index is calculated

Table 2-3. Estimated protein requirements in various disease states

Clinical condition	Protein requirements (g/kg ideal body weight per day)
Healthy, nonstressed	0.80
Bone marrow transplant	1.40–1.50
Liver disease without encephalopathy	1.00–1.50
Liver disease with encephalopathy	0.50–0.75 (advance as tolerated)
Renal failure without dialysis	0.60–1.00
Renal failure with dialysis	1.00–1.30
Pregnancy	1.30–1.50
Simplified estimates	
Mild metabolic stress (elective hospitalization)	1.00–1.10
Moderate metabolic stress (complicated postoperative care, infection)	1.20–1.40
Severe metabolic stress (major trauma, pancreatitis, sepsis)	1.50–2.50

Adapted from Nagel M. Nutrition screening: identifying patients at risk for malnutrition. *Nutr Clin Pract* 1998;8:171–175.

using the following equation:

$$CHI = \frac{\text{actual 24-hour creatinine excretion}}{\text{predicted creatinine excretion}}$$

where greater than 80% equals none to mild protein depletion, 60% to 80% equals moderate depletion, and less than 60% equals severe depletion.

II. **Administration of nutrition**
   A. **Indications.** The need for nutritional support should be assessed continually in all patients preoperatively and postoperatively. The majority of surgical patients do not require nutritional supplementation, and perioperative dietary supplements (e.g., Ensure) provide no clinical benefit (*Nutrition* 2000;16:723). Most patients have adequate fuel reserves to withstand common catabolic stresses and partial starvation for at least one week. For these patients, intravenous fluids with appropriate electrolytes and a minimum of 100 g glucose daily (to minimize protein catabolism) is adequate. However, even patients who were well nourished before a major operation or trauma but subsequently enter a prolonged hypermetabolic or severely catabolic period may require nutritional support (*Curr Probl Surg* 1995;32:833). Without nutritional intervention, these patients may have complications that are attributable to impaired immune function and poor wound healing as a result of depletion of visceral protein stores (see Chapter 9). Patients with a significant degree of preoperative malnutrition have less reserve, tolerate catabolic stress and starvation poorly, and are therefore at higher risk for postoperative complications.
   B. **Enteral nutrition.** In general, the enteral route is preferred over the parenteral route and should be the initial step in alimentation. Enteral feeding is simple, physiologic, relatively inexpensive, and well tolerated by most patients. Enteral feeding maintains the GI tract cytoarchitecture and mucosal integrity (through trophic effects), absorptive function, and normal microbial flora. This results in less bacterial translocation and endotoxin release from the intestinal lumen to the bloodstream (*Nutrition* 2000;16:606). **Enteral feedings are indicated** for patients who have a functional GI tract but are unable to sustain an adequate oral diet. **Enteral feedings may be contraindicated** in the patient with an intestinal obstruction, ileus, GI bleeding, severe diarrhea, vomiting, enterocolitis, or a high-output enterocutaneous fistula. Contraindications to enteral feeding are temporary in most cases. Choice of an appropriate feeding site, administration technique, and formula and appropriate equipment may circumvent many of these problems.
      1. **Feeding tubes.** Nasogastric, nasojejunal (e.g., Dobhoff), gastrostomy, and jejunal tubes are available for the administration of enteral feeding products. Percutaneous gastrostomy tubes can be placed using an endoscope or under fluoroscopy. Jejunal tubes are preferred for long-term use. The techniques for placement of these tubes and the common complications associated with their use are summarized in Chapter 7.
      2. **Enteral feeding products.** A variety of commercially available enteral feeding formulas are available. Standard solutions provide 1 kcal/mL; calorically concentrated solutions (>1 kcal/mL) are available for patients who require volume restriction. Currently available dietary formulations for enteral feedings can be divided into polymeric (blenderized and nutritionally complete commercial formulas), chemically defined formulas (elemental diets), and modular formulas (Table 2-4).
         a. **Blenderized tube feedings** can be composed of any food that can be blenderized. Caloric distribution of these formulas should parallel that of a normal diet.
         b. **Nutritionally complete commercial formulas** (standard enteral diets) vary in protein, carbohydrate, and fat composition. Several formulas use sucrose or glucose as carbohydrate sources and are suitable for lactose-deficient patients. Commercial formulas are convenient,

Table 2-4. Enteral formulas

Product	Description	kcal/mL	mOsm	Protein [g (% kcal)]	Carbohydrates [g (% kcal)]	Fat [g (% kcal)]	H$_2$O (mL)	Na (mEq)	K (mEq)	Ca (mg)	PO$_4$ (mg)	Vitamin K (mg)
Standard												
Ensure®	Lactose-free, low residue	1.06	470	37.2 (14)	145 (54.5)	37.2 (31.5)	845	36.8	40	530	530	43
Osmolite®	Isotonic, lactose-free, low residue	1.06	300	37.2 (14)	145 (54.6)	38.5 (31.4)	841	27.6	25.9	530	530	43
Jevity®	Isotonic, lactose-free, high dietary fiber (14.4 g/L), high nitrogen content	1.06	310	44.4 (16.7)	151.7 (53.3)	36.8 (30)	833	40.4	40	909	756	61
Glucerna®	Lactose-free, low carbohydrates, high fiber (14.4 g/L)	1	375	41.8 (16.7)	93.7 (33.3)	55.7 (50)	873	40.3	40	703	703	57
Low volume												
Ensure Plus®	Lactose-free, low residue	1.5	690	54.9 (14.7)	200 (53.3)	53.3 (32)	769	45.9	49.7	704	704	57
Magnacal®	Lactose-free, low residue	2	590	70 (14)	250 (50)	80 (34)	690	43.5	32	1000	1000	300
Low volume, high nitrogen												
Ensure Plus HN®	Lactose-free, low residue	1.5	650	62.6 (16.7)	199.9 (53.3)	50 (30)	769	51.5	46.5	1056	1056	85

Per 1,000 mL

(continued)

Table 2-4. (continued)

Product	Description	kcal/mL	mOsm	Per 1,000 mL Protein [g (% kcal)]	Carbohydrates [g (% kcal)]	Fat [g (% kcal)]	H_2O (mL)	Na (mEq)	K (mEq)	Ca (mg)	PO_4 (mg)	Vitamin K (mg)
Perative®*	Lactose-free, low residue	1.3	425	66.6 (20.5)	177 (54.5)	37.3 (25)	789	45.2	44.3	867	867	70
Very high nitrogen												
Replete with Fiber®	Lactose-free, high fiber (14 g/L)	1	300	62.5 (25)	113 (45)	34 (30)	840	21.7	40	1000	1000	80
Sustacal®	Lactose-free, low residue	1.01	650	61 (24)	140 (55)	23 (21)	840	40	54	1010	930	240
Elemental												
Vivonex TEN®	Elemental, low fat, low residue	1	630	38.2 (15.3)	205.6 (82.2)	2.77 (2.5)	845	20	20	500	500	22.3
Pudding (per 5-oz serving)												
Ensure® Pudding	Contains lactose	250		6.8	34.0	9.7		10.4	8.5	200	200	12
Modulars (analysis per tablespoon)												
Polycose® Liquid	Glucose polymer	30			7.5							
ProMod®	Protein supplement	17		3	0.4	0.4		0	1	15.6	15.6	
Microlipid®	Fat supplement	67.5				7.5						
MCT Oil®	MCT supplement	115.5				14						

sterile, and inexpensive. They are recommended for patients experiencing minimal metabolic stress who have normal gut function.

c. **Chemically defined formulas** are commonly called *elemental diets*. The nutrients are provided in predigested and readily absorbed form. They contain protein in the form of free amino acids or polypeptides. Amino acid (elemental) and polypeptide diets are efficiently absorbed in the presence of compromised gut function. However, they are more expensive than nutritionally complete commercial formulas and are hyperosmolar, which may cause cramping and diarrhea.

d. **Modular formulations** include special formulas that are used for specific clinical situations (e.g., pulmonary, renal, or hepatic failure or immune dysfunction).

3. **Enteral feeding protocols.** In the past, elaborate protocols for initiating tube feedings were used. Currently, it is recommended that feedings be started with full-strength formula begun at a slow rate and steadily advanced. This reduces the risk of microbial contamination and achieves full nutrient intake earlier. This approach can also be used with high-osmolarity or elemental products. Conservative initiation and advancement rates are recommended for patients who are critically ill, those who have not been fed for some time, and those who are receiving a high-osmolarity or calorie-dense formula.

a. **Bolus feedings** are reserved for patients with nasogastric or gastrostomy feeding tubes. Feedings are administered by gravity and begin at 50 to 100 mL every 4 hours and are increased in 50-mL increments until the intake goal is reached (usually 240 to 360 mL every 4 hours). Tracheobronchial aspiration is a potentially serious complication, particularly with prepyloric (gastric) feeding tubes. To reduce the risk of aspiration, the patient's head should be elevated to 30 to 45 degrees during feeding and for 1 to 2 hours after each feeding. The gastric residual volume should be measured before administration of the feeding bolus. If this volume is greater than 50% of the previous bolus, the next feeding should be held. The feeding tube should be flushed with approximately 30 mL water after each use. Free water volume can be increased as needed to treat hyponatremia or euvolemic hypernatremia.

b. **Continuous infusion** administered by a pump is generally required for nasojejunal, gastrojejunal, or jejunal tubes. Feedings are initiated at 20 mL per hour and increased in 10- to 20-mL-per-hour increments every 4 to 6 hours until the desired goal is reached. The feeding tube should be flushed with approximately 30 mL water every 4 hours. Advancement of feedings should be slowed or feedings should be held if the patient develops abdominal distension or pain. For some patients, the entire day's feeding volume can be infused over an 8- to 12-hour period at night to allow the patient to be disconnected from the infusion pump during the day.

c. **Conversion to oral feeding.** When indicated, an oral diet is resumed gradually. In an effort to stimulate appetite, enteral feeding can be modified by the following measures:

(1) **Providing fewer feedings**
(2) **Holding daytime feedings**
(3) **Decreasing the volume of feedings.** When oral intake provides approximately 75% of the required calories, tube feedings can be discontinued.

d. **Administration of medications.** Many oral medications can be administered through feeding tubes. The elixir form is preferred but is not always available. Medications that are not suitable for administration through a feeding tube include the following:

(1) Enteric-coated medications
(2) Drugs in gelatinous capsules

(3) Medications that are designed for sublingual use
(4) Most sustained-release medications
4. **Complications**
   a. **Metabolic complications.** Abnormalities in serum electrolytes, calcium, magnesium, and phosphorus can be minimized through vigilant monitoring. **Hyperosmolarity** (hypernatremia) may lead to the development of mental lethargy or obtundation. The treatment for this is the administration of free water by giving either D_5W intravenously or additional water in the tube feedings. Volume overload and subsequent congestive heart failure may occur as a result of **excess sodium administration**, observed especially in patients with impaired ventricular function or valvular heart disease. **Hyperglycemia** may occur in any patient but is particularly common in individuals with preexisting diabetes or sepsis. The serum glucose level should be determined frequently, and regular insulin administered accordingly.
   b. **Clogging** can usually be prevented by careful attention to routine flushing of the feeding tube. Wire stylets should not be used to unclog a feeding tube because of the risk of tube perforation and injury to the esophagus or stomach. Installation of carbonated soda, cranberry juice, pancreatic enzyme replacement, or meat tenderizer (1 teaspoon papain in 30 mL water) is sometimes useful for unclogging feeding tubes. Tubes that are refractory to these remedies, as well as those with cracks, leaks, or defective connectors, should be replaced.
   c. **Tracheobronchial aspiration** of tube-feeding solutions may occur with patients who are fed into the stomach or proximal small intestine and may lead to the development of pneumonia. Patients at particular risk are those with central nervous system abnormalities and those who are sedated. Testing tracheal aspirates with glucose strips or adding methylene blue (1 mL/L) to the tube-feeding solutions aids in assessing for aspiration. Historically, jejunal feeding has been the preferred route for patients who are at risk for aspiration; however, one comparison of tube feeding via jejunal and gastric routes found no difference in rates of aspiration pneumonia or other complications (*JPEN J Parenter Enteral Nutr* 2000;24:103).
   d. **High gastric residuals** of tube feedings as a result of outlet obstruction, dysmotility, intestinal ileus, or bowel obstruction may limit the usefulness of nasogastric or gastrostomy feeding tubes. Treatment of this problem should be directed at correcting the underlying cause. Gastroparesis frequently occurs in diabetic or head-injured patients. Promotility agents such as metoclopromide or erythromycin may aid in gastric emptying. If gastric retention prevents the administration of sufficient calories and intestinal ileus or obstruction can be excluded, a nasojejunal or jejunostomy feeding tube may be necessary.
   e. **Diarrhea** is a potential consequence of enteral feeding, occurring in 10% to 20% of patients; however, other causes of diarrhea (e.g., *Clostridium difficile* colitis) should be considered. Diarrhea may result from numerous causes: too rapid an increase in the volume of hyperosmolar tube feedings, certain medications (e.g., metoclopramide), a diet high in fat content, or the presence of components not tolerated by the patient (e.g., lactose). If other causes of diarrhea can be excluded, the volume or strength of tube feedings should be diminished. If no improvement occurs, a different formula should be used. Antidiarrheal agents such as loperamide should be reserved for patients with severe diarrhea. In surgical patients, *C. difficile* is a frequent cause of diarrhea due to the common use of perioperative antibiotics. Diagnosis can be confirmed with a *C. difficile* toxin assay or colonoscopy. Treatment includes stopping unnecessary antibiotics, followed by either metronidazole (Flagyl; oral or intravenous) or vancomycin orally or as a retention enema.

C. Parenteral nutrition is indicated for patients who require nutritional support but cannot meet their nutritional needs through oral intake and for whom enteral feeding is contraindicated or not tolerated.

1. **Peripheral parenteral nutrition (PPN)** is administered through a peripheral intravenous catheter. The osmolarity of PPN solutions generally is limited to 1,000 mOsm (approximately 12% dextrose solution) to avoid phlebitis. Consequently, unacceptably large volumes of solution (>2,500 mL) are necessary to fulfill the typical patient's total nutritional requirements. Temporary nutritional supplementation with PPN may be useful in selected patients but typically is not indicated.

2. **Total parenteral nutrition (TPN)** provides complete nutritional support (*Surgery* 1968;64:134). The solution, volume of administration, and solution additives are individualized for the patient and based on an assessment of the nutritional requirements.

   a. **Access.** TPN solutions must be administered through a central venous catheter. A dedicated single-lumen catheter or a multilumen catheter can be used. Catheters should be replaced for unexplained fever or bacteremia.

   b. **TPN solutions.** TPN solutions generally are administered as a 3-in-1 admixture of protein, as amino acids (10%; 4 kcal/g); carbohydrate, as dextrose (70%; 3.4 kcal/g); and fat, as a lipid emulsion of soybean or safflower oil (20%; 9 kcal/g). Alternatively, the lipid emulsion can be administered as a separate intravenous "piggyback" infusion. Standard preparations of TPN are used for most patients (Table 2-5). Special solutions that contain low, intermediate, or high nitrogen concentrations as well as varying amounts of fat and carbohydrate are available for patients with diabetes, renal or pulmonary failure, or hepatic dysfunction.

   c. **Additives.** Other elements can be administered in conjunction with the basic caloric and protein solutions.

      (1) **Electrolytes** (i.e., sodium, potassium, chloride, acetate, calcium, magnesium, and phosphate) that are added to the TPN solution should be adjusted daily. A suggested formulation often is listed on a prewritten order sheet, and the concentrations are designed for the patient whose current serum electrolytes and renal function are normal. The number of cations and anions must balance; this is achieved by altering the concentrations of chloride and acetate. If the serum bicarbonate is low, the solution should contain more acetate. The calcium:phosphate ratio must be monitored to prevent salt precipitation.

      (2) **Medications** such as albumin, H_2-receptor antagonists, heparin, iron, dextran, insulin, and metoclopramide can be administered in TPN solutions. However, not all medications are compatible with 3-in-1 admixtures. Regular insulin should initially be administered subcutaneously according to a sliding scale, based on a determination of the blood glucose level. After a stable insulin requirement has been established, insulin can be administered in the TPN solution, generally at two-thirds of the daily subcutaneous insulin dosage.

      (3) **Other additives.** Trace elements are added to the TPN solution daily using a commercially prepared mixture (e.g., 1 mL trace element-5: 1 mg copper, 12 μg chromium, 0.3 μg manganese, 60 μg selenium, and 5 mg zinc). Multivitamins generally are added daily to the TPN solution using a commercially prepared mixture (e.g., 10 mL MVI-12). Vitamin K is not included in most multivitamin mixtures and must be added separately (10 mg once a week). Vitamins A and C and zinc are particularly important for proper wound healing.

   d. **Routine physiologic and laboratory monitoring** should occur on a scheduled basis. This can be performed less frequently for patients

Table 2-5. Barnes-Jewish Hospital parenteral nutrition form

Date Due _____   Bag No _____
Calories to the nearest 100 kcal/24 hours _____

Check One	Standard solutions	% Total kcal provided as AA/Dex/Fat	Grams/1000 kcal of AA/Dex/Fat	mL/1000 kcal
	a) Intermediate Nitrogen	16/60/24	40/176/27	786
	b) High Nitrogen	20/55/25	50/162/28	843
	c) Very High Nitrogen	24/56/20	60/165/22	946
	d) Low Nitrogen	12/65/23	30/191/26	680
	e) Peripheral	16/32/52	40/94/58	1429
	f) Amino Acid/Dextrose	10% Amino acid _____ mL 70% Dextrose _____ mL		
	Lipids (as separate infusion)	Circle one: 100mL, 250mL, 500mL, 20% intralipid _____ mL/hr		

Electrolytes	Suggested amount	Amount ordered	Other additives	Suggested amount	Amount ordered
Na	60–120 mEq		MVI–12	10 mL/day	
K	30–80 mEq		Trace Element-5	1 mL/day	
Cl	80–140 mEq		Vitamin K	10 mg/week	
Acetate	*	Balance	Regular Insulin		units
Ca	4.6–9.2 mEq		Pepcid		mg
Mg	8.1–24.3 mEq				
PO$_4$	12–24 mmol				

AA, amino acids; Dex, dextrose; MVI, multivitamin.
*Cations (sodium and potassium) must be balanced by anions (chloride and acetate). In patients with normal electrolytes, the acetate:chloride ratio should be approximately 1:2.

whose postoperative course has stabilized and who are receiving a consistent TPN regimen. The initial frequency of monitoring includes vital signs and serum glucose every 6 hours; weight, serum electrolytes, and blood urea nitrogen daily; and triglycerides, complete blood cell count, prothrombin time, liver enzymes, and bilirubin weekly.

  e. **Administration of TPN.** Orders, written daily, should reflect the patient's dynamic nutritional status and biochemical profile (Table 2-5).

   (1) **Introduction of TPN** should be gradual. For example, approximately 1,000 kcal is provided the first day. If there is metabolic stability (i.e., normoglycemia), this is increased to 1,500 kcal the second day. The amount is increased by 500 kcal per day until the caloric goal is reached.

   (2) **TPN solutions** are delivered most commonly as a continuous infusion. A new 3-in-1 admixture bag of TPN is administered daily at a constant infusion rate over 24 hours. Additional maintenance intravenous fluids are unnecessary, and total infused volume should be kept constant while nutritional content is increased.

   (3) **Cyclic administration of TPN** solutions may be useful for selected patients, including (1) those who will be discharged from the hospital and subsequently receive home TPN; (2) those with limited intravenous access who require administration of other medications, such as chemotherapeutic agents; and (3) those who are metabolically stable and desire a period during the day when they can be free

of an infusion pump. Cyclic TPN is administered for 8 to 16 hours, most commonly at night. This should not be done until metabolic stability has been demonstrated for patients on standard, continuous TPN infusions.

(4) Discontinuation of TPN should take place when the patient can satisfy 75% of his or her caloric and protein needs with oral intake or enteral feeding. The calories provided by TPN can be decreased in proportion to calories from the patient's increasing enteral intake. To discontinue TPN, the infusion rate should be halved for 1 hour, halved again the next hour, and then discontinued. Tapering in this manner prevents rebound hypoglycemia from hyperinsulinemia. It is not necessary to taper the rate of TPN infusion if the patient is receiving less than 1,000 kcal per day.

f. Complications associated with TPN

(1) Catheter-related complications can be avoided by strict aseptic technique and routine catheter care (*Surg Clin North Am* 1985;65:835).

(2) Metabolic complications. A large parenteral sodium load in a severely malnourished patient may precipitate congestive heart failure. Without daily monitoring and correction, electrolyte abnormalities can occur rapidly; the consequences of various imbalances are discussed in Chapter 4. Hyperglycemia and hyperosmolarity may lead to coma or death. In addition, hyperglycemia may be the first indication of occult infection. As noted in section II.C.2.d, the serum glucose level should be monitored frequently. Strict maintenance of serum glucose level below 110 mg/dL improves mortality and reduces infectious complications (*New Engl J Med* 2001;345:1359). Table 2-6 depicts the standard insulin regimen used in the intensive care units at Barnes-Jewish Hospital.

(3) Refeeding syndrome occurs when TPN is administered to a severely malnourished patient, resulting in anabolism, a dramatic shift of extracellular ions into the intracellular space, and rapid depletion of remaining stores of ATP. Refeeding syndrome can present insidiously as respiratory failure. For this reason, frequent monitoring and additional supplementation of K, Mg, and PO_4 is required in severely malnourished patients.

(4) Hepatic dysfunction is a common manifestation of long-term TPN support. Steatosis is associated with mild elevations of the transaminases, alkaline phosphate, and bilirubin. Cirrhosis is the end result.

(5) Cholecystitis, particularly the acalculous type, may occur in patients who receive TPN for extended periods. Cholecystostomy or cholecystectomy is indicated for symptomatic patients. To avoid cholestasis and prevent this complication, gallbladder contraction can be stimulated with the C-terminal octapeptide of cholecystokinin, 0.02 μg/kg introvenously per day.

D. Specialized substrates. Promise has been shown for "nutritional pharmacology," in which interventions with cytokines, hormones, and substrates can augment basic nutritional repletion.

1. Cytokines such as IL-1, IL-6, and TNF-α contribute to the acute-phase response of inflammation, loss of skeletal muscle protein, and use of exogenous nutrients. Pharmacologic manipulation of these agents may reverse their deleterious effects (*Cancer* 1997;79:1828).

2. Exogenous **growth hormone** has been shown to increase amino acid uptake, decrease nitrogen loss, and hasten weaning from mechanical ventilation (*Am J Surg* 1996;171:576). Ongoing clinical trials are exploring indications for its use in critically ill patients.

3. Immunonutrition is the use of nutritional substrates to modulate a patient's immune response. Arginine and glutamine stimulate immune

Table 2-6. Barnes-Jewish Hospital insulin infusion orders

1. Mix insulin infusion: 1 unit/mL (100 units regular insulin in 100mL 0.9% saline)
2. Maintenance IV fluid: Dextrose 5% with lactated Ringer's at _____ mL/hr or
Other maintenance IV Fluid:
3. Select regular insulin infusion from below (check appropriate box):

Blood Sugar mg/dL	☐ Conservative Regimen for patients using <30 units/day or oral agents only, and who have glucose <250	☐ Moderate Regimen for patients using >30 units/day, or whose most recent glucose is >250	☐ Aggressive Regimen for patients failing to respond to other regimens. **Consider this regimen if on high dose inotropes.**	☐ Custom Regimen
<70	Stop infusion; give 25 mL of 50% dextrose IV; notify MD; recheck glucose in 15 minutes			
80–100	None	0.8 units/hr	1 unit/hr	
101–20	0.5 units/hr	1 unit/hr	1.5 units/hr	
121–150	1 unit/hr	1.5 units/hr	3 units/hr	
151–200	1.5 units/hr	2 units/hr	4 units/hr	
201–250	2 units/hr	3 units/hr	6 units/hr	
251–300	3 units/hr	5 units/hr	8 units/hr	
301–350	4 units/hr	6 units/hr	10 units/hr	
351–400	5 units/hr – call MD	8 units/hr – call MD	12 units/hr – call MD	

4. Frequency of blood sugar measurements:
  a. q1hr until stable, then q2hrs (stable is no change in insulin, and glucose 120–180)
  b. q1hr when increasing or weaning inotropes
  c. If patient's blood sugar remains **higher than 200 mg/dL** for 2 hours, contact MD
  d. If patient's blood sugar remains **70–100 mg/dL** for 2 hours, contact MD
5. Start oral glycemic control medications when tolerating ADA diet.

response and may improve gut integrity, thereby preventing bacterial translocation. Synthetic nucleotides also can enhance host defenses. The immunologic effect of omega-3 fatty acids is unclear. Recent meta-analyses demonstrated nutrition-related reductions in infectious complications and length of hospital stay but failed to show any improvement in mortality among complex surgical and critical care patients (*Ann Surg* 1999;229:467; *JAMA* 2001;286:944).
 E. **Disease-specific nutrition**
  1. **Thermal injury** has a tremendous impact on metabolism because of prolonged, intense neuroendocrine stimulation. The increase in metabolic demands following thermal injury correlates with the extent of ungrafted body surface area. Decreasing the intensity of neuroendocrine stimulation by providing analgesia and thermoneutral environments lowers the accelerated metabolic rate in many of these patients and helps to decrease catabolic protein loss until the burned surface can be grafted (*Compr Ther* 1991;17:47).
  2. **Diabetes** often complicates nutritional management. Complications associated with TPN administration (e.g., catheter-related sepsis) are more

common with prolonged hyperglycemia. Unopposed glycosuria may cause osmotic diuresis, loss of electrolytes in urine, and nonketotic coma. As stated in section **II.C.2.f.(2)**, the goal in glucose-intolerant patients is to maintain the serum glucose within the normal range; even mild hyperglycemia has deleterious effects. Hypoglycemia can result in shock, seizures, or vascular instability. This can be avoided by adjusting the insulin dosing, with the understanding that insulin requirements will decrease as the patient recovers from the initial stress that is associated with the illness.

3. **Difficulty weaning** a patient from mechanical ventilation can be caused by excessive administration of carbohydrate. Patients with marginal pulmonary reserve who are ventilator dependent may be particularly difficult to wean (*JAMA* 1980;243:1444). The respiratory quotient (**RQ**) is given by:

$$RQ = \frac{\dot{V}_{CO_2}}{\dot{V}_{O_2}}$$

The RQ represents the balance between CO_2 production and O_2 consumption and is a general indicator of metabolism. It can be measured using indirect calorimetry. Patients administered only lipids will have an RQ of 0.67, while the RQ equals 1.0 in those receiving only carbohydrates. Importantly, patients with excess caloric intake (i.e., overfed) will begin producing fat and have an RQ greater than 1.0. A higher RQ reflects increased relative CO_2 production, which can impair weaning from the ventilator.

4. **Renal failure** may be associated with glucose intolerance; negative nitrogen balance (resulting from increased losses through dialysis); loss of protein, with decreased protein synthesis; hyperkalemia; and diminished excretion of phosphorus. Dialysis should be adjusted accordingly, and these patients should be nutritionally replenished according to their calculated needs. Patients who receive peritoneal dialysis absorb approximately 80% of the dextrose in the dialysate fluid (assuming a normal serum glucose level). These factors must be considered when designing a nutritional support strategy.

5. **Hepatic failure** may result in wasting of lean body mass, fluid retention, vitamin and trace metal deficiencies, anemia, and encephalopathy. It may be difficult or impossible to limit the amount of nitrogen that a patient receives each day yet still provide adequate nutritional support. Branched-chain amino acids are metabolized by skeletal muscle and serve as an energy source during periods of stress. These amino acids are available enterally or parenterally to decrease the levels of aromatic amino acids and, therefore, the severity of encephalopathy; however, their efficacy has not been proved (*JPEN J Parenter Enteral Nutr* 1990;14:225).

6. **Cancer-related cachexia** is a syndrome of lean muscle wasting, peripheral insulin resistance, and increased lipolysis. More than two-thirds of patients with cancer experience significant weight loss during their illness, and it can develop at any time in the disease course (*JPEN J Parenter Enteral Nutr* 200226:S63). Antineoplastic therapies, such as chemotherapy, radiation therapy, or operative extirpation, can worsen preexisting malnutrition. Although the addition of TPN to these modalities in clinical studies has shown improvement in weight, nitrogen balance, and biochemical markers, there is little evidence to suggest better response rates or survival. Megestrol acetate (Megace) improves food intake, fat gain, and patient mood but does not alter outcome.

7. **Short-bowel syndrome** occurs in patients with less than 180 cm of functional small bowel. It may result from mesenteric ischemia, Crohn disease, or necrotizing enterocolitis. The estimated length of small bowel that is

required for adult patients to become independent of TPN is greater than 120 cm without colon or greater than 60 cm with some colonic continuity. Salvage of the ileocecal valve improves outcome. Dietary management includes consuming frequent small meals, avoiding hyperosmolar foods, restricted fat intake, and limiting consumption of foods high in oxalate (precipitates nephrolithiasis). Intestinal adaptation may occur in some patients. Uniquely formulated diets supplemented with glutamine and growth hormone show promise for accelerating this process (*Ann Surg* 1995;222:243).

8. **Patients with AIDS** develop protein-calorie malnutrition and lose weight. Malnourished AIDS patients require 35 to 40 kcal and 2.0 to 2.5 g protein/kg per day. In addition to the required electrolytes, vitamins, and minerals, they should receive glutamine, arginine, nucleotides, omega-3 polyunsaturated fats, branched-chain amino acids, and trace metal supplements. Those with normal gut function should be given a high-protein, high-calorie, low-fat, lactose-free oral diet. Patients with compromised gut function require an enteral (amino acid–enriched, polypeptide-enriched, or immunoenhancing) diet or TPN.

Life Support

Sekhar Dharmarajan and Bradley D. Freeman

The **time** from cardiopulmonary arrest to the initiation of **basic life support (BLS)** and **advanced cardiac life support (ACLS)** is critical to outcome. The following guidelines were developed by the American Heart Association (AHA) to standardize treatment for adults (*Circulation* 2000;102(Suppl I)). These guidelines do not preclude specific interventions based on individual characteristics.

LIFE SUPPORT AND CARDIOPULMONARY ARREST ALGORITHMS

I. **BLS.** The ABCDs of BLS—*a*irway, *b*reathing, *c*irculation, and early *d*efibrillation—are critical to successful resuscitative efforts. This algorithm has been recently updated to include BLS and ACLS in one format and can be represented in either simplified (not shown) or detailed forms (Fig. 3-1 and Table 3-1). After a person collapses, the following initial procedures are recommended:

- **Determine unresponsiveness** by gently tapping or shaking the victim and asking, "Are you okay?" **Do not shake the victim's head or neck** unless trauma to these areas has been excluded.
- **Call for help if there is no response.** In the field, activate the emergency medical service system by calling the local emergency telephone number (e.g., 911). Call for a defibrillator.

A. **Airway**
1. **Position the patient** supine on a firm, flat surface. While the patient is being moved, the head and neck should remain in the same plane as the torso, and the patient's body should be moved as a unit.
2. **Open the airway.** If there is no evidence of head or neck trauma, the head-tilt, chin-lift maneuver is used. For the patient with a suspected neck injury, the neck tilt should be avoided, and the modified jaw thrust should be used.

B. **Breathing**
1. **Assess for the presence of spontaneous respirations** with the patient's airway open. The rescuer should listen and feel for airflow while observing for movement of the patient's chest. Maintenance of an open airway may suffice for spontaneous respirations to resume.
2. **Perform rescue breathing** if spontaneous respirations are not present. Gently occlude the patient's nose, make a tight seal over the patient's mouth, and ventilate twice with slow, full breaths (1 to 2 seconds each, with a 2-second pause between breaths). Adequate ventilation is indicated by observing the chest rise and fall and hearing and feeling the air escape during exhalation. If the patient cannot be ventilated, his or her head should be repositioned, and ventilation should be attempted again. If these attempts are still unsuccessful, the foreign body–airway obstruction maneuver should be performed. In the hospital setting, **bag-mask ventilation** is the first choice and most effective method of basic life support ventilation. One hundred percent inspired oxygen should be delivered by the mask, preferably with an adjunctive oropharyngeal or nasopharyngeal airway.
3. **Foreign body–airway obstruction management.** If an unconscious patient cannot be ventilated after two attempts at repositioning the airway,

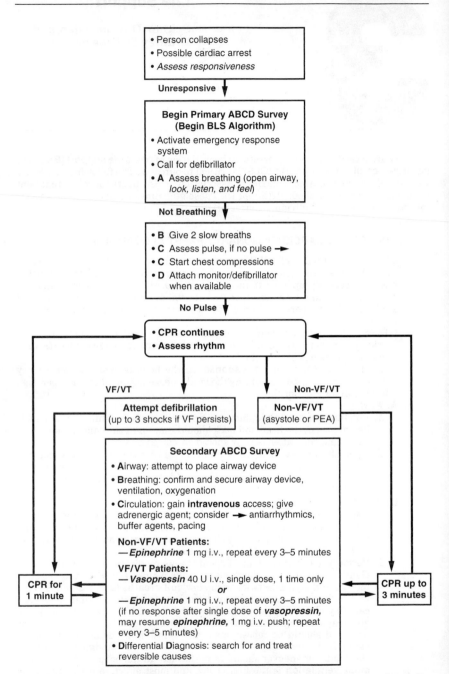

Figure 3-1. Comprehensive emergency cardiovascular care algorithm for the evaluation and management of persons after collapse. BLS, basic life support; CPR, cardiopulmonary resuscitation; PEA, pulseless electrical activity; VF, ventricular fibrillation; VT, ventricular tachycardia. (Adapted with permission from *A guide to the international ACLS algorithms. Circulation* 2000;102(Suppl I):I-142–I-157.)

Table 3-1. Primary ABCD Survey

Primary ABCD survey
(Begin basic life support algorithm)
Activate emergency response system.
Call for defibrillator.
A Airway: Open airway; assess breathing (open airway, look, listen, feel).
B Breathing: Give two slow breaths.
C Cardiopulmonary resuscitation: Check pulse; if no pulse
C Start chest compressions.
D Defibrillator: Attach automatic external defibrillator or monitor/defibrillator when available.

Secondary ABCD survey
A Intubate as soon as possible.
B Confirm tube placement; use two methods to confirm.
   Primary physical examination criteria *plus*
   Secondary confirmation device (qualitative and quantitative measures of end-tidal carbon dioxide)
B Secure tracheal tube.
   Prevent dislodgment; purpose-made tracheal tube holders are recommended over tie-and-tape approaches.
   If the patient is at risk for transport movement, cervical collar and backboard are recommended.
B Confirm initial oxygenation and ventilation.
   End-tidal carbon dioxide monitor
   Oxygen saturation monitor
C Oxygen, i.v., monitor, fluids, rhythm-appropriate medications
C Vital signs: temperature, blood pressure, heart rate, respirations
D Differential diagnoses

Adapted with permission from A guide to the international ACLS algorithms. *Circulation* 2000;102 (Suppl I):I-142—I-157.

abdominal thrusts (Heimlich maneuver) should be performed. After 6 to 10 quick thrusts, the victim's mouth is opened, and a finger sweep is performed to remove any debris. Ventilation is then attempted, and if unsuccessful, the sequence of abdominal thrusts and finger sweep are repeated. Cricothyroidotomy and transtracheal ventilation should be performed if effective ventilation cannot be established.

   C. Circulation
   1. **Assess for the presence of a pulse** by palpating the carotid artery. If a carotid pulse is present, rescue breathing should be continued at a rate of 10 to 12 breaths per minute until spontaneous respiration resumes.
   2. In the absence of a carotid pulse, **deliver chest compressions** at a rate of 80 to 100 per minute. During **one-rescuer BLS,** 15 compressions are delivered before ventilating twice. For **two-rescuer BLS,** the compression-ventilation ratio is 5:1, and the rescuer responsible for airway management should assess the adequacy of compressions by palpating periodically for the carotid pulse. Once the patient is intubated, ventilation can be given at a rate of 12 to 15 breaths per minute without pausing for compressions.
   D. Defibrillation
   1. **Early electrical defibrillation** is the single greatest determinant of survival for victims of cardiac arrest due to **ventricular fibrillation (VF),** **the most common presenting arrhythmia** in adult cardiac arrest. The

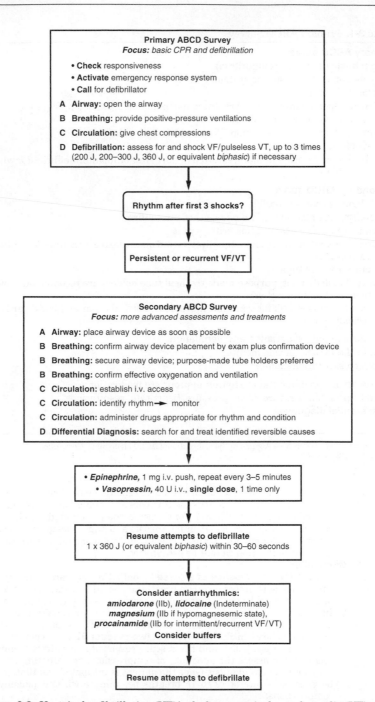

Figure 3-2. Ventricular fibrillation (VF)/pulseless ventricular tachycardia (VT) algorithm. CPR, cardiopulmonary resuscitation. (Adapted with permission from A guide to the international ACLS algorithms. *Circulation* 2000;102(Suppl I):I-142–I-157.)

success of defibrillation is dependent on the time from the moment of collapse to attempt at defibrillation. The chance for survival decreases 7% to 10% for every minute of delay, and after 10 minutes only 2% to 5% of patients survive. The AHA goal is a collapse-to-shock interval of less than 3 minutes, for this offers the best chance of survival.

2. **Defibrillation** can be performed with manual or automatic external units. Quick-look paddles on the manual defibrillator can be used initially to avoid delay. If VF or pulseless ventricular tachycardia (VT) is present, defibrillation should be performed immediately (Fig. 3-2). Asystole should be confirmed in at least two leads or monitor paddle positions, because fine VF can be mistaken for asystole in a single-lead or monitor paddle position.

3. **Automatic external defibrillators (AEDs)** have proved to be of significant value, especially for use by untrained individuals. AEDs require 5 to 15 seconds to analyze the electrocardiographic rhythm and then recommend whether defibrillation is appropriate for the situation. The use of AEDs is contraindicated in patients younger than 8 years of age or less than 25 kg and for any patient who is wet, lying in water, or in contact with a metal surface. Patients with a pacemaker, an automatic implantable cardioverter-defibrillator, or transdermal medication patches can be defibrillated externally without injury if a defibrillation paddle or electrode is not placed directly over the device.

4. **BLS should be stopped** for 5 seconds after four cycles of compressions and ventilation and every 2 to 3 minutes thereafter to assess whether the patient has resumed spontaneous breathing or circulation. If a pulse is present, ventilation should be continued as needed. When the defibrillator is available, it should be used immediately. Otherwise, BLS should not be stopped for more than 5 seconds except to intubate or defibrillate.

5. **"Compression-only" CPR** is an acceptable alternative specifically when a rescuer is unwilling or unable to perform mouth-to-mouth ventilation for an adult victim of cardiac arrest.

II. ACLS. Properly performed BLS is critical to the successful performance of ACLS, which is a team effort that depends on effective supervision by a team leader. The leader should ensure that the ABCDs of ACLS are expediently executed by the team.

A. Airway

1. **Proper airway management** is essential to the resuscitative effort. Endotracheal intubation remains the procedure of choice for the unconscious and/or apneic patient. When tracheal intubation is not possible, several alternative airway ventilation methods, such as the **laryngeal mask airway** or the **esophageal-tracheal combitube**, may provide more effective ventilation than a bag-mask apparatus. For the rescuer with little experience with intubation or alternative airway methods, continued bag-mask ventilation is recommended pending the arrival of personnel more experienced in airway management.

B. Breathing

1. If endotracheal intubation is performed, confirmation of tracheal intubation should be directly assessed by visualization of the tube passing through the vocal cords, auscultation of breath sounds bilaterally, and absence of gastric insufflation by auscultation over the epigastrium. Additional confirmation of endotracheal tube placement should be determined by an **end-tidal carbon dioxide detector** or an **esophageal detector device**. Once appropriate position is confirmed, the endotracheal tube should be secured to prevent dislodgment.

C. Circulation

1. Adequate **intravenous access** should be obtained expediently. The antecubital vein should be the first target for access, but if central venous catheterization is required to obtain access, the femoral vein usually provides the easiest and fastest access.

2. **Normal saline** is the recommended intravenous fluid vehicle as it offers the advantages of effective intravascular volume expansion, long shelf life, and low cost. A bolus of intravenous fluid should follow administration of intravenous medications, as this enhances delivery to the central circulation.

3. Appropriate monitor leads should be attached and rhythms and rates identified. A noninvasive measurement of blood pressure should be obtained if possible. If intravenous access cannot be established, **epinephrine, lidocaine,** and **atropine** can be administered via the endotracheal tube.

  D. Differential Diagnosis

  1. The critical question that must be asked and answered is, what caused the arrest? The purpose of the differential diagnosis is to search for, identify, and treat reversible causes of cardiopulmonary arrest with specific therapy. The differential diagnosis of cardiopulmonary arrest can be generally divided into three broad categories of shock, **hypovolemic, cardiogenic,** and **distributive,** the etiologies and therapies of which are discussed in further detail in Chapter 10.

III. **Universal algorithm of adult emergency cardiac care** (Fig. 3-1 and Table 3-1)

  A. Institute BLS protocols.

  1. **Assess responsiveness, breathing, and circulation.**

  2. **Defibrillate early** for VF or pulseless VT.

  B. Institute ACLS and arrhythmia-specific algorithm.

  1. **VF or pulseless VT** (Fig. 3-2)

  a. There are **two phases in the algorithm** for this dysrhythmia: The first involves electrocardioversion, and the second involves pharmacologic cardioversion and electrocardioversion. In the first phase, sequentially defibrillate three times at 200 J, 200 to 300 J, and 360 J in rapid succession for refractory VF or VT. Do *not* pause for a pulse check if the monitor clearly displays persistent VF or VT.

  b. There are **four guidelines for the second phase**: Follow a **drug-shock, drug-shock** sequence, shock within 30 to 60 seconds of drug administration, assess for a pulse after each shock, and maximize one antiarrhythmic before administering another to limit proarrhythmic drug-drug interactions.

  c. First-line antiarrhythmic medications are either **epinephrine**, 1 mg intravenously every 3 to 5 minutes, or **vasopressin**, 40 units intravenously once. After the administration of vasopressin, 10 to 20 minutes should elapse before epinephrine can be given. **Epinephrine** increases myocardial and cerebral blood flow during cardiopulmonary resuscitation, principally because of its α-adrenergic receptor–stimulating properties. There is no evidence to support the use of high-dose or escalating doses of epinephrine in VF or/pulseless VT. **Vasopressin (arginine vasopressin)** has vasoconstrictive properties at pharmacologic doses and may have a more favorable side effect profile than epinephrine. Vasopressin has not been found to be superior to epinephrine for resuscitation from VF or pulseless VT in recent randomized, controlled trials, although there is evidence that vasopressin followed by epinephrine may be more effective than epinephrine alone in the treatment of refractory cardiac arrest (*Lancet* 2001;358:105, *N Engl J Med* 2004;350:105).

  d. Antiarrhythmic drugs are used as second-line medications for the treatment of persistent or refractory VF or/pulseless VT. **Amiodarone** has been shown in recent trials to be superior to lidocaine and placebo in improving survival to hospital admission in patients with shock-refractory VF or/pulseless VT (*N Engl J Med* 1999;341:871, *N Engl J Med 2002;*346:884). Amiodarone affects the sodium, potassium, and calcium channels and is an α- and β-adrenergic antagonist. Amiodarone is initially administered as an intravenous bolus of 300 mg in 20 to 30 mL of D5W, and a second dose of 150 mg can be used in case of recurrence. With return of a spontaneous perfusing rhythm, an amiodarone drip is administered, consisting of 150 mg over the first 10 minutes, followed by 1 mg per minute over the next 6 hours, and finally a maintenance infusion of 0.5 mg per minute over the next 18 hours.

    e. Other antiarrhythmics that may be of benefit in refractory or persistent cases include **lidocaine** and **procainamide**. The initial dose of **lidocaine** for VF is 0.50 to 0.75 mg/kg intravenously every 5 to 10 minutes, with electrocardioversion attempts after the medication. The maximal dosage is 3 mg/kg. With return of a spontaneous perfusing rhythm, a lidocaine drip can begin with a loading dose of 1.0 to 1.5 mg/kg followed by a continuous infusion of 1 to 4 mg per minute. **Central nervous system symptoms**, especially seizure, are an early manifestation of lidocaine toxicity. **Procainamide** is loaded at 30 mg per minute up to a total of 17 mg/kg (1.2 g for a 70-kg patient), followed by a maintenance infusion of 1 to 4 mg per minute. Procainamide may induce hypotension, heart block, or even cardiac arrest.

    f. **Magnesium sulfate** is the treatment of choice in patients with **torsades de pointes** (polymorphic VT). For torsades de pointes, higher doses (up to 5 to 10 g) may be used. Rapid administration of magnesium can cause flushing, sweating, mild bradycardia, and hypotension. Depressed reflexes, flaccid paralysis, circulatory collapse, respiratory paralysis, and diarrhea may occur with hypermagnesemia.

    g. **A solitary precordial thump** can convert pulseless VT and, less often, VF to sinus rhythm. This should be used only for witnessed arrests when a defibrillator is not available and the patient is pulseless. A precordial thump should not be used in patients with VT who have a pulse because it may convert a pulse-forming into a pulseless rhythm (asystole, VF, or electromechanical dissociation).

2. **Pulseless electrical activity (PEA)** (Fig. 3-3)
    a. **PEA** is almost uniformly fatal unless an underlying cause can be identified and treated, usually because it represents a preterminal rhythm. Resuscitation rates from PEA are only 20%, with only 4% to 5% surviving to hospital discharge. Potentially reversible causes follow the acronym 5H 5T:
      (1) **Hypovolemia**, especially resulting from hemorrhage, is the most common cause of pulseless electrical activity.
      (2) **Hypoxia**
      (3) **Hypothermia**
      (4) **Hydrogen ions** (severe acidosis)
      (5) **Hyperkalemia or hypokalemia**
      (6) **Tablets/toxins**
      (7) **Tension pneumothorax**, evidenced by tracheal deviation and decreased ipsilateral breath sounds, should be treated by insertion of a large-bore angiocatheter (14-gauge) into the pleural space in the second intercostal space in the ipsilateral midclavicular line, followed by a thoracostomy tube.
      (8) **Pericardial tamponade** is treated by pericardiocentesis during cardiac arrest.
      (9) **Thrombosis of coronary vessels** (acute coronary syndromes)
      (10) **Thrombosis of pulmonary vessels** (pulmonary embolism)
    b. **Sodium bicarbonate** may be beneficial in patients with preexisting metabolic acidosis, hyperkalemia, or tricyclic or phenobarbital overdose. When bicarbonate is used, 1 mEq/kg should be given as the initial dose, with one-half this dose administered every 10 minutes thereafter. One ampule of sodium bicarbonate contains 8.4% bicarbonate (50 mEq/50 mL).
    c. **Calcium** is indicated for the treatment of myocardial instability secondary to hypocalcemia or hyperkalemia. A 10% calcium chloride solution may be given as an intravenous bolus of 2 to 4 mg/kg.

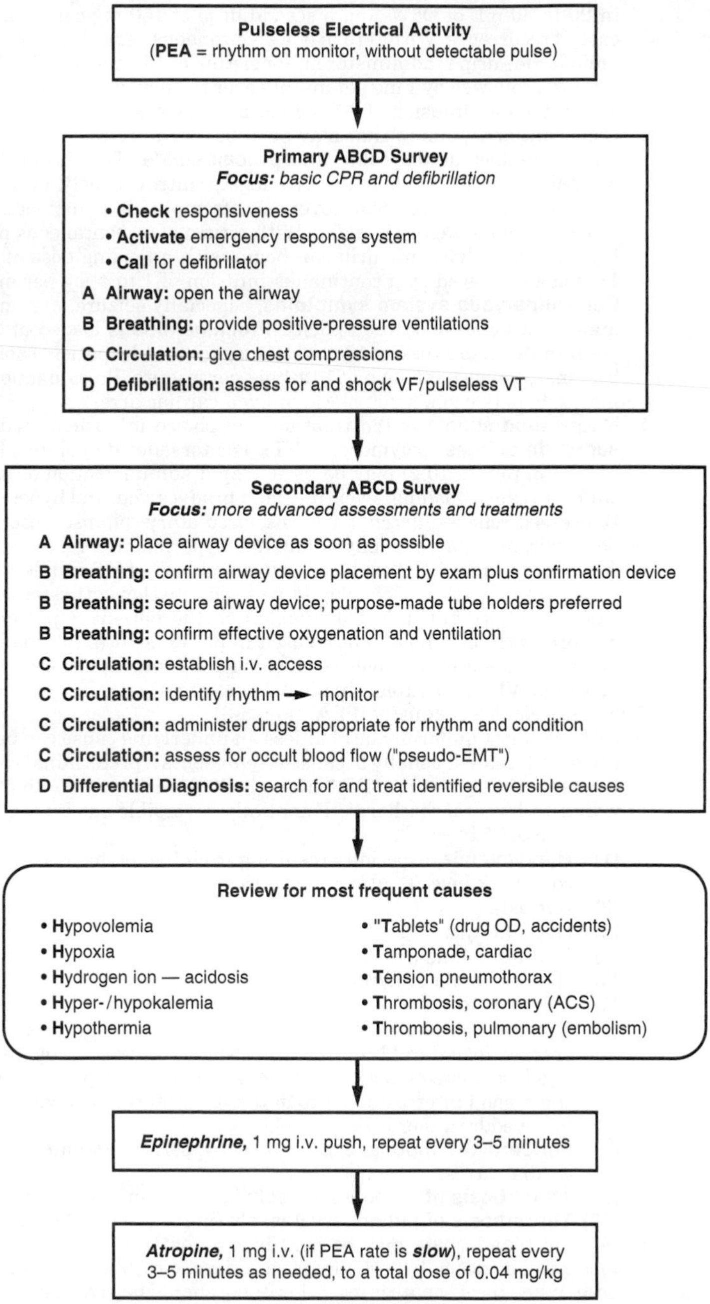

Pulseless Electrical Activity
(**PEA** = rhythm on monitor, without detectable pulse)

Primary ABCD Survey
Focus: basic CPR and defibrillation

- **Check** responsiveness
- **Activate** emergency response system
- **Call** for defibrillator

A **Airway:** open the airway

B **Breathing:** provide positive-pressure ventilations

C **Circulation:** give chest compressions

D **Defibrillation:** assess for and shock VF/pulseless VT

Secondary ABCD Survey
Focus: more advanced assessments and treatments

A **Airway:** place airway device as soon as possible

B **Breathing:** confirm airway device placement by exam plus confirmation device

B **Breathing:** secure airway device; purpose-made tube holders preferred

B **Breathing:** confirm effective oxygenation and ventilation

C **Circulation:** establish i.v. access

C **Circulation:** identify rhythm → monitor

C **Circulation:** administer drugs appropriate for rhythm and condition

C **Circulation:** assess for occult blood flow ("pseudo-EMT")

D **Differential Diagnosis:** search for and treat identified reversible causes

Review for most frequent causes

- **H**ypovolemia
- **H**ypoxia
- **H**ydrogen ion — acidosis
- **H**yper-/hypokalemia
- **H**ypothermia
- **"T**ablets" (drug OD, accidents)
- **T**amponade, cardiac
- **T**ension pneumothorax
- **T**hrombosis, coronary (ACS)
- **T**hrombosis, pulmonary (embolism)

Epinephrine, 1 mg i.v. push, repeat every 3–5 minutes

Atropine, 1 mg i.v. (if PEA rate is *slow*), repeat every 3–5 minutes as needed, to a total dose of 0.04 mg/kg

Figure 3-3. Pulseless electrical activity (PEA) algorithm. ACS, acute coronary syndrome; CPR, cardiopulmonary resuscitation; EMT, emergency medical treatment; OD, overdose; VF, ventricular fibrillation; VT, ventricular tachycardia. (Adapted with permission from A guide to the international ACLS algorithms. *Circulation* 2000;102(Suppl I):I-142–I-157.)

3. **Asystole** (Fig. 3-4)
   a. **Asystole** is associated with a dismal prognosis in resuscitation, with survival rates of only 1% to 2%. Asystole should be confirmed in two leads because fine VF might be difficult to distinguish from asystole. If the rhythm is unclear, the presence of fine VF should be assumed. **Transcutaneous pacing** may be useful if the asystolic period is brief. **Epinephrine, vasopressin,** and **atropine** are the mainstays of pharmacologic therapy. A recent clinical trial indicates that vasopressin is superior to epinephrine in the resuscitation of patients from asystolic cardiac arrest (*N Engl J Med* 2004;350:105).
      (1) **Atropine** may have some benefit in the treatment of asystole (1.0 mg every 3 to 5 minutes intravenously). A total dose of 3 mg may result in full vagal blockade and should not be exceeded. The denervated transplanted heart does not respond to atropine and requires pacing, catecholamine infusion, or both. Anticholinergic syndrome comprising delirium, tachycardia, coma, flushed and hot skin, ataxia, and blurred vision can occur with excessive doses of atropine.
   b. **Asystole most often represents a confirmation of death rather than a rhythm to be treated**. Just as important as knowledge of the treatment algorithms presented in this chapter is the knowledge of when resuscitative efforts should be terminated. With the exception of cardiac arrests in special situations such as hypothermia, electrocution, and drug overdose, team leaders can cease resuscitation efforts when:
      (1) **Asystole** persists for at least 10 minutes after CPR has been performed.
      (2) VF, if present, has been eliminated.
      (3) Successful endotracheal intubation has been accomplished and confirmed.
      (4) Adequate ventilation has been provided as determined by oxygen saturation and, if possible, end-tidal CO_2 monitoring.
      (5) A successful intravenous line has been established and rhythm-appropriate medications have been administered.
4. **Bradycardia** (Fig. 3-5)
   a. The indications for treatment of bradycardia include associated signs and symptoms (e.g., chest pain, shortness of breath, decreased level of consciousness, hypotension, or congestive heart failure). It should be remembered that some athletes and patients on beta-blockers may have a resting heart rate of less than 60. The sequential intervention sequence is the following:
      (1) **Atropine,** 0.5 to 1.0 mg intravenously every 3 to 5 minutes, up to a 3-mg total dose.
      (2) **Transcutaneous pacing** is indicated in patients with hemodynamically unstable bradycardia unresponsive to pharmacologic treatments (e.g., atropine, dopamine). Transcutaneous cardiac pacing is the initial method of choice because of the speed with which it can be initiated and because it is widely available. Transvenous pacing is best instituted in the postresuscitation period.
      (3) **Dopamine infusion,** 5 to 20 μg/kg intravenously per minute, may be used for symptomatic bradycardia not responding to atropine if transcutaneous pacing is not immediately available. At lower doses of dopamine, the α_1- and β-adrenergic effects cause increased myocardial contractility, cardiac output, heart rate, and blood pressure. The infusion may be increased to 20 μg/kg per minute for a predominant α-adrenergic effect if hypotension is associated with the bradycardia.
      (4) **Epinephrine,** 2 to 10 mg intravenously per minute
      (5) **Isoproterenol,** 2 to 10 μg intravenously per minute. Isoproterenol may be harmful because it causes increased myocardial oxygen

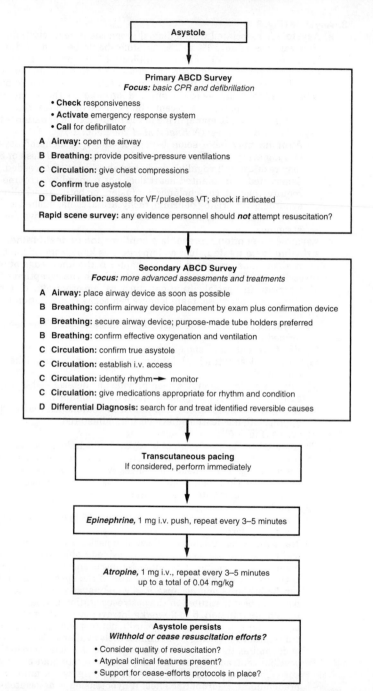

Figure 3-4. Asystole, the silent heart algorithm. CPR, cardiopulmonary resuscitation; VF, ventricular fibrillation; VT, ventricular tachycardia. (Adapted with permission from A guide to the international ACLS algorithms. *Circulation* 2000;102(Suppl I): I-142–I-157.)

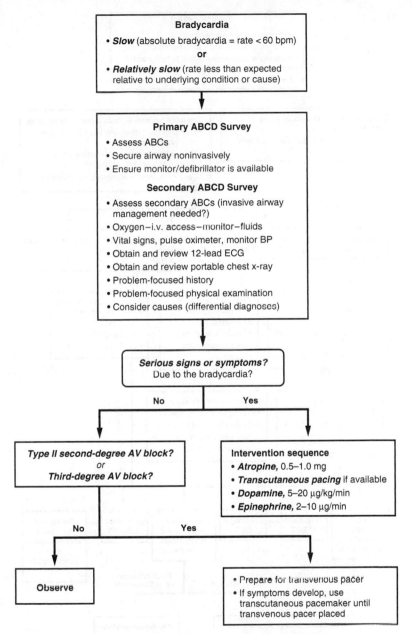

Figure 3-5. Bradycardia algorithm. AV, atrioventricular; BP, blood pressure; ECG, electrocardiogram. (Adapted with permission from A guide to the international ACLS algorithms. *Circulation* 2000;102(Suppl I):I-142–I-157.)

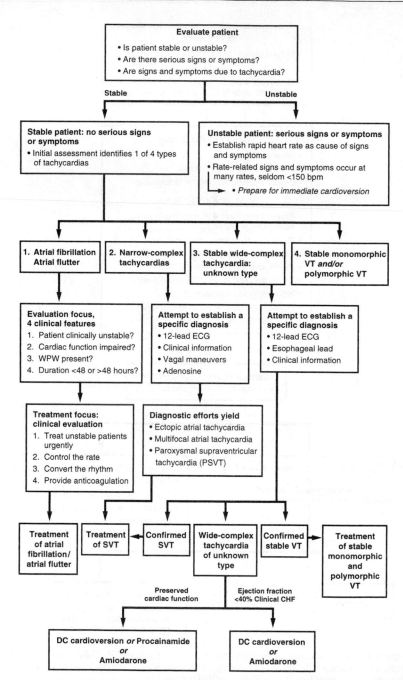

Figure 3-6. The tachycardia overview algorithm. CHF, congestive heart failure; DC, direct current; ECG, electrocardiogram; SVT; supraventricular tachycardia; VF, ventricular fibrillation; VT, ventricular tachycardia; WPW, Wolff-Parkinson-White syndrome. (Adapted with permission from The tachycardia algorithms. *Circulation* 2000;102(Suppl I):I-158–I-165.)

demand and peripheral hypotension. It is solely a temporary measure until transcutaneous or transvenous pacing is available.
5. **Tachycardia** (Fig. 3-6).
   a. Unstable patients with serious signs or symptoms (e.g., chest pain, shortness of breath, decreased level of consciousness, hypotension, pulmonary edema, or acute myocardial infarction) attributable to the tachycardia are treated initially with cardioversion if the ventricular rate is more than 150 beats per minute.
      (1) **Necessary equipment** includes an oxygen saturation monitor, oral suction equipment, intravenous access, sedation, and possibly analgesics.
      (2) **Synchronized cardioversion for VT** should be performed starting at 100 J and increasing to 200, 300, and 360 J, if necessary. Synchronized cardioversion starting with 50 J is appropriate for atrial dysrhythmias. If the patient's condition becomes critical, then unsynchronized cardioversion may be used.
IV. **Postresuscitation management** depends on the underlying disease process and the continued maintenance of hemodynamic and electrical stability. All patients should be transferred to an intensive care unit for continued care.
   A. The ultimate goal of resuscitation is not merely to restore spontaneous circulation but to achieve long-term neurologically intact survival. Two recent clinical trials suggest that treatment of patients successfully resuscitated from cardiac arrest with **mild to moderate therapeutic hypothermia** improves outcomes, increases the rate of a favorable neurologic outcome, and reduces mortality (*N Engl J Med* 2002;346:549, *N Engl J Med* 2002;346:557). The routine use of hypothermia in the management of postarrest patients awaits additional confirmatory studies.
V. **Long-term survival** among persons who have undergone successful early defibrillation after cardiac arrest is similar to that for matched patients who did not suffer cardiac arrest. The quality of life of survivors is similar to that of the general population (*N Engl J Med* 2003;348:2626).

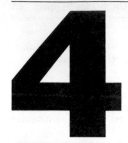

Fluid, Electrolyte, and Acid-Base Disorders

Felix G. Fernandez and Timothy G. Buchman

DIAGNOSIS AND TREATMENT OF FLUID, ELECTROLYTE, AND ACID-BASE DISORDERS

I. **Definition of body fluid compartments.** Water constitutes 50% to 70% of lean body weight. Total body water content is slightly higher in men, is most concentrated in skeletal muscle, and declines steadily with age. Total body water is divided into an intracellular fluid compartment, comprising 40% of total body weight, and an extracellular fluid compartment, comprising 20%. The extracellular fluid compartment consists of a plasma or intravascular compartment, comprising 5% of total body weight, and an interstitial compartment, comprising 15%. The extracellular and intracellular compartments have distinct electrolyte compositions. The principal extracellular cation is Na^+, and the principal extracellular anions are Cl^- and HCO_3^-. In contrast, the principal intracellular cations are K^+ and Mg^{2+}, and the principal intracellular anions are phosphates and negatively charged proteins.

II. **Osmolality and tonicity.** *Osmolality* refers to the number of osmoles of solute particles per kilogram of water. Total osmolality is composed of both effective and ineffective components. Effective osmoles cannot freely permeate cell membranes and are restricted to either the intracellular or extracellular fluid compartments. The asymmetric accumulation of effective osmoles in either extracellular fluid (e.g., Na^+, glucose, mannitol, glycine) or intracellular fluid (e.g., K^+, amino acids, organic acids) causes transcompartmental movement of water. Because the cell membrane is freely permeable to water, the osmolalities of the extracellular and intracellular compartments are equal. The effective osmolality of a solution is equivalent to its tonicity. Ineffective osmoles, in contrast, freely cross cell membranes and therefore are unable to effect shifts in water between fluid compartments. Such ineffective solutes (e.g., urea, ethanol, and methanol) contribute to total osmolality but not to tonicity. For example, the plasma of uremic patients may be hyperosmolar but not hypertonic because the concentration of urea is equally distributed between the intracellular and extracellular fluid compartments. *Tonicity*, not osmolality, is the physiologic parameter that the body attempts to regulate.

III. **Common electrolyte disorders**
   A. **Sodium**
      1. **Physiology.** The normal individual consumes 3 to 5 g NaCl (130 to 217 mmol Na^+) per day. Balance is maintained primarily by the kidneys. Normal Na^+ concentration is 135 to 145 mmol/L (310–333 mg/dL). Potential sources of significant Na^+ loss include sweat, urine, and GI secretions (Table 4-1). Na^+ concentration largely determines the plasma osmolality (P_{osm}), which can be approximated by the following equation:

$$P_{osm}(mOsm/L) = 2 \times serum\ [Na^+(mmol/L) + K^+(mmol/L)] + \frac{glucose\ (mg/dL)}{18} + \frac{BUN\ (mg/dL)}{2.8}$$

Normal P_{osm} is 290 to 310 mOsm/L. In general, hypotonicity and hypertonicity coincide with hyponatremia and hypernatremia, respectively. However, Na^+ concentration and total body water are controlled by

Table 4-1. Composition of gastrointestinal secretions

Source	Volume (mL/24 hr)[a]	Na+ (mmol/L)[b]	K+ (mmol/L)[b]	Cl- (mmol/L)[b]	HCO3- (mmol/L)[b]
Salivary	1,500 (500–2,000)	10 (2–10)	26 (20–30)	10 (8–18)	30
Stomach	1,500 (100–4,000)	60 (9–116)	10 (0–32)	130 (8–154)	0
Duodenum	(100–2,000)	140	5	80	0
Ileum	3,000	140 (80–150)	5 (2–8)	104 (43–137)	30
Colon	(100–9,000)	60	30	40	0
Pancreas	(100–800)	140 (113–185)	5 (3–7)	75 (54–95)	115
Bile	(50–800)	145 (131–164)	5 (312)	100 (89–180)	35

[a] Average volume (range).
[b] Average concentration (range).
Reprinted with permission from Faber MD, Schmidt RJ, Bear RA, et al. Management of fluid, electrolyte, and acid-base disorders in surgical patients. In: Narins RG, ed. *Clinical disorders of fluid and electrolyte metabolism.* New York: McGraw-Hill, 1994:1424.

independent mechanisms. As a consequence, hyponatremia or hyper-natremia may occur in conjunction with hypovolemia, hypervolemia, or euvolemia.

2. **Hyponatremia**
   a. **Causes and diagnosis.** The diagnostic approach to hyponatremia is illustrated in Figure 4-1. Hyponatremia may occur in conjunction with hypertonicity, isotonicity, or hypotonicity. Consequently, it is necessary to measure the serum osmolality to evaluate patients with hyponatremia.
      (1) **Isotonic hyponatremia.** Hyperlipidemic and hyperproteinemic states result in an isotonic expansion of the circulating plasma volume and cause a decrease in serum Na+ concentration, although total body Na+ remains the same. The reduction in serum sodium (mmol/L) can be estimated by multiplying the measured plasma lipid concentration (mg/dL) by 0.002 or the increment in serum protein concentration above 8 g/dL by 0.25. Isotonic, sodium-free solutions of glucose, mannitol, and glycine are restricted initially to the extracellular fluid and may similarly result in transient hyponatremia [see section **III.A.2.c.(5)**].
      (2) **Hypertonic hyponatremia.** Hyperglycemia may result in transient fluid shift from the intracellular to the extracellular compartment, thus diluting the serum Na+ concentration. The expected decrease in serum Na+ is approximately 1.3 to 1.6 mmol/L (2.99 to 3.68 mg/dL) for each 100-mg/dL increase in blood glucose above 200 mg/dL. Rapid infusion of hypertonic solutions of glucose, mannitol, or glycine may have a similar effect on Na+ concentration [see section **III.A.2.c.(5)**].
      (3) **Hypotonic hyponatremia** is classified on the basis of extracellular fluid volume. Hypotonic hyponatremia generally develops as a consequence of the administration and retention of hypotonic fluids (e.g., D5W, 0.45% NaCl) and rarely from the loss of salt-containing fluids alone.
         (a) **Hypovolemic hypotonic hyponatremia** in the surgical patient most commonly results from replacement of sodium-rich fluid losses (e.g., from the GI tract, skin, or lungs) with an insufficient volume of hypotonic fluid (e.g., D5W, 0.45% NaCl).

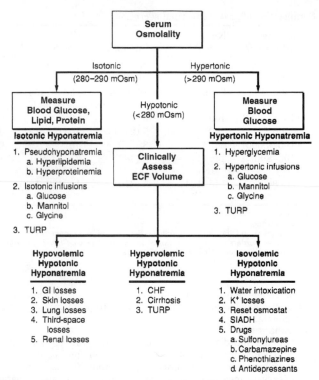

Figure 4-1. Diagnostic approach to hyponatremia. CHF, congestive heart failure; ECF, extracellular fluid; GI, gastrointestinal; SIADH, syndrome of inappropriate antidiuretic hormone secretion; TURP, transurethral resection of the prostate. (Adapted with permission from Narins RG, Jones ER, Stom MC, et al. Diagnostic strategies in disorders of fluid, electrolyte, and acid-base homeostasis. *Am J Med* 1982;72:496–520.)

(b) **Hypervolemic hypotonic hyponatremia.** The edematous states of congestive heart failure, liver disease, and nephrosis occur in conjunction with inadequate circulating blood volume. This serves as a stimulus for the renal retention of sodium and of water. Disproportionate accumulation of water results in hyponatremia.

(c) **Isovolemic hypotonic hyponatremia**

   (i)   **Water intoxication** typically occurs in the patient who consumes large quantities of water and has mildly impaired renal function (primary polydipsia). Alternatively, it may be the result of the administration of large quantities of hypotonic fluid in the patient with generalized renal failure.

   (ii) **K$^+$ loss**, either from GI fluid loss or secondary to diuretics, may result in isovolemic hyponatremia due to cellular exchange of these cations.

   (iii) **Reset osmostat.** Normally, the serum "osmostat" is set at 285 mOsm/L. In some individuals, the osmostat is "reset" downward, thus maintaining a lower serum osmolality. Several chronic diseases (e.g., tuberculosis and cirrhosis) predispose to this condition. Patients thus affected respond normally to water loads with suppression of antidiuretic hormone (ADH) secretion and excretion of free water. In contrast to the syndrome of inappropriate ADH secretion (SIADH), the administration of exogenous water does not worsen the hyponatremia.

(iv) SIADH is characterized by plasma hypo-osmolality; urine osmolality that exceeds 100 to 150 mOsm/kg; urine Na^+ concentration of greater than 20 mmol/L (46 mg/dL); normal adrenal, renal, and thyroid function; normal serum K^+ concentration; and normal acid-base balance. The major causes of SIADH include pulmonary disorders (e.g., atelectasis, empyema, pneumothorax, respiratory failure), central nervous system disorders (e.g., trauma, meningitis, tumors, subarachnoid hemorrhage), drugs (e.g., cyclophosphamide, cisplatin, nonsteroidal antiinflammatory drugs), and ectopic ADH production (e.g., small cell lung carcinoma).

(4) Transurethral resection syndrome refers to hyponatremia in conjunction with cardiovascular and neurologic manifestations, which infrequently follow transurethral resection of the prostate. This syndrome results from intraoperative absorption of significant amounts of irrigation fluid (e.g., glycine, sorbitol, or mannitol). Isotonic, hypotonic, or hypertonic hyponatremia may occur. Management of these patients may be complicated.

b. Clinical manifestations. Symptoms associated with hyponatremia are predominantly neurologic and result from hypo-osmolality. A decrease in P_{osm} causes intracellular water influx, increased intracellular volume, and cerebral edema. Symptoms include lethargy, confusion, nausea, vomiting, seizures, and coma. The likelihood that symptoms will occur is related to the degree of hyponatremia and to the rapidity with which it develops. Chronic hyponatremia is often asymptomatic until the serum Na^+ concentration falls below 110 to 120 mEq/L (253 to 276 mg/dL). An acute drop in the serum Na^+ concentration to 120 to 130 mEq/L (276 to 299 mg/dL), conversely, may produce symptoms.

c. Treatment

(1) Isotonic and hyperotonic hyponatremia correct with resolution of the underlying disorder.

(2) Hypovolemic hyponatremia can be managed with administration of 0.9% NaCl to correct volume deficits and replace ongoing losses.

(3) Water intoxication responds to fluid restriction (1,000 mL per day).

(4) For **SIADH**, water restriction (1,000 mL per day) should be attempted initially. This may be performed in conjunction with the administration of a loop diuretic (furosemide) or an osmotic diuretic (mannitol) in refractory cases.

(5) Hypervolemic hyponatremia may respond to water restriction (1,000 mL per day) to return Na^+ to greater than 130 mmol/L (299 mg/dL). In cases of severe congestive heart failure, optimizing cardiac performance may assist in Na^+ correction. If the edematous hyponatremic patient becomes symptomatic, plasma Na^+ can be increased to a safe level by the use of a loop diuretic (furosemide, 20 to 200 mg intravenously every 6 hours) while replacing urinary Na^+ losses with 3% NaCl. A reasonable approach is to replace approximately 25% of the hourly urine output with 3% NaCl. Hypertonic saline should not be administered to these patients without concomitant diuretic therapy. Administration of synthetic brain natriuretic peptide (BNP) is also useful therapeutically in the setting of acute heart failure, as it inhibits Na^+ reabsorbtion at the cortical collecting duct and inhibits the action of vasopressin on water permeabilty at the inner medullary collecting duct. This natriuresis and diuresis help restore a normal Na^+ and water balance.

(6) In the presence of symptoms or extreme hyponatremia [Na^+ <110 mmol/L (253 mg/dL)] hypertonic saline (3% NaCl) is indicated. Serum Na^+ should be corrected to approximately 120 mmol/L (276 mg/dL). The quantity of 3% NaCl that is required to increase serum Na^+ to 120 mmol/L (276 mg/dL) can be estimated by calculating the Na^+ deficit:

$$Na^+ \text{ deficit (mmol)} = 0.60 \times \text{lean body weight (kg)} \times [120 - \text{measured serum } Na^+\text{(mmol/L)}]$$

(Each liter of 3% NaCl provides 513 mmol Na^+.) The use of a loop diuretic (furosemide, 20 to 200 mg intravenously every 6 hours) may increase the effectiveness of 3% NaCl administration. Central pontine demyelination occurs in the setting of correction of hyponatremia. The risk factors for demyelination are controversial but appear to be related to the chronicity of hyponatremia (>48 hours) and the rate of correction. The serum Na^+ should be increased by no more than 12 mmol/L (27.6 mg/dL) over the first 24 hours of treatment [i.e., Na^+ <0.5 mmol (1.15 mg/dL) per hour]. For acute hyponatremia (<48 hours), the serum Na^+ may be corrected more rapidly [i.e., Na^+ = 1 to 2 mmol (2.3 to 4.6 mg/dL) per hour]. The patient's volume status should be carefully monitored over this time, and the serum Na^+ should be determined frequently (every 1 to 2 hours). Once the serum Na^+ concentration reaches 120 mmol/L (276 mg/dL) and symptoms have resolved, administration of hypertonic saline can be discontinued. Increasing serum sodium levels rapidly to normal values is not necessary.

3. **Hypernatremia**
    a. **Diagnosis.** Hypernatremia, which is less common in surgical patients, is uniformly hypertonic and typically the result of water loss in excess of solute. Patients are categorized on the basis of their extracellular fluid volume status. The diagnostic approach to hypernatremia is illustrated in Figure 4-2.
        (1) **Hypovolemic hypernatremia.** Any net loss of hypotonic body fluid results in extracellular volume depletion and hypernatremia. Common causes in the surgical patient include diuresis as well as GI, respiratory (especially patients with tracheostomies who are breathing unhumidified air), and cutaneous (particularly burn) fluid loss. Chronic renal failure and partial urinary tract obstruction also may cause hypovolemic hypernatremia.
        (2) **Hypervolemic hypernatremia** in the surgical patient is most commonly iatrogenic and results from the parenteral administration of hypertonic solutions (e.g., $NaHCO_3$, saline, medications, and nutrition).
        (3) **Isovolemic hypernatremia**
            (a) **Hypotonic losses.** Constant evaporative losses from the skin and respiratory tract, in addition to ongoing urinary free water losses, require the administration of approximately 750 mL electrolyte-free water (e.g., D5W) daily to parenterally maintained afebrile patients. Inappropriate replacement of these hypotonic losses with isotonic fluids is the most common cause of isovolemic hypernatremia in the hospitalized surgical patient.
            (b) **Diabetes insipidus** is characterized by isovolemic hypernatremia in association with the production of large volumes of hypotonic urine (urine osmolality <200 mOsm/kg). *Central diabetes insipidus* (CDI) describes a defect in hypothalamic secretion of ADH and may occur after head trauma or hypophysectomy. CDI may occur as a result of intracranial tumors, infections, vascular disorders (aneurysms), hypoxia, or medications (e.g., clonidine, phencyclidine). *Nephrogenic diabetes*

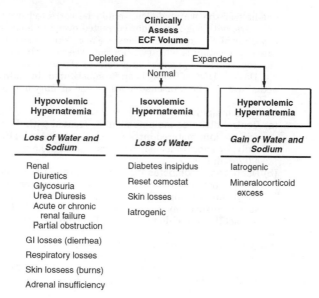

Figure 4-2. Diagnostic approach to hypernatremia. ECF, extracellular fluid; GI, gastrointestinal. (Adapted from Narins RG, Jones ER, Stom MC, et al. Diagnostic strategies in disorders of fluid, electrolyte, and acid-base homeostasis. *Am J Med* 1982;72:496–520.)

insipidus (NDI) describes renal insensitivity to normally secreted ADH. NDI may be familial or drug-induced (e.g., lithium, demeclocycline, methoxyflurane, glyburide) or may occur as a result of hypokalemia, hypercalcemia, or intrinsic renal disease. If CDI and NDI are not distinguishable clinically, they can be differentiated by dehydration testing.

(c) Deliberate hypernatremia by administration of **hypertonic saline** for osmolar therapy to control elevated intracranial pressure and cerebral edema after head injury. Apart from osmotic properties, hypertonic saline also has hemodynamic, vasoregulatory, and immunomodulatory effects after traumatic brain injury. Primary theoretical concerns with this therapy include development of central pontine myelinolysis; rapid shrinking of brain, with shearing of bridging veins leading to subarachnoid hemorrhage; renal failure; and rebound intracranial hypertension.

b. **Clinical manifestations.** Symptoms of hypernatremia that are related to the hyperosmolar state are primarily neurologic. These **initially** include lethargy, weakness, and irritability and may progress to fasciculations, seizures, coma, and irreversible neurologic damage.

c. **Treatment**

(1) **Water deficit** associated with hypernatremia can be estimated using this equation:

$$\text{Water deficit (L)} = 0.60 \times \text{total body weight (kg)} \times [(\text{serum Na}^+ \text{ in mmol/L}/140) - 1]$$

Rapid correction of hypernatremia can result in cerebral overhydration and permanent neurologic damage. Consequently, only one-half of the water deficit should be corrected over the first 24 hours, with the remainder corrected over the following 2 to 3 days. Serial Na^+ determinations are necessary to ensure that the rate of correction is adequate but not excessive. Oral fluid intake is acceptable for replacing water deficits. If oral intake is not possible, D5W or D5/0.45% NaCl can be substituted. In addition to the actual water deficit, insensible losses and urinary output must be replaced.

   (2) Diabetes insipidus

      (a) Central diabetes insipidus can be treated with desmopressin acetate administered intranasally [0.1 to 0.4 mL (10 to 40 μg) daily] or subcutaneously or intravenously [0.5 to 1 mL (2.0 to 4.0 μg) daily].

      (b) Nephrogenic diabetes insipidus treatment requires removal of any potentially offending drug and correction of electrolyte abnormalities. If these measures are ineffective, dietary sodium restriction in conjunction with a thiazide diuretic may be useful (hydrochlorothiazide, 50 to 100 mg per day orally).

B. Potassium

  1. Physiology. K^+ is the major intracellular cation, with only 2% of total body K^+ located in the extracellular space. The normal serum concentration is 3.3 to 4.9 mmol/L (12.9 to 19.1 mg/dL). Approximately 50 to 100 mmol (195 to 390 mg/dL) K^+ is ingested and absorbed daily. Ninety percent of K^+ is renally excreted, with the remainder eliminated in stools.

  2. Hypokalemia

    a. Causes. K^+ depletion from inadequate intake alone is rare. Common causes of K^+ depletion in the surgical patient include GI losses (e.g., diarrhea, persistent vomiting, nasogastric suctioning), renal losses (e.g., diuretics, fluid mobilization, amphotericin B), and cutaneous losses (e.g., burn). Other causes of hypokalemia include acute intracellular K^+ uptake (associated with insulin excess, metabolic alkalosis, myocardial infarction, delirium tremens, hypothermia, and theophylline toxicity). Hypokalemia may also occur in the malnourished patient after the initiation of total parenteral nutrition (the refeeding syndrome), caused by the incorporation of K^+ into rapidly dividing cells.

    b. Clinical manifestations. Mild hypokalemia [K^+ >3.0 mmol/L (11.7 mg/dL)] is generally asymptomatic. The symptoms present with severe K^+ deficiency [K^+ <3.0 mmol/L (11.7 mg/dL)] are primarily cardiovascular. Early electrocardiogram (ECG) manifestations include ectopy, T-wave depression, and prominent U waves. Severe depletion increases susceptibility to re-entrant arrhythmias.

    c. Treatment. In the absence of factors that cause redistribution, the relationship between the degree of hypokalemia and the extent of total body K^+ depletion is relatively predictable. For a decrement in the serum K^+ concentration from 4.0 mmol/L (15.6 mg/dL) to 3.0 mmol/L (11.7 mg/dL), total body K^+ stores decrease by 100 to 200 mmol (390 to 780 mg/dL). For a decrease from 3.0 mmol/L (11.7 mg/dL) to 2.0 mmol/L (7.8 mg/dL), total body K^+ stores may decrease by 200 to 400 mmol (780 to 1,560 mg/dL). When serum K^+ concentration falls below 2.0 mmol/L (7.8 mg/dL), the total body deficit may exceed 1,000 mmol (3,900 mg/dL). In mild hypokalemia, oral replacement is suitable. Typical daily therapy for the treatment of mild hypokalemia in the patient with intact renal function is 40 to 100 mmol (156 to 390 mg) KCl orally in single or divided doses. Parenteral therapy is indicated in the presence of severe depletion, significant symptoms, or oral intolerance. K^+ concentrations (administered as chloride, acetate, or phosphate) in peripherally administered intravenous fluids should not exceed 40 mmol/L (156 mg/dL), and the rate of administration should not exceed 20 mmol (78 mg) per hour. However, higher K^+ concentrations

[60 to 80 mmol/L (234 to 312 mg/dL)] administered more rapidly (with cardiac monitoring) are indicated in cases of severe hypokalemia, for cardiac arrhythmias, and in the management of diabetic ketoacidosis. Administration of high K^+ concentrations via subclavian, jugular, or right atrial catheters should be avoided because local K^+ concentrations may be cardiotoxic. Hypomagnesemia frequently accompanies hypokalemia and generally must be corrected to replenish K^+.

3. **Hyperkalemia**

   a. **Causes and diagnosis.** Hyperkalemia may occur with normal or elevated stores of total body K^+. Pseudohyperkalemia is a laboratory abnormality that reflects K^+ release from leukocytes and platelets during coagulation. Spurious elevation in K^+ may result from hemolysis or phlebotomy from a strangulated arm. Abnormal redistribution of K^+ from the intracellular to the extracellular compartment may occur as a result of insulin deficiency, β-adrenergic receptor blockade, acute acidemia, rhabdomyolysis, cell lysis (after chemotherapy), digitalis intoxication, reperfusion of ischemic limbs, and succinylcholine administration.

   b. **Clinical manifestations.** Mild hyperkalemia [K^+ = 5.0 to 6.0 mmol/L (19.5 to 23.4 mg/dL)] is generally asymptomatic. Signs of significant hyperkalemia [K^+ >6.5 mmol/L (25.4 mg/dL)] are, most notably, ECG abnormalities: symmetric peaking of T waves, reduced P-wave voltage, and widening of the QRS complex. If untreated, severe hyperkalemia ultimately may cause a sinusoidal ECG pattern. ECG changes are more likely to develop with rapid increases in K^+.

   c. **Treatment**

      (1) **Mild hyperkalemia** [K^+ = 5.0 to 6.0 mmol/L (19.5 to 23.4 mg/dL)] can be treated conservatively by the reduction of daily K^+ intake and the possible addition of a loop diuretic (e.g., furosemide) to promote renal elimination. Any medication that is capable of impairing K^+ homeostasis (e.g., nonselective β-adrenergic antagonists, angiotensin-converting enzyme inhibitors, K^+-sparing diuretics, nonsteroidal anti-inflammatory drugs) should be discontinued, if possible.

      (2) **Severe hyperkalemia** [K^+ >6.5 mmol/L (25.4 mg/dL)]

         (a) **Temporizing measures** produce shifts of potassium from the extracellular to the intracellular space.

            (i) **NaHCO$_3$** [1 mmol/kg or 1 to 2 ampules (50 mL each) of 8.4% $NaHCO_3$] can be infused intravenously over a 3- to 5-minute period. This dose can be repeated after 10 to 15 minutes if ECG abnormalities persist.

            (ii) **Dextrose** (0.5 g/kg body weight) infused with insulin (0.3 units of regular insulin per gram of dextrose) transiently lowers serum K^+ (the usual dose is 25 g dextrose, with 6 to 10 units of regular insulin given simultaneously as an intravenous bolus).

            (iii) **Inhaled beta-agonists** [e.g., albuterol sulfate, 2.0 to 4.0 mL of 0.5% solution (10 to 20 mg) delivered via nebulizer] have been shown to lower plasma K^+, with a duration of action of up to 2 hours. Although only modest increases in heart rate and blood pressure have been reported when the nebulized form of this drug is used, caution is warranted in patients with known or suspected cardiovascular disease.

            (iv) **Calcium gluconate 10%** (5 to 10 mL intravenously over 2 minutes) should be administered to patients with profound ECG changes who are not receiving digitalis preparations. Calcium functions to stabilize the myocardium.

         (b) **Therapeutic measures** decrease total body potassium by increasing potassium excretion.

      (i) **Sodium polystyrene sulfonate** (Kayexalate), a Na^+-K^+ exchange resin, can be administered orally (20 to 50 g of the resin in 100 to 200 mL 20% sorbitol every 4 hours) or rectally (as a retention enema, 50 g of the resin in 50 mL 70% sorbitol added to 100 to 200 mL water every 1 to 2 hours initially, followed by administration every 6 hours) to promote K^+ elimination. A decrease in serum K^+ level typically occurs 2 to 4 hours after administration.

      (ii) **Hydration** with 0.9% NaCl in combination with a **loop diuretic** (e.g., furosemide, 20 to 100 mg intravenously) should be administered to patients with adequate renal function to promote renal K^+ excretion.

      (iii) **Dialysis** is definitive therapy in severe, refractory, or life-threatening hyperkalemia.

C. Calcium

1. **Physiology.** Serum calcium (8.9 to 10.3 mg/dL or 2.23 to 2.57 mmol/L) exists in three forms: ionized (45%), protein-bound (40%), and complexed to freely diffusible compounds (15%). Only free ionized Ca^{2+} (4.6 to 5.1 mg/dL or 1.15 to 1.27 mmol/L) is physiologically active. Daily calcium intake ranges from 500 to 1,000 mg, with absorption varying considerably. Normal calcium metabolism is under the influence of parathyroid hormone (PTH) and vitamin D. PTH promotes calcium resorption from bone and reclamation of calcium from the glomerular filtrate. Vitamin D increases calcium absorption from the intestinal tract.

2. **Hypocalcemia**

    a. **Causes and diagnosis.** Hypocalcemia most commonly occurs as a consequence of calcium sequestration or vitamin D deficiency. Calcium sequestration may occur in the setting of acute pancreatitis, rhabdomyolysis, or rapid administration of blood (citrate acting as a calcium chelator). Transient hypocalcemia may occur after total thyroidectomy, secondary to vascular compromise of the parathyroid glands, and after parathyroidectomy. In the latter case, serum Ca^{2+} reaches its lowest level within 48 to 72 hours after operation, returning to normal in 2 to 3 days. Hypocalcemia may occur in conjunction with Mg^{2+} depletion, which simultaneously impairs PTH secretion and function. Acute alkalemia (e.g., from rapid administration of parenteral bicarbonate or hyperventilation) may produce clinical hypocalcemia with a normal serum calcium concentration due to an abrupt decrease in the ionized fraction. Because 40% of serum calcium is bound to albumin, hypoalbuminemia may decrease total serum calcium significantly. A fall in serum albumin of 1 g/dL decreases serum calcium by approximately 0.8 mg/dL (0.2 mmol/L). Ionized Ca^{2+} is unaffected by albumin. As a consequence, the diagnosis of hypocalcemia should be based on ionized, not total serum, calcium.

    b. **Clinical manifestations.** Tetany is the major clinical finding and may be demonstrated by Chvostek's sign (facial muscle spasm elicited by tapping over the branches of the facial nerve). Additionally, hypocalcemia can be associated with QT-interval prolongation and ventricular arrhythmias.

    c. **Treatment**

      (1) **Parenteral therapy.** Asymptomatic patients, even those with moderate hypocalcemia (calcium = 6.0 to 7.0 mg/dL or 1.5 to 1.75 mmol/L), do not require parenteral therapy. Symptoms such as overt tetany, laryngeal spasm, or seizures are indications for parenteral calcium. Approximately 200 mg elemental calcium is needed to abort an attack of tetany. Initial therapy consists of the administration of a calcium bolus (10 to 20 mL of 10% calcium gluconate over 10 minutes) followed by a maintenance infusion of 1 to 2 mg/kg elemental calcium per hour. Calcium chloride contains

three times more elemental calcium than calcium gluconate. One 10-mL ampule of 10% calcium chloride contains 272 mg (13.6 mEq) elemental calcium, whereas one 10-mL ampule of 10% calcium gluconate contains only 90 mg (4.6 mEq) elemental calcium. The serum calcium level typically normalizes in 6 to 12 hours with this regimen, at which time the maintenance rate can be decreased to 0.3 to 0.5 mg/kg per hour. In addition to monitoring calcium levels frequently during therapy, one should check Mg^{2+}, phosphorus, and K^+ levels and supplement as necessary. Calcium should be administered cautiously to patients who are receiving digitalis preparations because they may potentiate digitalis toxicity. Once the serum calcium level is normal, patients can be switched to oral therapy.

(2) Oral therapy. Calcium salts are available for oral administration (calcium carbonate, calcium gluconate). Each 1,250-mg tablet of calcium carbonate provides 500 mg elemental calcium (25.4 mEq) and a 1,000-mg tablet of calcium gluconate has 90 mg (4.6 mEq) elemental calcium. In chronic hypocalcemia, with serum calcium levels of 7.6 mg/dL (1.9 mmol/L) or higher, the daily administration of 1,000 to 2,000 mg elemental calcium alone may suffice. When hypocalcemia is more severe, calcium salts should be supplemented with a vitamin D preparation. Daily therapy can be initiated with 50,000 IU calciferol, 0.4 mg dihydrotachysterol, or 0.25 to 0.50 μg 1,25-dihydroxyvitamin D_3 orally. Subsequent therapy should be adjusted as necessary.

3. Hypercalcemia
  a. Causes and diagnosis. Causes of hypercalcemia include malignancy, hyperparathyroidism, hyperthyroidism, vitamin D intoxication, immobilization, long-term total parenteral nutrition, thiazide diuretics, and granulomatous disease. The finding of an elevated PTH level in the face of hypercalcemia supports the diagnosis of hyperparathyroidism. If the PTH level is normal or low, further evaluation is necessary to identify one of the previously cited diagnoses.
  b. Clinical manifestations. Mild hypercalcemia (calcium >12.0 mg/dL or 3.0 mmol/L) is generally asymptomatic. The hypercalcemia of hyperparathyroidism is associated infrequently with classic parathyroid bone disease and nephrolithiasis. Manifestations of severe hypercalcemia include altered mental status, diffuse weakness, dehydration, adynamic ileus, nausea, vomiting, and severe constipation. The cardiac effects of hypercalcemia include QT-interval shortening and arrhythmias.
  c. Treatment of hypercalcemia depends on the severity of the symptoms. Mild hypercalcemia (calcium >12.0 mg/dL or 3.0 mmol/L) can be managed conservatively by restricting calcium intake and treating the underlying disorder. Volume depletion should be corrected if present, and vitamin D, calcium supplements, and thiazide diuretics should be discontinued. The treatment of more severe hypercalcemia may require one or more of the following measures.
  (1) NaCl 0.9% and loop diuretics may rapidly correct hypercalcemia. In the patient with normal cardiovascular and renal function, 0.9% NaCl (250 to 500 mL per hour) with furosemide (20 mg intravenously every 4 to 6 hours) can be administered initially. The rate of 0.9% NaCl infusion and the dose of furosemide should be subsequently adjusted to maintain a urine output of 200 to 300 mL per hour. Serum Mg^{2+}, phosphorus, and K^+ levels should be monitored and replaced as necessary. The inclusion of KCl (20 mmol) and $MgSO_4$ (8 to 16 mEq or 1 to 2 g) in each liter of fluid may prevent hypokalemia and hypomagnesemia. This treatment may promote the loss of as much as 2 g calcium over 24 hours.

    (2) Salmon calcitonin, in conjunction with adequate hydration, is useful for the treatment of hypercalcemia associated with malignancy and with primary hyperparathyroidism. Salmon calcitonin can be administered either subcutaneously or intramuscularly. Skin testing by subcutaneous injection of 1.0 IU is recommended before progressing to the initial dose of 4 IU/kg intravenously or subcutaneously every 12 hours. A hypocalcemic effect may be seen as early as 6 to 10 hours after administration. If this dose is unsuccessful after 48 hours of treatment, it can be doubled. The maximum recommended dose is 8 IU/kg every 6 hours.

    (3) Pamidronate disodium, in conjunction with adequate hydration, is useful for the treatment of hypercalcemia associated with malignancy. For moderate hypercalcemia (calcium = 12.0 to 13.5 mg/dL or 3.0 to 3.38 mmol/L), 60 mg pamidronate diluted in 1 L of 0.45% NaCl, 0.9% NaCl, or D5W should be infused over 24 hours. For severe hypercalcemia, the dose of pamidronate is 90 mg. If hypercalcemia recurs, a repeat dose of pamidronate can be given after 7 days. The safety of pamidronate for use in patients with significant renal impairment is not established.

    (4) Plicamycin (25 μg/kg, diluted in 1 L of 0.9% NaCl or D5W, infused over 4 to 6 hours each day for 3 to 4 days) is useful for treatment of hypercalcemia associated with malignancy. The onset of action is between 1 and 2 days, with a duration of action of up to 1 week.

D. Phosphorus

  1. Physiology. Extracellular fluid contains less than 1% of total body stores at a concentration of 2.5 to 4.5 mg/dL (0.81 to 1.45 mmol/L). Phosphorus balance is regulated by a number of hormones that control calcium metabolism. As a consequence, derangements in concentrations of phosphorus and calcium frequently coexist. The average adult daily consumes 800 to 1,000 mg phosphorus, which is predominantly renally excreted.

  2. Hypophosphatemia

   a. Causes

    (1) Decreased intestinal phosphate absorption results from vitamin D deficiency, malabsorption, and the use of phosphate binders (e.g., aluminum-, magnesium-, calcium-, or iron-containing compounds).

    (2) Renal phosphate loss may occur with acidosis, alkalosis, diuretic therapy (particularly acetazolamide), during recovery from acute tubular necrosis, and during hyperglycemia as a result of osmotic diuresis.

    (3) Phosphorus redistribution from the extracellular to the intracellular compartment occurs principally with respiratory alkalosis and administration of nutrients such as glucose (particularly in the malnourished patient). This transient decrease in serum phosphorus is of no clinical significance unless there is a significant total body deficit. Significant hypophosphatemia may also occur in malnourished patients after the initiation of total parenteral nutrition (refeeding syndrome) as a result of the incorporation of phosphorus into rapidly dividing cells.

    (4) Hypophosphatemia may develop in **burn patients** as a result of excessive phosphaturia during fluid mobilization and incorporation of phosphorus into new tissues during wound healing.

   b. Clinical manifestations. Moderate hypophosphatemia (phosphorus = 1.0 to 2.5 mg/dL or 0.32 to 0.81 mmol/L) is usually asymptomatic. Severe hypophosphatemia (phosphorus <1.0 mg/dL or 0.32 mmol/L) may result in respiratory muscle dysfunction, diffuse weakness, and flaccid paralysis.

   c. Treatment. Hypophosphatemia can be corrected by the administration of oral or intravenous phosphate salts. Potassium phosphate or sodium phosphate salts are available for phosphorus repletion. Phosphorus

Table 4-2. Phosphorus repletion protocol

Phosphorus level	Weight 40–60 kg	Weight 61–80 kg	Weight 81–120 kg
<1.0 mg/dL	30 mmol Phos IV	40 mmol Phos IV	50 mmol Phos IV
1.0–1.7 mg/dL	20 mmol Phos IV	30 mmol Phos IV	40 mmol Phos IV
1.8–2.2 mg/dL	10 mmol Phos IV	15 mmol Phos IV	20 mmol Phos IV

If the patient's potassium is <4.0 use Potassium Phosphorus
If the patient's potassium is >4.0 use Sodium Phosphorus

Kg, kilogram; Mg, milligram; Dl, deciliter; Phos, phosphorus, IV, intravenous.
Adapted with permission from Taylor BE, Huey WY, Buchman TG, Boyle WA, Coopersmith CM.
Effectiveness of a protocol based on patient weight and serum phosphorus levels in repleting
hypophosphatemia in a surgical ICU. *J Am Coll Surg*, in press.

replacement should begin with intravenous therapy, especially for moderate (1.0 to 1.7 mg/dL) or severe (<1.0 mg/dL) hypophosphatemia. The amount of phosphorus administered depends on the serum phosphate level and patient weight (see Table 4-2). Risks of intravenous therapy include hyperphosphatemia, hypocalcemia, hypotension, hyperkalemia (with potassium phosphate), hypomagnesemia, hyperosmolality, metastatic calcification, and renal failure. The hypophosphatemic patient may require intravenous replenishment for 5 to 7 days before intracellular stores are corrected. Once the serum phosphorus level exceeds 2.0 mg/dL (0.65 mmol/L), the patient can be switched to oral therapy. Oral therapy can be initiated with a sodium-potassium phosphate salt [e.g., Neutra-Phos, 250 to 500 mg (8 to 16 mmol phosphorus) orally four times a day; each 250-mg tablet of Neutra-Phos contains 7 mmol each of K^+ and Na^+].

3. **Hyperphosphatemia**
   a. **Causes** include impaired renal excretion and transcellular shifts of phosphorus from the intracellular to the extracellular compartment (e.g., tissue trauma, tumor lysis, insulin deficiency, or acidosis). Hyperphosphatemia is also a common feature of postoperative hypoparathyroidism.
   b. **Clinical manifestations**, in the short term, include hypocalcemia and tetany. In contrast, soft tissue calcification and secondary hyperparathyroidism occur with chronicity.
   c. **Treatment** of hyperphosphatemia, in general, should eliminate the phosphorus source, remove phosphorus from the circulation, and correct any coexisting hypocalcemia. Dietary phosphorus should be restricted. Urinary phosphorus excretion can be increased by hydration (0.9% NaCl at 250 to 500 mL per hour) and diuresis (acetazolamide, 500 mg every 6 hours orally or intravenously). Phosphate binders (aluminum hydroxide, 30 to 120 mL orally every 6 hours) minimize intestinal phosphate absorption and can induce a negative balance of more than 250 mg phosphorus daily, even in the absence of dietary phosphorus. Hyperphosphatemia secondary to conditions that cause phosphorus redistribution (e.g., diabetic ketoacidosis) resolves with the treatment of the underlying condition and requires no specific therapy. Dialysis can be used to correct hyperphosphatemia in extreme conditions.

E. **Magnesium**
   1. **Physiology.** Mg^{2+} (1.3 to 2.2 mEq/L or 0.65 to 1.10 mmol/L) is predominantly an intracellular cation. Renal excretion and retention play the major physiologic role in regulating body stores. Mg^{2+} is not under direct hormonal regulation.
   2. **Hypomagnesemia**
      a. **Causes.** Hypomagnesemia on the basis of dietary insufficiency is rare. Common etiologies include excessive GI or renal Mg^{2+} loss. GI loss may

result from diarrhea, malabsorption, vomiting, or biliary fistulas. Urinary loss occurs with marked diuresis, primary hyperaldosteronism, renal tubular dysfunction (e.g., renal tubular acidosis), or chronic alcoholism or as a drug side effect (e.g., loop diuretics, cyclosporine, amphotericin B, aminoglycosides, cisplatin). Hypomagnesemia may also result from shifts of Mg^{2+} from the extracellular to intracellular space, particularly in conjunction with acute myocardial infarction or alcohol withdrawal or after receiving glucose-containing solutions. After parathyroidectomy for hyperparathyroidism, the redeposition of calcium and Mg^{2+} in bone may cause dramatic hypocalcemia and hypomagnesemia. Hypomagnesemia is usually accompanied by hypokalemia and hypophosphatemia and is frequently encountered in the trauma patient.

b. **Clinical manifestations.** Symptoms of hypomagnesemia are predominantly neuromuscular and cardiovascular. With severe depletion, altered mental status, tremors, hyperreflexia, and tetany may be present. The cardiovascular effects of hypomagnesemia are similar to those of hypokalemia and include T-wave and QRS-complex broadening as well as prolongation of the PR and QT intervals. Ventricular arrhythmias most commonly occur in patients who receive digitalis preparations.

c. **Treatment**

(1) **Parenteral therapy** is preferred for the treatment of severe hypomagnesemia (Mg^{2+} <1.0 mEq/L or 0.5 mmol/L) or in symptomatic patients. In cases of life-threatening arrhythmias, 1 to 2 g (8 to 16 mEq) $MgSO_4$ can be administered over 5 minutes, followed by a continuous infusion of 1 to 2 g per hour for the next several hours. The infusion subsequently can be reduced to 0.5 to 1.0 g per hour for maintenance. The normal range of Mg^{2+} (1.3 to 2.2 mEq/L or 0.65 to 1.10 mmol/L) probably is below its physiologic optimum. Thus, except in cases of renal failure, vigorous correction of either severe or symptomatic hypomagnesemia is warranted. In less urgent situations, $MgSO_4$ infusion may begin at 1 to 2 g per hour for 3 to 6 hours, with the rate subsequently adjusted to 0.5 to 1.0 g per hour for maintenance. Mild hypomagnesemia (1.1 to 1.4 mEq/L or 0.5 to 0.7 mmol/L) in an asymptomatic patient can be treated initially with the parenteral administration of 50 to 100 mEq (6 to 12 g) $MgSO_4$ daily until body stores are replenished. Treatment should be continued for 3 to 5 days, at which time the patient can be switched to an oral maintenance dose. Intravenous $MgSO_4$ remains the initial therapy of choice for torsades de pointes (polymorphologic ventricular tachycardia). Furthermore, it is used to achieve hypermagnesemia that is therapeutic for eclampsia and for preeclampsia.

(2) **Oral therapy.** Magnesium oxide is the preferred oral agent. Each 400-mg tablet provides 241 mg (20 mEq) Mg^{2+}. Other formulations include magnesium gluconate [each 500-mg tablet provides 27 mg (2.3 mEq) Mg^{2+}] and magnesium chloride [each 535-mg tablet provides 64 mg (5.5 mEq) Mg^{2+}]. Depending on the level of depletion, oral therapy should provide 20 to 80 mEq Mg^{2+} per day in divided doses.

(3) **Prevention of hypomagnesemia** in the hospitalized patient who is receiving prolonged parenteral nutritional therapy can be accomplished by providing 0.35 to 0.45 mEq/kg Mg^{2+} per day [i.e., by adding 8 to 16 mEq (1 to 2 g) $MgSO_4$ to each liter of intravenous fluids].

(4) **Serum Mg^{2+} levels should be monitored during therapy.** In patients with renal insufficiency, the dose of Mg^{2+} should be reduced.

3. Hypermagnesemia
   a. Causes. Hypermagnesemia occurs infrequently, is usually iatrogenic, and is seen most commonly in the setting of renal failure.
   b. Clinical manifestations. Mild hypermagnesemia (Mg^{2+} = 5.0 to 6.0 mEq/L or 2.5 to 3.0 mmol/L) is generally asymptomatic. Severe hypermagnesemia (Mg^{2+} >8.0 mEq/L or 4.0 mmol/L) is associated with depression of deep tendon reflexes, paralysis of voluntary muscles, hypotension, sinus bradycardia, and prolongation of PR, QRS, and QT intervals.
   c. Treatment. Cessation of exogenous Mg^{2+} is necessary. Calcium gluconate 10% (10 to 20 mL over 5 to 10 minutes intravenously) is indicated in the presence of life-threatening symptoms (e.g., **hyporeflexia**, respiratory depression, or cardiac conduction disturbances) to antagonize the effects of Mg^{2+}. NaCl 0.9% (250 to 500 mL per hour) infusion with loop diuretic (furosemide, 20 mg intravenously every 4 to 6 hours) in the patient with intact renal function promotes renal elimination. Dialysis is the definitive therapy in the presence of intractable symptomatic hypermagnesemia.
IV. Parenteral fluid therapy. The composition of commonly used parenteral fluids is presented in Table 4-3.
   A. Crystalloids, in general, are solutions that contain sodium as the major osmotically active particle. Crystalloids are relatively inexpensive and are useful for volume expansion, maintenance infusion, and correction of electrolyte disturbances.
      1. Isotonic crystalloids (e.g., lactated Ringer solution, 0.9% NaCl) distribute uniformly throughout the extracellular fluid compartment so that after 1 hour only 25% of the total volume infused remains in the intravascular space. Lactated Ringer solution is designed to mimic extracellular fluid and is considered a balanced salt solution. This solution provides a HCO_3-precursor and is useful for replacing GI losses and extracellular fluid volume deficits. In general, lactated Ringer solution and 0.9% NaCl can be used interchangeably. However, 0.9% NaCl is preferred in the presence of hyperkalemia, hypercalcemia, hyponatremia, hypochloremia, or metabolic alkalosis.
      2. Hypertonic saline solutions alone and in combination with colloids, such as dextran, have generated interest as a resuscitation fluid for patients with shock or burns. These fluids are appealing because, relative to isotonic crystalloids, smaller quantities are required initially for resuscitation. However, the intravascular hypertonic benefit rapidly dissipates as the fluid redistributes between the intravascular and extravascular spaces. Side effects of hypertonic solutions include hypernatremia, hyperosmolality, hyperchloremia, hypokalemia, and central pontine demyelination with rapid infusion. These solutions should be used with caution in all patients, in particular those with impaired renal function.
   B. Hypotonic solutions (D5W, 0.45% NaCl) distribute throughout the total body water compartment, expanding the intravascular compartment by as little as 10% of the volume infused. For this reason, hypotonic solutions should not be used for volume expansion. They are used to replace free water deficits.
   C. Colloid solutions contain high–molecular-weight substances that remain in the intravascular space. Early use of colloids in the resuscitation regimen may result in more prompt restoration of tissue perfusion and may lessen the total volume of fluid required for resuscitation. However, there are no situations in which colloids have unequivocally been shown to be superior to crystalloids for volume expansion. Because colloid solutions are substantially more expensive than crystalloids, their routine use in hypovolemic shock remains controversial. The use of colloids is indicated when crystalloids fail to sustain plasma volume because of low colloid osmotic pressure (e.g., increased protein loss from the vascular space, as in burns

Table 4-3. Composition of common parenteral fluids[a]

Solutions	Volumes[b]	Na$^+$	K$^+$	Ca^{2+}	Mg^{2+}	Cl$^-$	HCO$_3$ (as lactate)	Dextrose (g/L)	mOsm/L
Extracellular fluid	—	142	4	5	3	103	27	—	280–310
Lactated Ringer	—	130	4	3	—	109	28	—	273
0.9% NaCl	—	154	—	—	—	154	—	—	308
0.45% NaCl	—	77	—	—	—	77	—	—	154
D5W	—	—	—	—	—	—	—	50	252
D5/0.45% NaCl	—	77	—	—	—	77	—	50	406
D5LR	—	130	4	3	—	109	28	50	525
3% NaCl	—	513	—	—	—	513	—	—	1,026
7.5% NaCl	—	1,283	—	—	—	1,283	—	—	2,567
6% hetastarch	500	154	—	—	—	154	—	—	310
10% dextran 40	500	0/154[c]	—	—	—	0/154[c]	—	—	300
6% dextran 70	500	0/154[c]	—	—	—	0/154[c]	—	—	300
5% albumin	250, 500	130–160	<2.5	—	—	130–160	—	—	330
25% albumin	20, 50, 100	130–160	<2.5	—	—	130–160	—	—	330
Plasma protein fraction	250, 500	145	—	—	—	145	—	—	300

[a]Electrolyte concentrations in mmol/L.
[b]Available volumes (mL) of colloid solutions.
[c]Dextran solutions available in 5% dextrose (0 Na$^+$, 0 Cl) or 0.9% NaCl (154 mmol Na$^+$, 154 mmol Cl).
D5LR, 5% dextrose in lactated Ringer solution; D5/0.45% NaCl, 5% dextrose per 0.45% NaCl; D5W, 5% dextrose in water.

and peritonitis). Synthetic and human-derived colloids carry a minimal risk of transmitting infection.

1. **Albumin preparations** ultimately distribute throughout the extracellular space, although the initial location of distribution is the vascular compartment. Preparations of 25% albumin (100 mL) and 5% albumin (500 mL) expand the intravascular volume by an equivalent amount (450 to 500 mL). However, 25% albumin is indicated in the edematous patient to mobilize interstitial fluid into the intravascular space. The cost per liter of albumin is more than that of other colloid solutions and 30 times the cost of the intravascular volume–equivalent amount of crystalloid solutions. Consequently, albumin preparations should be used judiciously. They are not indicated in the patient with adequate colloid oncotic pressure (serum albumin >2.5 mg/dL, total protein >5 mg/dL), for augmenting serum albumin in chronic illness (cirrhosis or nephrotic syndrome), or as a nutritional source.

2. **Dextran** is a synthetic glucose polymer that undergoes predominantly renal elimination. In addition to its indications for volume expansion, dextran also is used for thromboembolism prophylaxis and promotion of peripheral perfusion. Dextran solutions expand the intravascular volume by an amount equal to the volume infused. Side effects include renal failure, osmotic diuresis, coagulopathy, and laboratory abnormalities (i.e., elevations in blood glucose and protein, interference with blood cross-matching). Preparations of 40 kD and 70 kD dextran are available (dextran 40 and dextran 70).

3. **Hydroxyethyl starch (hetastarch)** is a synthetic molecule resembling glycogen that is available as a 6% solution in 0.9% NaCl. Hetastarch, like 5% albumin, increases the intravascular volume by an amount equal to or greater than the volume infused. Hetastarch is less expensive than albumin and has a more favorable side effect profile than dextran formulations, making it an appealing colloid preparation. Hextend is a recently FDA approved colloid that contains 6% hetastarch, balanced electrolytes, a lactate buffer, and physiologic levels of glucose. Relative to hetastarch in saline, Hextend seems to have a more beneficial coagulation profile, less antigenicity, and antioxidant properties.

   a. **Indications** include use as a plasma volume–expanding agent in shock from hemorrhage, trauma, sepsis, and burns. Urine output typically increases acutely secondary to osmotic diuresis and must not be misinterpreted as a sign of adequate peripheral perfusion in this setting.

   b. **Elimination** is hepatic and renal. Patients with renal impairment are particularly subject to initial volume overload and tissue accumulation of hetastarch with repeated administration. In these patients, initial volume resuscitation accomplished with hetastarch should be maintained with another plasma volume expander, such as albumin or crystalloid.

   c. **Laboratory abnormalities** include elevations in serum amylase to approximately twice normal without associated alteration in pancreatic function.

   d. **Dosing** of hetastarch 6% solution is 30 to 60 g (500 to 1,000 mL), with the total daily dosage not exceeding 1.2 g/kg (20 mL/kg) or 90 g (1,500 mL). In hemorrhagic shock, hetastarch solution can be administered at a rate of 1.2 g/kg per hour (20 mL/kg per hour). Slower rates of administration generally are used in patients with burns or septic shock. In individuals with severe renal impairment (creatinine clearance <10 mL per minute), the usual dose of hetastarch can be administered, but subsequent dosage should be reduced 50% to 75%.

D. **Principles of fluid management.** A normal individual consumes an average of 2,000 to 2,500 mL water daily. Daily water losses include approximately 1,000 to 1,500 mL in urine and 250 ml, in stool. The minimum amount of urinary output that is required to excrete the catabolic end products of metabolism is approximately 800 mL. An additional 750-mL insensible

Table 4-4. Estimation of intraoperative fluid loss and guide for replacement

Preoperative deficit	Maintenance IVF × hr n.p.o., plus preexisting deficit related to disease state
Maintenance fluids	Maintenance IVF × duration of case
Third-space and insensible losses	1–3 mL/kg per hr for minor procedure (small incision)
	3–7 mL/kg per hr for moderate procedure (medium incision)
	9–11 mL/kg per hr for extensive procedure (large incision)
Blood loss	1 mL blood or colloid per 1 mL blood loss, or 3 mL crystalloid per 1 mL blood loss

IVF, intravenous fluids.

water loss occurs daily via the skin and respiratory tract. Insensible losses increase with hypermetabolism, fever, and hyperventilation.
1. **Maintenance.** Maintenance fluids should be administered at a rate that is sufficient to maintain a urine output of 0.5 to 1.0 mL/kg per hour. Maintenance fluid requirements can be approximated on the basis of body weight as follows: 100 mL/kg per day for the first 10 kg, 50 mL/kg per day for the second 10 kg, and 20 mL/kg per day for each subsequent 10 kg. Maintenance fluids in general should contain Na^+ (1 to 2 mmol/kg per day) and K^+ [0.5 to 1.0 mmol/kg per day (e.g., D5/0.45% NaCl + 20 to 30 mmol K^+/L)].
2. **Preoperative management.** Preexisting volume and electrolyte abnormalities should be corrected before operation whenever possible. Consideration of duration and route of loss provides important information regarding the extent of fluid and electrolyte abnormalities.
3. **Intraoperative fluid management** requires replacement of preoperative deficit as well as ongoing losses (Table 4-4). Intraoperative losses include maintenance fluids for the duration of the case, hemorrhage, and "third-space losses." The maintenance fluid requirement is calculated as detailed above (see section **IV.D.1**). Acute blood loss can be replaced with a volume of crystalloid that is three to four times the blood loss or with an equal volume of colloid or blood. Intraoperative insensible and third-space fluid losses are dependent on the size of the incision and the extent of tissue trauma and dissection and can be replaced with an appropriate volume of lactated Ringer solution. Small incisions with minor tissue trauma (e.g., inguinal hernia repair) result in third-space losses of approximately 1 to 3 mL/kg per hour. Medium-sized incisions with moderate tissue trauma (e.g., uncomplicated sigmoidectomy) result in third-space losses of approximately 3 to 7 mL/kg per hour. Larger incisions and operations with extensive tissue trauma and dissection (e.g., pancreaticoduodenectomy) can result in third-space losses of approximately 9 to 11 mL/kg per hour or greater.
4. **Postoperative fluid management** requires careful evaluation of the patient. Continued sequestration of extracellular fluid into the sites of injury or operative trauma can continue for 12 hours or more after operation. Urine output should be monitored closely and intravascular volume replenished to maintain a urine output of 0.5 to 1.0 mL/kg per hour. Gastrointestinal losses that exceed 250 mL per day from nasogastric or gastrostomy tube suction should be replaced with an equal volume of crystalloid. Mobilization of perioperative third-space fluid losses typically begins 2 to 3 days after operation. Anticipation of postoperative fluid shifts should prompt careful evaluation of the patient's volume status and, if needed, consideration of diuresis before the development of symptomatic hypervolemia.

V. Acid-base disorders
   A. Diagnostic approach
      1. General concepts
         a. Acid-base homeostasis represents equilibrium between the concentration of H^+, P_{CO_2}, and HCO_3^-. In clinical practice, H^- concentration is expressed as pH.
         b. Normal pH is 7.35 to 7.45. **Acidemia** refers to pH of less than 7.35, and **alkalemia** refers to pH of more than 7.45.
         c. Acidosis and alkalosis describe processes that cause the accumulation of acid or alkali, respectively. The terms *acidosis* and *acidemia* and the terms *alkalosis* and *alkalemia* are often used interchangeably, but such usage is inaccurate. A patient, for example, may be acidemic while alkalosis is occurring.
         d. Laboratory studies that are necessary for the initial evaluation of acid-base disturbances include arterial pH, P_{aCO_2} (normal is 35 to 45 mm Hg), and serum electrolytes [HCO_3^- (normal is 22 to 31 mmol/L)]. Although base excess or base deficit calculations can be made, this information does not add substantially to the evaluation.
      2. Compensatory response to primary disorders. Disorders that initially alter P_{aCO_2} are termed *respiratory acidosis* or *alkalosis*. Alternatively, disorders that initially affect plasma HCO_3^- concentration are termed *metabolic acidosis* or *alkalosis*. Primary metabolic disorders stimulate respiratory responses that act to return the ratio of P_{CO_2} to HCO_3^- (and therefore the pH) toward normal. Similarly, primary respiratory disturbances elicit countervailing metabolic responses that also act to normalize pH. As a general rule, these compensatory responses do not normalize pH because to do so would remove the stimulus for compensation. By convention, these compensating changes are termed *secondary* or *respiratory* or *metabolic* compensation for the primary disturbance. The amount of compensation to be expected from either a primary respiratory or metabolic disorder is presented in Table 4-5. Significant deviations from these expected values suggest the presence of a mixed acid-base disturbance.
   B. Primary metabolic disorders
      1. Metabolic acidosis results from the accumulation of nonvolatile acids, reduction of renal acid excretion, or loss of alkali. The most common causes of metabolic acidosis are listed in Table 4-6. Metabolic acidosis has few specific signs. The appropriate diagnosis depends on the clinical setting and laboratory tests.

Table 4-5. Expected compensation for simple acid-base disorders

Primary disorder	Initial change	Compensatory response	Expected compensation
Metabolic acidosis	HCO_3^- decrease	P_{CO_2} decrease	P_{CO_2} decrease = 1.2 × ΔHCO_3^-
Metabolic alkalosis	HCO_3^- increase	P_{CO_2} increase	P_{CO_2} increase = 0.7 × ΔHCO_3^-
Respiratory acidosis	P_{CO_2} increase	HCO_3^- increase	Acute: HCO_3^- increase = 0.1 × ΔP_{CO_2} Chronic: HCO_3^- increase = 0.35 × ΔP_{CO_2}
Respiratory alkalosis	P_{CO_2} decrease	HCO_3^- decrease	Acute: HCO_3^- decrease = 0.2 × ΔP_{CO_2} Chronic: HCO_3^- decrease = 0.5 × ΔP_{CO_2}

Table 4-6. Causes of metabolic acidosis

Increased anion gap
Increased acid production
  Ketoacidosis
    Diabetic
    Alcoholic
    Starvation
  Lactic acidosis
  Toxic ingestion (salicylates, ethylene glycol, methanol)
Renal failure

Normal anion gap (hyperchloremic)
Renal tubular dysfunction
  Renal tubular acidosis
  Hypoaldosteronism
  Potassium-sparing diuretics
Loss of alkali
  Diarrhea
  Ureterosigmoidostomy
  Carbonic anhydrase inhibitors
Administration of HCl (ammonium chloride, cationic amino acids)

---

    a. Anion gap (AG; normal is 3 to 11 mmol/L) represents the anions, other than Cl^- and HCO_3^-, that are necessary to counterbalance Na^- electrically:

$$AG\ (mmol/L) = Na^+(mmol/L) + [Cl\ (mmol/L) + HCO_3^-(mmol/L)]$$

It is useful diagnostically to classify metabolic acidosis into increased or normal AG metabolic acidosis.
    (1) Increased AG metabolic acidosis (see Table 4-6)
    (2) Normal AG (hyperchloremic) metabolic acidosis (see Table 4-6)
    b. Treatment of metabolic acidosis must be directed primarily at the underlying cause of the acid-base disturbance. Bicarbonate therapy should be considered in patients with moderate to severe metabolic acidosis, only after the primary cause has been addressed. The HCO_3^- deficit (mmol/L) can be estimated using the following equation:

$$HCO_3\text{-}deficit\ (mmol/L) = body\ weight\ (kg) \times 0.4 \times$$
$$[(desired\ HCO_3^-[mmol/L]) - (measured\ HCO_3^-[mmol/L])]$$

This equation serves to provide only a rough estimate of the deficit because the volume of HCO_3^- distribution and the rate of ongoing H^+ production are variable.
    (1) Rate of HCO_3^- replacement. In nonurgent situations, the estimated HCO_3^- deficit can be repaired by administering a continuous intravenous infusion over 4 to 8 hours [a 50-mL ampule of 8.4% $NaHCO_3$ solution (provides 50 mmol HCO_3^-) can be added to 1 L D5W or 0.45% NaCl]. In urgent situations, the entire deficit can be repaired by administering a bolus over several minutes. The **goal of HCO_3^- therapy** should be to raise the arterial blood pH to 7.20 or the HCO_3^- concentration to 10 mmol/L. One should not attempt to normalize pH with bicarbonate administration because the risks of bicarbonate therapy (e.g., hypernatremia, hypercapnia, cerebrospinal fluid acidosis, or overshoot alkalosis) are likely to be increased. Serial arterial blood gases and serum electrolytes should be obtained to assess the response to HCO_3^- therapy.

Table 4-7. Causes of metabolic alkalosis

Associated with extracellular fluid volume (chloride) depletion
Vomiting or gastric drainage
Diuretic therapy
Posthypercapnic alkalosis

Associated with mineralocorticoid excess
Cushing syndrome
Primary aldosteronism
Bartter syndrome

Severe K^+ depletion

Excessive alkali intake

---

            (2) Lactic acidosis. Correction of the underlying disorder is the primary therapy for lactic acidosis. Reversal of circulatory failure, hypoxemia, or sepsis reduces the rate of lactate production and enhances its removal. Because the use of $NaHCO_3$ in lactic acidosis is controversial, no definite recommendations can be made.

   2. Metabolic alkalosis (Table 4-7)

      a. Causes

         (1) Chloride-responsive metabolic alkalosis in the surgical patient is typically associated with extracellular fluid volume deficits. The most common causes of metabolic alkalosis in the surgical patient include inadequate fluid resuscitation or diuretic therapy (e.g., contraction alkalosis), acid loss through GI secretions (e.g., nasogastric suctioning, vomiting), and the exogenous administration of HCO_3^- or HCO_3^- precursors (e.g., citrate in blood). Posthypercapnic metabolic alkalosis occurs after the rapid correction of chronic respiratory acidosis. Under normal circumstances, the excess in bicarbonate that is generated by any of these processes is excreted rapidly in the urine. Consequently, maintenance of metabolic alkalosis requires impairment of renal HCO_3^- excretion, most commonly due to volume and chloride depletion. Because replenishment of Cl^- corrects the metabolic alkalosis in these conditions, each is classified as Cl-responsive metabolic alkalosis.

         (2) Chloride-unresponsive metabolic alkalosis is encountered less frequently in surgical patients and usually results from mineralocorticoid excess. Hyperaldosteronism, marked hypokalemia, renal failure, renal tubular Cl^- wasting (Bartter syndrome), and chronic edematous states are associated with chloride-unresponsive metabolic alkalosis.

      b. Diagnosis. Although the cause of metabolic alkalosis is usually apparent in the surgical patient, measurement of the urinary chloride concentration may be useful for differentiating these disorders. A urine Cl^- concentration <15 mmol/L suggests inadequate fluid resuscitation, ongoing GI loss from emesis or nasogastric suctioning, diuretic administration, or posthypercapnia as the cause of the metabolic alkalosis. A urine Cl^- concentration >20 mmol/L suggests mineralocorticoid excess, alkali loading, concurrent diuretic administration, or the presence of severe hypokalemia.

      c. Treatment principles in metabolic alkalosis include identifying and removing underlying causes, discontinuing exogenous alkali, and repairing Cl^-, K^+, and volume deficits. Because metabolic alkalosis generally is well tolerated, rapid correction of this disorder usually is not necessary.

(1) **Initial therapy** should include the correction of volume deficits (with 0.9% NaCl) and hypokalemia. Patients with vomiting or nasogastric suctioning also may benefit from H_2-receptor antagonists or other acid-suppressing medications.

(2) **Edematous patients.** Chloride administration does not enhance HCO_3^- excretion because the reduced effective arterial blood volume is not corrected by this therapy. Acetazolamide (5 mg/kg per day intravenously or orally) facilitates fluid mobilization while decreasing renal HCO_3^- reabsorption. However, tolerance to this diuretic may develop after 2 to 3 days.

(3) **Severe alkalemia** ($HCO_3^- >40$ mmol/L), especially in the presence of symptoms, may require more aggressive correction. The infusion of acidic solutions is occasionally indicated in the patient with severe refractory metabolic alkalosis and chloride loss, typically due to massive nasogastric drainage or complete prepyloric obstruction. Ammonium chloride (NH_4Cl) is hepatically converted to urea and HCl. The amount of NH_4Cl that is required can be estimated using the following equation:

$$NH_4Cl \text{ (mmol)} = 0.2 \times \text{weight (kg)} \times [103 - \text{serum } Cl^-(\text{mmol})]$$

NH_4Cl is prepared by adding 100 or 200 mmol (20 to 40 mL of the 26.75% NH_4Cl concentrate) to 500 to 1,000 mL of 0.9% NaCl. This solution should be administered at a rate that does not exceed 5 mL per minute. Approximately one-half of the calculated volume of NH_4Cl should be administered, at which time the acid-base status and Cl^- concentration should be repeated to determine the necessity for further therapy. NH_4Cl is contraindicated in hepatic failure.

(4) **HCl** (0.1 N(normal), administered intravenously) corrects metabolic alkalosis more rapidly. The amount of H^+ to administer can be estimated using the following equation:

$$H^+(\text{mmol}) = 0.5 \times \text{weight (kg)} \times [103 - \text{serum } Cl^-(\text{mmol/L})]$$

To prepare 0.1 N HCl, mix 100 mmol HCl in 1 L sterile water. The calculated amount of 0.1 N HCl must be administered via a central venous catheter over 24 hours. The HCO_3^- concentration can be safely reduced by 8 to 12 mmol/L over 12 to 24 hours.

(5) **Dialysis** can be considered in the volume-overloaded patient with renal failure and intractable metabolic alkalosis.

C. **Primary respiratory disorders**

1. **Respiratory acidosis** occurs when alveolar ventilation is insufficient to excrete metabolically produced CO_2. Common causes in the surgical patient include respiratory center depression (e.g., drugs, organic disease), neuromuscular disorders, and cardiopulmonary arrest. Chronic respiratory acidosis may occur in pulmonary diseases, such as chronic emphysema and bronchitis. Chronic hypercapnia may also result from primary alveolar hypoventilation or alveolar hypoventilation related to extreme obesity (e.g., pickwickian syndrome) or from thoracic skeletal abnormalities. The diagnosis of acute respiratory acidosis usually is evident from the clinical situation, especially if respiration is obviously depressed. Appropriate therapy is correction of the underlying disorder. In cases of acute respiratory acidosis, there is no indication for $NaHCO_3$ administration.

2. **Respiratory alkalosis** is the result of acute or chronic hyperventilation. The causes of respiratory alkalosis include acute hypoxia (e.g., pneumonia, pneumothorax, pulmonary edema, bronchospasm), chronic hypoxia (e.g., cyanotic heart disease, anemia), and respiratory center stimulation

Table 4-8. Common causes of mixed acid-base disorders

Metabolic acidosis and respiratory acidosis
Cardiopulmonary arrest
Severe pulmonary edema
Salicylate and sedative overdose
Pulmonary disease with superimposed renal failure or sepsis

Metabolic acidosis and respiratory alkalosis
Salicylate overdose
Sepsis
Combined hepatic and renal insufficiency

Metabolic alkalosis and respiratory acidosis
Chronic pulmonary disease, with superimposed
 Diuretic therapy
 Steroid therapy
 Vomiting
 Reduction of hypercapnia by mechanical ventilation

Metabolic alkalosis and respiratory alkalosis
Pregnancy with vomiting
Chronic liver disease treated with diuretic therapy
Cardiopulmonary arrest treated with bicarbonate therapy and mechanical
 ventilation

Metabolic acidosis and alkalosis
Vomiting superimposed on
 Renal failure
 Diabetic ketoacidosis
Alcoholic ketoacidosis

(e.g., anxiety, fever, Gram-negative sepsis, salicylate intoxication, central nervous system disease, cirrhosis, pregnancy). Excessive ventilation may also cause respiratory alkalosis in the mechanically ventilated patient. Depending on its severity and acuteness, hyperventilation may or may not be clinically apparent. Clinical findings are nonspecific. As in respiratory acidosis, the only effective treatment is correction of the underlying disorder.

D. **Mixed acid-base disorders.** When two or three primary acid-base disturbances occur simultaneously, a patient is said to have a mixed acid-base disorder. As summarized in Table 4-5, the respiratory or metabolic compensation for a simple primary disorder follows a predictable pattern. Significant deviation from these patterns suggests the presence of a mixed disorder. Table 4-8 lists some common causes of mixed acid-base disturbances. The diagnosis of mixed acid-base disorders depends principally on evaluation of the clinical setting and on interpretation of acid-base patterns. However, even normal acid-base patterns may conceal mixed disorders.

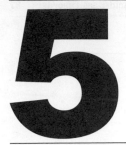

Hemostasis and Transfusion Therapy

Cassandra M. Kelleher,
John A. Curci, and Morey
A. Blinder

I. **Hemostasis**
   A. **Mechanisms of hemostasis.** Coagulation is a complex equilibrium between thrombotic, anticoagulant, and fibrinolytic processes. The disruption of these processes can lead to severe hemorrhagic or thrombotic complications.
      1. **Platelets** serve a primary role in hemostasis by filling defects in the vessel wall and through the release of thrombotic mediators. Exposure of platelets to subendothelial tissue allows platelet adhesion directly to collagen, or via interaction of tissue von Willebrand factor (vWF) with platelet glycoprotein Ib/IX. Adherance of platelets to collagen or exposure to thrombin causes local platelet activation. Activation of platelets precipitates release of vasoactive agents, including adenosine diphosphate, thromboxane A_2, and serotonin, leading to additional platelet recruitment. Activation also increases platelet glycoprotein IIb/IIIa's affinity for fibrinogen, causing platelet aggregation and thrombus formation.
         a. **Endogenous antiplatelet agents**
            Prostacyclin, produced by endothelial cells, inhibits resting and activated platelet aggregation. Disruption of the endothelial surface at the site of vessel injury results in augmented platelet plug formation owing to the loss of prostacyclin.
            Nitric oxide is produced by endothelium and platelets and downregulates P-selectin and glycoprotein IIb/IIIa expression, thereby decreasing platelet aggregation. Chronic cigarette smoking decreases platelet nitric oxide production and may lead to a propensity for thrombosis.
      2. **Coagulation cascade** is a series of reactions involving activation of serine proteases (factors), which eventually leads to formation of the cross-linked fibrin and platelet thrombus. Two types of events can initiate the coagulation cascade, activation of the intrinsic or extrinsic pathway (Fig. 5-1). The **extrinsic pathway** begins with exposure of circulating factor VIIa to tissue factor, a lipoprotein found in extravascular tissues. The **intrinsic pathway** is initiated by activation of factor XII to XIIa by contact with activated cellular surfaces (platelets, endothelial cells) or subendothelial tissue. The extrinsic pathway appears more important in initiating coagulation than the intrinsic pathway, but both pathways are required for normal hemostasis. The extrinsic and intrinsic pathways merge in the production of factor Xa, the first enzyme of the common pathway. In the final step of the cascade, fibrin is produced by the action of thrombin on fibrinogen, and this insoluble fibrin then is cross-linked by activated factor XIII (factor XIIIa). In addition to the enzymatic clotting factors, cofactors (e.g., factors V and VIII), phospholipids from platelet and endothelial cell surfaces, and calcium are required for normal coagulation. Deficiencies of any of the coagulation factors (except factor XII, high–molecular-weight kininogen, and prekallikrein) can lead to abnormal bleeding.

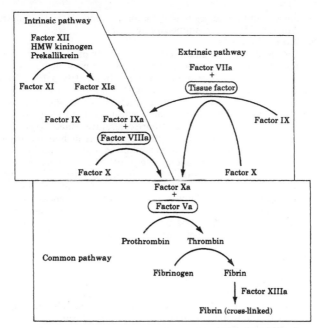

Figure 5-1. Blood coagulation cascade. Plasma zymogens are sequentially converted to active proteases (*arrows*). Nonenzymatic protein cofactors (*ovals*) are required at several stages of the cascade. Factors IX and X and prothrombin are activated on phospholipid surfaces. Thrombin cleaves fibrinogen, yielding fibrin monomers that polymerize to form a clot. HMW, high molecular weight. (Reprinted with permission from Ewald GS, McKenzie CR, eds. *Manual of Medical Therapeutics.* 28th ed. Boston: Little, Brown, 1995.)

    B. **Endogenous anticoagulants** are important to restrict coagulation to the specific area of vascular injury. Deficiencies in these anticoagulants can lead to thrombosis.

        1. **Antithrombin (AT; previously known as antithrombin III)** is an important inhibitor of the coagulation cascade. AT binds several clotting factors, including thrombin, factor Xa, and other activated proteases, producing complexes that are cleared from the circulation. Heparin markedly accelerates AT-induced factor inhibition, increasing factor clearance and leading to anticoagulation.

        2. **The thrombomodulin–protein C–protein S system** is also important in the regulation of hemostasis. Protein C, a vitamin K–dependent proenzyme, is cleaved by thrombin to form activated protein C. Activated protein C is a serine protease that inactivates factors Va and VIIIa in the presence of protein S. Activation of protein C is enhanced by thrombomodulin on intact endothelial cell surfaces.

    C. **Fibrinolytic system.** Once formed, fibrin can be degraded by plasmin, which allows for natural dissolution or remodeling of a clot. Plasmin is generated from fibrin-bound plasminogen by tissue plasminogen activator or from circulating plasminogen by urokinase or streptokinase. Naturally occurring inhibitors of plasmin include plasminogen activator inhibitor,

α_2-antiplasmin, and α_2-macroglobulin, along with the pharmacologic agents aprotinin and ϵ-aminocaproic acid.

II. **Evaluation of hemostasis**
   A. **History and physical examination.** A history of prolonged bleeding after injury, childbirth, or surgical or dental procedures should be sought from each patient before operation and can help identify patients at increased risk for surgical bleeding. Patients with a platelet disorder typically have signs of skin or mucosal bleeding, such as petechiae, frequent bruising, epistaxis, menorrhagia, and prolonged bleeding after minor injuries. Patients with deficiencies in one or more coagulation factors typically describe delayed development of soft-tissue hematomas or hemarthroses. The use of medications that affect platelet function and coagulation (e.g., aspirin, nonsteroidal anti-inflammatory drugs, ethanol, contraceptives, or anticoagulants) should be determined. A family history of bleeding disorders should be elicited. The physical examination should include an inspection of the patient's skin, oral mucosa, and joints for evidence of occult bleeding, liver or kidney disease, malignancy, or malnutrition. A personal or family history of venous thrombosis, particularly occurring in those younger than age 50 years, may also point to an increased perioperative risk of venous thromboembolism.
   B. **Laboratory evaluation**
      1. **Platelet testing**
         a. **Platelet count** (140,000 to 400,000/μL) usually is determined as part of an automated blood count. A low platelet count should be confirmed by a review of the blood smear, since platelet clumping may occur in vitro and lead to artifactually low platelet counts.
         b. **Bleeding time** (2.5 to 9.0 minutes) is an assay of platelet function and is only helpful in patients with normal platelet counts. Qualitative platelet disorders, von Willebrand disease (vWD), vasculitides, and connective tissue disorders can prolong the bleeding time; however, the sensitivity and specificity of this test in predicting surgical bleeding is poor, and therefore it is not a reliable predictor of surgical bleeding. The recently developed platelet function screen (PFA-100) has become widely available and may prove to be a better test of platelet function and vWD under most circumstances.
         c. **Platelet aggregometry** can be used to classify congenital platelet disorders but is less useful in the evaluation of acquired platelet dysfunction.
         d. **vWF assays** include the ristocetin cofactor assay, which is based on the ability of ristocetin to agglutinate platelets in the presense of vWF; vWF antigen (ELISA, which uses antibodies to the collagen-binding site for quantitation); the factor VIII:C test, which assesses coagulant activity of factor VIII; and vWF multimer analysis, which detects the quantity and structure of vWF and allows for the classification of vWD.
      2. **Coagulation factor activity** is measured as the time that it takes citrate-anticoagulated plasma (blue top tube) to clot after the addition of calcium, phospholipid, and the appropriate activating agent. Proper specimen collection and prompt performance of testing must be ensured for accuracy. Polycythemia (Hct >55) creates an elevated anticoagulant:plasma ratio, thereby artificially prolonging the clotting times. Clotting factor deficiencies, heparin, fibrin degradation products (FDPs), or coagulation factor inhibitors can prolong clotting times as well.
         a. **Prothrombin time (PT)** is the clotting time measured after the addition of thromboplastin, phospholipids, and calcium to citrated plasma. This test assesses the factors of the extrinsic and common pathways and is most sensitive to factor VII deficiency. In most laboratories, the normal PT is 10 to 13 seconds, but variability occurs

between facilities. Test reagents used vary in their responsiveness to warfarin-induced anticoagulation; therefore, the **international normalized ratio (INR)** is used to standardize PT reporting between laboratories. The INR is the ratio of the measured PT to a mean laboratory control PT corrected for the sensitivity of testing reagents. The PT may be prolonged in patients with liver disease, vitamin K deficiency, or dessiminated intravascular coagulation (DIC). The PT to INR is used to follow patient anticoagulation with warfarin.

b. **Partial thromboplastin time (PTT)** (26 to 36 seconds)is the clotting time for plasma that is preincubated in particulate material (causing contact activation) and to which phospholipid and calcium are then added. Inhibitors or deficiencies of factors in the intrinsic or common pathways cause prolongation of the PTT. A prolonged PTT should be evaluated by a 50:50 mixture with normal plasma. Factor deficiencies are corrected by the addition of normal plasma, whereas prolongation due to inhibitors is not. The PTT is used to follow patient anticoagulation with heparin.

c. **Activated clotting time (ACT)** assesses the clotting time of whole blood. A blood sample is added to a diatomate-containing tube, leading to activation of the intrinsic pathway. The ACT is used to follow coagulation in patients who are undergoing percutaneous coronary interventions, cardiopulmonary bypass, or vascular surgical procedures and who require high doses of heparin. Automated systems are available for bedside use, allowing accurate and rapid determinations of the state of anticoagulation during procedures. Normal ACT is 150 to 180 seconds, with therapeutic target values ranging from 300 to 500 seconds for cardiac bypass procedures and 250 to 350 seconds for other vascular procedures (Ann Pharm 1995;29:1015–1020).

d. **Thrombin time (TT)** (11 to 18 seconds) is the clotting time for plasma after the addition of thrombin. Patients with a fibrinogen level <100 mg/dl or with abnormal fibrinogen will have a prolonged TT. The presence of FDPs such as DIC or heparin can also elevate the TT. Prolongation of the TT by heparin can be confirmed by the addition of protamine sulfate to the assay, resulting in normalization of the test.

e. **Factor assays**
   Fibrinogen level (150 to 360 mg/dL) can be measured directly by functional or immunologic quantitative assays.
   FDP elevations (>8 μg/mL, >8mg/L) occur in many disease states with increased fibrinogen turnover, including DIC, in association with thromboembolic events and during administration of fibrinolytic therapy. **D-dimer** levels reflect fibrinolysis, and a negative test has been particularly useful in excluding patients with venous thromboembolism.
   Specific factor assays measure the ability of a patient's plasma to correct specific factor-deficient plasma clotting times so that each factor can be determined individually. Appropriate tsting is usually guided by abnormalities in the PT or PTT. The normal range for most factors is 60% to 160% of the activity of normal pooled plasma.

III. **Bleeding disorders**
   A. **Platelet disorders**
      1. **Thrombocytopenia** is defined as a platelet count of less than 140,000/μL. Significant bleeding usually does not occur with platelet counts greater than 50,000/μL, and severe spontaneous bleeding rarely occurs with platelet counts greater than 10,000/μL, provided that platelet function is normal. Efforts should be made to maintain platelet counts greater than 50,000/μL during surgical procedures, using platelet transfusions or other appropriate therapy administered at the start of surgery. In cases of serious hemorrhage, however, platelet

Table 5-1. Commonly used drugs affecting platelet number and function

Drugs causing decreased platelet production
Thiazide diuretics
Amrinone
Ethanol
Estrogens
Trimethoprim-sulfamethoxazole
Chemotherapeutic agents

Drugs causing increased platelet destruction
Heparin
Quinidine
Quinine
Gold salts
Rifampin
Sulfonamides
Penicillins
Valproic acid

Drugs affecting platelet function
Nonsteroidal anti-inflammatory drugs
Aspirin
Dipyridamole

transfusions should be administered to achieve platelet counts greater than $100,000/\mu L$ wherever possible. Intramuscular injections and rectal examinations, suppositories, or enemas should be limited in patients with severe thrombocytopenia ($<10,000/\mu L$). Drugs that are known to inhibit platelet function (e.g., nonsteroidal anti-inflammatory drugs and aspirin) should be discontinued. Thrombocytopenia is caused by decreased platelet production, increased platelet destruction, or platelet sequestration. An isolated thrombocytopenia in which the red blood cell (RBC) and white blood cell (WBC) counts are normal typically occurs with platelet destruction rather than other etiologies.

a. **Drug-induced thrombocytopenia.** Many drugs can affect platelet production or cause increased platelet destruction (Table 5-1) and are associated with bleeding. Increased destruction of platelets is most commonly the result of an immune mechanism in which platelets are destroyed by complement activation by drug-antibody complexes. **All nonessential drugs should be discontinued until the cause of the thrombocytopenia is identified.** Drug-induced thrombocytopenia typically resolves within 7 to 10 days after cessation of the offending agent. Occasionally, the thrombocytopenia may be long-lived if the responsible medication is not cleared rapidly from the body (e.g., gold salts). Prednisone (1 mg/kg per day orally) may facilitate recovery of platelet counts.

b. **Heparin-induced thrombocytopenia (HIT)** is a unique form of drug-induced thrombocytopenia that results in potentially life-threatening venous and arterial thromboembolic events. Two forms of HIT have been recognized. A mild thrombocytopenia (platelet count $>100,000/\mu L$) that occurs 2 to 10 days after the initiation of heparin therapy is not immune mediated and does not require cessation of heparin (Type I HIT) (*J Thromb Haemost* 2003;1:1471–1478). A severe immune-mediated syndrome caused by heparin-dependent antiplatelet antibodies (Type II HIT) occurs 4 to 15 days after initial exposure to heparin but within hours after reexposure. In 10%

to 50% of cases, thromboembolic events ensue, including extensive arterial thrombosis. Bleeding complications are rare, despite the thrombocytopenia. Diagnosis can be confirmed by radiolabeled serotonin release studies or via an enzyme-lined immunosorbent assay. This phenomenon is not type, dose, or route dependent, so heparin flushes and heparin-coated lines may cause or contribute to the reaction and must be discontinued or removed. Anticoagulation with a direct thrombin inhibitor (lepirudin or argatroban) is recommended. **If HIT is present, he use of warfarin is contraindicated and is associated with the development of venous limb gangrene.** Warfarin therapy may be used 5 to 7 days after thrombosis is controlled with a direct thrombin inhibitor and the platelet count recovers, then continued long-term.

  c. **Immune thrombocytopenic purpura may be either idiopathic or related to an underlying viral infection (e.g., HIV, Epstein-Barr virus), autoimmune disease (e.g., systemic lupus erythematosus), or medication.**

  d. **Thrombotic thrombocytopenic purpura (TTP) and hemolytic uremic syndrome (HUS)** are syndromes of microangiopathic hemolytic anemia, consumptive thrombocytopenia, and organ ischemia. TTP is more often associated with neurologic complications whereas HUS is associated with renal insufficiency, although multiple organs may be involved. These entities can occur spontaneously or in association with pregnancy, malignancy, infection, chemotherapy, or transplantation. The presence of schistocytes on the peripheral blood smear, along with a low platelet count, should suggest this diagnosis. Effective therapy consists of daily plasma exchange therapy with fresh frozen plasma (FFP) until the platelet count recovers. Platelet transfusion is not indicated unless the patient has severe bleeding. Additional treatment, including immunosuppressive therapy and splenectomy, are often used, but their role is not well defined for the prevention of disease relapse or in treatment of refractory disease.

  e. **Dilutional thrombocytopenia** can occur with rapid blood product replacement for massive hemorrhage. No formula predicts accurate platelet requirements in this setting. Therefore, frequent platelet counts should be used to guide platelet transfusion therapy. In the setting of ongoing hemorrhage, empiric platelet transfusion is appropriate.

  f. **Other causes of thrombocytopenia** include DIC, sepsis, and hematopoietic disorders, and therapy should be directed at the underlying disorder. Platelet transfusions should be considered prophylactically for a platelet count $<10,000/\mu L$ or in cases of bleeding with a platelet count $<5,000/\mu L$.

2. **Thrombocytosis** is defined as a platelet count $>600,000/\mu L$. It occurs primarily with myeloproliferative disorders, or secondarily after splenectomy, with iron deficiency, malignancy, or chronic inflammatory disease. Essential thrombocythemia is a myeloproliferative disorder that can cause either a thrombotic or hemorrhagic syndrome. Treatment with hydroxyurea (15 mg/kg per day orally) or anagrelide (1 to 4 mg per day orally in 2 to 4 divided doses) lowers platelet counts and decreases the associated risk of thrombosis and bleeding. Treatment to control the platelet count is recommended for patients with a previous thrombotic or hemorrhagic event or those at high risk for such an event, including patients who are over 60 years old, have a platelet count $>1,500,000$, or have coronary artery disease. Aspirin therapy (81 mg per day orally) is useful in the treatment of thrombotic events in patients with myeloproliferative disorders and in decreasing fetal loss in pregnant women. Secondary thrombocytosis is generally not associated with an increased thrombotic risk and requires no specific therapy.

3. **Qualitative platelet dysfunction**
   a. **Acquired defects** (e.g., those that result from uremia, liver disease, or cardiopulmonary bypass or from the use of such drugs as aspirin, nonsteroidal anti-inflammatory drugs, and β-lactam antibiotics) account for most qualitative platelet disorders. Treatment is aimed at the underlying cause. Because the effect of aspirin on platelets is irreversible, this medication should be discontinued about 1 week before elective nonvascular operations to allow new, functional platelets to form. For severe bleeding, platelet transfusions may be necessary. Desmopressin acetate (DDAVP, 0.3 μg/kg intravenously 1 hour before operation) may limit bleeding from platelet dysfunction, particularly in uremic patients. Conjugated estrogens (0.6 mg/kg per day intravenously for 5 days) also can improve hemostatic function.
4. **von Willebrand Disease** is a disorder characterized by a prolonged bleeding time secondary to a qualitative or quantitative deficiency of vWF. Identification of vWD subtype in each patient is strongly recommended, as therapy varies depending on the subtype. Type 1 (mild quantitative deficiency) accounts for 80% to 90% of cases of vWD. DDAVP (0.3 μg/kg every 12 to 24 hours intravenously or 300 μg intranasally given in a divided dose) stimulates endothelial release of vWF and is usually effective prophylaxsis for minor surgery in patients with type 1 vWD. Type 2A, 2B, and 3 vWD are generally treated with vWF replacement therapy. If replacement therapy is necessary to treat bleeding, factor VIII concentrates containing vWF (e.g., Humate-P) have high concentrations of vWF. Cryoprecipitate (1 to 2 bags per 10 kg body weight intravenously) also corrects bleeding times in patients with vWD but carries a small risk of viral transmission, similar to that of RBCs (*Clin Chem* 2000; 46:1260–1269).
5. **Congenital platelet disorders**, such as Bernard-Soulier syndrome, Glanzmann's thrombasthenia, and storage pool defects, are rare and are generally treated with platelet transfusions to control bleeding.

B. **Disorders of coagulation**
   1. **Inherited factor deficiencies**
      a. **Hemophilia** is an X-linked recessive disease of either factor VIII (hemophilia A) or factor IX (hemophilia B, Christmas disease) and can present with spontaneous hemarthroses, hemorrhage, or prolonged bleeding after injury or operation. Severity of the disease is dependent on the factor activity level. Patients with 5% to 35% of normal factor activity (mild hemophilia) rarely experience spontaneous bleeding but may bleed extensively during surgery or after trauma. Patients with 1% to 5% activity (moderate hemophilia) have prolonged bleeding with minor injuries but rarely develop spontaneous hemarthroses. In patients with less than 1% activity, hemarthroses and spontaneous bleeding episodes frequently occur. The diagnosis is suggested by patient history and an elevated PTT, normal PT, and normal bleeding time. Factor activity assays confirm the diagnosis.
         (1) **Treatment of hemophilia A** is based on the degree of bleeding and the severity of the disease.
         (2) **Minor bleeding** can often be controlled locally without the need for factor replacement therapy. DDAVP (0.3 μg/kg every 12 to 24 hours intravenously or 300 μg intranasally) stimulates the release of vWF into the circulation, increasing the factor VIII levels two to sixfold. This may control minor bleeding in patients with mild disease (*Semin Thromb Hemost* 2003;29:101–105). For dental procedures, ϵ-aminocaproic acid (EACA) (3 to 4 g orally or intravenously every 4 hours for 3 days), an inhibitor of fibrinolysis, can be used in conjunction with 50% factor replacement for control of bleeding. EACA should not be used for the treatment of hematuria.

(3) **Major bleeding** (e.g., during surgical procedures) requires factor VIII replacement. Factor VIII activity should be restored to 100% immediately before operation and be maintained at least to 50% for 3 to 5 days afterward. Neurosurgical patients and those with head trauma should be restored immediately to 100% activity and be maintained for 5 days at greater than 80%. The usual dosing scheme to maintain factor levels at 50% to 100% is 50 U/kg loading dose, followed by 25 U/kg every 12 hours. Plasma-purified and recombinant factor VIII are equally effective in preventing and controlling bleeding episodes, but product availability and cost may affect the choice of treatment. Available data suggest that these products are free of viral contamination. Cryoprecipitate contains factor VIII, vWF, and fibrinogen and can be used to treat patients with suspected hemophilia A for control of bleeding, but it is rarely used. FFP is not recommended for the treatment of hemophilia A.

(4) **Treatment of hemophilia B.** The treatment of choice for factor IX replacement therapy is purified factor IX. The initial dose to achieve ∼100% activity is 100 U/kg, followed by 50 U/kg every 24 hrs. FFP can be used for minor bleeding. Cryoprecipitate and DDAVP are not useful in the treatment of factor IX deficiency.

(5) **Factor inhibitors.** Antibodies to factor VIII and factor IX occur in up to 15% of patients with hemophilia A and 1% to 2% of those with hemophilia B, and their presence represents a challenge to health care providers. Patients with persistently low titers of antibodies can respond to factor replacement therapy in higher than normal doses. Patients with high levels of antifactor antibodies or those with a demonstrated anamnestic response are at risk for a severe uncontrolled bleeding disorder. They should not receive factor replacement therapy for minor episodes of bleeding. Hemorrhage in high-titer patients should be considered life-threatening, and any surgery should be undertaken with extreme caution. Recombinant human factor VIIa (90 mg/kg intravenously every 2 to 4 hours) has been approved for treatment in this setting for patients with hemophilia. Prothrombin complex concentrates can be used, but their use may be complicated by thromboembolism. Porcine factor VIII can also be used to treat patients with factor VIII inhibitors but may lead to the formation of alloantibodies.

b. **Other inherited factor deficiencies** account for fewer than 10% of severe inherited factor deficiencies. Deficiencies of factors XII, high–molecular-weight kininogen, or prekallikrein do not cause bleeding and require no treatment. Factor XI deficiency (hemophilia C) may lead to bleeding with operation or injury. In general, factor XI deficiency or other factor deficiencies can be corrected with FFP, if required for bleeding diatheses.

2. **Acquired factor deficiencies**
   a. **Vitamin K deficiency** leads to the production of inactive, noncarboxylated forms of prothrombin; factors VII, IX, and X; and proteins C and S. The diagnosis should be considered in a patient with a prolonged PT that corrects with a 50:50 mixture of normal plasma. Vitamin K deficiency can occur in patients without oral intake within 1 week, with biliary obstruction, and with malabsorption and in those receiving antibiotics or warfarin.

   Prophylaxis. Patients on nothing-by-mouth status should receive vitamin K_1 subcutaneously (10 mg once per week). Vitamin K can also be added as a supplement in total parenteral nutrition.

   Treatment. For mild deficiencies, vitamin K_1 (10 to 15 mg every 1 to 3 days subcutaneously or intravenously) corrects the deficit. Severe deficiencies (e.g., with warfarin overdose) might require much higher doses and longer duration of therapy. If patients have a PT that is greater than 1.5 times the control caused by vitamin K deficiency or warfarin therapy and have ongoing hemorrhage or require emergent surgery, FFP (2 to 4 units intravenously) should be used for correction along with vitamin K. Further FFP therapy is guided by the degree of bleeding and the PT.

   b. **Liver dysfunction** leads to complex alterations in coagulation through decreased synthesis of all clotting factors and inhibitors except vWF. The coagulopathy can be worsened by thrombocytopenia from associated hypersplenism. Spontaneous bleeding is infrequent, but coagulation defects should be corrected prior to invasive procedures. Parenteral vitamin K_1 administration (10 to 15 mg every 1 to 3 days subcutaneously or intravenously) infrequently corrects the coagulopathy. FFP administration often improves the hemostatic defect transiently (6 to 24 hours), and platelet transfusion can be used to augment the platelet count (*Semin Liver Dis* 2002;22:83–96).

3. **Disseminated intravascular coagulation (DIC)** has many inciting causes, including sepsis (particularly associated with Gram-negative bacteria, meningococcemia, Rocky Mountain spotted fever, and viral infections), extensive trauma or burns, necrotic tissue, intravascular antibody-antigen immune reactions, hematologic and other malignancies, liver failure, obstetric complications, intravascular prosthetic devices, and toxins or venoms. The pathogenesis of DIC generally is due to the inappropriate generation of thrombin within the vasculature leading to the formation of fibrin thrombi, platelet activation, and fibrinolytic activity. Often, DIC presents with complications from microvascular thrombi that involve the vascular beds of the kidney, brain, lung, and skin. In some patients, the consumption of coagulation factors, particularly fibrinogen and platelets, and the activation of the fibrinolytic pathway can lead to bleeding. Laboratory findings in DIC include thrombocytopenia, hypofibrinogenemia, increased FDPs (or D-dimer), and prolonged TT and PTT. Therapy begins with treatment of the underlying cause. Conscientious management of hemodynamics and oxygenation are critical. Correction of coagulopathy with platelet transfusions, FFP, and cryoprecipitate should be undertaken for bleeding complications only and should not be given empirically. Although not well defined, prophylactic anticoagulation with heparin (500 to 1,000 units per hour intravenously) should be considered in patients with DIC. Systemic anticoagulation should only be used in patients with evidence of arterial or venous thromboembolism.

IV. **Hypercoagulable states**
   A. **Inherited hypercoagulable disorders**
      1. **Antithrombin (AT) deficiency** is an autosomal dominant disorder that presents with recurrent venous thromboembolism, usually in the second decade of life. A family history of recurrent thromboses should be determined. Assays for AT levels typically are decreased in the setting of acute thrombosis and while the patient is receiving heparin. Treatment of acute thromboembolism is with heparin (or low–molecular-weight heparin, LMWH), which is usually effective at prolonging the PTT if the AT level is greater than 50% of normal. Antithrombin concentrate can also been used to treat venous thrombosis in patients who have difficulty achieving adequate anticoagulation with heparin, as is seen in patients with AT levels <50%. Patients with AT deficiency and an episode of thrombosis should subsequently receive lifelong oral anticoagulation. Women with AT deficiency should receive unfractionated heparin or LMWH anticoagulation during pregnancy to prevent the risk of deep venous thrombosis (DVT) (*J Thromb Haemos* 2003;1:1429–1434). AT-deficient patients should have the AT level restored to more

than 80% of normal activity with AT concentrate prior to operation or delivery.

2. **Protein C deficiency and protein S deficiency** are risk factors for venous thrombosis. In a state of protein C or S deficiency, factors Va and VIIIa are not adequately inactivated, thereby allowing unchecked coagulation. Besides the inherited type, protein C deficiency is encountered in patients with liver failure and in those who are receiving warfarin therapy. Initial treatment for symptomatic patients includes heparin (or LMWH) anticoagulation followed by warfarin therapy. In individuals with diminished protein C activity, effective heparin anticoagulation must be confirmed before the initiation of warfarin because warfarin transiently lowers protein C levels further and potentially worsens the hypercoagulable state. Patients with protein C or protein S deficiency but with no personal history of thrombosis do not require prophylactic anticoagulation in most circumstances.

3. **Activated protein C resistance (factor V Leiden)** is a genetic mutation in factor V that renders it resistant to breakdown by activated protein C. This mutation occurs in approximately 5% of people with a European heritage. The relative risk of venous thromboembolism in heterozygotes is 5- to 10-fold and in homozygotes up to 80-fold compared with individuals without the mutation. Research to date suggests that routine preoperative screening in asymptomatic patients is unnecessary. Therapy for venous thromboembolism consists of anticoagulation with heparin followed by warfarin therapy. The role of long-term anticoagulation with warfarin or LMWH for heterozygous patients with a single thrombotic event is undefined.

4. **Hyperhomocystinemia** in adults is defined as a plasma homocysteine level above the 95th percentile (2.5 mg/L, 18.5 μmol/L). Etiologies include genetic alterations in the enzymes involved in homocysteine metabolism and dietary deficiency of vitamin B_{12} or B_6, required to convert homocysteine to cysteine. Case-control studies have shown that hyperhomocysteinemia is an independent risk factor for atherosclerotic disease of the carotid and coronary arteries and for venous thromboembolism. Treatment with folate and vitamin B_{12} is effective in lowering homocysteine levels.

5. **Prothrombin gene mutation** occurs in approximately 2% of Caucasians and is associated with a two- to threefold increased risk of venous thromboembolic disease. When coinherited with factor V Leiden, the risk of venous thrombosis is considerably higher.

B. **Acquired hypercoagulable disorders**
1. **Antiphospholipid antibodies** are IgG, IgA, or IgM immunoglobulins that are targeted against antigens composed in part of platelet and endothelial cell phospholipids. Antiphospholipid antibody disorders may be detected by **a lupus anticoagulant, an anticardiolipin antibody, or other antiphospholipid antibodies.** Patients with these antibodies are at risk for arterial and venous thrombosis, recurrent miscarriages, and thrombocytopenia. The antibodies may be detected in patients with systemic lupus erythematosus or other autoimmune disorders, in those with infections (e.g., HIV), or in those who receive predisposing medications (e.g., chlorpromazine, dilantin, or hydralazine). However, up to 90% of patients with antiphospholipid antibodies have no identifiable predisposing condition. The diagnosis is suggested by history of unexplained thrombosis and can be confirmed using specific tests, such as Russell's viper venom clotting time (for lupus anticoagulant) and anticardiolipin antibody immunoassay. Treatment of patients with antiphospholipid antibodies using warfarin seems to be associated with a higher failure rate than occurs with other thrombotic states, so other approaches such as use of antiplatelet agents or long-term LMWH may be warranted. Prophylactic treatment for patients without thrombotic

Table 5-2. Relative contraindications to anticoagulation therapy

Ongoing bleeding
Recent surgical or invasive procedure
Recent severe trauma
Bleeding tendency (e.g., hemophilia, thrombocytopenia)
Intracranial hemorrhage
Malignant hypertension
Patients prone to falling
Pericarditis or pericardial effusion
Inadequate laboratory facilities
Noncompliant patient

episodes remains controversial but is generally not recommended except in pregnancy.

2. **Other acquired hypercoagulable states** include sepsis, malignancies, pregnancy or the use of estrogen therapy, intravascular hemolysis (e.g., hemolytic anemia or after cardiopulmonary bypass), and the localized propensity to thrombosis in arteries that have recently undergone endarterectomy or angioplasty or in new prosthetic vascular grafts. Along with effective anticoagulation therapy, treatment should be directed at any identified underlying risk factor.

V. Therapy

   A. Anticoagulation therapy

   1. **Principles and indications.** Anticoagulation is used to prevent and treat thrombosis and thromboembolic events. Before therapy is instituted, careful consideration must be given to the risk of thromboembolism and to anticoagulation-induced bleeding complications. Specific indications for antithrombotic therapy are discussed in detail in other chapters; they include atrial fibrillation, mechanical prosthetic heart valves, venous thromboembolism, stroke prevention, and acute arterial or graft occlusion. Relative contraindications to anticoagulation therapy are listed in Table 5-2.

   2. **Heparin and related therapy**

      a. **Unfractionated heparin** (MW 10,000 to 20,000) acts by potentiating the action of AT, leading to accelerated inhibition of thrombin, factor Xa, and other coagulation proteases by clearance of circulating AT protrease complexes.

      Administration. Heparin is administered parenterally, either subcutaneously or intravenously. Prophylaxis against venous thrombosis (typically 5,000 units subcutaneously) should be administered before surgery and every 8 to 12 hours thereafter. Treatment of venous thrombosis requires a higher daily dose, typically given as an 80-U/kg intravenous bolus, followed by 1,000 to 2,000 units per hour (or 18 U/kg per hour) continuous intravenous. The heparin concentration is typically prepared as a 25,000 U/250-mL bag of intravenous fluid to prevent errors. PTT should be measured before initiation of heparin and 6 hours after the initial bolus or at each change in dosing. A therapeutic PTT of 1.5 to 2.5 times the control (approximately 50 to 80 seconds) should be maintained. Platelet counts should be measured daily when initiating heparin therapy and periodically thereafter. The development of unexplained thrombocytopenia ($<100,000/\mu$L) should prompt discontinuation of heparin therapy and evaluation for HIT. **Complications** that occur with heparin therapy include bleeding and HIT. If bleeding occurs, heparin should be discontinued and immediate assessment of the PT, PTT, and CBC should be undertaken. Gastrointestinal (GI) bleeding that occurs while a patient is therapeutically anticoagulated suggests an occult source and warrants further evaluation. Heparin-induced thrombocytopenia is an uncommon but potentially devastating complication of heparin therapy and must be recognized early, with alternative therapy started to avoid life-threatening complications (see "Bleeding Disorders," section **III.A**).

Heparin clearance is rapid, occurring with a half-life of about 90 minutes. Reversal can be achieved more quickly with intravenous protamine sulfate. Each milligram of protamine sulfate reverses 100 units of heparin. For patients previously receiving continuous intravenous heparin infusion, enough protamine sulfate should be administered to neutralize approximately one-half of the preceding hour's dose by slow intravenous infusion (i.e., <50 mg/10 min). The PTT or activated clotting time can be used to assess the adequacy of the reversal. Anaphylactic reactions can occur to protamine, especially in diabetic patients who have received protamine-insulin [neutral protamine Hagedorn (NPH)] preparations, so this should be used with caution.

b. LMWH preparations (enoxaparin, dalteparin, and tinzaparin) are depolymerized, yielding fragments of 3,000 to 7,000 daltons. The anticoagulant effect of LMWH is predominantly due to factor Xa inhibition, and LMWH results in less thrombin inhibition than does unfractionated heparin. The advantages of LMWH include a more predictable anticoagulant effect, less platelet interaction, and a longer half-life. Dosing is based on weight, and laboratory monitoring is not typically needed. In prevention of postoperative DVT and pulmonary embolism (PE), LMWH (e.g., enoxaparin 40 mg subcutaneously each day) and low-dose unfractionated heparin (5,000 units subcutaneously two or three time each day) have equivalent effectiveness in moderate risk patients (general or thoracic surgery and age >40). LMWH has been shown to be *more effective* for DVT prophylaxis in patients undergoing orthopedic procedures or after multiple trauma or spinal injury (*Arch Int Med* 2003;163:759–768). Fixed-dose subcutaneous regimens of LMWH (e.g., enoxaparin 1 mg/kg subcutaneously 2 times each day) are as effective as adjusted-dose intravenous unfractionated heparin in the initial treatment of established DVT or PE that does not require fibrinolysis or surgery. LMWH may also be used for longer term therapy in patients with a contraindication to oral anticoagulant treatment (e.g., pregnant patients who cannot take warfarin). Because LMWH has a longer half-life and no effective antidote, it must be used with caution in surgical patients or in those in whom a bleeding risk has been substantiated.

3. Direct thrombin inhibitors are a class of compounds that bind to free and fibrin-bound thrombin. These agents inhibit thrombin activation of clotting factors, fibrin formation, and platelet aggregation.

a. Hirudin, an anticoagulant originally derived from leeches, has been formulated as lepirudin and bivalirudin. Lepirudin, recombinant hirudin, binds irreversibly to thrombin, providing effective anticoagulation. The drug is approved in patients with HIT but may be considered in other severe clotting disorders. Lepirudin is cleared unmodified by the kidney, so extreme care should be used in patients with renal insufficiency. Monitoring of anticoagulation is by the PTT, similar to heparin. Bivalirudin is a truncated form of recombinant hirudin that targets only the active site of thrombin. Bivalirudin is FDA approved for use during percutaneous coronary angioplasty and stenting

b. Argatroban is a synthetic thrombin inhibitor that is also approved for treatment of HIT.

    c. Oral direct thrombin inhibitors (ximelagatran) have been used in place of warfarin in a variety of settings and may become widely available.

4. **Warfarin** is a vitamin K antagonist that causes anticoagulation by inhibiting vitamin K–mediated carboxylation of factors II, VII, IX, and X as well as proteins C and S. The vitamin K–dependent factors decay with varying half-lives, so the full anticoagulant effect of warfarin is not apparent for 5 to 7 days. Therefore, when immediate anticoagulation is necessary, heparin or another agent must be used initially.

    a. Administration. Warfarin usually is initiated at 5.0 to 10.0 mg per day for 2 days, followed by dosage adjustment based on daily INR results. Use of the INR provides a standard for the assessment of anticoagulation by warfarin and should be used in place of the PT or a PT ratio. Elderly patients, those with hepatic insufficiency, and those who are receiving parenteral nutrition or broad-spectrum antibiotics should be given lower initial doses of warfarin. A daily dose of warfarin needed to achieve therapeutic anticoagulation usually ranges from 2 to 15 mg per day. An INR of 2 to 3 is therapeutic for most indications, but patients with prosthetic heart valves should be maintained with an INR of 2.5 to 3.5. Once a stable INR is obtained, it can be monitored biweekly or monthly.

    b. Complications. The bleeding risk in patients who are treated with warfarin is estimated to be approximately 10% per year, with major or fatal hemorrhagic events developing in 0.5% to 1.0% of patients annually. The risk of bleeding correlates directly with the INR. Warfarin-induced skin necrosis, caused by dermal venous thrombosis, occurs rarely when warfarin therapy is initiated in patients who are not already anticoagulated and is often associated with hypercoagulability caused by protein C deficiency. **Warfarin can produce significant birth defects and fetal death and therefore should not be used during pregnancy.** Changes in medications and diet that affect warfarin or vitamin K levels (Table 5-3) require more vigilant INR monitoring and dosage adjustment.

    c. Reversal of warfarin-induced anticoagulation requires up to a week after discontinuation of therapy. Vitamin K administration can be used to reverse warfarin anticoagulation within 1 to 2 days. The appropriate vitamin K dosage depends on the INR and the urgency with which correction must be accomplished. For patients with an INR of 6 to 10 and no serious bleeding, 0.5 to 1.0 mg vitamin K administered intravenously can be used. In patients with an INR of 10 to 20, 3 to 5 mg vitamin K is generally recommended to improve the coagulopathy. For patients with bleeding or an INR of more than 20, 10 mg of vitamin K should be administered. Serial INR should be followed every 6 hours. In addition, FFP (2 to 4 units intravenously) is administered to patients with a coagulopathy and ongoing hemorrhage. Recombinant human factor VIIa has also been used (90 μg/kg) along with FFP in cases of life-threatening bleeding.

5. **Indirect factor Xa inhibitors (Fondaparinux)** are small synthetic heparin-like molecules that enhance AT-mediated inhibition of factor Xa. Fondaparinux has been shown to be as effective in preventing DVT after hip and knee replacement as LMWH. The dosage is 2.5 mg subcutaneously each day starting 6 to 8 hours after surgery and continued for 5 to 8 days. Higher doses (5.0 to 10.0 mg subcutaneously each day) have been used for initial treatment of venous thromboembolic events (VTEs). Monitoring of coagulation parameters is usually not necessary. Bleeding complications occur, and no specific antidote is currently available, although stopping the drug and treating with FFP should be considered.

Table 5-3. Commonly used drugs that affect the INR in patients receiving oral anticoagulation

Prolong INR
Anabolic steroids
Cimetidine
Clofibrate
Dipyridamole
Disulfiram
Erythromycin
Fluconazole
Metronidazole
Oral hypoglycemic agents
Quinidine
Second- and third-generation cephalosporins
Trimethoprim-sulfamethoxazole

Shorten INR
Antihistamines
Cholestyramine
Haloperidol
Oral contraceptives
Penicillins
Phenobarbital
Rifampin
Spironolactone
Vitamin K

B. **Antiplatelet therapy**
1. **Aspirin** irreversibly acetylates cyclooxygenase, inhibiting platelet synthesis of thromboxane A_2 and causing decreased platelet function. It is useful in the prevention and treatment of acute transient ischemic attacks, stroke, myocardial infarction, and coronary and vascular graft occlusion. The optimal dose of aspirin for platelet inhibition is not well defined, but 80 to 160 mg per day orally is recommended, as higher doses do not have higher efficacy and may increase bleeding complications. Chronic aspirin use can lead to the development of peptic ulcers and elevation of the blood urea and uric acid. Use of aspirin in patients who are receiving anticoagulant therapy predisposes to increased bleeding complications and should be done with caution.
2. **Thienopyridines** irreversibly inhibit platelet function by binding the ADP receptor that promotes aggregation and secretion. **Clopidogrel** (75 mg orally each day) has been shown to be more efficacious in decreasing thrombotic events in high-risk patients than aspirin. Clopidogrel with aspirin treatment is more effective in preventing ischemic complications after percutaneous stenting and in patients with unstable angina than aspirin alone. Although the half-life of clopidogrel is 8 hours, the bleeding time remains prolonged over 3 to 7 days, reflecting the fact that complete recovery of platelet function takes 5 days. Therefore, **patients should discontinue clopidogrel therapy 7 days prior to elective operations** to decrease the risk of bleeding complications. **Ticlopidine** (250 mg orally twice a day) has been shown to lower the stroke, myocardial infarction, and vascular death rate of patients who have had a previous stroke. However, ticlopidine is associated with reversible neutropenia, pancytopenia, and agranulocytosis, so the use of clopidogrel is

generally favored. Expanded applications for clopidogrel are currently being explored, and more widespread use is likely in the future.

3. **Dextran** decreases platelet aggregation and adhesion, but the mechanism of this action is not completely understood. Dextran can be used to reduce thrombotic events in the perioperative period (bypass graft occlusion, DVT) but is not proven effective in long-term follow-up.

4. **Glycoprotein IIb/IIIa inhibitors** (abciximab, tirofiban, eptifibatide) bind to the fibrinogen receptor, blocking platelet adhesion to fibrin. Abciximab (ReoPro) is a chimeric anti-GP IIb/IIIa monoclonal antibody; tirofiban (Aggrastat) and epitifibatide (Integrilin) are synthetic agents that selectively inhibit GP IIb/IIIa. All three agents are efficacious in preventing coronary artery thrombosis after coronary angioplasty. Tirofiban and epitifibate are also approved for use in unstable angina. GP IIb/IIIa inhibitors are given intravenously during a coronary intervention or for 24 to 48 hours during unstable angina. Longer intravenous use and oral preparations are associated with increased bleeding complications. Abciximab occasionally causes severe thrombocytopenia, and therefore platelet counts should be monitored during therapy. GP IIb/IIIa inhibitor use in patients undergoing failed percutaneous transluminal coronary angioplasty (PTCA) or with unstable angina has led to increased blood loss during emergency coronary artery bypass graft (CABG). Although these agents have relatively short half-lives (0.5 to 2.5 hours), the bleeding time may remain elevated for longer periods. It is recommended that surgery be delayed 12 hours after discontinuing abciximab and 4 hours after discontinuing tirofiban or eptifibatide. Platelet transfusion should be given only if excessive bleeding is encountered. Standard heparin therapy during bypass is indicated. Zero-balance ultrafiltration may be beneficial in patients who need immediate surgical interventions (*Perfusion* 2002;17:33–37).

C. **Fibrinolytic therapy**

1. **Indications and contraindications.** Thrombolytic therapy is most often used for iliofemoral DVT; superior vena caval thrombosis; PE resulting in a hemodynamically unstable patient; acute thrombosis of peripheral, mesenteric, and coronary arteries; acute vascular graft occlusion; thrombosis of hemodialysis access grafts; and occlusion of venous catheters. Contraindications to fibrinolytic therapy are listed in Table 5-4.

Table 5-4. Contraindications to fibrinolytic therapy

Absolute contraindications
Intolerable ischemia (for arterial thrombosis)
Active bleeding (not including menses)
Recent (<2 mo) stroke or neurosurgical procedure
Intracranial pathology such as neoplasm

Relative contraindications
Recent (<10 days) major surgery, major trauma, parturition, or organ biopsy
Active peptic ulcer or recent gastrointestinal bleeding (within 2 wk)
Uncontrolled hypertension (BP >180/110)
Recent cardiopulmonary resuscitation
Presence or high likelihood of left heart thrombus
Bacterial endocarditis
Coagulopathy or current use of warfarin
Pregnancy
Hemorrhagic diabetic retinopathy

2. **Dosage** depends on the agent and the indication. Tissue plasminogen activator (alteplase) or a recombinant analogue (reteplase), as well as urokinase (Abbokinase), are used for lysis of catheter, venous, and peripheral arterial thrombi.

VI. **Anemia, Transfusions, and Hemostatic Agents**

   A. **Anemia**

      1. **Evaluation.** *Anemia* is a decreased circulating red blood cell (RBC) mass and is defined as a hemoglobin level of less than 12 g/dL in women and less than 14 g/dL in men. In addition to hemoglobin and hematocrit, peripheral blood smear, measurement of the reticulocyte count, and mean cellular volume help to evaluate and identify the cause of the anemia. The blood smear is used to identify abnormalities in RBC size and shape, white blood cells (WBCs), and platelets. The reticulocyte count assesses the bone marrow response to anemia. A normal or low reticulocyte count in the presence of anemia suggests an inadequate bone marrow response. The mean cellular volume and reticulocyte count help to classify an anemia and determine its cause.

      2. **Causes of anemia** (Table 5-5)

         a. **Anemias associated with increased RBC destruction**

            (1) Bleeding is the most frequently encountered cause of RBC destruction. Most surgical patients have an obvious etiology for blood loss; however, sources of occult bleeding include the GI tract, uterus, urinary tract, and retroperitoneum.

            (2) Hemolytic anemias

               (a) Hereditary hemolytic anemias include the hemoglobinopathies (e.g., sickle cell disease), RBC membrane abnormalities (e.g., hereditary spherocytosis), and the RBC enzymopathies (e.g., glucose 6-phosphate dehydrogenase deficiency). Sickle cell disease is caused by abnormal hemoglobin that polymerizes under decreased oxygen tension. Dehydration and hypoxia must be avoided to prevent sickling. This is particularly

---

Table 5-5. Classification of anemia based on red blood cell (RBC) kinetics

Anemias associated with impaired RBC production
Aplastic anemia
Iron-deficiency anemia
Thalassemia
Myelodysplastic syndromes and sideroblastic anemia
Megaloblastic anemia
Anemia of chronic renal insufficiency
Anemia of chronic disease
Zidovudine- and cancer chemotherapy–induced anemia

Anemias associated with increased RBC loss or destruction
Bleeding
Hereditary hemolytic anemias
  Hemoglobinopathies (e.g., sickle cell disease)
  Primary disorders of RBC membrane
  RBC enzymopathies (e.g., glucose 6-phosphate dehydrogenase)
Acquired hemolytic anemias
  Autoimmune hemolytic anemia
  Drug-induced hemolytic anemia
  Microangiopathic hemolytic anemia
  Traumatic hemolytic anemia
Paroxysmal nocturnal hemoglobinuria

true in patients with sickle cell disease who undergo general anesthesia. Preoperative transfusion to increase hemoglobin levels to 10 g/dL had been proven effective in reducing complications after major operations.

   (b) **Acquired hemolytic anemias** include autoimmune hemolytic anemia, drug-induced hemolytic anemia, microangiopathic hemolytic anemia (MAHA), and traumatic hemolytic anemias, such as those induced by malfunctioning prosthetic aortic valves or vascular bypass grafts. The direct Coombs test usually identifies autoimmune hemolytic anemia, and RBC schistocytes are present in all forms of MAHA. Idiosyncratic drug-induced hemolytic anemia rarely occurs with a range of medications, but cefotetan-induced hemolysis is noteworthy becaue of its frequency and severity.

b. Anemias associated with decreased RBC production

   (1) **Aplastic anemia** is an acquired defect of bone marrow stem cells and is associated with pancytopenia. The majority of cases are idiopathic or autoimmune, but approximately 20% are drug-related (e.g., phenylbutazone, gold, chemotherapeutics, anticonvulsants, sulfonamides, chloramphenicol, benzene), and some are associated with an antecedent viral infection (e.g., hepatitis, Epstein-Barr virus, cytomegalovirus). A bone marrow biopsy is needed to establish the diagnosis. Initial treatment is supportive, with cessation of any possibly offending agents. Stem cell transplantation or immunosuppressive therapy often is required.

   (2) **Iron deficiency anemia** is most commonly caused by blood loss from either menstrual bleeding or occult GI blood loss. Sources of GI blood loss include peptic ulcer disease, gastritis, hemorrhoids, angiodysplasia, and colon adenocarcinoma. In postmenopausal women and in men with iron-deficiency anemia, a complete GI evaluation for a potential source of blood loss is strongly recommended. Iron requirements for women are increased during pregnancy owing to the transfer of iron to the fetus. Iron uptake by the intestine may be diminished in patients who have had a partial or total gastrectomy, patients with achlorhydria, and patients with chronic diarrhea or intestinal malabsorption. The diagnosis is suggested by hypochromic microcytic anemia, low serum iron levels (<60 μg/dL), increased total iron-binding capacity (>360 μg/dL), and low serum ferritin levels (<14 ng/L). A bone marrow biopsy that demonstrates absence of iron staining or a response to a trial of iron therapy establishes the diagnosis definitively. Oral iron replacement (ferrous sulfate, 325 mg orally 3 times a day between meals) is usually sufficient; it is generally administered with a stool softener, such as docusate sodium, to prevent constipation. Iron polysaccharide (150 mg orally 2 times a day) appears to be a better tolerated alternative. Iron dextran also can be administered intramuscularly (100 mg per day) or as a single-dose intravenous preparation (1 to 2 g over 3 to 6 hours) in patients with malabsorption, poor compliance, or intolerance of oral preparations.

   (3) **Megaloblastic anemias** are associated with a deficiency of cobalamin (vitamin B_{12}) or folic acid. These deficiencies cause decreased DNA synthesis in all cells but primarily manifest in the hematopoietic tissue. Cobalamin, derived in the diet from meat and dairy products, is dependent on intrinsic factor (IF) for absorption. IF is produced by gastric parietal cells, and IF-cobalamin complex is absorbed in the terminal ileum. Therefore, along with pernicious anemia in which anti-IF antibodies occur, gastrectomy, ileal resection or ileitis, intestinal parasites, and

bacterial overgrowth can lead to vitamin B_{12} deficiency. However, because only a small portion of the body's stores is used each day, vitamin B_{12} deficiency takes several years to manifest. In addition to anemia, vitamin B_{12} deficiency often causes a neuropathy with paresthesias of the extremities, weakness, ataxia, and poor finger coordination. In contrast to cobalamin deficiency, folic acid deficiency can develop within weeks from decreased intake (e.g., alcohol abuse), malabsorption, or increased use (e.g., pregnancy or hemolysis). The serum vitamin B_{12} level (<100 pg/mL, 77.4 pmol/L) and the serum folate level (<4 ng/mL, 9.1 nmol/L) are used to establish the diagnosis. The RBC folate level is a more sensitive measure than the serum level (<150 ng/mL). Therapy for vitamin B_{12} deficiency involves replacement with cyanocobalamin (1 mg per day intramuscularly for 7 days, then weekly for 1 to 2 months, then monthly indefinitely). Folic acid is replenished (1 mg orally per day) until the deficiency is corrected. An incomplete response to therapy might indicate a coexisting iron deficiency, which occurs in one-third of patients with megaloblastic anemia.

(4) **Other anemias** associated with decreased RBC production include anemia due to renal insufficiency, chronic disease, chemotherapy, and the thalassemias. Anemia from renal failure is treated effectively with erythropoietin (50 to 100 U/kg subcutaneously 3 times a week).

VII. **Transfusion therapy.** The **risks and benefits** of transfusion therapy must be considered carefully in each situation. **Informed consent** should be obtained before blood products are administered, if possible, and the indications for transfusion should be noted in the medical record. Before elective operations that are likely to require blood transfusion, the available options of autologous or directed blood donation should be discussed with the patient in time to allow for the collection process.

A. **RBC transfusion**

1. **Indications.** RBC transfusions are used to treat anemia to improve the oxygen-carrying capacity of the blood. A hemoglobin level of 7 to 8 g/dL is adequate for tissue oxygenation in most normovolemic patients. However, therapy must be individualized based on the patient's age and cardiovascular and pulmonary status, the type of transfusion considered (i.e., homologous versus autologous), and the expectation of further blood loss. Correctable causes of anemia, such as folate, vitamin B_{12}, and iron deficiencies, must be identified because these patients typically do not require blood transfusion. Chronic anemia, particularly anemia due to renal disease, is usually treated with erythropoietin (50 to 100 U/kg subcutaneously 3 times a week) rather than with RBC transfusions.

2. **Preparation.** RBCs are most commonly administered as packed RBCs. When available, whole blood can be used for blood volume replacement associated with recent hemorrhage (i.e., in GI bleeding, major surgery, or trauma). Packed RBCs may be stored for approximately 1 month after collection. Before administration, both donor blood and recipient blood are tested to decrease transfusion reactions. Blood typing tests the recipient's RBCs for antigens A, B, and Rh and screens the recipient's serum for the presence of antibodies to a panel of known RBC antigens. Each unit to be transfused is then cross-matched against the recipient's serum to check for preformed antibodies against antigens on the donor's RBCs. In an emergency situation, type O/Rh-negative blood that has been prescreened for reactive antibodies may be administered prior to blood typing and cross-matching. After blood typing, type-specific blood can be given. Patients receiving transfusions must be monitored closely for evidence of a transfusion reaction, and the transfusion should be discontinued immediately if such a reaction occurs.

3. **Administration.** Proper identification of the blood and patient is necessary to prevent transfusion errors, particularly in the operating room. Packed RBCs should be administered through a standard filter (170 to 260 μm) and an 18-gauge or larger intravenous catheter. One unit of packed RBCs raises the hemoglobin level approximately 1 g/dL and the hematocrit approximately 3%. The rate of transfusion is determined by the clinical situation; typically, however, each unit of blood must be administered within 4 hours. Patients are monitored for adverse reactions during the first 5 to 10 minutes of the transfusion and frequently thereafter. Those who need chronic transfusion therapy and organ transplant patients should be administered leukocyte-depleted blood. Immunocompromised patients and those receiving blood from first-degree relatives should be given irradiated blood to prevent graft versus host disease.

4. **Complications**
   a. **Infections.** Despite the institution of aggressive testing of the blood supply, the spread of transmissible agents is still a concern with homologous blood. However, the use of polymerase chain reaction–based testing of blood products has greatly reduced transmission rates of viral diseases. Currently, the risk of HIV or hepatitis C transmission from blood transfusion is in the range of 1 in 1.5 million to 2 million units transfused. There have only been 4 cases of transfusion-related HIV infection identified since 1999. Risk of transmission of human T-cell lymphoma virus and parvovirus B 19 also exists. Recently, transmission of West Nile virus from a transfusion has also been confirmed. Cytomegalovirus (CMV) transmission is a risk in CMV-negative immunocompromised patients and can be lowered by using either leukocyte-depleted or CMV-negative blood products. Bacteria and endotoxins can be infused with blood products, particularly those that are stored for prolonged periods or at room temperature. Parasitic infections also can be transmitted, although rarely, with blood products.
   b. **Immune reactions**
      (1) **Acute hemolytic reactions** are caused by preformed recipient antibodies to transfused RBC antigens. These reactions result in intravascular hemolysis and usually are produced by ABO or Rh incompatibility. Initial symptoms in an awake patient may include restlessness, anxiety, flushing, chest or back pain, tachypnea, tachycardia, and nausea. These symptoms can progress to shock and renal failure with hemoglobinuria. In anesthetized or comatose patients, the first signs of a transfusion reaction may be excessive incisional bleeding or oozing from the mucous membranes. When a transfusion reaction is suspected, the infusion should be stopped immediately, and all intravenous tubing should be changed. A check of the identity of the donor unit and recipient is required because most ABO reactions today are the result of clerical error. A repeat of the cross-match should be performed with samples of the recipient's serum and the remaining donor unit. Plasma hemoglobin should be determined as well as serum bilirubin and blood coagulation parameters. Treatment includes maintenance of intravascular volume, hemodynamic support as needed, and preservation of renal function. Urine output should be maintained at greater than 100 mL per hour using volume resuscitation, diuretics, and mannitol, if needed. Alkalinization of the urine to a pH of more than 7.5 by adding sodium bicarbonate to the intravenous fluids (2 to 3 ampules of 7.5% sodium bicarbonate in 1,000 mL D5W) helps prevent precipitation of hemoglobin in the renal tubules.

(2) **Delayed hemolytic transfusion reactions** result from an anamnestic antibody response to antigens to which the recipient has been previously exposed. Transfused RBC survival is normal initially, but 1 to 25 days later the RBCs are lysed rapidly. A decline of hemoglobin and an elevated bilirubin suggest this diagnosis. Specific treatment rarely is necessary, but severe cases should be treated like acute hemolytic reactions, with volume support and maintenance of urine output.

(3) **Nonhemolytic immune transfusion reactions** usually are caused by reactions to transfused WBCs, platelets, or plasma antigens. Fever, chills, urticaria, pruritus, and respiratory distress are consequences of these reactions. To avoid these reactions, most patients should be treated before transfusion with acetaminophen and diphenhydramine unless they are specifically contraindicated. Patients with antibodies against WBCs and platelets can receive RBCs from which the WBCs have been removed by filters. Patients with IgA deficiency can develop antibodies to IgA, resulting in a severe anaphylactic reactions to infusions of blood that contains IgA. These patients should receive blood products from IgA-deficient donors or washed RBCs. Symptomatic treatment for nonhemolytic reactions includes acetaminophen and diphenhydramine (25 to 50 mg orally or intravenously), epinephrine, and glucocorticoid therapy. Meperidine (25 to 100 mg) is particularly helpful for shaking chills associated with transfusion reactions. Prophylaxis with acetaminophen, diphenhydramine, and hydrocortisone (100 to 150 mg intravenously) should be used before future transfusions in patients who have experienced severe reactions.

(4) **Noncardiogenic pulmonary edema** is caused by preformed antileukocyte antibodies in the donor unit and occurs shortly after a transfusion [also known as transfusion-related acute lung injury (TRALI)]. This condition is often severe but transient and is managed with supportive care.

(5) **Graft versus host disease (GVHD)** can occur after transfusion of immunocompetent T cells into immunocompromised recipients or human leukocyte antigen–identical family members. GVHD presents with a rash, elevated liver function tests, and pancytopenia and has an associated mortality of more than 80%. Irradiation of donor blood from first-degree relatives of immunocompetent patients and all blood for immunocompromised patients prevent this complication.

(6) **Volume overload after blood transfusion** can occur in patients with poor cardiac or renal function. Careful monitoring of the volume status and judicious administration of diuretic therapy can reduce the risk of this complication.

(7) **Massive transfusion,** usually defined as the transfusion of blood products that are greater in volume than a patient's normal blood volume in less than 24 hours, creates several risks not encountered with a lesser volume or rate of transfusion. **Coagulopathy** might arise as a result of platelet or coagulation factor depletion. Transfusion of platelets, FFP, or cryoprecipitate should be based on the clinical situation and laboratory values rather than empirically based. **Hypothermia** can result from massive volume resuscitation with chilled blood products but can be prevented by using blood warmers. Hypothermia can lead to cardiac dysrhythmias and coagulopathy. **Citrate toxicity** can develop after massive transfusion in patients with hepatic dysfunction. Hypocalcemia can be treated with 10 mL 10% calcium gluconate administered

intravenously. **Electrolyte abnormalities,** including acidosis and hyperkalemia, occur rarely after massive transfusions, especially in patients with preexisting hyperkalemia.

5. **Alternatives to homologous transfusion** exist and may provide advantages in safety and cost when used in elective procedures with a high likelihood of significant blood loss. However, it must be stressed that meticulous surgical technique can in itself allow significant reductions in transfusion requirements.

   a. **Autologous predonation** is the preferred alternative for elective transfusions and has become standard practice for some high-risk procedures. Up to 20% of patients still require allogeneic transfusion, however, and transfusion reactions may result from clerical errors in storage. Despite its intrinsic advantages, predonation is not cost-effective when the risk of transfusion is moderate or low.

   b. **Isovolemic hemodilution** is a technique in which whole fresh blood is removed and crystalloid is simultaneously infused in the immediate preoperative period. The blood is stored at room temperature and reinfused after acute blood loss has ceased. Moderate hemodilution (hematocrit 32% to 33%) is as effective as autologous predonation in reducing the need for allogeneic transfusion but is much less costly.

   c. **Intraoperative autotransfusion,** wherein blood from the operative field is returned to the patient, can decrease allogeneic transfusion requirements. Equipment to separate and wash recovered RBCs is required in most cases, and contraindications include neoplasm and enteric or purulent contamination.

   d. **Erythropoietin** may be effective in decreasing allogeneic transfusion requirements when given preoperatively. Appropriate dosages (1,000 to 3,500 U/kg) can be calculated based on anticipated transfusion requirements and are administered weekly over 2 to 4 weeks. Adjunctive use with autologous predonation has not consistently been shown to be effective.

B. **Platelet transfusion**

1. **Indications.** Platelet transfusions are used to control bleeding that is caused by thrombocytopenia (or occasionally due to platelet dysfunction) and to prevent spontaneous bleeding in situations of severe thrombocytopenia. For ongoing hemorrhage and before major operations, platelet counts greater than $100,000/\mu L$ ($100 \times 10^9/L$) should be the goal; however, platelet counts greater than $50,000/\mu L$ ($50 \times 10^9/L$) usually are sufficient for minor surgical procedures if the platelet function is normal. In patients with severe thrombocytopenia, platelet counts should be maintained above $10,000/\mu L$ ($10 \times 10^9/L$) with prophylactic platelet transfusions to prevent spontaneous bleeding.

2. **Administration.** Random donor platelets (pooled from 5 to 8 units of donated whole blood) are used routinely, but in patients who require long-term platelet replacement and those who are refractory to random donor platelet transfusions, single-donor transfusions (obtained by platelet apheresis) may be more effective in increasing the platelet count. Generally, a "six pack" of random donor platelets or 1 unit of single-donor platelets increases the platelet count by 30,000 to $60,000/\mu L$ ($60 \times 10^9/L$).

3. **Complications associated with platelet transfusions**

   a. **Alloimmunization** occurs in 50% to 75% of patients receiving repeated platelet transfusions and presents as a failure of the platelet count to increment significantly after a transfusion. Single-donor platelets might result in a better response than would random-donor platelet products. In patients who likely will need long-term platelet therapy, human leukocyte antigen–matched single-donor platelets slow the onset of alloimmunization.

    b. **Posttransfusion purpura** is a rare complication of platelet transfusions seen in previously transfused individuals and multiparous women. It is usually caused by antibodies that develop in response to a specific platelet antigen Pl^{A1} from the donor platelets. This condition presents with severe thrombocytopenia, purpura, and bleeding occurring 7 to 10 days after platelet transfusion. Fatal bleeding can occur. Plasmapheresis or an infusion of intravenous IG is often helpful, and the disease is usually self-limiting. Platelet transfusions are ineffective and not recommended.

C. **FFP** is the fluid portion of whole blood and contains all the coagulation factors. However, factors V and VIII may not be stable through the thawing process and are not reliably recovered from FFP. Therefore, it can be used to correct coagulopathies that are due to deficiencies of any other coagulation factor and is particularly useful when multiple factor deficiencies exist (e.g., liver disease or massive transfusion). Under most circumstances, 10 to 15 mL/kg of FFP will be adequate factor replacement. Dosing frequency varies depending on the half-life of the deficient factor. Deficiencies of factors VIII and IX are best treated with their specific factor concentrates.

D. **Cryoprecipitate** is the cold-insoluble precipitate of fresh plasma and is rich in factor VIII and vWF as well as fibrinogen, fibronectin, and factor XIII. Cryoprecipitate may be used as second-line therapy in replacing vWF in vWD but is most often used to correct fibrinogen deficiency in DIC or during massive transfusion. Typical replacement therapy consists of 1 U/10 kg body weight.

E. **Recombinant human factor VIIa (rhFVIIa)** is a recently approved product used primarily in the treatment of patients with factor VIII inhibitors. However, it may be considered for other patients with difficult bleeding problems for which therapy is inadequate or not available. Possible uses include CNS bleeding in the presence or absence of warfarin, thrombocytopenia with bleeding, or multiple coagulation factor deficiencies.

VIII. **Local hemostatic agents** can aid in the intraoperative control of bleeding from needle punctures, vascular suture lines, or areas of extensive tissue dissection. Anastomotic bleeding usually is best controlled with local pressure or a simple suture. Local hemostatic agents promote hemostasis by providing a matrix for thrombus formation.

A. **Gelatin sponge** (e.g., Gelfoam) can absorb many times its weight of whole blood by capillary action and provides a platform for coagulation. Gelfoam itself is not intrinsically hemostatic. It resorbs in 4 to 6 weeks without a significant inflammatory reaction.

B. **Oxidized cellulose** (e.g., Surgicel) is a knitted fabric of cellulose that allows clotting by absorbing blood and swelling into a scaffold. Its slow resorption can create a foreign body reaction.

C. **Collagen sponge** (e.g., Helistat) is produced from bovine tendon collagen and promotes platelet adhesion. It is only slowly resorbed and creates a foreign body reaction similar to that of cellulose.

D. **Microfibrillar collagen** (e.g., Avitene, Hemotene) can be sprayed onto wounds and anastomoses for hemostasis, particularly in areas that are difficult to reach. It, too, stimulates platelet adhesion and promotes thrombus formation. Because microfibrillar collagen can pass through autotransfusion device filters, these adjuncts should be avoided during procedures that involve cell-saver devices.

E. **Topical thrombin** can be applied to the various hemostatic agents or to dressings and placed onto bleeding sites to achieve a fibrin-rich hemostatic plug. Topical thrombin, usually of bovine origin, is supplied as a lyophilized powder and can be applied directly to dressings or dissolved in saline and sprayed onto the wound. Repeated use of bovine thrombin may result in formation of inhibitors to thrombin or factor V, which is not usually associated with a clinical bleeding disorder, although there may be dramatic alterations in the coagulation testing. Topical thrombin can be used effectively in anticoagulated patients.

F. Gelatin matrices (e.g., FloSeal) are often used in combination with topical thrombin intraoperatively. Typically, bovine thrombin (5,000 units) is sprayed onto the matrix, which is then applied to the site of bleeding.

G. Other agents include topical cryoprecipitate, which can be sprayed onto the wound with topical thrombin for a fibrin-rich coagulum, as well as topical EACA and topical aprotinin.

Anesthesia

**Elbert Y. Kuo and
Richard S. Hotchkiss**

PREPARING THE PATIENT

I. Patient preparation for operation
   A. Preoperative evaluation
   1. A **comprehensive preoperative evaluation** is critical to the safe administration of anesthetic care.
      a. A **thorough history**, including medication usage and prior anesthetic usage, should be obtained.
      b. An **examination of airway,** vascular access, and other pertinent anatomy tailored to the anticipated operation should be undertaken.
   2. For **patients without preexisting disease**, preoperative screening and testing are determined primarily by age.
      a. **Hemoglobin or hematocrit** may be the only test required in healthy patients younger than 40 years.
      b. A **serum pregnancy test** should be obtained for female patients of childbearing age.
      c. A **screening chest x-ray and electrocardiogram (ECG)** are obtained for patients who are 50 years or older, unless an indication is found from the history or physical examination, or both.
   3. **Additional testing** may be required when clinically indicated.
      a. **Serum electrolytes** must be evaluated in patients with diabetes or renal insufficiency and in patients who are taking diuretics.
      b. **Coagulation studies** (prothrombin time, partial thromboplastin time, bleeding time) must be evaluated in patients who are receiving anticoagulation therapy or have a personal or family history that is suggestive of abnormal bleeding.
      c. **Additional testing or consultation** may be required in patients with evidence of severe coexisting disease, especially those with cardiac, pulmonary, or renal compromise.
   4. Unstable or uncontrolled medical conditions, upper respiratory infections, and solid food ingestion within 6 hours of surgery are **indications to cancel or postpone elective surgery.**
   5. **American Society of Anesthesiologists (ASA) criteria** (see Table 6-1)
   B. Nothing by mouth (n.p.o.) status
   1. For all patients, it is customary to abstain from any oral intake except for medications with sips of water for 8 hours before elective surgery. However, for adult patients who are not considered to be at increased risk for aspiration of gastric contents, the following **aspiration prophylaxis regimens** can be used.
      a. **Solid food** is permitted until 6 hours before surgery.
      b. **Clear liquids** (which do not include milk or juices containing pulp) are permitted until 2 hours before surgery (*Anesthesiology* 1999;90:896–905).
   2. **Patients with slowed or incomplete gastric emptying** (e.g., those who are morbidly obese, diabetic, or on narcotic therapy) **may require longer fasting periods and additional pretreatment with metoclopramide, histamine H$_2$-receptor antagonists, or sodium citrate.** Rapid-sequence induction can be considered in these patients. Maintenance intravenous fluids should be started in n.p.o. inpatients.

Table 6-1. American Society of Anesthesiologists criteria

ASA Grade	Description
I	There is no organic, physiological, biochemical, or psychiatric disturbance. The pathological process for which the operation is to be performed is localized and is not a systemic disturbance.
II	Mild to moderate systemic disturbance caused either by the condition to be treated or by other pathophysiologic processes.
III	Severe systemic disturbance or disease for whatever cause, even though it may not be possible to define the degree of disability.
IV	Indicative of the patient with severe systemic disorder already life-threatening and not always correctable by the operative procedure.
V	The moribund patient who has little chance of survival but is submitted to operation in desperation.

Note. An E is added after grade to indicate emergency surgery (e.g., IVE).

C. Medications
1. Patients can receive **benzodiazepines or narcotics** to alleviate preoperative anxiety.
2. **Cardiovascular or other pertinent medications** usually are administered on the morning of surgery with small sips of water. Inpatients who normally receive scheduled insulin doses should instead be placed on sliding-scale insulin, with blood sugars checked frequently every 2 to 6 hours while n.p.o., depending on difficulty of their diabetic control. Outpatients should be instructed to take one half to one third of their regular insulin dose the morning of surgery and to check blood sugars frequently. **It is essential to avoid hypoglycemia.**

TYPES OF ANESTHESIA
I. **Local anesthetics** are categorized into two groups. **Esters** include tetracaine, procaine, cocaine, and chloroprocaine. **Amides** include lidocaine, mepivacaine, bupivacaine, and etidocaine. Characteristics of commonly used local anesthetic agents are summarized in Table 6-2.
   - A. **Mechanism of action**
     1. **Local anesthetics** work by diffusing through the nerve plasma membrane and causing blockade of sodium channels. The nerve cell is unable to depolarize, and axonic conduction is inhibited.
     2. **Local tissue acidosis** (e.g., from infection) slows the onset and decreases the intensity of analgesia by causing local anesthetic molecules to become positively charged and less able to diffuse into the neuron.
   - B. **Toxicity** (dose dependent, except for allergic reactions)
     1. **Central nervous system (CNS) toxicity**

Table 6-2. Local anesthetics for infiltration

Agent	Maximum Dose (mg/kg) Plain	With Epinephrine*	Length of Action (h) Plain	With Epinephrine*
Procaine	—	8.0	0.25–1.0	0.5–1.5
Lidocaine	5.0	7.0	0.5–1.0	2–6
Mepivacaine	5.0	7.0	0.75–1.5	2–6
Bupivacaine	2.5	3.0	2–4	3–7
Tetracaine	1.5		24	

*1:200,000.

a. Signs and symptoms include mental status changes, dizziness, perioral numbness, a metallic taste, tinnitus, visual disturbances, and seizures. Seizures resulting from inadvertent intravascular injection usually last only minutes. Continuous infusion of local anesthetics may result in high plasma levels and prolonged seizures.

b. Treatment involves airway support and ventilation with 100% oxygen, which should always be available. Prolonged seizures may require administration of benzodiazepines (midazolam, 1 to 5 mg intravenously; diazepam, 5 to 15 mg intravenously; or lorazepam, 1 to 4 mg intravenously). Intubation may be required to ensure adequate ventilation.

2. Cardiovascular toxicity

a. Signs and symptoms range from decreased cardiac output to hypotension and cardiovascular collapse. Most local anesthetics cause CNS toxicity before cardiovascular toxicity. Bupivacaine is an exception, and its intravascular injection can result in severe cardiac compromise.

b. Treatment includes fluid resuscitation, administration of vasopressors, and cardiopulmonary resuscitation, if necessary.

3. Hypersensitivity reactions, although rare, have been described with ester-based local anesthetics and are attributed to the metabolite *p*-aminobenzoic acid. True amide-based local anesthetic anaphylactic reactions are questionable.

a. Signs and symptoms can range from mild to life-threatening. These include urticaria, bronchospasm, hypotension, and anaphylactic shock.

b. Treatment is similar to that for hypersensitivity reactions from other etiologies. Urticaria responds to diphenhydramine, 25 to 50 mg intravenously. Bronchospasm is treated with inhaled bronchodilators (e.g., albuterol) and oxygen. Hypotension is treated with fluid resuscitation and vasopressors [e.g., phenylephrine hydrochloride (Neo-Synephrine)] as required. Anaphylactic cardiovascular collapse can be treated with epinephrine, 0.5 to 1.0 mg administered as an intravenous bolus.

C. Epinephrine (1:200,000, 5 μg/mL) is mixed with local anesthetic solutions to prolong the duration of neural blockade and reduce systemic drug absorption. Its use is contraindicated in areas where arterial spasm would lead to tissue necrosis (e.g., nose, ears, fingers, toes, penis).

II. Regional anesthesia

A. In the operating room

1. General considerations

a. The importance of preoperative communication between anesthesiologist and surgeon cannot be overemphasized. The extent and duration of the procedure must be appreciated by the anesthesiologist so that the appropriate area and duration of analgesia can be achieved. If the possibility of a prolonged or involved operative procedure is likely, a general anesthetic may be more appropriate. Certain surgical positions are poorly tolerated by awake patients (e.g., steep Trendelenburg may cause respiratory compromise); in these instances, a general anesthetic is appropriate.

b. Supplements to regional anesthesia. No regional anesthetic technique is foolproof, and various degrees of failure may occur because of inexperience or adverse anatomy. Local infiltration by the surgeon may be required if there is an incomplete block or one that is slow to set up fully. Intravenous sedation using short-acting benzodiazepines, narcotics, barbiturates, or propofol can also be helpful. General anesthesia may be required when a regional technique provides inadequate analgesia.

c. n.p.o. status. Because any regional anesthetic may progress to a general anesthetic, n.p.o. requirements for regional and general anesthetics are identical.

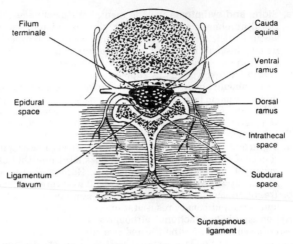

Figure 6-1. Anatomy for epidural and spinal anesthesia.

    d. Monitoring requirements are no different from those for general anesthesia. Heart rhythm, blood pressure (BP), and arterial oxygen saturation should be monitored regularly during regional or general anesthesia. Other monitoring may be indicated, depending on coexisting disease states.

2. Types of regional anesthesia

    a. Spinal anesthesia involves the injection of small volumes of local anesthetic solution into the subarachnoid space at the level of the lumbar spine.

      (1) Anatomy and placement (Figure 6-1)

        (a) With the use of sterile technique and after local anesthetic infiltration of the skin and subcutaneous tissues, a small (22- to 27-gauge) **spinal needle is passed between two adjacent lumbar spinous processes**. The needle is passed through the following structures: supraspinous ligament, interspinous ligament, ligamentum flavum, dura mater, and arachnoid mater. Cerebrospinal fluid (CSF) is aspirated, and the appropriate local anesthetic solution is injected.

        (b) The needle can be removed (single-shot method) or a catheter can be placed to allow repeated dosing for potentially longer procedures (continuous spinal).

      (2) Level of analgesia

        (a) Multiple variables affect the spread of analgesia. The **baricity** of the agent (solution density compared to that of CSF) and the position of the patient immediately after injection are major determinants of level. The **total dose injected** (increased dose results in higher spread) and the **total volume injected** (increased volume results in higher spread) are also important determinants of anesthetic level.

        (b) Older patients tend to have greater spread of anesthesia by a few dermatomes, but this difference may or may not be clinically significant.

      (3) Onset and duration of analgesia

        (a) The **specific characteristics of the local anesthetic** used and the **total dose injected** are the primary determinants of onset and duration of action. Epinephrine added to the solution increases the duration of analgesia.

(b) **The variability in length of analgesia** is significant, ranging from as little as 30 minutes (lidocaine) to up to 6 hours (tetracaine with epinephrine).

(4) Complications

(a) **Hypotension** may occur as a result of sympatholytic-induced vasodilation and bradycardia. It may be more severe in hypovolemic patients or in those with preexisting cardiac dysfunction. Treatment includes volume resuscitation (crystalloid, 500 to 1,000 mL), vasopressors (epinephrine, 5 to 10 μg intravenously for adults; phenylephrine hydrochloride, 50 to 100 μg intravenously), and positive chronotropic drugs. It is advisable to administer 500 to 1,000 mL of crystalloid prior to spinal block to avoid hypotension due to spinal anesthesia.

(b) **High spinal blockade.** Inadvertently high levels of spinal blockade may result in hypotension, dyspnea (loss of chest proprioception or intercostal muscle function), or apnea (decreased medullary perfusion secondary to hypotension). Respiratory dysfunction may necessitate intubation and ventilatory support.

(c) **Headache** after spinal anesthesia or diagnostic lumbar puncture is encountered with higher frequency in young or female patients. This is usually the result of leakage of CSF from the puncture site. A postural component is always present (i.e., symptoms worsened by sitting up or standing). The recent use of smaller-gauge spinal needles has reduced the frequency of this complication. Treatment includes oral or intravenous fluids, oral analgesics, and caffeinated beverages. Severe refractory headache may require placement of an epidural blood patch to prevent ongoing leakage of CSF.

(d) **CNS infection** after spinal anesthesia, although extremely rare, may result in meningitis, epidural abscess, or arachnoiditis.

(e) **Permanent nerve injury** is exceedingly rare and is seen with the same frequency as in general anesthesia.

(f) **Urinary retention with bladder distention** occurs in patients with spinal anesthesia whose bladders are not drained by urethral catheters. Catheters should remain in place until after the spinal anesthesia has been stopped and full sensation has returned.

(5) Contraindications

(a) **Absolute contraindications** to spinal anesthesia are localized infection at the planned puncture site, increased intracranial pressure, generalized sepsis, coagulopathy, and lack of consent.

(b) **Relative contraindications** include hypovolemia, preexisting CNS disease, chronic low back pain, platelet dysfunction, and aortic stenosis.

b. Epidural anesthesia

(1) Anatomy and placement (Figure 6-1)

(a) Inserting an epidural needle is similar to placing a spinal needle except that the **epidural needle is not advanced through the dura**. No CSF is obtained. The tip of the epidural needle lies in the epidural space between the ligamentum flavum posteriorly and the dura mater anteriorly. Local anesthetic solution can then be injected.

(b) Either the **needle is removed** (single-shot method) or, more commonly, **a flexible catheter is passed through the needle** into the space and the needle is withdrawn over the catheter (continuous catheter technique). Local anesthetics or opiates can be dosed intermittently or infused as needed.

(2) Level of analgesia
  (a) Once injected into the epidural space, the local anesthetic solution diffuses through the dura and into the spinal nerve roots, resulting in a **bilateral dermatomal distribution of analgesia.**
  (b) The spread of nerve root blockade is primarily determined by the **volume** of injection and, to a lesser degree, by patient **position and age** and by **area of placement.**

(3) Onset and duration of analgesia
  (a) Epidural anesthesia develops more slowly than does spinal anesthesia, because the local anesthetic solution must diffuse farther. The rate of onset of sympathetic blockade and hypotension also is slowed, enabling more precise titration of hemodynamic therapy compared with spinal anesthesia.
  (b) The **dosing interval** depends on the agent used.

(4) Complications are similar to those encountered with spinal anesthesia.
  (a) Spinal headache may result from inadvertent perforation of the dura.
  (b) Epidural hematoma is rare and usually occurs with coexisting coagulopathy. Emergent laminectomy may be required to decompress the spinal cord and avoid permanent neurologic injury.

c. Combined spinal and epidural anesthesia
  (1) Anatomy and placement
    (a) A **small-gauge spinal needle** is placed through an epidural needle once the epidural space has been located. The dura is punctured only by the spinal needle, and placement is verified by CSF withdrawal. Subarachnoid local anesthetics or narcotics can then be administered via the spinal needle.
    (b) The **spinal needle** is withdrawn after the initial dosing, and an epidural catheter is threaded into the epidural space through the existing epidural needle.
  (2) Onset and duration. This procedure combines the quick onset of spinal analgesia with the continuous dosing advantages of epidural analgesia.
  (3) Complications are similar to those seen in spinal and epidural anesthesia.

d. Comparison of spinal or epidural anesthesia with general anesthesia. Although the incidence of thromboembolic complications and total blood loss is reduced in certain surgical procedures with spinal or epidural anesthesia, there is no evidence that long-term mortality is reduced compared with general anesthesia (*Br J Anaesth* 1986;58:284).

e. Brachial plexus blockade. Injection of local anesthetic solution into the sheath surrounding the brachial plexus results in varying degrees of upper extremity blockade. This technique is indicated for any procedure involving the patient's shoulders, arms, or hands. The approach taken depends on the distribution of blockade desired.
  (1) Axillary block. The needle is placed into the brachial plexus sheath from the axilla. Blockade above the patient's elbow is unreliable.
  (2) Supraclavicular blockade. The needle is directed caudally from behind the posterior border of the inner one third of the clavicle. This technique reliably blocks the entire upper extremity, sparing the patient's shoulder. The risk of pneumothorax is low.
  (3) Interscalene blockade involves the cervical as well as brachial plexus and reliably blocks the patient's shoulder. There is a high incidence of phrenic nerve block, which increases the risk of pulmonary complications in patients with chronic obstructive

pulmonary disease. This also serves as a contraindication to bilateral blockade.

  f. Cervical plexus blockade blocks the anterior divisions of C1 to C4 and is the anesthetic method of choice for carotid endarterectomy at many institutions. Inadvertent blockade of neighboring structures does occur.

  (1) Phrenic nerve blockade may result in transient diaphragmatic paralysis. Simultaneous bilateral cervical plexus blockade is therefore contraindicated.

  (2) Ipsilateral cervical sympathetic plexus blockade may result in Horner syndrome, producing transient ptosis, miosis, and facial anhidrosis.

B. Outside the operating room

  1. Intercostal nerve block is indicated after thoracotomy or before chest tube placement.

  a. Anatomy and placement (Figure 6-2)

  (1) The **posterior axillary line is identified,** and with the use of sterile technique a 23-gauge needle is placed perpendicular to the patient's skin until contact is made with his or her rib. The needle is then walked caudad off the patient's rib and advanced several millimeters. After negative aspiration, 5 mL of bupivacaine 0.25% to 0.50% with epinephrine (1:200,000) is injected.

  (2) Usually, **five interspaces** (including two above and two below the interspace of interest) are injected.

  b. Complications include pneumothorax and intravascular injection causing arrhythmias. Injection into the nerve sheath with retrograde

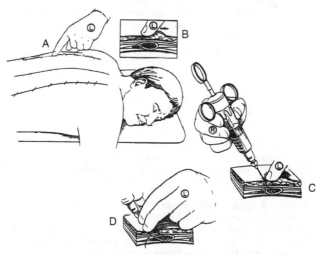

Figure 6-2. Anatomy and placement for intercostal nerve block. **A.** The anesthesiologist's hand closest to the patient's head (cephalic) first locates the target interspace and then **(B)** retracts the skin over the rib above. **C.** The hand closest to the patient's feet (caudad) places the needle and attached syringe containing local anesthetic through the skin onto the rib at approximately a 30-degree angle, with the needle bevel directed cephalad. **D.** The cephalic hand then grasps the needle while maintaining contact with the patient and allows the tension of the retracted skin to walk the needle off the inferior edge of the rib and advance 2 to 3 mm.

spread back to the spinal cord can produce a high spinal or epidural block [see section **II.A.2.a.(4)(b)**].
   2. **Digital block** is indicated for minor procedures of the fingers.
      a. **Anatomy and placement**
         (1) From the **dorsal surface of the hand**, a 23-gauge needle is placed on either side of the metatarsal head and inserted until the increased resistance of the palmar connective tissue is felt. An injection of 1 to 2 mL of lidocaine 1% to 2% is made as the needle is withdrawn.
         (2) **Supplemental injection** of 0.5 to 1.0 mL of lidocaine 1% to 2% in the interdigital web on either side may be required.
      b. Epinephrine is contraindicated.
   C. **Local infiltration**
      1. **In the operating room**, the area of incision can be infiltrated before incision or at the conclusion of the operation. Some evidence suggests that infiltration before incision is associated with less postoperative discomfort and reduced analgesic use (*Anesth Analg* 1992;74:495). Bupivacaine is frequently used.
      2. **Outside the operating room**, local anesthetic infiltration may also be useful during wound débridement, central venous catheter placement, or repair of minor lacerations. The agent of choice is lidocaine 1% to 2% due to its quick onset and low toxicity. The area of interest should be injected liberally. Frequent aspiration helps to avoid intravascular injection. Injection should be repeated as necessary.
      3. **Epinephrine should not** be used in areas at risk for vascular compromise from arterial spasm (e.g., nose, ears, fingers, toes, penis).
III. **General anesthesia provides hypnosis (unconsciousness), analgesia, amnesia, and skeletal muscle relaxation.**
   A. All patients who are undergoing general anesthesia require an appropriate **preoperative evaluation** and optimization of any coexisting medical problems (see "Preparing the Patient," sections **I.A.1** and **I.A.2**).
   B. **Monitoring.** Basic monitoring requirements for general anesthesia are similar to those for regional anesthesia (see section **II.A.1.d**).
   C. **Induction of general anesthesia.** Intravenous agents are most widely used owing to rapid onset and ease of administration.
      1. **Thiopental**, a barbiturate (3 to 5 mg/kg intravenously), has a rapid onset and redistribution. However, there often is an associated decrease in cardiac output, BP, and cerebral blood flow. It should be used with caution in patients with hypotension or active coronary ischemia.
      2. **Propofol**, a phenol derivative (1 to 3 mg/kg intravenously), is used for both induction and maintenance of anesthesia. Onset of action is immediate. It has hemodynamic properties that are similar to those of thiopental but is associated with a low incidence of postoperative nausea and vomiting. The pharmacokinetics are not changed by chronic hepatic or renal failure.
      3. **Etomidate**, an imidazole derivative (0.3 mg/kg intravenously), has an onset of 30 to 60 seconds and only mild direct hemodynamic depressant effects.
      4. **Ketamine**, a phencyclidine derivative (1 to 4 mg/kg intravenously), increases cardiac output and BP in patients who are not catecholamine depleted. Ketamine raises intracranial pressure and **is not** used in patients with head trauma. The **use of ketamine is limited** owing to the emergence of delirium and nightmares.
   D. **Airway management.** Ventilation during general anesthesia may be spontaneous, assisted, or controlled.
      1. **Mask ventilation** with spontaneous respiratory effort can be used during limited (usually peripheral) procedures that do not require neuromuscular relaxation. Because the airway is unprotected, this technique is contraindicated in patients at risk for aspiration.
      2. **Endotracheal intubation** secures the airway, allows control of ventilation, and protects against aspiration. Although frequently performed orally

with the laryngoscope, intubation can also be accomplished nasally and, in anatomically challenging patients, can be performed with the aid of a fiberoptic bronchoscope via oral or nasal routes.

E. Neuromuscular blockade facilitates tracheal intubation and is required for many surgical procedures. It provides the surgeon with improved working conditions and optimizes ventilatory support. Agents that produce neuromuscular blockade act on postsynaptic receptors in the neuromuscular junction to antagonize the effects of acetylcholine competitively. Agents are categorized as either depolarizing or nondepolarizing (Table 6-3).

1. **Succinylcholine** is a rapid-acting (60 seconds), rapidly metabolized depolarizing agent that allows return of neuromuscular function in 5 to 10 minutes. This agent causes a transient mild hyperkalemia that may be exaggerated in patients with severe burns, trauma, or paralysis; patients on prolonged bed rest; or patients with other neuromuscular disorders. In addition, it can cause increases in intraocular, intracranial, and gastric pressures.

2. **Nondepolarizing muscle relaxants** can be divided into short-, intermediate-, and long-acting agents. Associated hemodynamic effects and elimination pathways vary.

   a. **These agents are often used in an intensive care setting** when paralysis is necessary for adequate ventilation of an intubated patient. Such patients must have adequate sedation and analgesia before and

Table 6-3. Agents producing neuromuscular blockade

Agent	Initial Dose (mg/kg)	Duration (min)	Elimination	Associated Effects
Depolarizing				
Succinylcholine	1.0–1.5	3–5	Plasma cholinesterase	Fasciculations, increase or decrease in heart rate, transient hyperkalemia, known malignant hyperthermia trigger agent
Nondepolarizing				
Mivacurium	0.15	8–10	Plasma cholinesterase	Flushing, decrease in BP
Atracurium	0.2–0.4	20–35	Ester hydrolysis	Histamine release
Cisatracurium	0.1–0.2	20–35	Ester hydrolysis	–
Vecuronium	0.1–0.2	25–40	Primarily hepatic	–
Rocuronium	0.6–1.2	30	Primarily hepatic	–
d-Tubocurare	0.5–0.6	75–100	Primarily renal	Histamine release, decrease in BP
Pancuronium	0.04–0.1	45–90	Primarily renal	Increase in heart rate, mean arterial BP, and cardiac output
Doxacurium	0.050.08	90180	Primarily renal	Decrease in BP

BP, blood pressure.

during paralysis. Dosage should be monitored by train-of-four stimulus every 4 hours, with one out of four twitches the goal. Corticosteroids, aminoglycosides, and long-term use of neuromuscular blockers potentiate the risk of a critical level of neuromyopathy.

   b. **Reversal of neuromuscular blockade** for patients who are receiving nondepolarizing muscle relaxants usually is performed before extubation to ensure full return of respiratory muscle function and protective airway reflexes. The diaphragm is less sensitive to muscle relaxants than are the muscles of the head and neck. A spontaneously ventilating patient **may be unable to protect the airway.** The definitive test for assessing the degree of remaining paralysis is to have the patient raise the head from the bed for 5 seconds or more. **Anticholinesterases** (neostigmine, 0.06 to 0.07 mg/kg, and edrophonium, 0.1 mg/kg) act to increase the availability of acetylcholine at the neuromuscular junction. They reverse the blockade by reducing the binding frequency of the nondepolarizing muscle relaxant (a competitive acetylcholine antagonist).

F. Maintenance of anesthesia
   1. The **goal of anesthesia** is to provide unconsciousness, amnesia, analgesia, and, usually, muscle relaxation. Balanced anesthesia involves the combined use of inhalational agents, narcotics, and muscle relaxants to attain this goal.
   2. **Inhalational agents**
      a. All inhalational agents provide varying degrees of unconsciousness, amnesia, analgesia, and muscle relaxation.
      b. **Isoflurane** is the most commonly used inhalational agent due to its low rate of metabolism. It causes less cardiovascular depression than other agents. Enflurane, halothane, sevoflurane, and desflurane are also used.
      c. **Halothane** has a rapid onset of action. Its use is excellent for asthmatics because of its bronchial smooth muscle–relaxing properties. However, it does sensitize the myocardium to catecholamines, increasing the rate of ventricular arrhythmias. Halothane should also be used with caution in patients with brain lesions because it is a potent vasodilator and can increase cerebral perfusion and intracranial pressure. It is used extensively as an induction agent for pediatric patients because of the decreased irritating effects of halothane on the airway. Sevoflurane is also used in children for the same reason.
      d. **Nitrous oxide** by itself cannot provide surgical anesthesia. When combined with other inhalational agents, it reduces the required dose and subsequent side effects of the other agents. Nitrous oxide is extremely soluble and readily diffuses into any closed gas space, increasing its pressure. As a result, this agent should not be administered to patients with intestinal obstruction or suspected pneumothorax.
   3. **Intravenous agents**
      a. **Narcotics** can be administered continuously or intermittently. These agents provide superior analgesia but unreliable amnesia. Commonly used narcotics include fentanyl, sufentanil, alfentanil, remifentanil, morphine, and meperidine.
      b. **Hypnotics, benzodiazepines, and propofol.** Propofol infusion provides excellent hypnosis (unconsciousness) but insignificant analgesia and unreliable amnesia. The rapid dissipation of its effects and the low incidence of postoperative nausea have contributed to its widespread use in outpatient surgery. The maintenance dose is 0.1 to 0.2 mg/kg per minute.
      c. **Ketamine** by itself can provide total anesthesia. The associated emergence of delirium and nightmares limits its use.

G. Recovery from general anesthesia. The goal at the conclusion of surgery is to provide a smooth, rapid return to consciousness, with stable hemodynamics and pulmonary function, protective airway reflexes, and continued analgesia.

    1. Preparation for emergence from anesthesia usually begins before surgical closure, and communication between the surgeon and anesthesiologist facilitates prompt emergence of the patient at the procedure's termination.

    2. Patients recover from the effects of sedation or general or regional anesthesia in the **postanesthesia care unit.** Once they are oriented, comfortable, hemodynamically stable, ventilating adequately, and without signs of anesthetic or surgical complications, they are discharged to the appropriate ward or to home.

H. Complications of general anesthesia

    1. Malignant hyperthermia is a hypermetabolic disorder of skeletal muscle that is characterized by intracellular hypercalcemia and rapid adenosine triphosphate consumption. This condition is initiated by exposure to one or more anesthetic-triggering agents, including desflurane, enflurane, halothane, isoflurane, sevoflurane, and succinylcholine. Its incidence is approximately 1 in 50,000 in adults in 1 in 15,000 in children.

        a. Signs and symptoms may occur in the operating room or more than 24 hours postoperatively and include tachycardia, tachypnea, hypertension, hypercapnia, hyperthermia, acidosis, and skeletal muscle rigidity.

        b. Treatment involves immediate administration of dantrolene (1 mg/kg intravenously up to a cumulative dose of 10 mg/kg). This attenuates the rise in intracellular calcium. Repeat doses are given as needed if symptoms persist. Each vial commonly contains 20 mg dantrolene and 3 g mannitol and must be mixed with 50 mL sterile water. Acidosis and hyperkalemia should be monitored and treated appropriately. Intensive care monitoring for 48 to 72 hours is indicated after an acute episode of malignant hyperthermia to evaluate for recurrence, acute tubular necrosis, pulmonary edema, and disseminated intravascular coagulation.

    2. Laryngospasm

        a. During emergence from anesthesia, noxious stimulation of the vocal cords can occur at light planes of anesthesia. Additionally, blood or other oral secretions can irritate the larynx. As a result, the vocal cords may be brought into forceful apposition, and the flow of gas through the larynx may then be restricted or prevented completely.

        b. Treatment involves the use of positive-pressure ventilation by mask to break the spasm. Such therapy usually is sufficient. Succinylcholine may be required in refractory cases to allow successful ventilation.

    3. Nausea and vomiting

        a. Cortical (pain, hypotension, hypoxia), **visceral** (gastric distention, visceral traction), **vestibular,** and **chemoreceptor trigger zone** (narcotics) afferent stimuli all can play a role in postoperative nausea and vomiting. The overall incidence is approximately 30%. It is more common in preadolescents 11 to 14 years old, women, and obese patients. Narcotics, etomidate, and isoflurane have been implicated.

        b. Treatment includes avoiding gastric distention during ventilation as well as administering prochlorperazine (Compazine), an antidopaminergic agent, 10 mg intravenously or orally every 4 to 6 hours as needed. For severe cases of postoperative nausea and vomiting, ondansetron (Zofran), 4 mg intravenously, can be given. The dosing can be repeated every 6 to 8 hours if symptoms persist.

    4. Urinary retention

        a. Although very common with spinal anesthesia [see section **II.A.2.a.(4)(f)], urinary retention occurs in only 1% to 3% of cases involving general anesthesia.** It most commonly occurs after pelvic operations and in conjunction with benign prostatic hypertrophy.

b. Treatment ranges from conservative (early ambulation, having patient sit or stand while attempting to micturate) to aggressive (bladder catheterization).
5. Hypothermia
    a. General anesthesia induction causes **peripheral vasodilation**, which leads to internal redistribution of heat, resulting in an increase in peripheral temperature at the expense of the core temperature. The core temperature then decreases in a linear manner until a plateau is reached. Such hypothermia is more pronounced in the elderly.
    b. Treatment includes passive warming during an operation by insulation of all exposed surfaces. Additionally, active warming with forced-air convective warmers is effective, but care should be taken in using warmers with patients with vascular insufficiency (warmers should not be used on ischemic extremities).
6. Nerve injury
    a. Nerve palsies can occur secondary to improper positioning of the patient on the operating table or insufficient padding of dependent regions. Such palsies can be long-lasting and debilitating.
    b. Prophylactic padding of sensitive regions and attention to **proper positioning** remain the most effective therapies.

INTUBATION AND SEDATION

I. Emergent intubation by rapid-sequence induction
  A. Patients in respiratory distress outside the operating room may require intubation to ensure adequate oxygenation and ventilatory support. Whenever possible, an anesthesiologist should be alerted and present at the time of intubation to assist if necessary; however, intubation should not be unduly delayed while waiting for an anesthesiologist to arrive.
  B. Airway support with 100% oxygen mask ventilation should be initiated before intubation. In the emergent setting or with the hemodynamically unstable patient, rapid-sequence induction of anesthesia with etomidate followed by succinylcholine may be preferred. Succinylcholine should be avoided in patients with severe burns, intracranial bleeds, and eye trauma. Intubation can then be performed via laryngoscopy using an endotracheal tube of appropriate size—in general a size 8 tube for men and a size 7 tube for women. After inflation of the cuff, bilateral and equal breath sounds should be auscultated, end-tidal CO_2 and pulse oximetry measured, and a portable chest x-ray ordered to ensure proper placement. The patient should be continued on 100% oxygen until transfer to an intensive care setting.
II. Sedation for procedures
  A. Monitored anesthesia care
    1. In monitored anesthesia care or local standby cases, **an anesthesiologist is present** to monitor and sedate the patient during the procedure. The surgeon is responsible for analgesia, which is accomplished with local infiltration or peripheral nerve blockade. Sedating or hypnotic medications (e.g., propofol) provide sedation only and when given in conjunction with inadequate analgesia may result in a disinhibited, uncooperative patient.
    2. Monitoring is identical to that required for general or regional anesthesia. Supplemental oxygen is provided by face mask or nasal cannula.
    3. n.p.o. criteria are identical to those for general or regional anesthesia.
    4. Considerable variation exists regarding the response of patients to sedating medications, and protective airway reflexes may be diminished with even small doses.
  B. Local procedures in the operating room
    1. *Local* implies that **an anesthesiologist is not required** to monitor the patient or provide sedation. It still is advisable for the physician

Table 6-4. Medications for short-term sedation and analgesia during procedures

Agent	Route	Dose (as Needed)	Comments
Midazolam (Versed)	i.v.	1–2 mg q 5 min	Benzodiazepines provide sedation only
Meperidine (Demerol)	i.v.	25–50 mg q 10–15 min	Narcotics provide analgesia with unpredictable sedative effects
Fentanyl	i.v.	25–50 μg q 5–10 min	Narcotics provide analgesia with unpredictable sedative effects
Propofol (Diprivan)	i.v.	10–20 mg over 3–5 min q 10 min	May cause hypotension, especially with boluses

performing the procedure to monitor the ECG, arterial oxygen saturation, and BP even if sedation is not given.

2. **Painful stimuli** can increase vagal tone, resulting in bradycardia, hypotension, and hypoventilation.

C. **Sedation outside the operating room**

1. **Indications** are to relieve patient anxiety and avoid potentially detrimental hemodynamic sequelae during invasive procedures or diagnostic tests.

2. **Oxygen** should be supplied by nasal cannula or face mask when sedation is given. When benzodiazepines and narcotics are combined, even healthy patients breathing room air may become hypoxic.

3. **Monitoring** should include pulse oximetry, continuous ECG, and BP.

4. **Agents.** All medications should be titrated, with adequate time between doses to judge clinical effects. The end result should be a calm, easily arousable, cooperative patient. Oversedation may result in hypoventilation, airway obstruction, or disinhibition. Dosages of commonly used sedatives are summarized in Table 6-4.

5. **Side effects** that result from benzodiazepine administration include oversedation, respiratory depression, and depressed airway reflexes. Flumazenil (Romazicon), a benzodiazepine antagonist, can be used to reverse such effects. A dose of 0.2 mg intravenously should be administered and repeated every 60 seconds as required to a total dose of 1 mg. It can produce seizures and cardiac arrhythmias. Sedation can recur after 30 to 60 minutes, requiring repeated dosing.

POSTOPERATIVE MEDICATION AND COMPLICATIONS

I. **Postoperative analgesia** is provided to minimize patient discomfort and anxiety, attenuate the physiologic stress response to pain, enable optimal pulmonary toilet, and enable early ambulation. Analgesics can be administered by the oral, intravenous, or epidural route.

A. **Intravenous route.** Many patients are unable to tolerate oral medications in the immediate postoperative period. For these patients, narcotics can be administered intravenously by several mechanisms.

1. **As needed (p.r.n.)**

a. **Narcotics**

(1) The **intermittent administration of intravenous or intramuscular narcotics by nursing staff** has the disadvantage that the narcotics may be given too infrequently, too late, and in insufficient amounts to provide adequate pain control. This may be the only choice in patients who are functionally unable to operate a patient-controlled analgesia device.

(2) Morphine, 2 to 4 mg intravenously every 30 to 60 minutes, or **meperidine,** 50 to 100 mg intravenously every 30 to 60 minutes, should provide adequate analgesia for most patients. Orders should be written to withhold further injections for a respiratory rate of less than 12 breaths per minute or in cases of oversedation.

b. Nonsteroidal anti-inflammatory drugs (NSAIDs)

(1) Ketorolac is an NSAID that is available in oral and in injectable forms and is an effective adjunct to opioid therapy. The usual adult dose is 30 mg intramuscularly, followed by 15 to 30 mg every 6 hours.

(2) Ketorolac shares the potential side effects of other NSAIDs and should be used cautiously in the elderly and in patients with a history of peptic ulcer disease, renal insufficiency, steroid use, or volume depletion.

2. Patient-controlled analgesia (PCA)

a. With PCA, the patient has the ability to self-deliver analgesics within **preset safety parameters.**

b. Patients initially receive either **morphine** (100 mg in 100 mL, with each dose delivering 1 mg), **hydromorphone** (50 mg in 100 mL, with each dose delivering 0.25 mg), or **meperidine** (1,000 mg in 100 mL, with each dose delivering 20 mg), with a maximum of one dose every 10 minutes. If this treatment provides inadequate pain control, the concentration of the drug can be increased and/or the lockout time period can be reduced.

3. Continuous "basal" narcotic infusions are used rarely to treat patients who require sustained high serum narcotic concentrations. Continuous infusions should be used **with great caution** and only in patients with adequate monitoring and supervision to prevent respiratory depression and oversedation. Respiratory arrest can occur with the "buildup" of narcotic levels.

B. Epidural infusions are useful for treating postoperative pain caused by thoracotomy, extensive abdominal incisions, or orthopedic lower-extremity procedures. Narcotics, local anesthetics, or a mixture of the two can be infused continuously through catheters placed in the patient's lumbar or thoracic epidural space.

C. Oral agents. There are multiple oral agents and combination analgesics.

D. Side effects and complications

1. Oversedation and respiratory depression

a. Arousable, spontaneously breathing patients should be given supplemental oxygen and be monitored closely for signs of respiratory depression until mental status improves. Medications for pain or sedation should be decreased accordingly.

b. Unarousable but spontaneously breathing patients should be treated with oxygen and naloxone (Narcan). One vial of naloxone (0.4 mg) should be diluted in a 10-mL syringe, and 1 mL (0.04 mg) should be administered every 30 to 60 seconds until the patient is arousable. Adequate ventilation should be confirmed by arterial blood gas measurement. Current opioid administration should be stopped and the regimen decreased. In addition to continuous pulse oximetry, the patient should be monitored closely for potential recurrence of sedation as the effects of naloxone dissipate. Naloxone must be used carefully in patients with a history of coronary artery disease.

2. Apnea

a. Treatment involves immediate intubation and ventilation.

b. Naloxone, 0.2 to 0.4 mg intravenously, should be given immediately.

3. Hypotension and bradycardia

a. Local anesthetics administered via lumbar epidurals decrease sympathetic tone to the abdominal viscera and lower extremities and greatly increase venous capacitance. Thoracic epidurals can additionally block the cardioaccelerator fibers, resulting in bradycardia.

b. The **treatment** of choice for any of these situations (excluding brady-cardia) is volume resuscitation. Epinephrine can be used to raise BP acutely; 10 mg is diluted in 100 mL and given intravenously 1 mL at a time. If needed, this mixture can be infused intravenously starting at 15 mL per hour (25 μg per minute). Bradycardia can be treated with atropine, 0.4 to 1.0 mg intravenously, or glycopyrrolate given intravenously in 0.2-mg increments every 3 to 5 minutes as needed.

4. **Nausea and vomiting**
   a. **Naloxone** in small doses (0.04 to 0.1 mg intravenously as needed)
   b. **Metoclopramide** (10 mg intravenously every 6 hours)
   c. **Zofran** (4 mg intravenously every 6 to 8 hours)
   d. **Compazine** (10 mg intravenously or orally every 4 to 6 hours)

5. **Pruritus**
   a. **Naloxone**, 0.04 to 0.1 mg intravenously, is effective.
   b. **Diphenhydramine**, 25 to 50 mg intravenously as needed, may provide symptomatic relief.

6. **Monoamine oxidase inhibitors** (e.g., isocarboxazid, phenelzine) may **interact adversely with narcotics**, resulting in severe hemodynamic swings, respiratory depression, seizures, diaphoresis, hyperthermia, and coma. Meperidine has been most frequently implicated and should be avoided. Although morphine and fentanyl are believed to be safe, narcotics should be avoided whenever possible.

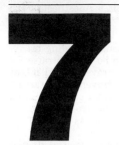

Vascular Access, Tubes, and Drains

Celine Buckley, David M. Hovsepian, and Surendra Shenoy

VENOUS ACCESS DEVICES

I. Indications. Indications for central venous access devices (CVADs) typically include (1) administration of fluids, blood products, and irritant medications such as vancomycin, potassium chloride, and cancer chemotherapy drugs; (2) monitoring of intravascular volume; (3) parenteral nutrition; (4) hemodialysis; (5) temporary transvenous cardiac pacing; and (6) blood sampling, when peripheral vein cannulation is not possible.

II. Sites of CVAD insertion. The internal jugular and subclavian veins are the most common sites for CVAD insertion.

   A. Internal jugular vein access. For elective central access, the right internal jugular vein remains the access route of choice. Reasons for this preference include its superficial position, its large size, the lower incidence of pneumothorax, the straight course to the superior vena cava, and the lower likelihood of malposition. Compared with subclavian vein access, stenoses involving internal jugular cannulation are less likely to cause morbidity, and the adjacent carotid artery can be directly compressed if inadvertently punctured. In addition, subclavian catheterization should be avoided in patients with severe hypoxemia, as these patients have little reserve to tolerate a pneumothorax. Specifically relevant to dialysis patients, subclavian access jeopardizes the use of present or future shunts on that side. The right internal jugular route of access is preferred for this group of patients.

   B. Subclavian vein access. The Centers for Disease Control (CDC) published guidelines in 2002 that recommend the use of subclavian access when possible in some subsets of patients, such as intensive care patients, who are at higher risk for CVAD infection when the CVAD is placed in the neck.

   C. Femoral vein access. Femoral veins may be used in emergent situations, but drawbacks include an even higher risk of infection from groin bacteria, problems with catheter kinking and malfunction, the development of deep venous thrombosis, and impairment of ambulation.

   D. Percutaneous placement. Venous access is gained percutaneously using the Seldinger ("over-the-guidewire") technique (see also Chapter 42, section I.) Portable ultrasound units, such as the Site-Rite (Dymax Corp, Pittsburgh, Pa), aid in safe and reliable needle insertion. Contrast injection through a peripheral intravenous line or fluoroscopic guidance using bone landmarks can aid subclavian vein access.

III. Preoperative evaluation. Before placement of a CVAD, the patient should be evaluated for previous central venous lines, the presence of a transvenous pacemaker, and signs of central venous obstruction, such as collateral veins about the shoulder and neck. Active site infection, an open wound, a tracheostomy, and tumors of the head and neck can influence the type and route chosen for catheter insertion. For example, women who have undergone axillary lymph node dissection during breast cancer surgery should have a CVAD inserted on the contralateral side to avoid the potential morbidity that can result from catheter-related central venous thrombosis.

Pertinent laboratory tests include coagulation parameters, hematocrit, and platelet count. For maximum safety, we recommend a minimum platelet count of 50,000 platelets/mL and an international normalized ratio (INR) below 2.25 for placement of a tunneled catheter. For placement of peripheral and nontunneled lines, these parameters are relaxed to a platelet count above 25,000/mL and an INR as high as 4.25, as bleeding complications can be readily identified and addressed, often with compressive dressings alone.

IV. **Types of catheters.** The terminology used to identify the different types of catheters refers to a variety of features. These include the number of lumen (single, double, triple), the location (artery or vein), the lifespan (temporary, intermediate-term, or long-term), the site of insertion (subclavian, femoral, internal jugular, peripheral), the presence or absence of a tract under skin (e.g., tunneled, nontunneled), the catheter length (arm's-length, to superior vena cava, to cavoatrial junction), specific characteristics (Dacron and/or antibiotic cuff, impregnated with heparin or antibiotic), and the structure of the tip (valved, nonvalved).

A. **Short-term (nontunneled) CVADs.** The advantages of single-lumen and multilumen nontunneled catheters include low cost, bedside placement and removal, and easy exchange of damaged catheters over a guidewire. The disadvantages arise from the inherent lack of durability (catheter displacement or infection) of these devices, as they are designed only for short-term use. Examples include the **triple-lumen catheter**, the **Quinton dialysis catheter** (now the **Mahurkar catheter**, Kendall, Mansfield, Minn), and the **Hemo-Cath pheresis catheter** (Medcomp, Harleysville, Pa).

B. **Intermediate-term, peripherally inserted CVADs.** Peripherally inserted central catheters (PICCs) are composed of Silastic or polyurethane, can be kept in place for up to 6 months, are commonly used for home total parenteral nutrition (TPN) or intravenous antibiotic (e.g., vancomycin for endocarditis or osteomyelitis) administration (4 to 12 weeks). PICC lines can be inserted using local anesthetic by a trained nurse at the bedside via the cephalic, basilic, or median cubital veins. They have a low risk of insertion-related complications, such as pneumothorax, and cost less to insert. They are associated with a lower infection rate by virtue of fewer skin bacteria on the arm compared to the chest wall (10^5 fewer bacteria per cm^2). The inherent disadvantages of these catheters result from their small size and long length (40 to 60 cm), including problems with withdrawal occlusion and a significant risk for thrombophlebitis (*JVIR* 2000;11:1309–1314).

C. **Intermediate-term, nontunneled CVADS.** The **Hohn catheter** is the prototypical CVAD of this type and can be placed at the bedside. Yet, it is better to perform this insertion procedure in a sterile setting using image guidance (ultrasound, fluoroscopy, and/or venography). Although no true tunnel is constructed, the addition of a silver-impregnated gelatin cuff (Vitacuff) just beneath the skin at the point of entry serves as a temporary barrier to infection. The gelatin dissolves within a short time, and there is no incorporation into the tissues, making removal easy. They are ideal for TPN, intermediate-term treatment, such as for bacterial endocarditis or induction chemotherapy, but can stay in for up to 6 months. Removal, as with other nontunneled central lines, consists of releasing the anchoring sutures, withdrawing the catheter, and applying gentle compression over the venotomy site for several minutes.

D. **Long-term, tunneled CVADS.** Tunneled catheters enable indefinite venous access for prolonged nutritional support, chemotherapy, antibiotics, or hemodialysis. They are typically tunneled subcutaneously from the chest wall to the subclavian or internal jugular vein and threaded into the superior vena cava. The subcutaneous portion of the catheter contains a double cuff (bicuff) that functions to induce scar formation, anchoring the catheter in place and preventing bacterial migration from skin. The antibacterial-coated (e.g., chlorhexidine) bicuffs are designed to lower the incidence of catheter-related bloodstream infections. Most tunneled catheters are manufactured using silicone, which is inherently more flexible and durable than other plastic used for catheters. Examples include the **Hickman** and

Broviac catheters (Bard Access Systems), which are smaller and intended for pediatric patients. The **Groshong catheter** differs by the presence of a slit valve at the tip, which seals it from the bloodstream. Unlike other venous catheters, which require heparinized saline injections daily or weekly, it only requires flushing with normal saline. This device is thus especially well suited for patients with a history of heparin allergy or heparin-induced thrombocytopenia. Hemodialysis catheters frequently are constructed using polyurethane because they can be made with thinner walls that allow for higher flow rates. Patients with exhausted upper extremity veins require different approaches such as translumbar, transhepatic, intercostal, and lower-extremity venous access.

E. **Implanted venous ports.** Ports were introduced in the early 1980s. They are used primarily for chronic therapy that lasts longer than 6 months and for which only intermittent access is needed. Common indications include chemotherapy and frequent hospitalization (e.g., patients with sickle cell disease or cystic fibrosis), and they are also used for cosmesis. Implanted ports are similar to tunneled catheters and are placed using the same techniques. Access is preferably obtained via the internal jugular vein and a reservoir placed in a subcutaneous pocket created in the infraclavicular fossa. Smaller port devices (e.g., **PASport**, Sims-Deltec, St. Paul, Minn) are designed for upper-extremity implantation. Most models contain a silicone or polyurethane catheter connected to a metal or plastic reservoir with a dense silicone septum for percutaneous needle access. Advantages of ports over other CVADs include a lower incidence of infection if not accessed too frequently and less maintenance (monthly heparin flushes when not in use). Plastic ports are magnetic resonance scan compatible (e.g., **MRI port**, Bard Access Systems) and are as durable as ports with reservoirs constructed of metal. Port access requires skin puncture using a special noncoring (Huber) needle to prevent deterioration of the septum. Ports are therefore inappropriate for daily access. Moreover, a port and its septum may be difficult to localize in large patients, especially when the pocket has been created along a deep or angled plane, which predisposes to cutaneous extravasation of infusate. Deep venous thrombosis complicates approximately 2% to 6.5% of ports but is usually asymptomatic when internal jugular access has been used.

V. **Catheter maintenance.** Proper care of access sites and devices is crucial to their long-term function. Short-term and tunneled CVADs require sterile, occlusive, transparent dressings that are changed weekly by trained personnel using meticulous technique. More frequent dressing changes may be needed for those patients who are immune compromised. Application of topical antibiotic beneath an occlusive dressing may provide a moist culture medium for bacterial growth. Catheter lumens should be flushed on a regular basis to prevent thrombosis, as outlined below.

A. **Venous access device care**
   1. **Aspirate contents of catheter lumen.**
   2. **Flush with saline** (10 mL normal saline).
   3. **Administer medications, fluids, and other infusates.**
   4. **Flush with saline** (10 mL normal saline).
   5. **Heparin lock per the following** (clamp while gently infusing the last 0.5 mL):
      a. **Hickman catheter** (2.5 mL/lumen): heparin, 100 units/mL
      b. **Implanted port** (5.0 mL/lumen): heparin, 100 units/mL
      c. **Hohn catheter** (2.0 mL/lumen): heparin, 100 units/mL
      d. **Plasmapheresis or dialysis catheter** (1.5 mL/lumen): heparin, 1,000 units/mL
      e. **PICC** (2.5 mL/lumen): heparin, 100 units/mL
      f. **Groshong catheter** (10 mL/lumen): normal saline

VI. **Complications.** Factors determining the risk of complications include (1) catheter-related features such as material, heparin, antiseptics, and antibiotic coating; (2) patient-related issues, such as underlying disease, anatomy, medications, and immune system competence; (3) central venous access site; and (4) catheter use and care by medical and nursing staff. Early complications of CVAD placement are often due to injury to anatomic structures during blind needle-sticks and passage of guidewires and catheters. Vein localization with ultrasound and fluoroscopically guided catheter placement has greatly reduced complications such as pneumothorax and catheter tip malposition.

VII. Mechanical complications

A. Pneumothorax. The incidence of pneumothorax for subclavian vein lines ranges from 1% to 4%, depending on operator experience, and accounts for one-fourth to one-half of reported early access complications. Fewer than half require tube thoracostomy. Asymptomatic pneumothoraces, occupying less than 30% of hemithoracic volume, usually only require observation and serial chest imaging. Increasing shortness of breath, rapid progression to a large pneumothorax, or signs of mediastinal shift should prompt insertion of a chest tube. Hemothorax usually requires insertion of a large-bore chest tube through a lateral thoracostomy. Small, apical pneumothoraces can be drained with a Heimlich valve (Becton-Dickinson and Company, Franklin Lakes, NJ) attached to an Angiocath or small-bore drainage tube (e.g., No. 8 Fr.). Pneumothorax complicates internal jugular access with an average incidence of 0.2% to 0.5% (*Acta Anesthesiol Scand* 1982;26:485); such cases usually result from skin puncture too close to the clavicle (*Anesthesiology* 1982;56:321).

B. Bleeding. Sudden decompensation during central CVAD insertion almost always indicates mediastinal hematoma, hemothorax, or pericardial tamponade from perforation. Although rare, bleeding due to perforation of the central venous system or heart by the guidewire, sheath, or catheter represents the most common cause of access-related mortality.

C. Arterial puncture. Anatomic variations in the relative positions of the internal jugular vein and the carotid artery are well known. Troianos et al. demonstrated that the carotid artery lies posterior to the internal jugular vein in a significant percentage of patients, predisposing it to injury if both walls of the vein are traversed (*Anesthesiology* 1996;85:43–48). Carotid artery puncture complicates internal jugular cannulation in 3% to 10% cases, representing 80% to 90% of all complications. Although carotid artery puncture is usually a benign event, it can be life-threatening when it results in inadvertent intra-arterial cannulation, stroke, hemothorax, carotid artery–internal jugular fistula, or airway compromise due to a neck hematoma. Subclavian artery puncture occurs in 0.5% to 1% of cases, constituting one-fourth to one-third of all complications. Femoral artery puncture occurs in 5% to 10% of femoral vein cannulations, with major hematomas forming in 1% of these patients. Even in the presence of coagulopathy, only rare reports document life-threatening thigh or retroperitoneal hemorrhage. The risk of arterial puncture can be significantly reduced using real-time ultrasound-guided cannulation, especially in infants and young children (*Anesthesiology* 1999;91:71–77). Other factors that predispose to arterial injury include small vein diameter and the relative positioning of the head, which can influence the location of the internal jugular vein during attempted internal jugular access. Return of pulsatile or bright-red blood from the introducer needle indicates probable arterial cannulation. In a hypoxemic or hypotensive patient, extension tubing with three-way stopcock can be attached to the catheter. Noting pulsatile flow in the tubing when it is held upright well above the level of the heart unequivocally demonstrates arterial cannulation. In patients with severe CHF and/or severe tricuspid regurgitation, blood may not necessarily be pulsatile but will rise to the end of tubing. When the artery is punctured, the needle should be withdrawn and sufficient pressure applied to tamponade the arteriotomy without overstimulating the carotid body and causing a vagal response. If a carotid arteriotomy is dilated and a sheath is placed, there is a significant risk for cerebrovascular events. If arterial puncture is diagnosed after the dilator has been threaded, it should be kept in place and a vascular surgeon consulted.

D. Catheter tip malposition. The catheter tip should ideally be located at the cavoatrial junction. The cavoatrial junction lies approximately 5 cm below the right tracheobronchial angle, which is the most reliable fluoroscopic landmark. This distance remains relatively constant regardless of patient gender and body habitus. Accurate placement can be documented by fluoroscopy or chest x-ray. Positioning of the catheter tip deep within the right atrium or into the right ventricle can be complicated by arrhythmias, intraventricular thrombus formation, perforation of the heart, cardiac tamponade, and death. Conversely, catheters placed too high in the superior vena cava or in the brachiocephalic veins will malfunction more frequently, particularly if inserted from the left side (*Chest* 1992;101:1633–1638). For lower-extremity CVADs, the confluence of the iliac veins represents the ideal position. Malpositioned catheters are best addressed by safe repositioning under fluoroscopic guidance

E. Air embolism. Venous air embolism is a rare but life-threatening complication that may occur during insertion, manipulation, or removal of a central venous catheter. One hundred cubic milliliters of air per second can enter the central venous system through a 14-gauge needle, even with a pressure gradient as low as 5 cm H_2O (*Ann Surg* 1974;179:479–481). Air embolism most commonly occurs as a catheter is being inserted through a peel-away sheath. Placing the patient in Trendelenburg position and performing Valsalva maneuver to increase the intrathoracic pressure often avoids air embolism. Applying occlusive dressing over the catheter exit site prevents air entry into the venous system through well-formed catheter tracts. Air embolus should be suspected in any patient with indwelling or recently discontinued CVAD in whom sudden unexplained hypoxemia or cardiovascular collapse develops. A large, sudden volume of air may generate an "air lock" in the chambers of the right heart or at the level of the pulmonary circulation, reducing forward blood outflow and causing rapid cardiovascular collapse. A characteristic mill wheel heart murmur may be auscultated over precordium. "Paradoxical" air embolism into the arterial circulation may occur through a patent foramen ovale or any other right-to-left shunt (*Crit Care Med* 2000;28:1621–1625). Treatment involves placing the patient in the Trendelenburg position with the right side up (to trap the air pocket), attempting to aspirate the air by attaching a syringe and withdrawing from the catheter, and providing supplemental oxygen.

F. Catheter embolism, breakage, and pinch-off syndrome. Risk of CVAD breakage occurs most commonly following extensive catheter manipulation during a difficult insertion procedure. A subclavian catheter may get compressed by the costoclavicular ligament and subclavius muscle, close to the junction of the first rib and clavicle. Repetitive compression in this area may cause catheter fatigue and fracture, which has been termed "pinch-off syndrome." The central catheter fragment can embolize to the right heart (*AJR Am J Roentgenol* 2002;179:309–318). Catheter fracture or separation of the reservoir and catheter may be suspected when a CVAD suddenly fails to function, especially if there is associated pain or swelling or a new arrhythmia develops. Any detached catheter fragment should be retrieved, which is usually easily done by radiological techniques.

G. Extravasation. Leakage of infusate from a vein into the subcutaneous tissue can occur as a result of CVAD dislocation, displacement of a port access needle, or separation of a catheter from its reservoir. Development of a fibrin sheath around a catheter may force infusate to flow back along the catheter outside the vein. Extravasation may result in pain or swelling, or both, and the severity of tissue injury depends on the amount and type of infusate. Chemotherapy agents are particularly irritating and can produce

substantial soft-tissue necrosis, requiring extensive débridement and, occasionally, reconstructive surgery.
H. **Thrombosis and stenosis.** More than 50,000 instances of deep venous thrombosis occur per year, 30% to 40% associated with central venous catheters. Partial and complete catheter blockage is evidenced by difficulty in aspirating blood or infusing fluid. Catheter blockage may be due to kinking of the catheter in the subclavian vein, occlusion of the catheter tip on the vessel wall, or luminal thrombosis. The spectrum of thrombotic complications ranges from fibrin sleeve formation around the catheter to mural or occlusive thrombus. Although only 3% to 5% of central venous catheters develop clinically significant thromboses, ultrasonography with color Doppler imaging has been found to detect venous thrombosis in 33% to 67% of patients when the indwelling time of the CVAD was greater than a week (*Chest* 1998;113:165–171). A negative Doppler ultrasound in a symptomatic patient should be followed by venographic assessment, as thrombi in the central upper venous system (superior vena cava, brachiocephalic, and subclavian veins) are better detected by venography. Multiple factors predispose to thrombus formation.
   1. **Patient-related risk factors** include prothrombotic states associated with underlying genetic coagulation disorders, malignancy, chronic disease, hydration state, nutritional status, and prior history of CVAD placement
   2. **Infusate-related risk factors** include solution composition, osmolality, and pH.
   3. **Catheter-related risk factors** include size, position, infection, and duration of placement. Risk of catheter-related thrombosis varies according to site of insertion, with reported rates of 21.5% in femoral catheters compared to only 1.9% with subclavian access (*P* <0.001) (*JAMA* 2001;286:700–707). Catheters in the subclavian or innominate veins are at higher risk for producing symptomatic central venous stenosis than are those that are placed in the right internal jugular vein. More pliable and smoother catheter material, such as silicone, is less thrombogenic than stiffer catheter materials, such as polyurethane. Risk of infection strongly correlates to the presence of thrombus. Regular flushing protocols may reduce the incidence of thrombotic complications. Thrombolytic intervention with urokinase or alteplase is generally an effective and safe means of restoring CVAD function and blood flow without resorting to catheter replacement. If this procedure fails or there is symptomatic upper limb thrombosis, systemic anticoagulation may be indicated. Prophylactic use of low-dose warfarin has been advocated in patients with cancer, who often have associated hypercoagulable syndromes, to prevent catheter-related venous thrombosis (*Ann Intern Med* 1990;112:423–429).
VIII. **Complications: infections.** Catheter-related bloodstream infection (CRBSI) occurs with a prevalence ranging from 3% to 7% and has a mortality rate of 15% (*Infect Control Hosp Epidemiol* 2000;21:375–380). Catheter colonization —or bacterial growth from the catheter tip—occurs in 20% of central venous catheters (*J Clin Microbiol* 19900;28:2520–2525).
   A. **Epidemiology.** Catheter-related bloodstream infections (CRBSIs) are generally caused by coagulase-negative staphylococci (~37%), followed by enterococci (13.5%), coagulase-positive *Staphylococcus aureus* (12.6%), and *Candida albicans* (8%). Treatment of these organisms has become increasingly difficult now that more than 50% of *S. aureus* isolates and more than 80% of coagulase-negative *Staphylococcus* isolates are resistant to oxacillin. The percentage of enterococcal isolates resistant to vancomycin has also increased, from 0.5% in 1989 to 25.9% in 1999 (*MMWR* 2002;51:1–29). For lower-extremity CVAD, Gram-negative rods represent the most frequent organisms, along with enterococci. Sixty-eight percent of catheter

infections are monomicrobial, and the remaining 32% are polymicrobial (*Arch Surg* 1998;133:1241–1246).

B. Pathogenesis. Infection of indwelling vascular catheters occurs from two routes. First, endogenous skin flora at the insertion site migrate along the external surface of the catheter and colonize the intravascular tip. Second, pathogens from contamination at the hub colonize the internal surface of the catheter and are washed into the bloodstream when the catheter is infused. Occasionally, catheters may become hematogenously seeded from another focus of infection. Rarely, infusate contamination leads to CRBSI. Important pathogenic determinants of catheter-related infection are as follows.

   1. Catheter material. Studies have demonstrated that catheters made of polyvinyl chloride or polyethylene are less resistant to adherence of microorganisms than are catheters made of Teflon, silicone elastomer, or polyurethane. Additionally, certain catheter materials are more thrombogenic than others, a characteristic that also might predispose to catheter colonization and CRBSI.

   2. Virulence of the infecting organism. The adherence properties of a given organism are important in the pathogenesis of CRBSI. *S. aureus* can adhere to host proteins such as fibronectin, which is commonly deposited on catheters. Also, coagulase-negative staphylococci adhere to polymer surfaces more readily than other surfaces and more readily than do other pathogens. Additionally, certain strains of coagulase-negative staphylococci produce an extracellular polysaccharide layer referred to as "biofilm" or "slime."

C. Definitions and diagnosis. Catheter colonization is defined as >15 colony-forming units of microorganisms on semiquantitative culture. Exit site infection presents with erythema, tenderness, induration, or purulence within 2 cm of the exit site of the catheter. The definition of CRBSI requires bacteremia or fungemia in a patient with CVAD and meeting of the following criteria: (1) clinical signs of infection (fever, chills, tachycardia, hypotension, leukocytosis), (2) no identifiable source for bloodstream infection other than the CVAD, and (3) isolation of the same organism from semiquantitative culture of the catheter and from the blood (drawn from a peripheral vein taken within 48 hours of each other) (*Clin Infect Dis* 2001;32:1249–1272). Diagnosis of CRBSI with coagulase-negative staphylococci requires two positive blood cultures.

D. Presentation. Catheter infections may manifest with local, regional, or systemic signs.

   1. Local catheter-related infections. Exit site infections may present with erythema and drainage locally. In the absence of systemic signs and negative blood cultures, treatment consists of routine antibiotics for skin flora and more frequent dressing changes and care. Catheter removal is required in only 10% of cases.

   2. Regional catheter infections. Tunnel infections or pocket infections present with erythema, induration, and tenderness along the catheter tract or over the pocket, often with a clear demarcation of the affected area. Often there are systemic or laboratory signs of bacteremia. If the diagnosis of a regional infection is made, the CVAD usually needs to be removed, and in some cases the tunnel or pocket may need to be débrided. Antibiotic treatment alone is rarely successful.

   3. Bacteremia or sepsis. Sepsis is the most severe manifestation of a catheter-related infection. Although the conservative approach necessitates removal of all CVADs in septic patients, in patients with limited access and other potential sources for infection, broad-spectrum antibiotics can be initiated and continued for 10 to 14 days. If the fever resolves, the catheter usually can be left in place unless evidence of a tunnel or pocket infection develops. Worsening septicemia or failure to resolve requires catheter removal. One exception is the presence of fungemia, which requires the catheter to be removed, with immediate initiation of antifungal treatment.

E. **Risk factors.** Several factors increase the risk of CVAD-related infections, including neutropenia, malignancy, parenteral feeding, ICU admission, mechanical ventilation, hyperalimentation, increasing number of catheter lumens, and thrombus. The risk for infection varies with the catheter insertion site, with the femoral vein associated with a much higher infection rate than subclavian vein access (19.8% versus 4.5%) (*JAMA* 2001;286:700–707). Jugular venous catheterization carries an intermediate risk of infection. The likelihood of infection clearly correlates to dwell time. For catheters in from 3 to 7 days, the cumulative infection risk doubles from 5% to 10% over that period of time. The presence of thrombus or a fibrin sleeve promotes the adherence of bacteria (mainly *S. aureus* and *S. epidermidis*) and mycetes (mainly *C. albicans*).

F. **Antimicrobial-impregnated catheters.** Antimicrobial-coated catheters, ionic silver cuffs, antibiotic-impregnated hubs, and intraluminal antibiotic locks have all been shown to reduce the incidence of CRBSI in critically ill patients. In a multicenter randomized trial, CVADs impregnated on the external and internal surfaces with minocycline/rifampin were associated with lower rates of CRBSI than the first-generation chlorhexidine/silver sulfadiazine–impregnated catheters (*N Eng J Med* 1999;340:1–8). The emergence of resistant organisms resulting from the use of antimicrobial-impregnated catheters remains a potentially important concern.

Routine (elective) catheter replacement. The clear correlation between catheter indwelling time and risk of infections spurred the practice of routine replacement of CVADs. However, studies in which CVAD were replaced every 3 to 7 days reported no decrease in infection rates, and routine replacement had the added disadvantage of increasing the mechanical complication rates (*N Eng J Med*, 1992;327:1062–1068). No study to date has demonstrated any benefit of *de novo* replacement at 7 days. Bacteremia is usually due to colonization of the skin tract between the insertion site and the vein; therefore, replacement over a guidewire is likely to result in recontamination. A new site for access should be chosen when possible.

VASCULAR ACCESS FOR DIALYSIS

The success of hemodialysis depends on the rate of blood flow through the dialyzer. Flow rates of between 350 mL and 450 mL per minute are required to provide adequate dialysis within a reasonable time frame (3 to 4 hours). The dialysis access is a port or site in the body that provides the necessary blood flow for dialysis. The access should be easy to cannulate and last for years with minimal maintenance. The incidence of complications, such as infection, stenosis, pseudoaneurysm formation, thrombosis, and outflow deterioration, should also be low. To date, no access type fulfills all of these criteria.

I. **Indications**

A. **Temporary hemodialysis access** provided with short- or intermediate-term CVADs is indicated when acute short-term dialysis is needed, as in (1) acute renal failure, (2) overdose or intoxication, (3) end-stage renal disease needing urgent hemodialysis without available mature access, (4) peritoneal dialysis patients with peritonitis, and (5) transplant recipients needing temporary hemodialysis during severe rejection episodes.

B. **Permanent hemodialysis access** is provide by surgical creation of subcutaneous conduits having high blood flows when long-term hemodialysis is needed, as in (1) long-term treatment of chronic renal failure and (2) patients awaiting deceased donor renal transplantation.

II. **Nomenclature**

A. **Dialysis access catheters**

1. **Nontunneled central venous catheters.** Short-term dialysis access includes percutaneous catheters in internal jugular, subclavian, or femoral

veins. The **Quinton catheter** provides access for short-term hemodialysis in acute renal failure, when established access fails and corrective action must be delayed for a short period, or as an alternative to peritoneal dialysis in patients who have undergone recent abdominal surgery. Noncuffed, double-lumen catheters can be percutaneously inserted at the bedside and provide acceptable blood flow rates (250 mL/min) for temporary hemodialysis—no more than 3 weeks for internal jugular or 5 days for femoral catheters due to considerations of infection and dislodgement.

   2. **Tunneled central venous silicone dialysis catheters.** Tunneled catheters (e.g., **Tesio, Ash Split** (Bard Access Systems), **and Duraflow catheters** (AngioDynamics)) have cuffs that anchor them to the subcutaneous tissues. Some indications for placement include need for access for longer than 3 weeks, exhaustion of all other access options, maturing primary arteriovenous (AV) fistula, and bridge to transplant in living-donor candidates. Tunneled, cuffed venous catheters should be placed preferentially in the right internal jugular vein because this site offers a more direct route to the cavoatrial junction and a lower risk of complications than other potential catheter insertion sites. Advantages of tunneled catheters include the ability to insert into a variety of sites, no maturation time requirement, no hemodynamic consequences, ease and cost of catheter placement and replacement, and a lifespan of the access of months to years. Disadvantages of tunneled, cuffed venous catheters include potential morbidity due to thrombosis, infection, risk of permanent central venous stenosis or occlusion, and lower blood flow rates than for AV grafts and fistulas.

   3. **Subcutaneous Hemodialysis ports.** The FDA has recently approved the LifeSite Hemodialysis Access System (Vasca, Inc., Tewksbury, Mass) as an acceptable subcutaneous venous access system that allows transcutaneous venous hemodialysis. The device consists of a valve, typically implanted below the clavicle, and a silicone cannula preferably tunneled to the right internal jugular vein. Access with a 14-gauge dialysis needle (Medisystems, Seattle, Wash) actuates an internal pinch clamp inside the valve. With needle removal, the pinch clamp closes, stopping flow. Two devices are typically implanted, one for withdrawal and one for return of blood during hemodialysis. The use of a 14-gauge needle enables the maintenance of a high flow rate with no increase in hemolysis. Another benefit of this access system resides in the ability to disinfect *in vivo* the valve, tissue pocket, and buttonhole before and after each use with an antimicrobial agent. This along with its subcutaneous placement decreases the rate of infectious complications. Indications for this device are similar to those for intermediate-term catheters—as a bridge for fistula maturation or in patients who have exhausted all other access options.

B. **Catheter complications**
   1. **Early dysfunction** usually occurs secondary to either malposition or intracatheter thrombosis.
   2. **Late dysfunction (>5 days).** Almost all catheters inserted into a central vein develop a fibrin sleeve after insertion. They are usually clinically silent until they obstruct the ports at the distal end of the catheter. They can also serve as a nidus for infection.
   3. **Central vein stenosis, thrombosis, or stricture.** Central vein stenosis arises from endothelial injury at the site of catheter-endothelial contact. Incidence increases with the use of nonsilicone catheters, with the use of a subclavian approach, and with a history of prior catheter-related infections. Removal of the CVAD may not improve the underlying problem and, by definition, sacrifices the access. Systemic anticoagulation remains the primary therapy.

C. Arteriovenous (AV) access nomenclature
   1. **Conduit. An autogenous conduit** is a subcutaneous native vein that is in situ, transposed, or translocated. An **autogenous AV access (also known as an AV fistula, a native vein fistula, and a primary fistula)** is an access created by connecting a native vein to an adjacent artery. A **nonautogenous conduit** is a prosthetic graft placed subcutaneously to connect an artery to a vein. **A nonautogenous AV access (also known as an AV graft or a graft fistula)** uses grafts that are either synthetic or biologic. **Synthetic grafts** include expanded polytetrafluoroethylene (ePTFE, e.g., Gore-Tex or Impra) and polyester (e.g., Dacron) grafts. **Biologic grafts** include bovine heterografts, human umbilical veins, and cryo-preserved allogeneic human vein grafts.
   2. **Configuration. A direct access** often connects a native vein to an adjacent artery. An **indirect access** uses an autogenous or prosthetic material placed subcutaneously between the artery and vein. All prosthetic accesses, therefore, constitute indirect configurations by definition. The course of the subcutaneous prosthesis may be **looped** (loop graft) or **straight** (straight graft).

III. Preoperative evaluation
   A. Timing. Ideally, any patient with renal insufficiency should be referred for surgical evaluation approximately 1 year before the anticipated need for dialysis. This point is reached when the creatinine clearance is less than 25 mL per minute or the serum creatinine rises above 4 mg/dL. This provides ample opportunity and time for appropriate access planning, and efforts can be instituted to ensure preservation of the native veins for later AV fistula creation.
   B. Preservation of access sites. All end-stage renal disease (ESRD) patients should protect their forearm veins from venipuncture and intravenous catheters. Likewise, hospital staff should be instructed to avoid damaging these essential veins. The nondominant arm is preferred for initial access creation. The sites in the dorsum of the hand should be frequently rotated in ESRD patients requiring routine venipuncture. Subclavian vein cannulation should be avoided at all costs, as this may induce central venous stenosis, which could preclude later use of an entire arm.
   C. History. A detailed assessment for the presence of peripheral vascular disease, diabetes mellitus, cardiopulmonary disease, and coagulation disorders best determines the type of vascular access needed for a particular patient. Any conditions that suggest stenosis or occlusion of the venous or arterial system should be elicited, as these may limit options for dialysis access. These include prior central venous line; transvenous pacemaker; previous surgery; trauma; or radiation treatment to the chest, neck, or arm. Evidence of early cardiac dysfunction or volume overload indicates a patient at risk for congestive heart failure following fistula creation due to increased preload. Comorbid conditions that limit life expectancy, such as severe coronary artery disease or malignancy, may render a cuffed catheter the best option.
   D. Physical examination
   1. **Pulse examination.** The axillary, brachial, radial, and ulnar artery pulses are carefully palpated in both upper extremities, and, when indicated, the femoral, popliteal, and pedal arteries are palpated. Residual scars from previous central venous catheters or surgery should also be carefully assessed.
   2. **Cardiovascular status.** Evaluation involves determining capillary refill, the presence of edema, unequal extremity size, and collateral veins on the chest wall. A tourniquet, gravity, and gentle percussion are used to distend the forearm and upper arm veins. Their patency and continuity can be addressed by palpation and detection of a fluid thrill.

3. **Segmental blood pressure measurements.** Discrepancies between the two upper extremities should be noted.
4. **Allen test.** This is intended to assess the integrity of the palmar circulatory arches and allow assessment of the dominant blood supply to the hand.

E. **Duplex ultrasound scanning.** Duplex ultrasound scan can determine the diameter of the artery and the adequacy of the superficial and deep veins. For venous evaluation, tourniquets are placed on the patient's midforearm and upper arm. Details of the venous lumen, such as webs, sclerosis, and occlusion, can be visualized. Doppler venous studies may also identify suitable veins for AV fistula creation that are not readily visible on the surface anatomy, especially in heavier patients.

F. **Diagnostic imaging.** History or physical findings suggestive of central venous stenosis or previous complicated vascular access warrant further diagnostic imaging.
1. **Contrast venography.** Venography is the gold standard for determining the patency and adequacy of the superficial and deep venous systems, particularly the central veins.
2. **Conventional arteriography or magnetic resonance angiography.** Angiography also remains the gold standard for the evaluation of a suspected arterial inflow stenosis or occlusion. When in doubt as to the adequacy of the donor artery or the runoff, it is advisable to obtain an arteriogram that shows the entire arterial system from the origin of the subclavian artery to the distal branches. Magnetic resonance angiography can also be used for the same purpose and is particularly useful when severe contrast allergy, vascular disease, or poor renal function preclude arteriography.

G. **Laboratory studies.** Hyperkalemia and acidosis are the most common electrolyte abnormalities seen in ESRD patients. Therefore, preoperative testing should include evaluation of serum electrolytes and glucose to avoid possible procedural or anesthesia-related complications.

IV. **Native vein AV fistulas**
A. **Characteristics.** Native vein fistulas are created by connecting a vein to the adjacent artery, usually the radial or brachial artery. These are the safest and longest lasting permanent means of vascular access, with the highest 5-year patency rates and minimum requirements for intervention. Disadvantages include a long maturation time of weeks to months to provide a flow state adequate to sustain dialysis. Revision of the outflow vein and hand exercises to increase flow to the extremity can accelerate fistula maturation. The patient's arterial and venous anatomy remains the most significant limitation, as diseased vessels (e.g., due to diabetes or atherosclerosis) can hinder normal maturation or may preclude the creation of a fistula altogether. Of the ESRD population in the United States, approximately 30% have AV fistulas as their permanent dialysis access (*Kidney Int* 2000;58:2178–2185). The Kidney Disease Outcomes Quality Initiative (K/DOQI) guidelines recommend a 50% fistula placement rate for first-time access in ESRD patients.
B. **Location.** The Brescia-Cimino fistula at the wrist (creating an end-to-side anastomosis between the cephalic vein and radial artery) and the Gratz fistula at the elbow (i.e., anastomosing the cephalic vein to the brachial artery) are the two most commonly performed autogenous AV fistulas. Flow of arterial blood under pressure distends the outflow vein to produce the subcutaneous conduit. The nondominant arm should preferentially be used to facilitate self-dialysis and limit rare consequences of any functional disability. Peripheral sites should be used first, moving to more central sites as the former sites fail.
C. **Construction.** Most procedures can be performed on an outpatient basis, using only conscious sedation administered intravenously and local analgesia. The end of a superficial vein, usually the cephalic, is anastomosed to

the side of the artery. The side-to-side anastomosis that is performed some-times can result in venous hypertension and swelling in the distal extremity due to higher venous pressures. An end-to-end anastomosis performed in a radial artery fistula has the advantage of providing limited flow, thereby re-ducing a hypercirculatory state. The disadvantage is that the anastomosis is technically challenging and has the risk of hand ischemia. This risk is particularly high in elderly and diabetic patients. The length (diameter) of the anastomosis dictates the blood flow in fistulas based on larger arter-ies (e.g., the brachial artery), making it an important determinant in the development of vascular steal symptoms in distal extremity.

V. AV graft

   A. Characteristics. AV grafts consist of biologic or synthetic conduits that connect an artery and a vein and are tunneled under the skin and placed in a subcutaneous location. PTFE material allows in-growth of host tissue and formation of a pseudointimal lining, which resists infection and self-seals after needle puncture. The advantages of AV grafts over AV fistulas include (1) large surface area, (2) easy cannulation, (3) short maturation time, and (4) easy surgical handling. However, the long-term patency of AV grafts remains inferior to that of AV fistulas, despite a fourfold increase in salvage procedures. Synthetic grafts require 3 to 6 weeks before they can be used; this period allows sufficient time for the material to incorporate into the surrounding subcutaneous tissues and for the inflammation and edema to subside.

   B. Location. AV grafts are typically placed between the brachial artery and the cephalic or brachial vein in the antecubital fossa and arranged in a loop configuration in the forearm. Upper arm grafts can also be created between the brachial artery and basilic or axillary veins. When all upper-extremity sites are exhausted, attention is turned to the lower extremity, where loop grafts typically connect the superficial femoral artery and femoral or saphe-nous veins.

   C. Placement. AV grafts are placed under local anesthesia with conscious sedation. Prophylactic antibiotics (e.g., second-generation cephalosporins) are commonly administered immediately prior to the surgery.

VI. Complications of AV access

Complications related to AV access account for 19% of all hospitalizations in hemodialysis patients, and their management requires a multidisciplinary approach (*Kidney Int* 1993;43:1091–1096).

   A. Stenosis. Pseudointimal hyperplasia within a synthetic graft or neointimal hyperplasia in a native AV fistula or outflow vein of a graft constitutes the most common cause of dysfunction. Approximately 85% of graft thromboses result in hemodynamically significant stenosis (*J Vasc Surg* 1997;26:373–380). Arterial inflow lesions are less common but can lead to low flow as well as elevated recirculation, making it more difficult to distinguish them from outflow lesions. Elevated venous pressures, increased recirculation, abnormal physical findings, or recurrent thrombosis necessitate a fistulo-gram and treatment of any underlying lesion(s) by angioplasty or surgical revision. Stenoses in long segments (>30% after angioplasty) or those that recur within a short interval require surgical intervention.

   B. Thrombosis. Thrombosis occurring within a month of placement is often due to anatomic or technical factors, such as a narrow outflow vein, misplaced suture, or graft kinking. Early thrombosis of native vein fistulas often results in permanent loss of the access. Prolonged hypotension during and after dialysis occasionally precipitates thrombosis, as can trauma from needle puncture or excessive compression after needle removal following hemostasis. By 24 months, 96% of grafts require thrombectomy, angioplasty, or surgical revision. Therefore, primary graft survival rates are quite low (*Am J Kidney Dis* 2000;36:68–74). Prosthetic AV shunt thrombosis can be managed by pharmacological thrombolysis, mechanical maceration, or surgical thrombectomy, either separately or in combination.

Fistulography at the time of treatment usually reveals the precipitating cause, allowing immediate intervention. Surgical thrombectomy should be followed by fistulography to detect stenosis not fully appreciable during standard balloon thrombectomy. The rate of secondary graft patency after intervention reaches only 65% at 1 year and 51% at 2 years (*Am J Kidney Dis* 2000;36:68–74).

C. **Infection.** Infection and bacteremia in dialysis patients are usually caused by *S. aureus*. The type of access constitutes the major risk factor for infection, with a relative risk of 1.29 for grafts in comparison to primary fistulas and 7.64 for catheters (*ASAIO J* 2000;46:S6–S12). AV fistula infections usually respond to a prolonged course (6 weeks) of antibiotic therapy. If septic embolization occurs, the fistula should be revised or taken down. AV graft infections occur in approximately 5% to 20% prosthetics placed and present a more challenging problem. Antibiotic treatment should cover Gram-positive organisms (including enterococci) as well as Gram-negative organisms (e.g., *E. coli*). A superficial skin infection not involving the graft may respond to antibiotics alone. Focal graft infections can be salvaged with resection of the infected portion of the graft, but extensive infections and those that involve newly constructed, unincorporated grafts should be managed with complete excision. Evidence of bacteremia, pseudoaneurysm formation, or local hemorrhage should prompt graft removal, with placement of a new access at a different site.

D. **Pseudoaneurysm formation.** Pseudoaneurysms result from destruction of the vessel wall and replacement by biophysically inferior collagenous tissue, usually after repetitive puncture of the same vessel segment. Laplace's law predicts that the aneurysm will progress, as wall stress increases with increasing diameter. A downstream stenosis predisposes to upstream aneurysm formation. Major complications include rupture, infection (which is promoted by intra-aneurysmal thrombus), and, rarely, antegrade or retrograde embolization. Before any intervention is embarked on, imaging is absolutely indispensable for identification of thrombus and assessment of the venous anastomosis and outflow. Aneurysmal dilations of AV fistula can be often treated by surgical correction, including partial or complete resection of the aneurysmal sac, repair of accompanying stenoses, and reconstruction of an adequate lumen. Aneurysm in an AV graft calls for replacement of the weakened graft segment.

E. **Arterial "steal" syndrome.** All AV accesses divert or "steal" blood from the distal circulation to a certain extent. A clinical syndrome resulting from this decrease in distal circulation occurs when the various local compensatory mechanisms fail; this syndrome is reported to occur in approximately 1% of patients with distal AV accesses (*Surgery* 1991;110:664–670). The clinical presentations of arterial insufficiency in the tissues distal to the fistula may include ischemic pain, neuropathy, ulceration, and gangrene. Patients with diabetes, prior AV access, or atherosclerotic disease are at a higher risk. Patients with mild ischemia complain of subjective coldness and paresthesias without sensory or motor loss and can be managed expectantly with increasing exercise tolerance. Failure of these symptoms to improve may require surgical correction with banding or ligation. Severe ischemia requires immediate surgical intervention to avoid irreversible nerve injury.

F. **Venous hypertension.** Venous hypertension can be caused by the presence or development of outflow vein obstruction. It manifests as swelling, skin discoloration, and hyperpigmentation in the access limb. In chronic cases, ulceration and pain may develop. Management consists of correction of stenosis and disconnecting the veins that are responsible for retrograde flow and pressure transmission.

G. **Congestive heart failure.** Venous return to the heart, cardiac output, and myocardial work can significantly increase after AV fistula or graft placement, leading to cardiomegaly and congestive heart failure in some patients. Hypercirculation ensues if the outflow resistance is too low and the anastomosis is too wide. This problem is more common with ePTFE grafts and brachial artery fistulas. Operative correction involves narrowing the proximal shunt or graft with either a prosthetic band or suture ligature. Occasionally, a new access must be constructed using a smaller-diameter conduit or tapered prosthetic material.

VII. Vascular access monitoring

A. Angiography (fistulogram) remains the gold standard for the evaluation of access problems. However, the need for frequent evaluations and the invasive nature of angiography do not make it a practical option for routine surveillance.

B. Doppler ultrasound measures access flow and correlates with the presence and severity of stenoses detected by angiography. Blood flow below a critical level (750 mL per minute) or a reduction in flow over time (>15%) predict the presence of stenosis and the development of thrombosis.

MANAGEMENT OF SURGICAL TUBES AND DRAINS

Surgical tubes are used to evacuate fluid from or to instill fluid into a body cavity, a visceral organ, or an organ with its own internal "circulation," such as the biliary tree and urinary tract. Placement and management are specific for each type of tube. To avoid misidentification of a tube or drain, a label should be attached immediately upon placement, a detailed description should be included in the procedure note, and complete instructions for use should be placed among the order sheets.

I. GI tubes. Nasogastric or intestinal intubation is used to decompress the stomach for treating gastric atony, ileus, or obstruction; to remove ingested toxins; to obtain a sample of gastric contents for analysis (volume, acid content, blood); and to supply nutrients through tube feeding. Tube feedings may be required to meet some or all of a patient's nutritional needs. Enteral nutrition is indicated when oral intake is less than two-thirds of the daily requirement, despite a functional GI tract.

A. Nasogastric (NG) and orogastric (OG) tubes. NG and OG tubes cross the nares and mouth, respectively, and course down the esophagus into the stomach.

1. **Indications for placement of an NG or OG tube:**
   a. Decompression of stomach and/or small bowel
   b. Administration of medications
   c. Enteral nutrition
   d. Gastric lavage

2. **Contraindications for NG tube placement:**
   a. Documented or suspected facial bone fractures. In this situation, an **OG tube** provides an alternative that avoids the potential complication of inadvertent intracranial penetration.
   b. Severe, uncorrectable coagulopathy (otherwise coagulopathy may be considered a relative contraindication)
   c. Esophageal strictures or a history of alkali ingestion, due to the potential risk of esophageal perforation

3. **Single lumen: Levin tube.** With its large internal diameter, this tube is mostly useful for diagnostic aspiration of stomach contents or administration of therapeutic agents. The tube has to be connected to low intermittent suction to prevent gastric mucosa aspiration into the open end of the catheter, which may obstruct the lumen and potentially injure the gastric mucosa.

4. **Dual lumen**
   a. **Argyle Salem Sump** (Sherwood Medical, St. Louis, Mo). The second lumen of these tubes remains vented to air and thus prevents suction injury. Such tubes can accordingly be placed to gravity, continuous, or intermittent suction.

b. Ewald tube. This dual lumen tube is most commonly used for evacuation of blood, toxic agents, medications, or other substances. Gastric contents are suctioned via the 36F lumen and irrigated through the 18F lumen.

5. **Placement.** NG and OG tubes can be inserted at the bedside.
   a. Gastric intubation in adults requires approximately 40 to 50 cm of tube length.
   b. Position the patient upright or supine with the head of the bed at a 45-degree angle and the neck flexed.
   c. A small amount of water-based lubricant (e.g., Surgilube) facilitates placement.
   d. A topical local anesthetic gel, such as viscous lidocaine, may provide additional relief from discomfort during passage of the tube. Further benefit may be gained by spraying the back of the throat with an anesthetic (e.g., Cetacaine).
   e. Instruct the patient to swallow as the tube is passed across the hypopharynx and upper esophageal sphincter. Having the patient sip water, if alert and cooperative, and swallowing while the tube is advanced can facilitate passage into the stomach.
   f. A patient who is gasping for air or coughing or who is unable to speak warns of inadvertent nasotracheal intubation.
   g. Tip location can be inferred by aspiration of gastric contents. When the pH of the aspirate is less than 4, the tip of the tube will be in the stomach in 95% of cases. The location of the tube can also be confirmed by injecting 30 to 60 mL of air and auscultating a rumbling sound in the left upper quadrant.

6. **Confirmation of correct tube placement**
   a. Most tubes are easily visualized on abdominal radiographs and have a radiopaque stripe that is interrupted at the most proximal side hole to confirm intragastric location of all of the side holes.
   b. NG tubes placed at the time of surgery should have their position confirmed by palpation before abdominal closure.

7. **Tube maintenance**
   a. Saline or water tube irrigation (30 mL) every 4 to 8 hours ensures patency.
   b. The air port of sump tubes should also be injected at similar intervals with 30 mL of air.
   c. Clogging can usually be remedied by injection of several milliliters of carbonated soda or meat tenderizer into the main lumen.
   d. All medications in pill or capsular form should be ground up and suspended in water before injecting through an NG or OG tube.

8. **Complications**
   a. Passage of an NGT in a patient with nasopharyngeal trauma and suspected anterior basilar skull fracture can result in perforation into the brain through the cribriform plate.
   b. Tracheal and pulmonary placements are more common in intubated or unconscious patients or those with an impaired gag reflex.
   c. NG and OG tubes frequently compromise the function of the lower esophageal sphincter and may lead to gastroesophageal reflux and bronchial aspiration of gastric contents, esophagitis, and esophageal stricture.
   d. Perforations of the esophagus, stomach, and duodenum are rare but can have serious and potentially life-threatening sequelae.
   e. Necrosis of the nasal skin can result from prolonged pressure or traction on the nares.
   f. Sinusitis can result from blockage of normal drainage of the paranasal sinuses and bacterial overgrowth.
   g. If needed for long-term enteral feeding, a soft single-lumen **Dobhoff**-type tube (e.g., Entriflex, Sherwood Medical) should be used instead.

B. Nasojejunal [nasoenteric (NET)] feeding tubes.
1. **Indications.** Intragastric feeding may be more physiologic, but small-bowel feeding is more reliable in critically ill patients, especially in those with gastroesophageal reflux, gastroparesis, and gastric ileus. However, present data are insufficient to show a significant decreased risk of aspiration with small-bowel feeding. Despite this, many experts believe that deep duodenal or jejunal feeding offers a significant theoretical advantage, especially when combined with gastric decompression.
2. **Contraindications.** These include patients with intestinal obstruction or for those in whom intestinal function is severely compromised. Metabolic management may not be possible for patients with peritonitis, intractable vomiting, paralytic ileus, or severe diarrhea. Relative contraindications, depending on the clinical scenario, include severe pancreatitis, enterocutaneous fistulas, and gastrointestinal ischemia
3. **Techniques** for achieving NET placement include unguided bedside insertion or fluoroscopic, endoscopic, or direct surgical guidance.
4. **Placement.** Tube placement without radiologic assistance in the ICU can be successful when using the following protocol:
   a. Administer metoclopramide intravenously over 1 to 2 minutes approximately 10 minutes before tube insertion.
   b. If the NG tube or OG tube is in place, obtain aspirate, noting color and pH; clamp the NG of OG tube.
   c. Set the hub of the stylet securely into the main port of the feeding tube. Close the cap on the medication port.
   d. Flush the tube with approximately 10 mL tap water to check for patency or leaks and to activate the hydrophilic outer coating.
   e. Elevate the head of the bed as tolerated.
   f. As with an NG tube, insert into the nostril and advance through the nasopharynx into the esophagus. Flexion of the neck and having the patient swallow can facilitate passage of the tube into the esophagus.
   g. Advance the tube to 55 to 60 cm and auscultate over the epigastric area. Attempt to aspirate the gastric contents, comparing aspirate with previous NG aspirate if available. Gastric aspirate is often bilious in appearance. The pH may range from 1 to 7, depending on the use of antacids.
   h. Continue to advance the small-bowel feeding tube slowly with a gentle touch. Infuse approximately 60 cc of air slowly starting at 70 to 75 cm to help open the pylorus. Never force the tube; if resistance is met, pull back and attempt to readvance. Continue to advance to the 100-cm mark.
   i. Aspirate and check the pH and color of the output when the tube is at the 100-cm mark. The color of the small-bowel aspirate is generally yellow and has a pH of 7+.
   j. When the tube is in position, remove the inner stylet and secure with tape.
5. **Placement confirmation.** Air instillation and auscultation are helpful but not wholly accurate methods of validating position. Misplacement is often not obvious until a radiograph is obtained.
6. **Complications** are similar to NG or OG tube placement and include the following:
   a. **Malposition.** Placement in tracheal, pulmonary, or pleural position can result in pneumothorax and pulmonary or pleural formula infusion.
   b. **Dislodgement.** Nasoenteric tubes may migrate in or out or be inadvertently withdrawn during transport, physical therapy, or routine nursing care.
   c. **Mechanical malfunction.** Causes of malfunction include cracking, breaking, or kinking of tubing. Clogging is related to a number of factors, including tube length, narrow caliber, inadequate irrigation

with water, continuous (as opposed to bolus) infusion, and the types of medication and infusate being administered.

7. Maintenance
  a. Flush the tube with 20 to 30 mL saline or tap water before and after each use and as often as every 4 hours as needed when not in use.
  b. Enteral feedings cannot be given as a bolus because they are hypertonic. They must be administered as a slow, continuous infusion to avoid osmotic fluid shifts and diarrhea.
  c. Occluded tubes can be usually be unclogged with injection of several milliliters of carbonated soda or meat tenderizer through a small-bore syringe (e.g., 1 to 3 mL).

C. Long (decompressive) intestinal tubes are used to intubate the small bowel, most often for the management of small-bowel obstruction caused by postoperative adhesions, although an NG tube often suffices for this purpose (*Ann Surg* 1987;206:126–133).
  1. Types
    a. Gowen decompression tube (Wilson-Cook, Winston Salem, NC) offers the advantage of a sump lumen and is placed endoscopically in the distal duodenum or proximal jejunum, obviating the need for serial radiographs during initial advancement.
    b. Cantor tube (Rush, Inc., Duluth, Ga) has only a single lumen and a balloon at the tip that is filled with 3 mL of mercury after insertion to weight it sufficiently for advancement along the GI tract through peristalsis.
    c. Miller-Abbott tube (Rush, Inc.) is a dual-lumen tube; one lumen is placed to intermittent suction, and the other has a weighted tip, which eliminates the need for mercury.
  2. Placement
    a. The tubes can be passed manually at the time of surgery, inserted radiologically or endoscopically, or placed at the bedside.
    b. Once placed in the patient's stomach, the tube should be taped to the forehead with 10 to 15 cm of slack to allow forward motion. As the tube advances, it should be periodically retaped with additional laxity. Serial abdominal radiographs should document the progression of the tube.
    c. Once in position, the tube can be placed to suction drainage. Water-soluble contrast can be injected through the tube to delineate the point of obstruction.
  3. Removal. The balloon should be deflated and, in the reverse of stepwise advancement, 10 to 15 cm of length should be gently withdrawn every 3 to 4 hours until the tip is in the patient's stomach. This technique is intended to prevent intussusception by too rapid removal.

D. Sengstaken-Blakemore (S-B) tubes (Rush, Inc.). These tubes are equipped with esophageal and gastric balloons for tamponade and ports for aspiration.
  1. Indication. S-B tubes provide a lifesaving measure for dealing with acute bleeding from gastroesophageal varices that are refractory to sclerotherapy and medical management. It can serve as a bridge until a transjugular intrahepatic portosystemic shunt (TIPS) or bypass surgery can be performed. It should not be used in cases of a suspected Mallory-Weiss tear because of the risk of esophageal disruption. It is also ineffective for treating bleeding gastric varices alone or portal gastropathy because the gastric balloon only tamponades the gastric cardia.
  2. Insertion
    a. Before an S-B tube is placed, the patient should be in an ICU, with endotracheal intubation, and undergo gastric lavage.
    b. The tube can be passed intranasally or orally.
    c. Confirm intragastric location by inflating the gastric balloon with 100 cc of air and applying gentle traction on the tube until resistance indicates placement at gastroesophageal junction.

    d. Document proper position with a portable radiograph.

    e. Insufflate an additional 100 to 150 cc of air in the gastric balloon to tamponade the varices.

    f. Affix the tube with 1- or 2-lb weight traction via a pulley system.

    g. Inflate the esophageal balloon with air to between 24 and 45 mm Hg.

    h. Insert an NG tube above the esophageal balloon to aspirate oral secretions and monitor for persistent or recurrent bleeding.

    i. Obtain a completion radiograph of the abdomen to document accurate positioning.

    j. After 24 hours, release the weights and deflate the balloons (sooner if signs of chest or abdominal discomfort develop).

    k. Remove the tube after an additional 24 hours if there is no further bleeding.

  3. Complications include recurrent hemorrhage after balloon deflation, esophageal perforation, tracheobronchial aspiration, and ischemic necrosis of the esophagus.

E. Nasobiliary (NB) tubes. These typically have a single lumen and are manufactured from soft silicone (Silastic) material.

  1. Indications

    a. Cholangitis. For patients who require decompression of the biliary tree, NB tubes are inserted across the sphincter of Oddi into the common hepatic or common bile duct. They drain externally and thus provide a more favorable pressure gradient than an internal drain.

    b. Biliary imaging. An NB tube also provides a means of performing diagnostic cholangiography and can be used to opacify the biliary tree during percutaneous transhepatic drainage.

  2. Placement. Insertion is performed using endoscopic guidance, and the tube is connected to gravity drainage.

  3. Complications typically result from traumatic placement, malposition, or dislodgement.

F. Gastrostomy (G) and gastrojejunostomy (GJ) tubes.

  1. Enteral access options

    a. Surgical gastrostomy (SG) or gastrojejunostomy. This procedure is most frequently performed on patients already undergoing laparotomy. For gastrojejunostomy, also sometimes referred to as *transgastric jejunostomy,* a feeding tube is advanced into the stomach and through the duodenum into the jejunum.

    b. Percutaneous endoscopic gastrostomy (PEG). PEG tubes are made from silicone or polyurethane tubing and are available in diameters from 18F to 28F. An internal retention bolster is designed to prevent accidental dislodgment. PEG placement is best accomplished by the pull, or Ponsky-Gauderer, technique, which was introduced in the 1980s. The feeding tube is advanced through the patient's mouth into the stomach and brought out through the abdominal wall over a guidewire that has been snared through a direct gastric puncture site. Later modifications of the original technique include placement using a variety or "push" methods, in which the stomach is directly punctured and a catheter is advanced into the stomach over a guidewire, with or without T-fastener gastropexy. Advantages of PEG over surgical gastrostomy include lower cost and shorter procedure time. However, the overall complication rates of PEG and surgical gastrostomy, when performed on a regular basis, are roughly equal (*Gastrointest Endosc* 1990;36:1–5)

    c. Percutaneous endoscopic gastrojejunostomy (PEG-J). A PEG-J is created by insertion of a jejunal extension tube through a preexisting or concurrently placed PEG. The theoretical merit of PEG-J is its ability to provide gastric decompression while supplying enteral alimentation. PEG-J may be indicated for patients who do not tolerate gastric feeding and/or are at perceived increased risk for aspirating gastric feeding formula. Although the initial technical success is high, the long-term success for feeding is lower because of problems with retrograde migration of tubes back into the stomach, often during vomiting, and tube malfunction caused by kinking or obstruction.

d. Radiologic percutaneous gastrostomy (RPG). Gastrostomy tubes can also be placed under fluoroscopic guidance, and it has been suggested that radiologic placement of enterostomy tubes is less expensive than both surgical and endoscopic placement. RPG access procedures can be performed safely and comfortably with local anesthesia. In high-risk patients with cardiopulmonary disease, RPG offers a significant advantage over endoscopic gastrostomy and surgical gastrostomy, which usually require heavy conscious sedation and general anesthesia, respectively. The technique is similar to PEG placement, with fluoroscopically guided needle access into a stomach filled with air via an NG tube in place of using transillumination to provide a safe target for gastric puncture. The gastrostomy tube is pulled or pushed over a fluoroscopically placed guidewire.

2. Indications

a. Pediatric and adult patients with an intact, functional gastrointestinal tract who are unable to consume sufficient calories to meet metabolic needs

b. Neurologic conditions associated with impaired swallowing (e.g., patients recovering from a cerebrovascular accidents and complex maxillofacial or neck surgery or trauma)

c. Obstructive neoplasms of the oropharynx, larynx, and esophagus

d. The need for supplemental nutrition in patients with a variety of catabolic conditions, including burns, wasting syndromes, and cystic fibrosis

e. Delivery of hydration and medications and for gastric decompression

f. Malignant gastric outlet obstruction that cannot be managed by endoscopic stent insertion

g. Gastroesophageal reflux or gastroparesis places patients at increased risk for aspiration of gastric contents. Combining a decompressive gastrostomy and feeding jejunostomy tube allows simultaneous aspiration of gastric contents and continuous jejunal feeding.

3. Contraindications

a. Absolute contraindications for PEG include severely limited life expectancy, inability to bring the anterior gastric wall in apposition to the anterior abdominal wall, colonic interposition, high (intrathoracic) position of stomach, complete pharyngeal or esophageal obstruction, peritonitis, and uncorrectable coagulopathy. Gastrointestinal obstruction also contraindicates the enteral route for use in feeding.

b. Relative contraindications include proximal small-bowel fistula, massive ascites, portal hypertension, peritoneal dialysis, hepatomegaly, large hiatal hernia, and prior subtotal gastrectomy. Neoplastic, inflammatory, and infiltrative diseases of the gastric and abdominal walls also constitute relative contraindications.

4. Complications

a. Minor complications include tube occlusion, maceration from leakage of gastric contents around tube, and peristomal pain. Minor complication rates vary from 14% to 43% for SG, 6% to 43% for PEG (*Arch Surg* 1998;133:1076–1083), and 0.7% to 12% for RPG (*J Vasc Interv Radiol* 2000;11:239–246).

b. Major complications are reported in 3% to 8.4% of cases for PEG and 0.5% to 6% for RPG, and they include wound infections, necrotizing fasciitis, aspiration, bleeding, perforation, peritonitis, ileus, injury to internal organs, and gastrocolic fistula (*Gastrointest Endosc* 2002;55:794–797). The mortality rates for SG, PEG, and RPG placement are respectively 3% to 16%, 0% to 2%, and 0.8%.

c. Placement of a jejunal tube though a gastrostomy can be complicated by balloon migration and potential pyloric or small-bowel obstruction, recoil of the jejunal tube into the duodenum or stomach, and trauma to the gastric and duodenal mucosa, with ulceration.

5. Management

a. **Enteral nutrition** is generally administered in a bolus fashion though G tubes, whereas GJ tubes require continuous jejunal feeding to avoid diarrhea.

b. **Tube replacement.** Time to tract maturation varies from 1 to 2 weeks for silicone or rubber catheters and up to 6 weeks for polyurethane. The tube is best changed over a guidewire under fluoroscopic guidance to lessen the chance of malpositioning or loss of access.

c. G and GJ tubes can be removed in the office or at the bedside. Most G sites close spontaneously in a day or two. Only rarely do they require operative closure at the fascial level.

G. Jejunostomy tubes

1. Indications. Jejunostomy tubes are used to provide enteral nutrition for those patients who cannot tolerate gastric feedings or who are at significant risk for aspiration of gastric feeding solution. This includes persons with severe gastroesophageal reflux, gastroparesis, repeated aspiration of gastric contents, an insufficient gastric remnant after surgery, and an unresectable cancer with gastric outlet obstruction and persons who have undergone major intestinal surgery.

2. Placement

a. **Surgical.** These tubes are placed through an incision in the anterior abdominal wall. The tube is secured in the jejunum with either a purse-string suture or by imbricating the serosa of the jejunum over the tube to create a Witzel tunnel.

b. **Direct percutaneous endoscopic jejunostomy (DPEG).** The DPEJ technique represents a modification of PEG placement. A long endoscope is advanced into the small bowel. Endoscopic transillumination is performed from within the jejunum. A trocar is passed through the anterior abdominal wall directly into the jejunum. Once this direct access is achieved, a standard "pull-type" gastrostomy tube is inserted. Although similar to PEG placement, DPEJ placement is considerably more technically challenging to perform. Technical success is reported in 72% to 88% of patients.

c. **Percutaneous radiological jejunostomy.** Feeding catheters can also be placed percutaneously under fluoroscopic guidance. The procedure is facilitated by prior surgery or conditions that result in relative fixation of otherwise freely mobile intestinal loops. T-fastener enteropexy may be a useful adjunct to anchor a bowel loop for tract dilatation and catheter placement.

3. Maintenance. As with other enteral feeding tubes, maintenance consists of flushing the tube with 20 to 30 mL of tap water or saline before and after each use and as often as every 4 to 6 hours when not in use. Tubes that have not been permanently sutured to the bowel or abdominal wall can be removed with gentle traction once a mature tract has formed.

4. Complications

a. **Surgical jejunostomy complications** can result from dislodgment before tract maturation, bowel perforation by the catheter, and technical problems that lead to traumatic or incorrect placement. Intestinal obstruction can result from inspissated feedings, volvulus of the bowel around the tube, intussusception, or partial occlusion of the bowel by the catheter itself, especially if the catheter is balloon-tipped.

b. **DPEJ complications** often result from inability to transilluminate the bowel or luminal obstruction preventing passage of the endoscope. Major complications requiring surgery occur in 2% of patients and include bleeding, abdominal wall abscesses, and colon perforations.

Less severe peristomal infections develop in 7% of patients, enteric ulcers in 5%, and leakage in 8%.

c. Percutaneous radiological jejunostomy. The most common problem is failure to place the catheter due to inability to puncture into the small-bowel lumen when the intestinal loops are very compliant and/or moving. The catheter-related complications listed in 4a and 4b apply to all enteral feeding catheters, regardless of insertion technique.

H. T tubes

1. **Surgical placement.** T tubes are exteriorized T-shaped tubes placed into the common bile duct, often through or adjacent to the cystic duct following cholecystectomy and common bile duct exploration, biliary anastomosis after liver transplantation, or some other form of biliary surgery.

2. **Management.** T tubes are usually connected to gravity drainage and can be used to perform cholangiography or provide access for the passage of interventional instruments. If there is no evidence of biliary obstruction, the tube can be removed with gentle traction once the tract has matured (usually within a few weeks).

3. **Complications** include cholangitis (tube malfunction in the setting of bile duct obstruction), leakage at the site of insertion, and biloma or abscess formation. Catheter fracture during removal is a very rare complication.

I. Cholecystostomy tubes

1. **Indications.** Cholecystostomy is a well-established procedure for rapid decompression of an inflamed gallbladder in patients who are deemed unsuitable for urgent cholecystectomy (*J Am Coll Surg* 2003;197:206–211). Interval laparoscopic cholecystectomy can be safely performed once sepsis and acute infection has resolved for those patients considered at high risk for general anesthesia and/or conversion to open cholecystectomy.

2. **Placement.** The gallbladder is most commonly approached subcostally, either by operative or radiological technique.

3. **Management.** Gravity drainage suffices for resolution of the acute inflammation. If the bile is very viscous, patency of the tube can be optimized by irrigation with 3 to 5 mL of sterile saline once a day, or more frequently as required. General recommendations prior to cholecystostomy tube removal include (1) drainage tract maturation to prevent intraperitoneal biliary leakage after removal (7 to 10 days); (2) absence of symptoms; (3) cystic duct patency verified by cholangiography; (4) consideration of percutaneous gallstone extraction. Acalculous cholecystitis can be successfully treated by cholecystostomy drainage alone, and the tube can later be removed when cholangiography has demonstrated patency of the cystic duct and a well-formed drainage tract.

4. **Complications.** Bile leakage, hemorrhage, colonic injury, and vasovagal reactions are among the percutaneous procedure–related complications. Catheter dislodgment has been reported in 5% to 10% of patients. The transhepatic approach is purported to minimize the risk of intraperitoneal bile leak and inadvertent injury to the hepatic flexure of the colon, but it carries the inherent risks of pneumothorax, intrahepatic bleeding, and hemobiliary fistula.

J. Cecostomy tubes

1. **Characteristics.** A cecostomy represents an artificial stoma formed between the cecum and the abdominal wall.

2. **Indications.** Historically, cecostomy tubes have been used for colonic irrigation in an unprepared, obstructed colon prior to resection of the obstructing lesion and primary anastomosis; for fecal diversion in patients with a large-bowel obstruction who are poor operative candidates; and occasionally for perforated appendicitis. They are also advocated for children who have large-bowel dysmotility or fecal incontinence syndromes (*Endoscopy* 1999;31:501–503) and for selected patients with spina bifida, spinal cord injury, anorectal anomalies, and severe neurologic handicaps.

3. **Placement.** The cecum is drained through the anterior abdominal wall using either an operative or radiological approach. The Malone procedure is performed by resecting the appendix with a cuff of the cecum. The remaining cecum is then reversed and sutured to the skin. In the modified Malone procedure, the appendix is left *in situ* and sutured to the skin. A circular flush stoma is created either at the appendiceal tip or the reversed cecum, followed by an antireflux procedure. A 10-Fr. catheter is left across the conduit for 2 weeks. This procedure is usually done via a laparotomy but can be attempted laparoscopically if the appendix is intact. In the radiological approach, a percutaneous cecostomy is inserted under fluoroscopic guidance. After bowel cleansing, the location of the viscera is identified by ultrasound. Through a self-retaining catheter in the rectum, the cecum and the proximal ascending colon are insufflated with air. Access to the cecum is obtained with a trocar, with or without T-fastener gastropexy. The tract is dilated, and a 10-Fr. locking loop catheter (Cook Inc., Bloomington, Ind) is inserted and secured to the anterior abdominal wall.

4. **Management.** The tube is left to gravity drainage and should be irrigated with 30 mL of saline periodically to prevent obstruction. If removal is desired, the tube can be taken out after the tract has healed (in approximately 4 to 6 weeks).

5. **Complications.** Complications of surgical cecostomy include stomal stenosis, stoma leakage, appendiceal necrosis, and peritonitis from a leak at the insertion site. Complications with percutaneous placement include granulation tissue formation (treated with silver nitrate cauterization), local infection, and dislodgement of the cecostomy tube into the subcutaneous tissues.

K. **Rectal tubes.** Rectal tubes are indicated in bedridden patients who have diarrhea or frequent loose stools in order to prevent maceration of the skin of the perineum. The tubes can be placed at the bedside and connected to gravity drainage. They are available with or without a balloon tip. The tubes should not be left in place for more than a week to prevent pressure necrosis.

II. **Thoracostomy tubes** are used to drain fluid from the pleural or mediastinal space. The use of thoracostomy tubes is described in Chapter 36.

III. **Urinary catheters** are used to relieve urinary retention, irrigate the bladder, instill medication or radiographic contrast, obtain urine for examination, and measure residual urine volume.

A. **Indications for long-term catheterization**
   1. Bladder outlet obstruction not correctable medically or surgically
   2. Intractable skin breakdown caused or exacerbated by incontinence
   3. Neurogenic bladder and urinary retention
   4. Patients at risk for contamination of perineal burns, trauma, or surgical wounds
   5. Patients with hematuria who require bladder irrigation for clot removal
   6. Palliative care for terminally ill or incontinent patients poorly responsive to specific treatments

B. **Indications for short-term catheterization**
   1. Urologic surgery or surgery on adjacent structures
   2. Urine output monitoring in critically ill patients
   3. Acute urinary retention

C. **Contraindications**
   1. Urethral trauma
   2. High riding prostate

D. **Foley catheters**
   1. **Catheter characteristics**
      a. **Size.** Foley catheters are available in sizes from 12-Fr. to 30-Fr. Rarely is a catheter larger than 18-Fr. required, and a 14-Fr. or 16-Fr. catheter usually suffices. In most patients, it is best to minimize bladder irritation by using a catheter with a 5-mL balloon that is inflated with 5 to 10 mL of fluid.

b. Lumens. Dual-lumen catheters have one channel for drainage and one for inflating the balloon. Triple-lumen catheters have an additional channel for irrigating the bladder and are used most commonly when hematuria is problematic, such as after transurethral resection of the prostate (TURP).

c. Material: Silastic (silicone) catheters have been recommended for short-term catheterization after surgery. Compared with latex catheters, Silastic catheters have a decreased incidence of urethritis and, possibly, urethral stricture. Because of its lower cost and other considerations that pertain to long-term use, latex is the material of choice for long-term catheterization, provided the patient is not allergic to it.

d. Antibiotic coating. Antimicrobial agents include silver oxide, silver hydrogel (silver alloy), nitrofurazone, and combinations of minocycline and rifampin. The combination of silver alloy and nitrofurazone appears to reduce bacteriuria for up to 2 weeks.

E. Difficult urethral catheterization

1. Causes include meatal stricture, urethral stricture or obstruction, and prostatic hypertrophy.

2. Solutions

a. Lubricate catheter with viscous lidocaine.

b. Use an angled-tip catheter coudé (Fr. "elbow"). The curved shape helps to guide it over the bladder neck.

c. If unsuccessful, obtain a urological consultation.

F. Complications

1. Urinary catheter blockage

a. Etiology. Patients who tend to develop catheter occlusions often excrete more calcium, protein, and mucin and have a higher urine pH. *Proteus mirabilis* has a potent urease that splits ammonia and alkalinizes urine, which in turn precipitates crystals of struvite and apatite in the catheter lumen. *P. mirabilis* often forms cultures with other bacteria, including *Enterococcus faecalis, Escherichia coli, Enterobacter aerogenes, Pseudomonas aeruginosa,* and *Providencia stuartii.* Methenamine preparations may be beneficial in reducing episodes of obstruction.

b. Management

(1) Maximize patient hydration.

(2) Irrigation may prevent repeated obstructions that are not responsive to increased fluid intake and urine acidification.

(3) Evaluate for UTI if frequent catheter blockage.

(4) Change catheter if no urine flow in 4 to 8 hours.

2. Urinary catheter leakage

a. Etiology. Bladder spasms commonly occur in patients with long-term catheterization, and the force generated can create leakage around the catheter.

b. Management

(1) Do not increase catheter diameter.

(2) Evaluate for catheter blockage (above).

(3) Evaluate for catheter-associated UTI.

(4) Antispasmodics, such as oxybutynin (Ditropan) and flavoxate (Urispas), can be effective in alleviating spasm due to detrusor instability.

3. Bacteriuria

a. Etiology. Bacteria often gain access to the urinary tract from periurethral colonization by colonic flora. Bacteria may then migrate along the catheter and uroepithelium into the bladder and invade the upper urinary tract. Rarely, uropathogens are introduced through loss of integrity of the collecting system in the upper urinary tract.

Bacteria almost always eventually colonize a chronically indwelling urinary catheter, but rarely does significant infection ensue

  b. **Pathogens.** Bacteriuria associated with short-term catheterization usually involves a single pathogen, most commonly *E. coli*. Bacteriuria associated with long-term catheterization is characteristically polymicrobial, usually with two to five isolates, including *E. coli, P. mirabilis, Klebsiella pneumoniae, Enterococcus* species, *P. stuartii,* and *Morganella morganii.* Gram-positive bacteria are responsible for approximately 15% of urinary tract infections, and *Candida* species are also a rising source of infection

  c. **Epidemiology.** The incidence of bacteriuria in catheterized patients is directly related to the duration of catheterization; the daily rate of acquiring bacteriuria is approximately 3% to 10%.

  d. **Complications.** The most common complication of catheter-related bacteriuria is symptomatic infection. In patients with bacteriuria, 10% to 25% will develop symptoms of local urinary tract infection, and about 3% will develop bacteremia (*Arch Intern Med* 2000;160:678–682). Classic signs of urinary tract infection, such as frequency of urination and pain and burning on urination, may not be present in patients with indwelling urinary catheters. Thus fever, suprapubic pain, leaking, and persistent obstruction may be more appropriate indicators of infection. Other serious complications of bacteriuria include pyelonephritis and urosepsis. In addition, long-term catheterization may give rise to urethritis, urinary calculi, epididymitis, vesicoureteral reflux, chronic pyelonephritis, and chronic tubulointerstitial nephritis with scarring of the renal parenchyma.

G. **Alternatives to indwelling urinary catheters**
  1. **Intermittent catheterization** for dysfunctional voiding
  2. **External catheter** (condom catheter)
    a. **Indication.** Incontinent men without obstructive uropathy.
    b. **Advantage.** Lower incidence of bacteriuria.
    c. **Disadvantage.** Increased incidence of skin breakdown.
  3. **Suprapubic catheterization**
    a. **Indications** include adjunctive use in gynecologic, urologic and other surgeries, or inability to catheterize the urethra for any reason.
    b. **Advantages** include decreased risk of infection due to decreased bacterial colonization of abdominal wall compared to perineum. In addition, catheters can be clamped to test for adequate voiding.
    c. **Disadvantages** include the risk of skin cellulitis, often present when leakage occurs, or hematoma at the puncture site.
  4. **Nephrostomy tubes.** Nephrostomy tubes are discussed in Chapter 40.
IV. **Surgical drains.** Catheters are also used to allow drainage of fluid or pus from a body cavity. Selection of the appropriate tube or drain for a particular situation is based on the type, viscosity, and volume of fluid to be evacuated.
  A. **Open drains.** Open drains are used to establish a tract from a body cavity to the skin surface. The most common open drain is the Penrose drain, made from 0.25- to 1.0-in. soft latex rubber tubing. Placed at the time of surgery, it acts as a wick and can effectively drain pus, serum, blood, or other fluid from virtually any body cavity. Dependent positioning facilitates drainage. The drain should be secured at the skin level to prevent retraction into the wound. A gauze sponge or ostomy appliance bag can be used to contain or collect drainage. Removal of this type of drain usually consists of withdrawal in increments during convalescence.
  B. **Closed suction drains.** Closed systems drain fluid into a collection container, sparing the skin from becoming macerated. They are placed at the time of surgery or postoperatively if there is a continued leak, particularly at the site of anastomotic breakdown. Large silicone (Silastic) catheters, such as the multi–side hole **Jackson-Pratt drain** (Allegiance Healthcare Corp.,

Waukegan, Ill) and the fluted **Blake drain** (Ethicon, Inc.), are the most commonly used closed systems placed intraoperatively, and they are usually attached to bulb suction. The output from the drain and the quality of the drainage fluid can be monitored easily. Analysis of the fluid may aid in the diagnosis of anastomotic leak. Closed suction drains are usually removed when the drainage has decreased to less than 30 mL in 8 hours. If the drain was placed after creation of a GI anastomosis, it is left in place until an oral diet has been resumed. Potential complications include erosion of the drain into an adjacent structure, fracture of the drain (often during attempted removal), and infection or superinfection.

C. **Sump drains.** Sump drains are large-caliber, multilumen tubes that provide continuous irrigation and aspiration. They are generally placed operatively for drainage of intra-abdominal spaces that might benefit from continuous postoperative irrigation, in anticipation of large volumes of drainage and/or large particulate material (e.g., pancreatic abscess).

D. **Abscess drainage catheters.** Typically made of polyurethane or similar thin-walled polymer plastic, these drains are inserted percutaneously using ultrasound, fluoroscopic, or computed tomography (CT) guidance. A wide variety of sizes and configurations are available. Gravity drainage usually suffices, but these catheters can also be connected to suction. After a period of defervescence, contrast injection is performed to delineate the size of the abscess cavity and to look for connections with the GI tract or other organs. After drainage of an infected collection, the catheter can be removed once the output has decreased to 10 mL per day or less. A flushing regimen of 3 to 10 mL per shift or per day (depending on catheter size and fluid viscosity) may be needed to ensure optimal performance. If the output drops off sharply despite flushing, or the patient fails to improve as determined by laboratory and physical parameters, a CT scan should be done to assess the situation.

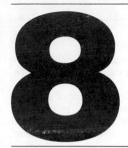

Minimally Invasive Surgery

Valerie J. Halpin
and Mary E. Klingensmith

Minimally invasive endoscopic surgery is a rapidly advancing and expanding field of surgical access and therapy. Minimally invasive surgical techniques are now routinely used for many operations in the abdominal cavity and retroperitoneum (laparoscopy), thorax (thoracoscopy), and joint spaces (arthroscopy). Percutaneous techniques are quickly developing for the treatment of vascular diseases. Novel applications (beyond the scope of this text) are continually being developed, such as axillary dissection, thyroidectomy, parathyroidectomy, minimally invasive coronary bypass, saphenous vein harvest for coronary artery bypass, ligation of penetrating veins associated with varicosities, celiac plexus block for pain palliation, and anterior spine surgery (*Mastery of Endoscopic and Laparoscopic Surgery*. Philadelphia: Lippincott Williams & Wilkins, 2000).

LAPAROSCOPY AND THORACOSCOPY

An overview of these areas is provided below. For consideration of individual disease processes, readers are referred to the relevant chapters in this volume.

I. **Laparoscopy**
   A. **Advantages** (compared with traditional laparotomy) include less pain, fewer systemic and wound-related complications, shorter hospital stay, quicker return to full activity and work, and potential overall cost savings.
   B. **Contraindications**
      1. **Absolute contraindications** include the inability to tolerate general anesthesia and uncorrectable coagulopathy.
      2. **Relative contraindications** include the following and require an increased level of laparoscopic experience.
         a. **Prior abdominal surgery**, which may require alternative port locations to avoid intra-abdominal adhesions and laparoscopic adhesiolysis to improve exposure
         b. **Peritonitis**, which may limit access secondary to adhesions
         c. **First- and third-trimester pregnancy.** The second trimester is the optimal time, but surgery should be undertaken in consultation with the mother's obstetrician. Intraoperative fetal monitoring is recommended. Close monitoring of end-tidal carbon dioxide is essential. Open insertion of the initial port and consideration of alternative port sites may be required to prevent iatrogenic injury to the gravid uterus. Later in pregnancy, it is important to position the patient in a left lateral decubitus (Sims) position to avoid inferior vena cava compression and preserve venous outflow from the lower extremities.
         d. **Severe cardiopulmonary disease** may be exacerbated by hypercarbia that occurs secondary to insufflation of carbon dioxide and changes in pulmonary and cardiovascular mechanics during periods of increased intra-abdominal pressure. These effects can be minimized by using lower intra-abdominal pressures (8 mm Hg) in conjunction with abdominal wall lift devices.
         e. **Massive abdominal distention,** due to increased risk of iatrogenic bowel injury.

C. Limitations inherent in laparoscopy
1. **Video imaging** of the operative field requires development of precise video-hand-eye coordination as well as clear communication between surgeon, assistant, and camera operator.
2. **Monocular two-dimensional imaging** requires development of artificial three-dimensional skills by the laparoscopic surgeon.
3. **Long rigid instruments** that are placed through ports fixed at the abdominal wall restrict movement, limit dexterity, decrease tactile sensation, and increase fatigue.
4. **Magnification** provides good visualization in tight areas but also may lead to misidentification of structures and obscured visualization from only small amounts of bleeding.

D. Laparoscopic procedures
1. **Basic.** Diagnostic and staging laparoscopy, cholecystectomy, appendectomy, and inguinal and abdominal wall herniorrhaphy.
2. **Advanced.** Gastric bypass for obesity, operations at the esophageal hiatus for gastroesophageal reflux and hiatal hernia, segmental bowel resection, gastrojejunostomy, gastrectomy, biliary bypass, common bile duct (CBD) exploration, adrenalectomy, nephrectomy, and splenectomy.
3. **Anecdotal experience.** Laparoscopic or minimally invasive procedures for peptic ulcer; esophagectomy; liver resection; pancreatic resection; bladder resection, augmentation, or replacement; aortobifemoral bypass; and anterior spinal fixation continue to expand the range of possible applications.

E. Technique of laparoscopy
1. **Consent** for laparoscopic procedures, similar to that for open operations, requires an understanding of the risks, benefits, and alternatives to the proposed laparoscopic procedure as well as the possibility of conversion to an open procedure at the discretion of the operating surgeon. It should be emphasized that long-term outcome studies for many of the minimally invasive procedures are not yet complete.
2. **Patient preparation.** The patient is fasted overnight, and his or her stomach is decompressed with an orogastric tube. The need for preoperative mechanical bowel preparation is dictated by the procedure. A urinary catheter is placed while the patient is in the operating room, although this can be omitted if the operation involves only the upper abdomen, the operation is expected to be brief, and the patient voids immediately preoperatively. An H_2-receptor antagonist is administered, and compression stockings are applied to the lower extremities. Because the operating table position is manipulated intraoperatively to displace intra-abdominal organs by gravity, the patient must be secured to the table and padded to prevent iatrogenic compression injuries; a beanbag is helpful. A laparotomy tray should be readily available before the procedure is started.
3. **Pneumoperitoneum.** A working space is created in the patient's abdomen using carbon dioxide via either a closed or open technique.
   a. **Closed technique.** A Veress needle is placed most commonly at the umbilicus through a small skin-stab incision. Two serial clicks are heard as the needle penetrates the fascia and peritoneum, respectively. The surgeon aspirates the needle with a 10-cc syringe partially filled with saline to look for blood or enteric contents. The surgeon injects 3 to 5 cc of saline through the needle. If any resistance is met, the syringe is most likely in the abdominal muscle or omentum and should be repositioned. If no resistance is met, the surgeon aspirates the syringe again and removes the plunger. Observing the saline pass freely into the abdomen with gravity (drop test) confirms proper intra-abdominal placement. The abdominal cavity is insufflated with an automatic pressure-limited insufflator to 10 to 15 mm Hg. The initial intra-abdominal pressure should be less than 10 mm Hg. As the abdomen expands, pneumoperitoneum is confirmed with percussion. After insufflation, the abdominal

wall is stabilized manually, and the initial trocar and port are inserted blindly and away from all critical abdominal structures.

(1) **Elevated pressure** with low flow (1 L/per minute) on insufflation usually indicates placement of the Veress needle into a closed space (e.g., pre- or retroperitoneal, within the omentum).

(a) The surgeon first verifies that the port's insufflation valve is open.

(b) If it is, the surgeon removes and reinserts the Veress needle and performs tests for placement.

(c) If the **needle position is in doubt**, the surgeon should use an open insertion technique.

(2) **Return of blood, cloudy or bilious fluid, or enteric contents** after Veress needle placement mandates needle repositioning.

(3) **Gas embolism is life-threatening.** With right ventricular outflow obstruction, expired end-tidal carbon dioxide falls, with concomitant hypotension and a "mill wheel" heart murmur.

(a) The surgeon should stop insufflation and release the pneumoperitoneum.

(b) The patient should be placed in a steep Trendelenburg position with the right side up to float the gas bubble up toward the right ventricular apex and away from the right ventricular outflow tract.

(c) Air from the right ventricle is aspirated through a central venous catheter.

(4) **Brisk bleeding** after trocar insertion warrants emergent conversion to open laparotomy. The trocar should not be removed until proximal and distal control of the injured vessel is achieved.

b. **Open insertion** of the initial port uses a direct cutdown through the abdominal fascia. A Hasson (wedge-shaped) port is placed under direct vision and secured to the abdominal fascia with stay sutures.

c. **Alternatives to carbon dioxide pneumoperitoneum** have been advocated because of the potentially deleterious effects of hypercapnia. Alternative pneumoperitoneum gases, such as nitrous oxide, helium, and argon, have been evaluated experimentally. Increased intra-abdominal pressure can occur with any insufflation gas. Compression of the vena cava can cause decreased venous return to the heart, with resulting hypotension, and decreased renal blood flow and diminished urinary output. External abdominal wall lift devices are available to create a working space without pneumoperitoneum.

4. **Port placement.** The location of ports has been standardized for most procedures, and several general rules for port placement have been established. All additional ports should be placed under direct video monitoring. Prior to inserting the port, the surgeon indents the abdominal wall manually and identifies the location with the video camera. Transilluminating the abdominal wall identifies significant vessels to avoid. The skin and peritoneum are anesthetized locally. The surgeon makes a small stab incision with a no. 11 blade. The trocar is introduced in a direct line with the planned surgical target to minimize torque intraoperatively. The tip of the trocar should be visualized as it passes through the peritoneum. If there is difficulty in passing the trocar, the adequacy of the size of the skin incision should be checked.

a. The **camera port** should be behind and between the surgeon's two operative ports to maintain proper orientation.

b. **Working ports** are placed lateral to the viewing port, with the operative field ahead. All ports should be at least 8 cm apart to avoid the interference of instruments with one another. Ports should be approximately 15 cm from the operative field for the site to be reached comfortably by standard 30-cm instruments and to maintain a 1:1 ratio of hand-instrument tip movement.

F. **Suturing and knot tying** are essential skills for the surgeon to master before attempting advanced laparoscopic procedures. It is important to remember and anticipate suturing when considering port placement.

1. **Extracorporeal knotting techniques** are generally simpler to perform and are recommended for more durable tissues that can tolerate the pulling through of the excess suture material (e.g., the gastric wall or diaphragmatic crura). Extracorporeal techniques usually require more than 32 cm of suture and use a "knot pusher" to advance the throw down the port and make the knot snug. To avoid disruption, the knot pusher should be envisioned as an extension of the surgeon's finger while the knot is pushed down to the tissue. Tension should be maintained on the other arm of the suture without pulling up on the tissue. An air leak occurs whenever suture is introduced or withdrawn through the introducer sheath. An assistant can reduce any air leak by occluding the reducer orifice with a fingertip.

2. **Loop ligatures** provide preformed sliding knots on a thin stylet to allow rapid ligation of structures. A grasping instrument is placed through the loop and grasps the tissue or vessel. The loop is then closed and tightened around the pedicle.

3. **Intracorporeal suturing** is preferred for delicate tissues, such as the intestine, bile duct, or esophagus. Sutures should be 8 to 12 cm long. Laparoscopic instrument tying is similar to that of open surgery. A variety of specific techniques have been developed to accomplish knot tying. The surgeon should be facile with at least one technique and be able to tie a square knot without undue tissue trauma or time. The square knot is performed similarly to an instrument tie performed in open surgery.

G. **Exiting the abdomen.** The surgeon should survey the abdomen at the conclusion of the procedure to detect any visceral injury or hemorrhage. The operative site is irrigated, and hemostasis is obtained. Inspection of the peritoneal side of all port sites as the trocars are removed allows verification of hemostasis. **Port site fascial incisions** that are larger than 5 mm should be closed with permanent or long-term absorbable suture to avoid the risk of incisional herniation. This can be done through the port site incision or under video guidance with a fascial closure device (also known as a "suture passer"). The suture passer is particularly helpful in obese patients.

H. **Converting to open surgery.** A laparoscopic case may need to be converted either electively or emergently. There are a number of reasons a surgeon should convert to an open procedure.

1. **Elective conversion**
   a. **Surgeon experience** is critical. The surgeon's threshold for conversion should be low while gaining experience.
   b. **Failure to progress** is the most common reason to convert. This can be secondary to adhesions, inflammatory changes, poor exposure, or altered or aberrant anatomy. In cases of unclear anatomy, avoiding injuries (e.g., to the bile duct) should take precedence over avoiding laparotomy.
   c. The surgeon may discover **a disease not appropriate for minimally invasive methods,** such as gallbladder cancer or colon cancer invading adjacent organs.
   d. **Technical problems or instrument malfunction** may occasionally require conversion. The surgeon must check that all equipment is in working order prior to starting the operation.

2. **Emergent conversion** should be performed in the event of severe bleeding or complex bowel injuries if repair is beyond the skill level of the surgeon.

I. **Postoperative management** for most laparoscopic procedures is similar to that for open procedures, although in-hospital and recuperative time are generally shorter.

1. **Urinary catheters and nasogastric tubes** can generally be removed in the operating room. This enhances patient comfort and encourages early ambulation.
2. **Drains and postoperative antibiotics** are used as needed.
3. **Analgesics** are usually administered as needed.
4. **Diet** is generally advanced on the first postoperative day, depending on the operative procedure.
5. **Physical activity** usually is not restricted, and patients can return to work in approximately 1 week.

II. **Thoracoscopy**
   A. **Diagnostic thoracoscopy** (*Surg Gynecol Obstet* 1922;34:289)
      1. **Video-assisted thoracoscopic surgery (VATS)** is performed in patients after thoracentesis and percutaneous pleural biopsy have failed to provide a diagnosis of suspected pleural disease. VATS frequently is used to diagnose malignancy in a solitary peripheral nodule. It is contraindicated in patients with extensive intrapleural adhesions or those who are unable to tolerate single-lung ventilation.
      2. **VATS is approximately 95% accurate** for diagnosis of pleural disease.
   B. **Therapeutic thoracoscopy**
      1. **VATS has been performed** for peripheral lung biopsy, closure of leaking blebs, parietal pleurodesis, pericardiectomy, and excision of mediastinal cysts. Fewer lobectomies, pneumonectomies, and esophagectomies have been performed owing to concern about adequacy of complete tumor resection, and therefore they should be considered investigational procedures at this time.
         a. **Absolute contraindications** include extensive intrapleural adhesions or the inability to tolerate single-lung anesthesia.
         b. **Relative contraindications** include previous thoracotomy, tumor involvement of the hilar vessels, and previous chemotherapy or radiotherapy for lung or esophageal tumors.
      2. The **patient is placed** in the lateral decubitus or semioblique position. Thoracoscopy requires selective intubation to allow collapse of the ipsilateral lung and to create a working space within the thorax (thus, insufflation gases are not needed). For most procedures, three incisions are required. The thoracoscope is placed through a port in the seventh or eighth intercostal space in the midaxillary line. Working ports for instruments generally are at the fourth or fifth intercostal space in the anterior axillary line and posteriorly near the border of the scapula. The endoscopic stapler, electrocautery, or laser can be used for resection. A chest tube is generally placed through one of the port sites.
      3. **Complications** include hemorrhage, perforation of the diaphragm, air emboli, prolonged air leak, and tension pneumothorax.
      4. **Postoperative thoracoscopy management**
         a. **A chest x-ray** is taken and checked for residual air or fluid.
         b. **Chest tubes**, if any, are usually removed in 1 to 2 days.
         c. **Analgesia** is provided by patient-controlled anesthesia or orally administered medication as needed.
         d. **Diet** is usually advanced by postoperative day 1.
         e. **Physical activity** is as tolerated with a chest tube. Depending on the procedure and diagnosis, patients can return to work in approximately 1 week.

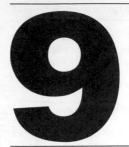

Wound Healing and Care

F. Jay Quayle and
Thomas Tung

Wound healing is the normal body response to injury, various disease states, and aging. The goal of modern wound care is to promote the timely restoration of the body to a previous state of normal form and function. Wound healing is often classified as "normal" (acute wound healing) or "abnormal" (chronic wound healing). A*cute wound healing* is the normal orderly process that occurs after a typical injury and requires minimal practitioner intervention. *Chronic wound healing* often necessitates a variety of interventions to correct and shift the healing process toward a more normal state of wound healing. An understanding of the basic processes found in normal or acute wound healing allows for a better understanding of how alterations of these processes lead to abnormal wound healing and how interventions can result in restoration of normal healing.

ACUTE WOUND HEALING

    I. Physiology of the acute wound. The disruption of the integrity of tissues, whether surgical or traumatic, stimulates a series of events that attempt to restore the injured tissue to a normal state. The process of wound healing occurs in an orderly fashion and strikes a fine balance between repair and regeneration of tissue. Normal wound healing is affected by the extent of injury, tissue type, and the existence of comorbid conditions in the patient. The steps of wound healing can be grouped into early, intermediate, and late stages.

    A. Early wound healing

        1. This stage involves the **establishment of hemostasis** (day 1 of wounding) and the onset of inflammation (days 1 to 4 postwounding). With the onset of injury, blood vessels are disrupted, with subsequent hemorrhage. Severed blood vessels with any smooth muscles in their walls immediately constrict, and within minutes the coagulation cascade is initiated and produces the end-product fibrin, which plays an important role in the formation of clot and in wound healing. Fibrin forms the initial matrix for early wound healing. In later phases of wound healing, the fibrin-formed matrix facilitates cell attachment and migration. It also serves as a reservoir for cytokines. With the production of fibrin, platelets are activated, and they bind to and aggregate on the fibrin lattice to form the clot that is necessary to achieve hemostasis.

        2. The **inflammatory phase** (days 1 to 4 postwounding) is the initial response of the body to injury. It is recognized at the skin level by the cardinal signs of inflammation—*rubor* (redness), *calor* (heat), *tumor* (swelling), and *dolor* (pain), which result from changes in the microcirculation. As hemostasis is established, leukocytes begin to migrate out of the intravascular space through gaps between endothelial cells and bind to the provisional wound matrix. Polymorphonuclear leukocytes (PMNs) are the dominant inflammatory cells in the wound for the first 24 to 48 hours, and they phagocytize bacteria, foreign material, and damaged tissue. They also release cytokines that stimulate fibroblasts and keratinocytes.

           a. The inflammatory phase progresses with the infiltration of **monocytes** into the wound. Monocytes migrate into the extravascular space through capillaries and differentiate into **macrophages** under the influence of cytokines and fibronectin. Macrophages are activated by several cytokines and are essential for normal healing because of their important role in the coordination of the healing process. They function to phagocytize bacteria and damaged tissue, secrete enzymes for the degradation of tissue and extracellular matrix, and release cytokines for inflammatory cell recruitment and fibroblast proliferation.

  b. The inflammatory phase lasts a well-defined period of time in primarily closed wounds (approximately 4 days), but it continues indefinitely to the endpoint of complete epithelialization in wounds that close by secondary or tertiary intention. Foreign material or bacteria can change a normal healing wound to one with chronic inflammation.

B. Intermediate wound-healing events involve mesenchymal cell migration and proliferation, angiogenesis, and epithelialization. Two to 4 days after wounding, chemotactic cytokines influence fibroblasts to migrate into the wound from undamaged tissue. Movement of cells occurs on the extracellular matrix, consisting of fibrin, fibronectin, and vitronectin.

  1. While the wound is infiltrated by mesenchymal cells, **angiogenesis** takes place to restore the vasculature that has been disrupted by the wound.

  2. **Epithelialization** is the third critical aspect of intermediate wound-healing events. It restores the barrier between the wound and the external environment. Epithelialization of wounds occurs via the migration of epithelial cells from the edges of the wound and from remaining epidermal skin appendages. Migration of epithelial cells occurs at the rate of 1 mm per day in clean and open wounds. Primarily closed wounds have a contiguous epithelial layer at 24 to 48 hours.

C. Late wound-healing events involve the deposition of collagen and other matrix proteins and wound contraction. After being present in the wound, the primary function of the fibroblast becomes protein synthesis. Fibroblasts produce several proteins that are components of the extracellular matrix, including collagen, fibronectin, and proteoglycans. Glucocorticoids inhibit protein production by fibroblasts.

  1. Collagen is the main protein secreted by fibroblasts. It provides strength and structure and facilitates cell motility in the wound. Collagen is synthesized at an accelerated rate for 2 to 4 weeks, greatly contributing to the tensile strength of the wound. Oxygen, vitamin C, α-ketoglutarate, and iron are important cofactors for the cross-linkage of collagen fibers. If they are not present, the wound healing may be poor.

  2. Wound contraction, another aspect of late wound healing, is a decrease in the size of the wound without an increase in the number of tissue elements that are present. It involves movement of the wound edge toward the center of the wound. It is differentiated from contracture, which is the pathologic and movement-limiting result of prolonged wound contraction across a joint. Wound contraction begins 4 to 5 days after wounding and continues for 12 to 15 days or longer if the wound remains open.

D. The final wound-healing event is **scar remodeling**. It begins at approximately 21 days after wounding. At the outset of scar remodeling, collagen synthesis is downregulated, and the cellularity of the wound decreases. During scar remodeling, collagen is broken down and replaced by new collagen that is denser and organized along the lines of stress. By 6 months, the wound reaches 80% of the bursting strength of unwounded tissue. It is important to note that a well-healed wound never achieves the strength of unwounded tissue. This process reaches a plateau at 12 to 18 months, but it may last indefinitely.

CHRONIC WOUND HEALING

  I. Physiology of the chronic wound. A chronic wound is a wound that fails to heal in a reasonable amount of time given the wound's etiology, location, and tissue type. Prolonged or incomplete healing occurs as a consequence of a disruption in the normal process of acute wound healing, which leads to a poor anatomic and functional result. Most chronic wounds are slowed or arrested in the inflammatory or proliferative phases of healing and have marked increased levels of matrix metalloproteinases, which bind up or degrade the various cytokines and growth factors at the wound surface. Most often, there are definable causes of the failure of these wounds to heal, and treatment of these causes, along with maximal medical management of the patient's medical problems, leads to a restoration of more normal healing processes. Therefore, treating a patient with a chronic wound involves investigation into the cause(s) of delayed healing and improving the intrinsic (within the wound itself) and extrinsic (systemic) patient factors that lead to poor wound healing.

A. Intrinsic or local factors are abnormalities within the wound that prevent normal wound healing. These factors include the presence of a foreign body, necrotic tissue, repetitive trauma, hypoxia/ischemia, venous insufficiency, infection, growth factor deficit, excessive matrix protein degradation, and radiation. Factors that can be controlled by the surgeon include the blood supply to the wound; the temperature of the wound environment; the presence or absence of infection, hematoma, or seroma; the amount of local tissue trauma, and the technique and suture material used to close the wound. It should be noted that the technique and suture material are important only after other local factors have been addressed.

1. Ischemia and hypoxia are common contributing causes of nonhealing wounds. Atherosclerosis or local damage to vessels in the form of trauma or vasculitis causes ischemia and subsequent hypoxia in the wound. Hypoxia leads to impaired collagen synthesis, prevents fibroblast migration, and increases the susceptibility of the wound to infection. Essential to normal wound healing, molecular oxygen is needed for the hydroxylation reaction that cross-links collagen fibers. Molecular oxygen also contributes to the ability of the host's defense to kill pathogens. Sickle cell anemia may lead to vascular occlusion, with subsequent ischemia and tissue ulceration.

2. Infection in the wound delays healing. Infection is considered to be present when the bacterial count of a quantitative tissue culture $>10^5$ organisms per gram of tissue. The critical factors in determining the susceptibility to infection are concentration of organisms, virulence, and host resistance. The host's resistance can be impaired by diabetes, malnutrition, malignancy, steroids, or other immunosuppressive therapies. If allowed to persist, wound infections lead to increased tissue destruction and alter the effect of cytokines on wound healing. Clinical signs of infection are pyrexia, erythema, swelling, and purulence. Treatment must involve drainage, local débridement, and systemic antibiotics.

3. The **presence of foreign bodies and necrotic tissue** can contribute to delayed wound healing. Their presence prolongs the inflammatory phase of wound healing until they are removed. Such factors also predispose a wound to infection. The combined presence of infection and a foreign body or devitalized tissue within the wound necessitates the removal of the latter by débridement before eradication of the infection can be achieved. Hematomas, seromas, devascularized bone, and sequestrum are all factors that can increase the susceptibility of a wound to infection.

4. Chronic venous insufficiency leads to persistent venous hypertension and chronic edema in the lower extremities. These factors in turn lead to pericapillary fibrosis, tissue ischemia, and the liberation of superoxide radicals, which are thought to result in delayed wound healing in extremities with chronic venous insufficiency.

5. Ionizing radiation to the wound leads to abnormal wound healing. Early manifestations include erythema, edema, and hyperpigmentation, but the chronic effects of tissue ischemia, atrophy, and fibrosis cause radiation-exposed wounds to enter a chronic course.

6. Edema. Acute swelling, especially around joints, can lead to skin breakdown and full-thickness skin loss. Chronic swelling often leads to fibrofatty tissue deposition in underlying skin, which develops verrucous changes and at times irregular crevices and folds. Such skin is prone to breakdown and to development of infection. Infection leads to further lymphatic blockage and obliteration, and the problem gets chronically worse. Patients need to adopt an aggressive program of limb elevation, external compression, and medical management of the edema.

7. The **microenvironment of the chronic wound** has been shown to be different from that of the acute wound in investigational settings. Studies have implicated a decrease in the endogenous levels of certain growth factors in wounds with impaired healing. Other studies have established that an imbalance in the synthesis and degradation of extracellular matrix proteins is central to the establishment and maintenance of chronic wounds. This occurs through inadequate synthesis of extracellular matrix proteins, increased degradative enzymes, decreased regulation of degradative enzymes, or a combination of these causes.

B. **Extrinsic or systemic factors** also contribute to abnormal wound healing. These factors are primarily linked to the underlying general health of the patient.

1. **Malnutrition** alters normal healing through the indirect and the direct effects of vitamin and mineral deficiency. An example is the patient with clinical or subclinical scurvy (vitamin C deficiency); such an individual produces inadequately hydroxylated collagen, and the healed wound becomes significantly weakened as a result.

2. **Diabetes mellitus** is believed to affect healing adversely at every level and in every phase of the healing process. The lack of insulin (and its poorly understood trophic effects on healing tissues), hyperglycemia (by adversely affecting the migratory and phagocytic functions of inflammatory cells and the proliferation of fibroblasts and endothelial cells), neuropathy, and the vascular disease that occurs in diabetic patients all contribute to poor healing.

3. **Steroids and antineoplastic drugs** can markedly diminish the speed and quality of the healing process. The exact effects of steroids are not yet understood. Vitamin A, by poorly understood mechanisms, seems to cause a partial reversal of the detrimental effects of steroids on healing. Chemotherapeutic agents alter wound healing by decreasing mesenchymal cell proliferation and inducing a leukopenic state that reduces the inflammatory cells available for wound healing. Immunosuppression from AIDS or other diseases may also affect various phases of wound healing.

4. **Smoking** contributes to delayed wound healing by causing cutaneous vasoconstriction, decreasing the oxygen-carrying capacity of hemoglobin, and contributing to atherosclerosis.

5. **Collagen vascular diseases** often are accompanied by a vasculitic component, which needs to be controlled before healing can begin. The medicines that are used to treat collagen vascular diseases may impair cell migration and collagen deposition. Adjustment of dosage may lead to improved wound healing.

6. **Cleansing agents** [such as chlorhexidine gluconate (Hibiclens) or povidone-iodine (Betadine)] **or chemicals** may impair wound healing by affecting cell migration.

7. **Repetitive trauma**, intentional or otherwise, from shearing or pressure forces often leads to a failure in healing. Wound areas over pressure points often require stabilization of the overlying skin envelope with external taping or splinting.

8. **Renal disease and liver disease—patients with renal and/or liver disease** often heal their wounds more slowly.

9. **Hematopoietic disorders.** Sickle cell disease, with its high incidence of ankle wounds and leukoclastic and granulomatous processes, and mycosis fungoides are associated with poorly healing wounds. Maximal medical treatment for the underlying disorder is needed to effect meaningful healing.

II. Evaluation and management of the chronic wound

A. History and physical examination. Evaluation and management of a chronic wound must begin with a thorough history and physical examination.

1. During the **history**, one must establish whether the wound is new or recurrent, how long it has been present, how it started, how quickly it developed, and whether it is improving or worsening. The patient must be questioned about existing comorbidities, with a focus on potential causes for immunosuppression (HIV, steroids, chemotherapy), undiagnosed diabetes mellitus, peripheral vascular disease, coronary artery disease, rheumatologic disorders, and radiation exposure. Smoking and alcohol use must also be documented.

2. The **physical examination** must evaluate the size, depth, and location of the wound and tissues that are involved. Signs of infection (erythema, purulence, tenderness, warmth, swelling) must also be evaluated, and a good pulse examination for extremity wounds must be performed. Serum chemistries may aid with the diagnosis of diabetes and renal or hepatic dysfunction. A complete blood cell count may indicate infection with elevated white cell count or white cell abnormalities. Radiography can be performed to determine underlying bony pathology. Doppler evaluation of the extremities should be carried out for suspected arterial insufficiency.

B. Management of the chronic wound must focus on the optimization of host and local factors.

1. **Adequate nutrition** is necessary for appropriate wound healing. Sufficient calories, protein, vitamins, minerals, and water are necessary to aid in the healing of chronic wounds. Patients who have severe malnutrition or whose gastrointestinal tract cannot be used should be placed on parenteral nutritional support.

2. **Underlying factors** that affect wound healing, such as chemotherapy, steroids, alcohol consumption, cigarette smoking, and blood glucose levels, must be modified as necessary to aid in the wound-healing process.

3. **Effective local wound care** is essential for the resolution of a chronic wound. Eradication of infection, aggressive débridement, and drainage of abscesses from the wound are important steps in local control.

4. **Antibiotics.** Systemic antibiotics should be administered to treat active infection such as cellulitis. Topical antibiotics applied to the wound are effective in lowering the bacterial count.

5. **Proper dressings** are an essential aspect of local care by helping to provide the appropriate environment for healing. Frequent wet-to-dry dressings are used when infection and drainage predominate. With the development of healthy granulation tissue, dressings should provide adequate protection and moisture to facilitate healing.

6. **Edema control** is often necessary for wounds of the lower extremity due to venous insufficiency. Elevation and wrapping in an elastic bandage reduce edema and venous hypertension. Unna boot, Jobst compression garments, and pneumatic compression devices can also be used.

7. **Surgical therapy** may be necessary to aid in the healing of a chronic wound. This may occur through surgical débridement of infected or necrotic wounds and skin grafting on a healthy bed of granulation tissue. Revascularization procedures may be necessary to provide adequate blood flow to distal circulation that supplies a nonhealing/or chronic wound.

III. Special categories of chronic wounds.
Chronic wounds are a heterogeneous group. Chronic wounds associated with diabetes, pressure necrosis, and radiation therapy are frequently encountered, cause great disability within the population, and place a great burden on the health care system.

A. Diabetic foot ulcers

1. **Differential diagnosis.** The three most common causes of lower-extremity ulcers are arterial insufficiency, venous stasis, and diabetes mellitus.

Venous stasis ulcers most often occur on the medial aspect of the patient's lower leg or ankle and are associated with the chronic edema and hyperpigmentation seen with venous insufficiency. Arterial insufficiency ulcers tend to occur distally on the tips of the patient's toes, but they can also occur at or near the lateral malleolus. The surrounding skin exhibits the thin, shiny, hairless characteristics that have been well described in these patients, and these individuals typically relate symptoms of claudication or rest pain. Peripheral pulses are diminished or absent. Diabetic ulcers are believed to be secondary to the severe neuropathy seen in these patients and to a lesser extent the vasculopathy as well (see the following). They are typically associated with very thick callus and most often occur on the patient's heels or on the plantar surface of the metatarsal heads.

2. **Causes**
   a. **Neuropathy**
      (1) **Peripheral neuropathy** is believed to be the most significant contributor to the development of lower-extremity ulcers in diabetic patients through impaired detection of injury from poorly fitting shoes or trauma. Diabetic motor neuropathy is also associated with abnormal weightbearing. The motor neuropathy results in abnormalities such as hammer toes or hallux valgus, which shifts weightbearing more proximally than normal on the metatarsal heads. Additionally, the dorsum of the toes at the posterior interphalangeal joints is often traumatized by ill-fitting shoes in patients with hammer toes.
      (2) **Autonomic neuropathy** leads to failure of sweating and inadequate lubrication of the skin. Dry skin leads to mechanical breakdown that initiates ulcer formation. Autonomic neuropathy also contributes to failure of autoregulation in the microcirculation; therefore, arterial blood will shunt past capillaries into the venous blood flow. This reduces the nutritive blood flow to the skin in the diabetic foot and predisposes to ulcer formation.
   b. **Ischemia.** The microvascular disease seen in diabetic patients also contributes to the development and progression of lower-extremity ulcers. These patients should be evaluated for proximal atherosclerotic disease, which may be amenable to intervention, thus improving the chances of healing of the ulcer or healing of an amputation.
3. **Evaluation and treatment**
   a. **Examination.** The quality of the peripheral circulation, the extent of the wound, and the degree of sensory loss should be assessed. Web spaces should be examined for evidence of mycotic infection, which may lead to fissuring of the skin and subsequent infection. Mal perforans ulcers occur on the plantar surface of the metatarsals and extend to the metatarsal head, leaving exposed cartilage. Osteomyelitis of the phalanx or metatarsal is common.
   b. **Treatment. Clean wounds** are treated with conservative débridement and dressing changes, with careful trimming of the calluses and nails. Close follow-up is essential. **Infected wounds** are diagnosed clinically; wound cultures are unreliable unless derived from actual tissue samples. Plain films may show osteomyelitis or gas in the soft tissues. The progression of infectious processes in diabetic patients can occur with extreme rapidity, and thus these patients require hospitalization and aggressive wound care, with broad-spectrum antibiotics at initial presentation. Abscess cavities must be completely drained and all dead tissue débrided; daily whirlpool treatments help cleanse the wound mechanically. Absolute nonweightbearing is crucial for healing.
   c. **Prevention** remains one of the single most important elements in the management of the diabetic foot. Meticulous attention to hygiene and daily inspection for signs of tissue trauma prevent the progression

of injury. Podiatric appliances or custom-made shoes are helpful in relieving pressure on weightbearing areas and should be prescribed for any patient who has had neuropathic ulceration.

B. Leg ulcers
1. When **arterial ulcers** are suspected, a vascular evaluation should be instituted. Due to the tissue ischemia, antibiotics are often indicated when there are any signs of cellulitis.
2. **Venous stasis ulcers** are one of the most common types of leg ulcers and typically occur on the medial leg in the supramedial malleolar location. A patient with a venous stasis ulcer typically has a history of ulceration and associated leg swelling or of deep venous thrombosis. The ulcer may appear as a relatively superficial and extremely painful wound with irregular borders and an inflamed wound bed that bleeds fairly easily or as a partial-thickness wound with a dense, whitish-yellow fibrotic base. There may be multiple wounds and they may be surrounded with a varying degree of inflammatory dermatitis. Cleansing the wound, providing a dressing that absorbs the wound drainage, leg compression, and leg elevation are the mainstays of treatment. After excluding significant ischemia, which can be present in up to 15% of patients, one can often use a multilayered compression dressing. This is changed on a weekly or biweekly basis until the wound heals. Aggressive medical treatment is often required to control the peripheral edema, which in some patients is quite marked. More advanced methods of wound management such as skin grafting or the use of skin substitutes can be used, but only after the leg edema is controlled. External leg compression pumps and massage therapy are also useful in some patients. Wounds that are present for some time and exhibit increased drainage or pain are often infected. Treatment of infected wounds requires the addition of antibiotics.

C. Skin tears are often seen in the elderly with skin that is markedly thinned and in the chronic steroid-using patient. The hypermobile skin, with its poor subcutaneous connections, is prone to rip under shearing forces, and patients often present with a flap of skin that is torn away from its wound bed. One should follow the principles outlined above, with this exception: the skin flap should be trimmed of obvious necrotic portions, and the remaining flap should be secured in place over the wound bed only to the extent that it can be without tension. It is rare that such a wound should be sutured closed, because the flap will most likely necrose under the tension of the swelling that occurs over the following 2 to 4 days. Topical management of the area that is intentionally left open is often easily achieved with a hydrogel dressing (see "Wound Care," section **III.D** below).

D. Pressure ulcers
1. **Pathophysiology.** Prolonged pressure applied to soft tissue over bony prominences, usually caused by paralysis or the immobility associated with severe illness, predictably leads to ischemic ulceration and tissue breakdown. Muscle tissue seems to be the most susceptible. The particular area of breakdown depends on the patient's position of immobility, with ulcers most frequently developing in recumbent patients over the occiput, sacrum, greater trochanter, and heels. In immobile patients who sit for prolonged periods on improper surfaces without pressure relief, ulcers often develop under the ischial tuberosities. Pressure ulcers are described by stages (Table 9-1). Such wounds do not necessarily proceed through each one of these stages during formation but can present at the advanced stages. Likewise, as these wounds heal, they do not go backward through the stages despite their present depth (e.g., a nearly healed stage IV ulcer does not become a stage II ulcer but rather a healing stage IV ulcer, signifying that the tissues of the healing wound are abnormal). When a full-thickness injury to the skin has occurred, one cannot adequately stage the wound until the eschar is incised and the actual depth is determined.

Table 9-1. National Pressure Ulcer Advisory Panel classification scheme

Stage	Description
I	Nonblanchable erythema of intact skin; wounds generally reversible at this stage with intervention
II	Partial-thickness skin loss involving epidermis or dermis; may present as an abrasion, blister, or shallow crater
III	Full-thickness skin loss involving damage or necrosis of subcutaneous tissue but not extending through underlying structures or fascia
IV	Full-thickness skin loss with damage to underlying support structures (i.e., fascia, tendon, or joint capsule)

2. **Prophylaxis**
   a. **Skin care.** The patient's skin should be inspected and cleansed at least daily with application of moisturizers and barrier creams as necessary. Patients need to have a complete skin assessment and risk assessment done at the time of admission. All patients should be placed on the optimal support surface. Pressure-reducing support can be classified as static or dynamic. Static systems include mattresses filled with air, water, gel, or foam; dynamic support systems include low–air-loss mattresses and air-fluidized beds. Urinary and fecal continence needs to be maintained to prevent maceration and skin breakdown.
   b. **Nutrition.** Nutritional deficits should be assessed and treated appropriately. Supplementation with vitamin C or vitamin A, or both, may be necessary if the patient is malnourished or is taking steroids.
   c. **Mobility.** Bedridden patients should be turned and repositioned with a minimum frequency of every 2 hours. Heel protectors, pillows, and foam wedges can be used to diffuse pressure from bony prominences across greater areas.
3. **Treatment.** Most pressure ulcers heal spontaneously when pressure is relieved. This remains the most important factor in their healing. The healing process may require up to 6 months. Unless the patient was only temporarily immobilized, recurrences are common. Surgical management may include simple closure, split-thickness skin grafting, or musculocutaneous flap, but these measures should be reserved for well-motivated patients in whom a real reduction of risk factors for recurrence is possible. Healing of perineal and sacral wounds can be facilitated by urinary and fecal diversion, which reduces soiling and maceration of the wound bed.
E. **Ionizing radiation**
   1. Although ionizing radiation is a useful mode of cancer therapy, it produces detrimental local effects on tissue in the field of radiation and impairs normal wound healing. Radiation injures target and surrounding cells by direct damage to DNA or indirectly through free radicals or reactive species. Radiation has a negative impact on wound healing by harming the cellular elements that play a prominent role in various phases of wound healing. For instance, radiation alters wound healing by decreasing the proliferative capacity of cells, particularly those of endothelial, mesenchymal, and epithelial origin. Radiation also harms wound healing by decreasing the vascularity of the wound, leading to the development of ischemia and hypoxia. Decreased vascularity occurs through the occlusion and thrombosis of small blood vessels and capillaries and the mechanisms for angiogenesis are limited due to poor endothelial cell proliferation.
   2. The **early epithelial changes** that are characteristic of acute radiation injury include ulceration, edema, and sustained inflammation. Late

changes include parenchymal degeneration, epithelial and dermal atrophy, decreased vascularity, fibrosis, and tissue necrosis. Like the healing wound, the skin has characteristic changes that are associated with radiation exposure. The skin is affected in a dose-dependent manner. Acute changes associated with the skin include erythema from dilation of blood vessels in the dermis, dry desquamation at moderate doses, or moist desquamation in conjunction with the eradication of the cells of the epidermis. Late manifestations include hyper- or hypopigmentation, fibrosis of the skin and subcutaneous tissues, telangiectasia, sebaceous and sweat gland dysfunction, alopecia, and necrosis.

3. The **timing of radiation therapy** as it relates to operative therapy has been an important aspect of oncologic care. The primary factors that determine the effects of preoperative radiation therapy on wound healing are the timing and dose. These vary from tissue to tissue. Postoperative radiation therapy has no effect on healing if it is administered 1 week after wounding. The intentional (surgical) wounding of a previously irradiated wound needs careful planning and consideration. Many of the cells in such an area have been permanently damaged; therefore, their proliferative capacity is decreased. In addition, the wound has decreased vascularity, which creates a relative state of hypoxemia. Furthermore, the dermis of such a wound is more susceptible to bacterial invasion. The combined factors place a previously irradiated area at extreme risk for abnormal wound healing if it is subjected to surgical intervention.

4. It has long been realized for the above reasons that **radiation-damaged skin and wounds heal poorly**. Local measures that must be undertaken with wounds affected by radiation follow the same principles of good wound care. These measures include infection control through aggressive débridement and systemic antibiotics, topical antibiotics to promote epithelialization, moist dressings, and lubrication of dry skin. Optimal nutritional status must also be emphasized. Other methods, such as hyperbaric oxygen, have been used to increase the oxygen tension of irradiated wounds. Experimental therapies are currently under investigation. The use of the growth factors TGF-β and PDGF has shown promise for treatment in radiation wound models in animals.

WOUND CLOSURE AND CARE

I. Timing of wound healing
   A. **Primary intention** occurs when the wound is closed by direct approximation of the wound margins or by placement of a graft or flap. Direct approximation of the edges of a wound provides the optimal treatment on the condition that the wound is clean, the closure can be done without undo tension, and the closure can occur in a timely fashion. Wounds that are less than 6 hours old are considered in the "golden period" and are less likely to develop into chronic wounds. At times, rearrangement of tissues is required to achieve tension-free closure. Directly approximated wounds typically heal as outlined above provided that there is adequate perfusion of the tissues and no infection. *Primary intention* also describes the healing of wounds created in the operating room that are closed at the end of the operative period.
   B. **Secondary intention**, or spontaneous healing, occurs when a wound is left open and is allowed to close by epithelialization and contraction. Contraction is a myofibroblastmediated process that aids in wound closure by decreasing the circumference of the wound (myofibroblasts are modified fibroblasts that have smooth muscle cell–like contractile properties). This method is commonly used in the management of wounds that are treated beyond the "golden period" (initial 6 hours) or of contaminated infected wounds with a bacterial count $>10^5$ per/gram of tissue. These wounds are characterized by prolonged inflammatory and proliferative phases of healing that continue until the wound has completely epithelialized or been closed by other means.

C. Tertiary intention, or delayed primary closure, is a useful option for managing wounds that are too heavily contaminated for primary closure but appear clean and well vascularized after 4 to 5 days of open observation so that the cutaneous edges can be approximated at that time. During this period, the normally low Pao_2 at the wound surface rises, and the inflammatory process in the wound bed leads to a minimized bacterial concentration, thus allowing a safer closure than could be achieved with primary closure and a more rapid closure than could be achieved with secondary wound healing.

II. Wound closure materials and techniques

A. Skin adhesives. Topically applied adhesives (Dermabond) can be used to maintain skin edge alignment in wounds that are clean, can be closed without tension, and are in areas not subject to motion or pressure.

B. Steri-Strips. Skin tapes are the least invasive way to close a superficial skin wound; however, because they provide no eversion of wound edges, the cosmetic result may be suboptimal. Additionally, skin tapes tend to loosen if moistened by serum or blood and therefore are seldom appropriate for all but the most superficial skin wounds in areas of minimal or no tension. Their most frequent use is in support of a skin closure after suture or staple removal.

C. Suture

1. Needles. Curved needles are designed for use with needle holders, whereas straight (Keith) needles can be used with or without a holder. Two types are in common usage: circular (tapered, noncutting) and triangular (cutting). Cutting needles are preferable for closure of tough tissue, such as skin, and noncutting needles are preferable for placing sutures in delicate tissues, such as blood vessels or intestine.

2. Suture material. Several characteristics differentiate the various suture materials. They include the following.

   a. Absorbable versus nonabsorbable. Among the absorbable materials, wide variability is found with regard to tensile strength, rate of absorption, and tissue reaction.

   b. Monofilament versus braided. Braided suture has better handling characteristics than does monofilament suture, but the interstices between the braided strands that compose the suture are easily colonized by bacteria and thus pose an infection risk.

   c. Natural versus synthetic.

3. Staples allow for quick closure. In areas of lower cosmetic sensitivity, such as the thick skin of the back or anterior abdominal wall, staples may produce cosmetic results approximating those of sutures. They are particularly useful for closure of scalp wounds.

D. Skin suture technique

1. Basic surgical principles apply: closure without tension, elimination of dead space, aseptic technique, and (when closing skin) eversion of the skin margins. A dog-ear occurs when unequal bites are taken on opposing sides of a wound or incision, causing the tissue to bunch up as the end of the wound is approached. This can be prevented by carefully aligning the wound at the time of deep tissue closure (elimination of dead space) with interrupted absorbable sutures and by taking equal bites of tissue on both sides of the wound.

2. Suture removal. Suture scars occur when stitches are left in place too long, allowing epithelialization of the suture tracts. This complication can be minimized by timely suture removal. Facial sutures should be removed at days 3 to 5; elsewhere, days 7 to 10 are appropriate. These guidelines should be modified for the individual patient. Application of skin tapes after suture removal provides further support.

III. Open wound care options (see also Table 9-4)

A. Topical ointments. Petroleum-based ointments that contain one or several antibiotics prevent adherence of dressings to the wound and, by maintaining

Table 9-2. Summary of Immunization Practices Advisory Committee recommendations for tetanus prophylaxis in routine wound management

Tetanus	Clean minor wounds		Tetanus-prone wounds	
Immunization	Td^a	TIG^b	Td	TIG
Unknown or less than three doses	Yes	No	Yes	Yes
Three doses or more	No (yes if >10 yr since last dose)	No	No (yes if >5 yr since last dose)	No

Td, tetanus-diphtheria toxoid (adult type); TIG, tetanus immune globulin.
^{a}Adsorbed tetanus and diphtheria toxoids, 0.5 mL i.m. For children younger than 7 years, diphtheria-polio-tetanus is recommended.
^{b}TIG (human), 250 units i.m., given concurrently with the toxoid at separate sites. Heterologous antitoxin (equine) should not be given unless TIG is not available within 24 hours and only if the possibility of tetanus outweighs the danger of adverse reaction.
Reprinted with permission from Centers for Disease Control and Prevention. Tetanus United States, 1987 and 1988. *MMWR* 1990;39(3):37.

moisture of the wound environment, accelerate epithelialization and healing of primarily approximated wounds.

B. **Impregnated gauze.** Gauze that is impregnated with petrolatum is used for the treatment of superficial, partial-thickness wounds to maintain moisture, prevent excessive loss of fluid, and, in the case of Xeroform, provide mild deodorizing. It can also be used as the first layer of the initial dressing on a primarily closed wound. The use of this type of gauze is contraindicated when infection of the wound is suspected and inhibition of wound drainage would lead to adverse consequences.

C. **Gauze packing.** The practice of packing an open wound with gauze prevents dead space, facilitates drainage, and provides varying degrees of débridement. The maximum amount of débridement is seen when the gauze is packed into the wound dry and removed after absorption and evaporation have taken place, leaving a dry wound with adherent gauze, which on removal also extracts superficial layers of the wound bed (dry-to-dry dressing). This dressing is seldom indicated. Wounds that are in need of great amounts of débridement usually benefit most from sharp débridement in the operating room or at the bedside; dry-to-dry dressings are painful and violate the principle of maintaining a moist environment for the wounds. Moist-to-dry dressings provide a much gentler débridement, are less painful, and can include sterile normal saline or various additives. Dakin solution [in full (0.5% sodium hypochlorite), half, or quarter strength] or acetic acid is used to pack infected open wounds when the antimicrobial action of these additives is desirable. Improvement of the foul odor that often emanates from drained abscesses and other infected open wounds is an added benefit of using these additives.

D. **Hydrogels.** These water- or glycerin-based gels (e.g., IntraSite) can be used in shallow or deep open wounds. The gel promotes healing by gently rehydrating necrotic tissue, facilitating its débridement, and absorbing exudate that is produced by the wounds, as well as maintaining a moist wound environment. A nonadherent, nonabsorbent secondary dressing is applied over the gel; dressings should be changed every 8 hours to 3 days, depending on the condition of the wound.

E. **Hydrocolloids.** These occlusive, adhesive wafers provide a moist and protective environment for shallow wounds with light exudate. They can remain in place for 3 to 5 days and can be used under compression dressings to treat venous stasis ulcers.

F. **Alginates.** Complex carbohydrate dressings composed of glucuronic and mannuronic acid, derived from brown seaweed, are formed into ropes or pads that are highly absorbent (e.g., Kaltostat). Alginates are absorbable and are useful for the treatment of deep wounds with heavy exudate because they form a gel as they absorb wound drainage.

G. Adhesive films. These plastic membranes (e.g., Tegaderm) are self-adhering and waterproof yet permeable to oxygen and water vapor. They are appropriate for partial-thickness wounds, such as split-thickness skin graft donor sites or superficial abrasions. They can also be used as secondary dressings on wounds that are being treated with hydrocolloids or alginates.

H. Collagen-containing products. A number of collagen-containing products are available in powder, sheet, or fluid form. They are available as pure collagen, typically types 1 and 3, or combined with other materials such as calcium alginate (Fibracol). Some wounds respond better to collagen than to other dressing materials.

I. Hydrofibers represent a newer dressing category of strands; they are some of the most absorptive materials available for packing in a heavily draining wound.

J. Growth factors. Human recombinant PDGF is the only U.S. Food and Drug Administration approved clinically available growth factor. Topically applied to a granulating wound, it promotes granulation tissue formation, angiogenesis, and epithelialization. A saline-moistened gauze dressing is applied daily at midday to help keep the wound bed moist. Although initial approval was for the treatment of diabetic plantar foot ulcers, the drug is mostly used on other wound types. EGF is presently in clinical trials for the treatment of venous stasis ulcers.

K. Skin substitutes. Cultured dermis and epidermis are available clinically for treatment of wounds as 5-cm^2 circular sheets (Apligraft). Wounds must have a good granulating wound bed and low bacterial counts, and hemostasis must be meticulous. Trials are underway on the use of topically applied quick-frozen fibroblasts on wounds.

L. Vacuum-assisted closure. Negative pressure created by vacuum-assisted closure devices (Wound VAC) appears to stimulate capillary ingrowth and the formation of granulation tissue in open wounds while keeping a relatively clean wound environment. V.A.C. therapy is effective in the management of wounds as diverse as diabetic foot wounds, sacral ulcers, mediastinal dehiscence, and wounds including prosthetic mesh. V.A.C. therapy is contraindicated where enteric fistulization is possible or where there are exposed major blood vessels, exposed bone, or cancer within the wound, and it is relatively contraindicated in anticoagulated patients.

IV. Care of wounds in the emergency room

A. History and physical examination. A careful history and physical examination of the whole patient should be performed, with attention to the time and mechanism of injury, initial treatments given, and prior or associated injuries. Medical, surgical, and immunization history and all known medication allergies should be documented. It is critically important that all injuries be identified, with appropriate prioritization of administered treatment plans. Careful neurologic and vascular examination should be performed distal to the site of injury and before administration of any anesthetics that could limit a later assessment.

B. Anesthesia. Lidocaine (Xylocaine) in concentrations from 0.5% to 2.0% is generally chosen for its rapidity of action (1 to 2 minutes). If longer duration is desired, bupivacaine (Marcaine) can be used; however, it may require up to 10 minutes to full onset. A 1:1 mixture of 1% lidocaine and 0.25% bupivacaine provides a rapid and reasonably long acting local anesthetic to improve hemostasis and prolong the effect of the anesthetic. This mixture should not be used to treat wounds on distal extremities (nose, earlobes, fingers, toes, penis) because the profound vasoconstriction may lead to ischemic tissue loss. Whenever local anesthetics are used, care should be taken to avoid intravascular injection by aspirating before infiltration. The maximum safe amount of anesthetic that can be administered to the patient should be calculated before starting treatment. Patients with an allergy to amide anesthetics should be treated with ester anesthetics. The addition of sodium bicarbonate to lidocaine in a 1:9 ratio adjusts the acidic pH of the anesthetic so that its administration is less painful.

C. **Wound cleansing.** After adequate anesthesia is administered, the wound and surrounding skin should be cleansed in a gentle fashion. This is best accomplished with a standard wound-cleansing solution (e.g., Saf-Clens, Shur-Clens). It should be remembered that many standard scrub solutions are extremely toxic to all living cells; thus, they should never be used to wash the wound itself. A good rule to follow is that one should never place a solution in a wound that one would not place in one's own eye. Wounds are best irrigated with saline or lactated Ringer solution with pressures of 8 to 15 psi. An 18- or 19-gauge intravenous catheter or needle on a 35- to 60-mL syringe provides 8 psi irrigating pressure, which is adequate to irrigate most wounds. Battery-powered irrigation systems, available for portable use, deliver pressures of up to 15 psi and are easier to use when irrigating a wound with several liters of fluid. Abrasions should be scrubbed carefully with a gloved hand during cleansing to remove foreign material that might lead to traumatic skin tattooing.

D. **Wound hemostasis and exploration.** Direct pressure, elevation, and even the use of a blood pressure cuff as a tourniquet are effective means of limiting blood loss in the emergency setting. Electrocautery, suture ligation, or hemostat clamping of a bleeding site is best done by a practitioner who is familiar with the anatomy of the area, because major nerves often lie adjacent to major arteries, and any imprecision can lead to an iatrogenic injury worse than the initial trauma. Wounds should be explored carefully for foreign bodies and to determine the extent of injury. Multiplane x-ray views of the soft tissues of the wounded area can prove to be useful in locating radiopaque objects. If the wound contains difficult-to-locate or numerous foreign bodies, it can best be explored in the operating room.

E. **Débridement.** Traumatic breaks of the skin are often irregular, and the force of impact leaves a zone of surrounding skin and underlying tissue injury that is often best treated by judicious sharp débridement. All foreign material and devitalized tissue must be removed before wound closure is attempted. The goal of débridement is to obtain a clean wound with a bleeding skin margin that overlies healthy, viable tissue.

F. **Wound closure.** The decision to close a wound depends largely on the amount of contamination present and the amount of time that the wound has been open. Wounds that are older than 6 to 8 hours, puncture wounds, human bites, and wounds with gross infection should not be closed, with the possible exception of facial wounds, for in these the superior vascular supply can often overcome otherwise major contamination. At a microscopic level, wounds with >10^5 bacteria per gram of tissue are considered too heavily contaminated to close safely. Dog and cat bites often can be closed safely after thorough irrigation and débridement, with administration of appropriate antibiotics.

G. **Additional considerations**
   1. **Tetanus prophylaxis.** Tetanus is a potentially fatal disorder that is characterized by uncontrolled spasms of the voluntary muscles. It is caused by the neurotoxin of the anaerobic bacterium *Clostridium tetani*. A tetanus-prone wound has one or more of the following characteristics: (1) more than 6 hours old; (2) deeper than 1 cm; (3) contaminated by soil, feces, or rust; (4) stellate configuration (burst-type injury with marked soft-tissue injury); (5) caused by missile, crush, burn, or frostbite; (6) contains devitalized or denervated tissue; and (7) caused by an animal or human bite (*Emerg Med Clin North Am* 1992;10:531). Current recommendations for tetanus prophylaxis are summarized in Table 9-2.
   2. **Antibiotics.** Antibiotic use does not allow closure of a wound that would otherwise be left open to heal secondarily, and it is not a substitute for good wound cleansing and débridement. Antibiotics should be chosen

Table 9-3. Rabies postexposure prophylaxis treatment guide

Species	Condition of animal	Treatment[a]
Domestic cat or dog	Healthy and available for at least 10 days of observation	None; however, treatment should be initiated at the first sign of rabies[b]
	Suspected rabid[b]	Immediate
	Unknown	Contact public health department
Wild skunk, bat, fox, coyote, raccoon, or other carnivore	Regard as rabid; animal should be killed and tested as soon as possible	Immediate; however, discontinue if immunofluorescence test is negative

[a](1) Human rabies immune globulin, 20 IU/kg [if feasible, infiltrate half of dose around the wound(s), the rest i.m. in gluteal area]; and (2) human diploid cell vaccine (HDCV), 1.0 mL i.m. in deltoid area (never in gluteal area) on days 0, 3, 7, 14, and 28. If the patient has previously been immunized, give booster HDCV only on days 0 and 3.
[b]Any animal suspected of being rabid should be killed and its brain studied with a rabies-specific fluorescent antibody.
Adapted with permission from Immunization Practices Advisory Committee. Rabies Prevention United States, 1991. *MMWR* 1991;40(RR-3):1.

based on the indication (prophylactic or therapeutic), the location and age of the wound, and the mechanism of injury. In addition, one should consider the likely pathogen(s) that are most involved under the circumstances. Prophylactic antibiotics are indicated for immunocompromised patients and those with prosthetic heart valves or other permanently implanted prostheses. Prophylactic antibiotics should also be used when intestinal or genitourinary tract contamination is present, when an infection is likely to develop, or when an infection has potentially disastrous consequences (*Surg Clin North Am* 1997;77:3). For wounds that are likely to become infected, obtaining good wound cultures at the time of injury helps to better target the specific organism(s) that failed to respond to initial broad-spectrum antibiotic treatment.

H. Bites. The treatment of a bite wound beyond the basic treatment of copious irrigation and débridement is most dependent on the source of the bite.

1. Human bites typically occur during interpersonal conflict. Because the wound often seems relatively trivial, such as a small puncture wound or a laceration in a patient who is very upset or intoxicated, the patient may delay seeking treatment, which increases the likelihood of the injury becoming infected. A particularly troublesome bite is a small skin injury that is seen over the metacarpophalangeal joint of a patient who punched someone else in the mouth and sustained a tooth cut of the skin overlying the fisted knuckle. Such injuries often require operative joint irrigation and parenteral antibiotics. Unintentional bites of the lip or tongue that are sustained in a fall or during a seizure may also occasionally come to the attention of a surgeon. The oral flora of humans include *Staphylococcus* and *Streptococcus* species, anaerobic bacteria, *Eikenella corrodens*, and anaerobic Gram-negative rods; antibiotic coverage should be directed initially toward these organisms.

2. Mammalian animal bites. As infection is the most common complication of domestic animal bites, these bites should be considered contaminated and their immediate closure deferred. Infections that are caused by dog bites are usually polymicrobial, and pathogens include viridans streptococci; *Pasteurella multocida*; and *Bacteroides, Fusobacterium*, and *Capnocytophaga* species. Because these wounds are often larger open lacerations, only about 5% of dog bites become infected. The oral flora of the domestic cat is believed to be less complex, with *P. multocida* found in up to 60% of wounds caused by cat bites. Since these are smaller puncture wounds, up to 80% of these will become infected. Local laws require the confinement of animals to ensure that they do not manifest rabies. Rabies, a routinely fatal disease of the central nervous system, is caused by the rabies virus, which is a member of the rhabdovirus group and contains a single strand of RNA. Thanks in large part to an intensive immunization program, the incidence of rabies in the United States has been reduced greatly, to approximately five cases per year. Today, the major risk comes from wild animal bites. The recommendations for rabies prophylaxis and treatment are summarized in Table 9-3.

3. **Snake bites.** Ten percent of the snakes in the United States are venomous. Determining whether a venomous snake caused the bite is critical in the early management of bite injuries. Pit vipers usually leave two puncture wounds, whereas nonvenomous snakes generally leave a characteristic U-shaped bite wound. Poisonous snake venom contains many polypeptides that are damaging to human tissues, including phospholipase A, hyaluronidase, adenosine triphosphatase, 5-nucleotidase, and nicotinic acid dehydrogenase. The degree of envenomation and the time from injury determine the clinical manifestations. Immediate signs of envenomation include regional edema, erythema, and intense pain at the site of the bite. Systemic manifestations can ensue rapidly, especially with greater envenomation. The hematocrit and platelet count may fall, with concomitant elevation of the prothrombin time, partial thromboplastin time, and bleeding times. Without treatment, severe envenomation may lead to pulmonary edema, peripheral vascular collapse, direct cardiotoxicity, and acute renal failure. Coral snake venom is less toxic locally but can lead to profound neurologic sequelae. Early symptoms include nausea, euphoria, salivation, paresthesias, ptosis, and muscle weakness leading to respiratory arrest.

Treatment is most successful if administered promptly. Extremity wounds should be immobilized and a tourniquet applied proximal to the bite site to minimize the spread of the venom. Although small amounts of venom can be removed by suction through small incisions over the bite wound, a wider surgical excision of the bite removes even more, provided that it can be done in a timely fashion. Polyvalent antivenin may help to neutralize the venom and should be administered intravenously as soon as possible after more severe bites or when systemic symptoms are noted. The species-specific dose of antivenin should correspond to the perceived severity of the envenomation. Larger doses of antivenin carry the risk of serum sickness. Shock is treated with circulatory support. Broad-spectrum antibiotics and tetanus prophylaxis are also indicated.

4. **Spider bites**
   a. The **black widow (_Latrodectus mactans_)** is found throughout the United States and prefers to inhabit dry, dark crevices. The female is distinguished by her shiny black body and a red hourglass mark on the abdomen. The actual bite may cause little pain, and victims often do not recall the event. The venom, a neurotoxin, causes muscular rigidity. Chest pain from muscular contraction follows upper-extremity bites, whereas lower-extremity bites may cause rigidity of the abdominal wall. Patients who present with abdominal wall rigidity, which might typically suggest an acute abdominal emergency, lack associated abdominal tenderness. Intense muscular spasms and pain are usually self-limiting and require no specific treatment. Severe cases may progress to respiratory arrest, which, along with shock, accounts for the observed mortality of approximately 5%. Therapy consists of respiratory and circulatory support, broad-spectrum antibiotics, narcotic analgesia, and muscle relaxants. Antivenin (_L. mactans_) is indicated for the very young or old and for patients with severe illness.

Table 9-4. Wound and skin care products

Product/trade name	Advantages	Limitations	Applications
Gauze			
Kerlix (roll gauze)	Debride mechanically	May disrupt viable tissue during change	Moderately/heavily exudating wounds
	Manages exudates by capillarity	May cause bleeding on removal	Partial- and full-thickness chronic wounds (Stages II, III, IV)
	Permeable to gases		
Gauze sponges	Fills deadspace	May cause pain on removal	Acute wounds
	Conformable	Particulate matter may be left in wound	Secondary dressing
	Adaptable	Permeable to fluids and bacteria	
		Limited thermal insulation	
		May dehydrate wound bed (if allowed to dry)	
		Wet to dry dressings contraindicated—Wound Ostomy Continence Nurses (WOCN) Society Standards of Care, 1992	
Transparent adhesive dressings			
Tegaderm (3M)	Manages exudates by moisture vapor	Manage light exudates only	IV entry sites
Opsite (Smith & Nephew)	Impermeable to fluids and bacteria	May disrupt fragile skin	Minor burns or lacerations
	Permeable to gases	Application may be difficult	Reduces surface friction in high-risk areas (Stage I)
	Visualization of wound		Lightly exudating partial-thickness chronic wounds (Stage II)

(*continued*)

Table 9-4. (continued)

Product/trade name	Advantages	Limitations	Applications
Hydrocolloids	Conformable		Over eschar to promote autolytic debridement
	Low profile		Cover dressing
Restore Hydrocolloid (Hollister)	Forms moist gel wound bed	Manages moderate exudates	Reduces surface friction in high-risk areas
DuoDerm (ConvaTec)	Impermeable to fluids and bacteria	Impermeable to gases	Partial- and full-thickness wounds
Comfeel Ulcer Care Dressing (Coloplast)	Manages exudates by particle swelling	May traumatize fragile skin	Moderately exudating wounds
Tegasorb (3M)		Do not use over eschar or puncture wounds	Venous stasis ulcers in conjunction with Unna boot
	Thermal insulation good	Use with extreme caution on diabetic ulcers	
	Conformable	Contraindicated in 3rd-degree burns	
Wound fillers	Wound filler	Not recommended in dry wounds or wounds with sinus tracts or tunnels	Absorbs moderate to minimal exudate
AcryDerm strands			
Absorbent Wound Dressing (AcryMed)	Absorbs exudate		May be used in combination with other wound dressing to increase absorption or fill shallow areas
	Forms moist wound bed		
Hydrogels	Forms moist wound bed	May dehydrate	Partial- and full-thickness chronic wound (Stages II, III)
Amorphous			
Restore Hydrogel (Hollister)	Conformable	Minimal absorption	

IntraSite Gel (Smith & Nephew)	Manages exudates by swelling	Requires secondary dressing	Partial- and full-thickness burns Diabetic ulcers Lightly exudating wounds
Enzymatic debriding agents			
Collagenase (Santyl, Smith & Nephew)	Liquefies necrotic tissue Contributes toward formation of granulation tissue and epithelialization of wounds	Conditions with pH higher or lower than 6–8 decreases enzyme activity	Debridement of chronic dermal ulcers and severely burned areas
Accuzyme (Healthpoint)	Does not attack healthy tissue or newly formed granulation tissue		
Absorbent dressings			
Bard Absorption Dressing (Bard Medical)	Manages exudates by osmotic action	Permeable to fluids and bacteria	Heavily exudating wounds
	Cleans debris	May increase pH beyond physiologic levels May sting on application Requires secondary dressing	Full-thickness chronic wounds (Stages III, IV) Malodorous wounds
	Reduces odor Maintains moist wound bed Permeable to gases Molds to wound contour Fills deadspace Extends life of secondary dressing Daily dressing change Inexpensive		

(continued)

Table 9-4. (Continued)

Product/trade name	Advantages	Limitations	Applications
Alginate			
Restore CalciCare (Hollister)	Forms moist gel in wound bed	Permeable to fluids and bacteria	Moderately/heavily exudating wounds
Sorbsan (Dow Hickman & Pharmaceuticals)	Manages exudates by capillarity	May produce burning sensation on application	Partial- and full-thickness wounds (Stages III, IV)
	Permeable to gases		Partial-thickness burns
Kaltostat (Convatec)	Molds to wound contour	Requires irrigation before removal if allowed to dry out	Skin donor sites
	Fills deadspace		
	Irrigates easily from wound bed		
	Reduces wound pain		
	Fibers left in wound are absorbed		
	May be used on clinically infected wounds		
	Nonirritating		
Solutions			
0.9% Normal saline	Noncytotoxic solution for wound care	Wound dehydrates if allowed to dry out	Partial- and full-thickness wounds
		If dressing saturated, may macerate periwound skin	Dressing changes 2–3 times daily
Hydrogen peroxide	Chemical debridement of necrotic tissue when used as an irrigating solution	Cytotoxic to fibroblasts	Wound irrigation—use only half strength and always rinse wound with normal saline
		Has been documented to result in air embolus if instilled into wound cavities under pressure	
Povidine-iodine (Betadine)	FDA has not approved for use in wounds	Cytotoxic to fibroblasts until diluted to 1:1,000	None for wound care

Product	Action	Precautions	Application
Antibacterial cream Silver sulfadiazine (Silvadene)	Broad-spectrum antibacterial (*S. aureus, E. coli, P. aeruginosa, P. mirabilis,* β-hemolytic streptococci)	May cause acidosis in burn patients Lasting systemic effects include cardiovascular toxicity, renal toxicity, hepatotoxicity, and neuropathy Impairs wound's ability to fight infection and increases potential for wound infection Never approved by FDA for wound management Do not use in presence of hepatic or renal impairment	Apply 1/8 inch to clean, debrided wound daily or twice daily
Platelet-derived growth factor Becaplermin (Regranex, Ortho-McNeil Pharmaceuticals)	May promote wound healing in otherwise recalcitrant neuropathic ulcer Very few side effects	Dressing protocol may be confusing Wound must have adequate blood supply Wound must be free of infection No osteomyelitis Wound must be free of necrotic tissue Complex dosing	Calculate dosage by multiplying length by width of wound in cm and divide by 4 Wound is irrigated with normal saline (NS) Apply precise amount of drug to wound, cover with NS dressing Leave in place for 12 hr Then irrigate wound with NS Pack wound with NS dressing Leave in place for 12 hr

Adapted with permission from Rolstad BS, Ovington LG, Harris A. Wound care product formulary. In: Bryand, RA (ed). *Acute and Chronic Wounds: Nursing Management.* 2nd ed. St. Louis: Mosby, 2000.

   b. The **brown recluse (*Loxosceles reclusa*)** is found throughout the central and southern United States, most often inhabiting dark, moist environments. It is 10 to 15 mm long, with a light tan to brown color, a flat
   body, and a violin-shaped band over the head and chest area of the back.
   Brown recluse venom is very locally toxic, containing hyaluronidase
   and other elements that lead to coagulation necrosis of the area around
   the wound. Systemically, hemolysis with hemoglobinuria, hemolytic
   anemia, and renal failure may develop. Pain at the time of the bite
   is an inconsistent symptom; however, several hours after the bite, a
   characteristic lesion is seen, with a central zone of pale induration surrounded by an erythematous border. By this time, pain is severe. After
   approximately 1 week, a black eschar develops, which soon sloughs,
   leaving an ulcer that may continue to enlarge, with extensive necrosis
   of the underlying fat and subcutaneous tissues. Systemic illness most
   often occurs in children, with fever, malaise, nausea, and vomiting.
   Therapy is supportive, and mortality is rare. Many of these wounds
   will heal spontaneously. If necessary, excision of the wound should be
   deferred until the ulcer is well demarcated; broad-spectrum antibiotics
   are recommended.

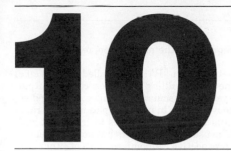

Critical Care

T. Philip Chung and Craig M. Coopersmith

Patients are admitted to intensive care units (ICUs) because of either the presence or the risk of organ dysfunction. This chapter focuses on routine monitoring of the critically ill patient, the three most common types of organ failure responsible for surgical ICU admissions (respiratory, circulatory, and renal failure), and sepsis. It also addresses adjunctive topics, including sedation and analgesia, prophylaxis against stress-induced upper gastrointestinal hemorrhage, and the role of transfusion and glucose control in the care of the critically ill.

I. **Monitoring of the critically ill patient**
   A. **Temperature monitoring.** Critically ill patients are at increased risk for temperature disorders as a result of debility and predisposition to infection. All critically ill patients should have their core temperatures measured at least every 4 hours. A rectal thermometer is the most accurate method of obtaining the core temperature. If contraindications exist to measuring temperature rectally, the oral route is preferable to the axillary route.
   B. **ECG monitoring.** Continuous ECG monitoring with computerized arrhythmia detection systems is standard in most ICUs. Aside from providing rapid assessment of heart rate and rhythm, continuous monitoring allows for rapid detection of dysrhythmias.
   C. **Arterial pressure monitoring**
      1. Indirect arterial pressure measurement with a sphygmomanometer should be performed at least hourly.
      2. **Direct arterial pressure measurement** with intra-arterial catheters offers continuous measurement of arterial pressures and waveforms and easy, painless access for arterial blood gas (ABG) measurement. Arterial cannulation is warranted in patients with hemodynamic instability and in those who require frequent blood gas analyses. The most common site of insertion is the radial artery, which is chosen because of its accessibility and generally good collateral blood flow. If this is unavailable, alternatives include femoral and less commonly dorsalis pedis or axillary artery catheterization. These should be avoided in infants, because occlusion may cause extremity ischemia and subsequent deformity.
      3. **Complications.** Arterial cannulation carries a low risk of complication. Thrombosis or clot formation in the artery occurs, most commonly in the smaller peripheral arteries, but usually recanalization occurs after catheter removal. The extremity distal to the catheter should be assessed frequently both prior to and after insertion, and the catheter should be removed immediately if there is evidence of ischemia. Infectious complications include local cellulitis and bacteremia, which may result from catheter colonization or from contamination of the fluid-filled monitoring system. Local infection and bacteremia generally resolve after catheter removal. Other complications include emboli from the catheter tip, hematoma at the insertion site, and hemorrhage from an open system.
   D. **Central venous pressure (CVP) monitoring.** Central venous catheters provide access to measure CVP and to administer vasoactive drugs and total

parenteral nutrition. For techniques of catheter insertion, refer to Chapter 42.

E. **Pulmonary artery (PA) catheterization.** PA (also called *Swan-Ganz*) catheters are used to determine cardiac filling pressures, cardiac output, pulmonary artery pressures, systemic vascular resistance, and mixed venous saturation (Svo_2). They may be used in unstable patients with rapid changes in hemodyanimic status to assess responses to treatment with fluid and cardioactive agents. The use of PA catheters has not been demonstrated to change mortality in prospective randomized trials of either elective high-risk surgical patients or those suffering from adult respiratory distress syndrome (ARDS).

1. **Continuous ECG and blood pressure monitoring and peripheral intravenous access** are required. An EKG must be checked prior to PA catheter placement to rule out left bundle branch block, since PA catheter placement can induce transient right bundle branch block. If a patient with left bundle branch block needs a PA catheter, a trancutaneous pacemaker must be placed prior to PA catheter placement.

2. **Complications** associated with central venous access are described in Chapter 7. PA catheter balloon rupture exposes the patient to the risk of air and balloon fragment emboli. **Balloon rupture** should be suspected when air inflated into the balloon does not return; the diagnosis is confirmed if blood can be aspirated from the balloon port. If either of these occurs, the catheter should be removed immediately. **Pulmonary infarction**, caused by peripheral migration of the catheter tip with persistent wedging of the tip in the PA, can be avoided by careful monitoring of PA waveforms and the daily chest x-ray (CXR) to document catheter position. **PA perforation** presents with hemoptysis, typically after balloon inflation. Management of this serious complication includes placement of the patient with his or her involved side in the dependent position emergent thoracic surgical consultation. **Thrombus** and central venous occlusion can occur and are rare causes of pulmonary embolism. Atrial and ventricular **arrhythmias** occur commonly during insertion of PA catheters and usually are self-limited. The most frequent persistent cardiac rhythm disturbance is catheter-induced right bundle branch block; hence, PA catheters are relatively contraindicated in patients with complete left bundle branch block. Catheter position should be assessed if catheter-induced ectopy persists; the catheter should be removed at any sign of hemodynamic compromise secondary to ventricular dysrhythmia.

3. **Esophageal dopplers** (CardioQ, Deltex Medical) have recently been introduced as a noninvasive alternative to PA catheters.

F. **Respiratory monitoring**

1. **Pulse oximetry** provides quantitative, continuous assessment of Sao_2 and closely correlates with Sao_2 obtained by ABG determination. Probe malposition, motion, hypothermia, vasoconstriction, and hypotension may result in poor signal detection and unreliable measurements. Nail polish, dark skin, and elevated serum lipids falsely lower the Sao_2 measurement, whereas elevated carboxyhemoglobin or methemoglobin falsely raise the measurements. Despite these caveats, pulse oximetry should be used in all critically ill patients.

2. **Capnography** provides quantitative, continuous assessment of expired CO_2 concentrations, and the gradient between $Paco_2$ and $ETco_2$ measurements can be used to follow trends. A rise in $ETco_2$ can indicate a decrease in alveolar ventilation or an increase in CO_2 production, as seen with overfeeding, sepsis, fever, exercise, or acute increases in CO. A fall in $ETco_2$ indicates either an increase in alveolar ventilation or an increase in dead space, as seen with massive pulmonary embolism or air embolism, endotracheal tube or main-stem bronchus obstruction, ventilator circuit leak, or a sudden drop in CO.

Table 10-1. Modified Ramsay sedation scale

Score	Characteristics
1	Anxious and agitated or restless, or both
2	Cooperative, oriented, and tranquil
3	Responding to commands only
4	Asleep, but responds to physical or auditory stimuli
5	Asleep, but responds sluggishly to physical or auditory stimuli
6	No response

II. **Sedation and analgesia.** Altered mentation, which can span the spectrum from delirium to coma, is a common manifestation of acute illness. The physician caring for the patient must also treat pain and emotional distress. Skillful control of pain and agitation in the ICU minimizes the threat of the patient to him- or herself and allows for the orderly conduct of resuscitative efforts.
   A. **Control of agitation.** The most frequently used agents are **benzodiazepines**, which are potent inducers of sedation, anxiolysis, and amnesia. The precise mechanism of action of benzodiazepines appears to be mediated through γ-aminobutyric acid, an inhibitory neurotransmitter.
      1. **Midazolam** has a short half-life (20 to 60 minutes) and therefore a rapid onset and offset of action. Titration of sedation and communication are simplified by the use of an objective scoring system, such as the modified Ramsay scale (Table 10-1). Effective doses of benzodiazepines may be higher in tolerant patients (e.g., those who have taken similar agents previously or who consume alcohol regularly). Patients older than 50 years or those with preexisting cardiopulmonary, hepatic, or renal dysfunction are particularly susceptible to benzodiazepines and their metabolites. In these patients, the initial doses should be reduced to avoid overdose (manifested clinically as cardiopulmonary collapse). Although midazolam has a short half-life, when it is given as a continuous infusion for a prolonged period of time, it accumulates in the body, and a patient, despite being off of all sedatives, may take a number of days to fully awaken while the agent is eliminated.
      2. **Lorazepam** has a longer half-life and a slower onset of action. Unlike midazolam, lorazepam does not have active metabolites. However, similar to midazolam, the drug accumulates with prolonged usage, and patients may remain sedated for a number of days after the agent is stopped. Despite this, either midazolam or lorazepam are acceptable alternatives for long-term sedation in the critically ill patient.
      3. **Flumazenil** antagonizes the pharmacologic actions of benzodiazepines but is limited by a very short half-life. Patients given this agent may experience side effects ranging from confusion and agitation to seizure and/or symptoms of benzodiazepine withdrawal.
      4. **Propofol** is a nonbenzodiazepine sedative-hypnotic that has an extremely short onset and offset of action and is usually delivered as a continuous infusion. It does not accumulate to the same degree as benzodiazepines and thus results in a shorter length of sedation after discontinuation. A major potential side effect of propofol is hypotension, especially in hypovolemic patients. Although more expensive that benzodiazepines, propofol is preferred for short-term sedation (<2 days) because of its rapid elimination.
      5. **Dexmedetomidine** is a new, relatively selective α_2-adrenoreceptor agonist that may be helpful for short-term sedation of mechanically ventilated critically ill patients. Patients treated with this agent are more easily arousable than those sedated with either propofol or benzodiazepine infusions. The main side effect is hypotension. Dexmedetomidine is approved for use for a maximum of 24 hours.

6. **Haloperidol** is also used short term to treat agitation, especially if it is accompanied by delirium. The combination of haloperidol and a benzodiazepine (midazolam or lorazepam) is particularly effective because smaller doses of each agent can be used, usually avoiding the extrapyramidal side effects of haloperidol. Major toxicities include hypotension, cardiac arrythmias, and prolongation of the QT interval. Therefore, the EKGs of patients on haloperidol should be checked daily.

B. **Control of pain.** Intravenous narcotics are used liberally in the surgical ICU. Morphine is administered most commonly for p.r.n. and patient-controlled dosing because of its low cost and familiarity. Fentanyl is the most commonly used opiate for continuous drips. It has a half-life of 30 to 60 minutes due to its rapid redistribution. Unlike morphine, fentanyl does not cause histamine release and therefore is less likely to cause hypotension. Hydromorphone is a viable option for patients who are allergic to morphine or fentanyl. Care should be used in patients with liver failure. Meperidine is used least frequently because of its side effects, which are most common in patients with renal insufficiency. Because all narcotics can cause respiratory depression and hypotension, care in the use of these agents is particularly important in patients with poorly compensated cardiopulmonary dysfunction (smaller than usual initial doses are safer). Thoracic or lumbar epidural catheters are usually well tolerated, decrease the need for intravenous narcotics, and can substantially improve compliance with respiratory therapy.

C. Regardless of which agents are used for sedation and anelgesia, the presence of a **sedation protocol** decreases both length of stay in the ICU and the length of time a patient requires mechanical ventilation compared with physician-directed sedation.

D. For patients who require **long-term sedation and analgesia,** daily interruption of sedation to wakefulness produces decreased time on mechanical ventilation and shorter ICU stays, according to a prospective, randomized controlled study (*N Engl J Med* 2000;342:1477). However, this study did not include surgical patients, who have higher analgesia requirements than typical medical ICU patients. Therefore, the applicability of a "daily wake-up" to surgical ICU patients is unclear.

III. **Acute respiratory failure**
A. **Etiology.** Respiratory failure results from inadequate exchange of oxygen and carbon dioxide. It may be caused by a failure of the gas-exchange mechanism [as in asthma, chronic obstructive pulmonary disease (COPD), ARDS, pneumonia, pulmonary embolism, and pulmonary edema] and a consequent ventilation-perfusion mismatch. Alternatively, it may be caused by a failure of the mechanical ventilatory apparatus (as in neuromuscular disease, inspiratory muscle fatigue, and airway obstruction), which results in hypoventilation and thereby hypercapnia and hypoxemia. Although the etiology (possibly multifactorial) is important for longer term treatment and prognosis, the early treatment of respiratory failure is similar regardless of the immediate cause.

B. **Diagnosis.** Signs or symptoms of respiratory impairment (e.g., tachypnea, dyspnea, or mental status changes) should prompt analysis of ABGs. Pulse oximetry monitoring results of <90% correspond to a PaO_2 of <60 mm Hg, which seriously compromises tissue oxygenation. An acute rise in $PaCO_2$ to >50 mm Hg, along with a pH of <7.35 (respiratory acidosis), implies a significant imbalance between carbon dioxide production and elimination (alveolar ventilation). Both of these laboratory abnormalities are consistent with respiratory insufficiency. In a patient with the aforementioned clinical signs of respiratory impairment, a diagnosis of respiratory failure is made.

C. **Treatment**
1. Securing and maintaining a **patent airway** is the first priority in an unstable patient (i.e., ABC's).

Table 10-2. Oxygen delivery systems

Type	FIO_2 capability	Comments
Nasal cannula	24–48%	At flow rates of 1–8 L/min; true FIO_2 uncertain and highly dependent on minute ventilation; simple, comfortable, and can be worn during eating or coughing
Simple face mask	35–55%	At flow rates of 6–10 L/min
High-humidity mask	Variable from 28% to nearly 100%	Flow rates should be 2–3 times minute ventilation; levels >60% may require additional oxygen bleed-in; excellent humidification
Reservoir mask		
Nonrebreathing	90–95%	At flow rates of 12–15 L/min; incorporates directional valves that reduce room air entrainment and rebreathing of expired air
Partial rebreathing	50–80%	At flow rates of 8–10 L/min
Ventimask	Available at 24%, 28%, 31%, 35%, 40%, and 50%	Provides controlled FIO_2; useful in chronic obstructive pulmonary disease patients to prevent depression of respiratory drive; poorly humidified gas at maximum FIO_2

FIO_2, fraction of inspired oxygen.

2. **Oxygen therapy.** The objective of supplemental oxygen administration is to increase the relative concentration of oxygen in the alveoli. This is accomplished most commonly by delivering oxygen through a nasal cannula, simple face mask, or face mask with a reservoir (Table 10-2). The inspired oxygen concentration varies depending on the percentage of entrained air: The more air that is entrained (with an ambient oxygen concentration of 0.21), the lower the fraction of inspired oxygen (FIO_2). When the required FIO_2 is high ($\sim$0.60), a high–air-flow system with oxygen enrichment via a jet-mixing or Venturi apparatus is used, and the oxygen is delivered by a tight-fitting mask with a reservoir (to minimize entrainment). Whenever possible, inspired oxygen should be humidified to prevent drying of the airways and respiratory secretions.

3. **Airway management.** The most common obstruction of the airway in a patient with an altered sensorium is the tongue. This is corrected easily by the chin-lift or jaw-thrust maneuver or by placing an oropharyngeal or nasopharyngeal airway. If uncertainty exists about whether the airway is patent or protected from aspiration, ET intubation is indicated. In most cases, intubation is not urgent. **Unless the physician is skilled in the placement of an artificial airway, the appropriate maneuver upon seeing a hypoxic patient is to give supplemental oxygen and to bag the patient if necessary until someone with airway expertise arrives.**

   a. **Oral and nasal ET intubation.** The oral route is usually the most expeditious. The nasal route can be used only when the patient is breathing spontaneously; significant skill is needed to direct the tip of the ET tube blindly past the vocal cords and into the trachea. Once the tube is in the trachea and the adequacy of bilateral ventilation has been established using auscultation and a carbon dioxide indicator, a CXR is required to document correct ET tube position.

b. Noninvasive ventilation. Biphasic positive airway pressure is a form of ventilation that is delivered by means of a tight-fitting nasal mask (no ET tube), which allows independent control of positive inspiratory and expiratory pressures. It is most useful as a bridge to aid respiratory efforts in patients with mild to moderate respiratory insufficiency of short duration [e.g., asthma or COPD exacerbations or pulmonary edema (*Am J Respir Crit Care Med* 1995;151:1799; *Chest* 1994;105:229)] and frequently can prevent the need for intubation in patients with rapidly reversible respiratory failure.

c. Tracheostomy should be considered in the presence of severe maxillofacial injury to ensure an adequate airway or if prolonged intubation (~2 weeks) is anticipated. Tracheostomy provides a more secure airway, improved patient comfort and oral hygiene, increased patient mobility, and enhanced secretion removal. Furthermore, it can reduce the work of breathing due to lower resistance compared with ET tubes and therefore may let patients wean off the ventilator more rapidly. **If a tracheostomy falls out before an adequate tract has formed, the patient should be reintubated orally rather than subjected to a blind attempt to replace the tracheostomy at the bedside.**

d. Cricothyroidotomy is useful in emergency situations when attempts to ventilate by bag-valve-mask and ET tube are unsuccessful. The technique is described in Chapter 42 (IV.B.2). Percutaneous cricothyoidotomy may also be performed if a kit is available and someone with expertise is present.

e. Complications. Immediate complications include passage of the ET tube into either the esophagus or the tissue surrounding the trachea. Either can lead to death if not promptly recognized. Of these, esophageal intubation is substantially more common. When an ET tube is placed in tissue surrounding the trachea (most comon when attempting to replace a tracheostomy that has fallen out), it can lead to hemorrhage, pneumothorax, pneumomediastinum, subcutaneous emphysema, and injury to the recurrent laryngeal nerve. Delayed complications of ET intubation include hemorrhage, which results, although rarely, from erosion of the tube into a prominent vessel (usually the brachiocephalic artery). Immediate orotracheal intubation, removal of the tracheostomy tube, insertion of the surgeon's finger into the tracheostomy site, and anterior compression of the brachiocephalic artery against the clavicle can be used treat the hemorrhage. ET tube cuff pressures should be monitored frequently and kept below capillary filling pressures (i.e., <25 mm Hg) to prevent tracheal ischemia, which, if untreated, can lead to tracheomalacia or tracheal stenosis.

4. Mechanical ventilation is indicated for the treatment of severe respiratory failure. The goal of treatment is to improve alveolar ventilation and oxygenation and to reduce the work of breathing while other therapies are instituted to treat underlying disease processes.

a. Modes of mechanical ventilation (*N Engl J Med* 1994;330:1056; *Chest* 1993;104:1833) can be divided into volume-limited and pressure-limited modes. The key to understanding the differences between these modes lies in the relationship of pressure to volume [i.e., pulmonary compliance, in which compliance equals the change in volume divided by the change in pressure ($C = V/P$)]. The goal of volume-limited modes is to deliver a set tidal volume to the patient at a rate that ensures adequate alveolar ventilation; airway pressure varies depending on compliance. In contrast, the goal of pressure-limited modes is to deliver a set airway pressure; tidal volume varies depending on compliance.

(1) Volume-limited modes

    (a) Assist-control (A/C) ventilation delivers a preset tidal volume at a set rate. As the machine senses each inspiratory effort by the patient, it delivers the set tidal volume. If the patient's respiratory rate is below the machine's set rate, ventilator-initiated breaths are delivered to make up the difference between the set rate and the patient's. A/C ventilation minimizes the work of breathing because the ventilator assists all breaths (hence, the term *full support*); however, for this reason, this mode is uncomfortable if the patient's breaths are dyssynchronous with those delivered by the ventilator. Respiratory alkalosis from hyperventilation may develop in agitated patients.

    (b) Intermittent mandatory ventilation (IMV), like A/C ventilation, delivers a preset tidal volume at a set rate. IMV does not assist spontaneous respiratory efforts. The tidal volume during these breaths differs from the A/C tidal volume for spontaneously breathing patients because the ventilator in the IMV mode is determined entirely by the strength of the patient's respiratory effort. To prevent the stacking of mechanical breaths on top of spontaneous breaths, positive-pressure breaths interjected by the ventilator are triggered by the patient's spontaneous efforts, allowing synchronization with the patient's ventilatory pattern. The gas for spontaneous breathing during IMV is provided by activation of either a flow-by valve in continuous-flow systems or a demand valve that opens a reservoir of fresh gas during inspiration. With demand-valve systems, often there is a significant lag between the start of the inspiratory flow (generated by the patient) and the arrival of fresh gas in the trachea. During this lag, the patient expends work in the effort to breathe, which may potentiate respiratory muscle fatigue (*Am Rev Respir Dis* 1986;134:902). This mode may be more comfortable than A/C for alert, robust patients because it allows unassisted breaths; however, for those with weak respiratory muscles, it is less comfortable because it makes them work harder for a given minute ventilation. Most ventilators allow low levels of pressure support [see section **III.C.1.b(2)**] to aid spontaneous ventilation and reduce the work imposed by these demand valves.

(2) Pressure-limited modes

    (a) Pressure-control ventilation delivers a preset inspiratory pressure (as opposed to tidal volume) at a set rate. This mode is used in patients with poor (low) lung compliance in whom high inspiratory pressures develop when they are ventilated with the more traditional modes described previously. Thus, the advantage of this mode is that it allows the physician to set the airway pressure and thereby minimize barotrauma. The disadvantage is that the tidal volume varies depending on compliance. The sudden development of an increase in airway resistance (coughing, thick secretions, a kink in the ET tube, a Valsalva maneuver), for example, increases airway pressures and decreases tidal volumes to dangerously low levels.

    (b) Pressure-support ventilation delivers a preset inspiratory pressure but at no set rate. Constant inspiratory pressure continues until the inspiratory flow of gas falls below a predetermined level and the exhalation valve opens. Thus, tidal volumes are generated only when the patient is breathing spontaneously. This allows the patient to maintain control of inspiratory and expiratory time and thus tidal volume; as a result, this mode is the most comfortable for spontaneously breathing patients. The disadvantages of pressure-support ventilation are that (1) all ventilation depends on patient effort and (2) sudden increases in airway resistance, as with pressure-control ventilation, decrease tidal volumes. Small amounts (5 to 8 cm H_2O) of pressure-support ventilation are used routinely to overcome the resistance to air flow caused by the ET tube and the inspiratory demand valves of the ventilator (*Am Rev Respir Dis* 1989;139:513).

(3) **High-frequency oscillatory ventilation** (HFOV) uses substantially faster rates (180 to 300 per minute) and smaller tidal volumes than conventional modes. The result is a relative decrease in diaphragmatic excursion, lung movement, and airway pressures. The physical mechanisms responsible for gas movement are complex and incompletely understood. Although HFOV has not been demonstrated to improve survival, it is associated with a trend toward decreased mortality in ARDS in a recent prospective, randomized trial [52% versus 37%, $P = 0.102$ (*Am J Respir Crit Care Med* 2002;166:801–808)] and represents a viable "rescue" therapy for those failing with conventional ventilation. HFOV may be considered when FIO_2 requirements exceed 70% and mean airway pressure is approaching 20 cm H_2O or higher or when there is a positive end-expiratory pressure of >15 cm H_2O in ARDS. It may also be useful in patients with severe damage of only one lung (using independent lung ventilation) or bronchopleural fistulas.

b. **Ventilator management**
   (1) **Choice of ventilator mode.** One of the most important duties of the intensivist is to match the needs of the patient with the appropriate ventilator mode. This is accomplished most easily by considering the advantages and disadvantages of each mode. Failure to do so results in patient agitation and a significant waste of patient energy spent "fighting the ventilator."
   (2) **FIO₂** should be adjusted to ensure adequate arterial oxygenation, which is a blood hemoglobin saturation of 92% in lighter-skinned individuals and 95% in darker-skinned patients (*Chest* 1990;97:1420). The lowest possible FIO_2 (ideally ≤ 0.40) should be used to achieve these levels of arterial saturation to prevent pulmonary oxygen toxicity and retrolental fibroplasia (in neonates). Warming and humidifying the inspired gas prevents drying of secretions and heat loss and promotes mucociliary clearance.
   (3) **Tidal volume.** There is no consensus on the optimal tidal volume for the postoperative patient who requires short-term mechanical ventilatory support. However, in ARDS, low tidal volumes are associated with improved survival. A recent multicenter, prospective, randomized trial, demonstrated improved survival in patients who were ventilated with low tidal volume (6 mL/kg predicted body weight) compared with high tidal volumes [12 mL/kg, 31.0% mortality versus 39.8%, respectively, $P = .007$ (*N Engl J Med* 2000;342:1301)]. As a result of this important study, the tidal volume should be adjusted to as low as 4 cc/kg to maintain plateau pressures at <30 cm H_2O to minimize barotrauma but >20 cm H_2O to minimize atelectasis.
   (4) **Ventilatory rate.** Once the tidal volume has been determined, the rate is chosen (typically 8 to 16 breaths per minute) to provide adequate minute ventilation (the product of rate and tidal volume). The rate is adjusted to optimize arterial pH and $PaCO_2$; an end-tidal CO_2 monitor is frequently useful in this regard.

(5) **Inspiratory-expiratory (I/E) ratio.** The normal I/E ratio is 1:2 to 1:3. Longer expiratory times allow patients with obstructive lung disease (high compliance) to exhale fully and prevent stacking of breaths. In contrast, longer inspiratory times, which decrease peak airway pressures, are useful in patients with low pulmonary compliance. Inverse ratio ventilation takes advantage of breath stacking, using I/E ratios from 1:1 to 4:1. Used only in patients with severe consolidating lung disease, inverse ratio ventilation is believed to improve gas exchange by progressive alveolar recruitment [mean airway pressures are higher, keeping a larger number of alveoli open for a greater percentage of the respiratory cycle (*Crit Care Med* 1995;23:224)]. Inverse ratio ventilation is used most commonly with pressure-control ventilation.

(6) **Positive end-expiratory pressure (PEEP)** increases functional residual capacity, increases lung compliance, and improves ventilation-perfusion matching by opening terminal airways and recruiting partially collapsed alveoli. Five-centimeter H_2O PEEP is considered physiologic; higher levels are used when hypoxemia is moderate to severe. PEEP significantly increases intrathoracic pressure and therefore decreases cardiac output (CO), reduces venous return to the heart, increases airway pressure, and alters pulmonary vascular resistance. PEEP levels of >15 cm H_2O significantly increase the risk of barotrauma and spontaneous pneumothorax. PEEP applied to the spontaneously ventilating patient without inspiratory ventilatory support is called *continuous positive airway pressure (CPAP)*.

(7) **Sedation and neuromuscular paralysis.** Sedation is often necessary in mechanically ventilated patients to control anxiety, to allow the patient to rest, and to synchronize breathing (*Am Rev Respir Med* 1993;147:234; *Chest* 1993;104:566). Paralysis rarely is necessary but is useful in patients with severe respiratory failure because it increases pulmonary compliance by decreasing the elastic recoil of the chest wall. If paralytics are necessary, they should be discontinued as soon as is practicable, because long-term use is associated with paresis, which may last for weeks to months after a patient is discharged from the ICU. Commonly used sedatives and paralytics and their dosages are listed in Chapter 6 (see Tables 6-3 and 6-4).

c. **Complications**
   (1) **ET tube dislodgment and patient self-extubation** can produce a medical emergency characterized by life-threatening hypoxia and hypercarbia in those who are profoundly ill. For this reason, restraint of the patient's upper extremities is frequently required. If a patient does self-extubate, he or she should be closely observed, as a surprising number of patients will be able to remain successfully extubated. If the patient shows any signs of persistent respiratory distress, however, he or she should be immediately reintubated or placed on noninvasive ventilation, depending on the clinical scenario.
   (2) **ET tube cuff leaks** should be suspected when there is an unexplained decrease in the returned expired volume associated with a fall in airway pressure. Because cuff leaks increase the risk of aspiration and decrease the efficiency of ventilation, the tube should be changed urgently if it is determined that the ET tube is in the correct position. A cuff leak may also indicate the ET tube is at or partially above the vocal cords, and the tube may be advanced using a bronchoscope if appropriate equipment and expertise are available.

(3) **Respiratory distress** may occur suddenly during mechanical ventilation, due either to an acute change in the patient's status or to ventilator malfunction. The first priority is to disconnect the ventilator and switch to bag ventilation using 100% oxygen to ensure adequate ventilation and oxygenation. Increased airway pressures may indicate obstruction of the tube with secretions or a kink in the tube, bronchospasm, pneumothorax, or migration of the ET tube into a main-stem bronchus. Check the ET tube for patency and suction; if there is a partial obstruction, use large-volume saline lavage to clear the tube. If the obstruction is complete, remove the ET tube and reintubate the patient. Listen closely for any change in breath sounds consistent with a pneumothorax, new lung consolidation, or pleural fluid collection. A less common but important cause of respiratory distress is pulmonary embolism.

(4) **Check the ventilator's function** and, if normal, return the patient to the ventilator, making any needed changes in ventilator settings to ensure adequate ventilation and oxygenation. The results of an ABG and a CXR frequently are helpful in identifying the cause of the change in respiratory status.

(5) **Barotrauma** from very high peak airway pressures (≥ 50 cm H_2O) can lead to subcutaneous emphysema, pneumomediastinum, and pneumothorax (*Crit Care Med* 1995;23:223). Whereas subcutaneous emphysema and pneumomediastinum usually are benign, a pneumothorax that develops while a patient is on positive-pressure ventilation is at high risk for becoming a tension pneumothorax and thus usually is treated emergently (tube thoracostomy).

(6) **Oxygen toxicity** refers to levels of intra-alveolar oxygen high enough to cause lung damage. The precise mechanism is not known but probably involves oxidation of cell membranes and generation of toxic oxygen radicals. An FIO_2 of 0.40 or less is considered safe even for long periods. Although experimental data demonstrate that microscopic damage to alveoli occurs after only a few hours of an FIO_2 of 1.0 in animals, convincing studies in patients are impossible to perform due to ethical consideration. It appears prudent, however, to keep the FIO_2 at 0.60 or less whenever possible, often using higher levels of PEEP (8 to 12 cm H_2O) to help reduce the FIO_2.

d. **Weaning off mechanical ventilation.** Although there are exceptions (e.g., immediate extubation of a healthy patient with normal lungs after general anesthesia), discontinuing mechanical ventilation may require weaning. In general, hemodynamic instability or high work of breathing (e.g., minute ventilation >15 L per minute) are contraindications to weaning. Reduction of the FIO_2 to 0.40 or less and of PEEP to 5 cm H_2O or less is accomplished first (see preceding section). Most relatively healthy patients tolerate rapid reduction in their ventilatory rate from full mechanical ventilatory support to spontaneous breathing as their mental status improves after general anesthesia. In contrast, the patient who has needed prolonged ventilatory support may require from several days to weeks to wean because of marginal respiratory muscle strength and the time required for the injured lungs to recover. The optimal strategy for weaning patients continues to be a topic of debate. The results of controlled clinical trials indicate that the method of weaning from ventilator support is most likely of little consequence for patients who have been on mechanical ventilatory support for 2 weeks or less, as the primary determinant of weaning success is simply resolution of the pathology that induced respiratory failure (*N Engl J Med* 1996;335:1864;

N Engl J Med 1995;332:345; *Am J Respir Crit Care Med* 1994;150:896). To aid spontaneous respiratory efforts, many intensivists wean a patient from the ventilator by keeping the patient on a low respiratory rate and providing a high level of pressure support, followed by decreasing the amount of pressure support supplied by the ventilator twice a day until the patient is ready for extubation. Others use short periods (30 to 60 minutes) of unassisted spontaneous ventilation with small amounts of CPAP (CPAP trials) to test muscle strength and recovery of pulmonary function. Much like sedation, the presence of a weaning protocol decreases patient time on the ventilator compared with physician-directed weaning.

IV. **Circulatory failure: shock**
   A. Shock is characterized by hypotension, and it occurs when either the supply of or the ability to use oxygen and other nutrients is insufficient to meet metabolic demands. If left uncorrected, shock inevitably leads to the death of cells, tissues, organs, and, ultimately, the patient. Understanding the **pathophysiology of shock** depends on an appreciation of the relationship of blood pressure [specifically, mean arterial pressure (MAP)] to CO and systemic vascular resistance (SVR): MAP is directly proportional to CO and SVR. Because CO is equal to stroke volume times heart rate, and stroke volume is directly proportional to preload, afterload, and myocardial contractility, MAP is directly proportional to heart rate, preload, afterload, and contractility. Compensatory changes in response to systemic hypotension include the release of catecholamines, aldosterone, renin, and cortisol, which act in concert to increase heart rate, preload, afterload, and contractility.
   B. **Classification and recognition of shock** (Table 10-3). The morbidity and mortality of circulatory shock are related not only to the underlying cause but also to the depth and duration of circulatory compromise. Early recognition and prompt intervention are therefore critical.
   1. **Hypovolemic shock** results from loss of circulating blood volume (usually at least 20%) caused by acute hemorrhage, fluid depletion, or dehydration; these three usually are distinguishable from one another by history. These patients typically are peripherally vasoconstricted, tachycardic, and oliguric and have low jugular venous pressure.
   2. **Cardiogenic shock** results from inadequate CO due to intrinsic cardiac failure (e.g., acute myocardial infarction, valvular stenosis, regurgitation or rupture, ischemia, arrhythmia, cardiomyopathy, or acute ventricular septal defect). These patients typically are peripherally

Table 10-3. Clinical parameters in shock

Shock classification	Skin	Jugular venous distention	Cardiac output	Pulmonary capillary wedge pressure	Systemic vascular resistance	Mixed venous oxygen content
Hypovolemic	Cool, pale	↓	↓	↓	↑	↓
Cardiogenic	Cool, pale	↑	↓	↑	↑	↓
Septic						
Early	Warm, pink	↑↓	↑	↓	↓	↑
Late	Cool, pale	↓	↓	↓	↑	↑↓
Neurogenic	Warm, pink	↓	↓	↓	↓	↓

vasoconstricted, tachycardic, and oliguric. Their jugular venous pressure typically is elevated.

3. **Obstructive shock** results from etiologies that prevent adequate cardiac output but are not intrinsically cardiac in origin. This type of shock may be caused by pulmonary embolus, tension pneumothorax, or cardiac tamponade. Jugular venous pressure is often elevated in these patients.

4. **Distributive shock** is characterized by a hyperdynamic state consisting of tachycardia, vasodilation (with decreased cardiac filling pressures), decreased SVR, and increased CO; however, some patients present with hypodynamic septic shock and have decreased CO and hypoperfusion. The most common causes of distributive shock include sepsis, the systemic inflammatory response syndrome (SIRS), adrenal insufficiency, and liver failure.

5. **Neurogenic shock** results from interruption of the spinal cord at or above the thoracolumbar sympathetic nerve roots, which also produces loss of sympathetic tone to the vascular system. During sepsis, vasodilation occurs secondary to vasoactive mediators released in response to infection. During neurogenic shock, vasodilation occurs secondary to loss of sympathetic tone. The cardiovascular response is the same: Patients are typically peripherally vasodilated (warm extremities), tachycardic, and oliguric. Jugular venous pressure is usually low.

6. **Interventions common to all types of shock.** The goal of therapy is to ensure adequate delivery of oxygen to the peripheral tissues. Because oxygen delivery is the arithmetic product of arterial oxygen saturation (Sao_2), hemoglobin concentration, and CO, each of these parameters should be optimized.

   a. **Sao_2.** It is necessary to administer supplemental oxygen, secure or provide an adequate airway, and check for adequate bilateral ventilation. A pulse oximetry (Sao_2) level that exceeds 92% should allow adequate delivery of oxygen at the periphery; however, levels should be maximized in the acute setting.

   b. **Hemoglobin concentration.** The hemoglobin concentration must be adequate to deliver oxygen to the tissues. One study has indicated that for most critically ill patients a transfusion trigger of 7 g/dL is appropriate, with the goal of keeping the hemoglobin concentration at 7.0 to 9.0 g/dL except in patients with an ongoing myocardial infarction or severe ischemic cardiomyopathy (*N Engl J Med* 1999;340:409). A tube of blood should be sent early to the blood bank for cross-matching to avoid delays in blood availability for transfusion.

   c. **Cardiac output.** The ECG tracing provides direct information about heart rate and several indirect clues about stroke volume. The atrial contraction provides approximately 25% of ordinary CO, so the atrioventricular dyssynchrony observed in atrial fibrillation or third-degree atrioventricular block predictably causes significant impairment of CO. Tachyarrhythmias decrease diastolic ventricular and coronary artery filling times. When severe (e.g., heart rate ~140 beats per minute), tachycardia predictably impairs preload, stroke volume, and CO. When treating tachycardia per se, it is imperative to distinguish between tachycardia as a compensatory response (e.g., sinus tachycardia secondary to hypovolemia) and tachycardia as a cause of shock (e.g., ventricular tachycardia). With the exception of the patient in pulmonary edema, *all* patients in circulatory shock should initially receive 10 to 20 mL/kg of a balanced salt solution, such as lactated Ringer solution (normal saline is not a balanced salt solution). The pace of volume infusion should reflect the depth of circulatory shock. To achieve rapid infusion rates, short, large-bore intravenous catheters (e.g., 14 or 16 gauge) in an antecubital vein are best. If this is not possible, a no. 8.5 French cordis (Swan-Ganz introducer) inserted into a central vein is effective. The stopcocks should be removed from the venous lines to reduce flow resistance and deliver *warmed* fluids. Hypothermia is aggravated by rapid infusion of room-temperature crystalloid and refrigerated blood, impairing the ability to unload oxygen from hemoglobin in the periphery and compromising all enzymatic processes, especially coagulation.

d. To assess the adequacy of resuscitation, peripheral pulses and urine output should be evaluated. Palpable pedal pulses or urine output that exceeds 1 mL/kg per hour usually indicates a cardiac index of >2 L/m^2 per minute. These two simple techniques can be used to estimate cardiac performance in many patients. Patients who do not improve with initial resuscitative measures may require invasive hemodynamic monitoring. All shock victims should be monitored with an indwelling bladder catheter. Metabolic acidosis, identified by an ABG determination and serum electrolytes, can reflect the depth of circulatory compromise and the adequacy of resuscitation; however, this is not true in patients acidotic with preexisting renal failure. Infusion of sodium bicarbonate should be reserved for patients with a pH of <7.15, because the sodium bicarbonate may actually worsen intracellular pH as the bicarbonate is converted to CO_2 at the tissue level.

7. **Specific therapy**
   a. **Cardiogenic shock.** It is critical to distinguish shock caused by intrinsic myocardial dysfunction from extrinsic processes that interfere with venous return to the heart. Diagnosis may require echocardiography and cardiac catheterization. Management is directed toward maintaining adequate myocardial perfusion and CO with volume expansion and vasopressors, inotropes, or chronotropes (Table 10-4). Initial treatment often is guided by CVP measurements or, in severe cases, PA catheter "wedge" pressure, while the precipitating cause of compromise is identified and treated. Mechanical support with intra-aortic balloon counterpulsation may be necessary before and during recovery from definitive surgical treatment (see Chapter 35). The two common thoracic processes that compromise venous return and cause pump failure are tension hemothorax or pneumothorax and pericardial tamponade (see Chapter 27), which require immediate mechanical rather than pharmacologic intervention.
   b. **Hypovolemic shock.** Therapy focuses on control of ongoing volume loss and restoration of intravascular volume. External hemorrhage should be controlled by direct pressure. Internal hemorrhage may require further diagnostic tests and/or surgical intervention. The degree of volume deficit (Table 10-5) determines the type and volume of resuscitative fluid. Patients with blood losses of up to 20% of their circulating blood volume can be resuscitated using crystalloid solutions alone, typically lactated Ringer solution. However, because salt solutions equilibrate with the interstitial space, volume replacement with these solutions alone requires three times the estimated volume deficit. Patients in whom diaphoresis, ashen facies, and hypotension develop have lost 30% or more of their blood volume and require urgent transfusion of blood. Individuals with severe dehydration often have profound metabolic and electrolyte abnormalities. Fluid administration should be modified once laboratory analysis of serum electrolytes is completed. With adequate volume resuscitation, vasoconstrictors and vasoactive agents can usually be avoided.
   c. **Distributive shock**
      (1) **Septic shock (see VI.C.2)**
      (2) **Adrenal insufficiency.** Critically ill patients in septic shock may have relative adrenal insufficiency, which may be indentified using a low-dose corticotropin stimulation test. A recent

Table 10-4. Vasoactive drugs and their specific actions

Class and drug	Blood pressure	Systemic vascular resistance	Cardiac output	Heart rate	Inotrope Low-dose	Inotrope High-dose	Renal blood flow	Coronary blood flow	Mvo₂
Alpha only									
Phenylephrine	↑↑	↑↑↑	→	→	±	±	↓↓↓	± ↑↑	↑
Alpha and beta									
Norepinephrine	↑↑↑	↑↑↑↑	↑↑↑	↑±	↑	↑	↓↓↓	↑↑	↑↑
Epinephrine	↑↑↑	↑↑↑↑	↑↑↑↑	↑↑↑	↑↑	↑↑↑	→ ±	↑↑	↑↑↑
Dopamine	↑↑	↑↑	↑↑↑	↑↑	±	↑↑	→ ↑↑↑	↑↑	↑↑
Beta only									
Dobutamine	±	↓↓↓	↑↑↑↑	↑↑	↑↑↑	↑↑↑	±	↑↑↑	↑↑↑
Beta-blocker									
Metoprolol	→	→	↓↓	↓↓↓	↓↓	↓↓↓	±	→ ↓	↓
Other									
Nitroglycerine	± ↓	↓↓	↑↑	±	±	±	± ↑	→	↓
Hydralazine	↓↓	↓↓↓	↑↑	↑↑	±	±	± ↑	→	↓
Nitroprusside	↓↓↓	↓↓↓	↑↑	±↑	±	±	↑↑	±	↓

Mvo₂, mixed venous oxygen saturation.

Table 10-5. Physiologic changes in hypovolemic shock

Blood loss (%)	<15	15–30	30–40	>40
Blood loss (mL)*	<750	750–1,500	1,500–2,000	>2,000
Heart rate (BPM)	Nl	>100	>120	>140
Blood pressure	Nl	SBP Nl	SBP↓	SBP↓↓
		DBP↑	DBP↓	DBP↓↓
Respiratory rate	Nl	↑	↑↑	↑↑↑
Urine output	Nl	↓	Oliguria	Anuria
Mental state	Minimal anxiety	Mild anxiety	Confusion	Lethargy

DBP, diastolic blood pressure; Nl, normal; SBP, systolic blood pressure.
*Based on a 70-kg male patient.

study showed that nonresponders to the corticotropin stimulation test had a modest decrease in mortality when treated with a 1-week course of hydrocortisone and fludrocortisone (*JAMA* 2002;288:862–871). Patients who respond appropriately to the stimulation test do not benefit from steroids.

(3) **SIRS** may result from noninfectious causes of inflammation (e.g., necrotizing pancreatitis, burns). Treatment is supportive, with volume infusion, mechanical ventilation, and the adminstration of pressors as needed until the inflammatory process resolves.

d. **Neurogenic shock.** As with septic shock, the initial intervention in neurogenic shock is volume infusion. A peripheral vasoconstrictor, such as phenylephrine or norepinephrine, is administered to increase vascular tone if hypotension is refractory to volume infusion alone. Dopamine is useful in patients with neurogenic shock and bradycardia. Because patients with spinal shock tend to equilibrate body temperature with their environment, fluids and ambient room temperature must be kept warm.

V. **Sepsis**
A. **Definition.** Sepsis is defined as SIRS resulting from infection. Severe sepsis is multiple organ dysfunction or hypoperfusion resulting from infection. The mortality of severe sepsis remains unacceptably high.
B. **Diagnosis**
1. **Appropriate cultures** should be obtained as part of the initial evaluation. Two or more blood cultures are recommended, one of which should be drawn percutaneously.
2. **Additional radiologic imaging and diagnostic procedures** should be performed as warranted.
C. **Treatment**
1. **Addressing the infection**
a. **Antibiotic therapy**
(1) **Broad-spectrum intravenous antibiotics** should be initiated within the first hour after obtaining appropriate cultures. Failure to do so results in significantly increased mortality from severe sepsis (*Chest* 2000;118:146–155). Inadequacy is defined as failing to cover a specific class of microorganisms and/or administering agents to which the causative microorganism is resistant.
(a) Patients with the following **risks for infection with antibiotic-resistant bacteria** should be treated appropriately.
(i) Prior treatment with antibiotics during the hospitalization
(ii) Prolonged hospitalization
(iii) Presence of invasive devices
(2) **Deescalation.** As soon as possible, antibiotic coverage should be focused on the causative organism.

        (a) No clear evidence exists that combination treatment of a single organism prevents subsequent resistance over monotherapy (*Crit Care* 2001;5:189–195). The use of double coverage with synergistic antibiotics for *Pseudomonas aeruginosa* is controversial.

        (b) Cycling of antibiotics by using a different antibiotic class to treat Gram-negative infections during each quarter may reduce the development of resistant organisms.

    b. Source control

      (1) Drainage, debridement, or removal of the infectious source as appropriate, through surgical or other means

2. Circulatory support

    a. Early goal-directed therapy involves adjustments of cardiac preload, afterload, and contractility to balance oxygen delivery with oxygen demand before the patient even arrives in the ICU. A recent study demonstrated a hospital mortality of 30.5% for patients treated with early goal-directed therapy compared with 46.5% for patients treated with standard therapy (*N Engl J Med* 2001;345:1368–1377).

    b. In the first six hours, the goals of resuscitation are as follows (*Intensive Care Med* 2004;30:536–555):

      (1) CVP 8 to 12 mm Hg

      (2) MAP $\geq$ 65 mm Hg

      (3) Urine output $\geq$ 0.5 mg/kg/hour

      (4) Mixed venous saturation $\geq$ 70%

    c. Vasoactive medications. To maintain CO, heart rate usually is increased. Septic patients who fail to achieve rapid hemodynamic stability with fluids and small doses of vasoconstrictors often undergo insertion of a PA catheter to optimize cardiac performance. Since PA catheters have not been demonstrated to improve outcome in either high-risk surgical patients or ARDS patients, placing this form of invasive monitoring should not be automatic, but should be decided on an individual basis. If a PA catheter is placed, higher filling pressures are typically needed (pulmonary capillary wedge pressure of 14 to 18 mm Hg) to optimize performance in the dilated, septic heart.

      (1) Dopamine and norepinephrine commonly are used to increase vascular tone and mean aortic pressure.

      (2) Circulatory concentrations of **vasopressin** increase intially, then decrease (*Crit Care Med* 2003;31:1752–1758), and they are lower in septic shock than in cardiogenic shock. Low-dose vasopressin increases MAP, SVR, and urine output in septic patients hyporesponsive to catecholamines. This may spare patients from high-dose vasopressor requirements, although its impact on survival is not clear.

3. Adjunctive treatments

    a. Activated protein C has recently been demonstrated to reduce mortality in a large-scale prospective, randomized trial (*New Engl J Med* 2001;344:699–709). Although this drug clearly improves survival in patients with severe sepsis and has a very short half-life, it is associated with an increase in serious bleeding and must be used with caution in patients in the immediate postoperative setting. Of note, activated protein C is approved for use in patients with APACHE II scores of >25 and has not been documented to help patients with less severe forms of sepsis.

VI. Upper gastrointestinal hemorrhage prophylaxis.

Patients in the ICU are at increased risk for stress-induced mucosal ulceration and resultant GI hemorrhage. Risk factors include head injury (Cushing ulcers); burns (Curling ulcers); requirement for mechanical ventilation; previous history of peptic ulcer disease; use of nonsteroidal anti-inflammatory drugs or steroids; and the presence of shock, renal failure, portal hypertension, or coagulopathy. Strong data exist to support the use of drugs to maintain mucosal integrity in these patients at increased risk. In an evidence-based review of discordant meta-analyses, H_2-receptor antagonists (cimetidine, ranitidine, famotidine) were found to reduce significantly the incidence of clinically important GI bleeding in critically ill patients (*JAMA* 1996;275:308). Proton pump inhibitors are useful in patients who bleed despite being on appropriate H_2-receptor antagonists, but they should not be used as first-line agents for GI prophylaxis in the ICU.

VII. **Renal dysfunction**
   A. **Etiology and diagnosis.** Renal dysfunction commonly presents as progressive oliguria in the setting of increased renal function indices [blood urea nitrogen (BUN) and serum creatinine]. This can progress to renal failure and anuria (urine output <100 mL per day), which require renal replacement therapy (approximately 5% of all ICU admissions). Renal insufficiency can also present as polyuria when decreased renal tubular function (fluid resorption) is not coupled with decreased glomerular filtration ("high-output" renal failure). Traditionally, the etiology of renal dysfunction has been divided into prerenal, intrarenal, and postrenal causes (*N Engl J Med* 1996;334:1448). A careful history and a review of the medical record are critical to making the correct diagnosis.
      1. **Prerenal.** The glomerular and tubular function of the kidneys is normal, but clearance is limited as a result of decreased renal blood flow. This is the most common cause of renal insufficiency in the surgical ICU, and it is usually the result of inadequate volume resuscitation. The rise in the BUN typically is greater than that of the serum creatinine (BUN/creatinine ratio >20). The concentrating ability of the kidneys is normal, and thus the urine osmolality (>500 mOsm) and the fractional excretion of sodium (FE_{Na} <1) are normal.
         a. **Abdominal compartment syndrome** results from massive tissue (bowel) edema within the abdominal compartment or retroperitoneal hemorrhage, frequently as a complication of severe trauma. Increased intra-abdominal pressure decreases renal perfusion and retards renal venous and urinary outflow, inducing renal injury by a combination of pre-, intra-, and postrenal insults. Assessment of urinary bladder pressure via a Foley catheter serves as an indirect but accurate measure of intra-abdominal pressure (*J Trauma* 1998;45:597). Pressure >25 cm H_2O demands intervention and typically reexploration (convert mm Hg to cm H_2O by multiplying mm Hg by 1.3).
      2. **Intrarenal.** Tubular injury is most often caused by ischemia or toxins. Nephrotoxins commonly encountered by ICU patients include aminoglycosides, intravenous radiocontrast agents, amphotericin, and chemotherapeutic drugs (e.g., cisplatin). Those with preexisting renal disease or diabetes are particularly susceptible. Intravenous hydration before and during the administration of nephrotoxins should be used to decrease the incidence of renal insufficiency in patients at risk (*N Engl J Med* 1994;331:1416). Because the concentrating ability of the tubules is compromised, the urine osmolality is low (<350 mOsm) and the FE_{Na} >1. Urinalysis and microscopic analysis of the urinary sediment may yield additional information about tubular pathology.
         a. **N-acetylcysteine,** an antioxidant, has recently been shown to prevent nephrotoxicity induced by intravenous dye (*N Engl J Med* 2000;343:180–184; *Am J Kidney Dis* 2004;43:1–9).
      3. **Postrenal.** Bilateral obstruction of urinary flow can be caused by direct intraoperative injury or manipulation, prostatic hypertrophy, coagulated blood, or extrinsic compression (e.g., tumors). Urinary catheter malfunction must always be ruled out, typically by flushing the catheter with sterile saline. Ultrasound examination of the urinary system is used to rule out hydronephrosis.

Table 10-6. Drugs commonly used in the intensive care unit

Drug	Dilution (concentration)	Loading dose	Initial maintenance dose	Comments
Diltiazem	125 mg/125 mL 0.9% NaCl or D5W (1 mg/mL)	0.25 mg/kg (followed by 0.35 mg/kg if needed)	5–10 mg/hr (max 15 mg/hr)	May cause hypotension
Dobutamine	250 mg/100 mL 0.9% NaCl (2,500 μg/mL)		2 μg/kg per min (max 20 μg/kg per min)	Selective inotropic (beta) effect; may cause tachycardia and arrhythmias
Dopamine	400 mg/250 mL 0.9% NaCl or D5W (1,600 μg/mL)		Dopa, 1–3 μg/kg per min; alpha, 3–10 μg/kg per min; beta, 10–20 μg/kg per min	Clinical response is dose- and patient-dependent; may cause arrhythmias and tachycardia
Epinephrine	5 mg/500 mL 0.9% NaCl or D5W, or 4 mg/100 mL 0.9% NaCl or D5W		14 μg per min	Mixed alpha and beta effects; use central line; may cause tachycardia and hypotension
Esmolol	2.5 g/250 mL 0.9% NaCl or D5W (10 mg/mL)	500 μg/kg per min for 1 min (optional)	50 μg/kg per min (max 300 μg/kg per min)	Selective beta1-blocker; T1/2 9 min; not eliminated by hepatic or renal routes; may cause hypotension
Heparin	25,000 units/250 mL 0.45% NaCl (100 units/mL)	60 units/kg	14 units/kg per h	Obtain PTT q4–6hr until PTT is 1.5–2.0 times control; may cause thrombocytopenia

Drug	Preparation	Bolus	Infusion	Comments
Lidocaine	2 g/500 mL D5W (4 mg/mL)	1 mg/kg (can repeat 2 times if needed)	1–4 mg per min	Dose should be decreased in patients with hepatic failure, acute MI, CHF, or shock
Nitroglycerin	50 mg/250 mL D5W (200 μg/mL)		5–20 μg per min	Use cautiously in right-sided MI
Nitroprusside	50 mg/250 mL D5W (200 μg/mL)		0.25–0.50 μg/kg per min (max 10 μg/kg per min)	Signs of toxicity include metabolic acidosis, tremors, seizures, and coma; thiocyanate may accumulate in renal failure
Norepinephrine	8 mg/500 mL D5W (16 μg/mL)		2–10 μg per min	Potent alpha effects; mainly beta1 effects at lower doses; use central line
Phenylephrine	10 mg/250 mL 0.9% NaCl or D5W (40 μg/mL)		10–100 μg per min	Pure alpha effects; use central line; may cause reflex bradycardia and decreased cardiac output
Vasopressin	20 units/100 mL NS (0.2 units/mL)		0.04 units/min per infusion	Do not titrate; higher doses may cause myocardial ischemia.

CHF, congestive heart failure; D5W, 5% dextrose in water; max, maximum; MI, myocardial infarction; PTT, partial thromboplastin time; QTc, electrocardiographic QT interval; T1/2, terminal half-life.

B. Treatment
  1. **Supportive measures.** Initial therapy should be directed at minimizing ongoing renal injury by optimizing renal perfusion and discontinuing potentially nephrotoxic agents. Optimization of renal perfusion is usually accomplished by judicious volume resuscitation. In the event that fluid resuscitation does not improve low urine output (<0.5 mL/kg per hour), measurement of CVP or pulmonary capillary wedge pressure can be used to guide fluid resuscitation and optimization of CO. Low-dose dopamine does not change progression to renal failure, nor does it change mortality. **There is no role for "renal dose" dopamine in the ICU.** The dosages or medications to be eliminated by the kidney should be adjusted for the degree of renal insufficiency. The treatment of the electrolyte (hyperkalemia) and acid-base disorders (metabolic acidosis) that accompany renal failure are covered in Chapter 4.
  2. **Renal replacement therapy.** Indications include complications of renal dysfunction that fail medical management, including hypervolemia, severe acidemia, refractory hyperkalemia, and uremia (pericarditis or encephalopathy). Decisions about when and how to initiate renal replacement therapy remain the subject of controversy and ongoing clinical trials.
     a. **Intermittent.** Because peritoneal dialysis is usually impractical in the surgical ICU, intermittent hemodialysis is the method of choice. Some hemodynamic impairment usually ensues as a result of rapid, large shifts of fluid from the intravascular compartment through the dialysis filter. This is usually well tolerated, but it can induce hemodynamic deterioration (hypotension or dysrhythmias) by decreasing myocardial preload.
     b. **Continuous** (*N Engl J Med* 1997;336:1303). Continuous venovenous hemodialysis (CVVHD) is used in patients with preexisting hemodynamic instability, usually in the setting of shock. CVVHD decreases the rate of fluid shifts and thus improves hemodynamic stability while permitting more precise control of fluid and electrolyte repletion. The disadvantage of this type of dialysis is that CVVHD requires constant systemic anticoagulation to prevent clotting of blood in the filter and continuous sophisticated nursing surveillance.
VIII. **Anemia.** It is not uncommon for patients in the ICU to receive multiple units of packed red blood cells during their critical illness.Concerns have arisen regarding morbidity from transfusion, most likely related to immunosuppression, and **transfusing all patients to a hemoglobin of 10 mg/dL either has no effect or may actually decrease survival in the critically ill** (*N Engl J Med* 1999;340:409–417). According to a recent report, patients started on recombinant erythropoietin on day 3 of ICU hospitalization were significantly less likely to undergo tranfusion (*JAMA* 2002;288:2827–2835), although whether this affects patient outcomes is unclear.
IX. **Tight blood glucose control.** A recent study of 1,548 patients randomly assigned to tight glucose control with intensive insulin therapy (sugar between 80 and 110 mg/dL) versus conventional control (blood glucose between 180 and 200 mg/dl and treatment only above 215 mg/dL) showed nearly a twofold decrease in mortality in the tight glucose control group. Intensive insulin therapy also reduced overall in-hospital mortality, bloodstream infections, acute renal failure, the median number of red-cell transfusions, and critical illness polyneuropathy (*New Engl J Med* 2001;345:1359–1367).
X. **Commonly used drugs.** Table 10-6 lists drugs that are commonly used in the ICU and their dosages.

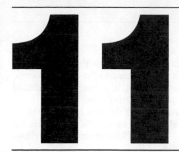

Esophagus

Ketan M. Desai and
Bryan F. Meyers

DISORDERS OF THE ESOPHAGUS

I. **Hiatal hernia.** The distal esophagus normally is held in position by a fusion of the endothoracic and endoabdominal fasciae at the diaphragmatic hiatus called the *phrenoesophageal membrane*. A hiatal hernia is present when a lax or defective phrenoesophageal membrane allows protrusion of the stomach up through the esophageal hiatus of the diaphragm.

A. **Epidemiology.** Hiatal hernia is the most common abnormality reported in upper gastrointestinal (GI) radiographic barium studies. An estimated 10% of the adult population in the United States has a hiatal hernia. The condition occurs most commonly in women in their fifth and sixth decades. Most hiatal hernias are asymptomatic; however, an estimated 5% of patients with a hiatal hernia have symptoms related to persistent gastroesophageal reflux disease (GERD).

B. The **type of hiatal hernia** is defined by the location of the gastroesophageal (GE) junction and the relationship of the stomach to the distal esophagus.

1. In **type I** or **sliding** hiatal hernia, the phrenoesophageal membrane is intact but lax, thereby allowing the distal esophagus and gastric cardia to herniate through the esophageal hiatus. The GE junction is therefore located above the diaphragm. This is the most common type and is usually asymptomatic.

2. A **type II** or **paraesophageal** hiatal hernia occurs when a focal defect is present in the phrenoesophageal membrane, usually anterior and lateral to the esophagus, which allows a protrusion of peritoneum to herniate upward alongside the esophagus through the esophageal hiatus. The GE junction remains anchored within the abdomen, whereas the greater curvature of the stomach rolls up into the chest alongside the distal esophagus. Eventually, most of the stomach can herniate. Because the stomach is anchored at the pylorus and cardia, however, the body of the stomach undergoes a 180-degree organoaxial rotation and ends up as an upside-down intrathoracic stomach when it is herniated.

3. **Type III** represents a **combination** of types I and II. This type is more common than a pure type II and is characterized by herniation of the greater curvature of the stomach and the GE junction into the chest. Patients thus affected are exposed to the problems and risks of both types of hernias.

4. A **type IV** hiatal hernia is defined as a condition in which abdominal organs other than or in addition to the stomach herniate through the hiatus. Typically, these hernias are large and contain colon or spleen in addition to the stomach within the chest.

C. **Symptoms and complications** in patients with **sliding** (type I) hiatal hernias are related to associated GE reflux (GER; see Section II). **Paraesophageal and combined** (types II, III, and IV) hernias frequently produce postprandial pain or bloating, early satiety, breathlessness with meals, and mild dysphagia related to compression of the distal esophagus by the adjacent herniated stomach. The herniated gastric pouch is susceptible to volvulus, obstruction, and infarction and can develop ischemic longitudinal ulcers (termed *Cameron ulcers*) with frank or occult bleeding.

D. Diagnosis and evaluation
1. **Chest x-ray.** The finding of an air-fluid level in the posterior mediastinum on the lateral x-ray suggests the presence of a hiatal hernia. Differential diagnosis includes mediastinal cyst, abscess, or a dilatated obstructed esophagus (as is seen in end-stage achalasia).
2. A **barium swallow** confirms the diagnosis and defines any coexisting esophageal abnormalities, including strictures or ulcers, and is the diagnostic study of choice. The positions of the GE junction and proximal stomach define the type of hiatal hernia.
3. **Esophagogastroduodenoscopy (EGD)** is indicated in patients with symptoms of reflux or dysphagia to determine the degree of esophagitis and whether a stricture, Barrett esophagus, or a coexisting abnormality is present. EGD also establishes the location of the GE junction in relation to the hiatus. A sliding hiatal hernia is present when 2 cm or more of gastric mucosa are present between the diaphragmatic hiatus and the mucosal squamocolumnar junction.
4. **Esophageal manometry** to evaluate esophageal motility is warranted in patients who are being considered for operative repair.

E. Management
1. **Asymptomatic sliding hernias** require no treatment.
2. **Patients with sliding hernias and GER with mild esophagitis** should undergo an initial trial of medical management.
3. **Patients who fail to obtain symptomatic relief with medical therapy or who have severe esophagitis** should undergo esophageal testing to determine their suitability for an antireflux procedure and hiatal hernia repair.
4. **Patients who do not experience reflux but have symptoms related to their hernia** (chest pain, intermittent dysphagia, or esophageal obstruction) should undergo hiatal hernia repair.
5. **All patients who are found to have a type II, III, or IV hiatal hernia and who are operative candidates should be considered for repair.** The management of asymptomatic paraesophageal hernias is a controversial issue. Some surgeons believe that all paraesophageal hernias should be corrected electively on diagnosis, irrespective of symptoms, to prevent the development of complications and avoid the risk of emergency surgery. Medically treated patients with a paraesophageal hernia, even when asymptomatic, have nearly a 30% incidence of death from the development of a catastrophic complication (*J Thorac Cardiovasc Surg* 1967;53:33). Despite these findings, "watchful waiting" has been suggested to be a reasonable alternative for the initial management of patients with asymptomatic or minimally symptomatic paraesophageal hernias (*Ann Surg* 2002;236:4). Operative repair, which can be performed using either an abdominal or thoracic approach, consists of reduction of the hernia, resection of the sac, and closure of the hiatal defect. In combined (type III) hernias, the esophagus frequently is shortened, and therefore a thoracic approach is preferred.
6. **Paraesophageal hiatal hernias** are associated with a 60% incidence of GER. Furthermore, the operative dissection may lead to postoperative GER in previously asymptomatic patients. Therefore, an antireflux procedure should be performed at the time of hiatal hernia repair.

II. Gastroesophageal reflux (GER)
A. Prevalence. GER is a normal event after a meal and during belching. Normally, refluxed gastric juice is cleared rapidly from the distal esophagus. Symptoms of heartburn and excessive regurgitation are relatively common in the United States, occurring in approximately 7% of the population on a daily basis and in 33% at least once a month. Often, these individuals have x-ray evidence of a hiatal hernia. Reflux and hiatal hernia are not necessarily related, and each can occur independently.

B. **Pathophysiology** in GER relates to abnormal exposure of the distal esophagus to refluxed stomach contents. In 60% of patients, a mechanically defective lower-esophageal sphincter (LES) is responsible for the GER. The sphincter function of the LES depends on the integrated mechanical effect of the sphincter's intramural pressure and the length of esophagus exposed to intra-abdominal positive pressure. Other etiologies of GER are inefficient esophageal clearance of refluxed material, fixed gastric outlet obstruction, functional delayed gastric emptying, increased gastric acid secretion, and inappropriate relaxation of the LES.

C. The classic **symptom** of GER is posturally aggravated substernal or epigastric burning pain that is readily relieved by antacids. Additional common symptoms include regurgitation or effortless emesis, dysphagia, and excessive flatulence. Atypical symptoms may mimic laryngeal, respiratory, cardiac, biliary, pancreatic, gastric, or duodenal disease.

D. **Diagnosis and evaluation**

1. **Contrast radiography (upper GI)** demonstrates spontaneous reflux in only approximately 40% of patients with GER. However, it documents the presence or absence of hiatal hernia; can demonstrate some complications of reflux, such as esophageal stricture and ulcers; and is an appropriate initial study. The study should include a full view of the esophagus as well as a complete evaluation of the stomach, pylorus, and duodenum.

2. **EGD** is indicated in patients with symptoms of GER to evaluate for esophagitis and the presence of Barrett changes. **Esophagitis** is a pathologic diagnosis, but an experienced endoscopist can readily distinguish the more advanced stages. Four general grades of esophagitis occur.

   a. **Grade I:** Normal or reddened mucosa

   b. **Grade II:** Superficial mucosal erosions and some ulcerations

   c. **Grade III:** Extensive ulceration with multiple, circumferential erosions with luminal narrowing; possible edematous islands of squamous mucosa present, producing the so-called cobblestone esophagitis

   d. **Grade IV:** Fibrotic peptic stricture, shortened esophagus, columnar-lined esophagus

3. **Esophageal manometric testing** is appropriate in the patient with reflux symptoms once surgery is being considered. Manometry defines the location and function of the LES and helps to exclude achalasia, scleroderma, and diffuse esophageal spasm from the differential diagnosis. Characteristics of a manometrically abnormal LES are (1) a pressure of less than 6 mm Hg, (2) an overall length of less than 2 cm, and (3) an abdominal length of less than 1 cm. These values are abnormal, and a patient with one or more of these abnormal values has a 90% probability of having reflux. Manometry also assesses the adequacy of esophageal contractility and peristaltic wave progression as a guide to the best antireflux procedure for the patient.

4. **Esophageal pH testing** over a 24-hour period is regarded as the gold standard in the diagnosis of GER. It is now used mainly when the data from the remainder of the evaluation are equivocal and diagnosis of reflux is in doubt. Twenty-four–hour pH testing can be performed on an outpatient or ambulatory basis: The patient has an event button to record symptoms and keeps a diary of body position, timing of meals, and other activities. This allows correlation of symptoms with simultaneous esophageal pH alterations. A score is derived based on the frequency of reflux episodes and the time required for the esophagus to clear the acid. Score values that fall outside two standard deviations from the mean of values obtained from normal volunteers are considered abnormal. This test has a 90% sensitivity and a 90% specificity for diagnosing or excluding reflux (*J Thorac Cardiovasc Surg* 1980;79:656).

5. **A gastric emptying study** can be useful in evaluating patients with reflux and symptoms of gastroparesis.
E. **Complications.** Approximately 20% of patients with GER have complications, including esophagitis, stricture, or Barrett esophagus. Other less common complications include acute or chronic bleeding and aspiration.
F. **Treatment**
1. **Medical treatment** aims to reduce the duration and amount of esophageal exposure to gastric contents and to minimize the effects on the esophageal mucosa.
   a. Patients are instructed to remain upright after meals, avoid postural maneuvers (bending, straining) that aggravate reflux, and sleep with the head of the bed elevated 6 to 8 inches.
   b. **Dietary alterations** are aimed at maximizing LES pressure, minimizing intragastric pressure, and decreasing stomach acidity. Patients are instructed to avoid fatty foods, alcohol, caffeine, chocolate, peppermint, and smoking and to eat smaller, more frequent meals. Obese patients are instructed to lose weight, avoid tight-fitting garments, and begin a regular exercise program. In addition, anticholinergics, calcium channel blockers, nitrates, beta-blockers, theophylline, alpha-blockers, and nonsteroidal anti-inflammatory medications may exacerbate reflux and should be replaced with other preparations or reduced in dosage if possible.
   c. **Pharmacologic therapy** is indicated in patients who do not improve with postural or dietary measures. The goal is to lower gastric acidity or enhance esophageal and gastric clearing while increasing the LES resting pressure.
      (1) **Antacids** neutralize stomach acidity and thus raise intragastric pH. Many patients self-medicate with these agents for many years before seeking professional attention.
      (2) **H_2-receptor antagonists** lower gastric acidity by decreasing the amount of acid that the stomach produces. **Proton pump inhibitors** act by selective noncompetitive inhibition of the H^+/K^+ pump on the parietal cell and are more effective than H_2 antagonists in healing esophagitis (*Aliment Pharmacol Ther* 1990;4:145).
      (3) **Prokinetic agents**, such as metoclopramide (dopaminergic antagonist), can decrease GER by increasing the LES tone and accelerating esophageal and gastric clearance.
   d. **Transoral endoscopic suturing** to plicate the gastroesophageal junction and **endoscopic application of radiofrequency energy** to the lower esophagus are two novel endoluminal therapies that can be performed on an ambulatory basis and generally with the patient under light sedation. These therapies, which were recently approved by the FDA, have been evaluated in several small, non-placebo-controlled trials with limited duration of posttreatment follow-up evaluation. Evidence of dysphagia, stricture, large hiatal hernia, and moderate to severe esophagitis generally has excluded patients from eligibilty for inclusion in these two endoluminal trials.
2. **Surgical treatment** should be considered in patients who have symptomatic reflux, have manometric evidence of a defective LES, and fail to achieve relief with maximal medical management. Alternatively, surgical therapy should be considered in symptomatic patients who have achieved relief with medical therapy but to whom the prospect of a lifetime of medicine is undesirable (i.e., because of cost, side effects, inconvenience, or compliance). Surgical treatment consists of either a transabdominal or transthoracic antireflux operation to reconstruct a competent LES and a crural repair to maintain the reconstruction in the abdomen.

a. A **laparoscopic, transabdominal approach** is preferred in most patients, except when a shortened esophagus is present because the shortened esophagus cannot be adequately pulled into the abdomen for the fundoplication. A shortened esophagus should be suspected when a stricture is present and in patients who have had a failed antireflux procedure. The transabdominal approach is recommended for patients with a coexisting abdominal disorder, a prior thoracotomy, or severe respiratory disorder.

(1) **Nissen fundoplication** is the most commonly performed procedure for GER. It consists of a 360-degree fundic wrap via open or laparoscopic technique. Long-term results in several series of open procedures are excellent, with 10-year freedom from recurrence of more than 90%. Short-term results of the laparoscopic approach are as good as the open-repair results for relief of GER symptoms, with concomitant shorter hospital stay, better respiratory function, and decreased pain postoperatively (*Br J Surg* 2000;87:873). The complete fundoplication in this repair is very effective at preventing reflux but, compared with the other procedures, is associated with a slightly higher incidence of inability to vomit, gas bloating of the stomach, and dysphagia. During surgery, care must be taken to ensure that the wrap is short, loose, and placed appropriately around the distal esophagus to minimize the incidence of these complications.

(2) The **Hill posterior gastropexy** anchors the GE junction posteriorly to the median arcuate ligament and creates a partial or 180-degree imbrication of the stomach around the right side of the intra-abdominal esophagus. Hill recommended using intraesophageal manometry during placement of the sutures to achieve a pressure of 50 mm Hg in the distal esophagus. With this technique, the incidence of recurrent hiatal hernia is low and the incidence of recurrent or persistent reflux is variable.

(3) The **Toupet fundoplication** is a partial 270-degree posterior wrap, with the wrapped segment sutured to the crural margins and to the anterolateral esophageal wall. For patients in whom esophageal peristalsis is documented to be abnormal preoperatively, a partial wrap or Toupet procedure has often been used as an alternative to lessen the potential for postoperative dysphagia.

b. A **transthoracic approach** is recommended in patients with esophageal shortening or stricture, coexistent motor disorder, obesity, coexistent pulmonary lesion, or prior antireflux repair.

(1) **Nissen fundoplication** can be done via a transthoracic approach, with results similar to those obtained with a transabdominal approach.

(2) The **Belsey Mark IV repair** consists of a 240-degree fundic wrap around 4 cm of distal esophagus. In cases of esophageal neuromotor dysfunction, it produces less dysphagia than may accompany a 360-degree (Nissen) wrap. Furthermore, the ability to belch is preserved, thereby avoiding the gas-bloat syndrome that may occur after a complete (360-degree) wrap. Careful 10-year follow-up demonstrates a good long-term result in 85% of patients (*J Thorac Cardiovasc Surg* 1967;53:33).

(3) **Collis gastroplasty** is a technique used to lengthen a shortened esophagus. To minimize tension on the antireflux repair, a gastric tube is formed from the upper lesser curvature of the stomach in continuity with the distal esophagus. The antireflux repair then is constructed around the gastroplasty tube. A gastroplasty should be considered preoperatively in patients with obvious or subtle esophageal shortening, such as those with gross ulcerative esophagitis or stricture, failed prior antireflux procedure, or

total intrathoracic stomach (*Ann Surg* 1987;206:473). However, in many of these patients the esophagus can be adequately mobilized to allow more than 3 cm of intra-abdominal esophagus and thereby avoid the need to lengthen the esophagus. Development of an angled endoscopic stapler has made laparoscopic Collis gastroplasty technically feasible.

III. **Barrett's esophagus** is defined as a metaplastic transformation of esophageal mucosa. Barrett's esophagus evolves as a result of chronic GER. To qualify as a case of Barrett's esophagus, the metaplastic epithelium must show, upon biopsy, intestinal-type metaplasia characterized by the prescence of goblet cells. The **specialized or intestinal type** has goblet cells scattered among the columnar epithelial cells, is the most common type, and has a high association with the subsequent development of adenocarcinoma. The columnar epithelium of Barrett's esophagus may replace the normal squamous epithelium circumferentially, or it may be asymmetric and irregular.

A. **Prevalence.** Barrett's esophagus is diagnosed in approximately 2% of all patients undergoing esophagoscopy and in 10% to 15% of patients with esophagitis. Autopsy studies suggest that the actual prevalence is much higher because many patients are asymptomatic and remain undiagnosed. Most patients diagnosed with Barrett's esophagus are middle-aged white men.

B. The **symptoms** of Barrett's esophagus are the result of GER. Approximately 50% of patients with endoscopically proven Barrett's have associated heartburn, 75% have dysphagia, and 25% have bleeding (*Ann Surg* 1983;198:554).

C. **Diagnosis.** The diagnosis of Barrett's esophagus may be suggested on x-ray by the presence of a hiatal hernia (associated with 80% of cases of Barrett's esophagus) with esophagitis and an esophageal stricture. Confirmation of the diagnosis requires endoscopy and careful correlation between the endoscopic appearance and the histologic findings of mucosal biopsies.

D. **Complications**

1. **Esophageal ulceration and stricture** are more likely to occur in patients with Barrett's esophagus than in those with GER alone. This most likely reflects the more severe nature of the GER in patients with Barrett's esophagus.

   a. **Barrett's ulcers** are distinctly different from the common erosions seen in esophagitis in that they penetrate the metaplastic columnar epithelium in a manner similar to that seen in gastric ulcers. They occur in up to 50% of patients with Barrett's esophagus and, like gastric ulcers, can cause pain, bleed, obstruct, penetrate, and perforate.

   b. **A benign stricture** occurs in 30% to 50% of patients with Barrett's esophagus. The stricture is located at the squamocolumnar junction, which in Barrett's esophagus is not the esophagogastric junction. Strictures secondary to Barrett's are located in the middle or upper esophagus, unlike peptic strictures not associated with Barrett's, which usually occur in the distal esophagus.

2. **Dysplasia.** The metaplastic columnar epithelium of Barrett's esophagus is prone to development of areas of dysplasia that can be detected only by biopsy. Pathologically, dysplasia is categorized as low or high grade, with high grade being pathologically indistinguishable from carcinoma *in situ*.

3. **Malignant degeneration** from benign to dysplastic to malignant epithelium has been demonstrated in Barrett's esophagus. Low-grade dysplasia is present in 5% to 10% of patients with Barrett's esophagus and can progress to high-grade dysplasia and malignancy.

4. **Adenocarcinomas** that arise within the esophagus above the normal GE junction are characteristic of malignant degeneration in Barrett's esophagus. The risk of development of adenocarcinoma in Barrett's esophagus is 50 to 100 times that of the general population. In several

long-term series, the incidence of malignant degeneration in Barrett's esophagus has been estimated at between 1 in 50 and 1 in 400 patient-years of follow-up.

E. Treatment

1. Uncomplicated Barrett's esophagus in **asymptomatic** patients requires no specific therapy, but endoscopic surveillance and biopsy should be performed at least annually. Neither medical nor surgical treatment of reflux has been demonstrated to reverse the columnar metaplasia of Barrett's esophagus. However, elimination of reflux with an antireflux procedure may halt progression of the disease, heal ulceration, and prevent stricture formation.

2. Uncomplicated Barrett's esophagus in **symptomatic** patients should be treated using the same principles that apply to patients with GER without Barrett's esophagus. In addition, symptomatic patients should have annual surveillance endoscopy with biopsy. After laparoscopic antireflux surgery, patients with Barrett's esophagus have symptomatic relief and reduction in medication use equivalent to non-Barrett's patients. Absence of progression to high-grade dysplasia or adenocarcinoma suggests that laparoscopic surgery is an effective approach for the management of patients with Barrett's esophagus (*Am J Surg* 2003; 186:6).

3. **Barrett's ulcers** usually heal with medical therapy. Frequently, 8 weeks of treatment with an H_2-receptor antagonist or proton pump inhibitor are necessary to achieve complete healing. Recurrence of ulcers is common after discontinuation of therapy. Ulcers that fail to heal despite 4 months of medical therapy are an indication for rebiopsy and antireflux surgery.

4. **Strictures** associated with Barrett's esophagus usually are successfully managed with periodic esophageal dilation combined with medical management. Recurrent or persistent strictures warrant an antireflux operation combined with intraoperative stricture dilation. After surgery, several dilations can be required to maintain patency during the healing phase. Rarely, undilatable strictures require resection.

5. **Dysplasia** on biopsy of Barrett's esophagus indicates that the patient is at risk for the development of adenocarcinoma.
   a. **Low-grade dysplasia** requires frequent (every 3 to 6 months) surveillance esophagoscopy and biopsy. Medical therapy for GER is recommended in these patients, even when asymptomatic.
   b. **High-grade dysplasia** is pathologically indistinguishable from carcinoma *in situ* and is an indication for esophagectomy. Patients who undergo esophagectomy for high-grade dysplasia have up to a 22% to 73% chance of having an unidentified focus of invasive carcinoma present in the resected esophagus. Cure rates of nearly 100% can be expected in patients whose cancer is limited to the mucosa and who undergo esophagectomy (*J Thorac Cardiovasc Surg* 1994;108:813).

6. **Adenocarcinoma** in patients with Barrett's esophagus is an indication for esophagogastrectomy. Early detection offers the best opportunity to improve survival after resection, which overall is 20% at 5 years.

IV. Esophageal carcinoma

A. Epidemiology. Carcinoma of the esophagus represents 1% of all cancers in the United States and causes 1.8% of cancer deaths. The two principal histologies are adenocarcinoma and squamous cell carcinoma.

1. **Risk factors** for squamous cell esophageal cancer include African American race, alcohol and cigarette use, tylosis, achalasia, caustic esophageal injury, Plummer-Vinson syndrome, nutritional deficiencies, and ingestion of nitrosamines and fungal toxins. Geographic location also represents a risk factor, likely as a result of local dietary customs, with a high incidence noted in certain areas of China, South Africa, Iran, France, and Japan.

2. **Risk factors** for adenocarcinoma of the esophagus include Caucasian race, chronic GERD, and Barrett's esophagus.

B. **Pathology**

1. **Squamous cell carcinoma** was previously the most common type of esophageal carcinoma. It tends to be multicentric and most frequently involves the middle third of the esophagus.

2. **Adenocarcinoma** now constitutes more than 50% of esophageal carcinomas and is the carcinoma with the greatest rate of increase in the United States. It is less likely to be multicentric, but it typically exhibits extensive proximal and distal submucosal invasion. Adenocarcinoma most commonly involves the distal esophagus.

3. **Less common malignant esophageal tumors** include small cell carcinoma; melanoma; leiomyosarcoma, and, rarely, other sarcomas; lymphoma; and esophageal involvement by metastatic cancer.

C. Most patients with early-stage disease are asymptomatic or may have symptoms of reflux. **Symptoms** of esophageal cancer are dysphagia, odynophagia, and weight loss. Symptoms that are suggestive of unresectability include hoarseness, abdominal pain, persistent back or bone pain, hiccups, and respiratory symptoms (cough, aspiration pneumonia), which suggest possible esophagorespiratory fistula formation. Approximately 50% of presenting patients have unresectable lesions or distant metastasis, which is largely responsible for the generally poor prognosis.

D. The **diagnosis** is suggested by a barium swallow and confirmed with esophagoscopy and biopsy or brush cytology.

E. **Staging.** A system for staging esophageal cancer allows assignment of patients to groups with similar prognosis, helps determine if local or systemic therapy is needed, and allows comparison of response to different types of therapy (Table 11-1). Evaluation for lymph node and distant-organ metastatic disease is often accomplished with CT scan. Whole body imaging with positron emission tomographic scanning has shown great promise, particularly for detection of metastatic disease (*Ann Thorac Surg* 1997;64:770). Endoscopic ultrasonography is more accurate in determining the depth of wall invasion and the involvement of peritumoral lymph nodes. Upper esophageal and midesophageal lesions require bronchoscopy to evaluate the airway for involvement by tumor.

F. **Treatment**

1. **Surgical resection** remains a mainstay of curative treatment for vigorous patients with localized disease. It offers the best opportunity for cure and provides substantial palliation when cure is not possible. Resection and esophageal replacement also offer reliable relief of dysphagia. The overall 5-year survival rate is 20% to 30%, with higher rates for patients with lower stages of disease (*J Thorac Cardiovasc Surg* 1993; 105:265).

   a. **Options for resection** include a standard transthoracic esophagectomy, a transhiatal esophagectomy, or an *en bloc* esophagectomy. Total esophagectomy with a cervical esophagogastric anastomosis and subtotal resection with a high intrathoracic anastomosis have become the most common resections and produce the best long-term functional results as well as the best chance for cure. Esophagogastrectomy with anastomosis to the distal half of the esophagus is seldom used because troublesome postoperative reflux symptoms are common.

   b. **Options for esophageal replacement** include the stomach, colon, and jejunum.

2. **Neoadjuvant therapy** with preoperative chemotherapy (cisplatin, vinblastine, and 5-fluorouracil) and 4,500-cGy radiotherapy has been shown to improve survival (*J Thorac Cardiovasc Surg* 1993;105:265; *N Engl J Med* 1996;335:462). This approach has not yet become the standard of care and is the focus of ongoing investigation.

Table 11-1. TNM (tumor, node, metastasis) staging system for esophageal cancer

Definition of TNM

T: Primary tumor

Tx	Primary tumor cannot be assessed (cytologically positive tumor not evident radiographically or endoscopically)
T0	No evidence of primary tumor (e.g., after treatment with radiation and chemotherapy)
Tis	Carcinoma *in situ*
T1	Tumor invades the submucosa
T2	Tumor invades the muscularis propria
T3	Tumor invades periesophageal tissue
T4	Tumor invades contiguous structures

N: Regional lymph nodes

Nx	Regional nodes cannot be assessed
N0	No regional node metastasis
N1	Regional node metastasis

M: Distant metastasis

Mx	Distant metastasis cannot be assessed
M0	No distant metastasis
M1a	Upper thoracic esophagus metastatic to cervical lymph nodes
	Lower thoracic esophagus metastatic to celiac lymph nodes
M1b	Metastases to nonregional lymph nodes or other distant sites

Stage Grouping

Stage 0	Tis	N0	M0
Stage I	T1	N0	M0
Stage IIA	T2	N0	M0
	T3	N0	M0
Stage IIB	T1	N1	M0
	T2	N1	M0
Stage III	T3	N1	M0
	T4	Any N	M0
Stage IVA	Any T	Any N	M1a
Stage IVB	Any T	Any N	M1b

Adapted with permission from Fleming ID, Cooper JS, Henson DE, et al., eds. *AJCC Cancer Staging Manual.* 5th ed. Philadelphia: Lippincott Raven, 1997:65–69.

3. **Radiotherapy** is used worldwide for attempted cure and palliation of patients with squamous cell esophageal cancer deemed unsuitable for resection. The 5-year survival rate is 5% to 10%. Palliation of dysphagia is successful temporarily in 80% of patients but rarely provides complete long-term relief. Combination therapy involving radiation and concurrent administration of 5-fluorouracil with mitomycin C or cisplatin has been suggested to improve results and has replaced radiation alone in most current protocols.

4. The goal of **palliative treatment** is the relief of obstruction and dysphagia.

   a. **Radiotherapy and chemotherapy** work best in patients with squamous cell carcinoma, particularly when it is located above the carina. Adenocarcinoma is less responsive to radiation, and the acute morbidity of external-beam irradiation of the epigastric area, in terms of nausea and vomiting, is substantial.

    b. **Esophageal bypass procedures** have been tried, but the morbidity
       and mortality of such procedures are excessive.
    c. **Intraluminal prostheses** have been developed to intubate the esoph-
       agus and stent the obstruction. Self-expanding wire-mesh stents, of-
       ten with a soft silicone (Silastic) coating, have been used with greater
       ease of insertion and satisfactory results. None of these prostheses al-
       low normal swallowing, and, in most cases, little more than a pureed
       diet can be tolerated. The two methods for insertion are (1) peroral
       (push technique) and (2) via a laparotomy (pull technique). Of these,
       the peroral route is associated with fewer complications. Potential
       complications include perforation, erosion or migration of the tube,
       and obstruction of the tube by food or proximal tumor growth.
    d. **Endoscopic laser techniques** can restore an esophageal lumen suc-
       cessfully 90% of the time, with only a 4% to 5% perforation rate.
V. **Esophageal perforation**
  A. **Causes** of esophageal perforation may be either intraluminal or extralu-
     minal and are associated with a 20% mortality rate.
    1. **Intraluminal causes**
      a. **Instrumental injuries** represent 75% of esophageal perforations and
         occur during endoscopy, dilation, sclerosis of esophageal varices,
         transesophageal echocardiography, and tube passage. The common
         sites are the normal anatomic sites of narrowing in the cervical and
         distal esophagus. Tumors that are located at the cardia pose a par-
         ticular risk for perforation during dilation, as a result of fixation and
         angulation of the esophagus at the GE junction that occur with this
         condition.
      b. **Foreign bodies** can cause acute perforation or commonly take a more
         indolent course, with late abscess formation in the mediastinum or
         development of empyema.
      c. **Ingested caustic substances**, such as alkali chemicals, can produce
         coagulation necrosis of the esophagus and perforation.
      d. **Cancer of the esophagus** may lead to perforation.
      e. **Barotrauma** induced by external compression (e.g., Heimlich maneu-
         ver), forceful vomiting (Boerhaave syndrome), seizures, childbirth, or
         lifting can produce esophageal perforation. Almost all of these perfo-
         rations occur in the distal esophagus on the left side.
    2. **Extraluminal causes**
      a. **Penetrating injuries** can occur from stab wounds or, more commonly,
         gunshot wounds.
      b. **Blunt trauma** may produce an esophageal perforation related to a
         rapid increase in intraluminal pressure or compression of the esoph-
         agus between the sternum and the spine.
      c. **Operative injury** to the esophagus during an unrelated procedure oc-
         curs infrequently but has been reported in association with thyroid
         resection, anterior cervical spine operations, proximal gastric vago-
         tomy, pneumonectomy, and laparoscopic fundoplication procedures.
  B. **Signs and symptoms** of esophageal perforation typically begin with dys-
     phagia, pain, and fever and progress to leukocytosis, tachycardia, respira-
     tory distress, and shock if the perforation is left untreated. Cervical per-
     forations may present with neck stiffness and subcutaneous emphysema,
     and an intrathoracic perforation should be suspected in patients with chest
     pain, subcutaneous emphysema, dyspnea, and a pleural effusion (right
     pleural effusion in proximal perforations, left effusion in distal perfora-
     tions). Intra-abdominal perforations usually present with peritonitis.
  C. The **diagnosis** of esophageal perforation is suggested by pneumomedi-
     astinum, pleural effusion, pneumothorax, atelectasis, and soft-tissue em-
     physema on chest x-ray or mediastinal air and fluid on CT scan and
     is followed with water-soluble or dilute barium contrast esophagogra-
     phy. Contrast studies carry a 10% false-negative rate for esophageal

perforations. Because esophagoscopy is used primarily as an adjunctive study and can miss sizable perforations, any discoloration or submucosal hematoma should be considered highly suspicious for perforation after trauma to the posterior mediastinum. Whenever an esophageal perforation is suspected, diagnosis and treatment must be prompt because morbidity and mortality increase in proportion to their delay.

D. Principles of management include (1) adequate drainage of the leak, (2) intravenous antibiotics, (3) adequate fluid resuscitation, (4) adequate nutrition, (5) relief of any distal obstruction, (6) diversion of enteric contents past the leak, and (7) restoration of GI integrity. Initially, patients are kept on nothing-by-mouth status, a nasogastric tube is placed carefully in the esophagus or stomach, and they receive intravenous hydration and broad-spectrum antibiotics.

E. Definitive management generally requires operative repair, although a carefully selected group of nontoxic patients with a locally contained perforation may be observed. Patients with an intramural perforation after endoscopic procedures or dilation have a characteristic radiographic finding of a thin collection of contrast material parallel to the esophageal lumen without spillage into the mediastinum. Management with a nasogastric tube and antibiotics almost always is successful in these patients.

  1. **Cervical and upper thoracic perforations** usually are treated by cervical drainage alone or in combination with esophageal repair.
  2. **Thoracic perforations** should be closed primarily and buttressed with healthy tissue, and the mediastinum should be drained widely. Even in operations on perforations that are more than 24 hours old, primary mucosal closure usually is possible. When primary closure is not possible, options include wide drainage alone or in combination with resection or with exclusion and diversion in cases of severe traumatic injury to the esophagus.
  3. **Abdominal esophageal perforations** typically result in peritonitis and require an upper abdominal midline incision to correct.
  4. **Perforations associated with intrinsic esophageal disease** (e.g., carcinoma, hiatal hernia, or achalasia) require addressing the perforation as described previously and surgically correcting the associated esophageal disease concomitantly.

VI. Esophageal diverticula are acquired conditions of the esophagus found primarily in adults. They are divided into traction and pulsion diverticula based on the pathophysiology that induced their formation.

A. A **pharyngoesophageal (or Zenker) diverticulum** is a pulsion diverticulum and is the most common type of symptomatic diverticulum. **Typical symptoms** are progressive cervical dysphagia, cough on assuming a recumbent position, and spontaneous regurgitation of undigested food, which may produce episodes of choking and aspiration. **Diagnosis** with a barium swallow should prompt **surgical correction** with cricopharyngeal myotomy and diverticulectomy or suspension. Notably, almost all patients with a pharyngoesophageal diverticulum have GER, which is thought to produce cricopharyngeal dysfunction and the resultant diverticulum.

B. A **traction or midesophageal or parabronchial diverticulum** occurs in conjunction with mediastinal granulomatous disease. Symptoms are rare, but when they are present, operative excision of the diverticulum and adjacent inflammatory mass usually corrects the problem. On rare occasions, these diverticula present with chronic cough from an esophagobronchial fistula.

C. An **epiphrenic or pulsion diverticulum** can be located at almost every level but typically occurs in the distal 10 cm of the thoracic esophagus. It is also a pulsion diverticulum and develops as a herniation of the mucosa through the muscular layers of the esophagus on the right side as a result of functional or mechanical esophageal obstruction. Many patients are asymptomatic at the time of diagnosis, and, in those who are symptomatic, it is difficult to determine whether the symptoms stem from the diverticulum or from the underlying esophageal disorder.

1. The **diagnosis** is made with a contrast esophagogram; however, endoscopic examination and esophageal function studies are essential in defining the underlying pathophysiology. In advanced disease, the diagnosis can be confused with achalasia owing to the dependency of the diverticulum and the lateral displacement and narrowing of the GE junction.

2. **Surgical treatment** is recommended for patients with progressive or incapacitating symptoms associated with abnormal esophageal peristalsis; it consists of diverticulectomy or diverticulopexy, with an extramucosal esophagomyotomy. The myotomy extends from the neck of the diverticulum down to the stomach. When the diverticulum is associated with a hiatal hernia and reflux, a concomitant nonobstructive antireflux procedure (Belsey Mark IV) is recommended. Any associated mechanical obstruction must be corrected.

VII. **Functional esophageal disorders.** This category includes a diverse group of disorders involving esophageal skeletal or smooth muscle.

   A. **Motor disorders of esophageal skeletal muscle** result in defective swallowing and aspiration. Potential causes can be classified into five major subgroups: neurogenic, myogenic, structural, iatrogenic, and mechanical. Most causes of oropharyngeal dysphagia are not correctable surgically. However, when manometric studies demonstrate that pharyngeal contractions, although weak, are still reasonably well coordinated, cricopharyngeal myotomy can provide relief.

   B. **Motor disorders of esophageal smooth muscle** can be subdivided into primary dysmotilities and disorders that involve the esophagus secondarily and produce dysmotility.

   1. **Primary dysmotility**

      a. **Achalasia** is rare (1/100,000 population) but is the most common primary esophageal motility disorder. It typically presents between the ages of 35 and 45 years. Chagas disease, caused by *Trypanosoma cruzi* and seen primarily in South America, can mimic achalasia and produce similar esophageal pathology. Achalasia is a disease of unknown etiology, characterized by loss of effective esophageal body peristalsis and failure of the LES to relax with swallowing, with resultant esophageal dilatation. LES pressure is often (but not invariably) elevated. The characteristic pathology is a deficiency of, or changes in, the ganglia of Auerbach plexus. Three clinical stages have been outlined and are characterized by symptomatology and diameter of the esophagus: stage I (esophagus <4 cm), stage II (esophagus 4 to 7 cm), and stage III (esophagus >7 cm).

         (1) **Symptoms** include progressive dysphagia, noted by essentially all patients; regurgitation immediately after meals (>70%); odynophagia (30%); and aspiration, with resultant bronchitis and pneumonia (10%). Some patients experience chest pain due to esophageal spasms.

         (2) The **diagnosis** is suggested by a chest x-ray, which often shows a fluid-filled, dilatated esophagus and absence of a gastric air bubble. A **barium esophagogram** demonstrates tapering ("bird's beak") of the distal esophagus and a dilatated proximal esophagus. The bird's beak deformity is not specific for achalasia and can be seen in any process that narrows the distal esophagus (e.g., benign strictures or carcinoma). **Esophageal manometry** is the definitive diagnostic test for achalasia. Characteristic manometric findings include the absence of peristalsis, mirror-image contractions, and limited or absent relaxation of the LES with swallowing. Endoscopy should be performed to rule out benign strictures or malignancy, so-called pseudoachalasia.

(3) Medical treatment is aimed at decreasing the LES tone and includes nitrates, calcium channel blockers, and endoscopic injection of botulinum toxin (blocks acetylcholine release from nerve terminals) in the area of the LES.

(4) Surgical treatment with a **modified Heller esophagomyotomy** has been shown to produce excellent results in 95% of patients, compared with only 65% excellent results using forceful **pneumatic bougienage** (*Gut* 1989;30:299). Many esophageal surgeons favor extending the myotomy onto the stomach and a concomitant antireflux procedure with the esophagomyotomy to avoid the two major causes of operative failure: (1) an incomplete myotomy due to inadequate mobilization of the esophagogastric junction and (2) late stricture due to GER disease caused by the incompetent LES combined with the inability of the aperistaltic esophagus to evacuate refluxed material. **Video-assisted thoracoscopic approaches** have been tried, with early results showing a higher incidence of postoperative GER than with the open procedure (*Ann Thorac Surg* 1993;56:680). More recently, **laparoscopic esophagomyotomy** combined with a partial fundoplication has been reported and is rapidly being adopted by most centers as the primary surgical option (*Surg Endosc* 2000; 14:746).

b. *Vigorous achalasia* is a term used to describe a variant of achalasia in which patients present with the clinical and manometric features of classic achalasia and diffuse esophageal spasm. These patients have spastic pain and severe dysphagia, likely because of residual disordered peristalsis ineffective in overcoming the nonrelaxed LES. Treatment is the same as for classic achalasia, except that consideration should be given to performing a longer esophagomyotomy (to the aortic arch). With relief of the obstruction caused by the nonrelaxing LES, the pain usually disappears.

c. **Diffuse esophageal spasm** is characterized by loss of the normal peristaltic coordination of the esophageal smooth muscle. This results in simultaneous contraction of segments of the esophageal body.

(1) The primary **symptom** is severe spastic pain, which can occur spontaneously and at night. Additionally, dysphagia, regurgitation, and weight loss are common.

(2) The **diagnosis** is confirmed with esophageal manometry, which usually demonstrates spontaneous activity, repetitive waves, and prolonged, high-amplitude contractions. Characteristic broad, multipeaked contractions with or without propagation are seen, and normal peristaltic contractions also may be present. Intravenous injection with the parasympathomimetic bethanechol (Urecholine) can provoke pain and abnormal contractions.

(3) **Treatment** with calcium channel blockers and nitrates can reduce the amplitude of the esophageal contractions but usually is not beneficial. Surgical treatment consists of a long esophagomyotomy, extending from the stomach to the aortic arch, and often a concomitant antireflux procedure.

d. **Nutcracker esophagus** refers to a condition characterized manometrically by prolonged, high-amplitude peristaltic waves associated with chest pain that may mimic cardiac symptoms. Treatment with calcium channel blockers and long-acting nitrates has been helpful. Esophagomyotomy is of uncertain benefit.

2. **Secondary dysmotility** represents the esophageal response to inflammatory injury or systemic disorders, such as scleroderma, multiple sclerosis, or diabetic neuropathy. Inflammation can produce fibrosis that can lead to partial or complete loss of peristalsis and esophageal contractility. The most common cause of secondary dysfunction is the reflux of gastric contents into the esophagus.

   a. Progressive systemic sclerosis, or scleroderma, has esophageal manifestations in 60% to 80% of patients, and often the esophagus is the earliest site of GI involvement. It is characterized by atrophy of the smooth muscle of the distal esophagus, deposition of collagen in connective tissue, and subintimal arteriolar fibrosis. Normal contractions are present in the striated muscle of the proximal esophagus.

   b. In a subset of patients with severe, long-standing GER disease, **complications**, including erosive esophagitis and stricture formation, occur as a result of the combination of a hypotensive incompetent LES and poor esophageal emptying secondary to low-amplitude, disordered peristaltic contractions. Intensive medical treatment of the reflux is essential before operation. Most surgeons prefer a Collis gastroplasty and a Belsey antireflux procedure for these patients because of the presence of esophageal shortening and weak peristalsis.

VIII. Esophageal strictures are either benign or malignant, and the distinction is critical. **Benign strictures** are either congenital or acquired.

   A. Congenital webs are the only true congenital esophageal strictures. They represent a failure of appropriate canalization of the esophagus during development and can occur at any level. An imperforate web must be distinguished from a tracheoesophageal fistula, although a perforate web may not produce symptoms until feedings become solid.

   B. Acquired strictures

   1. Esophageal rings or **webs** occur at all levels in relation to the etiology of the webbing process. An example is **Schatzki ring**, which occurs in the lower esophagus at the junction of the squamous and columnar epithelium. A hiatal hernia is always present, and the etiology is presumed to be GER. Esophagitis is rarely present. Treatment generally consists of medical management of reflux with periodic dilation for symptoms of dysphagia.

   2. Strictures of the esophagus can result from any esophageal injury, including chronic reflux, previous perforation, infection, or inflammation.

   C. Symptoms associated with a stricture consist of progressive dysphagia to solid food and usually begin when the esophageal lumen narrows beyond 12 mm.

   D. Evaluation and treatment of a stricture begins with the categorical **exclusion of malignancy**. The diagnosis usually is based on a barium swallow. Esophagoscopy is essential to assess the location, length, size, and distensibility of the stricture and to obtain appropriate biopsies or brushings. Because a peptic stricture secondary to reflux always occurs at the squamocolumnar junction, biopsy of the esophageal mucosa below a high stricture should demonstrate columnar mucosa. If squamous mucosa is found, the presumptive diagnosis of a malignant obstruction should be made, although strictures due to Crohn disease, previous lye ingestion, or monilial esophagitis are among alternative diagnoses. Most strictures are amenable to **dilation**, and this relieves the symptoms. Attention is then directed at correcting the underlying etiology. **Resection** can be required for recurrent or persistent strictures or if malignancy cannot be ruled out.

IX. Benign esophageal neoplasms are rare, although probably many remain undetected. The most common lesion is a stromal tumor (leiomyoma), followed by polyps. Less common lesions are hemangioma and granular cell myoblastoma.

   A. Clinical features depend primarily on the location of the tumor within the esophagus. **Intraluminal** tumors, such as polyps, cause esophageal obstruction, and patients present with dysphagia, vomiting, and aspiration.

Intramural tumors, such as leiomyomas, usually are asymptomatic but, if large enough, can produce dysphagia or chest pain.
B. **Diagnosis and evaluation** usually involve a combination of barium swallow, esophagoscopy, and perhaps CT scanning or MR scan studies.
C. **Treatment** for all symptomatic or enlarging tumors is surgical removal. Intraluminal tumors can be removed successfully via endoscopy, but if large and vascular, they should be resected via thoracotomy and esophagotomy. Intramural tumors, such as leiomyomas, can usually be enucleated from the esophageal muscular wall without entering the mucosa. This is done via a video-assisted thoracoscopic or open thoracotomy approach. Laparoscopic resection may be appropriate for distal lesions.
X. **Caustic ingestion.** Liquid alkali solutions (e.g., **Drano** and **Liquid-Plumr**) are responsible for most of the serious caustic esophageal and gastric injuries and can produce necrosis in both organs. Acid ingestion is more likely to produce isolated gastric injury.
   A. **Initial management** is directed at hemodynamic stabilization and evaluation of the airway and extent of injury.
      1. **Airway compromise** can occur from burns of the epiglottis or larynx and may require tracheostomy.
      2. **Fluid resuscitation** and **broad-spectrum antibiotics** should be instituted.
      3. **Vomiting should not be induced,** but patients should be placed on **nothing-by-mouth** status and given an **oral suction** device.
      4. **Steroids** are of no proven benefit.
   B. **Evaluation** with water-soluble contrast esophagography and gentle esophagoscopy should be done early to assess the severity and extent of injury and rule out esophageal perforation or gastric necrosis.
   C. **Management**
      1. **Without perforation,** management is supportive because acute symptoms generally resolve over several days.
      2. **Perforation, unrelenting pain, or persistent acidosis** mandate surgical intervention. A transabdominal approach is recommended to allow evaluation of the patient's stomach and distal esophagus. If necrotic, the involved portion of the patient's stomach and esophagus must be resected, and a cervical esophagostomy must be performed. A feeding jejunostomy is placed for nutrition, and reconstruction is performed 90 or more days later.
      3. **Late problems** include the development of **strictures** and an increased risk of **esophageal carcinoma** (1,000 times that of the general population).
XI. **Complications of esophageal surgery.** Esophageal surgery is fraught with potential complications, and consistently good results require meticulous attention to operative technique.
   A. **Postthoracotomy complications** can include atelectasis and respiratory insufficiency, pneumonia, atrial fibrillation, wound infections, and persistent postoperative pain.
   B. **Complications related to an esophageal anastomosis** consist primarily of leaks and strictures.
      1. Management of an **anastomotic leak** is based on the size of the leak, the location of the anastomosis, and the clinical status of the patient.
         a. A **cervical** anastomotic leak usually can be managed by opening the incision to allow drainage. Occasionally, the leak tracks below the thoracic inlet into the mediastinum, necessitating wider débridement and drainage. If a major leak occurs, esophagoscopy should be performed to rule out a significant ischemic injury to the stomach. If present, the anastomosis should be taken down, and a cervical esophagostomy should be performed. The necrotic portion of the stomach should be resected, and the remaining stomach should be returned to the abdomen, with placement of a gastrostomy and

feeding jejunostomy. Reconstruction with residual stomach or the colon is done at a later date.

   b. Intrathoracic anastomotic leaks are associated with a high mortality rate. Small, well-drained leaks can be treated conservatively, but large or poorly drained leaks require operative exploration.

   2. Strictures usually are the result of a healed anastomotic leak, relative ischemia of the anastomosis, or recurrent cancer. Most can be dilated successfully.

C. **Complications of antireflux repairs** generally result from **preoperative** failure to recognize a confounding abnormality, such as poor gastric emptying or weak esophageal peristalsis, or **operative** miscalculations that result in too tight a fundoplication or excessive tension on the repair. Most of these complications require operative revision.

   1. Postoperative dysphagia can result from a fundoplication that is too long or tight, a misplaced or slipped fundoplication that is positioned around the stomach rather than the distal esophagus, or a complete fundoplication in the setting of poor esophageal contractile function. It also can result from operative distortion of the GE junction, excessive narrowing of the diaphragmatic hiatus, or disruption of the crural closure and herniation of an intact repair into the chest.

   2. Persistent or recurrent reflux after surgery suggests an inadequate or misplaced fundoplication, disruption of the fundoplication, or herniation of the repair into the chest (*Ann Surg* 1999;229:669).

   3. Breakdown of an antireflux repair usually is recognized by a gradual recurrence of symptoms. Most commonly, disruption of a repair is due to inadequate mobilization of the cardia and excessive tension on the repair.

   4. Gas bloating or gastric dilation can occur if the fundoplication is too tight or if there is unrecognized gastric outlet obstruction or delayed gastric emptying.

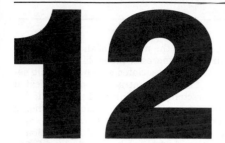

Stomach

Julie A. Margenthaler and
Mary E. Klingensmith

DISORDERS OF THE STOMACH

I. **Treatment of peptic ulcer disease** has changed dramatically over the past two decades with the development of antisecretory drugs (H_2 blockers and proton pump inhibitors) and the recognition of the role of *Helicobacter pylori* in its pathogenesis (*Gastroenterology* 2000;118(2 Suppl 1):S2–8). Intractability and recurrence of disease in adequately treated patients are quite rare, with surgical management reserved primarily for complications of ulcers (bleeding, perforation, gastric outlet obstruction). Cigarette smoking is a clear risk factor for **ulcerogenesis**, whereas the role of alcohol is less clear; diet and caffeine do not appear to be important. The use of nonsteroidal anti-inflammatory drugs must be determined when evaluating a patient with peptic ulcer disease.

   A. **Symptoms** of uncomplicated peptic ulcer disease include chronic, intermittent, gnawing, or burning epigastric pain. Ingestion of food may alleviate discomfort in patients with duodenal ulcers, whereas it may exacerbate pain in patients with gastric ulcers.

   B. **Differential diagnosis** is broad and includes acute cholecystitis, pancreatitis, reflux esophagitis, and gastric cancer.

   C. **Esophagogastroduodenoscopy (EGD)** is more sensitive and specific than contrast examination for peptic ulcer disease (*Ann Intern Med* 1984;101:538). In addition, EGD offers therapeutic options (ligation of bleeding vessels) and diagnostic options (biopsy for malignancy, antral biopsy for *H. pylori*). Right upper quadrant ultrasonography and serum amylase level are helpful in ruling out other causes of upper abdominal pain.

   D. *H. pylori* **infection** is associated with more than 90% of duodenal ulcers and 75% of gastric ulcers. The **cod liver oil (CLO) test** is a rapid, relatively inexpensive urease test performed on antral tissue obtained during endoscopy; **histology** is considered the gold standard. Noninvasive testing for infection includes **serum immunoglobulin** for *H. pylori* and the **labeled urea breath test**, which is the test of choice for confirming eradication. **Treatment** involves a 2-week course of triple therapy (omeprazole-amoxicillin-clarithromycin or omeprazole-metronidazole-clarithromycin). When *H. pylori* is eradicated, the 12-month recurrence rate of duodenal ulcer is less than 5%, compared to 15% with maintenance H_2-blocker therapy (*Arch Intern Med* 1995;155:1958).

   E. **Fasting serum gastrin level** should be obtained in patients with recurrent ulcer after adequate treatment, multiple ulcers, ulcers in unusual locations (such as the second and third portions of the duodenum), and complications of ulcers that require surgical therapy to rule out Zollinger-Ellison syndrome [normal gastrin level is <100 pg/mL (current units) or <100 ng/L (SI units)].

   F. **Classification of peptic ulcers** is based on location and has important treatment ramifications. **Duodenal ulcers** occur most frequently in the first portion of the duodenum and are associated with **acid hypersecretion**. Gastric metaplasia is common in the surrounding mucosa. Because there is minimal risk of malignancy as compared with gastric ulcers, excision of duodenal ulcers is not usually an important part of surgical strategy.

1. **Type I gastric ulcer** (55%) occurs near the junction of the parietal and antral mucosa on the lesser curvature where the inner oblique muscle is absent (usually near the incisura) and is associated with **normal acid secretion**. The surgical treatment of choice for intractable or complicated benign type I gastric ulcer is antrectomy with Billroth I reconstruction (recurrence rate 3%). Truncal vagotomy (TV) does not confer additional benefit. Alternatively, wedge excision of the ulcer with parietal cell vagotomy (PCV; vagotomy in which antral and pyloric vagal innervation is preserved) can be performed, although this can be technically difficult and is associated with a higher recurrence rate (up to 20%).

2. **Type II gastric ulcer** (25%) is located in the gastric body in combination with a duodenal ulcer and is associated with **acid hypersecretion**. Antrectomy (including the gastric ulcer) and truncal vagotomy with either Billroth I or II reconstruction is the procedure of choice for intractable type II gastric ulcer. Wedge excision of the gastric ulcer with PCV is also acceptable.

3. **Type III gastric ulcer** (15%) is prepyloric and is also associated with **acid hypersecretion**. Treatment is similar to that for type II gastric ulcer, but wedge excision with PCV is associated with a higher recurrence rate.

4. **Type IV gastric ulcer** (5%) is located on the lesser curve near the gastroesophageal junction and is associated with **normal acid secretion**. Excision of the ulcer may require a generous distal gastrectomy. An acid reduction procedure is not necessary.

II. **Complications** of peptic ulcer disease usually require surgical evaluation.

A. **Hemorrhage** is the leading cause of death due to peptic ulcer disease, with 5% to 10% mortality. Evaluation and management begin with aggressive resuscitation and correction of any coagulopathy, followed by EGD. Although spontaneous cessation of bleeding occurs in 70% of patients, endoscopy is especially warranted in individuals who present with hypotension, hematemesis, melena, age older than 60 years, multiple medical comorbidities, and inability to clear gastric blood with lavage, as these patients have a higher risk of recurrent bleeding. Individuals with endoscopic findings of a visible vessel or active bleeding are also at high risk, and endoscopic thermal coagulation with or without epinephrine injection is mandated in these cases (*JAMA* 1989;262:1369). Repeated episodes of bleeding, continued hemodynamic instability, an ongoing transfusion requirement of more than 6 units of packed red blood cells over 24 hours, and more than one unsuccessful endoscopic intervention are **indications for surgery**.

1. **Bleeding duodenal ulcers** are usually located on the posterior duodenal wall within 2 cm of the pylorus and typically erode into the gastroduodenal artery. Bleeding is controlled by duodenotomy and oversewing of the bleeding vessel. Patients who have failed medical therapy, have presented with shock, or have had other medical comorbidities but are otherwise stable should have a concomitant acid-reducing procedure, most commonly truncal vagotomy with pyloroplasty if this can be performed expeditiously. Occasionally, PCV can be considered in young, otherwise healthy, hemodynamically stable patients. Alternatively, some surgeons advocate *H. pylori* eradication rather than vagotomy after control of bleeding to reduce the risk of recurrent bleeding without the morbidity of vagotomy (*Br J Surg* 1991;77:1004).

2. **Bleeding gastric ulcers** are optimally treated by wedge resection to eliminate the bleeding site and exclude malignancy, with a concomitant acid-reduction procedure for type II and type III (high-acid) gastric ulcers in stable patients (truncal vagotomy with pyloroplasty). If wedge resection of the ulcer cannot be performed due to its juxtapyloric location, a gastrotomy or pyloroplasty incision is made, the bleeding site is oversewn, and multiple biopsies are taken. Partial gastrectomy or antrectomy is associated with high mortality and morbidity in the emergent setting and should be viewed with caution.

B. **Perforated peptic ulcer** typically presents with sudden onset of severe abdominal pain but can present less dramatically, particularly in hospitalized, elderly, and immunocompromised patients. The resulting peritonitis is often generalized but can be localized when the perforation is walled off by adjacent viscera and structures. Examination reveals low-grade fever, tachycardia, abdominal wall rigidity, and leukocytosis. Abdominal x-ray reveals free subdiaphragmatic gas in 80% to 85% of cases. **Nonoperative treatment of perforated duodenal ulcer** can be considered in cases in which the perforation has been present for more than 24 hours, the pain is well localized, there is no evidence of ongoing extravasation on upper GI water-soluble contrast studies, and the patient is reliable and can be examined frequently (*World J Surg* 2000;24:256). All patients with perforation should undergo aggressive fluid resuscitation and have broad-spectrum antibiotics instituted before **surgical management**.

1. **Perforated duodenal ulcers** are best managed by simple omental patching and peritoneal débridement, followed by *H. pylori* eradication. An acid-reducing procedure (preferably PCV) should be added in stable patients who are known to be *H. pylori* negative or have failed medical therapy.

2. **Perforated gastric ulcers** are best treated by wedge resection to eliminate the perforation and exclude malignancy, with a concomitant acid-reduction procedure (truncal vagotomy with pyloroplasty or PCV) in stable patients with type II and type III gastric ulcers. If wedge resection of the ulcer cannot be performed due to its juxtapyloric location, multiple biopsies of the ulcer are taken and omental patching is performed. Partial gastrectomy or antrectomy is associated with high mortality and morbidity in the emergent setting and is rarely indicated.

C. **Gastric outlet obstruction** can occur as a chronic process due to fibrosis and scarring of the pylorus and duodenum from chronic ulcer disease or as a consequence of acute inflammation superimposed on previous scarring of the gastric outlet. **Patients present** with recurrent vomiting of poorly digested food, dehydration, and hypochloremic hypokalemic metabolic alkalosis. **Initial management** consists of aggressive correction of volume and electrolyte abnormalities, nasogastric suction, and administration of intravenous antisecretory agents. Parenteral nutrition is occasionally required. EGD is necessary for evaluating the nature of the obstruction and for ruling out malignant etiology. Acute obstruction typically resolves in 3 to 4 days. One-third of patients have significant improvement with initial management, but eventually 75% of patients require surgical intervention. **Indications for surgical therapy** include persistent obstruction after 7 days of nonoperative management and recurrent obstruction. The goals of operative management are to relieve the obstruction and reduce acid secretion. PCV with gastrojejunostomy may be the treatment of choice, as peripyloric scarring, inflammation, and edema may make pyloroplasty difficult in the case of truncal vagotomy with pyloroplasty and may make closure of the duodenal stump difficult in the case of truncal vagotomy with antrectomy and Billroth II reconstruction. **Endoscopic balloon dilatation results in immediate symptomatic improvement in 80% of patients, but fewer than 40% have sustained improvement at 3 months (*Gastrointest Endosc* 1996;43:98), and it is reserved for patients who are high operative risks.

III. **Gastric adenocarcinoma** is the second most common cause of cancer mortality worldwide but only the seventh most frequent cause of cancer death in the United States (11,780 deaths in 2003). Its incidence in the United States (22,710 new cases in 2003) has decreased dramatically over the past 70 years (46/100,000 in 1930 to 7/100,000 at present in men and 37/100,000 in 1930 to 4/100,000 at present in women). The reasons for this decline are incompletely understood but may be related to changes in diet or food storage. Interestingly, proximal adenocarcinomas make up an increasing proportion of newly diagnosed cancers. The overall 5-year survival rate in the United States is 15%.

A. Risk factors for gastric cancer include *H. pylori* infection, male gender, chronic atrophic gastritis, pernicious anemia, adenomatous gastric polyps, Ménétrier disease, and previous gastric resection. Unlike colorectal carcinoma, the majority of gastric cancers do not arise from adenomatous polyps. Up to 12% of gastric ulcers may be cancerous.

B. Signs and symptoms of gastric cancer include abdominal pain, unexplained weight loss, anorexia, early satiety, anemia, and upper GI bleeding, but none of these is sensitive or specific. Similarly, the physical examination is usually nonspecific, occasionally revealing evidence of advanced or metastatic disease, such as abdominal mass, ascites, jaundice, temporal wasting, enlarged supraclavicular node (Virchow node), infiltration of the umbilicus (Sister Mary Joseph node), a mass in the pelvic cul-de-sac (Blumer shelf), or enlarged ovaries on pelvic examination (Krukenberg tumor).

C. Diagnosis is typically made by **EGD,** which permits visualization of the tumor, determination of its size and location, and biopsy and brushing of suspicious lesions. **Screening examination** by endoscopy or contrast studies is not cost-effective for the general U.S. population given the low incidence and high cost but may be warranted in high-risk individuals, such as patients more than 20 years post–partial gastrectomy, patients with pernicious anemia or atrophic gastritis, or immigrants from endemic areas (Russia, Asia).

D. Staging is important in selecting the appropriate treatment (Table 12-1). Abnormal findings on physical examination and chest x-ray may indicate metastatic spread.

    1. CT scan of the abdomen and pelvis may show ascites, metastatic spread to other organs, and lymphadenopathy. However, it is not uncommon for tumors to be either understaged due to failure to detect small peritoneal, omental, or hepatic metastases or incorrectly determined to be unresectable due to involvement of contiguous organs when evaluated by CT alone (*Gut* 1997;41:314).

    2. Endoscopic ultrasonography is superior to CT in delineating the depth of tumor invasion in the gastric wall and adjacent structures and identifying perigastric lymphadenopathy. Lesions that are confined to the mucosa or submucosa are known as **early gastric cancer** and account for 5% of gastric cancer cases. Tumors that are limited to the mucosa rarely metastasize to regional lymph nodes (1% to 4%) and are thus potentially amenable to endoluminal resection or local excision as opposed to radical resection.

    3. Laparoscopy significantly enhances the accuracy of staging, leading to a change in the preoperative staging in up to 58% of patients, with upstaging more common than downstaging (*Surg Endosc* 1997;11:1159), resulting in a change in management of up to 40% (*Endoscopy* 1999;31:3427). Laparoscopy may prevent unnecessary laparotomy or allow more accurate selection of those patients with locally advanced disease for investigational neoadjuvant therapies. It can be performed as a separate procedure or as part of a planned curative resection.

E. Surgery is indicated for potentially curable tumors and for palliation of patients who present with bleeding, obstruction, or perforation due to locally advanced, incurable cancers. The abdomen is thoroughly explored via an upper midline or Chevron incision to rule out metastatic disease and to determine the extent and mobility of the primary tumor.

    1. Curative resection is undertaken if the cancer appears to be confined to the primary tumor and the regional lymph nodes. The primary tumor is resected in its entirety with a normal stomach tissue margin of 5 to 7 cm, with adequacy of margins confirmed by frozen section. *En bloc* resection of adjacent structures, including the transverse colon, pancreas, liver, or spleen, may be required to obtain negative margins. As a consequence, most surgeons instruct their patients to undergo a mechanical

Table 12-1. TNM (tumor, node, metastasis) staging of gastric cancer

T: Primary tumor
T0 No evidence of primary tumor
Tis Carcinoma *in situ*
T1 Invasion of lamina propria or submucosa
T2 Invasion of muscularis propria or subserosa
T3 Penetration of serosa
T4 Invasion of adjacent structures

N: Regional lymph nodes
N0 No regional node metastasis
N1 Involved perigastric nodes within 3 cm of tumor
N2 Involved perigastric nodes >3 cm from tumor edge or involvement of left gastric, splenic, celiac, or hepatic nodes

M: Distant metastasis
M0 No distant metastases
M1 Distant metastases present

Stage Grouping		
Stage 0	Tis	N0	M0
Stage IA	T1	N0	M0
Stage IB	T1	N1	M0
	T2	N0	M0
Stage II	T1	N2	M0
	T2	N1	M0
	T3	N0	M0
Stage IIIA	T2	N2	M0
	T3	N1	M0
	T4	N0	M0
Stage IIIB	T3	N2	M0
	T4	N1	M0
Stage IV	T4	N2	M0
	Any T	Any N	Any M1

Adapted from Fleming ID, Cooper JS, Henson DE, et al., eds. *AJCC Cancer Staging Manual*. 5th ed. Philadelphia: Lippincott Williams & Wilkins, 1998.

and antibiotic bowel prep preoperatively. **The optimal extent of lymphadenectomy** is controversial. A D1 lymphadenectomy entails removal of perigastric nodes; a D2 lymphadenectomy includes removal of left gastric, hepatic, splenic, and celiac nodes. Even wider (D3 and D4) resections are practiced in Japan when involvement of those nodes is suspected, but they are rarely performed in the West. D2 dissection may improve the accuracy of staging and offers radical local clearance; it was shown to have survival benefit in patients with stage II and IIIA disease (*Ann Surg* 1998;228:449) but was found to be associated with increased morbidity and mortality and have no survival benefit in another study (*N Engl J Med* 1999;340:908).

2. **Reconstruction** is usually performed with an antecolic Roux-en-Y or Billroth II gastrojejunostomy in order to avoid having an anastomosis in the retroperitoneal bed, where recurrence leading to anastomotic obstruction can occur. Retrocolic anastomosis is associated with improved dependent gastric emptying and is usually preferred for resections for nonmalignant disease.

3. **Palliative resection** may prevent bleeding, obstruction, and perforation in patients with metastatic or otherwise unresectable cancer.

Alternatively, if gastric outlet obstruction is the primary symptom of an unresectable tumor, laparoscopic gastrojejunostomy can be performed at the time of staging laparoscopy, as it affords lower morbidity than open surgery. If laparotomy has been performed, however, open resection of the primary cancer results in a longer period of symptom palliation than does bypass alone (*Surg Oncol Clin N Am* 2002;11: 459).

F. **Adjuvant therapy**
   1. **Adjuvant chemotherapy** has not shown any consistent benefit in terms of disease-free interval or survival (*J Natl Cancer Inst* 1993;85:1839; *J Clin Oncol* 2002;21:2282).
   2. **Neoadjuvant chemotherapy** may reduce tumor size, enhancing the chance for resectability. Other theoretical benefits include the elimination of delayed administration of therapy due to prolonged postoperative recovery; prevention of nontherapeutic gastrectomy when disease is rapidly progressive during treatment; and administration of therapy when measurable disease is present to assess response, allowing treatment to continue only in those patients who respond to the regimen. Response to neoadjuvant chemotherapy has been associated with markedly improved survival after curative resection in phase II trials (*Ann Surg* 1999;229:303), warranting further investigation in the context of clinical trials.
   3. **Postoperative radiotherapy** with concomitant 5-fluorouracil may decrease locoregional recurrence in patients with advanced disease, but its use postoperatively and as a component of neoadjuvant treatment remains investigational (*Cancer* 1999;86:1657).
   4. **Hyperthermic intraperitoneal chemoperfusion with mitomycin C** was associated with improved peritoneal recurrence rates and long-term survival in patients with locally advanced cancer in a prospective, randomized trial (*Arch Surg* 2004;139:20) and is currently being investigated.

IV. **Primary gastric lymphoma (PGL)** accounts for fewer than 5% of gastric neoplasms. PGL, however, accounts for two-thirds of all primary GI lymphomas. It is usually B-cell, non-Hodgkin lymphoma. *H. pylori* has been shown to be associated with PGL, particularly with mucosa-associated lymphoid tissue tumors, and its eradication has been demonstrated to result in clinical regression of these tumors (*Ann Oncol* 199;10:637). Patients are typically in their 50s, and presentation is similar to that of gastric adenocarcinoma, with pain (68%), weight loss (28%), and bleeding (28%) the most common symptoms. Most PGLs are located in the distal stomach.

A. **Diagnosis of PGL** can be difficult. **Physical examination** is nonspecific and may reveal adenopathy, abdominal mass, or hepatosplenomegaly. **EGD** typically shows superficial stellate ulcers with extensive gastric wall infiltration. Endoscopic biopsy has a sensitivity of only 80% because obtaining adequate tissue can be difficult. The cod liver oil (CLO) test should be performed to assess *H. pylori* status. GI contrast studies cannot reliably differentiate lymphoma from adenocarcinoma. Occasionally, percutaneous CT-guided fine-needle biopsy can yield the diagnosis. Failure to establish a definitive pathologic diagnosis is an indication for surgery.

B. **Staging** via physical examination, complete blood count, lactic dehydrogenase, chest and abdominopelvic CT scan, and bone marrow biopsy that reveals no evidence of extragastric tumor is adequate to exclude metastatic disease. As with adenocarcinoma, endoscopic ultrasonography and laparoscopy can be helpful in more accurately determining staging information. Modified Ann Arbor stage IIIE and stage IV lymphoma must be ruled out, as their treatment is nonsurgical.

C. **Optimal treatment of PGL** has not been determined, as there are no large prospective trials with adequate numbers of patients. Some centers advocate gastric resection as the treatment of choice for stage IE or IIE PGL

(*Gastroenterology* 2000;119:1191), whereas others suggest reserving resection for those in whom chemotherapy fails (*Cancer* 2000;88:1979).

1. **Surgery** provides a good chance of cure for stage IE and IIE PGL and is the most effective treatment for complications such as bleeding, perforation, obstruction, or fistula formation. Additionally, resection affords accurate tissue diagnosis, staging, and grading and may prevent the development of the aforementioned complications during or after additional treatment. Of note, microscopically positive margins do not have a negative impact on survival if adjuvant treatment is given.

2. **Chemotherapy** consists of cyclophosphamide-doxorubicin-vincristine-prednisone or cyclophosphamide–nitrogen mustard–vincristine–procarbazine–prednisone and is used primarily for stage III and IV disease and as adjuvant treatment in patients with a high probability of recurrence.

3. **Radiotherapy** as adjuvant treatment is controversial but may improve survival if positive margins or gross disease remain after surgery (*World J Gastroenterol* 2004;10:5).

V. **Benign gastric tumors** account for fewer than 2% of all gastric tumors. They are usually located in the antrum or corpus. Presentation can be similar to that of peptic ulcer or adenocarcinoma, and diagnosis is made by EGD or contrast radiography.

A. **Gastric polyps** are classified by histologic findings. Endoscopic removal is appropriate if the polyp can be completely excised.

1. **Hyperplastic polyps** are regenerative rather than neoplastic and constitute 75% of gastric polyps. Risk of malignant transformation is minimal.

2. **Adenomatous polyps** are the second most common gastric polyp and are neoplastic in origin. The incidence of carcinoma within the polyp is proportionate to its size, with polyps of greater than 2 cm having a 24% incidence of malignancy. Patients with familial adenomatous polyposis have a 50% incidence of gastroduodenal polyps and require endoscopic surveillance. Surgical resection with a 2- to 3-cm margin of gastric wall can often be performed laparoscopically and is required if endoscopic excision is not possible.

VI. **Gastrointestinal stromal tumors (GISTs)** are most commonly found in the stomach and are usually benign (90%), although the true benign or malignant nature of the lesion is established by the lack of adjacent organ invasion or metastasis. Bleeding may arise from the erosion of the overlying mucosa, or these tumors may present secondary to mass effect. Endoscopy reveals an extraluminal mass with overlying normal or umbilicated mucosa. Treatment can be accomplished by wedge resection with a 2- to 3-cm histologically negative margin of gastric wall, although formal gastric resection may be required, depending on the location of the tumor.

VII. **Postgastrectomy syndromes** are caused by changes in gastric emptying as a consequence of gastric operations. Clearly defining the syndrome that is present in a given patient is critical to developing a rational treatment plan (*World J Surg* 2003;27:725). Most are treated nonoperatively and resolve with time. They may occur in up to 20% of patients who undergo gastric surgery, depending on the extent of resection, disruption of the vagus nerves, status of the pylorus, type of reconstruction, and presence of mechanical or functional obstruction. Denervation of the proximal stomach impairs its receptive relaxation and accommodation functions, resulting in a rapid rise in intragastric pressure, with consequent accelerated emptying of liquids. Because emptying of solids is normally regulated by antral innervation and function, distal stomach denervation usually results in an increased rate of emptying of solids.

A. **Dumping syndrome** is thought to result from the rapid emptying of a high osmolar carbohydrate load into the small intestine, caused by the loss of reservoir capacity (due to vagotomy or resection) and the loss of pylorus function (due to resection or pyloroplasty). It occurs most commonly after Billroth II reconstruction.

1. **Early dumping** occurs within 30 minutes of eating and is characterized by nausea, epigastric distress, explosive diarrhea, and vasomotor symptoms (dizziness, palpitations, flushing, diaphoresis). It is presumably caused by rapid fluid shifts in response to the hyperosmolar intestinal load and release of vasoactive peptides from the gut.

2. **Late dumping** symptoms are primarily vasomotor and occur 1 to 4 hours after eating. The hormonal response to high simple carbohydrate load results in hyperinsulinemia and reactive hypoglycemia. Symptoms are relieved by carbohydrate ingestion.

3. **Treatment** is primarily nonsurgical and results in improvement in nearly all patients over time. Meals should be smaller in volume but increased in frequency, liquids should be ingested 30 minutes after eating solids, and simple carbohydrates should be avoided. Use of the long-acting somatostatin analogue octreotide (25 to 100 μg subcutaneously before meals) results in significant improvement and persistent relief in 80% of patients when behavioral modifications fail (*Clin Endocrinol* 1999;51:619). If reoperation is necessary, conversion to Roux-en-Y gastrojejunostomy is usually successful. Other surgical options include conversion to Billroth I (gastroduodenostomy) and jejunal segment interposition.

B. **Alkaline reflux gastritis** is most commonly associated with Billroth II gastrojejunostomy and requires operative treatment more often than do other postgastrectomy syndromes. It is characterized by burning epigastric pain, nausea, and bilious emesis. The latter does not relieve the pain and is not associated with meals. Bile, not pancreatic enzymes or alkalinity, is responsible for damage to the gastric mucosa (*Ann Surg* 1995;180:648). Endoscopy reveals inflamed, beefy-red, friable gastric mucosa and can rule out recurrent ulcer as a cause of symptoms. Bile reflux into the stomach is occasionally seen. Enterogastric reflux can be confirmed by hepatic iminodiacetic acid (HIDA) scan, in which radiolabeled nucleotide is administered intravenously and excreted into the bile. Mechanical obstruction is absent, distinguishing alkaline reflux gastritis from loop syndrome.

1. **Nonoperative therapy** consists of feeding patients ursodeoxycholic acid and is only occasionally effective.

2. **Surgery** is the only proven treatment and consists of diversion of bile from the gastric mucosa. The creation of a long-limb (45-cm) Roux-en-Y effectively eliminates alkaline reflux (*Gastroenterol Clin North Am* 1994;23:281). However, symptoms are not always alleviated, and complications of operation include delayed gastric emptying, marginal ulceration, and the Roux stasis syndrome. Some authors advocate conversion to Billroth I gastroduodenostomy with biliary diversion using choledochojejunostomy via a 30- to 35-cm Roux-en-Y limb (*Arch Surg* 1997;132:245).

C. **Roux stasis syndrome** may occur in up to 30% of patients after Roux-en-Y gastroenterostomy (*Am J Surg* 2003;186:269) and is characterized by chronic abdominal pain, nausea, and vomiting that is worsened by eating. It results from a functional obstruction due to disruption of the normal propagation of pacesetter potentials in the Roux-en-Y limb from the proximal duodenum and altered motility in the gastric remnant. Near total gastrectomy to remove the atonic stomach can improve gastric emptying and is occasionally useful in patients with refractory Roux stasis. Use of an "uncut" Roux-en-Y reconstruction (*Am J Surg* 2001;182:52) may preserve normal pacemaker propagation and prevent the development of the syndrome.

D. **Loop syndromes** result from mechanical obstruction of either the **afferent** or **efferent** limb of the Billroth II gastrojejunostomy. The location and etiology of the obstruction are investigated by plain abdominal x-rays, CT scan, upper GI contrast studies, and endoscopy. Relief of the obstruction may require adhesiolysis, revision of the anastomosis, or, occasionally, bowel resection.

1. **Afferent loop syndrome** can be caused acutely by bowel kink, volvulus, or internal herniation, resulting in severe abdominal pain and nonbilious emesis within the first few weeks after surgery. Lack of bilious staining of nasogastric drainage in the immediate postoperative period suggests this complication. Examination may reveal a fluid-filled abdominal mass, and laboratory findings may include elevated bilirubin or amylase. **Duodenal stump blowout** may result from progressive afferent limb dilatation, producing peritonitis, abscess, or fistula formation. In the urgent setting, jejunojejunostomy can effectively decompress the afferent limb. A more **chronic form** of afferent loop syndrome results from partial mechanical obstruction of the afferent limb and causes postprandial right upper quadrant pain relieved by bilious emesis that is not mixed with recently ingested food. Stasis can lead to bacterial overgrowth and subsequent bile salt deconjugation in the obstructed loop, causing **blind loop syndrome** (steatorrhea and vitamin B_{12}, folate, and iron deficiency) by interfering with fat and vitamin B_{12} absorption.

2. **Efferent loop syndrome** results from intermittent obstruction of the efferent limb of the gastrojejunostomy, presenting as abdominal pain and bilious emesis months to years after surgery and behaving like a proximal small bowel obstruction.

E. **Postvagotomy diarrhea** has an incidence of 20% after truncal vagotomy and is thought to result from alterations in gastric emptying and vagal denervation of the small bowel and biliary tree. The diarrhea is typically watery and episodic. Treatment includes antidiarrheal medications (loperamide, diphenoxylate with atropine, cholestyramine) and decreasing excessive intake of fluids or foods that contain lactose. Symptoms usually improve with time and surgery is rarely indicated. Surgical alleviation involves placement of a 10- to 15-cm antiperistaltic jejunal segment 100 cm distal to the gastrojejunostomy.

F. **Nutritional disturbances** can occur in up to 30% of patients after gastric surgery, either as a result of functional changes or postgastrectomy syndromes. Prolonged **iron, folate, vitamin B_{12}, calcium, and vitamin D deficiencies** can result in anemia, neuropathy, dementia, and osteomalacia. These can be prevented with supplementation.

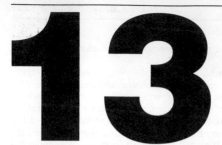

Small Intestine

Kim C. Lu and
David W. Dietz

The small intestine is the portion of the alimentary tract from the pylorus to the ileocecal valve. While the small intestine's absorptive functions are widely appreciated, it also has important immune and endocrine functions.

I. **Embryology**

A. **Embryologic origin.** The small intestine forms during the 4th week of fetal development. While the duodenum arises from the foregut, the jejunum and ileum derive from the fetal midgut. The endoderm forms the absorptive epithelium and the secretory glands. The splanchnic mesoderm gives rise to the rest of the intestinal wall, including the musculature and the serosa.

B. **Rotation of the small intestine.** During the 5th week of fetal development, the intestine elongates and herniates through the umbilicus. The intestine rotates 90 degrees around the axis of the vitelline duct and the superior mesenteric artery. By the 10th week, the intestine returns to the abdominal cavity and rotates another 180 degrees. This rotation places the ligament of Treitz in the left upper quadrant and the cecum into the right upper quadrant. Between the third and fifth months of development, the cecum descends to its customary position in the right lower quadrant.

C. **Formation of the lumen.** Between the 4th and 7th weeks of fetal development, the small intestine is lined by cuboidal cells. Rapid proliferation may lead to occlusion of the lumen, particularly in the duodenum. Due to apoptosis, the lumen becomes patent between the 9th and 10th weeks of development. Then, villi develop, starting from the duodenum and spreading caudad, even into the colon. Later, between the 10th and 12th weeks, crypts begin to form. The crypts are the sites for cell proliferation and give rise to the absorptive cells—the enterocytes—and the goblet cells, Paneth cells, and enteroendocrine cells.

II. **Anatomy**

A. **Gross anatomy.** The small intestine, which includes the duodenum, the jejunum, and the ileum, begins at the pylorus and extends to the ileocecal valve. The entire intestine measures between 270 and 290 cm.

The **duodenum** measures 20 cm. While the first portion, the bulb, is intraperitoneal, the second, third, and fourth portions are retroperitoneal. The second portion is particularly important, since biliary and pancreatic secretions enter at the ampulla of Vater. Pathology in this portion of the duodenum may require a pancreaticoduodenectomy for treatment.

The **jejunum** measures 100 to 110 cm, while the **ileum** measures 150 to 160 cm. Of interest, the jejunum and ileum together add up to approximately 160% of a patient's height. The jejunum and ileum can be differentiated by closely examining the mesenteric blood supply.

The mesentery of the jejunum has fewer, larger arcades and long vessels between the arcades and the bowel wall. In contrast, the mesentery of the ileum has many small arcades located close to the bowel wall. Further, the jejunum has many circumferential mucosal folds called *plicae circularis,* which are missing in the distal ileum.

B. **Vascular/lymphatic supply.** The pancreaticoduodenal arteries, which connect the gastroduodenal and superior mesenteric arteries, supply the duodenum. The superior mesenteric artery supplies the jejunum and ileum. The veins run parallel to the arteries. The superior mesenteric vein provides the venous drainage of the small bowel and joins the splenic vein to form the portal vein.

The **lymph drainage** begins in the submucosal Peyer patches, extends to the mesenteric lymph nodes, and parallels the course of the named blood vessels. Eventually, the lymph drainage accumulates at the subdiaphragmatic cysterni chyli and enters the chest through the cisterna chyli.

C. Nervous innervation. The vagus is the origin for all abdominal parasympathetic fibers. These fibers cross mesenteric ganglia, particularly the celiac ganglion, and innervate the myenteric ganglion cells within the walls of the small intestine. The parasympathetic innervation is important for intestinal secretions and motility.

Three sets of sympathetic nerves innervate the gut. They form a plexus around the superior mesenteric artery. They modulate intestinal blood supply, secretion, and motility. Further, afferent sympathetic nerves carry all the pain signals from the intestine.

D. Anatomy of the intestinal wall. The four layers of the intestinal wall include the mucosa, the submucosa, the muscularis propria, and the serosa.

1. The **mucosa** includes the epithelial layer, the lamina propria, and the muscularis mucosae.

a. The **epithelial layer** has both villi and crypts. The villi are protrusions of the epithelial layer into the lumen and dramatically increase absorptive capacity. The crypts are the sites of pluripotent cells that give rise to the absorptive enterocytes (over 95% of the epithelial layer), Paneth cells, goblet cells, and enteroendocrine cells. Paneth cells secrete lysozyme, tumor necrosis factor, and cryptidins, which function in nonspecific immunity. Goblet cells secrete mucus. There are over 10 different subpopulations of enteroendocrine cells. Secreted intestinal hormones include gastrin, secretin, cholecystokinin, somatostatin, enteroglucagon, motilin, neurotensin, and gastric inhibitory peptide. While the villi are the sites of absorption, the crypts provide proliferation and secretory functions. Of note, the crypts replace the entire intestinal lining every 3 to 5 days.

b. The **lamina propria** is the loose connective tissue layer between the epithelial lining and the muscularis mucosae. Of especial importance are the Peyer patches, collections of lymphocytes that span the lamina propria and submucosa and are crucial for mucosal immunity.

c. The **muscularis mucosae** is a single layer of muscle that separates the mucosa from the submucosa.

2. The **submucosa** is the connective tissue layer between the mucosa and the muscularis propria. Blood vessels and nerves run within this layer. In particular, the submucosal Meissner ganglion cells are located here. This is the strongest layer of the intestinal wall.

3. The **muscularis propria** consists of a thicker, inner circular layer and an outer longitudinal layer. The Auerbach (myenteric) ganglion cells are located between those layers.

4. The **serosa** is a single layer of flat mesothelial cells lining the walls of the anterior duodenum and the entire jejunum and ileum.

E. Anatomy of the absorptive enterocyte. Two particular structures enhance the absorptive area of an enterocyte. Below the apical side of the cell membrane, actin microfilaments form the scaffolding for apical protrusions or folds, **microvilli**, into the lumen. A **glycocalyx** coating outside the cellular membrane further increases the absorptive surface. Digestive enzymes, such as disaccharidases, and sodium-nutrient cotransporters are located in the apical membrane.

In the lateral membrane, tight junctions prevent crossing of intraluminal contents across the epithelial layer. Intermediate junctions and desmosomes also help maintain the barrier function of the intestinal epithelium. In the basal membrane, Na-K ATPases and passive nutrient transporters are located.

III. Physiology
A. Absorption.
1. **Water absorption.** Under normal circumstances, approximately 7 to 10 L of fluid enters the small intestine each day. Of this fluid, 2 L is derived from oral intake, 1 L from saliva, 2 L from gastric secretion, 2 L from pancreatic secretion, 1 L from bile, and 1 L from small-intestinal secretion. Only 600 to 1,500 mL fluid reaches the large bowel, indicating a net absorption of fluid. Alterations in small-bowel permeability, tonicity of enteric substances, or rate of transit can result in diarrhea and large volume losses.
2. **Electrolyte absorption.** The majority of electrolyte absorption occurs in the small intestine. The most important electrolytes absorbed are sodium, chloride, and calcium. Sodium absorption occurs through passive diffusion, countertransport with hydrogen, and cotransport with chloride, glucose, and amino acids. Chloride is absorbed in exchange for bicarbonate, which accounts for the alkalinity of the luminal contents. Calcium is actively absorbed in the proximal small intestine by a process that is stimulated by 1,25-dihydroxyvitamin D_3. Emesis, diarrhea, obstruction, and small-bowel ostomy effluent can result in impaired small-bowel electrolyte absorption.
3. **Vitamin or mineral absorption.** Bile salts and vitamin B_{12}–intrinsic factor complexes are absorbed in the terminal ileum. Thus, ileal resection that leaves less than 100 cm of the ileum results in bile acid deficiencies. This limits absorption of the fat-soluble vitamins A, D, E, and K. Further, vitamin B_{12} deficiency can result in chronic megaloblastic anemia.
4. **Nutrient absorption.** The absorption of carbohydrates, proteins, and fat are discussed in Chapter 2 and in the next section (III.B).
B. Digestion.
While macronutrient digestion by salivary, gastric, biliary, and pancreatic secretions has been covered in Chapter 2, this section will discuss digestion at the level of the enterocyte.
1. **Brush border.** Brush border peptidases and disaccharidases break down peptides and disaccharides into simple amino acids and monosaccharides.
2. **Active transport of amino acids and monosaccharides.** Na-K ATPases in the basolateral membrane of enterocytes keep the intracellular Na concentration very low. This sodium gradient enables Na-nutrient cotransporters to move amino acids and monosaccharides into enterocytes. The amino acids and monosaccharides then move across the basolateral membrane by facilitated transport.
3. **Passive transport of fats via micelles.** After digestion by pancreatic lipases, triglycerides and fatty acids form micelles with the bile salts. These micelles diffuse across the apical membrane. The smooth endoplasmic reticulum reconstitutes these fats into chylomicrons, which enter submucosal lymphatics.
C. Motility
1. **Types of contractions.**
   a. When the circular muscle contracts, **ring contractions** can accomplish one of two purposes. They can temporarily segment the intestine for better mixing. If they progress caudad, they can propel food antegrade.
   b. When the longitudinal muscle contracts, **sleeve contractions** shorten the intestinal length, which helps to propel food antegrade.
2. **Neurohumoral effects on contractions.**
   a. **Vagal cholinergic** input and hormones such as **motilin and CCK** stimulate contractions. Of note, pacemaker cells, called **interstitial cells of Cajal**, initiate peristalsis in the duodenum.
   b. **Sympathetic neurons** inhibit peristalsis.
3. **Fasting state.** During the fasting state, the **migrating motor (or myoelectric) complex (MMC)** performs the housekeeping function of

clearing the lumen of debris. Each cycle of the MMC has three phases. The first, resting phase has few contractions. This takes up 80% of a MMC cycle. The second phase (15% of the MMC cycle) has random contractions of moderate strength. The third phase (5% of the MMC cycle) is initiated by motilin. It consists of several, very strong contractions.

4. **Fed state.** During the fed state, contractions occur more frequently and last longer. Of interest, multiple areas of the small bowel may contract at the same time. From each stimulated site, peristalsis proceeds caudally for a varying distance.

D. **Immunity.** The small intestine provides two roles in the immune system, both as a barrier and in acquired immunity.

1. **Barrier.** Tight junctions between the enterocyte apical membranes prevent pathogens from crossing the epithelial layer. Further, mucosal plasma cells secrete IgA, which is transported across enterocytes via the polymeric immunoglobulin receptors. This IgA binds pathogens and further prevents microbes from entering enterocytes.

2. **M cells** are located in the epithelial layer over the Peyer patches. They facilitate the conveying of antigens directly to macrophages and lymphocytes and help initiate acquired immunity to luminal pathogens.

3. **$\gamma\delta$ T cells** can be located within vacuoles of M cells and seem to have immunosuppressive effects. This may explain nonreactivity to ingested food.

E. **Endocrine.** The small intestine is the largest endocrine organ and has multiple subpopulations of enteroendocrine cells.

1. **Cholecystokinin (CCK).** Duodenal and jejunal I cells and enteric nerves secrete CCK in response to intraluminal amino acids and medium- to long-chain fatty acids. CCK induces gallbladder contraction, pancreatic enzyme secretion, and relaxation of the sphincter of Oddi.

2. **Enteroglucagon** (glucagon-like peptide 1). Ileal and colonic L cells secrete enteroglucagon in response to intraluminal fat and bile acids. Of note, inflammatory processes, such as Crohn's disease and celiac sprue, can dramatically increase enteroglucagon secretion. Since enteroglucagon has a trophic effect on intestinal villi, early studies have tried this hormone, and the related GLP-2, in short-gut syndrome.

3. **Gastric inhibitory peptide** (glucose-dependent insulinotropic polypeptide). Duodenal and jejunal K cells secrete gastric inhibitory peptide (GIP) in response to active transport of monosaccharides, long-chain fatty acids, and amino acids. GIP inhibits HCl/pepsinogen secretion and gastric emptying but stimulates insulin release.

4. **Gastrin.** Duodenal G cells secrete gastrin in response to vagal stimulation and peptides. Gastrin stimulates HCl/pepsinogen secretion by the gastric fundus and body and increases gastric mucosal blood flow. Further, it has some trophic effects on gastric mucosa.

5. **Gastrin-releasing polypeptide** (similar to bombesin). In response to vagal stimulation, enteric neurons release gastrin-releasing polypeptide. Unlike somatostatin, it enhances exocrine and endocrine functions. It stimulates gastric acid secretion, gastric motility, and the release of all gastrointestinal hormones except secretin.

6. **Motilin.** Duodenal and jejunal M cells secrete motilin in response to duodenal acid, vagal stimulation, and gastrin-releasing peptide. Motilin initiates phase III of the migrating motor complexes during the fasting state.

7. **Neurotensin.** Ileal N cells secrete neurotensin in response to intraluminal fat. Neurotensin inhibits gastric HCl secretion, gastric antral motility, and gastric emptying. It stimulates pancreatic exocrine secretion, gallbladder contraction, mesenteric vasodilatation, and colonic motility. It may also stimulate the growth of intestinal mucosa.

8. **Secretin.** Duodenal and jejunal S cells release secretin in response to acid, bile salts, and fatty acids in the duodenum. Secretin increases

bicarbonate and water secretion from pancreatic ducts. It inhibits gastric acid secretion and gastric motility.
9. **Somatostatin.** Intestinal D cells and enteric neurons secrete somatostatin in response to intraluminal fat, protein, and acid. This hormone inhibits exocrine and endocrine functions. For example, it inhibits gallbladder contraction, gastric acid secretion, and small-bowel secretion of water and electrolytes. It also inhibits the secretion of pancreatic hormones.
10. **Vasoactive intestinal peptide (VIP).** Enteric neurons secrete VIP in response to vagal stimulation. VIP increases mesenteric blood flow, intestinal motility, and pancreatic/intestinal secretions.

IV. **Small-bowel obstruction** is one of the most common clinical problems faced by general surgeons.
A. **Etiology**
1. **Adhesions** are the most common cause of small-bowel obstruction in adults, accounting for 50% to 70% of all cases. Adhesions can be acquired from previous intra-abdominal surgery or inflammatory processes. They may also be congenital. Of note, 5% of patients with previous abdominal surgery may develop an adhesive obstruction during their lifetime.
2. **Incarcerated hernias** (e.g., inguinal, femoral, umbilical, incisional, parastomal, or internal) are the second most common cause of small-bowel obstructions in adults. They are the most common cause in children and in patients with no history of abdominal surgery.
3. **Neoplasms.** Primary small-bowel tumors can cause intraluminal obstruction, whereas metastases can cause external compression.
4. **Intussusception.** Tumors, polyps, enlarged mesenteric lymph nodes, or even a Meckel's diverticulum may serve as lead points, resulting in one portion of bowel, the intussusceptum, telescoping into another, the intussuscipiens.
5. **Volvulus** is often caused by adhesions or congenital anomalies such as intestinal malrotation. It is a more common cause of large-bowel obstruction.
6. **Strictures** secondary to ischemia, inflammation (Crohn's disease), radiation therapy, or prior surgery.
7. **Less common etiologies include these:**
   a. **Gallstone ileus.** Intense inflammation of the gallbladder results in fistulization between the biliary tree and the small bowel. Gallstones can travel into the small bowel and become lodged at or near the ileocecal valve, resulting in obstruction.
   b. **External compression** from tumors, abscesses, hematomas, or other fluid collections.
   c. **Foreign bodies,** such as bezoars.
   d. **Meconium ileus.** In cystic fibrosis, intestinal secretion of chloride and water is impaired. Thus, inspissated lumenal contents can cause an obstruction.
B. **Classifications**
1. **Mechanical obstruction** is the blockage of the intestinal lumen by an intrinsic or extrinsic lesion. The resulting obstruction can be partial, allowing some distal passage of gas or fluid, or complete, with total occlusion of the lumen.
   a. **Simple obstruction** implies that there is no vascular compromise of the involved bowel and that the occlusion has occurred at only one site.
   b. **A strangulated obstruction** means that the involved bowel has vascular compromise, which can ultimately lead to gangrene of the intestinal wall. A closed-loop obstruction occurs when a segment of bowel is occluded proximally as well as distally. Unfortunately, many studies have been unable to reliably find either clinical or laboratory values able to differentiate simple and strangulated obstructions.

2. **Paralytic ileus** implies failure of peristalsis secondary to a neurogenic disturbance. It can be caused by recent abdominal surgery, electrolyte disturbances, peritonitis, systemic infections, bowel ischemia, trauma, and medications.

C. **Diagnosis**
   1. **Signs and symptoms**
      a. **Vomiting. Proximal** small-bowel obstructions present with early bilious vomiting. During more **distal** obstructions, vomiting tends to be less, tends to occur later in the course, and can be thick and feculent.
      b. **Abdominal distention** typically increases the more distal the obstruction.
      c. **Abdominal pain,** characterized as crampy, intermittent, and colicky, is poorly localized.
      d. **Obstipation** occurs after the bowel distal to a complete obstruction is evacuated of gas and feces; thus, obstipation usually occurs later the more proximal the obstruction.
      e. **Dehydration.** With a persistent obstruction, hypovolemia progresses due to impaired absorption, increased secretion ("third spacing"), and vomiting. The patient may complain of palpitations, weakness, fatigue, and dark, concentrated urine.
      f. **Bloody bowel movements** should raise the level of suspicion that a strangulated bowel is present.
   2. **Physical examination**
      a. **Vital signs.** An elevated heart rate, low blood pressure, and low urine output may be signs of worsening dehydration. Although the preoperative diagnosis of a strangulated obstruction cannot be made or excluded reliably by any known clinical or laboratory parameter (*Am J Surg* 1983;145:176), one retrospective study suggests that shock is significantly associated with strangulation (*Am Surg* 2004; 70:40).
      b. **Abdominal exam.** The patient should be examined for abdominal distension, prior surgical scars, and hernias. Visible and audible peristaltic waves may be present. Palpation should determine the location and severity of tenderness and evaluate for the presence of peritoneal signs. Localized pain, guarding, or peritonitis is a sign of ischemic bowel. Digital rectal examination may reveal the presence of a rectal mass or impacted stool. A recent retrospective study suggests that peritonitis is significantly associated with strangulation (*Am Surg* 2004;70:40).
   3. **Laboratory evaluation.** In early stages of a small-bowel obstruction, laboratory values may be normal. As the obstruction progresses, patients tend to become dehydrated. Laboratory tests may reveal decreased levels of sodium, chloride, and potassium, accompanied by increased levels of bicarbonate, blood urea nitrogen (BUN), creatinine, and hematocrit. Serum amylase, released from small-bowel mucosa, can be elevated. A mild leukocytosis (WBC $>10,000$ cells/μL) is not unusual. An elevated WBC is significantly associated with strangulation (*Am Surg* 2004;70:40).
   4. **Radiologic evaluation**
      a. **Supine and upright abdominal plain films** that reveal dilated loops of small bowel (>3 cm in diameter), three or more air-fluid levels, and paucity of gas in the colon and rectum are characteristic findings of a small-bowel obstruction. These findings may be absent in proximal obstructions, early obstructions, or closed-loop obstructions. Thumbprinting, loss of mucosal pattern, and gas within the bowel wall or intrahepatic branches of the portal vein are suggestive of a strangulated obstruction. Free intra-abdominal air in an upright chest x-ray or a lateral decubitus film indicates perforation of a hollow viscus. The findings of air in the biliary tree and a radiopaque

gallstone in the right lower quadrant are pathognomonic of gallstone ileus. Paralytic ileus appears as gaseous distention uniformly distributed throughout the stomach, small intestine, and colon.

  b. **Contrast studies** (small-bowel follow-through [SBFT] or enteroclysis) can localize the site of obstruction and suggest an etiology (e.g., neoplasm). These studies may be particularly helpful in patients without prior abdominal surgery or a hernia. Water-soluble contrast should be used rather than barium. Should the bowel perforate, leakage of barium into the peritoneal cavity causes an intense inflammatory reaction, which can significantly increase morbidity and mortality. There may also be prognostic and therapeutic benefits to a water-soluble SBFT.

  c. **Abdominal/pelvic CT** is an excellent imaging modality for diagnosing small-bowel obstruction. It has the ability to localize and characterize the obstruction as either partial or complete. It can give information regarding the cause of obstruction (e.g., malignancy, inflammatory process, or extrinsic causes) and the presence of other intra-abdominal pathology. Evidence suggests that CT scanning can improve the preoperative diagnosis of strangulation (*Semin Ultrasound CT MR* 2003;24:336). CT findings of thickened bowel wall, pneumatosis, and mesenteric edema are all suggestive of strangulated bowel.

D. Differential diagnosis

  1. **Mesenteric vascular ischemia** can produce colicky abdominal pain, especially after meals. Acute occlusion often presents with marked leukocytosis and severe abdominal pain out of proportion to physical findings. Angiography confirms the diagnosis. This topic is discussed more fully in Chapter 21.

  2. A **colonic obstruction** can easily be confused with a distal small-bowel obstruction if the ileocecal valve is incompetent. A contrast enema would be helpful.

  3. **Paralytic ileus.** A thorough history, physical exam, and radiologic workup (e.g., ascertaining narcotic use, psychiatric medications, recent abdominal surgery, hypokalemia, gas throughout the entire GI tract on plain films) should differentiate ileus from obstruction.

  4. **Primary hypomotility disorders** are impairments of the small bowel's intrinsic nervous system or musculature. They can result from a congenital absence or an acquired absence due to systemic diseases such as scleroderma, lupus, diabetes mellitus, amyloidosis, or muscular dystrophy. As in paralytic ileus, on radiography there is air/gas throughout the entire GI tract, with particular distention of the small bowel. The treatment for this chronic disease is medical rather than surgical. Medical therapy includes the use of prokinetic drugs (e.g., metoclopramide or erythromycin) and dietary manipulation.

E. Treatment

  1. **Partial small-bowel obstructions** can be treated expectantly as long as the patient continues to be clinically stable. The cornerstone of treating any type of bowel obstruction is adequate fluid resuscitation to achieve a urine output of at least 0.5 mL/kg per hour. The patient is placed on nothing-by-mouth status, all electrolyte abnormalities are corrected, and a nasogastric tube is placed for gastrointestinal decompression. During this trial of nonoperative management, it is imperative that the patient undergo serial abdominal examinations every 4 to 6 hours and that daily abdominal plain films be obtained. If the abdominal exam worsens, peritonitis/shock develops, or the patient fails to improve after 48 hours of tube decompression, a laparotomy is indicated.

     In patients with a bowel obstruction secondary to an incarcerated hernia, attempts to reduce the hernia can be made with mild sedation and gentle force. After successful reduction, the patient should be monitored carefully for evidence of bowel infarction or perforation. Inability to reduce the hernia is grounds for an urgent operation.

Other situations that may warrant a trial of nonoperative therapy include early postoperative obstruction, multiple prior episodes of obstruction, a history of multiple previous abdominal operations with extensive adhesions, abdominal irradiation, Crohn's disease, and abdominal carcinomatosis.

2. **Complete bowel obstructions** are often associated with strangulation and are therefore managed with prompt surgical intervention. Mortality that is associated with gangrenous bowel can approach 30% if surgery is delayed beyond 24 to 36 hours. Once again, fluid/electrolyte resuscitation and tube decompression are crucial in the preoperative preparation of the patient.

   a. **Fluid replacement** should begin with an isotonic saline solution (0.9% NaCl). Potassium should be added only after adequate urine output (0.5 mL/kg per hour) is achieved. Bicarbonate should be given if the arterial pH is less than 7.1. Serum electrolyte values, hourly urine output, and central venous pressure can be monitored to assess adequacy of resuscitation. Monitoring of arterial blood pressure and measurement of serial arterial blood gases should be done when indicated. Intravenous antibiotics should be given if strangulation is suspected.

   b. **Operation.** After fluid resuscitation has been initiated and antibiotics have been administered, an exploratory laparotomy is performed. In the majority of cases, this is done through a midline incision. However, in the case of an incarcerated inguinal or femoral hernia, a standard groin incision can be used. Some surgeons have had success with a laparoscopic lysis of adhesions (*Am Surg* 2003;69:966). During the exploration, adhesions are lysed, any gangrenous bowel is resected, and the source of obstruction is identified. The viability of adjacent or compromised bowel must be assessed; various methods include inspection of bowel color, visualization of peristalsis in the bowel after several minutes of being wrapped in warm saline-soaked packs, and Dopplers of mesenteric arterial pulsations. Intravenous fluorescein injection followed by inspection of the bowel under ultraviolet (Wood's) light can also be used. A second-look operation within 24 to 48 hours should be planned if any doubt exists about the viability of the remaining bowel. This minimizes unnecessary resection. In cases in which the obstructing lesion cannot be resected, a bypass procedure should be performed. Placement of a gastrostomy tube for postoperative decompression may be considered if a prolonged ileus is expected.

F. **Prognosis.** The postoperative mortality from nonstrangulating obstruction is 2%. Obstructions that are associated with strangulated bowel carry a mortality of 8% if surgery is performed within 36 hours of the onset of symptoms. Mortality can approach 30% if operation is delayed beyond 36 hours.

V. **Meckel's diverticulum** is the most common congenital anomaly of the gastrointestinal tract. It occurs when the vitelline or omphalomesenteric duct fails to obliterate during the 5th or 6th week of fetal development. It is a true diverticulum that contains all layers of the bowel wall and is located on the antimesenteric border of the bowel. It can contain heterotopic mucosa, such as gastric (62%), pancreatic (6%), combined gastric and pancreatic (5%), jejunal (2%), and Brunner gland (2%) mucosa, although up to 50% contain normal ileal mucosa.

   A. **Rule of two's.** The incidence is 2%. Male/female incidence is 2:1. Patients typically present before the age of 2. It is located 2 feet from the ileocecal valve. The base is typically 2 inches in width and often contains two types of mucosa.

B. Diagnosis. The vast majority of Meckel's diverticula are asymptomatic and are diagnosed incidentally at surgery or during an autopsy. Two-thirds of patients who manifest symptoms present before the age of 2 years. Signs and symptoms occur only after a complication of Meckel diverticulum has occurred.

1. **Clinical presentation**
   a. **Bleeding** in the form of melena or bright red blood per rectum is the most common presenting symptom (30% to 50%). It tends to be painless and episodic. The source is typically a peptic ulcer on the adjacent normal ileal mucosa caused by the acid-secreting gastric mucosa that lines the diverticulum.
   b. **Intestinal obstruction** due to volvulus of the small bowel around a fibrous band connecting the diverticulum to the anterior abdominal wall, intussusception, or incarcerated internal hernia (Littré hernia) is the second most common presentation (30% to 35%).
   c. **Acute Meckel's diverticulitis** occurs in 20% of symptomatic patients and is often mistaken for acute appendicitis. It is caused by intraluminal obstruction of the diverticulum, which leads to inflammation, edema, ischemia, necrosis, and perforation.

2. **Radiologic evaluation.** The preoperative diagnosis of Meckel's diverticulum is very difficult. Therefore, it requires a high index of suspicion.
   a. A **technetium-99m sodium pertechnetate ("gastric" or "Meckel")** **scan** is able to identify the ectopic gastric mucosa present within the diverticulum. The sensitivity of the scan may be increased by the administration of an H_2-receptor antagonist. Of note, the sensitivity is 62% in adults (*South Med J* 2002;95:1338).
   b. **Contrast studies**, such as small-bowel follow-through or enteroclysis, occasionally may detect the presence of the diverticulum. They may also be helpful in detecting a small-bowel intussusception.
   c. **Angiography** can be helpful in finding the site of hemorrhage during episodes of active bleeding. Sixty-nine percent of Meckel's diverticula have a persistent vitellointestinal artery (*Am J Roentgenol* 1998;170:1329).

C. Differential diagnosis
1. Acute appendicitis
2. Diverticulitis
3. Crohn's disease

D. Treatment
1. **Surgical resection** is indicated in the symptomatic patient. For patients who present with obstruction, either from a fibrous band connecting the diverticulum to the anterior abdominal wall or from intussusception, simple diverticulectomy can be performed. Segmental resections should be performed for acute diverticulitis, a wide-based diverticulum, compromised bowel, or bleeding. When done for bleeding, the resection removes the diverticulum's ectopic gastric mucosa as well as the bleeding ileal ulcer.
2. **Incidental diverticulectomy** remains controversial. Morbidity and mortality associated with the presence of a Meckel's diverticulum are extremely low. However, different studies have cited varying postop morbidity and mortality after incidental resection. Current recommendations are to leave the diverticulum unless it's symptomatic. For example, if a patient is undergoing surgery for presumed appendicitis and the appendix is normal, the terminal ileum must be inspected for a Meckel's diverticulum. If present, the diverticulum should be resected.

VI. Small-intestinal bleed. While the workup of upper and lower gastrointestinal bleeding are discussed in Chapters 12 and 15 respectively, this section will discuss other modalities that may be required to diagnose small-intestinal hemorrhage. Small-intestinal bleeding requires significantly more diagnostic procedures than either upper GI bleeding or colonic bleeding.

A. Enteroscopy
   1. Push enteroscopy. This 400-cm-long enteroscope can visualize well into the jejunum, depending on the skill of the endoscopist. It can perform biopsy and therapeutic maneuvers.
   2. Extended small-bowel enteroscopy. Since this scope requires peristalsis to move distally, the procedure may require up to 8 hours to complete. Further, it has no biopsy or therapeutic capabilities. It may visualize as much as 70% of the small intestine and may be more sensitive than conventional enteroclysis.
   B. "Camera pill" (capsule endoscopy). In 2001, the FDA approved the "camera pill." This is a disposable camera that can be swallowed and can transmit images of bleeding. The published data are too limited to comment on its efficacy.
VII. Enteric fistulas are abnormal communications between intestinal segments. They can cause significant malabsorption either by bypass of intestine or by large loss of fluid, electrolytes, and nutrients. For example, **gastrocolic fistulas** cause malabsorption by diverting ingested food into the colon, which results in nutrients bypassing the small bowel. Also, these fistulas enable the colonic flora to reflux into the stomach, allowing bacterial overgrowth of the stomach and small bowel. Of note, Crohn's patients can develop enterocolic and enterocutaneous fistulas. Management of Crohn's inflammatory fistulas is discussed in Section IX. Additional discussion of fistulas is presented in Chapter 20.
VIII. Short-bowel syndrome after massive small-bowel resection results in serious nutritional and absorptive abnormalities. All patients should initially be started on total parenteral nutrition (TPN). Individuals with less than 100 cm of small bowel remaining will most likely require lifelong TPN. Patients with 1 to 3 m of small intestine may be able to meet their nutritional requirements with oral food intake, especially if the colon remains. Further discussion of short-gut syndrome is presented in Chapter 20.
   A. Medical therapy directed at increasing dietary fiber, inhibiting bowel secretion and motility, reducing gastric hypersecretion, binding bile salts, and preventing bacterial overgrowth can help to maximize intestinal absorption of nutrients, minimize fluid losses, and minimize the complications of malnutrition. Future therapies may include the use of the hormone **GLP-2.** In one small study, GLP-2 patients showed growth of intestinal mucosa (*Gastroenterology* 2001;120:806–815).
   B. Surgical therapy. Some centers have had successful case reports of intestinal transplantation from living donors. Such patients were able to discontinue parental nutrition postop (*Transplantation* 2001;71:569–571). At this time, this therapy should be considered experimental.
IX. Crohn's disease is an idiopathic, chronic, granulomatous inflammatory disease that can affect any part of the GI tract from the mouth to the anus. It is a slowly progressive disease characterized by episodes of exacerbation and remission, and there is no known cure at this time.
   A. Epidemiology. The incidence ranges from 2.7 to 5.0 per 100,000. The age distribution tends to be bimodal (ages 15 to 29 years and 55 to 70 years). The etiology of Crohn's disease is unknown but most likely involves bacterial infection, a defective mucosal barrier, and an abnormal intestinal immune response. There is a clear genetic component as well. Crohn's disease is 17 to 35 times more likely to develop in patients with a family history than in the general population, and a concordance rate of 58% has been found in monozygotic twins. Recent studies have also identified several susceptibility genes involved in Crohn's disease (NOD2/CARD15, DLG5, OCTN). Environmental factors such as smoking increase the risk of developing Crohn's disease.
   B. Gross and **microscopic pathology** are the keys to distinguishing Crohn's disease from ulcerative colitis. The management of these two diseases is distinctly different.

1. **Disease distribution.** The distal ileum is the most common site involved (75% of patients). In 15% to 30% of patients, disease is limited only to the small bowel. Twenty-five percent to 30% of patients have disease confined to the colon; 40% to 60% have disease that occurs in both the small bowel and the colon. The duodenum is involved in 1% to 7% of cases, and 3% of patients have anorectal disease only. Skip lesions occur in 15% of patients.

2. **Gross appearance.** Externally, diseased bowel is thickened, displays "creeping fat" and "corkscrew vessels," and has a shortened fibrotic mesentery containing enlarged lymph nodes. The mucosal lesions include pinpoint hemorrhages, aphthous ulcers, deep linear fissures, and, ultimately, cobblestoning. It is common for these lesions to occur segmentally along the intestine rather than being contiguous.

3. **Microscopic appearance.** Crohn's disease is characterized by full-thickness, transmural inflammation of the bowel wall. The inflammation begins adjacent to the crypts, which leads to the development of crypt abscesses, aphthous ulcers, and linear fissures. The transmural involvement can lead to sinus tracts and fistulas between crypt abscesses and adjacent segments of bowel. Granulomas are found in the bowel wall in 40% to 60% of patients, and they are detected in mesenteric lymph nodes in 25% of patients.

C. **Diagnosis**
1. **Clinical presentation**
   a. **Diarrhea** occurs in more than 90% of patients and usually is not bloody when only the small bowel is involved. However, if the colon is involved, up to one-third of patients have bloody diarrhea. With ileal disease, patients may be bile salt deficient, resulting in steatorrhea. Mucosal inflammation with decreased absorption and increased secretion results in diarrhea.
   b. **Abdominal pain** typically is intermittent, crampy, worse after meals, relieved by defecation, and poorly localized. Constant and localized pain suggests peritonitis. A mass caused by thickened bowel, a phlegmon, or an abscess may be palpable.
   c. **Weight loss** occurs as a result of decreased oral intake, malabsorption, protein-losing enteropathy, and steatorrhea. Children with Crohn's disease develop vitamin and mineral deficiencies and growth retardation.
   d. **Constitutional signs and symptoms,** such as malaise, fever, and anemia, occur.
   e. **Anorectal disease** is a common finding and may precede intestinal symptoms by several years. Such lesions include recurrent nonhealing anal fissures; large ulcers; complex anal fistulas; perianal abscesses; large, fleshy tags; and bluish skin discoloration. They are characterized by a multiplicity of lesions, lateral fissures, deep ulcers of the perianal skin and anal canal, and anal stricture. Thus, patients with recurrent or atypical anorectal pathology should be investigated for Crohn's disease.
   f. **Extraintestinal manifestations.** The eyes may develop conjunctivitis, iritis, and uveitis. The skin may develop pyoderma gangrenosum, erythema nodosum multiforme, and aphthous stomatitis. Musculoskeletal manesfestation include arthritis, ankylosing spondylitis, and hypertrophic osteoarthropathy. Finally, the associated sclerosing cholangitis can lead to cirrhosis.
2. A thorough **physical examination** with special attention to the abdominal and anorectal areas is performed. No physical signs are pathognomonic for Crohn's disease, but the presence of peritoneal signs or undrained perianal sepsis needs to be ruled out.
3. **Laboratory evaluation** is nonspecific and variable. A modestly elevated white blood cell count can indicate active disease; marked elevation

suggests an abscess or other suppurative complications. Anemia due to iron, vitamin B_{12}, or folate deficiency is common. Thrombocytosis can occur in active disease. Elevated sedimentation rate and hypoalbuminemia can be present.

4. **Imaging studies** are indicated when establishing the diagnosis of Crohn's disease or when a complication develops that requires surgical intervention.

   a. **Contrast x-rays,** which include **small-bowel follow-through, enteroclysis,** and **water-soluble contrast enema,** are very valuable in the diagnosis of Crohn's disease. **Air-contrast studies** give better mucosal detail and can detect aphthous ulcers, but single-contrast ("full-column") studies are more useful for detecting fistulas, strictures, and tumors. Small-bowel studies are helpful because they give an idea of the extent of disease, and contrast enemas can help determine whether the colon is involved.

   b. **Direct endoscopic visualization** is applicable to patients with terminal ileal and colonic disease. Colonoscopy can detect the presence of ulcers, deep fissures, and cobblestoning, and it allows for biopsies. The presence of granulomas is diagnostic for Crohn's disease. Colonoscopy is also important for cancer surveillance. As in patients with ulcerative colitis, those with long-standing (>10 years) Crohn's colitis are at increased risk for developing adenocarcinoma. These patients also have an increased incidence of small-bowel cancer.

   c. **CT scan** is useful for identifying abscesses, focal inflammation, and wall thickening. Abscesses can be drained percutaneously under CT guidance.

   d. **Nuclear medicine** studies using **indium-111–tagged granulocytes** or **technetium-99–labeled phagocytes,** for example, can identify the location, extent, and severity of intestinal inflammation. However, these studies are of limited utility.

D. **Complications** of Crohn's disease include intestinal obstruction, stricture, fistula, perforation, intra-abdominal abscess, and perirectal abscess and fistula. Toxic colitis is a surgical emergency that can occur in these patients. They also have an increased risk of cancer in those areas of the small bowel or colon involved in the disease process. Surgically bypassed loops of intestine are thought to be at a particularly high risk.

E. **Differential diagnosis**

   1. **Ulcerative colitis.** Patients with Crohn's disease generally have less severe diarrhea, usually without gross blood. Perianal lesions, nonconfluent skip lesions, transmural involvement, large mucosal ulcers and fissures, involvement of small intestine, rectal sparing, and the presence of granulomas all help to differentiate Crohn's disease from ulcerative colitis. Patients who cannot be clearly differentiated are diagnosed with indeterminate colitis.

   2. **Appendicitis.** Acute right lower quadrant abdominal pain due to Crohn's ileitis can mimic acute appendicitis.

   3. **Ileitis** due to *Shigella* species, amebas, *Giardia* species, or *Yersinia* species can mimic Crohn's disease, and the diagnosis is made by stool culture.

   4. **Intestinal lymphoma** often appears as diffuse involvement, with masses in the bowel wall, whereas Crohn's disease shows more localized involvement of the ileum, with ulcers and strictures.

   5. **Intestinal tuberculosis** most commonly involves the cecum and ileum.

   6. Other diseases, such as **ischemic enteritis, diverticulitis, pseudomembranous colitis, and irritable bowel syndrome,** can also mimic Crohn's disease.

F. **Treatment**

   1. **Medical management.** Crohn's disease has no cure. Therefore, treatment seeks to palliate symptoms, reduce bowel inflammation, and

correct nutritional disturbances. Therapeutic recommendations depend on the disease location, severity, and complications.

a. **Adequate nutritional intake** is essential in the treatment of disease flares and in the maintenance phase. Whenever possible, enteral feeds should be continued. A low-residue, high-protein, milk-free diet can often provide adequate nutritional support for patients with mild to moderate disease flares. Supplementation with iron, calcium, magnesium, folate, zinc, and vitamins B_{12}, D, and K may be necessary.

Nutritional requirements often need to be individualized given the disease location and history of surgery. Patients with bile salt deficiency due to ileal disease benefit from consuming of medium-chain fatty acids. Those with ileal resection or extensive small-bowel disease are prone to oxalate nephrolithiasis and should receive a low-oxalate, high-calcium diet. Patients with severe or unresponsive disease should be started on TPN and placed on complete bowel rest. Long-term TPN may be indicated for patients with short-gut syndrome.

2. **Medical therapy** is divided into **acute** and **maintenance phases**. Mild to moderate disease can be treated with an oral aminosalicylate (sulfasalazine, 3 to 6 g per day, or mesalamine (Pentasa), 1,000 mg four times a day). For ileal, colonic, or perianal disease, metronidazole, 500 mg three times a day, can be added. In patients with severe disease, steroid therapy should be initiated provided that an active infection or abscess has been excluded (prednisone, 40 to 60 mg orally per day in outpatients; hydrocortisone, 50 to 100 mg intravenously every 6 hours in inpatients). Response to therapy should become evident within 5 to 7 days of its initiation. Data have shown that infusions of infliximab (Remicaide), a monoclonal antibody against tumor necrosis factor, is effective for Crohn's flares and even Crohn's fistulas (*N Engl J* Med 2004;350:876). The patient must have no active source of infection and be PPD negative prior to receiving infliximab. Once a patient has recovered from an acute flare of the disease, the medical regimen should be simplified to prevent long-term complications of the medications. Steroids should be tapered as soon as possible (i.e., within 3 to 6 months). To help taper steroids, 6-mercaptopurine (1.5 mg/kg orally per day) has been used. However, onset to effect may take 8 to 17 weeks. Since this agent may cause leukopenia and thrombocytopenia, the patient's complete blood count should be closely monitored.

3. **Surgical therapy**
   a. **Indications.** Surgical therapy is directed against complications, including obstruction from fibrotic strictures, high-output fistulas, perforation, intra-abdominal abscess, fulminant or toxic colitis, carcinoma, bleeding (rare), and growth failure in children. Toxic colitis, free perforation, or peritonitis require emergent operations. Abdominal abscesses can usually be drained percutaneously, with an elective bowel resection following in 6 weeks. Approximately 70% to 80% of all patients with Crohn's disease require surgery at some point in their lifetime.
   b. **Surgical procedures.** During surgical therapy, the most important principle is to correct the complication while preserving bowel length to prevent short-gut syndrome. Resection to histologically negative margins does not significantly reduce the likelihood of disease recurrence; therefore, grossly normal margins of 2 cm are accepted. In the absence of free perforation, large abscesses, massively dilated bowel, or severe malnutrition, primary anastamosis is safe. Stapling should be avoided in thick-walled bowel; in this situation, a handsewn anastamosis is indicated. Recent series suggest that laparoscopic ileocolic resections were as effective but less morbid than open procedures (*Dis Colon Rectum* 2003;46:1129).

Specific issues that require special consideration are duodenal disease, multiple skip lesions, and chronic fibrotic strictures. Duodenal Crohn's disease usually presents surgically as obstruction secondary to stricture. Short strictures can be managed by strictureplasty. For more extensive involvement, gastrojejunostomy should be performed to bypass the duodenum. Controversy exists over the use of vagotomy in these patients, who are already prone to diarrhea. When multiple strictures are found that are separated by significant segments of normal bowel, strictureplasty may be used to conserve bowel length. Heineke-Mikulicz or Finney strictureplasties are the most commonly employed and have been shown to be as safe and effective as resection.

  c. Appendectomy. Patients who are being explored for presumed acute appendicitis and are found to have Crohn ileitis should have the appendix removed if the cecum is not inflamed. Conventional teaching has been that the terminal ileum should not be removed. This is controversial, however, given the low morbidity of ileocecal resection and the uncertainty of response to subsequent medical therapy.

  d. Perianal disease

    (1) Abscesses are treated by incision and drainage.

    (2) Fistulas are initially managed conservatively. **Fistulotomy** is permitted if *minimal* sphincter muscle is involved. However, more commonly, fistulas are treated by mucosal advancement flap repair, which has a success rate of 60% to 80%. Fibrin glue is a newer, less invasive option, albeit with modest success rates.

    Complex fistulas are treated with draining Silastic setons, sometimes indefinitely. Once the acute sepsis has resolved after drainage, infliximab may be useful. Ciprofloxacin, metronidazole, and cyclosporine have been shown to "heal" some fistulas. However, these fistulas often recur promptly after the medications are stopped. An important principle in the management of perianal disease is to treat and control synchronous intestinal disease to maximize the chance of success. Fecal diversion with or without proctectomy is reserved for severe cases.

    (3) Fissures, ulcers, and hemorrhoids. Do not operate!

G. Complications of surgery include anastomotic leaks, enterocutaneous fistulas, and sepsis related to intra-abdominal abscesses and wound infections. Overall, operative mortality is less than 5%.

H. Prognosis. Crohn's disease is a chronic panintestinal disease and currently has no cure. It usually recurs in the preanastomotic segments of bowel. The rate of reoperation is approximately 50% at 5 years and 75% at 15 years. Reoperation after strictureplasty is required in one-third of patients by 10 years. Drugs such as mesalamine, 6-mercaptopurine, and metronidazole only modestly delay the time to recurrence. Thus, Crohn's disease requires chronic, lifelong treatment, with surgery reserved for severe complications.

X. **Neoplasms** of the small intestine occur infrequently and account for fewer than 2% of all GI neoplasms. Tumors of the small intestine present insidiously with vague, nonspecific symptoms. Most benign tumors remain asymptomatic and are diagnosed incidentally during a laparotomy or at the time of an autopsy. However, they can act as lead points in an intussusception. On the other hand, the majority of malignant tumors eventually become symptomatic at late stages of the disease. Such symptoms include weight loss, abdominal pain, obstruction, perforation, and hemorrhage.

A. Benign tumors are much more common than malignant tumors.

  1. Adenomas account for up to 25% of all benign small-intestinal tumors. They can occur sporadically as solitary lesions or in association with familial polyposis syndrome or Gardner syndrome. Symptomatic lesions can cause fluctuating pain secondary to intermittent obstruction, intussusception, or bleeding. The three types of small-bowel adenomas are simple tubular adenomas, villous adenomas, and Brunner gland adenomas. The duodenum is the most common site for all three types of adenomas to occur. Tubular adenomas have a low malignant potential and can be treated with complete endoscopic polypectomy. Villous adenomas have significant malignant potential. If the polyp can be completely excised endoscopically (<2 cm), this is adequate treatment. If complete resection is not possible, transduodenal excision with adequate margins is needed. Villous adenomas of the jejunum or ileum should be resected with a segmental bowel resection. Brunner tumors represent hyperplasia of exocrine glands of the first part of the duodenum and have no malignant potential. Therefore, endoscopic resection is adequate for symptomatic lesions.

2. **Leiomyomas** account for up to 35% of benign small-intestinal neoplasms. They are the most common benign neoplasms of the small intestine and arise from the mesenchymal cells of the small bowel. They grow submucosally and project into the lumen of the small bowel. On a small-bowel contrast study, they appear as a smooth, eccentric filling defect with intact, normal-appearing mucosa. Histopathologic examination is needed to distinguish benign from malignant stromal tumors. Therefore, once a lesion is detected, treatment consists of a segmental small-bowel resection.

3. **Hamartomas** arise in patients with Peutz-Jeghers syndrome. This is an autosomal dominant inherited syndrome of mucocutaneous melanotic pigmentation and multiple gastrointestinal polyps. Surgery is indicated only for obstruction, intussusception, or bleeding. At surgery, all polyps larger than 1 cm should be resected. Due to an increased risk for adenocarcinoma, such patients need to be screened closely by endoscopy.

4. **Lipomas** account for about 15% of all benign small-intestinal neoplasms. They occur most often in the ileum. They have no malignant potential. On CT, they show fatty attenuation. They should only be resected for symptoms such as intussusception.

5. **Hemangiomas** account for about 10% of all benign small-intestinal neoplasms. They may be associated with Osler-Weber-Rendu disease and present with bleeding. Diagnosis can be made with enteroscopy, capsule endoscopy, or angiography.

6. **Neurofibromas and fibromas,** less common tumors, can cause intussusception. **Endometriosis**, appearing as puckered, bluish-red, serosally based nodules, can become implanted on the small bowel. They can cause gastrointestinal bleeding or obstruction.

B. **Malignant tumors**
1. **Adenocarcinoma** accounts for 50% of malignant small-bowel tumors. Forty percent of them occur in the duodenum (periampullary region), and their frequency decreases as one progresses distally along the small bowel. Risk factors for the development of adenocarcinoma include villous adenomas, polyposis syndromes, Crohn's disease, and hereditary nonpolyposis colorectal cancer (HNPCC).

   Patients often remain asymptomatic for long periods of time, and up to 80% of patients have distant metastases at the time of diagnosis. The presenting symptoms depend on the location of the primary tumor. Periampullary tumors can present with painless jaundice, duodenal obstruction, or bleeding. Jejunal or ileal tumors tend to present with abdominal pain and weight loss from progressive obstruction. Contrast studies, endoscopy with or without retrograde cholangiopancreatography, and CT can be used to make the diagnosis. Treatment consists of segmental resection of the small bowel and its adjacent mesentery. Any adherent structures should be resected *en bloc* if possible. Tumors of the terminal ileum should be resected along with the right colon. For carcinomas of the duodenum, a Whipple procedure is usually required. In completely resected duodenal adenocarcinoma, the 5-year survival rate is 56% and 83% for node-positive and node-negative disease, respectively (*Ann Surg Oncol* 2004;11:380). Distal duodenal, jejunal, and ileal lesions tend to present at a later stage and have a poorer prognosis. In patients with metastatic disease at the time of diagnosis, survival of more than 6 months is rare. Of note, 5-fluorouracil–based chemotherapy regimens have been tried. However, not enough data exist to comment on their efficacy (*Oncology* 2002;10:1364).

2. **Gastrointestinal stromal tumors** (leiomyosarcomas) account for 10% to 20% of small-bowel malignant neoplasms. These tumors express a mutated c-kit (CD117), a tyrosine kinase responsible for neoplastic growth. Thus, the diagnosis is made by immunohistochemical staining for c-kit. Malignant potential is determine histologically by the number of mitotic figures per high-powered field (mf/hpf).

   These tumors can arise from any one of the mesodermal-derived components of the small-intestinal wall, such as the connective tissue, fat, muscular, nervous, or vascular elements. They can be located anywhere throughout the small intestine, and their distribution is proportional to the length of each anatomic division (ileum > jejunum > duodenum). These tumors grow extraluminally and cause symptoms late in their course. Because of their vascular nature, when theses tumors outgrow their blood supply and develop necrosis, they may hemorrhage into either the peritoneum or the lumen of the bowel. The treatment for GI stromal tumors is surgical resection. Wide *en bloc* surgical resection to obtain tumor-free margins must be performed for curative therapy. Extensive lymph node resection is unnecessary because these tumors have a low potential for lymphatic spread.

   Chemotherapy and radiation therapy have not been shown to be effective in the treatment of metatstatic GI stromal tumors. However, a recent report has shown metastatic GI stromal tumors to respond to Gleevec (STI-571, imatinib mesylate). This targets the overactive tyrosine receptor c-kit found on all gastrointestinal stromal tumor (GIST) cells. Inhibition of this receptor has been shown to lead to radiographic and histologic regression of metastatic lesions (*N Engl J Med* 2001;344:1052). The benefit of resection of isolated pulmonary or hepatic lesions is unknown, but an aggressive approach is warranted in selected patients.

   Histologic grade, determined by the mf/hpf, and tumor size are the most important predictors of survival. After complete resection, the overall 5-year survival rate is 50%. In low-grade tumors (<10 mf/hpf), the survival rate is 60% to 80%, while in high-grade tumors (>10 mf/hpf), the survival rate is less than 20%. With local recurrence, the median length of survival is 9 to 12 months. With metastatic disease, the median length of survival is 20 months (*Br J Surg* 2003;90:1178). With imatinib mesylate, the rate of 2-year survival approached 78% in metastatic disease (*Eur J Cancer* 2004;40:689).

3. **Primary small-bowel lymphomas** account for approximately 15% of all small-bowel malignancies. The ileum is the most common location for lymphoma, since it has the largest amount of gut associated lymphoid tissue. Virtually all small-bowel lymphomas are non-Hodgkin's, B-cell lymphomas. Lymphomas can arise *de novo* in the lymphoid tissue of the small bowel or in association with a preexisting systemic condition such as celiac disease, Crohn's disease, or several forms of immunosuppression (pharmacologic immunosuppression, HIV).

   The presentation of these patients can range from nonspecific symptoms such as fatigue, malaise, weight loss, and abdominal pain to severe symptoms such as obstruction, intussusception, bleeding, and perforation. Imaging studies, such as CT scans or small-bowel contrast studies, can help with the diagnosis, but surgery is frequently required for histologic confirmation of the diagnosis.

Treatment of lymphoma localized to the small bowel involves wide resection of the affected segment of intestine and its associated mesentery. To stage the tumor accurately, the liver should be biopsied and the periaortic lymph nodes should be sampled. For widespread disease, resection of the affected small bowel should be performed to prevent complications. The role of adjuvant chemotherapy and radiotherapy remains controversial. The 5-year survival rate for patients with fully resected disease approaches 80%, but individuals with more advanced disease usually die within a year of surgery.

4. **Carcinoid tumors** account for up to 25% of small-bowel malignancies. They arise from the Kulchitsky or enterochromaffin cells of the intestinal crypts. Up to 80% of small-intestinal carcinoids occur within 2 feet of the ileocecal valve. Small-bowel carcinoid tumors tend to be much more aggressive than their appendiceal or rectal counterparts.

Most patients do not manifest signs or symptoms of the tumor until late in the course. Carcinoid tumors can produce symptoms locally by causing intestinal obstruction, pain, or bleeding, or they can produce systemic symptoms of the carcinoid syndrome. The tumor causes an intense mesenteric desmoplastic reaction that can lead to shortening and fibrosis of the mesentery. This reaction can cause obstruction due to kinking or narrowing of the bowel. The presence of the carcinoid syndrome implies the presence of hepatic metastases.

For tumors smaller than 1 cm in size, metastases are rare; tumors between 1 and 2 cm have a 50% rate of metastases, whereas up to 90% of tumors larger than 2 cm will have spread.

a. **Carcinoid syndrome** is caused by the tumor's oversecretion of hormones. Normally, hormones released by intestinal tumors are metabolized by the liver. However, with hepatic metastases, hormones are released directly into the systemic circulation. Classic symptoms include diarrhea and flushing of the face, neck, and upper chest, which can last for seconds to minutes. Tachycardia, hypotension, bronchospasm, and even coma can also occur. If the carcinoid syndrome has been long-standing, patients develop right heart endocardial and valvular fibrosis. The hormonal mediators responsible for the syndrome are unclear. Serotonin, bradykinin, substance P, histamine, dopamine, and prostaglandins have all been implicated. The diagnosis of carcinoid syndrome is confirmed by finding increased urinary excretion of 5-hydroxyindoleacetic acid, a metabolite of serotonin.

b. **Treatment**

(1) The management of carcinoid tumors is **surgical**. The type of surgery depends on the location and size of the tumor. The entire small bowel should be inspected because in 30% of cases synchronous lesions are present. Jejunal and ileal tumors should be treated with segmental resection including the adjacent mesentery. Small tumors (<1 cm) that are located in the third or fourth portions of the duodenum can be either locally excised or included in a segmental resection. For large duodenal tumors and periampullary tumors, a Whipple procedure should be performed. In the presence of locally advanced disease with involvement of adjacent organs or peritoneum, aggressive surgical resection should be undertaken. This can help delay the occurrence of mesenteric desmoplastic reaction, hepatic metastases, and carcinoid syndrome. Solitary and accessible liver lesions should be resected. Adjuvant cytotoxic chemotherapy and radiotherapy are of little benefit.

(2) The somatostatin analogue **octreotide** offers excellent palliation of carcinoid syndrome in patients with unresectable disease. Octreotide decreases the concentration of circulating serotonin and urinary 5-hydroxyindoleacetic acid and can relieve the diarrhea and flushing in 90% of patients.

  c. Carcinoids are slow-growing tumors, and **prognosis** depends on the stage of the tumor. The overall 5-year survival rate is 60%. Patients with local disease that is completely resected have a normal life expectancy. For patients with resectable node-positive disease, the median length of survival is 15 years. The median length of survival drops to 5 years with unresectable intra-abdominal disease, and it is 3 years for patients with hepatic metastases.

5. Peritoneal carcinomatosis is defined as diffuse studding of the peritoneal, mesenteric, and bowel surfaces by tumor nodules. Common neoplasms that are associated with peritoneal carcinomatosis include carcinomas of the pancreas, stomach, ovaries, and colon. The use of staging laparoscopy in pancreatic cancer before laparotomy enhances the sensitivity for detecting peritoneal carcinomatosis and hepatic metastases, which are frequently missed by more conventional staging modalities.

Surgical treatment is generally palliative, given the extremely poor prognosis. The exception is pseudomyxoma peritonei. Patients with this low grade malignancy may benefit from complete peritonectomy and intraperitoneal chemotherapy.

6. Metastases from cutaneous melanoma as well as carcinomas of the cervix, kidney, breast, and lung can spread to the small bowel. Small-bowel metastases are found in 50% of patients dying from malignant melanoma. Palliative surgical resection is performed for lesion-causing symptoms, such as obstruction or bleeding.

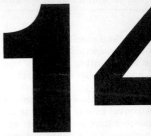

Acute Abdominal Pain and Appendicitis

Joseph J. Wizorek and Robb R. Whinney

ACUTE ABDOMINAL PAIN

Evaluation of the patient with acute abdominal pain requires a careful history and physical examination by a skilled physician in conjunction with selective diagnostic testing.

I. **Acute abdomen** is defined as a recent or sudden onset of unexpected abdominal pain.

   A. The **differential diagnosis** includes a variety of intra- and extraperitoneal processes.

   B. Acute abdomen **does not always** signify the need for surgical intervention.

II. **Epidemiology.** Acute abdomen is the most common general surgical problem presenting to the emergency department (ED).

III. **Pathophysiology**

   A. **Abdominal pain** is caused by irritation of the peritoneum. The peritoneal membrane consists of two layers, visceral and parietal, developmentally distinct areas with separate nerve supplies.

   1. **Visceral pain**

      a. **Visceral peritoneum** is innervated bilaterally by the autonomic nervous system. The bilateral innervation causes visceral pain that is midline, vague, deep, dull, and poorly localized (e.g., vague periumbilical pain of the midgut).

      b. Visceral pain is **triggered by inflammation, ischemia, and geometric changes** such as distention, traction, and pressure.

      c. Visceral pain signifies **intra-abdominal disease** but not necessarily the need for surgical intervention.

   2. **Parietal pain**

      a. **Parietal peritoneum** is innervated unilaterally via the spinal somatic nerves that also supply the abdominal wall. Unilateral innervation causes parietal pain to lateralize to one or more abdominal quadrants (e.g., inflamed appendix producing parietal peritoneal irritation).

      b. Parietal pain is **sharp, severe, and well localized.**

      c. Parietal pain is **triggered by irritation of the parietal peritoneum** by an inflammatory process (e.g., chemical peritonitis from perforated peptic ulcer or bacterial peritonitis from acute appendicitis). It may also be triggered by mechanical stimulation, such as a surgical incision.

      d. Parietal pain is **associated with physical examination findings of peritonitis** and frequently signifies the need for surgical treatment.

   3. **Embryologic origin** of the affected organ determines the level of visceral pain in the abdominal midline.

      a. **Foregut-derived structures** (stomach to second portion of duodenum, liver and biliary tract, pancreas, spleen) present with epigastric pain.

      b. **Midgut-derived structures** (second portion of duodenum to proximal two-thirds of transverse colon) present with periumbilical pain (e.g., early appendicitis–visceral irritation).

      c. **Hindgut-derived structures** (distal transverse colon to anal verge) present with suprapubic pain.

   4. **Referred pain** arises from a deep visceral structure but is superficial at the presenting site (Figure 14-1).

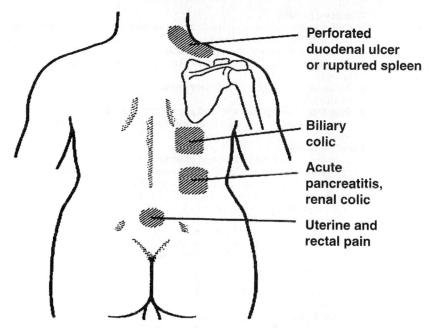

Figure 14-1. Frequent sites of referred pain and common causes.

    a. It results from **central neural pathways** in the spinal cord that are common to the somatic nerves and visceral organs.

    b. Examples include **biliary tract pain** (referred to the right inferior scapular area) as well as **diaphragmatic irritation** from any source, such as subphrenic abscess (referred to the ipsilateral shoulder).

IV. Evaluation. Pain that is severe and persists for longer than 6 hours should prompt a thorough surgical evaluation.

  A. History of present illness

    1. Onset and duration of pain

      a. Sudden onset of pain (within seconds) suggests perforation or rupture [e.g., perforated peptic ulcer or ruptured abdominal aortic aneurysm (AAA)]. Infarction, such as myocardial infarction or acute mesenteric occlusion, can also present with sudden onset of pain.

      b. Rapidly accelerating pain (within minutes) may result from several sources.

        (1) Colic syndromes, such as biliary colic, ureteral colic, and small-bowel obstruction

        (2) Inflammatory processes, such as acute appendicitis, pancreatitis, and diverticulitis

        (3) Ischemic processes, such as mesenteric ischemia, strangulated intestinal obstruction, and volvulus

      c. Gradual onset of pain (over several hours) increasing in intensity may be caused by one of the following:

        (1) Inflammatory conditions, such as appendicitis and cholecystitis

        (2) Obstructive processes, such as nonstrangulated bowel obstruction and urinary retention

        (3) Other mechanical processes, such as ectopic pregnancy and penetrating or perforating tumors

 2. **Character of pain**
   a. **Colicky pain** is severe, sharp pain accompanied by intervals when the pain is less severe or is absent.
   b. It occurs **secondary to hyperperistalsis of smooth muscle** against a mechanical site of obstruction (e.g., small-bowel obstruction, renal stone).
   c. An important exception is **biliary colic,** in which pain tends to be constant.
   d. **Pain that is sharp, severe, and persistent and increases in intensity** over time suggests an infectious or inflammatory process (e.g., appendicitis).
 3. **Location of pain**
   a. Pain caused by **inflammation of specific organs** may be localized [e.g., right upper quadrant (RUQ) pain caused by acute cholecystitis].
   b. Careful attention must be given to the **radiation of pain.** The pain of renal colic, for example, may begin in the patient's back or flank and radiate to the ipsilateral groin, whereas the pain of a ruptured aortic aneurysm or pancreatitis may be referred to the patient's back.
 4. **Alleviating and aggravating factors**
   a. Patients with **diffuse peritonitis** describe worsening of pain with movement (i.e., parietal pain); therefore, the pain is ameliorated by lying still.
   b. Patients with **intestinal obstruction** have visceral pain and usually experience a transient relief from symptoms after vomiting.
 5. **Associated symptoms**
   a. **Nausea and vomiting** frequently accompany abdominal pain and may hint at its etiology. Vomiting that occurs after the onset of pain may suggest appendicitis, whereas vomiting before the onset of pain is more consistent with the diagnosis of gastroenteritis or food poisoning. The sequence as well as the character of the emesis should be documented. Bilious emesis suggests a process distal to the pylorus.
   b. **Fever or chills** suggest an inflammatory or an infectious process, or both.
   c. **Anorexia** is present in the vast majority of patients with acute peritonitis.
 B. **Past Medical History, Surgical History, and Organ-System Review**
  1. **Pathologic medical conditions** may precipitate intra-abdominal pathology and pain
   a. Patients with a history of **peripheral vascular disease or coronary artery disease** and abdominal pain may have an AAA or mesenteric ischemia.
   b. Patients with a history of **cancer** may present with bowel obstruction from recurrence.
   c. **Major medical problems** are important to recognize early in the patient and may call for urgent surgical exploration.
  2. A **complete medical history and organ-system review** must be carried out to exclude various extra-abdominal causes of abdominal pain.
   a. Diabetic patients or patients with known **coronary artery disease or peripheral vascular disease** who present with vague epigastric symptoms may have myocardial ischemia as the cause of the abdominal symptoms.
   b. **Right lower lobe pneumonia** may present as RUQ pain in association with cough and fever.
  3. A **thorough menstrual history** must be obtained in women.
   a. **Pelvic inflammatory disease (PID)** typically occurs early in the cycle and may be associated with a vaginal discharge.
   b. **Ectopic pregnancy** must be considered in any woman of childbearing age with lower abdominal pain, especially if accompanied by a history of amenorrhea.

    c. Ovarian cysts can cause sudden pain by enlarging or rupturing. The timing in relation to the menstrual cycle is key. A ruptured follicular cyst pain occurs at midcycle (i.e., mittelschmerz), whereas the pain of a ruptured corpus luteum cyst develops around the time of menses.

    d. Abdominal pain that occurs monthly suggests **endometriosis.**

  4. Previous abdominal surgery in a patient with colicky abdominal pain may suggest **intestinal obstruction** secondary to adhesions, malignancy, or incarceration of an incisional hernia.

C. Medications

  1. Nonsteroidal anti-inflammatory medications, such as aspirin or ibuprofen, place patients at risk for the complications of peptic ulcer disease, including bleeding and perforation.

  2. Corticosteroids may mask classic signs of inflammation, such as fever and peritoneal irritation, making the abdominal examination less reliable.

  3. Antibiotics consumed by patients may aid or hinder diagnosis.

    a. Patients with **peritonitis** may have decreased pain.

    b. Patients who have diarrhea and abdominal pain may have **antibiotic-induced pseudomembranous colitis** caused by *Clostridium difficile.*

    c. Beware of the **elderly patient on immunosuppressants or antibiotics.**

D. Physical examination

  1. Overall appearance should be assessed.

    a. Patients with diffuse peritonitis appear acutely ill and tend to lie quietly on their side with their knees drawn toward their chest.

    b. Patients with colic tend to be restless and unable to find a comfortable position. Patients with ureteral colic may writhe in pain and walk around the examination room.

    c. Patients who are jaundiced may have biliary obstruction from periampullary cancer, a biliary stone, or ductal stricture.

    d. Patients who appear weak and lethargic may be septic.

  2. Vital signs are important indicators of a patient's overall condition.

    a. Fever suggests the presence of inflammation or infection. Marked fever ($>39°C$) suggests an abscess, cholangitis, or pneumonia.

    b. Hypotension or tachycardia, or both, may indicate hypovolemia or sepsis.

  3. The **abdominal examination** should be carried out thoroughly and systematically.

    a. The patient's abdomen should be inspected for **distention, surgical scars, bulges, and areas of erythema.**

    b. Auscultation may reveal the high-pitched, tinkling bowel sounds of obstruction or the absence of sounds due to ileus from diffuse peritonitis.

    c. Percussion of the patient's abdomen may reveal the tympanitic sounds of distended bowel in intestinal obstruction or the fluid shift that is characteristic of ascites. Percussion is also a useful tool for the delineation of localized tenderness and peritoneal irritation (deep palpation or rebound is usually unnecessary to determine peritoneal irritation).

    d. Palpation of the patient's abdomen should be performed with the patient in a supine position and with his or her knees flexed, if necessary, to relieve pain.

      (1) Begin the examination at a point remote from the site of pain.

      (2) Areas of tenderness and guarding should be noted. Rebound tenderness is not a very reliable sign of peritonitis. The presence of involuntary guarding (localized or diffuse) due to muscular rigidity from underlying peritoneal irritation is often a better sign of peritonitis. Peritonitis may also be elicited by rocking the patient's pelvis or shaking the bed to create friction between the abdominal wall and peritoneal viscera.

      (3) Pain out of proportion to physical examination findings may suggest mesenteric ischemia.

(4) A thorough search for **hernias,** including femoral hernias, must be carried out.

(5) Any **palpable masses** should be noted.

e. Rectal examination should be performed routinely in all patients with abdominal pain.

   (1) Tenderness or mass on the right pelvic side wall is sometimes seen in appendicitis.

   (2) A **mass in the rectum** may indicate obstructing cancer. Important details are the fraction of circumference involved, tumor mobility, and distance from the anal verge.

   (3) The presence of **occult blood in the stool specimen** may indicate GI bleeding from peptic ulcer disease. Beware of the positive Hemoccult following rectal examination.

f. Pelvic examination must be performed in all women of childbearing age who present with lower abdominal pain.

   (1) Cervical discharge and overall appearance of the cervix should be noted.

   (2) Bimanual examination should be performed to assess cervical motion tenderness, adnexal tenderness, or the presence of adnexal masses.

g. Specific physical examination findings should be sought in **the appropriate clinical setting.**

   (1) Murphy sign is inspiratory arrest while continuous pressure is maintained in the RUQ. Seen in acute cholecystitis, Murphy sign reflects the descent of an inflamed gallbladder with inspiration. When the inflamed gallbladder makes contact with the examiner's hand, the patient experiences pain, causing the inspiratory arrest. A sonographic Murphy sign may be elicited during ultrasound (US) palpation of the gallbladder with the US probe tip (this is secondary to direct pressure and is less reliable).

   (2) The **obturator sign** reflects inflammation adjacent to the internal obturator muscle (as is sometimes seen in appendicitis); it may also be present with an obturator hernia. While the patient is in a supine position with the knee and hip flexed, the hip is internally and externally rotated. The test is positive if the patient experiences hypogastric pain.

   (3) The **iliopsoas sign** is seen when an adjacent inflammatory process irritates iliopsoas muscle. It is classically observed in retrocecal appendicitis. The patient's thigh is usually already drawn into a flexed position for relief. The test is best performed with the patient lying on the left side. With the knee flexed, the thigh is hyperextended. The test is positive if the patient experiences pain on the right side with this maneuver.

   (4) Rovsing sign may also be seen in acute appendicitis. Indicative of an inflammatory process in the right lower quadrant (RLQ), Rovsing sign is RLQ pain from percussion in the left lower quadrant (LLQ).

E. Laboratory evaluation

   1. A **complete blood count** with cell count differential is important in the assessment of surgical conditions and should be done in every patient with acute abdominal pain.

   a. White blood cell (WBC) count elevation may indicate the presence of an infectious source (e.g., ruptured appendix).

   b. Left shift on the differential to more immature forms is often helpful because this may indicate the presence of an inflammatory source even if the WBC count is normal.

   c. Hematocrit elevation may be due to volume contraction from dehydration. Conversely, a low hematocrit may be due to occult blood loss.

2. An **electrolyte profile** may reveal clues to the patient's overall condition.
   a. **Hypokalemic, hypochloremic, metabolic alkalosis** may be seen in patients with prolonged vomiting and severe volume depletion. The hypokalemia reflects the potassium–hydrogen ion exchange occurring at the cellular level in an effort to correct the alkalosis.
   b. **Elevation of the blood urea nitrogen or creatinine** is also indicative of volume depletion.
3. **Liver function tests** may be performed in the appropriate clinical setting.
   a. **A mild elevation of transaminases** (<2 times normal), **alkaline phosphatase, and total bilirubin** is sometimes seen in patients with acute cholecystitis.
   b. **A moderate elevation of transaminases** (>3 times normal) in the patient with acute onset of RUQ pain is most likely due to a common bile duct (CBD) stone. Elevation of the transaminases often precedes the rise in total bilirubin and alkaline phosphatase in patients with acute biliary obstruction (e.g., from a CBD stone).
   c. **Markedly elevated transaminases** (i.e., >1,000 IU/L) in the patient without acute pain are more likely due to hepatitis or ischemia.
4. **Pancreatic enzymes** (i.e., amylase and lipase) should be measured if the diagnosis of pancreatitis is considered. It is important to note that the degree of enzyme elevation does not correlate with the severity of the pancreatitis.
   a. **Mild degrees of hyperamylasemia** may be seen in several situations, such as intestinal obstruction.
   b. **Elevation of lipase** usually indicates pancreatic parenchymal damage.
5. **Urinalysis** with microscopic examination is helpful in assessing urologic causes of abdominal pain.
   a. **Bacteriuria, pyuria, and a positive leukocyte esterase** usually suggest a urinary tract infection (UTI). Recurrent UTI in males should always elicit an evaluation for etiology, as this is unusual.
   b. **Hematuria** is seen in nephrolithiasis and renal and urothelial cancer.
6. *β*-**Human chorionic gonadotropin** must be obtained in any woman of childbearing age. A positive urine result should be quantitated by serum levels.
   a. **A low level** (<4,000 mIU) is seen in ectopic pregnancy.
   b. **Levels above 4,000 mIU** indicate intrauterine pregnancy (i.e., one that should be seen on US).
F. **Diagnostic imaging.** Radiologic evaluation of the patient with abdominal pain is a key element in the workup. However, it must be emphasized that the use of the various modalities available should be very selective to avoid the unnecessary cost and possible morbidity associated with some modalities.
1. **Plain abdominal films** often serve as the initial radiologic evaluation.
   a. Films should be obtained in **the supine and erect positions.**
   b. Free intraperitoneal air is best visualized on an **upright chest film** with both hemidiaphragms exposed.
      (1) If the patient is unable to assume an upright position, a **lateral decubitus film,** with the patient's left side down, should be obtained.
      (2) Free air may not be detectable in up to 20% of cases of **perforated viscus.**
   c. The **bowel gas pattern** should be assessed with regard to dilatation, air-fluid levels, and the presence of gas throughout the small and large intestine.
      (1) In **small-bowel obstruction,** one sees small-bowel dilatation (valvulae conniventes), air-fluid levels, and a paucity of gas in the colon or in the segment of bowel distal to the obstruction. The absence of air in the rectum suggests complete obstruction (beware of the presence of colonic gas following rectal examination).

(2) A **sentinel loop** (i.e., a single, dilated loop of bowel) may be seen adjacent to an inflamed organ (as in pancreatitis) and is due to localized ileus in that segment.
d. Calcifications should be noted.
  (1) The vast majority of **urinary stones** (90%) are visible on plain films, whereas only 15% of **gallstones** are calcified and therefore visible on plain films.
  (2) Calcifications in the region of the pancreas may indicate chronic pancreatitis.
  (3) Fecalith in the RLQ may suggest appendicitis in the appropriate clinical setting.
  (4) Calcification in the wall of the aorta may suggest an AAA.
  (5) The most common calcifications seen in the abdomen are "**phleboliths**" (benign calcifications of the pelvic veins). Phleboliths can be distinguished from renal stones by their central lucency, which represents the lumen.
e. The **presence of gas** in the portal or mesenteric venous systems, intramural gas in the GI tract, or gas in the biliary tree (in the absence of a surgical enteric anastomosis) may indicate an ominous condition in the appropriate clinical setting.
2. US may provide diagnostic information in some conditions. This modality has the advantages of being portable, relatively inexpensive, and free of radiation exposure. Unfortunately, US visibility is limited in settings of obesity, bowel gas, and subcutaneous air.
a. RUQ US is particularly useful in biliary tract disease.
  (1) Gallstones can be detected in up to 95% of patients.
  (2) Findings suggestive of **acute cholecystitis** include gallbladder wall thickening of greater than 3 mm, pericholecystic fluid, or a stone in the neck of the gallbladder.
  (3) Dilatation of the CBD (>8 mm, or larger in elderly patients), indicative of obstruction, may be detected.
  (4) Sonographic Murphy sign may be present, indicating gallbladder inflammation.
b. Pelvic or transvaginal US is particularly useful in women in whom ovarian pathology or an ectopic pregnancy is suspected.
c. US is also sometimes used in the evaluation of RLQ pain.
  (1) It may be helpful in the **diagnosis of appendicitis,** particularly in the pediatric population or in nonobese adults.
  (2) Its utility is operator-dependent.
3. Contrast studies, although rarely indicated in the acute setting, may be helpful in some situations.
a. In most instances, a **water-soluble contrast agent** (e.g., Hypaque) should be used to avoid possible barium peritonitis.
b. Contrast enema is particularly useful in differentiating adynamic ileus from distal colonic obstruction.
4. Computed tomographic (CT) scanning may provide a thorough evaluation of the patient's abdomen and pelvis in a relatively short period. Oral and intravenous contrast should be administered if not specifically contraindicated. CT scanning is the best single radiographic study in the patient with unexplained abdominal pain. It is of particular benefit in certain situations, including the following:
a. When **an accurate history cannot be obtained** (e.g., the patient is demented or obtunded or has an atypical history).
b. When a patient has **abdominal pain and leukocytosis and examination findings are worrisome but not definitive for peritoneal irritation.**
c. When a patient with a chronic illness (e.g., Crohn disease) experiences **acute abdominal pain.**

Table 14-1. Differential diagnosis for acute abdominal pain

Upper abdominal		Perforated peptic ulcer
		Acute cholecystitis
		Acute pancreatitis
Mid & lower abdominal		Acute appendicitis
		Acute diverticulitis
		Intestinal obstruction
		Mesenteric ischemia
		Ruptured AAA
Other	OB/ GYN	PID
		Ectopic pregnancy
		Ruptured ovarian cyst
	GU	Nephrolithiasis
		Pyelonephritis/cystitis
	Nonsurgical	Acute MI
		Gastroenteritis
		Pneumonia
		DKA

    d. When **evaluating retroperitoneal structures** (e.g., in a stable patient with a suspected leaking AAA).

    e. When evaluating patients with a history of **intra-abdominal malignancy.**

  5. Radionuclide imaging studies have few indications in the acute setting.

    a. Biliary radiopharmaceuticals, such as hepatic 2,6-dimethyliminodiacetic acid or diisopropyliminodiacetic acid, may be used to evaluate filling and emptying of the gallbladder in a patient who has suspected acute cholecystitis or has undergone a nondiagnostic US examination. Nonfilling of the gallbladder implies cystic duct obstruction and may indicate acute cholecystitis in the appropriate clinical setting. This test is especially valuable in the diagnosis of acalculous cholecystitis.

    b. Radioisotope-labeled red blood cell (RBC) or WBC scans are sometimes helpful in delineating sites of bleeding or inflammation, respectively.

    c. Technetium-99m pertechnetate may be used to detect a Meckel diverticulum because this isotope is concentrated in the ectopic gastric mucosa frequently seen within the diverticulum.

  6. Invasive radiologic techniques may have a role in some situations, including these:

    a. Angiographic diagnosis of **suspected mesenteric arterial occlusion.**

    b. Diagnosis and therapy of **acute GI bleeding.**

V. Differential diagnoses. See Table 14-1.

APPENDICITIS

  I. Epidemiology

    A. Appendectomy is the most common surgical procedure performed on an emergency basis.

    B. Acute appendicitis develops in approximately 10% of the population in Western countries.

    C. The **maximal incidence** occurs in an individual's teens and 20s.

    D. The **male-female ratio** of approximately 2:1 gradually shifts after age 25 until a 1:1 ratio is reached.

II. Pathophysiology

A. **Appendiceal obstruction** is the most common initiating event of appendicitis.

   1. **Hyperplasia** of the submucosal lymphoid follicles of the appendix accounts for approximately 60% of obstructions (most common in teens).

   2. In older adults and children, the **fecalith** is the most common etiology (35%).

B. **Intraluminal pressure** of the obstructed appendiceal lumen increases secondary to continued mucosal secretion and bacterial overgrowth; the appendiceal wall becomes thinned and lymphatic and venous obstruction occurs.

C. **Necrosis and perforation** develop when the arterial flow to the appendix is compromised.

III. Diagnosis.

The diagnosis of acute appendicitis is made by clinical evaluation. Although laboratory tests and imaging procedures can be helpful, they are of secondary importance.

A. **Clinical presentation**

   1. **Classic.** Appendicitis typically begins with progressive, persistent midabdominal discomfort caused by obstruction and distention of the appendix, which stimulates the visceral afferent autonomic nerves (T8–10 distribution). This is followed by anorexia and a low-grade fever (<38.5°C). As distention of the appendix increases, venous congestion stimulates intestinal peristalsis, causing a cramping sensation that is soon followed by nausea and vomiting. Ninety percent of patients are anorexic, 70% become nauseated and vomit, and 10% have diarrhea. Once the inflammation extends transmurally to the parietal peritoneum, the somatic pain fibers are stimulated, and the pain localizes to the RLQ. Peritoneal irritation is associated with pain on movement, mild fever, and tachycardia. One-fourth of patients present initially with localized pain and no prior visceral symptoms. The onset of symptoms to time of presentation is usually less than 24 hours for acute appendicitis and averages several hours.

   2. **Unusual presentations of appendicitis**

      a. When the appendix is **retrocecal or behind the ileum,** it may be separated from the anterior abdominal peritoneum, and abdominal localizing signs may be absent. Irritation of adjacent structures can cause diarrhea, urinary frequency, pyuria, or microscopic hematuria.

      b. When the appendix is **located in the pelvis,** it may simulate acute gastroenteritis, with diffuse pain, nausea, vomiting, and diarrhea. The diagnosis may be suspected if tenderness is present on digital rectal examination.

   3. **Pregnancy**

      a. Appendicitis is the most common nongynecologic surgical emergency during pregnancy. The **incidence of appendicitis** during pregnancy is 1 in 1,500 to 2,000 pregnancies. It occurs in the pregnant and the nonpregnant patient with equal frequency. Appendicitis is evenly distributed throughout the trimesters, but the incidence of perforation is highest in the third trimester.

      b. Appendicitis must be suspected in any pregnant woman with **abdominal pain.** The gravid uterus displaces the appendix superiorly and laterally toward the RUQ (Figure 14-2), thereby complicating the diagnosis of appendicitis. Separation of the visceral and parietal peritoneum due to the enlarging uterus limits localization of the pain by decreasing the somatic component of the pain. In addition, nausea and vomiting can be incorrectly attributed to the morning sickness that is common in the first trimester.

      c. **Operation** is indicated in a pregnant patient as soon as the diagnosis of appendicitis is suspected. Death of the fetus occurs in 1.5% to 3.0% of pregnant patients with uncomplicated appendicitis, but this figure can reach 35% when complicated by perforation and diffuse peritonitis. A negative laparotomy carries a risk of fetal loss of up to 3%.

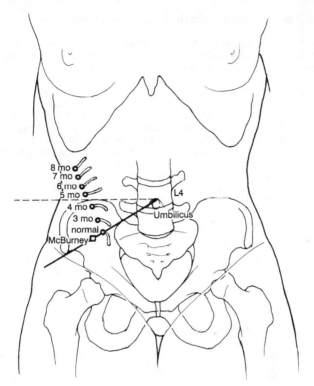

Figure 14-2. Changes in location and direction of the appendix during pregnancy. The normal and postpartum position of the base of the appendix is medial to McBurney point. At the 5th month, the appendix is at the level of the umbilicus and iliac crest. (Adapted from Baer Л, et al. *JAMA* 1932;98:1359.)

B. Physical examination

1. The examination begins by **assessing the patient's abdomen** in areas other than the area of suspected tenderness. Location of the appendix is variable. However, the base usually is found at the level of the S1 vertebral body, lateral to the right midclavicular line at McBurney point (two-thirds of the distance from the umbilicus to the anterosuperior iliac spine). The presence of pain in the RLQ during gentle finger percussion in the LLQ (Rovsing sign) indicates peritoneal irritation. The degree of direct tenderness is appreciated. The degree of muscular resistance to palpation parallels the severity of the inflammatory process. Cutaneous hyperesthesia is often present, overlying the region of maximal tenderness. Exacerbation of pain with passive stretching of the iliopsoas muscle (positive psoas sign) implies the presence of local inflammation in the area of the muscle (e.g., retrocecal appendicitis). A pelvic appendix may produce hypogastric pain with passive internal rotation, a positive obturator sign.

2. **Rectal examination** is performed to evaluate the presence of localized tenderness or an inflammatory mass in the pararectal area. It is most useful for atypical presentations suggestive of a pelvic or retrocecal appendix.

3. In women, a **pelvic examination** is performed to assess the presence of cervical motion tenderness and adnexal pain or masses.

4. **A palpable mass in the RLQ** suggests a periappendiceal abscess or phlegmon.
C. **Laboratory evaluation.** Complete blood cell count, serum electrolytes, and urinalysis should be obtained preoperatively for patients with suspected appendicitis. A serum pregnancy test also must be performed for all ovulating women.
   1. **Complete blood cell count.** A leukocyte count of greater than 10,000 cells/μL, with polymorphonuclear cell predominance (>75%), is common in the child and young adult with appendicitis. The total number of WBCs and the proportion of immature forms increase if there is appendiceal perforation. In older adults, the leukocyte count and differential are normal more frequently than in younger adults, as high as 10%. Pregnant women normally have an elevated WBC count that can reach 15,000 to 20,000 as their pregnancy progresses.
   2. **Urinalysis** is abnormal in 25% to 40% of patients with appendicitis. Pyuria, albuminuria, and hematuria are common. Large quantities of bacteria suggest UTI as the cause of abdominal pain. If the urinalysis shows more than 20 WBCs per high-power field or more than 30 RBCs per high-power field, it suggests UTI. Significant hematuria should prompt consideration of ureteral stones.
   3. **Serum electrolytes, blood urea nitrogen, and serum creatinine** are obtained to identify and correct electrolyte abnormalities caused by dehydration secondary to vomiting or poor oral intake.
D. **Radiologic evaluation.** Diagnosis of appendicitis usually can be made without radiologic evaluation. In complex cases, however, the following imaging can be helpful.
   1. **Abdominal x-rays** are not helpful in diagnosing appendicitis. One study demonstrated an appendicolith on only 1.14% of the plain films performed on patients with surgically proved appendicitis. Other suggestive radiologic findings include a distended cecum with adjacent small-bowel air-fluid levels, loss of the right psoas shadow, scoliosis to the right, and gas in the lumen of the appendix. A perforated appendix rarely causes pneumoperitoneum.
   2. **US** is most useful in women of childbearing age and in children because other causes of abdominal complaints can be demonstrated. Findings associated with acute appendicitis include an appendiceal diameter >6 mm, lack of luminal compressibility, and presence of an appendicolith. The perforated appendix is more difficult to diagnose and is characterized by loss of the echogenic submucosa and the presence of loculated periappendiceal or pelvic fluid collection. The quality and accuracy of US are highly operator dependent. In women, ovarian pathology may be identified or excluded.
   3. **Abdominal CT scan** is generally performed only in complex cases or in patients with atypical presentations. It is superior to US in these cases (*Am J Surg* 2000;179:379). CT findings of appendicitis include a distended thick-walled appendix with inflammatory streaking of surrounding fat, a pericecal phlegmon or abscess, an appendicolith, or RLQ intra-abdominal free air that signals perforation. CT scan is particularly useful in distinguishing between periappendiceal abscesses and phlegmon.
   4. **Barium enema (BE)** is rarely used to diagnose acute appendicitis. It may establish luminal patency of the appendix and may show mass effects on the colonic wall characteristic of appendicitis. If barium contrast completely fills the appendix, appendicitis is unlikely (10% to 20% of normal appendixes do not fill). BE may be helpful in differentiating right colonic or terminal ileal mucosal diseases that may simulate appendicitis, such as inflammatory bowel disease. However, this test must be avoided in patients with toxic colitis.
E. **Diagnostic laparoscopy** is most useful for evaluating ovulating women with an equivocal examination for appendicitis. In this subgroup, one-third of

women prove to have primary gynecologic pathology. The appendix may also be removed via the laparoscopic approach. Therefore, some surgeons advocate an initial laparoscopic approach in all ovulating women with suspected appendicitis.

F. Differential diagnosis
 1. **Gastrointestinal diseases**
    a. **Gastroenteritis** is characterized by nausea and emesis before the onset of abdominal pain, along with generalized malaise, high fever, diarrhea, and poorly localized abdominal pain and tenderness. Although diarrhea is one of the cardinal signs of gastroenteritis, it can occur in patients with appendicitis. Diarrhea is most common in young children. Additionally, the WBC count is less frequently elevated in patients with gastroenteritis.
    b. **Mesenteric lymphadenitis** usually occurs in patients younger than 20 years old and presents with middle, followed by RLQ, abdominal pain but without rebound tenderness or muscular rigidity. Nodal histology and cultures obtained at operation can identify etiology, most notably *Yersinia* species, *Shigella* species, and *Mycobacterium tuberculosis*. Mesenteric lymphadenitis is known to be associated with upper respiratory tract infections.
    c. **Meckel diverticulitis** presents with symptoms and signs indistinguishable from those of appendicitis, but it characteristically occurs in infants.
    d. **Perforated peptic ulcer disease, diverticulitis, and cholecystitis** can present clinical pictures similar to those of appendicitis.
    e. **Typhlitis** is characterized by inflammation of the wall of the cecum or terminal ileum. It is most commonly seen in immunosuppressed children who are being treated with chemotherapy for leukemia, and it can also occur in HIV-positive patients. Although management of typhlitis is usually nonsurgical, it is difficult to distinguish preoperatively between typhlitis and appendicitis in susceptible children.
 2. **Urologic diseases**
    a. **Pyelonephritis** causes high fevers, rigors, costovertebral pain, and tenderness. Diagnosis is confirmed by urinalysis with culture.
    b. **Ureteral colic.** Passage of renal stones causes flank pain radiating into the groin but little localized tenderness. Hematuria suggests the diagnosis, which is confirmed by intravenous pyelography or noncontrast CT. Abdominal plain films frequently show renal stones.
 3. **Gynecologic diseases**
    a. **PID** can present with symptoms and signs indistinguishable from those of acute appendicitis, but the two often can be differentiated on the basis of several factors. Cervical motion tenderness and milky vaginal discharge strengthen a diagnosis of PID. In patients with PID, the pain is usually bilateral, with intense guarding on abdominal and pelvic examinations. Transvaginal US can be used to visualize the ovaries and to identify tubo-ovarian abscesses.
    b. **Ectopic pregnancy.** A pregnancy test should be performed in all female patients of childbearing age presenting with abdominal complaints.
    c. **Ovarian cysts** are best detected by transvaginal or transabdominal US.
    d. **Ovarian torsion.** The inflammation surrounding an ischemic ovary often can be palpated on bimanual pelvic examination. These patients can have a fever, leukocytosis, and RLQ pain consistent with appendicitis. A twisted viscus, however, differs in that it produces sudden acute intense pain with simultaneous frequent and persistent emesis. This diagnosis can also be confirmed using US.

IV. Treatment
 A. **Preoperative preparation.** Intravenous isotonic fluid replacement should be initiated to achieve a brisk urinary output and to correct electrolyte

252 Ch. 14 Acute Abdominal Pain and Appendicitis

abnormalities. Nasogastric suction is helpful, especially in patients with peritonitis. Temperature elevations are treated with acetaminophen and a cooling blanket. Anesthesia should not be induced in patients with a temperature higher than 39°C. Preoperative antibiotic coverage is begun.

B. Antibiotic therapy. Broad-spectrum antibiotic coverage is initiated preoperatively to assist in controlling local and general sepsis and to reduce the incidence of postoperative wound infection. For acute appendicitis, this typically consists of a second-generation cephalosporin (cefotetan or cefoxitin). In patients with acute nonperforated appendicitis, therapy should not continue for more than 24 hours. Many studies have shown that a single preoperative dose is sufficient. Antibiotic therapy in perforated or gangrenous appendicitis should be continued for 3 to 5 days.

C. Appendectomy. With very few exceptions, the treatment of appendicitis is appendectomy. Patients with diffuse peritonitis or questionable diagnosis should be explored through a midline incision. The mortality after appendectomy is high in elderly patients. Equivocal diagnosis of appendicitis in this frail patient population warrants increased diagnostic effects before emergent appendectomy (*Ann Surg* 2001;233:4). In most patients, a transverse incision (e.g., Davis-Rockey, Fowler-Weir) provides the best cosmetic appearance and allows easy extension medially for greater exposure. The external and internal oblique and transversus abdominis muscle layers may be split in the direction of their fibers. After entering the peritoneal cavity, Gram stain and cultures are obtained if purulence is present. Once the cecum is identified, the anterior taenia can be followed to the base of the appendix. The appendix is gently delivered into the wound, with any surrounding adhesions broken carefully. If the appendix is normal on inspection (occurring in 5% to 20% of explorations), it is removed, and appropriate alternative diagnoses are entertained. The cecum, sigmoid colon, and ileum are carefully inspected for changes indicative of diverticular (including Meckel diverticulum), infectious, ischemic, or inflammatory bowel disease (e.g., Crohn disease). Evidence of mesenteric lymphadenopathy is sought. In women, the ovaries and fallopian tubes are inspected for evidence of PID, ruptured follicular cysts, ectopic pregnancy, or other pathology. Bilious peritoneal fluid suggests perforation either of a peptic ulcer or the gallbladder.

D. Laparoscopic appendectomy. Laparoscopic management of appendicitis has evolved from a purely diagnostic to a therapeutic modality. The surgical literature to date shows little or no patient benefit over the traditional open procedure. Laparoscopic appendectomy is more costly and offers no decrease in the length of stay or complications, with a slight decrease in wound infection but a slight increase in intra-abdominal infection (*Am J Surg* 2000;179:375).

E. Drainage of appendiceal abscess. Management of appendiceal abscesses remains controversial. Patients who have a well-localized periappendiceal abscess and are initially seen when symptoms are subsiding can be treated with systemic antibiotics and considered for percutaneous US- or CT-guided catheter drainage, followed by elective appendectomy 6 to 12 weeks later (*Radiology* 1987;163:23). This strategy is successful in more than 80% of patients. The appendix must be removed because the patient has a 60% risk of developing appendicitis again within 2 years. Alternatively, immediate appendectomy can shorten the duration of the illness and is as safe as catheter drainage and delayed appendectomy. Anatomically obscure or multiloculated appendiceal abscesses should be cultured and evacuated surgically. Appendectomy should be performed at this initial operation, with the wound left open. Systemic antibiotics are administered for at least 5 days or until the leukocyte count and temperature have returned to normal.

F. Incidental appendectomy is removal of the normal appendix at laparotomy for another condition. Although one study showed an increased risk of wound infection in patients older than 50 years undergoing routine cholecystectomy with incidental appendectomy, most studies demonstrate no evidence of adverse consequences after incidental appendectomy. The appendix must be easily accessible through the present abdominal incision, and the patient must be clinically stable enough to tolerate the extra time needed to complete the procedure. Because most cases of appendicitis occur in a patient's teens and 20s, the benefit of incidental appendectomy decreases substantially once a person is older than 30 years. Crohn disease involving the cecum, radiation treatment to the cecum, immunosuppression, and vascular grafts or other bioprostheses in place are contraindications for incidental appendectomy because of the increased risk of infectious complications or appendiceal stump leak.

V. **Complications of acute appendicitis**
  A. **Perforation** is accompanied by severe pain and fever. It is unusual within the first 12 hours of appendicitis but is present in 50% of appendicitis patients younger than 10 years and older than 50 years. Acute consequences of perforation include fever, tachycardia, generalized peritonitis, and abscess formation. Treatment is appendectomy, peritoneal irrigation, and broad-spectrum intravenous antibiotics for several days.
  B. **Postoperative wound infection risk** can be decreased by appropriate intravenous antibiotics administered before skin incision. The incidence of wound infection increases from approximately 3% in cases of nonperforated appendicitis to 4.7% in patients with a perforated or gangrenous appendix. Primary closure in the setting of perforation is unchanged from delayed closure (4.6%) and is not recommended (*Surgery* 2000;127:136). Wound infections are managed by opening, draining, and packing the wound to allow healing by secondary intention. Intravenous antibiotics are indicated for associated cellulitis or systemic sepsis.
  C. **Intra-abdominal and pelvic abscesses** occur most frequently with perforation of the appendix. Postoperative intra-abdominal and pelvic abscesses are best treated by percutaneous CT- or US-guided aspiration. If the abscess is inaccessible or resistant to percutaneous drainage, operative drainage is indicated. Antibiotic therapy can mask but does not treat or prevent a significant abscess.
  D. **Other complications**
    1. **Pyelophlebitis** is septic portal vein thrombosis, is usually caused by *Escherichia coli,* and presents with high fevers, jaundice, and eventually hepatic abscesses. CT scan demonstrates thrombus and gas in the portal vein. Prompt treatment (operative or percutaneous) of the primary infection is critical, followed by broad- spectrum intravenous antibiotics.
    2. **Enterocutaneous fistulas** from a leak at the appendiceal stump closure occasionally require surgical closure, but most close spontaneously.
  E. **Small-bowel obstruction** is four times more common after surgery in cases of perforated appendicitis than in uncomplicated appendicitis.

OTHER ETIOLOGIES OF ACUTE ABDOMINAL PAIN

I. **Acute cholecystitis**
  A. **Presentation**
    1. Most patients provide an **antecedent history of biliary colic** (i.e., epigastric or RUQ pain after consumption of a fatty meal).
    2. Typical presentation is **epigastric or RUQ pain, nausea, and vomiting** 4 to 6 hours after consumption of a meal.
  B. **Examination** is characterized by fever, RUQ tenderness, and a positive Murphy sign.
  C. **Ancillary studies**
    1. **Laboratory examination** reveals leukocytosis (with left shift) and a slight elevation of liver function tests (not always present).
    2. Helpful **radiographic studies** include US (may show the presence of gallstones, gallbladder wall thickening, pericholecystic fluid, and

sonographic Murphy sign) and diisopropyliminodiacetic acid scan (shows nonfilling of the gallbladder).
   D. It is important to consider the full spectrum of **biliary tract disease.**
II. **Acute pancreatitis**
   A. **Etiology**
      1. The most common cause is **alcohol consumption.**
      2. **Gallstones** account for the majority of remaining cases.
      3. **Other causes** include endoscopic retrograde cholangiopancreatography, certain medications, and hypertriglyceridemia.
   B. **Presentation and severity**
      1. Typically, acute pancreatitis presents as **severe epigastric pain** that radiates to the patient's back.
      2. Examination is characterized by **epigastric tenderness** and varying degrees of **tachycardia, fever, and hypotension,** depending on the severity of the attack.
      3. The spectrum of severity ranges from **mild edema** around the pancreas to **pancreatic necrosis with infection.**
   C. The **severity of the attack and the prognosis** may be estimated by various indicators (Ranson criteria).
   D. **Ancillary studies**
      1. **Laboratory examination** typically shows elevation of amylase, lipase, and serum transaminases, none of which correlate with severity.
      2. **Plain film** may reveal sentinel loop or pancreatic calcifications; **CT scan** with intravenous contrast is indicated in severe cases to determine the presence of pancreatic necrosis or fluid collection (optimal results are obtained after 3 days).
III. **Perforated peptic ulcer**
   A. **Duodenal ulcers** are more common than **gastric ulcers.**
   B. **Presentation**
      1. Perforated peptic ulcer is associated with the **chronic use of nonsteroidal anti-inflammatory medications.**
      2. Most patients provide a **history compatible with peptic ulcer disease.**
      3. Perforated peptic ulcer typically presents as sudden onset of **severe epigastric pain** that eventually involves the patient's entire abdomen.
   C. **Physical examination** is remarkable for diffuse abdominal tenderness, rigidity, and peritoneal signs.
   D. **Plain films** usually, but not always, reveal free intraperitoneal air.
   E. **Therapy** consists of fluid resuscitation, intravenous antibiotics, and emergent surgical exploration.
IV. **Intestinal obstruction**
   A. **Small-bowel obstruction**
      1. The most common cause is **adhesions from previous surgery;** others include hernias, cancer, intussusception, and volvulus.
      2. Usually presents as **sharp, crampy periumbilical pain** with intervening pain-free periods; associated symptoms include nausea and vomiting.
      3. **Examination** is marked by abdominal distention, high-pitched or tinkling bowel sounds, and a variable degree of abdominal tenderness.
      4. **Plain abdominal films** reveal dilatated loops of small bowel, air-fluid levels, and paucity of gas in the colon. Proximal small-bowel obstruction, however, may not be associated with dilatated bowel loops on plain films and often requires a contrast study for diagnosis.
   B. **Large-bowel obstruction**
      1. Large-bowel obstruction may be caused by **cancer, diverticulitis, volvulus, or impaction.**
      2. Presenting symptoms include **constipation, abdominal distention, and varying degrees of abdominal pain.**
      3. Examination may reveal **abdominal distention or a mass** (the latter revealed by rectal examination).

4. Plain abdominal films may reveal **colonic distention.** An enema with opaque contrast (e.g., Hypaque) is often necessary to rule out the presence of a mass (e.g., obstructing colon, rectal cancer).
5. The **risk of perforation** increases as the cecal diameter exceeds 12 to 13 cm.

V. **Mesenteric ischemia**

A. Mesenteric ischemia may result from **superior mesenteric artery thrombosis,** from severe vascular disease, or from superior mesenteric artery occlusion by embolus (e.g., atrial fibrillation).

B. It presents as **sudden onset of severe, constant abdominal pain** with associated emptying of bowel contents (vomiting and diarrhea).

C. **Examination** may reveal pain out of proportion to physical findings.

D. **Laboratory studies** are marked by leukocytosis and acidosis (secondary to accumulation of lactate).

E. **Angiography** may confirm the diagnosis; however, radiologic studies are not indicated if the patient is found to have peritonitis on physical examination.

VI. **Ruptured AAA**

A. A ruptured AAA presents as **sudden onset of abdominal pain** with varying degrees of radiation to the patient's flank or back, or both.

B. Patients with **free intra-abdominal rupture** rarely, if ever, survive until hospital arrival; those with contained rupture or leak may present in shock.

C. **Examination** is marked by the presence of a tender, pulsatile abdominal mass.

D. **Plain films** may reveal calcification in the aortic wall; CT scan is the gold standard for diagnosis (only performed in hemodynamically stable patients).

E. Patients with **hypotension from a known aneurysm** should be taken emergently to the operating room without further diagnostic studies. Anesthesia induction should be delayed until the patient is prepped and draped to avoid intubation-induced hypotension.

VII. **Surgical options**

A. **Exploratory laparotomy** is mandatory in any patient in whom a surgically correctable cause of acute abdomen is suspected or diagnosed.
1. **Diffuse peritonitis** (e.g., from a perforated viscus)
2. **Acute, high-grade intestinal obstruction**
3. **Ischemic or necrotic bowel**

B. **Laparoscopy** may be used as a diagnostic and a therapeutic tool in patients with a variety of acute abdominal conditions. It has the advantage of enabling a more thorough examination of the peritoneal cavity than is obtainable through a small (e.g., RLQ) surgical incision. Laparoscopy is not as useful in the visualization of retroperitoneal structures. Settings in which laparoscopy may be particularly beneficial include the following:
1. **Suspected but equivocal appendicitis** (e.g., RLQ pain in a young woman, in whom gynecologic pathology might easily confound the diagnosis); laparoscopy may be diagnostic and therapeutic because laparoscopic appendectomy can usually be carried out in patients with uncomplicated appendicitis.
2. **Critically ill patients** in whom a negative laparotomy may cause great morbidity.

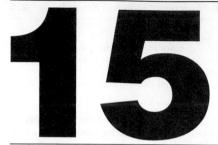

Colon, Rectum, and Anus

**Steven R. Hunt and
James W. Fleshman**

DISTURBANCES OF PHYSIOLOGY

I. **Normal colon function**
  A. **Water absorption.** Normal ileal effluent totals 900 to 1,500 mL per day, and stool water loss amounts to only 100 to 200 mL per day. Under maximum conditions, the colon can absorb 5 to 6 L of fluid a day, and only when large-bowel absorption is less than 2 L per day does an increase in fecal water content result in diarrhea. The majority of colonic absorption takes place in the right colon.
  B. **Electrolyte transport.** Sodium and chloride absorption occur by active processes in exchange for potassium and bicarbonate.
  C. **Nutrition.** Although absorption of nutrients is minimal in the colon, passive absorption of short-chain fatty acids produced by colonic bacteria can account for up to 540 kcal per day and provide much of the energy needed for electrolyte transport in normal colons. Colonic and rectal mucosa nutrition relies on the local delivery of short-chain fatty acids such as butyric acid. When absent from the lumen for a prolonged period of time, a "colitis" known as diversion colitis can occur.
  D. **Motility patterns of the colon** allow for mixing and elimination of intestinal contents. In part, these patterns result from the balance of excitatory parasympathetic input and inhibitory sympathetic input. A patient's emotional state, amount of exercise and sleep, amount of colonic distention, and hormonal milieu may all affect the three patterns of colonic motility.
    1. **Retrograde movements** occur mainly in the right colon. These contractions prolong the exposure of luminal contents to the mucosa and thereby increase the absorption of fluids and electrolytes.
    2. **Segmental contractions**, the most commonly observed motility pattern, represent localized simultaneous contractions of the longitudinal and circular colonic musculature in short colonic segments.
    3. **Mass movements** occur three to four times a day and are characterized by an antegrade, propulsive contractile wave involving a long segment of colon.
  E. **Microflora.** One-third of the dry weight of feces is normally composed of bacteria. Anaerobic *Bacteroides* species are most prevalent (10^{11}/mL), although *Escherichia coli* has a titer of 10^9/mL. Bacteria produce much of the body's vitamin K. Endogenous colonic bacteria also suppress the emergence of pathogenic microorganisms. Antibiotic therapy can alter the endogenous microflora, resulting in changes in drug sensitivity (warfarin) or infectious colitides due to pathogenic microbial overgrowth (*Clostridium difficile* colitis).
  F. **Colonic gas** (200 to 2,000 mL per day) is composed of (1) swallowed oxygen and nitrogen and (2) hydrogen, carbon dioxide, and methane produced during fermentation by colonic bacteria. Hydrogen and methane are combustible gases and may explode when electrocautery is used for polypectomy or biopsy. Adequate bowel cleansing is therefore necessary before the use of intracolonic electrocautery.

II. **Disorders of colonic physiology**
  A. **Constipation** is difficult to define and is often used by patients to describe a number of different defecatory symptoms (infrequent bowel movements, difficult or painful movements, etc.). Constipation is generally defined clinically as one or fewer spontaneous bowel movements or stools per week.
    1. **Etiologies** include medications (narcotics, anticholinergics, antidepressants, and calcium channel blockers), hypothyroidism, hypercalcemia, dietary factors (low fluid intake or low fiber intake), decreased exercise, neoplasia, and neurologic disorders (e.g., Parkinson disease and multiple sclerosis). Abnormalities of pelvic floor function (obstructed defecation), such as paradoxical puborectalis muscle function or intussusception of the rectum (internal or external rectal prolapse), may result in constipation, as may idiopathic delayed transit of feces through the colon (dysfunction of the intrinsic colonic nerves or colonic inertia).
    2. **Evaluation.** Change in bowel habits is a common presentation of colorectal neoplasia. Constipation should initially be evaluated with colonoscopy or proctoscopy with barium enema. If this workup is negative and the patient fails to respond to a trial of fiber supplementation and increased fluid intake, a colonic transit time study is indicated. On day 0, the patient ingests an enteric-coated capsule containing 24 radiopaque rings. Abdominal plain x-rays are obtained on day 3 and day 5. Normal transit results in 80% of the rings in the left colon by day 3 and 80% of all the rings expelled by day 5. The persistence of rings throughout the colon on day 5 indicates colonic inertia. When the rings stall in the rectosigmoid region, functional anorectal obstruction (obstructed defecation) may be present. This may be evaluated with cine defecography or anorectal manometry, or both; the task is to look for nonrelaxation of the puborectalis muscle or internal intussusception of the rectum.
    3. **Treatment** of colonic inertia initially includes laxatives (polyethylene glycol, 12 oz per day), fiber (psyllium 9 g per day), increased exercise, and avoidance of predisposing factors. If these prove unsuccessful and obstructed defecation has been ruled out, the patient may benefit from surgical therapy. In patients with long-standing, debilitating symptoms refractory to nonoperative measures, **total abdominal colectomy with ileorectal anastomosis** may prove curative. The risk of total intestinal inertia after surgery is significant, and the patient should understand this.
  B. **Colonic pseudo-obstruction** (Ogilvie syndrome), a profound colonic ileus without evidence of mechanical obstruction, is a diagnosis of exclusion. It most commonly occurs in critically ill or institutionalized patients. Initial treatment after confirmation of the absence of a fixed mechanical obstruction is conservative. Nasogastric decompression, rectal tube placement, an aggressive enema regimen (e.g., cottonseed and docusate sodium enema), correction of metabolic disorders, and discontinuation of medications that decrease colonic motility are the cornerstones of initial management. Hypaque enema is often therapeutic as well as diagnostic. Epidural injection of lidocaine at the T7 level will often relieve the pseudo-obstruction by blocking the sympathetic plexus to the colon. Neostigmine intravenous infusion (2mg/h) in a monitored setting has been shown to be useful in resistant cases.

  Rapid cecal dilation or a cecal diameter of 9 to 12 cm on plain abdominal x-rays requires prompt colonoscopic decompression. This is initially successful in 70% to 90% of cases, with a recurrence rate of 10% to 30% (recurrence is usually amenable to repeat colonoscopic decompression). Laparotomy should be reserved for patients with peritonitis, at which time a total colectomy with end ileostomy and rectal stump should be performed.

C. Volvulus is the twisting of an air-filled segment of bowel about its mesentery and accounts for nearly 10% of bowel obstruction in the United States.

   1. Sigmoid volvulus accounts for 80% to 90% of all volvulus and is most common in elderly or institutionalized patients and in patients with a variety of neurologic disorders. It is an acquired condition resulting from sigmoid redundancy with narrowing of the mesenteric pedicle.

   a. Diagnosis is suspected when there is abdominal pain, distention, cramping, and obstipation. **Plain films** often show a characteristic **inverted-U**, sausage-like shape of air-filled sigmoid pointing to the right upper quadrant. If the diagnosis is still in question and gangrene is not suspected, water-soluble **contrast enema** usually shows a **bird's beak deformity** at the obstructed rectosigmoid junction. This can be therapeutic.

   b. In the absence of peritoneal signs, **treatment** involves **sigmoidoscopy**, with the placement of a rectal tube beyond the point of obstruction. If a sigmoidoscope does not reach the obstruction, colonoscopic decompression may be useful. An elective sigmoid colectomy should be performed in an acceptable operative candidate. If **peritonitis** is present, the patient should undergo laparotomy and **Hartmann procedure** (sigmoid colectomy, end-descending colostomy, and defunctionalized rectal pouch). An alternative in the stable patient without significant fecal soilage of the peritoneal cavity is sigmoidectomy, on-table colonic lavage, and colorectal anastomosis with or without proximal fecal diversion (loop ileostomy).

   c. The **recurrence rate** after sigmoidoscopic decompression is approximately 40% once the rectal tube is removed. Therefore, if the patient's medical condition allows, an elective sigmoid colectomy with primary anastomosis should be performed after mechanical bowel preparation.

   2. Cecal volvulus occurs in a younger population than does sigmoid volvulus and is thought to occur secondary to congenital failure of retroperitonealization of the cecum (in axial volvulus) or a very redundant pelvic cecum that flops into the left upper quadrant to kink the right colon (in bascule volvulus).

   a. Diagnosis. Presentation is similar to that of distal small-bowel obstruction, with nausea, vomiting, abdominal pain, and distention. Plain films show a **kidney-shaped** air-filled cecum with the convex aspect extending into the left upper quadrant. A **Hypaque enema** may be performed, which shows a tapered cutoff (in axial volvulus) or sharp cutoff (in bascule volvulus) in the ascending colon.

   b. Management involves urgent laparotomy and right hemicolectomy. Ileocolostomy is preferred; otherwise, ileostomy and mucous fistula are performed if concern about patient stability or bowel viability exists. Cecopexy has also been advocated. This involves elevation of a retroperitoneal flap and suture of the cecum to this flap to eliminate the pathologic condition predisposing the patient to cecal volvulus. This technique is often a formidable undertaking in the setting of the acutely dilated and fragile cecum and is rarely indicated.

   3. Transverse volvulus is rare and has a clinical presentation similar to that of sigmoid volvulus. Diagnosis is made based on the results of plain films (which show a dilated right colon and upright U-shaped dilated transverse colon) and Hypaque enema (revealing a cutoff). Endoscopic decompression has been reported, but operative resection is usually required.

D. Diverticular disease

   1. General considerations. Colonic diverticula are **false diverticula** in which mucosa and submucosa protrude through the muscularis propria. This occurs at the mesenteric side of the antimesenteric taenia, where arterioles penetrate the muscularis. The **sigmoid colon** is most commonly affected, perhaps owing to decreased luminal diameter and increased luminal pressure. Diverticula are associated with a low-fiber diet and are rare before age 30 years (<2%), but the **incidence increases with age** to a 75% prevalence after age 80.

2. **Complications**
   a. **Infection (diverticulitis).** Microperforations can develop in long-standing diverticula, leading to fecal extravasation and subsequent peridiverticulitis.

   (1) **Presentation** is notable for left lower quadrant pain (which may radiate to the suprapubic area, left groin, or back), fever, altered bowel habit, and urinary urgency. Physical examination varies with severity of the disease, but the most common finding is localized left lower quadrant tenderness. The finding of a mass suggests an abscess or phlegmon.

   (2) **Evaluation** by a computed tomographic (CT) scan and complete blood count (CBC) is the standard of care. CT visualizes thickened bowel wall as well as abscess formation, which may be drained percutaneously under CT guidance. Neither sigmoidoscopy nor contrast enema is recommended in the initial workup of diverticulitis, owing to the risk of perforation or barium or fecal peritonitis, respectively.

   (3) **Treatment** is tailored to symptom severity.
      (a) **Mild diverticulitis** can be treated on an outpatient basis with a clear liquid diet and broad-spectrum oral antibiotics for 7 to 10 days.
      (b) **Severe diverticulitis** is treated on an inpatient basis, with complete bowel rest, intravenous fluids, narcotic analgesia using meperidine, and broad-spectrum parenteral antibiotics. If symptoms improve within 48 hours, a clear liquid diet is resumed, and antibiotics are given orally when the fever and leukocytosis resolve. A high-fiber diet is resumed after 1 week of pain-free tolerance of a liquid diet. Fiber supplements and stool softeners should be given to prevent constipation. A colonoscopy or water-soluble contrast study must be performed after 4 to 6 weeks to rule out colon cancer, inflammatory bowel disease, or ischemia as a cause of the segmental inflammatory mass. If resection is planned after a particularly severe, complicated initial attack of diverticulitis (abscess requiring drainage, fistula formation) or recurrent diverticulitis, clear liquids and/or parenteral nutritional supplementation are used for 2 to 3 weeks until operation to allow for a one-stage procedure.

   (4) The lifetime likelihood of **recurrence** is 30% after the first episode and more than 50% after the second episode of diverticulitis. Therefore, **resection** is considered 4 to 6 weeks after treatment of a complicated initial attack of diverticulitis or after treatment of the first recurrence if the condition of the patient permits.

   (5) **Elective resection** for diverticulitis usually consists of a sigmoid colectomy. The proximal resection margin is through uninflamed, nonthickened bowel, but there is no need to resect all diverticula in the colon. The distal margin extends distal to normal, pliable rectum, even if this means dissection beyond the anterior peritoneal reflection. Recurrent diverticulitis after resection is most frequently related to inadequate distal margin of resection.

   b. **Generalized peritonitis** is rare and results if diverticular perforation leads to widespread fecal contamination. Patients present with diffuse severe abdominal pain with voluntary and involuntary guarding; they require emergent laparotomy. In most cases, resection of the diseased segment is possible (**two-stage procedure**), and a Hartmann procedure is performed. The colostomy can then be taken down at a separate operation in the future. Colostomy closure is not a trivial procedure and has rates of morbidity of 20% to 30% (bleeding, anastomotic leak, abscess) and of mortality of 2% to 3%. An alternative in the management of the stable patient undergoing urgent operation for acute diverticulitis without significant fecal contamination or sigmoid stricture due to chronic diverticulitis is sigmoidectomy, on-table colonic lavage, and colorectal anastomosis with or without proximal fecal diversion (loop ileostomy).

c. **Diverticular abscess** is usually identified on CT scan. A **percutaneous drain** should be placed under **radiologic guidance**. This avoids immediate operative drainage, allows time for the inflammatory phlegmon to be treated with intravenous antibiotics, and turns a two- or three-stage procedure into a one-stage procedure. A low pelvic abscess may be drained into the rectum via a transanal approach.

d. **Fistulization** may occur between the colon and other organs, including the bladder, vagina, small intestine, and skin, owing to diverticulitis. Diverticulitis is the most common cause of enterovesical fistulas, which are more common in men. Colovaginal and colovesical fistulas usually occur in women who have previously undergone hysterectomy. Colocutaneous fistulas are uncommon and are usually easy to identify. Coloenteric fistulas are likewise uncommon and may be entirely asymptomatic or result in corrosive diarrhea.

(1) **The presentation of enterovesical fistula** involves frequent **urinary tract infections** and often is unsuspected until **fecaluria** or **pneumaturia** is noted. The best confirmatory test is CT scan, which reveals air in the uninstrumented bladder. Lower endoscopy, barium enema, intravenous pyelography, and cystoscopy often fail to demonstrate the fistula. A colovaginal fistula is usually suspected based on the passage of air or gas per vagina. The fistula may be difficult to identify on physical examination or the previously mentioned tests. Both fistulas may be identified by the ingestion of charcoal and the presence of charcoal in the urine or on a tampon inserted into the vagina. A Hypaque vaginogram is useful to confirm sigmoid colon involvement.

(2) **Immediate treatment** of the inflammatory mass adjacent to the bladder is as previously described for severe diverticulitis [Section II.D.2.a(3)(b)]. Colonoscopy is performed after 4 to 6 weeks to rule out other possible etiologies, including cancer or inflammatory bowel disease. After several weeks of antibiotics, sigmoid resection is performed after preoperative placement of temporary ureteral catheters. Ureteral catheters can be very helpful in identifying the distal ureter in the inflammatory pericolonic mass, thereby shortening the operative time, and in identifying ureteral injuries. Usually, the fistula tract can be broken using finger fracture, and the bladder defect does not typically require repair. A Foley catheter is left in place for 7 to 10 days to allow this defect to heal. A colovaginal fistula is managed in a similar fashion. It may be helpful to interpose omentum between the colorectal anastomosis and the bladder or vaginal defect.

E. **Acquired vascular abnormalities and lower gastrointestinal (GI) bleeding** are more common in elderly patients than in younger individuals. Most cases of massive lower GI hemorrhage stop spontaneously, but surgery is required in 10% to 25% of cases.

1. **Diverticulosis.** The media of the perforating artery adjacent to which the colonic diverticula protrude may become attenuated. If this erodes at the neck or dome of a diverticulum, massive intraluminal bleeding can result. This arterial bleeding usually is bright red and is not associated with previous melena or chronic blood loss. Bleeding most commonly

occurs from the left colon. Urgent resection of the affected colonic segment should be considered in patients with active ongoing bleeding (>6 units packed RBCs per 24 hours). Elective resection of the affected colonic segment should be performed in patients with recurrent bleeding or in those in whom recurrent bleeding may be poorly tolerated.

2. **Angiodysplasias** are small arteriovenous fistulas resulting from mucosal venule dilation followed by precapillary sphincter incompetence. They rarely occur before age 40 years and are more common in the right colon (80%). Diagnosis can be made by colonoscopy or angiographic features (early filling of a dilated venule).

3. **Massive lower GI bleeding** is defined as hemorrhage distal to the ligament of Treitz that requires more than 3 units of blood in 24 hours. **Management** consists of simultaneously restoring intravascular volume and identifying the site of bleeding so that treatment may be instituted.

   a. **Resuscitation** is performed using a combination of isotonic crystalloid solutions and packed RBCs as needed.

   b. **Diagnosing the site of bleeding** is more important initially than identifying the cause. A nasogastric tube must be placed to rule out an upper GI source of bleeding. Return of bilious fluid effectively eliminates an upper GI source. Proctoscopy is helpful for ruling out anorectal causes of bleeding. The choice of localizing study depends on the estimate of bleeding rate.

      (1) **Nuclear scan** using technetium-99m sulfur colloid or tagged RBCs can identify bleeding sources with rates in excess of 0.5 to 1.0 mL per minute. Tagged RBC scan can identify bleeding up to 24 hours after isotope injection, which may be important in patients who bleed intermittently. Although these scans can accurately demonstrate ongoing bleeding, they do not definitively identify the anatomic source of bleeding; hence, planning a segmental gastrointestinal resection based on this study is not entirely reliable. A rapidly positive scan indicates that angiography has a high likelihood of identifying the source, and immediate plans should be made to proceed with this study.

      (2) **Mesenteric angiography** should be performed in the patient with a positive nuclear medicine bleeding scan with massive lower GI bleeding to definitively identify the anatomic source of bleeding. Angiography can localize bleeding exceeding 1.0 mL per minute and allows either therapeutic vasopressin infusion (0.2 units per minute) or embolization, which together are successful in stopping the bleeding in 85% of cases. The advantage is that this can convert an emergent operation in an unstable patient with unprepared bowel to an elective one-stage procedure. Provocative angiography may also be useful in the patient with recurrent bleeding without a localized source. It is performed by administration of heparin to induce bleeding, followed by mesenteric angiography to localize the source. It is an infrequently performed procedure in selected patients with recurrent massive lower GI bleeding.

      (3) **Colonoscopy** is not effective when there are high rates of bleeding because of poor visualization and higher complication rates. With slower bleeding after the administration of an adequate bowel preparation over 2 hours, colonoscopy offers the therapeutic advantages of injecting vasoconstrictive agents (epinephrine), vasodestructive agents (alcohol, morrhuate, sodium tetradecyl sulfate), or thermal therapy (laser photocoagulation, electrocoagulation, heater probe coagulation) to control bleeding.

      (4) In the rare **patients who continue to bleed with no source identified**, laparotomy should be considered. Intraoperative small-bowel enteroscopy may be performed if the source is not obvious at the time of exploration. If the source is still not identified, **total**

colectomy with ileorectostomy or end ileostomy is performed. This is associated with an incidence of recurrent bleeding of less than 10%, but the mortality rate for patients who rebleed is 20% to 40%. It is now rare for a patient to undergo resection for lower GI bleeding without a localized source.

4. **Ischemic colitis** results from many causes, including venous or arterial thrombosis, embolization, iatrogenic ligation after abdominal aortic aneurysm repair, thromboangiitis obliterans, and polyarteritis nodosa. It is idiopathic in the majority of patients. Patients are usually elderly and present with low abdominal pain localizing to the left and melena or hematochezia. The rectum often is normal on proctoscopy, owing to its dual vascular supply. Contrast enema may show thumbprinting that corresponds to submucosal hemorrhage and edema. Diagnosis depends on the state of the mucosa on colonoscopy. Disease is present most frequently at the watershed areas of the splenic flexure and sigmoid colon (although it may occur anywhere in the colon). Once the diagnosis is made, bowel rest is instituted. In the presence of bowel necrosis or peritonitis, emergent resection is recommended, usually with proximal fecal diversion. Patients without peritonitis or free air and with fever or an elevated white blood cell count may be treated with bowel rest, close observation, and intravenous antibiotics. Repeat colonoscopy after 2 to 5 days or if there is a change in symptoms is helpful. Patients may develop focal colonic strictures in the future, particularly if the ischemic episode was severe. The strictures typically present in the descending colon and must be differentiated from a neoplastic process. Segmental resection with anastomosis is curative.

5. **Radiation proctocolitis** results from pelvic irradiation for uterine, cervical, bladder, prostate, or rectal cancers. Risk factors include dose >6,000 centigray (cGy), vascular disease, diabetes mellitus, hypertension, and advanced age. The early phase occurs within days to weeks; mucosal injury, edema, and ulceration develop, with associated nausea, vomiting, diarrhea, and tenesmus. The late phase occurs within weeks to years, is associated with tenesmus and hematochezia, and consists of arteriolitis and thrombosis, with subsequent bowel thickening and fibrosis. Ulceration with bleeding, stricture, and fistula formation may occur. Medical treatment may be successful in mild cases, with the use of stool softeners, steroid enemas, and topical 5-aminosalicylic acid products. Application of 4% formalin to affected mucosa may be efficacious if these measures fail in patients with transfusion-dependent rectal bleeding. With stricture or fistula, thorough evaluation is required to rule out locally recurrent disease or primary neoplasm. Strictures may be treated by endoscopic dilation but often recur. Surgical treatment consists of a diverting colostomy and is reserved for medical failures, recurrent strictures, and fistulas. Proctectomy is rarely required and is usually associated with unacceptable morbidity and mortality.

III. **Dysfunction of the anorectum**
   A. **Normal anorectal function**
      1. The **rectum functions as a capacitance organ**, holding 650 to 1,200 mL, whereas daily stool output is 250 to 750 mL.
      2. The **anal sphincter mechanism** allows defecation and continence. The internal sphincter (involuntary) accounts for 80% of resting pressure, whereas the external sphincter (voluntary) accounts for 20% of resting pressure and 100% of squeeze pressure. The internal anal sphincter relaxes periodically to sample rectal contents but is contracted at rest. The puborectalis muscle is contracted at rest and relaxes only during defecation. The external anal sphincter contracts in response to stimulation indicating the presence of stool in the rectum and relaxes during defecation.

3. **Defecation** has four components: (1) mass movement of feces into the rectal vault; (2) rectal-anal inhibitory reflex, wherein distal rectal distention causes involuntary relaxation of the internal sphincter; (3) voluntary relaxation of the external sphincter mechanism and puborectalis muscle; and (4) increased intra-abdominal pressure.

4. **Continence** requires normal capacitance, normal sensation at the transition zone above the dentate line, puborectalis function for solid stool, external sphincter function for fine control, and internal sphincter function for resting pressure. The puborectalis maintains the anorectal angle, and contraction prevents solid-stool passage.

B. **Incontinence** is the inability to prevent elimination of rectal contents.

1. **Etiologies** include (1) **mechanical defects,** such as sphincter damage from obstetric trauma, treatment of abscess or fistula by fistulotomy through a significant portion of the external sphincter in the anterior quadrant, and scleroderma affecting the external sphincter; (2) **neurogenic defects,** including spinal cord injuries, pudendal nerve injury due to birth trauma or lifelong straining, and systemic neuropathies such as multiple sclerosis; and (3) **stool content–related causes,** such as diarrhea and radiation proctitis.

2. **Evaluation** includes visual and digital examination observing for gross tone or squeeze abnormalities. **Anal manometry** quantitatively measures parameters of anal function, including resting and squeeze pressure, sphincter length, and minimal sensory volume of the rectum. **Electromyography** can be used to determine innervation abnormalities but has been supplanted by a combination of anorectal manometry, pudendal nerve latency testing, and endoanal ultrasound.

3. **Treatment** depends on the type and severity of the defect. Minor **mechanical anal sphincter defects** are treated using dietary fiber to increase stool bulk and biofeedback. Major anal sphincter defects require anal sphincter reconstruction in which the external sphincter is circularized and the perineal body is reconstructed using the overlapping muscle repair. Artificial anal sphincters may be used in patients without a reconstructible native anal sphincter. **Neurogenic defects** may be managed with biofeedback in mild cases. Severe denervations of an intact anal sphincter may be managed with sacral nerve stimulation or artificial sphincters.

C. **Obstructed defecation** (pelvic floor outlet obstruction) presents with symptoms of chronic constipation and straining with bowel movements.

1. **Physiologic evaluation** includes (1) **defecography** to evaluate maintenance of fixation of the posterior rectum to the sacrum as well as relaxation of the puborectalis and (2) **colonic transit study** to distinguish colonic inertia from anorectal malfunction.

2. **Anal stenosis** is a rare cause of obstructed defecation and presents with frequent thin stools and bloating. The most common etiologies include scarring after anorectal surgery (rare), chronic laxative abuse, radiation, recurrent anal ulcer, Crohn's disease, and trauma. Initial treatment is anal dilation, although advanced cases are treated with advancement flaps of normal perianal skin.

3. **Pelvic floor abnormalities**
   a. **Nonrelaxation of puborectalis** results in straining and incomplete evacuation. Diagnosis requires a normal colonic transit time and persistent puborectalis distortion on defecography. Biofeedback is the treatment of choice.
   b. **Internal intussusception** (see section III.D.1).
   c. **Problems associated with obstructed defecation** include **fecal impaction** and **stercoral ulcer** (mucosal ulceration due to pressure necrosis from impacted stool), which is treated with enemas, increased fiber, and stool softeners. **Descending perineum syndrome**

occurs when chronic straining causes pudendal nerve stretch and subsequent neurogenic defect. **Rectocele** results from a weak, distorted rectovaginal septum that allows the anterior rectal wall to bulge into the vagina. Attempts at correction of any of these conditions without addressing the underlying pathology are doomed to failure.

  D. Abnormal rectal fixation, which occurs in varying degrees, leads to internal or external prolapse of the full thickness of the rectum.

    1. Internal intussusception (internal rectal prolapse) presents with mucous discharge, hematochezia, tenesmus, and constipation. Proctoscopy is performed and can demonstrate a **solitary rectal ulcer** at the lead point of the internal prolapse. **Treatment** initially is increased bulk, stool softeners, and glycerin suppositories. **Indications for surgery** are chronic bleeding, impending incontinence, and lifestyle-changing symptoms. Surgical options are controversial. The most frequent procedure is transabdominal rectopexy (suture fixation of the rectum to the presacral fascia) and anterior resection of the sigmoid colon if constipation is prominent among the patient's complaints.

    2. External rectal prolapse is protrusion of full-thickness rectum through the anus. Symptoms include pain, bleeding, mucous discharge, and incontinence. Examination shows a prolapsed mass with concentric mucosal rings, in distinction from prolapsed hemorrhoids (rectal mucosal prolapse), with which they may be confused but which show deep radial grooves. **Risk factors** include increased age, female gender, institutionalization, antipsychotic medication, previous hysterectomy, and spinal cord injury. **Evaluation includes barium enema or colonoscopy** to rule out malignancy and **manometry and electromyography** to determine sphincter function. With a **normal sphincter**, the surgical strategy is to shorten the redundant rectosigmoid colon and reestablish posterior sacral attachment. In patients able to tolerate a general anesthetic and abdominal exploration, the procedure of choice is sigmoid resection and rectopexy. The lowest recurrence rates (7% to 8%) are obtained with transabdominal rectopexy with or without an anterior resection of the sigmoid colon (Goldberg-Frykman procedure). **Incontinent patients** regain continence in 60% to 70% of cases, and final continence may not be evident for up to a year after surgical correction of the prolapse. Patients unable to withstand a general anesthetic or major abdominal procedure may be managed with a perineal proctectomy (modified Altemeier procedure). In order for this procedure to be accomplished, there must be complete eversion of the distal rectum and anal canal. Although very well tolerated by the patient, it has a higher recurrence rate (~20%). This is also an attractive procedure for the rare young man with external rectal prolapse in whom potency is a concern.

  E. Hemorrhoids are vascular and connective tissue cushions that exist in three columns in the anal canal: right anterolateral, right posterolateral, and left lateral. **Internal hemorrhoids** are above the dentate line and thus covered with mucosa. These may bleed and prolapse, but they do not cause pain. **External hemorrhoids** are below the dentate line and covered with anoderm. These do not bleed but may thrombose, which causes pain and itching, and secondary scarring may lead to skin tag formation. Hard stools, prolonged straining, increased abdominal pressure, and prolonged lack of support to the pelvic floor all contribute to the abnormal enlargement of hemorrhoidal tissue.

    1. Internal hemorrhoids are **graded** as first degree (bleed only), second degree (bleed and prolapse but reduce spontaneously), third degree (bleed and prolapse and require manual reduction), and fourth degree (bleed and are fixed externally). Incarcerated-strangulated third- or fourth-degree hemorrhoids constitute an indication for urgent operation if accompanied by fever and elevated white blood cell (WBC) count.

2. **Treatment** is medical for first-degree and most second-degree hemorrhoids. It includes increased dietary fiber and water, stool softeners, and avoidance of straining during defecation. **Refractory second- and third-degree hemorrhoids** may be treated in the office by elastic ligation. The ligation must be 1 to 2 cm above the dentate line and be kept away from the anoderm to avoid pain and infection. One quadrant is ligated every 2 weeks in the office, and the patient is warned that the necrotic hemorrhoid may slough in 7 to 10 days, with bleeding noted at that time. Aspirin or other nonsteroidal anti-inflammatory drugs taken during this postoperative period increase the risk of bleeding with sloughing. Patients on anticoagulation should be treated with excisional hemorrhoidectomy instead of elastic ligation (see following section). Severe sepsis may occur after banding in immunocompromised patients or those who have had full-thickness rectal prolapse ligated by mistake. Patients present with severe pain, fever, and urinary retention within 12 hours of ligation. Patients with this life-threatening disorder should undergo examination under anesthesia, immediate removal of rubber bands, and débridement of any necrotic tissue, accompanied by broad-spectrum intravenous antibiotics.

3. **Excisional hemorrhoidectomy** is reserved for large third- and fourth-degree hemorrhoids, mixed internal and external hemorrhoids, and thrombosed, incarcerated hemorrhoids with impending gangrene. The procedure is performed with the patient in the **prone flexed position**, and the resulting elliptical defects are closed. Complications include a 10% to 50% incidence of urinary retention, bleeding, infection, sphincter injury, and anal stenosis from taking too much mucosa at the dentate line.

4. **Stapled hemorrhoidectomy** is an alternative to traditional excisional hemorrhoidectomy for large prolapsing, bleeding third-degree hemorrhoids with minimal external disease. This procedure is performed by a circumferential excision of redundant rectal mucosa approximately 5 cm superior to the dentate line using a specially designed circular stapler. Preliminary results have shown a decrease in postoperative pain and a quicker return to normal activity.

5. **Acutely thrombosed external hemorrhoids** are treated by excision outside the mucocutaneous junction, which can be done in the office or emergency room with the wound left open. If the thrombosis is more than 48 hours old, the patient is treated with nonsurgical management.

F. **Anal fissure** is a split in the anoderm. Ninety percent of anal fissures occur posteriorly, and 10% occur anteriorly. Symptoms include tearing pain with defecation (which lasts for hours afterward) and blood, usually on the toilet paper. Manometry and digital rectal examination demonstrate increased sphincter tone and muscular hypertrophy in the distal one-third of the internal sphincter. Repeated tearing results in a chronic anal ulcer that usually is accompanied by an external skin tag. Differential diagnosis includes Crohn's disease (often in the lateral location), tuberculosis, anal cancer, abscess or fistula, cytomegalovirus, herpes simplex virus, chlamydia, and syphilis. **Ninety percent heal with medical treatment** that includes increased fiber, steroid suppositories, stool softeners, and sitz baths. Topical nifedipine ointment (0.2%) has also been shown to promote healing. If surgery is required, lateral internal anal sphincterotomy is 90% successful. Recurrence and minor incontinence occur in fewer than 10% of patients.

INFECTIONS

I. **Colitis**

A. **Pseudomembranous colitis** is an acute diarrheal illness resulting from toxins produced by overgrowth of *C. difficile* after antibiotic treatment (especially the use of clindamycin, ampicillin, or cephalosporins). Antibiotics already have been stopped in one-fourth of cases, and symptoms can occur up to 6 weeks after the cessation of antibiotic use. **Diagnosis** is made by measurement of toxin or culture of bacteria in one of at least three stool samples. Treatment begins with stopping the offending antibiotic, followed by oral or intravenous metronidazole. Oral (but not intravenous) vancomycin is an alternate, but more expensive, therapy. For severe cases in patients unable to take oral medications, vancomycin enemas may be useful. Recurrence after treatment is 20%, but this disease usually responds to retreatment. Rarely, pseudomembranous colitis presents with severe peritoneal irritation and colonic distention with **toxic megacolon** or **perforation**. Emergency laparotomy with total colectomy and end-ileostomy is required.

- **B. Amebic colitis** results from invasive infection by the protozoan *Entamoeba histolytica*, which is spread by the fecal-oral route. It is most commonly encountered in patients who have traveled abroad. The cecum usually is affected with small ulcers that may perforate or form an inflammatory mass or **ameboma**. **Diagnosis** is made by examining stool for ova and parasites, which is 90% sensitive in identifying the trophozoites. **Treatment** is oral metronidazole and iodoquinol. Surgical treatment is reserved for perforation or for ameboma refractory to treatment.

- **C. Actinomycosis** is an abdominal infection that most commonly occurs around the cecum after appendectomy owing to the anaerobic Gram-positive *Actinomyces israelii*. An inflammatory mass often is present with sinuses to the skin that can drain **sulfur granules**. **Diagnosis** is confirmed by anaerobic culture (the organism may take up to a week to isolate), and **surgical drainage** combined with penicillin or tetracycline is required.

- **D. Neutropenic enterocolitis** after chemotherapy occurs most commonly in the setting of acute myelogenous leukemia after cytosine arabinoside therapy. It is also seen frequently in patients undergoing chemotherapy for stage III or IV colon cancer. Patients present with abdominal pain, fever, bloody diarrhea, distention, and sepsis. The cecum often dilates, and there may be pneumatosis. **Initial treatment** includes bowel rest, total parenteral nutrition, granulocyte colony–stimulating factor (G-CSF), and broad-spectrum intravenous antibiotics. Laparotomy with total colectomy and ileostomy is required only if peritonitis develops. If further chemotherapy is required, elective right colectomy is considered.

- **E. Cytomegalovirus colitis** presents with bloody diarrhea, fever, and weight loss. It affects 10% of patients with acquired immunodeficiency syndrome (homosexuals are more commonly affected) and is the most common cause for emergent abdominal surgery in patients with acquired immunodeficiency syndrome. Ganciclovir is the treatment of choice; emergent colectomy with ileostomy is reserved for toxic megacolon.

II. Infection of the anorectum

- **A. Anorectal abscess**
  - **1. Cryptoglandular abscess** results from infection of the anal glands in the crypts at the dentate line. Because the glands penetrate the internal sphincter, the initial abscess is in the intersphincteric space. Then infection can spread (1) superficially into the external sphincter into the perianal space, (2) through the external sphincter into the ischiorectal space (which in turn may connect posteriorly via the deep postanal space, resulting in a horseshoe abscess), or (3) deep in the external sphincter into the supralevator space.
    - **a. Diagnosis** usually is obvious, with severe anal pain and a palpable, fluctuant mass. An intersphincteric abscess yields only a bulge in the rectal wall with no external manifestations.
    - **b. Treatment** is surgical drainage, with the skin incision kept close to the anal verge to avoid the possible creation of a long fistula tract. Intersphincteric abscesses are drained by an internal sphincterotomy

over the entire length of the abscess. Perianal and ischiorectal abscesses are drained through the perianal skin with a cruciate incision to keep the abscess unroofed. Antibiotic therapy is not necessary unless the patient (1) is immunocompromised, (2) is diabetic, (3) has extensive cellulitis, or (4) has valvular heart disease. Immunocompromised patients may present with anal pain without fluctuance because of the paucity of leukocytes. The painful indurated region must still be drained, and the underlying tissue must undergo biopsy and culture.

    c. Outcome from drainage alone shows that 50% of patients are cured and 50% develop a chronic fistula. We do not advocate fistulotomy at the initial operation because the internal opening may not be evident and a complicated fistulotomy may result in sphincter injury.

  2. Necrotizing anorectal infection (Fournier's gangrene) occurs rarely but can result in massive, life-threatening tissue destruction. Patients present with systemic toxicity and perianal pain. There may be crepitance and extensive necrosis under relatively normal skin. Synergistic flora (including clostridial and streptococcal species) of anorectal and urogenital origin may be involved. Immediate wide surgical débridement of all nonviable tissue and intravenous antibiotics are mandatory. Early treatment is critical, but mortality is still approximately 50%.

  3. Fistula in ano represents the chronic stage of cryptoglandular abscess but also may be due to trauma, Crohn's disease, tuberculosis, cancer, or radiation.

    a. Patients **present** with persistent purulent perianal drainage from the external and the internal openings of the fistula. The location of the internal opening along the dentate line is approximated by using **Goodsall's rule**: fistulas with external openings anterior to a transverse plane through the anal canal penetrate toward the dentate line in a radial direction, whereas fistulas posterior to that plane curve so that the internal opening is in the posterior midline. One exception consists of fistulas in which the anterior opening is more than 3 cm from the anal margin; these tend to have an internal opening in the posterior midline.

    b. Treatment is fistulotomy of the tract outside the external sphincter with curette or cauterization of the granulation in the fistula tract and healing by secondary intention. Posterior transsphincteric fistulas are incised if there is adequate puborectalis external to the tract. Horseshoe fistulas have a high recurrence rate and require bilateral counterdrainage with mushroom catheters and fistulotomy of the posterior tract. Anterior transsphincteric and high complicated fistulas involving the majority of the external sphincter cannot be incised. Soft, loose seton placement allows slow scarring of the fistula tract until a definitive advancement mucosal flap can be performed. We prefer primary drainage, with delayed repair using an endorectal advancement flap.

B. Rectovaginal fistula

  1. The **diagnosis** of rectovaginal fistula is suspected from a history of passing flatus or stool per vagina. Diagnosis is usually made via speculum or anoscopic examination, but occasionally administration of methylene blue enema, which can contaminate a vaginal tampon, is necessary.

  2. Classification and etiology depend on location. Low fistulas are due to obstetric injuries, foreign body penetration, or Crohn's disease. Midlevel fistulas are due to ischiorectal abscess, Crohn's disease, radiation, or surgical excision of an anterior rectal tumor. High fistulas are due to diverticulitis, operative injury, radiation, or Crohn's disease. Carcinoma of the rectum, cervix, or vagina may result in fistulas at any level.

  3. Treatment depends on the cause. Fistulas due to obstetric injury are observed for 3 months before operative repair is attempted. Low and midlevel fistulas are treated with endorectal advancement (sliding) flap after full mechanical and antibiotic bowel preparation. High fistulas are best treated transabdominally with resection of the affected segment of rectum or colon. Nonhealing fistulas are biopsied to rule out cancer. Operative repairs of fistulas due to radiation rarely heal and should not be undertaken because the tissue is permanently damaged. Advancement flaps for anal fistulas due to perineal Crohn's disease are often successful if the Crohn's disease is in remission.

C. **Pilonidal disease** occurs secondary to infection of a hair-containing sinus in the postsacral intergluteal fold 5 cm superior to the anus. Patients present with pain, swelling, and drainage when the sinuses become infected. The disease is most prevalent in men in the second and third decades of life. Symptoms are distinguished from perianal abscess by the lack of anal pain, the more superior location of the fluctuant mass, and the presence of midline cutaneous pits. Treatment is incision, drainage, and curettage, with allowance for secondary closure when the sinus is acutely inflamed. The disease tends to recur, however, and once the active inflammation has resolved, the sinus can be excised electively, with primary closure and a higher chance of cure.

D. **Hidradenitis suppurativa** is an infection of the apocrine sweat glands and mimics fistula in ano except that involvement is external to the anal verge. The treatment of choice is wide incision of the involved skin.

E. **Pruritus ani** is a common symptom of hemorrhoids, fissure, rectal prolapse, rectal polyp, anal warts, Bowen disease, and Paget disease. Treatment is directed toward resolution of the underlying cause. Failure to find an underlying cause should prompt investigation of dietary factors (e.g., coffee, alcohol). Children should be evaluated for pinworms, which, if found, are treated with piperazine citrate.

F. **Proctitis and anusitis** present as a bloody mucous discharge with tenesmus. They may be inflammatory, owing to ulcerative colitis or Crohn's disease, or secondary to radiation. Treatment includes increased dietary fiber, hydrocortisone suppositories, and antispasmodics such as belladonna and opium suppositories.

G. **Condyloma acuminatum** is an anorectal and urogenital wart caused by infection with human papilloma virus. The disease is most commonly transmitted through anal intercourse and presents with visible perianal growth, often accompanied by pruritus, anal discharge, bleeding, and pain. Common treatments include topical trichloracetic acid, Aldara (imiquimod), or excision with electrocoagulation under local anesthesia. Smoke generated by coagulation contains viable organisms and must be completely evacuated. Anal canal warts must be destroyed at the same time as external warts.

INFLAMMATORY BOWEL DISEASE

I. **General considerations**

A. **Ulcerative colitis** is an inflammatory process limited to the colonic mucosa characterized by alterations in bowel function, most commonly bloody diarrhea with tenesmus. The disease always involves the rectum and may extend continuously to the proximal colon. Patients often have abdominal pain, fever, and weight loss, which correlate to the degree of intestinal inflammation. The disease has a male predominance. As the duration of the inflammation increases, pathologic changes progress. Initially, mucosal ulcers and crypt abscesses are seen. Later, mucosal edema and pseudopolyps (islands of normal mucosa surrounded by deep ulcers) develop, and the end-stage pathologic changes show a flattened, dysplastic mucosa. The lumen is normal in diameter.

B. **Crohn's disease** is a transmural inflammatory process that can affect any area of the GI tract from the mouth to the anus. The disease has a segmental distribution, with areas of normal mucosa interspersed between affected areas of bowel. Common symptoms include diarrhea, abdominal pain, nausea and vomiting, weight loss, and fever. There can be signs of an abdominal mass or of perianal fistulas on physical examination. The disease has a female predominance. Common pathologic changes include fissures and fistulas, transmural inflammation, and granulomas. Grossly, the mucosa shows aphthoid ulcers that often deepen over time and are associated with fat wrapping and bowel wall thickening. As this progresses, the bowel lumen narrows, and obstruction or perforation may result.

C. **"Indeterminate colitis"** is a term used for cases in which the pathologic pattern does not fall clearly into one or the other of the aforementioned patterns. The indeterminacy can be due either to inadequate tissue biopsy or to a truly indeterminate form of disease.

D. **Extraintestinal manifestations** of inflammatory bowel disease are common with ulcerative colitis and with Crohn's disease. Musculoskeletal, skin, eye, blood, and hepatic abnormalities predominate.

E. In the **chronic phase of inflammatory bowel disease**, pathologic patterns of ulcerative colitis differ from those of Crohn's disease. Ulcerative colitis shows dry granular mucosa, which may harbor severe dysplasia or malignancy. In Crohn's disease, there is bowel wall scarring and loss of reservoir function. The mucosa is less involved.

II. **Ulcerative colitis**
A. **Indications for surgery**
1. **Active disease is unresponsive to medical treatment.** Failure to wean from high-dose steroids after two successive tapers prompts evaluation for surgery.
2. The **risk of malignancy** is related to the extent and duration of the disease but not the intensity of the disease. The risk increases by 1% per year after 10 years of disease. Colonoscopy is performed 7 to 10 years after the diagnosis and every 1 to 2 years thereafter, with random biopsies every 10 cm and directed biopsies of mass lesions. If dysplasia is found, resection is recommended.
3. **Severe bleeding** that does not respond adequately to medical therapy requires resection for control.
4. **Acute severe fulminate colitis** (WBC >16K, fever, abdominal pain, and distention) initially is treated with bowel rest, antibiotics, steroids, and avoidance of contrast enemas, antidiarrheals, and morphine. If the patient develops worsening sepsis or peritonitis, abdominal colectomy is performed.

B. **Surgical management** aims at removing the colorectal mucosa while maintaining bowel function as much as possible. Because the disease is localized to the rectum and colon, curative resection is possible. Sphincter-sparing procedures are preferred because they preserve the functions of continence and defecation. However, they are associated with higher postoperative complication risk. Anal sphincter function is assessed with manometry to ensure normal function before contemplation of a sphincter-sparing procedure in a patient medically able to undergo the operation.
1. **Restorative proctocolectomy (ileal pouch–anal anastomosis)** maintains fecal stream through the anal sphincter mechanism and is the operation of choice in most patients. A total proctocolectomy is carried out to the anal transition zone. At this point, the rectum may be transected, leaving the sphincters and levators intact. A distal ileal pouch is constructed over a distance of 15 cm in a J configuration, pulled through the sphincters, and stapled or sutured to the rectal cuff. A stapled anastomosis leaving a 2-cm cuff of anal canal mucosa technically is easier but requires long-term surveillance of the residual mucosa. A protecting loop ileostomy is constructed and is taken down 3 months later, after healing of the distal anastomosis. **Complications** include increased stool frequency (five to seven times daily), nocturnal soiling (20%), pouch fistula

(10%), and pouchitis (28%), an intermittent inflammatory process that typically responds to metronidazole. Pouch capacity increases over time, and eventually the need to empty the pouch may be decreased to an average of four to five times daily. The pouch procedure can be performed laparoscopically.

2. **Total proctocolectomy and end ileostomy** is performed in patients who have perioperative sphincter dysfunction or incontinence and in high-risk patients who would not tolerate potential postoperative complications. Most patients do well with a well-placed **Brook ileostomy** that has a spigot configuration and empties into a bag appliance in an uncontrolled fashion. A **Kock pouch** or continent ileostomy does not empty spontaneously, does not require a permanent appliance, and requires cannulation six to eight times daily. These are more difficult to construct and prone to obstruction. This alternative is occasionally offered to patients who desire continence or who have severe skin allergies, which make ileostomy appliances problematic.

III. **Crohn's disease** is a chronic disease that is not surgically curable. Surgery should therefore be performed only for complications of the disease, with foreknowledge that recurrence is common and that the disease is segmental in nature. Complications of acute disease include perforation, fistulas, and phlegmon. Chronic disease results in a fibrotic phase in which strictures may form. When a patient presents with a complication requiring surgery, all attempts should be made to prepare the patient so that a single operation will suffice. With complications of acute disease, this may require bowel rest with total parenteral nutrition, antibiotics, anti-inflammatory medications, and, when indicated, percutaneous drainage of abscesses.

A. **Surgical management** of Crohn's disease involves resection of the diseased segment of intestine responsible for the complications requiring surgery. Resection is bounded by grossly normal margins; no attempt is made to obtain microscopically negative margins because outcome and recurrence are unaffected by this. If significant intra-abdominal infection or inflammation is encountered during surgery, a proximal ostomy is created to allow complete diversion of intestinal contents and resolution of the initial process. If no infection or inflammation is encountered, normal-appearing bowel can be primarily anastomosed. The surgical principle is to remove the diseased segment and preserve as much functional intestine as possible.

B. **Small-intestinal Crohn's disease** is covered in Chapter 13.

C. **Colonic Crohn's disease** often requires operation after a shorter duration of symptoms than is typical for patients with either small-intestinal or ileocolic Crohn's disease. Perforation can occur without dilation of the colon, secondary to thickening of the colonic wall. Surgical options include total abdominal colectomy with ileorectal anastomosis (which may be protected by a proximal loop ileostomy), total abdominal colectomy with an end ileostomy and maintenance of the rectum as a Hartmann pouch, or total proctocolectomy with permanent end ileostomy. Rarely, colonic strictures can occur in an isolated segment, causing obstruction. Segmental resection should then be considered. Stricturoplasty to salvage part of the colon should be avoided because the colon has no critical physiologic function.

D. **Rectal Crohn's disease** rarely occurs in isolation. Once the rectum has become so fibrotic that it loses its reservoir capacity, proctectomy should be considered. Precise intersphincteric dissection along the rectal wall should minimize complications in comparison with patients treated for rectal cancer, in which surrounding tissue must be included in the resection specimen.

E. **Anal disease** occurs in 35% of patients with Crohn's disease. Conservative therapy with anti-inflammatory agents, immunosuppressive agents, and metronidazole is the mainstay of treatment for anal Crohn's disease. Perianal sepsis should be controlled with local drainage. Proctectomy or diversion may eventually be the only way to return quality of life to the patient, but this should be the patient's decision.

F. Ileostomy construction
1. **Effluent from an ileostomy** is high-volume liquid and contains proteolytic enzymes. It is crucial to maintain a stoma appliance that protects the surrounding skin and seals to the base of the ileostomy.
2. **Stoma construction** of either a loop ileostomy or end ileostomy should include eversion of the functioning end to create a 2.5-cm spigot configuration. Precise apposition of mucosa and skin prevents serositis and obstruction.
3. **Ileostomy care** requires special attention to avoid dehydration and obstruction. The patient is encouraged to drink plenty of fluids and to use antidiarrheal agents as needed to decrease output volume. Patients should be warned to avoid fibrous foods, such as whole vegetables and citrus fruits, because these may form a bolus of indigestible solid matter that can obstruct the stoma. Irrigating the ostomy with 50 mL warm saline from a Foley catheter inserted beneath the fascia, in combination with intravenous fluids and nasogastric decompression, may relieve obstruction and dehydration. Alternatively, even if the obstruction is due to food blockage, water-soluble contrast enema may be diagnostic and therapeutic.

NEOPLASTIC DISEASE

I. The **etiology** of colorectal neoplasia has genetic and environmental components.
   A. **Familial cancer syndromes** account for 10% to 15% of colorectal cancers. The evaluation and treatment of these syndromes is discussed in Chapter 25.
   B. **Sporadic cancers** account for approximately 85% of colorectal neoplasia. Although no inherited genetic mutation can be identified, first-degree relatives of patients with colorectal cancer have a three- to ninefold increase in the risk of developing the disease. Overwhelming evidence suggests that colorectal carcinomas develop from precursor adenomas and are associated with an increasing number of genetic mutations. A single genetic mutation in the germ line of a patient may cause an adenoma to develop. Further mutation in either a tumor-suppressor gene or oncogene is responsible for further development of the adenoma and eventually transformation to neoplasia. Genes implicated in this journey from normal epithelium to carcinoma include *K-ras, DCC,* and *p53.*
   C. **Environmental factors** have also been proposed to play a significant role in the etiology of colorectal neoplasia. Dietary factors that have been shown to increase cancer risk include a diet high in unsaturated animal fats and highly saturated vegetable oils. Increased fiber decreases cancer risk in those on a high-fat diet. Epidemiologic studies indicate that people from less industrialized countries have a lower risk of colorectal cancer. This appears to be associated with a diet that is lower in processed foods and higher in natural fiber. This survival benefit disappears in people who immigrate to the United States.
   D. **Premalignant conditions.** The incidence of cancer in ulcerative colitis with pancolitis is 1% per year after 10 years or 10% after 20 years, and the risk of cancer being present when biopsies show dysplasia is 30%. The cancers tend to be more advanced (~35% are stage III or IV) when they present. Crohn's disease also has an increased cancer risk, which is as high as 7% at 20 years (although this risk might be primarily in patients who have excluded segments of bowel). There is a high cancer incidence at stricture sites, and biopsies are performed at the time of stricturoplasty. Squamous cell cancers and adenocarcinomas can develop in chronic fistula tracts.
II. **Detection. Surveillance** is the periodic complete examination of a patient with known increased risk. **Screening** is the limited examination of a population with the goal of detecting patients with increased risk.

A. Screening of the general population is of unproved cost-effectiveness. The American Cancer Society recommends yearly digital rectal examination and testing for fecal occult blood past age 40 years. Air-contrast barium enema with sigmoidoscopy or total colonoscopy should be offered to patients at the age of 50 years. These should be repeated every 10 years if normal or if the patient is not at high risk for colorectal neoplasia. Another screening algorithm calls for flexible sigmoidoscopy at age 50 years and repeat imaging every 3 to 5 years. Indications for colonoscopy in this algorithm are detection of fecal blood or polyp on sigmoidoscopy.

B. High-risk individuals should be in a surveillance program. Previous cancer or polypectomy increases the risk of metachronous cancer by a factor of 2.7 to 7.7. Routine surveillance has been shown to reduce the incidence of metachronous cancer, although its influence on survival is unknown. High-risk patients are those with (1) ulcerative colitis of more than 10 years' duration, (2) Crohn's disease with stricture, (3) a history or family history of polyps or cancer, or (4) a family history of adenomatous polyposis (FAP) or hereditary nonpolyposis colorectal cancer (HNPCC). Our surveillance algorithm calls for initial or perioperative colonoscopy followed by yearly examination until no lesions are detected, examination every 3 years until no lesions are detected, and then examination every 5 years.

III. Polyps

A. Nonadenomatous polyps

1. **Peutz-Jeghers syndrome** is an autosomal dominant condition characterized by hamartomatous polyps of smooth muscle throughout the GI tract and mucocutaneous pigmentation. It is associated with increased risk of malignancy in multiple organs and with a 2% to 13% incidence of GI malignancy. Symptoms include bleeding or obstruction secondary to intussusception. Treatment is polypectomy for polyps >1.5 cm in diameter. When symptomatic polyps require surgery, all polyps should be removed via intraoperative polypectomy and endoscopy. Surveillance colonoscopy and esophagogastroduodenoscopy (EGD) are recommended every 2 years as well as periodic screening for breast, cervical, testicular, ovarian, and pancreatic cancer.

2. **Juvenile polyps** are cystic dilations of glandular structures in the lamina propria without malignant potential that may result in bleeding or obstruction. There are two peaks in incidence of isolated juvenile polyps: in infants and at age 25 years. They are the most common cause of GI bleeding in children and should be treated with polypectomy. **Multiple polyposis coli** (diffuse juvenile polyps) is an autosomal dominant syndrome characterized by multiple juvenile polyps and increased risk for GI malignancy. These patients are considered for total abdominal colectomy or proctocolectomy with ileal pouch–anal anastomosis.

3. **Hyperplastic polyps** show epithelial dysmaturity and hyperplasia and are the most common colorectal neoplasm (10 times more common than adenoma). They have no malignant potential. Most are less than 0.5 cm in diameter and rarely need treatment.

B. Adenomas are benign neoplasms with unrestricted proliferation of glandular epithelium within the colonic mucosa but with no invasion of the basement membrane. It is generally accepted that adenomas are precursors to colorectal cancer in the majority of cases. The degree of differentiation decreases as a polyp becomes more like a cancer. *Severe atypia* refers to malignant cells in a polyp that have not invaded the muscularis mucosae (formerly known as *carcinoma in situ*). Adenomatous polyps fall into three broad categories.

1. **Tubular adenomas** are usually pedunculated and account for 65% to 80% of adenomas. They have a 5% risk of containing malignant cells.

2. **Tubulovillous adenomas** account for 10% to 25% of adenomas. They have a 22% risk of containing cancer.

3. **Villous adenomas** are usually sessile and account for 5% to 10% of adenomas. They have an increasing risk of containing cancer, a risk is influenced by size and palpable induration in the polyp. For example, a 4-cm sessile villous adenoma has a 40% risk of cancer and the same polyp with induration has a 90% risk.

C. **Treatment** consists of colonoscopic removal. Pedunculated polyps have a stalk of less than 1.5 cm and are removed using the cautery snare. Semisessile and sessile polyps have stalks or pedicles >1.5 cm and may require piecemeal extraction. The site of incomplete removal should be marked with 0.1 mL India ink for possible later intraoperative or repeat colonoscopic identification. For sessile or large polyps (>3 cm) that cannot be removed endoscopically, surgical resection is required.

   1. **The risk of metastatic cancer** in regional lymph nodes is 1% in a completely excised, pedunculated polyp in which cancer invades only the head of the polyp, unless there is lymphatic or vascular invasion. These cases may be treated with either colectomy or polypectomy with close follow-up. Invasion of the cancer down the stalk to the lower third requires colectomy.

   2. **Sessile polyps** containing cancer require colectomy, even if completely excised, because the risk of local recurrence and lymph node metastasis is greater than 10% to 20%.

   3. **Colonoscopic complications** include perforation and bleeding. Conservative therapy for perforation—close observation, intravenous antibiotics, and bowel rest—is possible if sepsis and peritonitis are absent. Otherwise, urgent laparotomy with colonic repair with or without proximal diversion (loop ileostomy) is required. An alternative is segmental colonic resection with primary anastomosis, especially attractive if the perforated segment harbors intraluminal pathology.

      Bleeding after colonoscopic polypectomy may be immediate or delayed 7 to 10 days. Angiography or colonoscopy is performed, depending on the rate of bleeding, followed by surgery if needed. Most post polypectomy bleeding abates spontaneously.

D. **Villous adenoma of the rectum** can present with watery diarrhea and hypokalemia. The risk of cancer in lesions >4 cm with induration is 90%, and transrectal ultrasonography should be used to determine the depth of invasion before excision. **Treatment** of favorable lesions is by transanal, full-thickness local excision followed by closure of the defect with suture. If the adenoma is large (>4cm), circumferential, invasive, or above the peritoneal reflection (generally 10 cm above the anal verge), a transabdominal proctectomy should be considered.

IV. **Colon cancer**

A. The **incidence** of colorectal cancer in the United States has been stable since the 1950s, with 131,000 new cases (94,000 colon and 37,000 rectal) each year and 58,000 deaths each year. It is the third most lethal cancer in men and women, with a slight female predominance in colon cancer and male predominance in rectal cancer. There is a 5% lifetime risk; 6% to 8% of cases occur before age 40 years, and the incidence increases steadily after age 50.

B. **Subacute presentation** of colon cancer depends on the location of the lesion. Many tumors are asymptomatic and discovered on routine screening colonoscopy. **Right colon** lesions occasionally cause hematochezia, but more often bleeding is occult, causing anemia and fatigue. **Left colon** lesions more often cause crampy abdominal pain, altered bowel habit, or hematochezia. Approximately 50% of patients with other symptoms complain of weight loss, but weight loss is almost never the sole manifestation of a colorectal tumor.

C. **Acute presentation.** Left colon cancer presents as large-bowel obstruction with inability to pass flatus or feces, abdominal pain, and distention in fewer than 10% of cases. Rarely, colon cancer presents as perforation with focal or diffuse peritonitis or as a fistula with pneumaturia or feculent vaginal discharge. These symptoms may be difficult to distinguish from those of diverticulitis. Metastatic disease is usually asymptomatic but may present with jaundice, pruritus, and ascites or with cough and hemoptysis.

D. **Diagnosis and staging**
   1. **Once the diagnosis is suspected based on history, physical examination, or screening tests**, every attempt should be made to obtain biopsy of the primary lesion and rule out synchronous cancer (3% to 5%). Colonoscopy to the cecum or flexible sigmoidoscopy and barium enema are acceptable. In patients presenting with obstructive symptoms, diagnosis is suggested on plain abdominal films, and water-soluble contrast is performed to assess the degree and level of obstruction.
   2. **Staging studies** to look for distant metastases include chest x-ray and abdominal CT scan. CT scan identifies liver metastases as well as adrenal, ovarian, pelvic, and lymph node metastases. Serum carcinoembryonic antigen (CEA) is a useful prognostic and surveillance tumor marker in colorectal cancer. CEA should be obtained preoperatively as part of the staging evaluation.

E. **Surgical treatment**
   1. **Bowel preparation** minimizes the titers of *E. coli* and *Bacteroides fragilis*, which are the primary sources of infection. Mechanical cleansing consists of Fleets Phospho-Soda (mono and dibasic sodium phosphate), which acts as a purgative when given in adequate volume (45 mL) and is accompanied by large volumes (24 oz) of clear liquids. Two doses are given, at 12 PM and at 6 PM, the day before surgery. Patients with cardiac or renal failure or severe hypertension on sodium restriction may have severe fluid and electrolyte abnormalities after administration of this mechanical bowel preparation. An alternate mechanical bowel preparation for these patients includes an isotonic lavage solution (GoLYTELY). Early on the preoperative day, 4 L is given orally within a 4-hour period, accompanied by a clear liquid diet. Broad-spectrum intravenous antibiotics are required to decrease the wound infection rate from 30% to less than 10%. In addition to a mechanical bowel preparation, some centers prefer a nonabsorbable oral antibiotic regimen with neomycin or erythromycin on the day before surgery.
   2. **Operative technique** begins with a thorough exploration that includes palpation of the liver. After mobilization of the involved segment, the main segmental vessels are then ligated and divided, and *en bloc* resection of colon and any adherent structure is carried out, including small bowel, ovaries, uterus, or kidney. If curative resection is not possible, palliative resection should be attempted, and if this cannot be done, bypass should be performed. For right colon cancer, resection includes the distal 10 cm of terminal ileum to the transverse colon, taking the ileocolic, right colic, and right branch of the middle colic vessels. A transverse colon lesion is resected with either an extended right colectomy or a transverse colectomy, taking only the middle colic vessels. Left colon lesions require dividing the inferior mesenteric artery (IMA) at its origin. If multiple carcinomas are present, or if a colon carcinoma with multiple neoplastic polyps is present, then a subtotal colectomy is performed. The specimen margin is inspected in the operating room to ensure at least a 2-cm margin (5 cm for poorly differentiated tumors). Laparoscopic colectomy is proving to be a safe and equally effective method for treating selected colon cancers (NEJM 2004;350:2050). If laparoscopic colectomy is performed, it should be guided by the same principles as a standard open colectomy.
   3. **Emergency operations** are undertaken without bowel preparation and have a higher incidence of wound infection. For obstruction, right

colectomy still can be performed with primary anastomosis and no diversion. Options with a left colon cancer include (1) resection with colostomy and either mucous fistula or Hartmann pouch, (2) resection with intraoperative lavage and primary anastomosis, (3) resection with primary anastomosis and proximal diverting ileostomy, (4) subtotal colectomy and ileosigmoidostomy, and (5) colostomy with staged resection of the tumor in an unstable patient with markedly dilated colon. In all but the subtotal colectomy, the proximal colon must be evaluated in the postoperative period for synchronous cancer.

F. Staging and prognosis. The American Joint Committee on Cancer TNM staging identifies the depth of invasion of the tumor (T), regional lymph node status (N), and presence of distant metastases (M). Stage I (T1 or T2, N0, M0) tumors do not involve the muscularis and have a 90% 5-year survival. Stage II (T3 or T4, N0, M0) tumors penetrate the muscularis and have a 60% to 80% 5-year survival. Stage III (Tx, N1 or N2, M0) tumors involve lymph nodes and have a 50% 5-year survival. Stage IV (Tx, Nx, M1) tumors have distant metastases and a 5-year survival of less than 5%. Unfavorable characteristics include poor differentiation, mucinous or signet-ring pathology, venous or perineural invasion, bowel perforation, aneuploid nuclei, and elevated CEA.

G. Adjuvant chemotherapy using 5-fluorouracil and leucovorin with oxaliplatin or irinotecan increases overall survival and disease-free survival in patients with stage III colon cancer. Chemotherapy has not been shown to offer a survival benefit to patients with stage II cancer, and adjuvant treatment in this population is controversial.

H. Follow-up is crucial in the first 2 years after surgery, when 90% of recurrences occur. Surveillance colonoscopy is recommended the first year after resection and then every 3 years until negative, at which time every 5 years is recommended. CEA should be checked in the first year, and rising levels should prompt a CT scan, a chest x-ray, and possibly a PET scan evaluation to detect recurrence. A PET scan allows differentiation of metabolically active tumor from scar tissue, which often appear similar on a CT scan.

V. Rectal cancer
  A. The **pathophysiology** of rectal cancer differs from that of colon cancer because of several anatomic factors: (1) confinement of pelvis and sphincters, making wide excision impossible; (2) proximity to urogenital structures and nerves, resulting in high levels of impotency in men; (3) dual blood supply and lymphatic drainage; and (4) transanal accessibility.
  B. Diagnosis and staging
    1. Local aspects. Digital rectal examination can give information on the size, fixation, ulceration, local invasion, and lymph node status. Rigid sigmoidoscopy and biopsy are crucial for precisely measuring the distance to the dentate line and for obtaining a tissue diagnosis. Flexible sigmoidoscopy cannot accurately assess the length of the tumor from the dentate line (which in turn determines the operative procedure to be performed) and so is not a useful diagnostic modality when staging rectal cancer. **Transrectal ultrasonography** is reasonably accurate in detecting the depth of invasion in rectal cancer and should be an integral part of the staging of rectal tumors. T1 lesions are limited to the mucosa and submucosa, T2 lesions are limited to the muscularis propria, T3 lesions penetrate the rectal wall, and T4 lesions invade adjacent structures. Transrectal ultrasonography is less accurate in detecting regional lymphadenopathy, but the negative predictive value is >90%.
    2. Regional aspects. Pelvic CT, MR scan, and transrectal ultrasound can yield information on the local extension of the tumor toward the bony pelvis. Pelvic examination is necessary to assess the possible fixation of the tumor to adjacent genitourinary structures. Cystoscopy may be required in some men to evaluate extension into the prostate or bladder.

3. **Distant spread** is evaluated (as with colon cancer) with chest x-ray, abdominal CT, and serum CEA. PET scanning is frequently helpful in identifying recurrent disease or disease outside of the liver or lung.

C. **Surgical treatment goals** are to remove cancer with adequate margins and perform an anastomosis only if there is good blood supply, absence of tension, and normal anal sphincters. If any of these conditions cannot be met, the entire rectum must be removed and the patient left with a permanent colostomy.

   1. **Bowel preparation** is the same as that for colon cancer.
   2. The **stoma sites on the abdominal wall should be marked** for possible colostomy on the left side or midline, avoiding bony prominences and scars and staying inside the rectus muscle at the summit of a fat fold. The right lower quadrant should also be marked in the event that a temporary loop ileostomy is necessary. Stoma sites should be marked even if the surgeon is anticipating performing an anastomosis.
   3. **Positioning and preparation.** If the patient has had previous pelvic surgery or the cancer is suspected to involve the bladder or ureter, ureteral stents should be placed after induction of anesthesia. The patient is placed in the dorsal lithotomy position, which gives access to the abdomen and perineum. A nasogastric tube, Foley catheter, and No. 34 French mushroom rectal catheter are placed, and the rectum is irrigated until clear with warm saline before instilling 100 mL povidone-iodine (Betadine).
   4. **Operative technique.** The patient's abdomen is explored through a midline incision. The left colon is mobilized using the embryonic fusion plane, reflecting the ureter and gonadal vessels laterally. The IMA is ligated at the aorta. The inferior mesenteric vein is ligated with the left colic artery or at the ligament of Treitz. The colon is transected at the descending and sigmoid junction with a purse-string suture, and an end-to-end anastomosis stapler anvil is placed in the proximal segment. Rectal dissection then proceeds posteriorly through the avascular presacral fascia, laterally through the vascular lateral ligaments, and finally anteriorly, with preservation of the seminal vesicles or vagina. Dissection continues distally well beyond the tumor so that transection allows at least a 2-cm distal margin and a full removal of the rectal mesentery transected at a right angle at the level of the distal intestinal margin.
   5. **Surgical options** at this point depend on the height of the lesion, the condition of the sphincters, and the condition of the patient. An abdominoperineal resection is performed for tumors that cannot be resected with a 2-cm distal margin or if sphincter function is questionable or destroyed. Low anterior resection using an intraluminal stapler is the operation of choice when technically possible for tumors that can be resected with an adequate distal margin. Hartmann resection is chosen if there is preoperative obstruction, sepsis, or intraoperative instability. Coloanal anastomosis with temporary proximal stoma may be elected in patients with benign neoplasms or carpet villous adenomas low in the rectum, for management of radiation-induced rectal injury, and for selected rectal cancers in the lower third of the rectum.
   6. **Complications**
      a. **Impotence** occurs in 50% of men and must be discussed preoperatively. The sites of nerve injury are the IMA origin, the presacral fascia, the lateral ligaments, and anteriorly at the level of the vagina and seminal vesicles. Prosthesis may be considered 1 year after surgery, once the pelvis is shown to be free of recurrence and the patient has had appropriate time to adapt to changes in body image.
      b. **Leakage** at the anastomosis occurs in up to 20% of patients, typically on postoperative days 4 to 7. Fever, elevated WBC count, increased or changed drain output, or abdominal pain during this period should

prompt in-depth physical examination and CT scan evaluation. Intravenous antibiotics and bowel rest are usually sufficient, but laparotomy and fecal diversion are necessary for large leaks.

    c. Massive presacral venous bleeding can occur at the time of resection. This is controlled either with a pledget of abdominal wall muscle sutured to the sacrum or by packing the pelvis for 24 to 48 hours.

7. Obstructive rectal cancer requires emergent laparotomy on an unprepared bowel. The type of procedure depends on whether presurgical adjuvant therapy is considered. A decompressing transverse colostomy can be made through a small upper midline incision. This may be a blowhole type if the colon is massively dilatated or it may be a loop colostomy over a rod. If preoperative radiotherapy is not given, options include Hartmann resection, total colectomy with ileorectostomy, and low anterior resection protected by proximal diversion.

8. Colostomy construction technique depends on whether the goal is decompression or diversion.

    a. A **decompressing colostomy** vents the distal and proximal bowel limbs while maintaining continuity between the limbs. A blowhole is used for massively dilated colon. The anterior wall of the transverse colon is sewn in two layers to the abdominal fascia and the skin. A loop colostomy is formed by bringing a loop of colon through the abdominal wall and suspending it on an ostomy rod. This colostomy also diverts for 6 weeks.

    b. Diverting colostomies, such as end colostomy and mucous fistula, are used for distal resection or perforation so that the distal limb is completely separated from the fecal stream. All colostomies are matured in the operating room. If a stoma rod is used, it is removed 1 week after surgery.

    c. Complications of colostomies include necrosis, stricture, and herniation. If the stoma becomes dusky, an anoscope is inserted. If necrosis does not extend below the fascia, it can be observed safely; otherwise, urgent revision is performed.

D. Adjuvant therapy for rectal cancer should routinely be considered because the overall 5-year survival rate for the disease is only 50% and the local recurrence rate is 20% to 30%.

1. Preoperative radiotherapy was shown to increase the 5-year survival rate and decrease local recurrences in all stages in a multicenter, prospective randomized trial and is now the standard of care (*N Engl J Med* 1997;336:980). Two dosage options that are biologically similar may be considered: (1) 2,000 cGy over 5 days preoperatively, followed by immediate operation, or (2) 4,500 cGy over 5 weeks, followed by a 7-week waiting period to allow for tumor shrinkage. Postoperative therapy has been advocated by some if the adequacy of the resection is in doubt and the patient did not receive preoperative radiotherapy. Postoperative radiotherapy is associated with a higher risk of complications, including injury to the small intestine and the colorectal anastomosis.

2. Neoadjuvant chemoradiation, including chemotherapy with a 5-fluorouracil–based regimen, results in a modest survival benefit and decreased local recurrence over radiation therapy alone in patients with stage II and stage III disease.

E. Nonresectional therapy is indicated in some early-stage cancers, patients with poor operative risk, and patients with widespread metastases. Options include transanal excision, electrocoagulation, endocavitary radiation, cryotherapy, and laser vaporization. Most recently, we have used combined external-beam and endocavitary radiation as the definitive treatment for favorable but invasive rectal cancers.

F. If the patient has **incurable cancer** and a life expectancy of less than 6 months, external beam radiation, with or without chemotherapy, combined with laser destruction, dilation, or stenting the rectum can prevent obstruction. If the life expectancy exceeds 6 months, resectional therapy is attempted.

G. The major cause of **locally recurrent rectal cancer** is a positive margin on the pelvic side wall (radial margin). Recurrences tend to occur within 18 months and grow back into the lumen, presenting with pelvic pain, mass, and rectal bleeding or a rising CEA level. Diagnosis is confirmed by examination and biopsy as well as CT or PET scan. Treatment is not highly satisfactory, and there is a 10% to 20% palliation rate. If chemoradiation has not been given previously, it is given at this point, and if distant metastases are again ruled out, low anterior resection, abdominoperineal resection, or pelvic exenteration (resection of rectum and urinary bladder) is performed based on whether the sphincters and the genitourinary organs are involved.

VI. Other colorectal tumors

A. Lymphoma is most often metastatic to the colorectum, but primary non-Hodgkin's colonic lymphoma accounts for 10% of all GI lymphomas. The GI tract is also a common site of non-Hodgkin's lymphoma associated with human immunodeficiency virus. The most common presenting symptoms include abdominal pain, altered bowel habit, weight loss, and hematochezia. Biopsies are often not diagnostic because the lesion is submucosal. The workup is similar to that for colon cancer but should include a bone marrow biopsy and a thorough search for other adenopathy. Treatment is resection with postoperative chemotherapy. Intestinal bypass, biopsy, and postoperative chemotherapy should be considered for locally advanced tumors.

B. Retrorectal tumors usually present with postural pain and a posterior rectal mass on physical examination and CT scan.
   1. The **differential diagnosis** includes congenital, neurogenic, osseous, and inflammatory masses.
   2. **Diagnosis** is suspected based on CT scan and physical findings. Biopsy should not be performed. Formal resection should be undertaken.

C. Carcinoid tumor
   1. **Colonic carcinoids** account for 2% of GI carcinoids. Lesions less than 2 cm in diameter rarely metastasize, but 80% of lesions >2 cm in diameter have local or distant metastases, with a median length of survival of less than 12 months. These lesions are treated with local excision if small and with formal resection if >2 cm.
   2. **Rectal carcinoid** accounts for 15% of GI carcinoids. As with colonic carcinoids, lesions less than 2 cm in diameter have low malignant potential and are well treated with transanal or endoscopic resection. Rectal carcinoids >2 cm in diameter are malignant in 90% of cases. Treatment of large rectal carcinoids is controversial, but low anterior resection or abdominoperineal resection is probably warranted.

VII. Anal neoplasms

A. Tumors of the anal margin
   1. **Squamous cell carcinoma** behaves like cutaneous squamous cell carcinoma, is well differentiated and keratinizing, and is treated with wide local excision and chemoradiation if large.
   2. **Basal cell carcinoma** is a rare, male-predominant cancer and is treated with local excision.
   3. **Bowen's disease** is intraepidermal squamous cell carcinoma. It is rare and usually slow growing. Treatment is wide local excision.

B. Anal canal tumors
   1. **Epidermoid carcinoma** is nonkeratinizing and derives from the anal canal up to 6 to 12 mm above the dentate line.
      a. **Epidermoid cancer** has a female predominance and usually presents with an indurated, bleeding mass. On examination, the inguinal lymph nodes should be examined specifically because spread below the dentate line passes to the inguinal nodes. Diagnosis is made by biopsy, and 30% to 40% are metastatic at the time of diagnosis.

b. Treatment involves chemoradiation following the **Nigro protocol**: 3,000-cGy external-beam radiation, mitomycin C, and 5-fluorouracil. Surgical treatment is reserved for locally persistent or recurrent disease only. The procedure of choice is abdominoperineal resection.

2. **Adenocarcinoma** is usually an extension of a low rectal cancer and has a poor prognosis.

3. **Melanoma** accounts for 1% to 3% of anal cancers and is more common in Caucasians in the 5th and 6th decades of life. Symptoms include bleeding, pain, and a mass, and the diagnosis is often confused with that of a thrombosed hemorrhoid. At the time of diagnosis, 38% of patients have metastases. Treatment is wide local excision, and the 5-year survival rate is less than 20%.

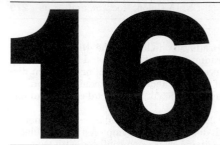

Pancreas

Nirmal K. Veeramachaneni
and David Linehan

I. **Acute pancreatitis**
   A. **Pathophysiology.** Acute pancreatitis is an inflammatory process of variable clinical severity in which the pancreatic injury ranges from mild edema to pancreatic and peripancreatic necrosis. Mechanisms of pathogenesis, which are not mutually exclusive, include the following:
      1. **Secretion** into an obstructed duct
      2. **Bile reflux** into the pancreatic duct
      3. **Duodenal reflux** into the pancreatic duct
      4. **Intracellular protease activation**
   B. **Causes.** Biliary disorder (gallstones) accounts for approximately 40% of cases, alcohol accounts for approximately 40%, and drugs (definite association: isoniazid, estrogens; probable association: thiazides, furosemide, sulfonamides, tetracycline, corticosteroids) account for approximately 5%. Iatrogenic causes, particularly endoscopic retrograde cholangiopancreatography (ERCP), may account for another 5% of cases. Other less common causes include scorpion stings, hypertriglyceridemia (especially types I and V), hypercholesterolemia, hypercalcemia, infectious diseases (mumps; orchitis; coxsackie virus B; Epstein-Barr virus; cytomegalovirus; rubella; hepatitis A, B, non-A, non-B; *Ascaris* species; and *Mycoplasma pneumoniae*), tumors, trauma, and idiopathic factors.
   C. **Diagnosis**
      1. **Clinical presentation.** Patients typically complain of upper abdominal pain, often radiating to the back. Tenderness is usually limited to the upper abdomen but may be associated with signs of diffuse peritonitis. Occasionally, irritation from intraperitoneal pancreatic enzymes results in impressive peritoneal signs, simulating other causes of an acute abdomen. Nausea, vomiting, and a low-grade fever are frequent, as are tachycardia and hypotension secondary to hypovolemia. Asymptomatic hypoxemia, renal failure, hypocalcemia, and hyperglycemia are evidence of severe systemic effects. Rarely, peripheral manifestations (e.g., subcutaneous fat necrosis or pancreatic arthritis) can be associated with acute pancreatitis. Subcutaneous fat necrosis is not necessarily associated with a worse prognosis, but when multiple sites are involved, mortality is high.
      2. **Laboratory studies**
         a. **Serum amylase** is the single most useful test. Levels rise within 2 to 12 hours of symptoms and may return to normal over the following 2 to 5 days. Persistent elevations of levels for longer than 10 days indicate complications, such as pseudocyst formation. Normal levels can indicate resolution of acute pancreatitis, pancreatic hemorrhage, or pancreatic necrosis. There is no correlation between amylase level and etiology, prognosis, or severity.
            Nonpancreatic causes of hyperamylasemia include renal failure, salivary gland disease, cirrhosis, hepatitis, common bile duct stones, acute cholecystitis, penetrating peptic ulcers, intestinal obstruction, afferent loop syndrome, diabetic ketoacidosis, lung cancer, pancreatic cancer, parotid tumors, ruptured ectopic pregnancy, endometritis, ruptured graafian follicle, and ovarian cysts and cancer. Amylase

isoenzymes and clinical signs and symptoms help differentiate between hyperamylasemia due to acute pancreatitis and other sources.
  b. **Serum lipase** generally is considered more specific for pancreatic disease and remains elevated longer, returning to normal after 3 to 5 days.
  c. **Urinary amylase** is increased in acute pancreatitis (usually >5,000 IU per 24 hours).
  d. **Serum calcium** levels may fall as a result of complexing with fatty acids (saponification) produced by activated lipases.
  e. **Discrimination between interstitial and necrotizing pancreatitis.** Some authors have demonstrated the usefulness of elevated serum levels of C-reactive protein and lactate dehydrogenase for early detection of necrotizing pancreatitis and for following the severity of the inflammatory response, but we have not found this to be helpful.
  f. **Trypsin-like immunoreactivity and elastase** levels may also be measured but do not add to the specificity of serum amylase or lipase.
3. **Radiology.** No single radiographic technique provides a perfect index of acute pancreatitis.
  a. **Computed tomographic (CT) scan** is superior to ultrasonography in evaluating the pancreas and is not limited by bowel gas. Contrast-enhanced CT scan has a sensitivity of 90% and a specificity of close to 100% for acute pancreatitis and also can provide prognostic information by assessing the amount of glandular necrosis. CT findings include parenchymal enlargement and edema, necrosis, blurring of fat planes, peripancreatic fluid collections, bowel distention, and mesenteric edema. While intravenous contrast-enhanced CT scan is helpful, it should not be performed in the setting of hypovolemia, due to the risks of nephrotoxicity. During the early course of treatment, a CT scan should often be deferred until the patient has had adequate resuscitation.
  b. **Plain films** can show pancreatic calcifications (best seen obliquely 15 degrees in either direction from the supine or prone position), gallstones, focal areas of small-bowel dilatation, segmental ileus (sentinel loop sign), ascites, and upper abdominal masses. Chest radiographs may reveal right or left pleural effusions, basilar atelectasis, or an elevated left hemidiaphragm.
  c. **Ultrasonography** sensitivity for pancreatitis ranges from 62% to 95%, whereas its specificity is greater than 95%. The pancreas is not visualized in up to 40% of patients due to overlying bowel gas.
4. **ERCP** is not indicated routinely for the evaluation of patients during an attack of acute pancreatitis. **Indications for ERCP** are as follows:
  a. **Preoperative evaluation** of patients with suspected traumatic pancreatitis, to determine whether the pancreatic duct is disrupted
  b. Patients with **suspected biliary pancreatitis and severe disease** who are not clinically improving by 24 hours after admission, so that endoscopic sphincterotomy and stone extraction may be performed. Randomized trials have shown improved outcome with early ERCP in this setting.
  c. **Patients older than age 40 years with no identifiable cause,** to rule out occult common bile duct stones, pancreatic or ampullary carcinoma, or other causes of obstruction
  d. **Patients younger than age 40 years** who have had cholecystectomy or have experienced more than one attack of unexplained pancreatitis
5. **Percutaneous transhepatic cholangiography** is typically used in situations in which ERCP cannot be performed due to clinical, technical, or anatomic restrictions and in which documented common bile duct obstruction is present.
D. **Prognosis** can be estimated by Ranson's criteria (Table 16-1).

Table 16-1. Ranson's criteria

Admission	
Age	>55 yr
White blood cell count	>16,000/μL
Blood glucose	>200 mg/dL
Serum lactate dehydrogenase	>350 IU/L
Aspartate aminotransferase	>250 IU/L
Initial 48 hr	
Hematocrit decrease	>10 %
Blood urea nitrogen elevation	>5 mg/dL
Serum calcium	<8 mg/dL
Arterial Po_2	<60 mm Hg
Base deficit	>4 mEq/L
Estimated fluid sequestration	>6 L

Mortality	
Number of Ranson's signs	Approximate mortality (%)
0–2	0
3–4	15
5–6	50
>6	70–90

 E. **Complications**
   1. **Necrotizing pancreatitis** refers to loss of pancreatic microcirculation resulting in the death of significant portions of the pancreas; it develops in 10% to 20% of cases. The prognosis for necrotizing pancreatitis is linked closely to the extent of necrosis.
   2. **Infected pancreatic necrosis** occurs in 5% to 10% of cases. Pancreatic infections are responsible for more than 80% of deaths. Gram-negative organisms are more common than Gram-positive organisms (typically *Pseudomonas*, *Escherichia coli*, *Klebsiella*, *Proteus*, *Enterobacter*, and *Staphylococcus* species). With the use of antibiotic prophylaxis, fungal infections are becoming increasingly more common.
   3. **Acute pseudocyst** (see Section VI)
 F. **Treatment**
   1. **Supportive care**
     a. **Gastric rest with nutritional support.** Patients are kept with empty stomachs to decrease neurohormonal stimulation of pancreatic secretion. Oral feeding is resumed once the attack has resolved. Often TPN is required. Postpyloric nasojejunal tube feeding has been shown to be as safe as TPN in the setting of pancreatitis.
     b. **Volume resuscitation** is done with isotonic fluids; urinary output is monitored with a Foley catheter. Central hemodynamic monitoring (central venous pressure or PA catheter) may be useful in guiding resuscitation. During the course of resuscitation, frequent monitoring of electrolytes, including calcium, is mandatory. Calcium depletion and other electrolyte deficiency should be corrected aggressively.
     c. **Analgesia.** Narcotics usually are required for pain relief.
     d. **Respiratory monitoring** and arterial blood gases should be done every 12 hours for the first 3 days in moderately severe pancreatitis to assess oxygenation and acid-base status. Hypoxemia is extremely common, even in mild cases of acute pancreatitis. Pulmonary complications occur in up to 50% of patients.
     e. **Alcohol withdrawal prophylaxis** is important during alcoholic pancreatitis.

f. Stress ulcer prophylaxis can be achieved through the use of H_2-blockers, antacids, and proton pump inhibitors.

g. Antibiotics are not effective in preventing septic complications in mild to moderate cases of pancreatitis. However, in several prospective, randomized trials, patients with severe pancreatitis who received prophylactic antibiotics had a significantly lower rate of septic complications (12% versus 30%), especially if the patient has evidence of necrosis on CT. Controversy exists as to whether this latter group of patients should proceed directly to surgical debridement.

h. Nasogastric tube decompression has **not** been shown to change the course of pancreatitis significantly, but it may be useful in the setting of intractable vomiting.

i. Somatostatin analogues are not useful in treating acute pancreatitis.

2. Surgical treatment

a. Diagnostic uncertainty. Exploratory laparotomy may be indicated if the diagnosis of pancreatitis is uncertain. Exploration is indicated for all patients who fail to improve, have significant clinical deterioration, or have suspected infected necrotic tissue.

b. Pancreatic drainage and debridement. For infected necrotizing pancreatitis, percutaneous drainage is futile. Wide debridement (necrosectomy), supplemented by either open packing or closed drainage, is effective. At our institution, the preference is for wide debridement and packing, and frequent debridement in the operating room. Marsupialization of the lesser sac facilitates rapid access to the pancreatic bed and facilitates daily dressing changes (usually done in the ICU).

c. Pancreatic resection. Because severe pancreatitis often leads to necrosis of large areas of the pancreas and peripancreatic fat, some have attempted to gain control of fulminant disease by resecting much or even all of the pancreas (partial or total pancreaticoduodenectomy). Radical resection procedures place greater stress on already severely ill patients; pancreaticoduodenectomy or total pancreatectomy is associated with very high mortality and is not recommended.

d. Gallstone-induced pancreatitis. Eradication of the biliary disease almost always prevents recurrent acute pancreatitis. Choledocholithiasis is found in only 25% of cases. Gallstones frequently produce pancreatitis due to transient obstruction of the ampulla of Vater and then pass spontaneously. Cholecystectomy should be carried out as soon as possible after recovery to prevent recurrent attacks of pancreatitis. During open or laparoscopic cholecystectomy, intraoperative cholangiography is mandatory.

II. Chronic pancreatitis

A. Etiology. In the Western Hemisphere, alcohol abuse accounts for more than 75% of cases. Causes for the remaining 25% include idiopathic, metabolic (hypercalcemia, hypertriglyceridemia , hypercholesterolemia, hyperparathyroidism, cystic fibrosis), drugs, trauma, and congenital abnormalities (sphincter of Oddi dysfunction or pancreas divisum). Chronic pancreatitis is characterized by diffuse scarring and strictures in the pancreatic duct and is often seen in association with endocrine or exocrine insufficiency. A history of recurrent acute pancreatitis is present in some but not all patients with chronic pancreatitis.

B. Diagnosis

1. History and physical examination. A complete history and physical examination should be complemented by the appropriate investigative studies. It is not possible to rely on clinical detection of known stigmas of pancreatic disease for the diagnosis of chronic pancreatitis (e.g., pancreatic insufficiency) because substantial glandular destruction must occur before secretory function is lost. Clinical examination should focus on a careful search for manifestations of hyperlipidemia, nutritional deficiencies, or signs of alcohol abuse. Physical findings include weight loss proportional to the severity of anorexia, as well as steatorrhea. Tenderness of the upper abdomen is common. An enlarged pancreas occasionally is palpable, especially in a thin person, but the findings of a mass may indicate the presence of a pseudocyst. Occasional findings include jaundice secondary to stricture of the common bile duct, enlarged spleen secondary to thrombosis of the splenic vein, or ascites secondary to a pancreaticoperitoneal fistula.

2. **Abdominal pain.** Upper midepigastric pain radiating to the back is the cardinal symptom and is present in 95% of cases. Early episodes mimic an attack of acute pancreatitis and may last for several hours to days. As the disease progresses, the attacks tend to be more frequent and prolonged.

3. **Malabsorption** due to exocrine insufficiency requires destruction of more than 90% of the pancreas parenchyma. This can result in weight loss, steatorrhea, asthenia, metabolic bone disease, clotting dysfunction, and vitamin deficiency, including in vitamins A, D, E, K, and B_{12}.

4. **Steatorrhea** occurs when lipase output by the pancreas is less than 10% of normal.

5. **Endocrine deficiency.** Pancreatic endocrine function should always be assessed when there is evidence of exocrine insufficiency. The islets of Langerhans have a greater resistance to injury by inflammation and fibrosis than do the exocrine tissues; most patients who develop diabetes already have pancreatic exocrine insufficiency and steatorrhea. Deficient insulin and glucagon secretion results in brittle diabetes mellitus.

6. **Laboratory tests**
   a. **Amylase and lipase levels** are elevated in acute pancreatitis but rarely are useful in chronic pancreatitis.
   b. **Pancreatic stimulation tests** (see Section V)
   c. **Pancreatic endocrine function.** Fasting and 2-hour postprandial blood glucose levels or glucose tolerance tests may be abnormal in 14% to 65% of patients with early chronic pancreatitis and in up to 90% of patients when calcifications are present.
   d. **Fecal fat** (see Section V)
   e. **Liver function tests** may suggest biliary obstruction from cicatricial narrowing of the lower common bile duct.

7. **Radiology studies**
   a. **Plain films** of the abdomen show diffuse calcification of the pancreas in approximately 30% of patients with relatively early stages of chronic pancreatitis and in 50% to 60% of cases of advanced disease.
   b. **Ultrasonography** is approximately 60% sensitive for the diagnosis of parenchymal or ductal disease.
   c. **CT scan** is approximately 75% sensitive for the diagnosis of parenchymal or ductal disease.
   d. **ERCP is often essential** to define the extent of disease and to optimize surgical management. It is 85% to 90% sensitive. It allows for evaluation of ductal anatomy. Brushings and biopsies of suspicious lesions can be performed as well as therapeutic interventions, including stenting and sphincterotomy.
   e. **Ultrasonography-** or **CT-guided fine-needle biopsies** may be useful in cases in which chronic pancreatitis cannot be distinguished from pancreatic cancer. By itself, however, a single biopsy finding of inflammatory changes is not sufficient to rule out carcinoma. A normal biopsy may also be the result of sampling error.

C. **Distinguishing between chronic pancreatitis and pancreatic cancer** is challenging. Factors favoring malignancy include the following:
   1. **ERCP signs suggestive of cancer**
   2. **Abrupt complete obstruction of an otherwise normal main pancreatic duct**
   3. **Encasement of a long segment of main pancreatic duct with normal ductal appearances on either side**

4. **Parenchymal filling of necrotic tumor areas**
5. **Double-duct sign of invasion of main pancreatic duct and common bile duct**
6. **Cytology** from pancreatic juice, duodenal aspirate, or fine-needle aspiration (CT-guided, ultrasonography-guided, or ERCP brushings and biopsies). Percutaneous biopsy should be reserved to prove the diagnosis in patients with apparent unresectable disease.
7. **Carbohydrate antigen (CA)** 19-9 is often elevated in pancreatic cancer, but it rarely detects small tumors and may also be elevated in pancreatitis. This is not useful in screening asymptomatic patients. Carcinoembryonic antigen, tissue polypeptide antigen, and CA 125 may be elevated in cystic pancreatic neoplasms but are not useful in periampullary carcinomas.

D. **Complications**
1. **Common bile duct obstruction**
   a. **Etiology** may be transient obstruction from pancreatic inflammation and edema or from stricture of the intrapancreatic common bile duct.
   b. **Strictures**
      (1) **Often long and smooth** (2 to 4 cm in length)
      (2) **Are present in 3%–29% of chronic pancreatitis**
      (3) **Must be distinguished from pancreatic carcinoma**
2. **Duodenal obstruction** as a result of
   a. **Acute pancreatic inflammation and edema**
   b. **Chronic fibrotic reaction**
   c. **Pancreatic pseudocyst**
   d. **Pancreatic cancer**
3. **Pancreaticoenteric fistulas** result from spontaneous drainage of a pancreatic abscess cavity or pseudocyst into the stomach, duodenum, transverse colon, or biliary tract. They are often asymptomatic but may become infected or result in hemorrhage.
4. **Pancreaticopleural fistulas** often have communication from the distal duct traversing the esophageal hiatus.
5. **Pseudocyst** (see Section VIA)
6. **Splenic vein thrombosis** results in left-sided portal hypertension and gastric varices. It can present with hematemesis, melena, anemia, abdominal pain, or splenomegaly. Splenectomy results in cure in 90% of patients.
7. **Pancreatic carcinoma.** Chronic pancreatitis has been suggested in some studies to increase the risk of pancreatic carcinoma by a factor of two or three.

E. **Treatment**
1. **Medical management**
   a. **Malabsorption or steatorrhea** (see Section V). There is some evidence that adequate oral pancreatic enzyme supplementation can improve pain control.
   b. **Diabetes** initially can be responsive to careful attention to overall good nutrition and dietary control; however, oral hypoglycemic agents or insulin therapy often are ultimately required. There is some propensity for hypoglycemic attacks. Diabetic ketoacidosis is not commonly seen except after major pancreatic resections.
   c. **Analgesia.** Narcotics usually are required for pain relief. Narcotic dependency is a frequent complication of therapy and correlates with higher mortality.
   d. **Abstinence** from alcohol and withdrawal prophylaxis are of paramount importance.
   e. **Cholecystokinin antagonists and somatostatin analogues** have been considered for treatment of chronic pancreatitis, but early studies have shown disappointing or only short-lived effects.

f. **Tube thoracostomy or repeated paracentesis** may be required for pancreatic pleural effusions or pancreatic ascites. Approximately 40% to 65% of patients respond to nonsurgical management within 2 to 3 weeks.

2. **Surgical principles**

a. **Indications for surgery** include severe intractable pain, multiple relapses, inability to rule out neoplasm, and complications of pancreatitis (pseudocyst, obstruction, fistula, infections, and portal hypertension).

b. **Surgical candidates.** Patients must have a trial of nonsurgical therapy, including abstinence. They must be willing and able to care for themselves after surgery, which may include an apancreatic state.

c. **Choice of procedure.** Surgical therapy must allow for drainage of the pancreatic duct and resection of the diseased pancreas. Choice of procedure is made based on structural changes found on ERCP, CT scan, and ultrasonography and those found during surgery. Drainage procedures are preferable because they allow for preservation of pancreatic tissue and function but require a dilatated pancreatic duct of at least 8 mm.

d. **Drainage procedures**

(1) **Longitudinal side-to-side pancreaticojejunostomy (Partington-Rochelle).** It is indicated in patients with functionally significant strictures along the pancreatic duct (chain of lakes on pancreatograms) and with ducts at least 8 mm in diameter.

(2) **Puestow** procedure includes a distal pancreatectomy with a distal pancreaticojejunostomy for drainage.

(3) **Frey** procedure incorporates a limited resection of the head of the pancreas.

e. **Pancreatectomy**

(1) **Distal subtotal pancreatectomy.** This technique is used for disease lateralized to the tail of the gland, cysts in the body and tail, severe disease in the body and tail with ductal obstruction at the neck of the gland, and previous ductal injury from blunt abdominal trauma with fracture of the pancreas and stenosis of the duct at the midbody level.

(2) **Total pancreatectomy** is performed only as a last resort in patients whose previous operations have failed and who appear capable of managing an apancreatic state.

(3) **Pancreaticoduodenectomy (Whipple procedure)** is indicated in cases in which the pancreatitis disproportionately involves the head of the pancreas, the pancreatic duct is of small diameter, or cancer cannot be ruled out in the head of the pancreas. For chronic pancreatitis, the pylorus-preserving technique is advocated. The use of vagotomy is controversial. This procedure, although more technically demanding, results in a higher degree of pain relief than does the distal resection.

(4) **The Beger procedure** is a duodenum-preserving resection of a portion of the pancreatic head. This operation preserves a small amount of pancreatic tissue within the C-loop of the duodenum and also in front of the portal vein. A jejunal loop is anastomosed to the proximal and the larger distal stumps of the remaining pancreas. This procedure should not be performed in the presence of cancer.

f. **Celiac plexus block.** Although transiently effective in some cases, nerve ablation procedures have a minimal role in the management of pain in patients with chronic pancreatitis because of their poor long-term results.

III. **Exocrine pancreatic cancer**

A. **Incidence and epidemiology.** Pancreatic cancer is the fifth most common cause of cancer death in women and the fourth most common cause of death in men. Despite advances in surgical technique and adjuvant therapy, few patients are resectable, and overall 5-year survival is <5%. Pancreatic cancer is associated with smoking, benzidine and β-naphthylamine exposure, alcohol, diet, recent-onset diabetes, chronic pancreatitis, and family history. Approximately 80% of pancreatic carcinomas are ductal cell adenocarcinomas, 4% are giant cell carcinomas, 3% are adenosquamous carcinomas, 2% are mucinous carcinomas, 1% are cystadenocarcinomas, 1% are acinar cell adenocarcinomas, and the remaining 9% are unclassified. Seventy percent of pancreatic cancers occur at the head, 20% in the body, and 10% in the tail. Other periampullary tumors, such as carcinomas of the distal bile duct, duodenum, and ampulla of Vater, are less common and constitute approximately one-third of resectable periampullary cancers.

B. Diagnosis
   1. **History and physical examination**
      a. **Abdominal pain.** Patients present with a typically progressive midepigastric dull ache that often radiates to the back. It is present in 80% of patients, especially if the tumor involves the body or tail of the pancreas.
      b. **Weight loss** occurs in approximately 70% of patients. Pancreatic cancer must be ruled out in patients older than 50 years who present with vague abdominal pain and weight loss.
      c. **Obstructive jaundice and pruritus** commonly are associated with cancer of the pancreatic head.
      d. **Weakness, fatigue, malaise, anorexia, and vague constitutional symptoms** present in 30% to 40% of patients.
      e. **Cholangitis** develops in approximately 10% of patients.
      f. **Courvoisier sign** (painless jaundice with a palpable gallbladder) usually is associated with pancreatic head tumors, periampullary carcinoma, and primary bile duct tumors.
      g. **Virchow node** (left supraclavicular) and **Sister Mary Joseph node** (umbilical) indicate metastatic disease.
      h. **Trousseau migratory thrombophlebitis** is a superficial thrombophlebitis that can be associated with pancreatic cancer.
   2. **Laboratory tests.** None is singularly diagnostic for pancreatic cancer.
      a. **Elevated serum bilirubin**
      b. **Elevated alkaline phosphatase**
      c. **Mild elevations of serum glutamic-oxaloacetic transaminase and serum glutamate pyruvate transaminase**
      d. **Tumor markers** (see Section II.C.7)
   3. **Radiologic studies**
      a. **Plain films** of the abdomen usually are of little benefit.
      b. **CT scan.** In periampullary carcinoma, dilatation of intrahepatic and extrahepatic ducts as well as the main pancreatic duct can be seen. Tumors larger than 2 cm generally can be detected.
      c. **ERCP** (see Section I.C.4.)
      d. **Upper gastrointestinal series.** This test can be of use in evaluating patients with duodenal and gastric outlet obstruction.
      e. **Percutaneous (CT- or ultrasonography-guided) needle biopsies** have a limited role. A percutaneous needle biopsy should be performed in patients who are not surgical candidates, to obtain a tissue diagnosis. A negative biopsy does not rule out carcinoma, however, and any biopsy risks seeding the peritoneal cavity.
      f. **Others.** Ultrasonography is not as sensitive as CT scan and is limited by the presence of bowel gas. MR scan may provide as much information as does CT scan but is costly, is limited in availability, and takes longer. Endoscopic ultrasonography can assess tumor size as well as portal and mesenteric vascular involvement and obtain tissue samples. Staging laparoscopy may be useful in identifying small liver metastasis and peritoneal implants.

C. Treatment

1. **Resectable tumors** have no evidence of metastasis, no involvement of the superior mesenteric artery, and patent superior mesenteric vein and portal vein confluence. While some surgeons consider any involvement of mesenteric vein or portal vein a contraindication to surgical resection, we favor resection and reconstruction of the venous structures.

2. **Unresectable tumors.** Patients preoperatively found to have unresectable disease or considered to be poor surgical candidates may be offered palliative nonsurgical treatment. Biliary bypass can be performed by percutaneous drainage or preferably with endoscopic stent placement. Gastric outlet obstruction can be palliated with a gastrojejunostomy or percutaneous gastrostomy tube.

3. **Surgical approach.** Initially, exploratory laparotomy or laparoscopy is performed to assess whether the disease is resectable. We advocate staging laparoscopy and biopsies to assess the primary tumor, local invasion, peritoneal implantation, and metastases to lymph nodes and the liver. Available data suggest that this technique, combined with preoperative spiral CT scanning, can reduce the incidence of unresectable disease at laparotomy to less than 10%.

   a. **Pancreaticoduodenectomy (Whipple procedure)** consists of *en bloc* resection of the head of the pancreas, distal common bile duct, duodenum, jejunum, and gastric antrum. Pylorus-sparing pancreaticoduodenectomy has been advocated by some, but there are no data demonstrating improved survival or lower morbidity. Extended lymphadenectomy, including nodes from the celiac axis to the iliac bifurcation and nodes from the portal vein and superior mesenteric artery, has not been shown to affect survival but has increased morbidity. There has been a sharp decline in morbidity and mortality in specialized centers, with a 30-day mortality of less than 5%.

   b. **Palliative bypass.** If the disease is considered unresectable at the time of surgery, palliative choledochojejunostomy or gastrojejunostomy can be performed to palliate or prevent biliary and gastric outlet obstruction.

4. **Postoperative considerations.** Delayed gastric emptying, pancreatic fistula, and wound infection are the three most common complications of the pancreaticoduodenectomy. Up to 10% of patients require a nasogastric tube for longer than 10 days, but delayed gastric emptying almost always subsides with conservative treatment. The incidence of delayed gastric emptying is increased with pylorus-preserving procedures. The rate of pancreatic fistula has been demonstrated to be reduced to <2% by meticulous attention to the blood supply of the pancreaticoenteric duct-to-mucosa anastomosis. While many surgeons routinely place abdominal drains, a prospective, randomized study showed no benefit and possible increased complications due to the presence of drains. Randomized studies have not demonstrated that the perioperative use of octreotide (a somatostatin analogue) can decrease pancreatic fistulas in patients undergoing pancreaticoduodenectomy.

5. **Radiotherapy and chemotherapy.** The use of adjuvant therapy has been investigated in prospective fashion, and clear conclusions are not evident. The available studies have been criticized for selection bias and small sample sizes. Given the high recurrence rate after resection, most patients are considered for some form of adjuvant therapy. The median survival for resectable patients is less than 20 months. Current regimens consist of radiation and 5-flurouracil. Newer agents incorporating gemcitabine or immunomodulation therapy utilizing a combination of radiation, conventional chemotherapy, and alpha interferon are under study.

6. **Prognosis.** Surgical resection can increase survival. Overall 5-year survival rates are 5% to 20% for patients after resection. In patients with

small tumors, negative resection margins, and no evidence of nodal metastases, the 5-year survival rate is as high as 40%. Mean length of survival for unresectable locally advanced disease is 3 to 10 months and for hepatic metastatic disease 6 months.

IV. Congenital abnormalities

  A. Pancreatic divisum. Failure of the ventral and dorsal pancreatic buds to fuse during the 6th week of development results in pancreatic divisum. The ventral bud normally forms the liver, gallbladder, and uncinate process of the pancreas. The common bile duct and duct of Wirsung originate from this ventral bud, while the normally smaller duct of Santorini and rest of the pancreas are derived from the dorsal pancreatic bud. In pancreas divisum, the normally minor duct of Santorini becomes the primary means of pancreatic drainage from the larger mass of pancreatic tissue. The condition is detected by ERCP, and the incidence is estimated to be 5%. Approximately 25% of affected patients develop pancreatitis secondary to obstruction or stenosis. However, the association between pancreatitis and pancreas divisum is controversial. Open sphincteroplasty of the minor papilla forming the orifice of the minor duct of Santorini and cholecystectomy is the procedure of choice for symptomatic patients. One should exclude other etiologies of pancreatitis before embarking on surgical intervention for pancreas divisum.

  B. Heterotopic (accessory) pancreas. Typical locations for ectopic pancreatic tissues include the stomach, duodenal or ileal wall, Meckel diverticulum, and umbilicus. Less common sites include the colon, appendix, gallbladder, omentum, and mesentery. Most ectopic pancreatic tissue is functional; islet tissue is most often present in the stomach and duodenum. Heterotopic pancreas may result in pyloric stenosis, disruption of peristalsis, peptic ulcers, or neoplasms.

  C. Annular pancreas. Malrotation of the ventral primordium during the 5th week results in a thin, flat band of normal pancreatic tissue surrounding the second part of the duodenum. The pancreatic tissue may be completely free from the duodenum or may invade the muscularis deeply. The annular pancreas usually contains a duct that connects to the main pancreatic duct. Annular pancreas may cause duodenal obstruction *in utero*, resulting in hydramnios. Approximately one-half of affected patients do not have symptoms until late in adulthood, however, and complaints usually relate to duodenal obstruction. Treatment of choice is duodenoduodenostomy for symptomatic patients.

V. Exocrine pancreatic insufficiency

  A. Etiology

    1. Pancreatic disease (acute and chronic pancreatitis)

    2. Pancreatic resection

    3. Cystic fibrosis

  B. Diagnosis

    1. History and physical examination

      a. Malabsorption and steatorrhea are the most common complaints associated with exocrine pancreatic insufficiency.

      b. Family history (particularly pancreatic disease or cystic fibrosis) and **social history** (particularly alcohol consumption and smoking) are relevant.

      c. Clinical examination should focus on a careful search for the following signs:

        (1) Manifestations of hyperlipidemia

        (2) Nutritional deficiencies

        (3) Signs of alcohol abuse

    2. Laboratory tests. Most of the available studies are labor intensive and not routinely performed.

      a. A 72-hour fecal collection for estimation of daily fecal fat is the most sensitive and specific stool test for exocrine insufficiency. Fat absorption has the most clinical significance, although fewer problems are associated with protein malabsorption. Carbohydrate malabsorption probably is unimportant. Malabsorption occurs only if more than 90% of pancreatic exocrine function is lost. In an individual ingesting 100 g fat per day, excretion of more than 7 g fat in a 24-hour period suggests pancreatic insufficiency. Neutral fat (Sudan stain) suggests pancreatic disease, whereas split fat suggests small-bowel disease.

b. Pancreolauryl test. Ingested fluorescein dilaurate is broken down by pancreatic esterase and excreted in the urine. Low levels of urinary fluorescein suggest exocrine insufficiency.

C. Treatment. Pancreatic enzyme supplements are extracted from animal pancreata and are used to treat malabsorption. Supplements also have been advocated in alleviation of pain in chronic pancreatitis, but their efficacy is not well established. A low-fat diet is combined with enzyme supplementation at each meal. The dosages and preparation depend on the diet and extent of the pancreatic insufficiency.

VI. Cystic diseases

A. Pancreatic pseudocysts

1. **General considerations.** A true cyst has an epithelial lining and does not communicate with the pancreatic ducts. A pseudocyst has no epithelial lining but communicates with the pancreatic ducts and thus contains elevated pancreatic enzyme concentrations. It is important to distinguish pseudocysts from tumors. An acute pancreatic fluid collection follows in approximately 25% of patients with acute pancreatitis. It is characterized by acute inflammation, cloudy fluid, a poorly defined cyst wall, and necrotic but sterile debris. This may resolve spontaneously, and in fact most "pseudocysts" that resolve are likely of this type. By definition, a fluid collection in the first 4 weeks is an *acute fluid collection*; after 4 weeks, it becomes an *acute pseudocyst.*

2. **Causes.** Pseudocysts develop after disruption of the pancreatic duct with or without proximal obstruction; they usually occur after an episode of acute pancreatitis. In children, most pseudocysts arise as a complication of blunt abdominal trauma.

3. **Diagnosis**

   a. **Clinical presentation.** The most common complaint is recurrent or persistent upper abdominal pain. Other symptoms include nausea, vomiting, early satiety, anorexia, weight loss, and jaundice. Physical examination is significant for upper abdominal tenderness and occasionally reveals an abdominal mass.

   b. **Laboratory tests**

      (1) **Amylase.** Serum concentrations are elevated in approximately one-half of cases. Urinary levels of amylase are elevated in up to 80% of cases.

      (2) **Liver function tests** occasionally are elevated and therefore are not of diagnostic use.

      (3) **Cystic fluid analysis** is discussed in Section VI.B.2.

   c. **Radiologic studies**

      (1) **CT scan** is the radiographic study of choice for initial evaluation of pancreatic pseudocysts and is twice as sensitive as ultrasonography in detection of pseudocysts. CT scan findings that determine prognosis include the following:

         (a) **Pseudocysts smaller than 4 cm** usually resolve spontaneously.

         (b) **Pseudocysts with wall calcifications** generally do not resolve.

         (c) **Pseudocysts with thick walls** are resistant to spontaneous resolution.

      (2) **Ultrasonography** detects approximately 85% of pseudocysts. The false-positive rate is 8.3%, and the false-negative rate is 8.5%. Its use is limited by obesity and bowel gases, but it may be used

in follow-up studies once a pseudocyst has been identified by CT scan.

d. ERCP allows for the determination of pancreatic duct anatomy and influences therapeutic intervention. Approximately one-half of pseudocysts have ductal abnormalities identified by ERCP, such as proximal obstruction, stricture, or communications with the pseudocyst. ERCP itself risks superinfection of a communicating pseudocyst.

4. Complications

  a. Infection is reported in 5% to 20% of pseudocysts and requires external drainage.

  b. Hemorrhage results from erosion into surrounding visceral vessels and occurs in approximately 7% of cases. The most common arteries are the splenic (45%), gastroduodenal (18%), and pancreaticoduodenal (18%) arteries. Immediate angiography has emerged as the initial treatment of choice.

  c. Obstruction. Compression can occur anywhere from the stomach to the colon. The arteriovenous system also can be subject to compression, including the vena caval and portal venous system. Hydronephrosis can result from obstruction of the ureters. Biliary obstruction can present as jaundice, cholangitis, and biliary cirrhosis.

  d. Rupture occurs in fewer than 3% of cases. Approximately one-half of patients can be treated nonsurgically, with total parenteral nutrition and symptomatic paracentesis or thoracentesis. Rupture is occasionally associated with severe abdominal pain and presents as a surgical emergency.

5. Treatment depends on symptoms, age, pseudocyst size, and the presence of complications. **Pseudocysts smaller than 6 cm and present for less than 6 weeks have low complication rates. The chance of spontaneous resolution after 6 weeks is low, and the risk of complications rises significantly after 6 weeks.**

  a. Nonoperative. If the pseudocyst is new, asymptomatic, and without complications, the patient can be followed with serial CT scans or ultrasonography to evaluate size and maturation of the pseudocyst. The majority of pseudocysts larger than 6 cm require surgery.

  b. Percutaneous drainage can be considered for patients in whom the pseudocyst does not communicate with the pancreatic duct and for those who cannot tolerate surgery. External drainage is indicated when the pseudocyst is infected and without a mature wall. Simple aspiration is the least effective of the percutaneous interventions. The duration of drainage ranges from several days to several months (usually 3 to 4 weeks). The results are variable, and the rate of complications (e.g., fistulas) may be high.

  c. Excision may be necessary in patients with symptomatic immature pseudocysts associated with complications or in those with mature distal pancreatic pseudocysts. Resection can require a Whipple procedure (pancreaticoduodenectomy) for pseudocysts at the head of the pancreas (rarely indicated) or distal pancreatectomy for pseudocysts in the body or tail of the pancreas.

  d. Internal drainage. Cystoenteric drainage is the procedure of choice in uncomplicated pseudocysts requiring surgical treatment. Options include Roux-en-Y cystojejunostomy, loop cystojejunostomy, cystogastrostomy, and cystoduodenostomy. It is always important to obtain a biopsy of the cyst wall to rule out cystic neoplasm. The recurrence rate after these procedures is approximately 10%. Typically, at least a 5-cm anastomosis is performed. Endoscopic cystogastrostomy or cystoenterostomy has been performed in some centers. There is an increased risk of perforation with this procedure, and an increased risk of recurrence due to inadequate drainage. At our institution, we favor the Roux-en-Y cystojejunostomy or cystogastrostomy in most patients.

B. True pancreatic cysts
1. **Histopathologic classification.** Serous cystic neoplasms tend to have a low malignant potential, as opposed to mucinous tumors, which have latent malignant tendency or overt malignancy.
   a. **Serous cystadenoma** is frequently located at the pancreatic head.
   b. **Mucinous cystadenoma** is usually located in the pancreatic body or tail.
   c. **Other cystic neoplasms** include **intraductal papillary mucinous tumor** (considered a premalignant lesion), **cystadenocarcinoma, acinar cell cystadenocarcinoma, cystic choriocarcinoma, cystic teratoma, and angiomatous neoplasms.**
2. **Laboratory tests/cystic fluid analysis**
   a. **Carcinoembryonic antigen** is elevated in mucinous cysts and is low in serous cysts and pseudocysts.
   b. **CA 125** is elevated in malignant cysts, low in pseudocysts, and variable in mucinous cystic neoplasms and serous cystadenoma. Very high levels suggests malignancy, but the association is not perfect.
   c. **CA 19-9** is nondiscriminatory in the evaluation of cystic neoplasms of the pancreas.
   d. **CA 72-4** is low in pseudocysts and serous tumors. Levels are elevated in benign mucinous cystadenomas, and very high in the setting of cystic malignancy.
   e. **Amylase** generally is high in pseudocysts and low in cystic tumors.
   f. **Lipase** generally is high in pseudocysts and low in cystic tumors.
   g. **Fluid viscosity** is elevated in mucinous tumors and low in pseudocysts and serous cystic tumors.
   h. **Percutaneous cytology** is useful in determining malignant tumors but limited in discriminating between pseudocysts and serous cystadenoma.
   i. **Percutaneous wall biopsy.** Full-thickness biopsy allows for discrimination between pseudocysts (which lack epithelial lining) and cystic neoplasms. It also can discriminate between serous (cuboidal epithelium) and mucinous (tall columnar epithelium and goblet cells). However, neoplastic cysts may have areas of cyst wall denuded of epithelium, which mimic pseudocysts.
3. **Radiographic characteristics of cystic neoplasms:**
   a. **Sharply circumscribed and encapsulated**
   b. **Multiple septations and cystic cavities**
   c. **Central calcifications with stellate pattern and multiple tiny cysts**, suggesting benign serous cystadenoma
   d. **Peripheral calcifications and larger cysts**, suggesting mucinous cystadenoma
   e. **Ultrasonography can reveal mixed echogenic fluid with septations.**
   f. **Angiography can show irregular tumor vessels, hypervascularity, and atrioventricular shunting.**
4. **Treatment relies on total extirpation.** Extent of resection depends on location and extent of the tumor. Aggressive therapy is warranted even in the presence of metastases. The role of adjuvant therapy has yet to be determined.
5. **Prognosis.** With curative resection, patients with mucinous cystadenocarcinoma have 5-year survival rate >60%.
6. **Miscellaneous cystic lesions**
   a. **True pancreatic cysts are congenital,** not premalignant, and usually are asymptomatic.
   b. **Hydatid cysts** are managed like other intraperitoneal hydatid cysts.
   c. **von Hippel-Lindau syndrome** can involve cystic lesions of the pancreas and nonfunctional islet cell pancreas tumors.

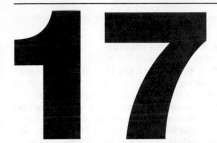

Surgical Diseases of the Liver

Udaya Liyanage and William Chapman

Advances in surgical techniques and critical care over the last 2 decades have made major hepatic surgery safer and more effective. This section reviews conditions affecting the liver that require or benefit from surgical intervention, including portal hypertension. Indications for and techniques of hepatic transplantation are discussed in Chapter 28.

RESECTION OF THE LIVER

I. **Hepatic resection** is used to treat a variety of benign or malignant neoplasms and some chronic diseases, such as cystic disorders. Resection of up to 80% of the liver is possible, as for the remaining liver regenerates rapidly to a normal liver volume in the noncirrhotic patient. By the 3rd postoperative week, liver function tests, including serum albumin, bilirubin levels, and prothrombin time, usually reflect restored physiology.

II. **Nomenclature**
   Although hepatic resections have become more common, more effective, and safer, the nomenclature remains redundant and confusing. In an effort to standardize descriptions, a modified nomenclature for hepatic structures and resections was introduced by the International Hepato-Pancreato-Biliary Association (*HPB* 2000;2:333) and has been embraced by hepatobiliary specialists. This system is predicated on the surgical anatomy of the liver, with the internal hepatic divisions delineated by the arterial and biliary anatomy.

   A. **Internal anatomy: first division.** The liver is divided into two almost equally sized *hemilivers*. The plane between the hemilivers is the *midplane* of the liver and runs from the gallbladder fossa to the inferior vena cava. Each hemiliver is supplied by one hepatic arterial branch, one bile duct, and one portal vein; those of the right hemiliver, for example, are referred to as the *right hepatic artery, right bile duct,* and *right portal vein.* A resection of a hemiliver is termed a *hepatectomy* or *hemihepatectomy* (e.g., right hepatectomy).

   B. **Internal anatomy: second division.** Further divisions of the liver are based on the internal course of the hepatic artery and bile duct. These structures retain a high order of bilateral symmetry, whereas the portal vein does not. Its asymmetry results from retained portions from the fetal circulation. The liver is thus divided into four nearly equal **sections:** the right anterior and posterior sections and the left medial and lateral sections. A vessel supplying a section is a sectional vessel (e.g., the right anterior sectional artery).

   C. **Internal anatomy: third division.** The liver is further subdivided into segments numbered I–VIII. These are the same as originally described by Couinaud. Resection of a segment is termed a *segmentectomy.* Resection of more than one segment can be precisely defined by the segments removed.

III. **Perioperative management of hepatic resections.** Preoperative management involves correction of anemia and coagulopathy, the administration of vitamin K in the presence of jaundice, optimization of nutrition, and administration of proper prophylactic antibiotics. **Operative conduct** for major liver resection consists of wide exposure through a bilateral subcostal incision. The vascular pedicles to the side of the liver to be resected are isolated. The same is done for the hepatic vein(s) draining the part of the liver to be resected. During transection, maintenance of a low central venous pressure (<5 mm Hg) and placement of the patient in the Trendelenburg position reduce blood loss. A small amount of positive end-expiratory pressure (5 cm H_2O) is used to prevent air embolism. Vascular control can be augmented by intermittent occlusion of all hepatic inflow (Pringle maneuver) or total vascular occlusion. Postoperatively, hypoglycemia may result in the absence of supplemental glucose, and therefore frequent blood sugar measurements should be obtained. Hyperbilirubinemia is unusual but may occur and persist for days to weeks. Hypoprothrombinemia develops but usually is not critical; if necessary, fresh frozen plasma is infused to keep the international normalized ratio (INR) at less than 2. Albumin infusion may be necessary to keep the serum albumin above 2 g/dL. The most common complication from liver resection is intra-abdominal abscess. Treatment usually consists of percutaneous drainage, although rarely some collections require an operative intervention. Another procedure-specific complication is a bile leak from the cut surface of the liver or a damaged biliary duct. This may manifest as a bile fistula or a *biloma*, a localized collection of bile. This can usually be managed by percutaneous drainage. Liver failure may result from insufficient residual functional hepatic parenchyma after extensive resections.

DISEASES OF THE LIVER

I. **Liver tumors**
   A. **Benign tumors**
      1. **Hemangioma** is the most common benign liver tumor, being reported in up to 7% of autopsies. It is also a form of hamartoma rather than neoplasm. Two forms predominate. The more frequently seen capillary form is often multiple, asymptomatic, and usually of no clinical significance. Cavernous lesions, on the other hand, are generally solitary, large, and sometimes symptomatic. A description of their qualities follows.
         a. **Pathology.** Size ranges from 1 to 2 cm up to the volume of a hemiliver or more. They are spherical, soft, and easily compressible. On sectioning, they are purple in color and spongelike. Microscopically, vascular spaces are lined with flat cuboidal cells and may show evidence of thrombotic congestion. Malignant degeneration does not occur.
         b. **Presentation.** Most hemangiomas are asymptomatic and are identified incidentally. Patients with large lesions are occasionally symptomatic, presenting as hepatomegaly, often in conjunction with upper abdominal fullness or penetrating abdominal or pleuritic pain. This discomfort may be positional. High-output cardiac failure has been reported, especially in the pediatric population. These lesions can also cause sequestration of platelets and clotting factors, which may result in a consumptive coagulopathy or purpura. Women are more frequently symptomatic (10:1 ratio) due to the larger average size of their lesions on presentation. Hemorrhage from free rupture into the peritoneal cavity is an extremely rare occurrence but can be precipitated by needle biopsy.
         c. **Diagnosis.** Laboratory abnormalities are rare. As these are vascular tumors, diagnostic biopsy is unnecessary and should be discouraged, as it can cause severe and even fatal hemorrhage. Ultrasound is highly sensitive but not specific and can identify an homogenous hyperechoic mass with pathognomonic compressibility. Contrast computed tomography (CT) scans show a low-density area with characteristic peripheral enhancement in the early phase. The specificity of CT scanning has rendered arteriography less useful. The most specific and sensitive tests are MR scan and tagged–red cell radionucleotide scan.
         d. **Treatment** consists of observation alone for most hemangiomas. One rare exception is the asymptomatic patient with a large mass who is at significant risk for a traumatic event. The preferred treatment for

symptomatic lesions is surgical extirpation. Hemangiomas can usually be enucleated under vascular control (intermittent Pringle maneuver). Formal anatomic resection (e.g., right hepatectomy) is used when the tumor has largely replaced a distinct anatomic unit. Regression after low-dose radiation therapy or embolization in select cases has been described but should be reserved for large unresectable lesions or for a patient unfit for surgery. In the rare case of spontaneous hemorrhage, control with vascular interventional embolization provides temporary help until a definitive surgical approach can safely be implemented after resuscitation.

2. **Hepatic adenoma.** An association with all the synthetic estrogen and progesterone preparations is known (*Toxicol Environ Health* 1979;5:231). With the introduction of oral contraceptive medication, the incidence of adenomas markedly increased in the 1960s and 1970s but has stabilized since, probably due to modification of these medications, including a decrease in their estrogen content.

   a. **Pathology.** Grossly, adenomas are soft, fleshy tumors with smooth surfaces. Microscopically, they are made up of monotonous sheets of hepatocytes containing glycogen. Portal triads are absent, and the vessels are thin walled. The lesions are separated from normal liver by a capsule.

   b. **Clinical manifestations.** Most cases present as a mass in the liver, often palpable. Approximately 33% of patients present with intraperitoneal bleeding, and others present with abdominal pain without rupture. Asymptomatic tumors noted either radiographically or at laparotomy are less frequent presentations. Rupture may occur during pregnancy due to rapid growth under the influence of estrogens. These lesions are premalignant.

   c. **Diagnostic studies.** Liver serology and a-fetoprotein (AFP) levels usually are normal. Ultrasonography or CT scan can identify lesions but cannot differentiate an adenoma from a malignant lesion. Some advocate needle biopsy as a method of differentiating benign from malignant lesions, although the accuracy is less than 100%. Technetium sulfur colloid scan is useful for distinguishing adenoma from focal nodular hyperplasia. The latter registers warm or hot, based on the uptake of sulfur by the abundant Kupffer cells, whereas the adenoma, which has few or no Kupffer cells, is cold. Hemangiomas can be confused with these entities and can be differentiated by a tagged red blood cell scan, as previously mentioned.

   d. **Treatment.** Some small, asymptomatic lesions regress with cessation of oral contraceptives. Lesions that do not regress should be excised unless they are small and centrally located or are multiple and dispersed throughout the liver. Resection is indicated for large, painful, or ruptured lesions or those larger than 5 cm in diameter. An anatomic resection is usually performed, although no normal liver tissue need be taken. Recurrence after resection has not been reported.

3. **Focal nodular hyperplasia (FNH)** represents a reaction to an injury rather than a true neoplasm. Although an association with oral contraceptives has been suggested, the correlations are much lower than are those for adenomas. FNH frequently occurs in women who are not on oral contraceptives, as well as in men.

   a. **Pathology.** The lesions usually are solitary and small and often are peripherally located near the edge of the liver. Histologically, they are composed of fibrous bands and normal liver tissue. The overall appearance resembles a regenerating nodule with a central stellate scar.

   b. **Clinical manifestations.** The large majority of lesions are found incidentally at laparotomy. Less commonly, patients present with a palpable mass or pain. Hemorrhage is not characteristic but has been reported. Malignant degeneration has not been reported.

    c. Diagnostic studies. Liver function tests, AFP levels, and hepatitis B serology usually are normal. The lesions are isodense on ultrasonography and CT examination. Angiography, however, can demonstrate a hypervascular tumor with large arteries and evidence of arteriovenous shunting in 85% of cases. There is a characteristic stellate distribution of the blood vessels and a central scar on CT scan. The lesions are warm or hot on technetium sulfur colloid scan, as previously mentioned.

    d. Treatment. Elective resection is not indicated in asymptomatic patients when studies differentiate FNH from adenoma or malignant lesions. Oral contraceptives should be stopped. There is no contraindication to pregnancy with this lesion.

4. Hamartoma is normal liver tissue in an abnormal arrangement. It is usually tiny and of no clinical significance. An exception is mesenchymal hamartoma, which can present as a rapidly growing mass in children and, in rare cases, in adults. Hamartomas may be solitary or multiple, with a firm and nodular gross appearance. Typically, they are white lesions 1 to 5 mm in diameter, but they may be larger. Resection may be indicated based on growth or obstructive symptoms; however, except for mesenchymal hamartomas, this is a very uncommon indication for resection.

B. Malignant tumors of the liver are classified as primary epithelial carcinomas [hepatocellular carcinoma (HCC), hepatoblastoma, and cholangiocarcinoma], mesenchymomas, mixed tumors, and sarcomas. Secondary tumors (metastases) are far more prevalent in Western countries.

1. Hepatoma (HCC)

    a. Incidence. There are wide geographic variations in the incidence of HCC. The annual incidence in the United States has been approximately 2 to 4 per 100,000 population. This has increased with an increase in the incidence of viral hepatitis. Some areas of Africa and Asia have incidences as high as 60 per 100,000 population. Although HCC occurs in all age groups, it is diagnosed mainly in the 5th and 6th decades. In Africans and Asians, however, the peak age is between 20 and 40 years. There is a 3:1 male predominance.

    b. Risk factors. A variety of etiologic factors have been implicated. These include ethanol, aflatoxin, chronic hepatitis B and C, hemochromatosis, Wilson's disease, α_1-antitrypsin deficiency, and Thorotrast (a radiocontrast agent). Because almost every type of experimentally induced cirrhosis transforms into carcinoma, a strong association exists between cirrhosis and the development of primary hepatic carcinoma. Malignant tumors of the liver occur in 4.5% of cirrhotic patients and in up to 10% when hemochromatosis is the inciting factor. Conversely, approximately 70% to 85% of primary HCC arises in the setting of cirrhosis.

    c. Viral hepatitis has a strong correlation with HCC. Serologic markers for hepatitis B virus or antibody to hepatitis C virus is detected in almost all patients with HCC in endemic areas. The question remains as to whether the viruses themselves are oncogenic or whether they lead to chronic active hepatitis and then to cirrhosis and finally cancer. The evidence for the association between hepatitis C and HCC, although weaker, appears to be established, and it is germane given that infection with hepatitis C is now more common than infection with hepatitis B. Hepatitis C viral RNA has been demonstrated within HCC tumor extracts.

    d. Pathology. Gross patterns of HCC include the nodular type (aggregate of clusters of nodules), the massive type (single large mass), and the diffuse type (widespread fine nodular pattern). The right hemiliver is involved more frequently than the left, except for the fibrolamellar variant, of which 75% of reported cases have been in the left lobe. Microscopically, the formation of giant cells is a feature of HCC. HCC cells frequently invade venous branches, causing vascular dilatation, which contributes to the nodular appearance of the liver. Fibrolamellar carcinoma has a distinctive feature: abundant fibrous stroma arranged in thin parallel bands.

e. **Clinical manifestations.** Eighty percent of patients experience weight loss and weakness. Approximately 50% (75% with fibrolamellar carcinoma) present with abdominal pain that usually is dull, persistent, and in the epigastrium or right upper quadrant. Acute severe abdominal pain has been associated with intraperitoneal hemorrhage due to rupture of a necrotic nodule or erosion of a blood vessel. This occurs infrequently (10% of patients) but may be lethal.

   Physical examination may reveal an enlarged but nontender liver. Splenomegaly as a result of portal hypertension may be present. Ascites is present in nearly half the patients but usually is mild. As it is often difficult to distinguish HCC from nodular areas of cirrhosis, a clinical picture with rapid acceleration of symptoms may suggest HCC. For instance, hypoglycemic intervals or amelioration of preexisting diabetes also suggests superimposed HCC.

f. **Diagnostic studies**

   (1) **Laboratory.** In cirrhotic patients, HCC may be associated with abnormal liver function tests due to hepatitis. In noncirrhotic patients, HCC is usually, but not always, associated with increases in alkaline phosphatase levels as well as elevations of transaminases and 5'-nucleotidase. Serum bilirubin usually is normal. AFP appears in the serum and is elevated in 75% of affected African patients but in only 30% of patients in the United States. AFP is also often elevated in chronic hepatitis and cirrhosis. A level greater than 200 ng/mL (normal less than 20 ng/mL) is suggestive of HCC, even in the cirrhotic patient.

   (2) **Radiologic studies**

      (a) **Ultrasonography** is noninvasive, relatively inexpensive, and can be highly accurate, when performed by a skilled sonographer, in the detection of HCC. The diagnostic accuracy is enhanced when ultrasound findings are coupled with concomitant AFP elevations.

      (b) **MR scan** can be useful in differentiating other small nodular masses from HCC. This is the most accurate imaging modality for distinguishing HCC from dysplastic or regenerative nodules in the cirrhotic patient.

      (c) **Spiral CT scan** with arterial and portal venous phase contrast imaging can identify liver masses. HCC enhances in the arterial and not usually in the portal venous phase. Its sensitivity may be enhanced with lipiodol (a lipid lymphographic agent that is selectively retained in HCC) when this is injected 2 hours before the scan.

      (d) **Needle biopsy.** Laparoscopic or image-guided percutaneous biopsies are used for obtaining a tissue diagnosis. A tissue diagnosis is not required before an attempt at surgical extirpation if other diagnostic modalities favor HCC as the diagnosis. Unresectable tumors may be biopsied to guide chemotherapy and confirm diagnosis.

g. **Treatment**

   (1) **Surgical resection.** The size and location of the HCC dictate the extent of hepatectomy. A macroscopic margin of 1 cm generally is regarded as adequate, although this may vary according to the size of the lesion. In some cases, resection entails a hemihepatectomy, although lesser liver-sparing segmental "anatomic" resections are preferred and have satisfactory results (*J Am Chem Soc* 1998;187:471) This is especially true in cases in which cirrhosis and associated morbidities pose a prohibitive risk for a major hepatic

resection. Repeat hepatic resection for recurrence has been demonstrated to be safe and effective in selected lesions.

   (2) **Liver transplantation** has become the surgical procedure of choice in patients with established cirrhosis and HCC who are not candidates for resection. To minimize recurrence, strict criteria for number and size of tumors exist in most centers (Milan Criteria). A single tumor up to 5 cm in size or up to 3 tumors with the largest less than 3 cm in size with no vascular invasion on imaging and absence of nodal and distant metastases is the criterion used by most centers. Transplantation for HCC is now performed in over 20% of cases in many areas of the United States.

   (3) **Radiation and chemotherapy** are not curative. Combining chemotherapy with surgery preoperatively or postoperatively has no benefit in terms of patient survival. Unresectable lesions or recurrences have been palliated with ablative techniques and chemotherpy.

   (4) **Ablative therapies** are effective for small HCCs and are the treatment of choice in patients who are not candidates for surgery because of advanced cirrhosis or other morbidities. In many Japanese centers, **percutaneous ethanol injection** has been reported to produce results as good as liver resection in lesions less than 3 cm in cirrhotic patients. Ethanol is injected into the tumor in one procedure or in staged procedures, depending on the size of the tumor. **Transarterial chemoembolization** combines devascularization of the tumor with administration of chemotherapy and is the primary therapy in many U.S. centers. **Radiofrequency ablation (RFA)** places RF electrodes in tumors and destroys them by heating the tumors to a temperature of between 60°C and 100°C. It is the newest modality and can also be performed percutaneously. All of the ablative modalities have been used to slow progression of tumors in patients who are on transplantation waiting lists.

 h. **Prognosis.** Unresected HCC has a very poor prognosis, with a median length of survival of 3 to 6 months after the diagnosis. Patients rarely survive beyond 4 months after the diagnosis. The 5-year survival rate after curative resection is 35% to 50%. The general assumption that fibrolamellar carcinoma (FLC) has a more favorable prognosis is no longer valid (*Hepatology* 1997;26: 877). FLC is often an aggressive tumor diagnosed at an advanced stage, and intrahepatic recurrence is common, occurring after 60% to 70% of resections. Indicators of poor outcomes include larger tumors, major vessel invasion, and serum AFP levels >2,000. In addition, resection in the setting of cirrhosis also demonstrates decreased long-term survival when compared with resection in noncirrhotics (*Ann Surg* 1999;229:790). Liver transplantation for extensive disease has achieved similar 5-year survival rates but probably has a much higher cure rate for tumors less than 5 cm and favorable histologic grade (*Ann Surg* 1998;228:479).

 2. **Metastatic neoplasms**
 a. **Pathology.** Metastatic disease of the liver is almost 20 times more common than primary carcinoma in the United States. Colorectal primaries frequently present with metastases confined within the liver. The metastatic lesion is usually more aggressive, with accelerated growth kinetics, than its extrahepatic primary. Operative resection is the only potentially curative approach, but it is applicable in only about 25% of patients who present with liver metastases. There have also been successful curative extirpations of metastatic lesions of breast, neuroendocrine, and melanoma derivation, although indications for such operations are limited.
 b. **Clinical manifestations.** Most patients are asymptomatic; however, with advanced disease, symptoms include fatigue, anorexia, weight

loss, dull pain, fullness in the epigastrium or a palpable mass, ascites, jaundice, and fever. With a carcinoid primary tumor, liver metastases are responsible for the carcinoid "flushing" syndrome, as serotonin byproducts are excreted directly into the systemic circulation from the liver without hepatic degradation.

c. **Diagnostic studies.** Although elevations in serum alkaline phosphatase, γ-glutamyl transpeptidase, lactate dehydrogenase, serum glutamic oxaloacetic transaminase, and 5'-nucleotidase levels may occur, they are neither sensitive nor specific for liver metastases. Serum AFP should be assessed to rule out a hepatoma, and the test is usually negative. In a patient with colorectal cancer, a **carcinoembryonic antigen (CEA) level** in excess of 5 ng/mL is the most sensitive blood test for detecting metastases. An elevation should prompt an abdominal CT scan or preferably a **positron emission tomogram (PET)** for more precise staging.

(1) **CT or MR scan** with arterial contrast enhancement is a sensitive preoperative imaging study, and T1-weighted MR scan is comparable to CT scan. However, small surface lesions frequently are missed by all preoperative imaging studies. Intraoperative ultrasonography with palpation is the most sensitive detector of liver metastasis.

(2) **PET** is the most sensitive test for liver metastases as well as extrahepatic metastases and may detect lesions in patients with elevated CEA and normal CT scan. It is based on the principle that metabolically active tumor cells have an increased avidity for glucose. Fluorodeoxyglucose is taken up by tumor cells but not metabolized, so that it accumulates in them. A glucose analogue–linked positron emitter is injected, and uptake is measured by nuclear scintigraphy. This technique is also extremely valuable in determining if tumor has recurred at the primary site, a condition that would preclude metastasectomy. Higher rates of resection and short-term survival have been reported following screening with this modality (*Ann Surg* 2001;233:293).

d. **Treatment of colorectal metastases.** Two conditions must be met for consideration of curative resection. First, control of the primary disease must be assured, and there should be no evidence of systemic disease. Second, the metastatic lesion must be suitable for local hepatic resection. When local factors include fewer than 5 tumors, and a 1-cm margin can safely be obtained, a formal anatomic liver resection should be performed. Outcomes are not as good if these parameters are not adhered to. For small solitary lesions that can safely be removed, a nonanatomic resection generally produces results similar to those of formal hepatectomy.

(1) **The timing of resection** is variable. If, during an uncomplicated initial colon resection, disease amenable to a wedge resection or a resection of segments II and III is identified, it can be resected without added morbidity. However, for lesions requiring hepatectomy or greater resections, a second operation is often performed after recovery from the primary operation (staged approach).

(2) **Hepatic resection** for colorectal cancer, when the preceding criteria are met, has a 30% to 35% 5-year survival rate and a 20% 10-year survival rate. Repeat hepatic resection for recurrent disease is safe and may be indicated in selected patients, yielding results similar to those of initial hepatic resection procedures. Adjuvant chemotherapy after liver resection is actively under investigation.

(3) **Regional chemotherapy** can be used to try to control microscopic disease in the liver, the primary site of failure following hepatic resection. Regional chemotherapy has been a focus of controversy

and has recently been utilized less as systemic chemotherapy has improved.

(4) The ablative technologies, **cryotherapy** and **RFA,** have also been used to treat unresectable metastatic tumors. RFA is a more convenient therapy and associated with fewer postoperative complications than cryoablation. RFA is used in combination with resection in selected patients who have metastases in both hemilivers.

II. Hepatic abscess. Liver abscesses may originate from bacterial, parasitic, or fungal pathogens. Bacterial abscesses predominate in the United States, whereas amebic (parasitic) abscesses are more common in younger age groups and in endemic areas.

A. Pyogenic abscesses in the liver

1. Etiology. Pyogenic liver abscesses generally occur secondary to other sources of bacterial sepsis in the abdomen, the two main sources being biliary sepsis and portal vein sepsis. Direct spread from biliary infections such as empyema of the gallbladder, from cholangitis, or after biliary tract surgery or instrumentation is uncommon but may be life-threatening. Bacterial abscesses from portal venous spread of infection from appendicitis, diverticulitis, or other enteric sources also are uncommon and may be difficult to diagnose. "Cryptogenic" hepatic abscesses have no identified primary infection and today are the most common abscesses. Other sources for hepatic contamination are distant infections, such as pneumonia, upper urinary tract infection, and endocarditis. Other rare bacterial liver abscess etiologies include superinfection of amebic or hydatid cyst lesions in the liver. The abscesses are solitary in approximately half of cases and curiously occupy the right hemiliver more frequently.

2. Diagnosis depends on clinical suspicion and is often delayed. Constitutional **symptoms** include fever, malaise, rigors, and weight loss. **Signs** include right upper quadrant or right costovertebral angle tenderness and a consistent, intermittent spiking fever. Jaundice is uncommon in the presence of the primary abscess, although it may accompany the associated primary biliary tract focus. The signs and symptoms typically reflect the nature of the primary bacterial source rather than the hepatic abscess. Useful imaging studies include ultrasonography and CT examination of the liver.

3. Treatment of bacterial liver abscess includes systemic antibiotic therapy and percutaneous drainage of the abscess cavity. The drain is removed when the cavity has collapsed. Drainage may be impossible, particularly if there are multiple small abscesses. Such cases represent a disproportionate percentage of the mortality associated with liver abscess. Operative drainage is used either when the patient requires laparotomy for management of the primary disease, such as appendicitis or cholecystitis, or when abscess drainage is not technically feasible via percutaneous techniques. Empiric antibiotic treatment should include coverage for bowel flora (Gram-negatives and anaerobic bacteria); once an isolate has been identified, appropriate treatment should be modified for the identified pathogens. Aggressive antibiotic therapy should continue for at least 1 week beyond the resolution of abscesses that can be imaged and beyond any overt evidence of systemic illness (i.e., resolution of fever and normalization of WBC).

B. Amebic abscess should be considered in every case of solitary hepatic abscess.

1. Etiology. Amebic abscess is caused by the organism *Entamoeba histolytica,* which travels from the GI tract to the liver via the portal venous system. The abscesses are most frequently solitary in the right hemiliver, and the contents are often necrotic, with a pasty consistency. The most concentrated area of amebic infiltration is at the edges of the abscess cavity.

2. Signs and symptoms of amebic abscess are similar to those of pyogenic abscess but may appear more indolent. Patients less frequently have chills, and symptoms may go on for a longer period before detection. Serologic tests for amebic infestation are positive in nearly 100% of affected patients. The imaging modalities that are most useful are CT scan and ultrasound of the liver.

3. **Management** requires systemic metronidazole (750 mg orally three times a day or 500 mg intravenously every 6 hours for 14 days). If there is no improvement in clinical systems within 48 hours of beginning antibiotics, a complicated amebic abscess must be considered.

4. **Complications** can include bacterial superinfection, erosion into surrounding structures, or free rupture into the peritoneal cavity. Percutaneous or operative drainage may then be necessary. Although mortality is infrequent in uncomplicated cases, complicated cases may carry a considerable mortality (as high as 40%).

III. **Hepatic cysts** can be divided into nonparasitic cysts and echinococcal cysts.

A. **Nonparasitic cysts** generally are benign. They can be solitary or multiple and typically are small and asymptomatic, often identified incidentally on imaging for other symptoms. Asymptomatic cysts require no treatment regardless of size. Large cysts may be symptomatic because of increased abdominal girth or compression of adjacent structures, and there may be vague pain. Bleeding, infection, or obstructive jaundice can occur but are infrequent. Such cysts can be unroofed operatively by either an open approach or, more recently, by laparoscopy. Infected cysts are treated in a similar manner to hepatic abscesses. If the cyst contains bile, communication with the biliary tree is assumed. It should be excised, enucleated, or drained, with the closure of the biliary communication.

Polycystic kidney disease sometimes is accompanied by **polycystic liver disease**, which usually is asymptomatic. If symptomatic, the symptoms generally are attributable to hepatomegaly from numerous cysts. Liver function is rarely impaired by the gross displacement of parenchyma by these massive cystic cavities. Symptomatic polycystic liver disease has been treated by drainage of the superficial cysts into the abdominal cavity and fenestration of deeper cysts into the superficial cyst cavities. Liver resection and retention of the least cystic areas of hepatic parenchyma may be more effective. Neoplastic cystic lesions, cystadenoma or cystadenocarcinoma, rarely occur in the liver. These lesions are distinguished from simple cysts by the presence of a mass or septa. They are treated by resection or enucleation (in the case of cystadenoma) to completely remove cyst epithelium.

B. **Echinococcal cysts** are the most common hepatic cystic lesions in areas outside the United States. Approximately 80% of hydatid cysts are single and in the right liver. The most common presenting symptoms and signs are right upper quadrant abdominal pain and palpable hepatomegaly. Imaging by nuclear medicine scan, ultrasonography, CT scan, or MR scan can demonstrate the abnormality. The cyst should not be aspirated as an initial test because aspiration can cause spillage of the organisms and spread the disease throughout the abdominal compartment. Useful laboratory tests include liver function tests, the results of which may be mildly elevated. In addition, a peripheral eosinophilia is often detected. Serologic tests include indirect hemagglutination and Casoni skin test, each of which is 85% sensitive.

Treatment is primarily operative, although percutaneous drainage after antihelminthic treatment is increasingly utilized in many centers in endemic regions. Operation is required for symptomatic and asymptomatic cysts, unless the asymptomatic cyst wall is completely circumferentially calcified. Small superficial or pendulous cysts may be excised. Larger cysts should be unroofed and the contents removed piecemeal. The abdomen is explored, and before unroofing, the cyst is isolated and excluded from the peritoneal cavity. Next, the cavity is aspirated with a closed system. If there is no evidence of bile in the cyst aspirate, a scolecoidal agent is instilled into the cavity. Choices include hypertonic saline, 80% alcohol, or 0.5% cetrimide.

A second cycle is performed after 5 minutes. In patients with biliary communication, only hypertonic sodium chloride (10% to 20%) or 0.5% sodium hypochlorite should be used as a scolecoidal agent because other agents may damage communicating bile ducts. Pericystectomy is excision of the cyst in the plane between the host pericyst and liver tissue. The advantage of this technique is that there is no residual cavity. Formal right or left hepatectomy is another alternative, particularly for larger multiple cysts, but it is rarely necessary. For those cysts with demonstrated communication with a biliary radical, drainage should be achieved with a Roux-en-Y hepaticoenterostomy. Postoperative therapy with mebendazole or albendazole has been advocated to prevent recurrence. In patients with disseminated echinococcosis or in those with systemic illnesses that prevent operative intervention, these agents are the cornerstone of therapy.

IV. **Portal hypertension** is the sequela of pre-, intra-, or posthepatic mechanical obstruction of the portal venous system.

  A. The **most common cause of portal hypertension** in the United States is *intrahepatic* obstruction of portal venous flow from cirrhosis (most commonly due to alcohol and/or hepatitis C but also due to nutritional, postnecrotic, and biliary causes); intrahepatic portal venous obstruction can also be due to hepatic fibrosis from hemochromatosis, Wilson disease, and congenital fibrosis. *Prehepatic* portal venous obstruction due to congenital atresia or portal vein thrombosis is far less common. *Posthepatic* obstruction (Budd-Chiari syndrome) is associated with lymphoreticular malignancy or a hypercoagulable state such as polycythemia vera. The prognosis is poor. Transjugular intrahepatic portosystemic stent-shunts (TIPS) or transplantation is recommended if no primary malignancy can be identified. The remainder of this section focuses on the management of portal hypertension caused by intrahepatic portal vein obstruction, primarily cirrhosis.

  B. **The manifestations of liver disease with portal hypertension result from hepatic insufficiency and the mechanical effects of portal venous hypertension.**

    1. **Hepatic insufficiency may result in hepatic encephalopathy,** which is a syndrome of disordered consciousness in patients with decreased hepatocellular function. The specific toxin that causes the encephalopathy has not yet been delineated. Potential agents include multiple toxins that normally are cleared by the liver, such as ammonia, γ-aminobutyric acid, mercaptans, and short-chain fatty acids. Factors associated with progressive hepatic encephalopathy include volume shifts due to medical treatment or renal failure, the use of medications that act on the central nervous system (e.g., benzodiazepines or opioids), protein load due to hemorrhage of blood in the GI tract, high dietary protein intake, worsening hepatocellular function, and the creation of central portosystemic shunts.

    2. **Manifestations of increased pressure** in the portal vein include increased blood flow through collateral venous beds and increased interstitial tissue hydrostatic pressure. The latter causes ascites. The collateral venous beds, which develop in cirrhosis, bypass the liver by connecting the portal circulation to the systemic circulation. The most clinically significant sites are those at the gastroesophageal junction that connect the left gastric vein (a part of the portal circulation) to the esophageal veins (systemic circulation), resulting in esophageal and gastric varices. Other common collaterals develop when a recanalized umbilical vein collateralizes to the abdominal wall veins or a superior hemorrhoidal vein collateralizes to middle and inferior hemorrhoidal veins. Left-sided (**sinistral**) portal hypertension can be caused by isolated splenic vein thrombosis. This is most often caused by adjacent pancreatitis. Thrombosis results in increased pressure in the splenic vein at the distal end of the pancreas and the development of collaterals through the short gastric vessels and gastric mucosa back to the liver, thus bypassing the thrombosed splenic

vein segment. This segmental area of portal hypertension typically causes gastric varices without esophageal varices. Cure is achieved by splenectomy in isolated splenic vein thrombosis.

3. **Mechanisms of ascites and edema** are salt and water retention by the kidneys, decreased plasma oncotic pressure, and increased lymphatic flow from increased portal venous hydrostatic pressure. Although the ascites can be massive, it is rarely life-threatening unless complications occur, such as umbilical hernia with erosion, infection and ascitic leak, respiratory embarrassment, and spontaneous bacterial peritonitis. Spontaneous bacterial peritonitis presents as abdominal pain, fever, ileus, and worsening encephalopathy; however, the signs are subtle, and diagnosis may be difficult. Diagnosis is made by paracentesis and is likely when ascitic fluid contains more than 250 polymorphonuclear leukocytes per μL and if a single organism is cultured. Bacterial cultures should be collected in blood culture bottles; the most common organisms are *Escherichia coli*, pneumococci, and streptococci.

C. **Management of portal hypertension**

1. **Elective reduction of portal venous pressure** can be accomplished by a variety of venous shunting procedures or by hepatic replacement with liver transplantation. The objective of these procedures is to reduce the pressure in the portal vein and thus decrease the flow through collateral venous beds. In addition, central shunts are effective in reducing ascites. Excellent results have been reported over the last decade with the use of surgical shunts in patients with preserved hepatic function (Child's grade A or B). Liver transplantation is the only treatment that addresses and reverses the primary defect of increased hepatic resistance to portal venous flow. This modality is reserved for those patients with chronic or acute hepatic failure.

   a. **Liver transplantation** should be considered for any patient with cirrhosis who has survived an episode of variceal hemorrhage and who has manifestations of end-stage liver disease (see Chapter 28). Patients who are likely candidates for liver transplantation probably should not undergo elective portosystemic shunt operations, if possible, because such shunts may make subsequent liver transplantation more technically demanding.

   b. **Total portosystemic shunt** operations include end-to-side, side-to-side, portacaval, mesocaval, and central splenorenal shunts. The end-to-side operation is the prototype and is the simplest portacaval shunt to perform. It involves disconnection of the portal venous circulation from the liver and connection of the intestinal end of the portal vein to the inferior vena cava. This bypasses all the portal circulation from the liver to the systemic circulation, thus decompressing any collateral venous beds. The other variations of this operation include a side-to-side portacaval anastomosis as well as anastomoses at sites more distant from the liver, such as mesocaval H-graft and central splenorenal shunts. The physiologic effects of all these shunts are similar because flow through the hepatic limb of the portosystemic shunt is nearly always away from the liver and toward the anastomosis. If a shunt is constructed, immediate and permanent protection from visceral bleeding occurs, as the venous collateral beds are decompressed. The primary complication of these operations is hepatic encephalopathy due to reduced hepatic blood flow. Attempts have been made to construct smaller side-to-side grafts to partly maintain hepatic flow and reduce the incidence of encephalopathy.

   c. **Selective shunts** were developed to decrease the pressure in a portion of the portal circulation while disconnecting from the remainder of the portal circulation. The classic procedure is the distal splenorenal (Warren) shunt, which involves dividing the splenic vein and anastomosing the splenic end of the vein to the left renal vein. The left gastric vein, the right gastroepiploic vein, and the veins in the splenocolic ligament are then all divided. This excludes the gastrosplenic portal circulation from the remainder of the portal circulation and selectively decompresses the gastroesophageal varices. This operation is more difficult and time consuming than the total shunt procedures, and it is appropriate only for elective treatment of patients with gastroesophageal varices and a history of bleeding. It is contraindicated in patients with ascites that cannot be controlled medically. Hepatic encephalopathy occurs less commonly with this approach. Over time, the shunt tends to become less selective as alternative collateral pathways develop that reconnect the main portal venous circulation to the gastrosplenic portal venous system; varices may redevelop at that time.

  d. **The Sugiura procedure** may occasionally be used in patients with recalcitrant variceal hemorrhage. In this procedure, the spleen is removed, the stomach and lower esophagus are devascularized, and the esophagus is transected and reanastomosed with a circular stapling device to disrupt the esophageal venous plexus. This procedure is rarely used in the United States but is popular in the Far East.

  e. The development of **TIPS** has provided a nonsurgical alternative for the treatment of portal hypertension. TIPS is a minimally invasive alternative to open surgical procedures and can temporarily and effectively reduce portal hypertension. It involves the intrahepatic placement of an expandable metallic stent between branches of the hepatic and portal venous circulation. Technical success rates approach 95%, with short-term success in controlling acute variceal hemorrhage observed in more than 80% of patients. Although TIPS is clearly indicated in cases of acute variceal bleeding that cannot be successfully managed with standard medical therapy (see the following section), TIPS stenoses require careful follow-up and revision procedures in a significant percentage of patients. Recently introduced polytetrafluoroethylene-covered stents have markedly decreased stenosis and improved long-term patency.

2. **Acute management of bleeding esophageal varices** is complex and requires multidisciplinary support of the bleeding patient. Because up to one-third of patients affected with bleeding esophageal varices die during the initial hospitalization for GI bleeding, an aggressive approach is necessary. Many patients experience a warning or "herald" episode of lesser severity before life-threatening exsanguination. Therefore, all patients with known or suspected esophageal varices and active GI bleeding should immediately be admitted to the intensive care unit for resuscitation and monitoring. Endotracheal intubation to protect the airway, prevent aspiration, and facilitate the safe performance of endoscopy and other procedures is nearly always indicated. Vascular access, including short, large-bore peripheral lines, and invasive monitoring of central venous pressure and arterial pressure should be achieved. Urinary bladder catheterization and initial volume resuscitation should ensue. Then the patient should have emergent upper endoscopy to document the source of hemorrhage. Because up to 50% of patients with known esophageal varices have upper GI hemorrhage from an alternative source, such as gastric or duodenal ulcer, a thorough endoscopy is required. Once varices are identified as the source, several therapeutic options exist, and one should be implemented.

  a. **Endoscopic sclerotherapy or banding** is performed at the patient's bedside in the intensive care unit at initial endoscopy. Sclerotherapy or band ligation can be effective in controlling primary hemorrhage and obliterating varices after primary hemorrhage is controlled. Recurrent bleeding occurs in as many as 50% of patients. Endoscopic variceal ligation (banding) is as effective as sclerotherapy in controlling active variceal bleeding and is associated with fewer complications and a lower rebleeding rate than endoscopic sclerotherapy.

b. **Intravenous octreotide** can be used simultaneously with other treatments. It can decrease flow through the esophageal varices and control hemorrhage but is less effective than variceal banding. The standard dosage is 50 μg intravenous bolus, followed by 50 μg/hr infusion continued until endoscopic management can be performed. Vasopressin became second line to octreotide after multiple clinical trials proved octreotide to be superior. A newer alternative not currently available in the United States is terlipressin (Glypressin), a synthetic analogue of vasopressin that appears to be equally effective but has fewer side effects.

c. **Balloon tamponade** is useful as a temporary remedy for variceal bleeding while more definitive therapy is planned. The specially designed balloon catheters include the Sengstaken-Blakemore tube, the Minnesota tube, and the Linton tube. Each has a gastric balloon; the Sengstaken-Blakemore and Minnesota tubes also have an esophageal balloon. For safe and effective use of these devices, the balloons must be carefully placed according to the manufacturer's directions. The position of the gastric balloon in the stomach must always be confirmed by x-ray before inflation because balloon inflation in the esophagus can be disastrous. Balloon pressure must be maintained as directed by the manufacturer to avoid the complications of mucosal ulceration and necrosis. This is not definitive therapy and should be used only as a temporizing measure, for no longer than 24 hours.

d. **TIPS** can be used in the acute management of patients with variceal bleeding. Once the patient has been stabilized enough to travel to an interventional radiology suite, the TIPS procedure may provide acute decompression of the esophageal varices and thus control bleeding that has been recalcitrant to endoscopic sclerotherapy. This may be particularly useful as a bridge to transplantation for appropriate candidates.

e. **Emergency portacaval shunt** generally is reserved for patients in whom other measures have failed and is almost never performed today. This operation carries significant in-hospital mortality and risk of hepatic encephalopathy, particularly because the patients selected to undergo the operation typically have not been successfully treated by other means and require multiple blood transfusions, often due to poor hepatic reserve. Only the technically simpler central portacaval shunts (end-to-side or side-to-side) should be used in the emergency setting because the other shunts require more dissection and operative time.

f. **After acute variceal hemorrhage is controlled,** the patient should be treated with chronic esophageal variceal sclerotherapy/banding. After initial control has been achieved, a second session is scheduled for 7 to 10 days later. A third treatment is scheduled approximately 1 month after the initial bleed and then at 3-month intervals thereafter until all varices are eliminated. This treatment regimen can decrease the rebleeding rate from 80% to 50% and has resulted in a 25% reduction in overall mortality in randomized trials. Patients who fail on chronic band ligation because of rebleeding should be considered for elective shunting procedures, TIPS, or liver transplantation, depending on their degree of hepatic reserve and other indications for liver transplantation.

3. **Management of ascites** must be cautious and gradual to avoid sudden changes in systemic volume status, which can precipitate hepatic encephalopathy, renal failure, or death.

a. **Salt restriction** is the initial treatment. Sodium intake should be limited to 1,000 mg per day. Stricter limitations are unpalatable, and most patients are non-compliant with such regimens.

b. Diuretic therapy should be gradually applied in patients in whom ascites is not controlled by salt restriction. Weight loss should rarely be more than 500 g per day to avoid significant side effects. Spironolactone is the initial diuretic of choice at 25 mg orally twice per day. This dosage may be increased to a maximum of 400 mg per day in divided doses. Furosemide (20 mg orally per day initially) may be added if spironolactone fails to initiate diuresis. Volume status must be monitored closely by daily weight check and frequent examinations during initial furosemide treatment.

c. Paracentesis is useful in the initial evaluation of ascites, when spontaneous bacterial peritonitis (SBP) is included in the differential diagnosis, and to provide acute decompression of tense ascites. Up to 10 L of ascites can be removed safely if the patient has peripheral edema, the fluid is removed over 30 to 90 minutes, and oral fluid restriction is instituted to avoid hyponatremia. Paracentesis can be used to provide acute relief of symptoms of tense ascites, including respiratory compromise, impending peritoneal rupture through an ulcerated umbilical hernia, or severe abdominal discomfort.

d. TIPS can be used for refractory ascites. Complete resolution of ascites has been reported in 57% to 74% of patients and partial response in another 9% to 22%.

e. A **peritoneal venous shunt** can be used in the minority of patients who have ascites refractory to all medical therapy. The LeVeen shunt, constructed of plastic, is placed with one end in the peritoneal cavity and the other end in the subclavian vein. The Denver shunt is a modification that includes a subcutaneous manual pump that can be used to transfer ascites intermittently from the abdomen to the subclavian vein. These shunts are particularly useful in patients with tense ascites and umbilical hernias because they can provide decompression of the ascites during the perioperative period of the hernia repair. The main complication of peritoneal venous shunting is disseminated intravascular coagulation, which can be fulminant after shunt placement and requires shunt occlusion. This rarely occurs if the peritoneal cavity is lavaged first. Shunts are **contraindicated** in patients with bacterial peritonitis, recent variceal hemorrhage, liver failure, advanced hepatorenal syndrome, or existing severe coagulopathy. The shunts tend to occlude with time and are used very rarely today.

4. Control of hepatic encephalopathy requires the limitation of dietary protein intake and the use of lactulose and oral antibiotics.

a. Dietary changes should be initiated first. Dietary protein should be eliminated while adequate nonprotein calories are administered. After clinical improvement, a 20-g-per-day protein diet may be administered, with increasing protein allowances of 10 g per day every 3 to 5 days if encephalopathy does not recur.

b. If the encephalopathy is not controlled by diet alone, **oral agents** can be added.

(1) Lactulose is a nonabsorbed synthetic disaccharide that produces an osmotic diarrhea, altering intestinal flora. The oral dosage is 15 to 45 mL two to four times a day. The dosage then is adjusted to produce two to three daily soft stools. Alternatively, a lactulose enema can be prepared with 300 mL lactulose and 700 mL tap water administered two to four times a day.

(2) Useful oral antibiotic preparations include neomycin (1 g orally every 4 to 6 hours or 1% retention enema every 6 to 12 hours) and metronidazole (250 mg orally every 8 hours). The oral antibiotics are used as second-line agents to lactulose because, although they are equally effective, neomycin carries some risk of ototoxicity and nephrotoxicity, and metronidazole carries some risk of neurotoxicity, albeit only with prolonged administration.

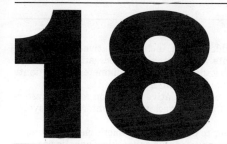

Biliary Surgery

Yolanda Y. L. Yang and
Steven M. Strasberg

I. **Cholelithiasis and its complications**
   A. **Incidence** of cholelithiasis increases with age. At age 60, approximately 25% of women and 12% of men have gallstones. In some countries (e.g., Sweden, Chile) and among certain ethnic groups (e.g., Pima Indians), the incidence of gallstones may approach 50%.
   B. **Pathogenesis and natural history.** People with gallstones can be divided into three groups: those who are asymptomatic, those with symptoms, and those who develop complications. This is generally a stepwise progression. The majority of people with gallstones never become symptomatic. Of the asymptomatic patients with gallstones, only 1% to 2% per year will manifest symptoms of biliary colic. It is unusual (<0.5% per year) for an asymptomatic patient to develop complicated gallstone disease without first suffering symptoms. Complications develop in ~3% of patients with symptomatic biliary colic per year. These complications include acute cholecystitis, choledocholithiasis, cholangitis, pancreatitis, and gallstone ileus.
      1. **Cholesterol gallstones** (85% of all stones) are associated with increasing age, female gender, obesity, and Western diet. The female to male ratio is 2:1, and the increased incidence among women is in part related to pregnancy and/or the use of oral contraceptives. Obesity is an independent factor increasing the prevalence of cholesterol gallstones by a factor of 3. Western diet is closely related, and stones are rare in vegetarians.
      2. **Pigment gallstones** (15% of all stones)
         a. **Black gallstones** are composed of calcium bilirubinate, calcium phosphate, and calcium carbonate, which may be complexed with other minerals or proteins. Risk factors include hemolytic disorders, cirrhosis, and ileal resection.
         b. **Brown gallstones** are associated with biliary stasis and infection (particularly with *Klebsiella* species). The stones are composed of bacterial cell bodies and also contain calcium bilirubinate and calcium palmitate.
   C. **Asymptomatic gallstones**
      1. **Diagnosis.** Asymptomatic gallstones are usually discovered on routine studies performed on healthy patients or patients being investigated for a symptom not related to the presence of gallstones. This may include radiopaque stones found on routine x-ray or gallstones visualized during obstetric ultrasonography. Common abdominal symptoms such as dyspepsia, bloating, eructation, or flatulence *without associated pain* are probably not caused by gallstones. Gallstones may also be discovered incidentally at laparotomy. In this situation, the patient's history and physical exam must be reviewed to determine whether the gallstones were truly asymptomatic.
      2. **Management.** There is no role for prophylactic cholecystectomy in most patients with asymptomatic gallstones, with a few exceptions.
         a. **High cancer risks.** Patients with a **porcelain gallbladder** (the rare occurrence of a calcified gallbladder *wall*) should have cholecystectomy because of a higher risk of malignancy (reported rates vary between 7% and 62%). Prophylactic cholecystectomy may also be warranted in other subgroups of patients with asymptomatic gallstones who are at

increased risk for gallbladder cancer, including Native American ad-
mixed populations, patients with anomalous pancreatic–biliary ductal junctions, patients with gallstones >3 cm in diameter, and patients
with solitary gallbladder polyps >1 cm in diameter.

b. Children with gallstones have a relative indication for cholecystectomy due to the general difficulty of declaring and interpreting symptoms in this population.

c. Diabetes mellitus. Whether to perform prophylactic cholecystectomy
in the diabetic patient with gallstones is debatable. Diabetic patients
are not more likely than other asymptomatic patients to become symptomatic with biliary colic or even to experience more severe complications without first presenting with biliary colic. However, the
consequences of complications are more severe in diabetic patients.
Therefore, there appears no reason to treat diabetic patients while
they are asymptomatic, but it is recommended that *symptomatic* diabetic patients have prompt surgery.

d. Patients debilitated with **spinal cord trauma** have an increased incidence of asymptomatic, symptomatic, and complicated cholelithiasis but are also at increased risk for perioperative morbidity with
cholecystectomy. Therefore, prophylactic cholecystectomy for uncomplicated gallstone disease in this population is *not* warranted, but
there should be a low threshold for cholecystectomy if complications
are suspected.

e. Patients with **sickle cell anemia** do *not* have an indication for prophylactic cholecystectomy for asymptomatic gallstones. However, elective
cholecystectomy is recommended for symptomatic patients or when
there has been difficulty discriminating between cholecystitis and
intrahepatic crisis. These patients require special perioperative attention to prevent anoxic injury and may need preoperative blood
transfusions, volume expansion, and oxygen therapy. After cholecystectomy, these patients may still form symptomatic common bile duct
stones.

f. Management of **gallstones discovered at laparotomy** remains controversial. The literature is conflicting with regard to the incidence of
biliary symptoms after surgery in patients in whom the gallbladder
is not removed and also with regard to the incidence of longer recovery time and perioperative complications in patients who do have
incidental cholecystectomy ("cholecystectomy *en passant*"). A clear-
cut role for prophylactic cholecystectomy for treatment of asymptomatic stones discovered during major abdominal surgery has yet
to be demonstrated. Cholecystectomy *en passant* is contraindicated
when vascular grafts are being placed concommitantly in the abdomen, when the cholecystectomy procedure is likely to be hazardous,
when the patient is unstable from the primary procedure, or when
long extensions of incisions are required to gain exposure of the gallbladder.

D. Symptomatic gallstones (biliary colic)

1. Diagnosis largely depends on correlating symptoms with imaging.
Differential diagnoses includes acute cholecystitis, peptic ulcer disease, renal colic, gastroesophageal reflux, irritable bowel syndrome,
and diseases based in the chest, including inferior wall myocardial is-
chemia/infarct or right lower lobe pneumonia. Appropriate auxiliary
testing is dictated by clinical suspicion of these entities.

a. Symptoms. Biliary colic is the main symptom and is initiated by impaction of a gallstone in the outlet of the gallbladder. Typical pain is
characterized by the following four attributes:

(1) Periodicity. The pain comes in distinct attacks lasting 30 minutes
to several hours, between which the patient is well.

(2) **Location.** The pain occurs in the epigastrium or right upper quadrant.

(3) **Severity.** The pain is steady and intense and may cause the patient to cry or restrict breathing. Frequently it is so severe that it prompts the patient to seek professional care immediately, and parenteral narcotics may be necessary for control.

(4) **Timing.** The pain occurs within hours of eating a meal; often, it awakens the patient from sleep.

Other related symptoms include back pain, left upper quadrant pain, nausea, and vomiting, but it is important to understand that these usually occur in addition to rather than in place of the pain as described. Although the pain may be atypical (varying in one or more of the four attributes), the less typical the pain, the more another cause should be suspected.

b. Physical signs include mild right upper quadrant tenderness, although there may be few abdominal findings during an attack of biliary colic. Jaundice is not typical.

c. Diagnostic imaging. Ultrasound diagnosis is based on the presence of echogenic structures in conjunction with posterior acoustic shadows. There is usually little or no associated gallbladder wall thickening or other evidence of cholecystitis. The biliary ducts must be assessed for evidence of dilatation or choledocholithiasis (gallstones in the common bile duct).

d. Pathology. Note that *chronic cholecystitis* is a pathological term and not a clinical diagnosis. Patients with symptomatic gallstones have chronic cholecystitis (chronic inflammatory cells, fibrosis) in the wall of the gallbladder.

2. Laparoscopic cholecystectomy is the appropriate treatment for the vast majority of patients with symptomatic gallstones (see Section I.F.1.).

E. Complications of cholelithiasis

1. Acute calculous cholecystitis is an inflammatory complication of cholelithiasis that involves the gallbladder to a variable degree. As in biliary colic, acute cholecystitis is initiated by obstruction of the cystic duct by an impacted gallstone. Persistance of stone impaction leads to inflammation, by incompletely understood mechanisms, but supersaturated bile seems important. Although the onset and character of the resulting pain resemble those of biliary colic, the pain is unremitting and may persist for days. In a limited number of cases, one of the complications of acute cholecystitis may develop, including empyema, gangrene, or contained or free perforation of the gallbladder with abscess formation.

a. Diagnosis of cholecystitis depends on the constellation of symptoms and signs and the demonstration of characteristic findings with diagnostic imaging.

(1) The **symptoms** of acute cholecystitis are similar to but more severe than those of biliary colic. Unlike in the case of biliary colic, the right upper quadrant pain is persistent. As the inflammatory process progresses to the parietal peritoneum, patients develop tenderness in the right upper quadrant or even more diffusely and are reluctant to move. Systemic complaints such as anorexia, nausea, and vomiting are common. Rigors may occur but are uncommon. Fever may or may not be present. **Murphy's sign** (inspiratory arrest during deep palpation of the right upper quadrant) is characteristic of acute cholecystitis and is most informative when the acute inflammation has subsided and direct tenderness is absent. Mild jaundice may be present, but severe jaundice is rare and suggests the presence of common bile duct stones, cholangitis, or obstruction of the common hepatic duct. Biliary obstruction

may occur as a result of external compression of the common bile duct by a large stone impacted in the Hartmann pouch and the associated intense pericholecystic inflammatory process; this is termed *Mirizzi syndrome.*

(2) **Laboratory abnormalities** may include leukocytosis (typically 12×10^3 to 15×10^3 cells/μL, or 12×10^9 to 15×10^9 cells/L), although often the white blood cell count is normal. Complications of cholecystitis, such as gangrene, perforation, or cholangitis, are suggested by an extremely high white blood cell count, more than 20×10^3 cells/μL (or 20×10^9 cells/L). Liver function tests, including serum bilirubin, alkaline phosphatase, and serum amylase tests, also may be abnormal. However, patients with acute cholecystitis often present with persistent right upper quadrant pain even in the absence of fever or leukocytosis.

(3) **Diagnostic imaging**

    (a) **Ultrasonography** is the best test for diagnosing acute cholecystitis. Findings indicative of acute cholecystitis include gallbladder wall thickening, pericholecystic fluid, and a sonographic Murphy sign (tenderness over the gallbladder when directly compressed by the ultrasound probe). In one meta-analysis, the sensitivity and specificity of ultrasonography for evaluating patients with suspected gallstones were 0.84 and 0.99, respectively. For the diagnosis of acute cholecystitis, the sensitivity was 0.88 and specificity 0.80 (*Arch Int Med* 1994;154:2573).

    (b) **Radionuclide cholescintigraphy** occasionally is useful when the diagnosis is still unclear after ultrasonography. Scintigraphic scanning with derivatives of iminodiacetic acid such as hepatic 2,6-dimethyliminodiacetic acid (HIDA) enables visualization of the biliary system. The radionuclide is concentrated and secreted by the liver, allowing visualization of the bile ducts and the gallbladder normally within 30 minutes. Because the test depends on hepatic excretion of bile, it may not be useful in jaundiced patients. Nonfilling of the gallbladder *after* 4 hours in the appropriate clinical setting is good evidence of acute cholecystitis. Administration of morphine may increase the sensitivity and specificity of the test by encouraging spasm of the sphincter of Oddi and thereby enhancing gallbladder filling.

    (c) **Computed tomographic (CT) scanning** occasionally is performed to evaluate the patient with abdominal pain and acute illness. CT scan can demonstrate gallstones, although it is less sensitive for these than is ultrasonography. Other signs of acute cholecystitis on CT scan may include gallbladder wall thickening, pericholecystic fluid and edema, and emphysematous cholecystitis (air in the gallbladder or gallbladder wall).

b. **Management**

    (1) **Initial management** for patients with acute cholecystitis includes hospitalization, intravenous fluid resuscitation, and parenteral antibiotics appropriate for the Gram-negative rods and anaerobes that are typical of bowel flora. Traditionally, the regimens have been (1) a third-generation cephalosporin with good anaerobic coverage, (2) a third-generation cephalosporin combined with metronidazole, and, less frequently, (3) an aminoglycoside with metronidazole. However, the recent introduction of fourth-generation cephalosporins with broad coverage has provided a simple, powerful alternative. Although enterococci are frequently cultured from the gallbladder in acute cholecystitis, it is not

necessary to cover these organisms separately because rarely are they solitary pathogens.

(2) Acute cholecystitis often resolves with nonsurgical initial management. However, the patient must be **reassessed frequently** with respect to fever curve, symptoms, physical signs of inflammation, and laboratory values. If the patient is deteriorating or not improving, alterations in management must be made. These include changing the antibiotic regimen, percutaneous cholecystostomy, or operative cholecystectomy or cholecystostomy.

(3) Patients with acute cholecystitis should have **cholecystectomy as definitive treatment** (see Section I.F). Controversy surrounds the timing of operation. Because most cases of acute cholecystitis resolve with antibiotic therapy, cholecystectomy may be performed in either an early or delayed fashion.

(a) **Early cholecystectomy** has the advantage of resolving the illness more quickly than delayed cholecystectomy. The operation is best performed within 48 hours after the onset of symptoms, when there is less inflammation around the base of the gallbladder. When cholecystectomy is performed during an episode of acute cholecystitis (as compared with symptomatic cholelithiasis), the rate of conversion from laparoscopic to open surgery increases from <1% to approximately 5% (*Am J Surg* 2002;184:254).

(b) If the patient presents well into the course of acute cholecystitis (>3 days of symptoms), **delayed cholecystectomy** ("interval cholecystectomy") is usually indicated to allow surrounding inflammation to subside before the operation.

(c) **Prospective, randomized trials** comparing early versus delayed (6 weeks) laparoscopic cholecystectomy for acute cholecystitis suggest no significant differences in the conversion rate to open cholecystectomy between the two types. This suggests that for most patients with acute cholecystitis, early laparoscopic cholecystectomy should be attempted, with conversion to an open procedure if necessary (*Br J Surg* 1998,85:764, *Ann Surg* 1998,227:468).

(4) **Tube cholecystostomy** should be performed in patients who have acute cholecystitis and who are failing systemic therapy but are not candidates for cholecystectomy because of severity of illness or concomitant medical problems. Although cholecystostomy can be performed operatively, these patients usually benefit from the less invasive percutaneous approach. Drainage and decompression of the gallbladder almost uniformly resolves the episode of acute cholecystitis. After resolution of the acute episode, the patient can eventually undergo either cholecystectomy or percutaneous stone extraction and removal of the cholecystostomy tube. Such nonoperative stone removal as definitive treatment is reasonable in very elderly or debilitated patients who cannot have a general anesthetic.

2. **Choledocholithiasis** generally is due to gallstones that originate in the gallbladder and pass through the cystic duct into the common duct ("secondary" bile duct stones). In Western countries, stones rarely originate in the hepatic or common ducts, although these "primary" stones are more prevalent in the Far East.

a. **Diagnosis.** The most common manifestation of uncomplicated choledocholithiasis is **jaundice**, with bilirubin typically between 3 and 10 mg/dL (51 and 170 μmol/L). Biliary colic is common and is similar to that previously described (see Section I.D.). On physical examination, signs may be limited to icterus. Ultrasonography is useful and usually demonstrates associated gallstones in the gallbladder and bile duct dilation. The bile duct stones are seen in only about 50% of cases. Frequently, gallstones in the *lower* common bile duct cannot be demonstrated by ultrasonography because of overlying bowel gas. The diagnosis often is confirmed by endoscopic retrograde cholangiopancreatography (ERCP) or percutaneous transhepatic cholangiography (PTC), which can opacify the biliary tree and demonstrate the intraductal stones. Occasionally, the diagnosis of choledocholithiasis is confirmed by intraoperative cholangiography at the time of cholecystectomy.

b. Management of choledocholithiasis depends on the available expertise.

(1) Initial management includes **ERCP with sphincterotomy and stone removal** in all patients who are not candidates for surgery or who have had prior cholecystectomy and in patients who are jaundiced with stones, including all patients with acute cholangitis. Patients with intrahepatic stones and those with many common duct stones are also usually treated with ERCP. Other patients with choledocholithiasis in whom cholecystectomy is indicated may have the stones removed by operative bile duct exploration with postoperative ERCP if necessary. ERCP with sphincterotomy carries a <1% risk of mortality and 5% to 10% risk of morbidity, principally acute pancreatitis. When the expertise for laparoscopic bile duct exploration is not available, ERCP may be used preoperatively to clear all stones.

(2) Definitive management includes **cholecystectomy with cholangiography**. Cholangiography is performed prior to bile duct exploration to localize stones. Intraoperative attempts to clear the common bile duct of stones includes use of irrigation, blind passage of balloon catheters or stone baskets, or passage of these devices via choledochoscope. If the bile duct cannot be cleared of stones by laparoscopic exploration or ERCP, open bile duct exploration may be required, but this is uncommon.

3. Gallstone ileus is an uncommon complication that results from obstruction of the intestine by a large gallstone. The gallstone erodes from the gallbladder into the adjacent duodenum and travels in the small bowel lumen until it lodges in the narrowest portion of the small bowel, just proximal to the ileocecal valve. Patients present with a small bowel obstruction and air in the biliary tree (from the cholecystoenteric fistula). Treatment is exploratory laparotomy and removal of the obstructing gallstone from the bowel by milking the stone back through an enterotomy made in healthy intestine. Rarely, segmental small bowel resection is needed because of erosion of the stone. The entire bowel should be searched diligently for other stones. Additional stones may be present in the gallbladder, which should be removed if the patient is stable and the inflammation is not too severe. If cholecystectomy is not possible, cholecystostomy with stone removal is indicated for large stones. Intraoperative ultrasound may aid in making the decision.

4. Biliary pancreatitis is caused by blockage of pancreatic secretion by passage of a gallstone into the common biliary-pancreatic channel that exists in most patients at the termination of these ducts. The greatest risk is carried by small (~2 mm) stones. Management of *severe* biliary pancreatitis includes ERCP with sphincterotomy. Otherwise, ERCP in the acute setting probably is not indicated, because most of the time the causative stone has passed. Once the acute episode of pancreatitis has resolved, the gallbladder should be removed while the patient is still hospitalized, or within 2 weeks, to prevent recurrent acute biliary pancreatitis. A longer delay may be justified in patients who have had severe pancreatitis and in whom local inflammation or systemic illness contraindicates surgery. An operative cholangiogram should *always* be done at the time of the cholecystectomy to confirm that the bile duct is free of stones.

F. **Surgical management of symptomatic cholelithiasis and acute cholecystitis**

   1. **Laparoscopic cholecystectomy** is performed following standard laparoscopic principles. The complication rate from this procedure is low, and the patient's recovery and return-to-work times are excellent. During the procedure, a standard method of identifying the cystic duct and artery should be used.

      a. **Indications.** Approximately 95% of patients with cholelithiasis are candidates for the laparoscopic approach. Contraindications include generalized peritonitis, cholangitis, concomitant diseases that prevent use of a general anesthetic, and the patient's refusal of open cholecystectomy should urgent conversion be required. Local inflammation in the triangle of Calot can prevent complete visualization of the appropriate structures and increases the risk of injury to the bile ducts or hepatic arteries.

      b. **Critical view technique.** To prevent biliary injury, the cystic duct and cystic artery must be identified before transection. To achieve proper identification, the triangle of Calot must be dissected free of fat as well as fibrous and areolar tissue, and, importantly, the lower end of the gallbladder must be dissected off of the liver bed. A complete dissection demonstrates only two structures (the cystic duct and artery) entering the gallbladder. This constitutes the "critical view of safety."

      c. **Intraoperative cholangiography** is indicated in patients with known choledocholithiasis, a history of jaundice, a history of pancreatitis, a large cystic duct and small gallstones, any abnormality in preoperative liver function tests, or dilated biliary ducts on preoperative sonography. In addition, an absolute indication is the need to confirm the ductal anatomy during laparoscopic cholecystectomy whenever the critical view is not achieved by dissection. The infundibular technique (in which identification of the cystic duct relies solely on the funnel-shaped juncture of the gallbladder with the cystic duct) should be avoided because it can be deceptive, especially in the presence of inflammation. If the infundibular technique is used, cholangiography is recommended for confirming the anatomy before placing clips and transecting the cystic duct.

      d. **Laparoscopic ultrasound** as an alternative method for the detection of common bile duct stones is highly accurate and has decreased operative time and cost in experienced hands (*Surg Clin North AM* 2000;80:1151).

      e. **Complications.** Laparoscopic cholecystectomy appears to be associated with a higher incidence of bile duct injury than open cholecystectomy, approximately 6/1,000 (*Surg Clin North Am* 1996;76:623). In addition, there are also risks to other structures, including the hepatic artery and the bowel. Unretrieved gallstone spillage can be the source of infrequent but serious long-term complications.

   2. **Open cholecystectomy** is performed in the minority of patients who have contraindications to laparoscopic cholecystectomy, in patients who require conversion from laparoscopic cholecystectomy because of inability to complete the laparoscopic procedure, or when necessary in conjunction with a laparotomy for another operation (e.g., Whipple procedure). The gallbladder is dissected free of the hepatic bed from the top down after identification but before division of the cystic structures. This allows definitive demonstration of the cystic duct and cystic artery and prevents damage to the remaining biliary tree or hepatic arterial circulation. As biliary and arterial anatomy is variable, a method for conclusive identification of the cystic duct and artery is recommended before each is

divided. Drains are infrequently necessary and are most often placed when there is concern about leakage from a biliary radical.

3. **Medical dissolution** of gallstones can sometimes be effected with oral bile acid therapy, but given the proven effectiveness of laparoscopic cholecystectomy, there is virtually no current application of medical dissolution. Development of gallstones after gastric bypass for morbid obesity is very common and may largely be prevented by bile acid therapy. The current optimal bile acid therapy for dissolution of gallstones is ursodeoxycholic acid (10 to 15 mg/kg per day).

II. **Acalculous cholecystitis and other biliary tract inflammations**

A. **Acalculous cholecystitis** typically occurs in severely ill hospitalized patients, especially with a history of hypotension. It is also associated with prolonged dependence on parenteral nutrition, with episodes of systemic sepsis, or during multiple organ system failure. The mortality rate is high, ranging from 10% to 50%.

1. A high index of suspicion is required to make the **diagnosis**.

a. **Presentation** depends largely on the patient's concurrent medical conditions. Alert patients typically complain of right upper quadrant or diffuse upper abdominal pain and tenderness. However, many of these patients may not be alert, and therefore pain and tenderness is absent in up to 75% of patients. Unexplained deterioration in severely ill patients as described above should lead to suspicion of this diagnosis.

b. Especially in patients who are sedated or those with altered consciousness, **laboratory data** may be the only indication of acalculous cholecystitis. Typically, a high white blood cell count is seen, and bilirubin, aspartate aminotransferase, and alkaline phosphatase levels may also be elevated.

c. Diagnostic **imaging** is essential for establishing the diagnosis of acalculous cholecystitis.

(1) **Ultrasonography** can be done at the bedside in the critically ill patient. Typical findings of acalculous or calculous cholecystitis include gallbladder wall thickening, pericholecystic fluid, or abscess formation in the right upper quadrant. Limitations include overlying bowel gas or concomitant abdominal wounds or dressings. False negatives are possible.

(2) **CT scan** is as sensitive as ultrasonography for acalculous cholecystitis and provides more complete imaging of the remainder of the abdominal cavity from the lung bases to the pelvis. CT scan can also reveal other intra-abdominal problems that may be a part of the differential diagnosis, particularly in postoperative patients. The principal disadvantage of CT scan is that it requires transfer of the patient to the radiology suite, which may be a prohibitive risk if the patient is critically ill.

(3) **Hepatobiliary scintigraphy** is a better test for excluding acute acalculous cholecystitis than for confirming it.

(4) In difficult cases, **percutaneous cholecystostomy** may be both diagnostic and therapeutic.

2. **Management** of acalculous cholecystitis must be tailored to the individual patient. Initial treatment involves decompression of the gallbladder. In severely ill patients not fit enough to tolerate an operation, PTC is the procedure of choice and resolves the cholecystitis in over 85% of patients (*Curr Gastroenterol Rep* 2003;5:302). The definitive treatment is interval cholecystectomy. Alternatively, if the absence of gallstones is confirmed, simple removal of the tube may be adequate treatment after the patient has fully recovered from the underlying illness. Additional principles of management include initiation of systemic antibiotics, maintenance of nothing-by-mouth status, and treatment of the associated illnesses that placed the patient at risk for this condition.

B. Acute cholangitis is a potentially life-threatning bacterial infection of the biliary tree. Cholangitis is typically associated with partial or complete obstruction of the biliary tree and concomitant infection. Although acute cholangitis is often associated with cholelithiasis and choledocholithiasis, other causes of biliary tract obstruction and infection, including benign and malignant strictures, biliary-enteric anastomoses, parasites, and indwelling tubes or stents, also have a causative relationship. ERCP without concommitant stenting in the presence of a stricture is also associated with cholangitis, and therefore patients should routinely be pretreated with antibiotics in case a stent cannot be placed.

1. **Diagnosis**
   a. Patients present with a spectrum of disease severity, ranging from subclinical illness to acute toxic cholangitis. Over 90% of patients with cholangitis present with fever. **Charcot's triad,** the combination of fever, jaundice, and right upper quadrant pain, remains the hallmark of this disease and is present in 50% to 70% of patients. The advanced symptoms of **Reynold's pentad** (Charcot's triad with hemodynamic instability and mental status changes) are seen on presentation in up to 10% of patients, especially in the elderly, and suggest a more toxic or suppurative course of cholangitis.
   b. **Laboratory data** supportive of acute cholangitis include elevations of the white blood cell count, bilirubin, alkaline phosphatase, and transaminases.
   c. Investigation of the biliary tree is mandatory to demonstrate and relieve the underlying etiology of the obstruction. Ultrasonography or CT scan may reveal gallstones and biliary dilatation, but **definitive diagnosis is made by ERCP or PTC.** These studies are both diagnostic and therapeutic, as they demonstrate the level of obstruction and allow culture of bile, removal of stones or indwelling foreign bodies, and placement of drainage catheters if necessary.

2. **Management**
   a. Initial management of cholangitis includes **intravenous antibiotics** appropriate for the coverage of the most commonly cultured organisms: *Escherichia coli, Klebsiella pneumoniae,* enterococci, and *Bacteroides fragilis.* In patients with acute toxic cholangitis or in patients who fail to respond to antibiotic therapy, **emergent decompression of the biliary tree** is required. Effective biliary drainage can be accomplished by either the endoscopic or percutaneous route. ERCP is more commonly used because it does not leave the patient with an uncomfortable external drain. If decompression by these means is not available or possible, operative intervention to decompress the biliary tree is indicated, though it should usually be limited to extraction of obvious stones and insertion of a T tube in the common bile duct. Patients who present with hemodynamic instability or who develop hemodynamic instability after emergent decompression of the biliary tree should be closely monitored and supported with fluids.
   b. Cholangitis in patients with indwelling tubes or stents generally requires stent removal and replacement.
   c. **Definitive operative therapy** for benign or malignant biliary tract strictures should be deferred until a later date.

C. **Oriental cholangiohepatitis,** also known as **recurrent pyogenic cholangitis,** is endemic to the Far East. It is usually due to infestation of the biliary tree with parasites (*Ascaris lumbricoides, Clonorchis sinensis*) that cause stasis, bacterial overgrowth, and brown stone formation. Typical findings include multiple intrahepatic and extrahepatic biliary ductal stones, strictures, and repeated bacterial infections of the biliary tract. Strictures may be found throughout the biliary tree but are more common in the main hepatic ducts. The left duct is more frequently and severely affected than is the right.

1. **Diagnosis**
   a. The **symptoms and signs** are those of recurrent cholangitis. The patients typically are young and thin and present with right upper quadrant pain, fever, and jaundice. The episodes can vary in severity, from chronic subclinical illness leading gradually to generalized symptoms of hepatic insufficiency and malnutrition to severe acute suppurative cholangitis with hypotension, alteration in mental status, acidosis, and even death when not recognized and treated in a timely fashion.
   b. **Diagnostic imaging** demonstrates the typical diffuse biliary findings and multiple stones.
      (1) **Ultrasonography** can show focal or general bile duct dilation, stones in the biliary tree, pneumobilia from infection with gas-forming organisms, and liver abscesses. Ultrasound is very good at demonstrating intrahepatic stones by their characteristic posterior acoustic shadowing. Conversely, ultrasonography is not sensitive for demonstrating strictures, although some may be evident with this test.
      (2) **CT scan** is similar to ultrasonography in the findings it can demonstrate. It is also valuable in delineating the hepatic anatomy and judging the amount of hepatic parenchyma that has been preserved in more advanced disease. In addition, it can help guide parameters for potential liver resection.
      (3) **ERCP and PTC** are the mainstays of imaging for Oriental cholangiohepatitis. As is the case with more conventional cholangitis, these studies can allow the diagnosis of biliary obstruction, define the level of biliary strictures and stones, and provide the opportunity for therapeutic decompression of the biliary tree in the acute setting.
2. **Management** of Oriental cholangiohepatitis is palliation of the biliary strictures and the provision of wide biliary drainage.
   a. During an acute episode of cholangitis, systemic supportive care, including intravenous antibiotics and generous hydration, is indicated. Temporary percutaneous or endoscopic drainage must be achieved to **decompress the biliary system** and alleviate the sepsis. In occasional patients with known Oriental cholangiohepatitis and documented lower duct strictures, acute surgical intervention with drainage of the common bile duct by T-tube placement is appropriate.
   b. In the chronic setting, the multiple biliary strictures and stones must be addressed, and this generally requires multiple percutaneous or endoscopic approaches to the biliary tree, with attempts at dilation. If these eventually fail, the patient should have **cholecystectomy and wide biliary drainage** above the level of obstruction in the common bile duct, such as a choledochoduodenostomy or a Roux-en-Y hepaticojejunostomy. When using this technique, the blind end of the limb should be sutured to the peritoneal surface of the abdominal wall and marked with a radiopaque ring to provide access to the biliary-enteric anastomosis for percutaneous removal of additional stones and treatment of intrahepatic strictures. Alternatively, the blind end of the limb can be brought out as a cutaneous stoma, which is later closed and buried subcutaneously after completion of therapy. In occasional cases, liver resection is appropriate if the damaged area is completely or mostly confined to one portion of the liver.

III. **Biliary dyskinesia** is seen in patients with *typical* symptoms of biliary colic, but without evidence of gallstones. These patients require extensive workup to exclude other causes of right upper quadrant pain. Cholecystokinin–Tc-HIDA scan is useful in evaluating biliary dyskinesia. After the gallbladder has filled with the labeled radionuclide, cholecystokinin is administered, and a gallbladder ejection fraction is calculated 20 minutes later. An ejection fraction of <35% is suggestive of biliary dyskinesia. The definitive treatment is cholecystectomy, and over 85% of patients report postoperative improvement or relief of symptoms.

IV. **Primary sclerosing cholangitis (PSC)** is a cholestatic disorder of unknown etiology characterized by progressive fibrous obliteration of bile ducts. Almost 70% of patients are men, and many are in the 5th decade of life. An association with inflammatory bowel disease exists. PSC is present in 1% to 5% of those with inflammatory bowel disease. However, the incidence of inflammatory bowel disease in patients with PSC is greater, between 25% and 75%. PSC is a risk factor for cholangiocarcinoma, which may occur in 4% to 20% of patients, although a higher prevalence is seen in autopsy studies (*Clin Liver Dis* 1999;3:529).

A. **Pathology.** The most consistent change on liver biopsy is periductal concentric fibrosis around the macroscopic bile ducts, which is seen in up to 50% of biopsy specimens. Obliterative fibrous cholangitis, or concentric fibrosis with obliteration of the small ducts, is virtually diagnostic but is seen in less than 10% of cases. Findings may be diffuse or segmental in the bile ducts. Additional findings may include cholestasis, inflammation (with accumulation of plasma cells, lymphocytes, and polymorphonuclear leukocytes), and secondary biliary sclerosis. In most patients, both intrahepatic and extrahepatic ductal segments are involved. The hepatic duct bifurcation is typically the area most severely involved.

B. **Diagnosis** is based on a combination of findings.

1. There are **no pathognomonic signs** of PSC. Although patients can be asymptomatic for up to 15 years, prolonged disease ultimately leads to progressive hepatic failure. The condition is characterized by relapses and remissions, with quiescent periods. Jaundice with pale stools and dark urine forms the initial clinical picture. With advanced disease, pain in the right upper quadrant, pruritus, fatigue, and weight loss often accompany the jaundice. Cholangitis with fever and rigors may ultimately occur. Physical exam commonly reveals jaundice, hepatomegaly, and splenomegaly.

2. **Diagnostic imaging.** The procedure of choice is ERCP. In some instances, the intrahepatic biliary tree may not be well visualized, and transhepatic cholangiography is complementary. The most common finding is a diffuse and irregular narrowing of the entire biliary tree. The strictures are short and annular, giving a beaded appearance. In progressive disease, the strictures become confluent, and diverticula of the ducts appear. Although cholangiography is the gold standard, scintigraphy, sonography, and CT scan also are useful in making the diagnosis.

3. **Laboratory data.** The alkaline phosphatase level is almost always elevated, usually out of proportion to the bilirubin level. Serum transaminases may be mildly elevated. Most patients are negative for hepatitis B surface antigen.

C. **Management.** Symptomatic improvements have been reported with the use of various drugs aimed at reversing a presumed autoimmune etiology. These include corticosteroids, immunosuppressive agents, methotrexate, and D-penicillamine. However, none of these alter the natural history of the disease. PSC has been effectively palliated with endoscopic or percutaneous dilation of strictures. Placement of stents after dilation can be a valuable preoperative adjunct. However, some form of operative intervention is required for most patients.

1. **Resection or bypass of localized strictures.** The role of nontransplant surgery in this disease is limited. Occasionally, however, the disease is focused in the extrahepatic bile ducts, and a dominant stricture exists that can be excised or bypassed by hepaticojejunostomy. The candidates

should be ideal, and the procedure should only be done in patients with good residual liver function.

2. Extensive, diffuse stricture disease with end-stage cirrhosis is an indication for orthotopic **liver transplantation**. If the patient has undergone a previous decompressive operation, transplantation is technically more challenging but not contraindicated. Decompressive procedures are performed less commonly now than in the past, and patients are referred and listed for transplantation sooner.

3. Because PSC is a risk factor for cholangiocarcinoma, **close surveillance** of patients is needed. The diagnosis is difficult because cholangiocarcinomas also masquerade as strictures. A dominant biliary stricture should raise the suspicion of cholangiocarcinoma in a PSC patient and suggests the need for further evaluation. An elevated CA 19-9 may be helpful in diagnosing malignancy. Rapid clinical deterioration is also highly suggestive.

D. Prognosis. Many patients have a course that progresses to cirrhosis and liver failure despite early palliative interventions. Liver transplantation likely improves survival and quality of life, and early referral for liver transplantation is indicated to decrease the risk of developing cholangiocarcinoma. Overall, the median lengh of survival from diagnosis to death or liver transplantation is 10 to 12 years.

V. **Choledochal cysts** are congenital dilations of the biliary tree. They may occur in any bile duct but characteristically involve the common hepatic duct and common bile duct. They are more frequently identified in women (3:1 ratio) and those of Asian descent. Sixty percent are diagnosed in patients under the age of 10 years. Diagnosis and treatment are essential because the cysts predispose to jaundice, choledocholithiasis, cholangitis, portal hypertension, and cholangiocarcinoma.

A. Anatomic classification. These are not cystic lesions per se but rather dilations of the bile duct. In addition, the majority of choledochal cysts are associated with an unusually long common channel where the biliary and pancreatic ducts join much higher than usual ("anomalous biliary-pancreatic junction"). A **classification scheme** has identified five distinct types. Type I cysts are fusiform dilations of the common bile duct and are by far the most common (65% to 90%). Type II cysts are rare, isolated saccular diverticula of the common bile duct. Type III cysts, also termed *choledochoceles,* are localized dilations within the intraduodenal part of the common bile duct. Most lesions thought to be choledochoceles are in fact duodenal duplications. Type IV cysts are characterized by multiple cystic areas of the biliary tract, both inside and outside of the liver. Finally, type V cysts are single or multiple lesions based only in the intrahepatic portion of the tract (Caroli disease).

B. Diagnosis. The classic triad of right upper quadrant pain, jaundice, and a palpable abdominal mass is present only a minority of the time. Pain may mimic biliary colic. Neonates frequently present with biliary obstruction, whereas older youths suffer from jaundice and abdominal pain. Rarely, pancreatitis or duodenal obstruction can be caused by a choledochocele. Cirrhosis, sepsis from cholangitis, or free intraperitoneal rupture occur infrequently as late complications. Initial diagnosis is often made with ultrasonography and/or CT scan. An apparent increase in incidence of these lesions has paralleled advances in and use of these modalities. Further evaluation of the cyst should be obtained with specific biliary imaging such as ERCP.

C. Treatment is primarily surgical, as medical therapies are not successful. Cholangiocarcinoma develops in up to 30% of cysts and usually presents in the fourth decade of life. Cyst excision with a Roux-en-Y hepaticojejunostomy reconstruction is the treatment of choice for types I and IV. Simple excision of the rare type II cyst has been performed. Local cyst excision with sphincteroplasty through a transduodenal approach is effective for type III disease. Endoscopic excision is now being evaluated. Caroli disease can be treated with hemihepatectomy when confined to one side of the intrahepatic tract. More often, bilateral disease is present with associated liver damage and mandates orthotopic liver transplantation.

VI. **Tumors of the bile ducts**
  A. **Benign tumors of the bile ducts**, usually adenomas, are rare and arise from the ductal glandular epithelium. They are characteristically polypoid and rarely are larger than 2 cm. Most are found adjacent to the ampulla, with the common bile duct being the next most common site. The malignant potential of these uncommon lesions is unclear.
    1. Most patients present with **intermittent obstructive jaundice**, often accompanied by right upper quadrant pain. This presentation may be confused with choledocholithiasis. The lesions often are detected by intraoperative cholangiography, choledochoscopy, or ultrasonography. Lesions near the ampulla may be visible via endoscope.
    2. **Treatment** should involve complete resection of the tumor with a margin of duct wall. High recurrence rates have been reported after simple curettage of the polyps. Lesions situated at the ampulla can usually be managed by transduodenal papillotomy or wide local excision.
  B. **Cholangiocarcinoma** arises from the bile duct epithelium and can occur anywhere along the course of the biliary tree. Cholangiocarcinoma is an uncommon malignancy (9,000 cases per year in the United States). These tumors tend to be locally invasive, and when they metastasize, they usually involve the liver and the peritoneum. They characteristically spread along the bile ducts microscopically for long distances beyond the palpable end of the tumor (1.5 cm). Frequently, their proximity to critical structures such as the hepatic artery or portal vein precludes curative resection. The median age of onset is approximately 60 years, and men are afflicted more frequently than women. Associations exist with primary sclerosing cholangitis, choledochal cysts, intrahepatic stones, certain parasitic infestations, and previous exposure to the radiocontrast agent Thorotrast (no longer in use).
    1. **Classification and staging.** Cholangiocarcinoma has been classified into three main types according to anatomic location: intrahepatic (20%), extrahepatic upper duct (also called *hilar* or *Klatskin tumor*, 40%), and extrahepatic lower duct (40%). This simple classification dictates preferred surgical treatment (see Section VI.B.3). Staging of cholangiocarcinoma follows the TNM system of the American Joint Committee on Cancer (AJCC). Stage I tumors are limited to the bile duct mucosa or muscular layer, stage II tumors invade periductal tissues, stage III tumors have regional lymph node metastases, and stage IV tumors either invade adjacent structures or have distant metastases.
    2. **Diagnosis**
      a. **Jaundice**, followed by weight loss and pain, are the most frequently encountered signs and symptoms at presentation.
      b. **Diagnostic imaging**
        (1) **Magnetic resonance imaging (magnetic resonance cholangiopancreatography)** can be used for an all-purpose investigation of cholangiocarcinoma. It provides cholangiography, can demonstrate the tumor and its relationship to key vessels, and can detect intrahepatic metastases. It is rapidly supplanting older diagnostic approaches.
        (2) **Ultrasonography** can demonstrate bile duct masses and bile duct dilatation and provide rudimentary information on the extent of tumor involvement within the liver. Duplex ultrasonography also can demonstrate the relationship to critical vascular structures.

Some reports indicate that ultrasonography is more than 80% accurate in predicting portal vein involvement.

(3) **CT scan** may also be helpful in delineating the mass and defining its relation to the liver. Advanced scanners can provide information similar to that offered by MR scan. Using both types of imaging in conjunction is not necessary.

(4) **ERCP** is the most valuable diagnostic tool for cholangiography of lower duct tumors. Distal lesions may be indistinguishable from small pancreatic carcinomas on preoperative evaluation, and the distinction is often not made until final pathologic analysis. It is also valuable for upper duct tumors, but if obstruction is complete, the upper limit of the tumor cannot be delineated. Since the advent of MR cholangiography, ERCP is increasingly being used for preoperative therapeutic decompression of the biliary tree, which is controversial. Preoperative decompression of the biliary tree has the advantage of improving liver function prior to resection but has the risk of cholangitis and increased postoperative infection. It is not usually used unless the bilirubin is >10 mg/dL (>170 μmol/L). When used, only the less affected hemiliver should be decompressed so that it will hypertrophy while the undrained side (the side to be resected) atrophies.

(5) **PTC** has been used when ERCP cannot delineate the tumor completely. Under PTC guidance, fine-needle aspiration cytology can provide a tissue diagnosis in approximately 75% of patients. However, if a tumor is resectable, prolonged efforts to obtain a tissue diagnosis before resection are not indicated.

(6) **Endoscopic ultrasound (EUS)** is a new and very important endoscopic investigation in lower bile duct strictures. It is useful for determining if small masses are present around the bile duct and for obtaining tissue diagnosis by endoscopic needle biopsy.

3. **Assessment of tumor resectability and treatment.** Resection remains the primary treatment for cholangiocarcinoma and provides the only opportunity for cure. Adjuvant radiation and chemotherapy have been attempted, but clinical trials are limited by the paucity of eligible patients. The most efficacious chemotherapeutic agent to date is 5-fluorouracil, with response rates of up to 15%.

a. **Intrahepatic tumors** are best treated with hepatic resection. Resectability is assessed as for other solitary primary tumors or secondary colorectal metastases arising in otherwise normal livers. The tumor is resected provided that it can be completely removed while at least 30% of functioning liver mass can be retained. If resection of more than 60% of the hepatic parenchyma is required, preoperative portal vein embolization can be used to cause atrophy of the affected hemiliver and hypertrophy of the liver segments that will remain. Unfortunately, these tumors often present at an advanced stage, often with bilateral hepatic spread, and only 15% to 20% are resectable.

b. **Extrahepatic upper duct (hilar) tumors.** Resection of hilar tumors includes the bile duct bifurcation and the caudate lobe (which should always be resected *en bloc* with a mass in this area because of the proximity to caudate lobe bile ducts). In addition, ipsilateral hemihepatectomy is necessary in most cases in order to obtain an R0 resection (resection with negative margins). Up to 70% of the liver, the affected extrahepatic ducts, and portions of extrahepatic vessels can be resected. Subsequent biliary reconstruction is performed as a Roux-en-Y hepaticojejunostomy. Resection is usually excluded by the following findings: (1) bilateral intrahepatic bile duct spread of the disease, (2) involvement of the main trunk of the portal vein (depending on extent), (3) bilateral involvement of hepatic arterial and/or portal venous branches, and (4) a combination of vascular involvement with cholangiographic evidence of extensive contralateral ductal spread. Intraoperative findings of gross lymph node or omental/peritoneal metastases (distant spread) also preclude resection. Staging laparoscopy may be useful to evaluate for distant spread before formal laparotomy. Vascular involvement is not an absolute contraindication to resection, since it is possible to resect and reconstruct portal venous segments. Arterial reconstructions are more difficult.

   c. Some lesions situated in the **middle of the extrahepatic bile duct** may be approached with an excision of the supraduodenal extrahepatic bile duct, cholecystectomy, and portal lymphadenectomy. These lesions may be clinically indistinguishable from a tumor of gallbladder origin, and in fact most malignant strictures in the mid bile duct are due to local invasion of a gallbladder cancer rather than cholangiocarcinoma.

   d. **Extrahepatic lower duct tumors.** The considerations are the same as for carcinoma of the head of the pancreas, although vascular involvement is much less common. When it occurs, it usually involves the portal vein at the top of the pancreas. Staging laparoscopy may be useful. In contrast to more proximal tumors, approximately 80% of lower duct tumors are resectable by pancreaticoduodenectomy. Survival data are also more favorable, with the 5-year survival rate ranging from 17% to 39%. Tumors derived from the bile duct have a slightly better prognosis than those of pancreatic origin in the same region, probably reflecting a more favorable biologic behavior.

4. **Palliation** for patients with disseminated or unresectable disease involves surgical, radiologic, or endoscopic biliary decompression. When unresectability is demonstrated preoperatively or at staging laparoscopy, the first choice for biliary decompression is via endoscopic or percutaneous internal stenting. When unresectable disease is encountered at laparotomy, internal biliary drainage is best achieved by choledochojejunostomy for lower duct lesions. Intrahepatic bypasses are rarely performed.

5. **Prognosis** is highly dependent on resectability of the tumor at presentation. Patients with resectable cholangiocarcinoma with microscopically negative margins and negative lymph node status have a 5-year survival rate of approximately 35%. In contrast, median length of survival for patients with unresectable cholangiocarcinoma is only 3 to 6 months, even with palliative procedures or adjuvant treatment.

C. **Gallbladder cancer**, like cholangiocarcinoma, is an uncommon cancer (9,000 cases per year in the United States) with a poor prognosis. It is relatively more aggressive than cholangiocarcinoma. The incidence increases with age, peaking at 70 to 75 years, with a 3:1 female to male ratio. There is a strong correlation with gallstones (95%). Histologically, nearly all gallbladder cancers are adenocarcinomas, and concomitant cholecystitis is frequently present. Gallbladder cancer spreads primarily by direct extension into segments IV and V of the liver, adjacent to the gallbladder fossa. The cancer also spreads via lymphatics along the cystic duct to the common bile duct. Only a small percentage of patients with a preoperative diagnosis of gallbladder cancer are resectable for potential cure.

1. **Staging** by the AJCC TNM system is as follows: Stage I tumors include *in situ* disease confined to the gallbladder wall (T1a, not penetrating the muscularis) and also early disease (T1b, with invasion into the gallbladder muscularis). Stage II disease includes tumors with invasion into the perimuscular connective tissue. Stage III tumors extend up to 2 cm into the liver and may have regional node metastases. Stage IV tumors extend >2 cm into the liver and/or two or more adjacent organs and have more distant nodal spread or distant metastatic disease.

2. Diagnosis. Approximately one-third of these tumors are diagnosed incidentally during cholecystectomy, and cancer is found in 0.3% to 1% of all cholecystectomy specimens. Symptoms of stage I and II gallbladder cancer are often directly caused by gallstones rather than the cancer and include right upper quadrant pain in >80% of patients. Stage III and IV cancers present with jaundice due to bile duct obstruction and exhibit the signs and symptoms of advanced cancers, including weight loss, hepatomegaly and/or a palpable mass, and ascites. Ultrasound findings suggestive of gallbladder cancer may include thickening or irregularity of the gallbladder, or a polypoid mass. Porcelain gallbladder seen on diagnostic imaging carries a risk of cancer of approximately 25%.

3. Treatment

  a. *In situ* **disease** confined to the gallbladder wall (stage I, T1a) is often identified after laparoscopic cholecystectomy for gallstone disease. Because the overall 5-year survival rate approaches 100%, cholecystectomy alone with negative resection margins (including the cystic duct margin) is adequate therapy. Patients with a preoperative suspicion of gallbladder cancer should undergo open cholecystectomy, since port site recurrences and late peritoneal metastases (associated with bile spillage) have been reported even with *in situ* disease.

  b. Early disease (stage I, T1b) may be treated by radical cholecystectomy that includes the gallbladder and the gallbladder bed of the liver.

  c. Stage II or III disease with invasion through the muscularis of the gallbladder or the presence of lymph node metastases requires more radical resection. Depending on the extent of local invasion, extirpation may range from wedge resection of the liver adjacent to the gallbladder bed to resection of 75% of the liver. Due to the three-dimensional characteristics of the gallbladder fossa, hepatic wedge resection in this area is technically difficult and has the risk of entry into the tumor plane. Therefore, segmental liver resection (usually segments IV and V) is recommended. Dissection in continuity of the portal, paraduodenal, and hepatic artery lymph nodes should accompany the liver resection. Survival advantages have been demonstrated after radical resection. Because of the aggressive nature of this malignancy, adjuvant chemoradiation is often recommended, but no proof of efficacy is available.

  d. Most gallbladder cancers have invaded the liver or extend into the porta hepatis before clinical diagnosis. **Extensive liver involvement or discontiguous metastases** preclude surgical resection as a reasonable option. Patients thus affected often are symptomatic, with pain, jaundice, nausea and vomiting, and weight loss. Jaundice may be palliated by percutaneous or endoscopically placed biliary stents. Duodenal obstruction can be surgically bypassed if present. Radiotherapy can decrease tumor bulk and temporarily relieve obstruction, but no survival benefits have been demonstrated. As with most malignancies of hepatobiliary origin, there are no effective chemotherapeutic agents.

4. Prognosis is stage dependent. Patients with completely resected T1a tumors have a 5-year survival rate approaching 100%. However, the 5-year survival rate for patients with completely resected T1b tumors is only 72%, and patients with resectable later stage tumors have 5-year survival rates of 20% to 40%. Since most patients present with advanced, unresectable disease, the overall 5-year survival rate is less than 15%, and patients who present with stage IV disease have a median length of survival of only 1 to 3 months.

VII. Benign strictures and bile duct injuries occur in association with a number of conditions, including pancreatitis, choledocholithiasis, Oriental cholangiohepatitis, primary sclerosing cholangitis, prior hepatic transplantation, trauma, or iatrogenic injury after biliary instrumentation or operations on the upper

GI tract. Laparoscopic cholecystectomy is by far the leading cause of iatrogenic bile duct injuries and benign strictures. Iatrogenic injuries can be quite morbid and are often associated with litigious action.

A. Risk factors for injury during cholecystectomy include the following:

   1. **Lack of training or experience**, especially when operating in the face of acute edema
   2. Local factors of acute or chronic **inflammation**
   3. **Cholecystectomy technique.** The best approach to preventing bile duct injuries is described by the aforementioned "critical view of safety" (see Section I.F.1.b), where a complete dissection demonstrates only two structures (the cystic duct and artery) entering the gallbladder. In addition, cholangiography before transection of any structures should be performed when the anatomy is unclear.
   4. **Aberrant anatomy** is common in the porta hepatis and may predispose toward injuries to both the biliary systems and the hepatic vasculature.

B. Classification. A classification scheme has been proposed and is now widely accepted. Type A injuries are cystic duct leaks or leaks from small ducts in the liver bed. Type B and C injuries involve an aberrant right hepatic duct. Type B represents an occluded segment, whereas Type C involves open drainage from the proximal draining duct not in continuity with the common duct. Type D injuries are *lateral* injuries to the extrahepatic bile ducts. Type E injuries (I–V) are derived from the Bismuth classification of common bile duct injuries and represent circumferential injury (transections or occlusions) at various levels of the common bile duct.

C. Diagnosis

   1. **Presentation** depends on the type of injury. Approximately 25% of major bile duct injuries are recognized at the time of the initial procedure. Intraoperative signs of a major bile duct injury include unexpected bile leakage, abnormal intraoperative cholangiogram, or delayed recognition of the anatomy after transection or injury of important structures. If an injury is not recognized intraoperatively, the patient usually presents with symptoms within 1 week and almost always within 3 to 4 weeks after the initial procedure. Patients with a bile leak often present with right upper quadrant pain, fever, and sepsis secondary to biloma and may have bile drainage from a surgical incision. Patients with occlusion of the common bile duct without a bile leak present with jaundice. Occasionally, a delayed presentation of months or years is seen.
   2. **Diagnostic imaging.** CT scan is the best imaging test to demonstrate an intra-abdominal bile collection, which should then be percutaneously drained. Ongoing bile leaks can also be diagnosed by HIDA scan. ERCP is also useful to demonstrate biliary anatomy, and therapeutic stent placement is often possible for bile duct leaks. In the case of occlusion of the common bile duct, PTC can demonstrate the proximal biliary anatomy, can define the proximal extent of the injury, and can be used for therapeutic decompression of the biliary tree. MRI with MRCP can demonstrate the bile ducts both above and below an obstruction and is now often used for the initial investigation.

D. Management depends on the type and timing of the presentation.

   1. If the injury is identified at the time of the initial procedure, the surgeon should proceed directly to open exploration and repair only if qualified and comfortable with complex techniques in hepatobiliary surgery or to control life-threatening hemorrhage. If the surgeon is not prepared to perform a definitive repair, he or she should place a drain in the right upper quadrant, and the patient should be immediately **referred to a specialist hepatobiliary center**.
   2. **Immediate management.** Many of the simpler injuries can be successfully managed with ERCP and sphincterotomy, stenting, or both. Occlusive lesions require decompression of the proximal drainage systems via PTC. In general, if an injury requires operative repair and the patient

is stable, the repair should be done within the first few days after the initial procedure while inflammation is at a minimum. If this is not possible due to delayed diagnosis, longer term temporization (at least 8 weeks) is required to allow the acute inflammation to resolve. In addition, if there is a concern about a vascular injury along with the bile duct injury, definitive repair should be delayed in order to more easily identify ischemic areas of bile duct. These ischemic areas should not be incorporated in the repair.

3. Control of sepsis, percutaneous drainage, and adequate nutrition should be **optimized before definitive repair**.

4. **Operative repair**, when indicated, is best achieved by means of a Roux-en-Y hepaticoenterostomy, in which the bile duct is dissected and débrided back to viable tissue. All bile ducts must be accounted for, and an adequate blood supply must be apparent for each. A mucosa-to-mucosa anastomosis constructed with fine absorbable suture and no tension is desired. Excellent long-term outcomes have been described, with anastomotic stricture the most common, yet infrequent, complication (*Arch Surg* 1999;134:604). Rarely, liver transplantation may be necessary for those patients who suffer profound hepatic insufficiency secondary to the injury.

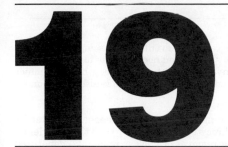

Spleen

Emily R. Winslow and
L. Michael Brunt

SPLENIC ANATOMY AND PHYSIOLOGY

I. Splenic Anatomy

A. Macroscopic anatomy

1. The spleen is located in the **left upper quadrant of the abdomen** and is in close proximity to the 9th to 11th ribs. The costodiaphragmatic recess of the left pleural cavity extends as far as the inferior border of a normal spleen.

2. The **normal spleen** is 12 cm in length, 7 cm in width, and 4 cm in thickness and weighs about 150 g.

3. The spleen is **intimately related** to the colon (i.e., the splenic flexure), the greater curvature of the stomach, the left kidney, and the pancreatic tail. The tail of the pancreas extends laterally to within 1 cm of the splenic hilum in most patients and is in direct contact with the spleen in up to 30% of patients.

4. **Peritoneal reflections** in the region surrounding the spleen form the fibrous suspensory "ligaments" through which most of the principal vascular structures course. The pancreas is partially invested in the leaves of the splenorenal ligament, just inferior to the contained splenic artery and its branches.

5. The **splenic artery** is a branch of the celiac trunk and follows a serpiginous path along the superior border of the pancreas. The terminal branching pattern into the spleen is most commonly distributive, and the main trunk arborizes into multiple arterial branches that enter the hilum broadly over its surface. Less commonly, the arterial supply has a magistral configuration, with one dominant splenic artery entering over a narrow and compact area.

6. **Accessory spleens** occur in 10% to 20% of patients and are most commonly found at the splenic hilum, the gastrosplenic omentum, and near the pancreatic tail. However, accessory splenic tissue can be found throughout the abdomen and pelvis.

B. Microscopic anatomy

1. The **spleen consists** primarily of red pulp but has interspersed areas of white pulp.

    a. The **white pulp** has three components: periarteriolar lymphoid sheaths, lymphoid nodules, and the marginal zone. T-cells predominate in the lymphoid sheaths, and B-cells predominant in the lymphoid nodules.

    b. The **red pulp** is highly vascular and is composed of large branching, thin-walled sinuses, with intervening areas filled with phagocytic cells and blood cells, known as splenic cords.

2. Although this view is controversial, the spleen is thought to have both an **open and a closed circulation.**

    a. The **closed circulation** refers to that part of the spleen in which the arterioles branch into capillaries that are contiguous with the venous sinuses within the red pulp.

    b. The **open circulation** refers to that part of the spleen in which the capillaries drain freely into the splenic parenchyma and the cellular

elements flow through the red pulp, eventually passing through the fenestrations in the venous sinuses and back into the bloodstream.
II. **Splenic function.** In its normal physiologic state, the spleen has two major functions. It is a part of the reticuloendothelial system and is also a component of the immune system.
   A. **Reticuloendothelial/filtration system**
      1. The red pulp of the splenic parenchyma serves as a **mechanical filter** for the removal of senescent erythrocytes (called *culling*) and the remodeling of healthy red cells, including removal of nuclear remnants, denatured hemoglobin, and iron granules (called *pitting*). The splenic macrophages and reticular cells then phagocytose these filtered particles.
      2. Another minor hematologic function of the spleen is to serve as a **reservoir for platelets.** In certain disease states (e.g., myelofibrosis), the adult spleen becomes a major site of extramedullary hematopoiesis.
   B. **Immune system**
      1. The white pulp is a **nonspecific filter** and removes blood-borne pathogens (e.g., bacteria and viruses) that are coated with complement.
      2. The spleen also participates in the **specific immune response** by producing antibody, plasma cells, and memory cells in response to specific trapped antigens.
      3. **Encapsulated bacteria** are also effectively removed from the circulation, likely via prolonged contact with macrophages in the splenic parenchymal cords, where the transit time is slow.
      4. The spleen also **manufactures opsonins,** namely, properdin and tuftsin.

INDICATION FOR SPLENECTOMY

I. **General indications**
   A. The primary therapy for most nontraumatic splenic disorders is medical. In general, splenectomy is warranted only after failure of medical therapy or as an adjunct to medical therapy. With time, the role of surgery in many disorders has fluctuated. Because the intended effect of splenectomy varies from diagnosis to cure, it important to understand the specific goal of surgery when evaluating each patient.
   B. The **goals of splenectomy** can be broadly classified into one of the following groups:
      1. **Cure or palliation of hematologic disease.** Immune thrombocytopenia (ITP) and hemolytic anemias are the most common indications for splenectomy. Splenectomy may also be used to palliate other disease states [e.g., chronic lymphocytic leukemia (CLL), chronic myelogenous leukemia (CML), and Felty syndrome], primarily via the control of cytopenias.
      2. **Palliation of hypersplenism.** Patients with refractory cytopenias due to hypersplenism that require frequent transfusion or significantly limit the delivery of cytotoxic therapy may benefit from splenectomy.
      3. **Relief from symptomatic splenomegaly.** Patients with a massively enlarged spleen can develop early satiety, vague abdominal pain, and weight loss. Removing the spleen can dramatically improve symptoms due to the spleen's mass effect within the abdomen.
      4. **Diagnosis of splenic pathology.** Solid mass lesions in the spleen can be an indication for splenectomy, particularly if a malignant diagnosis is suspected. Splenectomy may be necessary to establish a diagnosis of lymphoma in the absence of more easily accessible tissue but is no longer indicated for the staging of lymphomas.
      5. **Control of splenic hemorrhage.** Although splenic injury is increasingly managed nonoperatively, splenectomy is the definitive treatment for patients with ongoing traumatic splenic hemorrhage. Splenic hemorrhage may also rarely occur spontaneously in disease states such as infectious mononucleosis.

Table 19-1. Indications for splenectomy

Hematologic splenic pathology
  Thrombocytopenias
    Immune thrombocytopenic purpura (ITP)
    Thrombotic thrombocytopenic purpura (TTP)
  Anemias
    Hereditary hemolytic anemias (hereditary spherocytosis)
    Acquired warm autoimmune hemolytic anemias
    Congenital hemoglobinopathies (sickle cell anemia)
  Myeloproliferative and myelodysplastic disorders
    Chronic myelogenous leukemia
    Polycythemia vera
    Myelofibrosis or myeloid metaplasia
    Essential thrombocytosis
    Myeloproliferative disorder not otherwise specified
  Lymphoproliferative disorders
    Chronic lymphocytic leukemia
    Hairy-cell leukemia
    Non-Hodgkin's lymphoma
    Hodgkin's lymphoma
  Neutropenias
    Felty syndrome
Nonhematologic splenic disorders
  Splenic abscess
  Splenic cyst/pseudocyst
  Storage diseases
Other disorders
  Trauma
  Incidental splenectomy
  Vascular problems (splenic artery aneurysm, splenic vein thrombosis)

II. **Specific indications** (see Table 19-1)
  A. **Hematologic splenic pathology**
    1. **Thrombocytopenias**
      a. **Idiopathic (immune) thrombocytopenic purpura (ITP)** is the most common indication for elective splenectomy. It is an acquired disorder caused by the destruction of platelets exposed to antiplatelet IgG antibodies. The spleen is the major site for the production of antiplatelet antibodies and serves as the principal site of platelet destruction. ITP is characterized by a low platelet count, normal or increased megakaryocytes in the bone marrow, and the absence of other potential causes of thrombocytopenia. Management varies depending on the degree of the thrombocytopenia and the age of the patient.
        i. **Children** usually present with acute ITP, often associated with a recent viral syndrome. In 90% of cases, the disease spontaneously remits within 6 to 12 months. Only those few patients with refractory cases despite medical treatment require splenectomy.
        ii. **Adults** typically present with a more chronic form of ITP that is much less likely to spontaneously remit. Asymptomatic patients with platelet counts >50,000/mm^3 may simply be followed without specific therapy. Symptomatic patients or those with counts <30,000/mm^3 should be treated. The initial therapy is medical treatment with oral glucocorticoids (1 mg/kg dosing). About 20% of patients respond after several weeks of treatment. Those who

fail medical treatment are candidates for splenectomy, which results in a complete and durable remission in nearly two-thirds of patients. Indications for more urgent splenectomy in patients with ITP include profound refractory thrombocytopenia or a major or life-threatening bleed, including CNS hemorrhage. The majority of patients who respond to splenectomy do so within the first 10 postoperative days.

   iii. Patients who fail splenectomy or relapse after an initial response should be investigated for **accessory splenic tissue.** If accessory splenic tissue is found by imaging studies or is strongly suspected based on the red cell morphology on a peripheral smear (absent Howell-Jolly bodies), reexploration for an accessory spleen should be considered.

  b. Thrombotic thrombocytopenic purpura (TTP) is characterized by the pentad of hemolytic anemia, consumptive thrombocytopenia, mental status changes, renal failure, and fever. Its pathogenesis is related to endothelial damage resulting in platelet aggregation and microvascular occlusions.

   i. First-line therapy for this condition is medical, with plasmapheresis and steroid administration. Other therapies include aspirin, vincristine, and IVIG.

   ii. Splenectomy is occasionally indicated in patients who do not respond to medical therapy and those who relapse after an initial response. Plasmapheresis must be continued for several days postoperatively after a response is observed.

2. Anemias

  a. Hereditary hemolytic anemias constitute a group of disorders in which splenectomy is almost universally curative.

   i. Hereditary spherocytosis is an autosomal dominant disorder in which there is a defect in the red cell membrane protein spectrin. This defect leads to small, spherical, and relatively rigid erythrocytes that are unable to deform adequately to traverse the splenic microcirculation, which results in their sequestration and destruction in the splenic red pulp. In addition to anemia, patients may have jaundice and splenomegaly. The diagnosis is made by the typical appearance of the cells on a peripheral smear, a positive osmotic fragility test, and a negative direct Coombs test. Splenectomy is indicated in nearly all cases but should be delayed to age 6 in children to minimize the risk of overwhelming postsplenectomy sepsis, unless growth retardation, severe anemia, or aplastic crisis is present. Prior to splenectomy, patients should have a right upper quadrant ultrasound, and if gallstones are present (usually pigment stones from hemolysis), a cholecystectomy should be performed concomitantly.

   ii. Hereditary elliptocytosis is an autosomal dominant disorder in which an intrinsic cytoskeletal defect causes the red blood cells (RBCs) to be elliptical. The majority of patients have an asymptomatic and mild anemia that does not need specific treatment. Patients with symptomatic anemia should undergo splenectomy to correct the anemia by prolonging RBC survival.

  b. Acquired autoimmune hemolytic anemias are characterized as either warm or cold, depending on the temperature at which they interact with antibody.

   i. Warm autoimmune hemolytic anemia results from splenic sequestration and destruction of RBCs coated with autoantibodies that interact optimally with their antigens at 37°C. Anti-IgG antiserum causes agglutination of the patient's RBCs (positive direct Coombs test). Etiologies include chronic lymphocytic leukemia, non-Hodgkin's lymphoma, collagen vascular disease, and drugs, although most cases are idiopathic. Presentation is similar to other hemolytic anemias, and primary treatment is directed against the underlying disease. If treatment of the primary disease is unsuccessful, the mainstay of therapy is corticosteroids. Nonresponders or patients requiring high steroid doses respond to splenectomy in 60% to 80% of cases.

ii. **Cold autoimmune hemolytic anemia** is characterized by fixation of C3 to IgM antibodies that bind RBCs with greater affinity at temperatures approaching 0°C. Hemolysis occurs either immediately by intravascular complement–mediated mechanisms or via removal of C3-coated RBCs by the liver. Splenectomy has no therapeutic benefit.

c. **Congenital hemoglobinopathies**

i. **Sickle-cell anemia** is due to the homozygous inheritance of the S variant of the hemoglobin beta chain. The disease is usually associated with autosplenectomy due to repeated vaso-occlusive crises, but splenectomy can be required for those patients with acute splenic sequestration crisis, evidence of hypersplenism, splenic abscess, and symptomatic splenomegaly.

ii. **Thalassemias** are hereditary anemias caused by a defect in hemoglobin synthesis wherein an insufficient amount of hemoglobin polypeptide is produced. β-Thalassemia major is primarily treated with iron chelation therapy, but in severe cases splenectomy can be required, usually to treat symptomatic splenomegaly or pain from splenic infarcts.

3. **Myeloproliferative and myelodysplastic disorders**

a. **Chronic myelogenous leukemia** is a myelodysplastic disorder characterized by the *bcr-abl* fusion oncogene, known as the *Philadelphia chromosome*. Treatment is primarily medical and ranges from hydroxyurea to high-dose chemotherapy with bone marrow transplantation. Splenectomy is indicated only for palliation of symptomatic splenomegaly or hypersplenism that significantly limits therapy.

b. **Myelofibrosis and myeloid metaplasia** are incurable myeloproliferative disorders that usually present in patients older than 60 years. The condition is characterized by bone marrow fibrosis, leukoerythroblastosis, and extramedullary hematopoiesis, which can result in massive splenomegaly. Indications for splenectomy in this group of patients include massive symptomatic splenomegaly and transfusion-dependent anemias. Although the compressive symptoms are effectively palliated with splenectomy, the cytopenias frequently recur. In addition, these patients are at increased risk for postoperative hemorrhage and thrombotic complications after splenectomy.

4. **Lymphoproliferative disorders**

a. **Chronic lymphocytic leukemia**, a B-cell leukemia, is the most common of the chronic leukemias and is characterized by the accumulation of mature but nonfunctional lymphocytes. Primary therapy is medical, with splenectomy indicated for those patients with symptomatic splenomegaly and severe hypersplenism. Although the use of splenectomy in such cases is controversial, data from at least one study demonstrated that early splenectomy in some patient subgroups was associated with improved survival.

b. The **non-Hodgkin's lymphomas** are a diverse group of disorders with a wide range of clinical behaviors, ranging from indolent to highly aggressive. As with other malignant processes, splenectomy is indicated for symptomatic splenomegaly and palliation of hypersplenism. However, splenectomy does play an important role in the diagnosis and staging of patients with isolated splenic lymphoma (known as *malignant lymphoma with prominent splenic involvement*). In these cases, improved survival has been shown in those patients undergoing splenectomy.

c. **Hodgkin's lymphoma.** Splenectomy currently has a limited role in the diagnosis and treatment of Hodgkin's lymphoma due to refinements in imaging techniques and progress in the methods of treatment. The important guiding principal for the surgeon today is that staging laparotomy should only be considered in those patients for whom the outcome with significantly affect therapy. This small subgroup includes primarily those patients with stage I or II disease whose therapy will be tailored based on the results at laparotomy (e.g., stage I patients with favorable predictors who will receive only mantle radiation if the laparotomy is negative, and stage II patients with favorable predictors will receive chemotherapy if the laparotomy is positive).

d. **Hairy cell leukemia** is a rare disease of elderly men that is characterized by B lymphocytes with membrane ruffling. Splenectomy was previously regarded as the primary therapy for this disease, but progress with systemic chemotherapy has significantly changed the role of splenectomy, which is now reserved for patients with massive splenomegaly and those with disease that is refractory to medical therapies.

5. **Neutropenias**
   a. **Felty's syndrome** is characterized by rheumatoid arthritis, splenomegaly, and neutropenia. The primary treatment is steroids, but in refractory cases splenectomy may be required to reverse the neutropenia. In addition, patients with recurrent infections and significant anemia may benefit from splenectomy. The clinical course of the arthritis is not affected.

B. **Nonhematologic splenic disorders**
   1. **Splenic cysts** are uncommon and can be parasitic or nonparasitic. Most are located in the lower pole in a subcapsular position.
      a. **Parasitic cysts** make up more than two-thirds of splenic cysts worldwide but are rare in the United States. The majority are hydatid cysts caused by *Echinococcus* species. They are typically asymptomatic but may rupture or cause symptoms due to splenomegaly. The primary treatment is splenectomy, with careful attention not to spill the cyst contents. The cyst may be aspirated and injected with hypertonic saline prior to mobilization if concern about rupture exists.
      b. **Nonparasitic cysts** can be true cysts or pseudocysts.
         i. **Pseudocysts** lack an epithelial lining and make up more than two-thirds of nonparasitic cysts. They typically result from traumatic hematoma formation, with subsequent absorption. Symptomatic splenic pseudocysts may present with left upper quadrant pain radiating to the shoulder. Pseudocysts smaller than 5 cm can be followed safely with ultrasonography and often resolve spontaneously. Larger cysts may rupture and require excision with splenorrhaphy or partial excision and marsupialization. Splenectomy is indicated if splenic salvage is not possible. Percutaneous aspiration is associated with a high incidence of infection and reaccumulation and is not indicated.
         ii. **True cysts** have an epithelial lining and are most often congenital. Other rare true cysts include epidermoid and dermoid cysts. They are typically asymptomatic and are found during radiologic examinations or surgery. Generally, no treatment is needed. For cysts that become symptomatic, splenic salvage can be attempted for cysts less than one-half the size of the organ; otherwise, splenectomy is indicated.
   2. **Splenic abscesses** are rare but potentially lethal. Approximately two-thirds are due to seeding from a distant bacteremic focus, most commonly endocarditis or urinary tract infection. Other etiologies include posttraumatic events, hemoglobinopathies, and contiguous spread. Fever is present in nearly all cases, and abdominal discomfort and splenomegaly occur in one-half of all patients.

a. **CT scanning and ultrasonography** are the best diagnostic modalities for splenic abscess. CT scans typically show an area of low homogeneous density with edges that do not intensify with intravenous contrast.

b. **Antibiotic therapy** should be instituted immediately after blood cultures are obtained. Nearly 60% of identified infectious agents are aerobes, with one-half being *Staphylococcus* and *Streptococcus* species. Unilocular abscesses may be amenable to treatment by percutaneous drainage and antibiotics. Splenectomy in combination with postoperative antibiotics is the definitive therapy. Fungal abscesses, however, can often be treated with antifungal agents alone, without splenectomy or drainage.

C. **Other forms of splenic pathology**

1. *En bloc* **oncologic resections** for colon, pancreatic, or gastric cancers may require splenectomy if the tumor invades the spleen. Splenectomy should then be performed as part of the *en bloc* resection. If this is anticipated preoperatively by imaging studies, the patient should be vaccinated as with planned splenectomy.

2. **Incidental splenectomy** occurs when the spleen is injured iatrogenically during another abdominal operation. This can occur either by damage from a retractor in the left upper quadrant or, more commonly, from mobilization of the splenic flexure in colon resection. Capsular tears can often be treated with topical hemostatic agents and even with use of the argon beam coagulator, but if significant hemorrhage results that cannot be controlled expeditiously, splenectomy is indicated.

3. **Splenic artery aneurysms** account for the majority of visceral artery aneurysms and have a particular tendency to affect women, with rupture occurring with increased frequency during pregnancy. Asymptomatic aneurysms less than 2.0 cm in size in patients in whom pregnancy is not anticipated can be followed closely with serial imaging. Those with larger aneurysms or symptomatic aneurysms or those in whom pregnancy is anticipated should have the aneurysms approached operatively.

a. For proximal and middle-third aneurysms, the aneurysms may be simply excised with distal ligation, with the splenic blood supply then coming predominantly from the short gastric vessels.

b. For distal third aneurysms, resection with splenectomy is usually performed.

c. More recently, less invasive techniques, such as transcatheter embolization and laparoscopic excision, have been reported.

TECHNICAL CONSIDERATIONS IN SPLENECTOMY

I. **Preoperative preparation.** The decision to perform splenectomy should be made jointly by the surgeon, hematologist, and patient. All preoperative diagnostic tests and studies should be reviewed to ensure an accurate diagnosis.

A. **Vaccinations**

1. **Polyvalent pneumococcal vaccine.** Pneumovax covers 85% to 90% of pneumococcal types and should be administered at least 2 to 3 weeks preoperatively to all patients older than 2 years. The vaccine should be repeated 5 years after splenectomy.

2. **Meningococcal vaccine** can be given as a one-time vaccination to patients older than 2 years. Some physicians reserve meningococcal vaccination for the pediatric age group.

3. **Haemophilus influenzae type B** conjugate vaccine should be considered if the patient did not receive it during infancy.

4. **Influenza vaccination** should be considered.

B. **Considerations for transfusion**

1. **Patients with hematologic disease,** particularly those with autoimmune phenomena, often have autoantibodies and are difficult to crossmatch. Thus, blood should be typed and screened at least 24 hours prior to

the scheduled operative time. Patients with splenomegaly should have 2–4 units of packed red blood cells crossmatched and available for surgery.

2. **Patients with severe thrombocytopenia** (particularly those with counts <10,000/μL) should have platelets available for transfusion but these should be withheld until the splenic artery is ligated so they will not be quickly consumed by the spleen.

C. **Preoperative imaging**

1. Either **ultrasound or CT** may be necessary in patients with malignancy or suspected splenomegaly to help determine the optimal operative approach.

2. **Right upper quadrant ultrasound** is indicated preoperatively for those who are at high risk for developing gallstones (hemolytic anemias, sickle cell anemia) so that cholecystectomy may be performed concomitantly if needed.

3. **Technetium-99–sulfur colloid liver-spleen scanning** can be used to identify accessory splenic tissue but has not been shown to be particularly useful prior to splenectomy. However, in patients with recurrence of thrombocytopenia after initial splenectomy, this may be a useful imaging technique.

D. **Other considerations**

1. If the **patient has been receiving steroids** in the preoperative period, administration of stress-dose steroids should be considered.

2. As with other major intra-abdominal operations, **patients at high risk for cardiovascular disease** should undergo appropriate evaluation and treatment prior to undertaking elective surgery.

3. Patients who are to undergo a laparoscopic splenectomy should be counseled preoperatively about the possibility of **conversion to open splenectomy** and should be prepared identically to those patients for whom an open procedure is planned.

II. **Operative approach**

A. **Open splenectomy**

1. **The incision used** is surgeon-dependent, but the operation can be performed through either an upper midline incision or a subcostal incision. When significant splenomegaly is present, a midline incision is usually preferred.

2. **A drain is not routinely required** unless it is suspected that the pancreatic tail may have been injured during the hilar dissection.

3. A search for **accessory splenic tissue** should be conducted, particularly if the patient has a hematologic indication for splenectomy.

B. **Laparoscopic splenectomy** has been increasingly adopted as the primary mode of resection for patients with normal-size spleens and has become the preferred approach for patients with ITP and hemolytic anemias. More recently, laparoscopic splenectomy is being increasingly used for selected patients with splenomegaly.

1. **Contraindications** to laparoscopic splenectomy are presented in Table 19-2.

Table 19-2. Contraindications to laparoscopic splenectomy

Absolute contraindications	Difficult cases
Massive splenomegaly (>30 cm length)	Moderate splenomegaly (>20–25 cm)
Portal hypertension	Severe uncorrectable cytopenia
Splenic trauma, unstable patient	Splenic vein thrombosis
	Splenic trauma, stable patient
	Bulky hilar adenopathy
	Morbid obesity

2. **Splenomegaly** complicates the laparoscopic approach because of the difficulty of manipulating the organ atraumatically and achieving adequate exposure of the ligaments and hilum.
   a. Although the size limits for attempting laparoscopic or laparoscopic-assisted splenectomy are still evolving, most moderately enlarged spleens (<1000 g weight or 15 to 20 cm in length) can be removed in a minimally invasive fashion, often without a hand-port device.
   b. For spleens between 1,000 and 3,000 g, the use of a hand-port should be considered if a laparoscopic procedure is attempted.
   c. In general, spleens >28 cm in craniocaudal length or those >3,000 g should not be attempted laparoscopically because of the low success rate.
3. **Outcomes of laparoscopic splenectomy.**
   a. Several large series of laparoscopic splenectomy with good results have been published to date. In a recent meta-analysis examining the complications of splenectomy (*Surgery* 2003;134:647), laparoscopic splenectomy was associated with significantly fewer complications overall, primarily as a result of fewer wound and pulmonary complications.

COMPLICATIONS OF SPLENECTOMY

I. **Intraoperative complications**
   A. **Bowel injury**
      1. **Colon.** Because of the close proximity of the splenic flexure to the lower pole of the spleen, it is possible to injure the colon during mobilization. Some surgeons have advocated bowel preparation because of this potential complication, but that has not been our practice.
      2. **Stomach.** Gastric injuries can occur by direct trauma or can result from devascularization when the short gastric vessels are being taken down. Use of cautery too close to the greater curvature of the stomach can result in a delayed gastric perforation.
   B. **Vascular injury.** The most common intraoperative complication of splenectomy is hemorrhage, which can occur either during the hilar dissection or from a capsular tear during retraction of the spleen. The incidence of this complication is 2% to 3% during open splenectomy but is nearly 5% using the laparoscopic approach. Bleeding during laparoscopic splenectomy may necessitate conversion to an open procedure or to a hand-assisted approach.
   C. Clinical evidence of **pancreatic injury** occurs in 1% to 3% of splenectomies but would be much more common if postoperative amylase levels were checked routinely (*Surg Endosc* 2001;15:1273). The most common manifestation is mild asymptomatic hyperamylasemia, but clinical pancreatitis, pancreatic fistulas, and peripancreatic fluid collections can develop.
   D. **Diaphragmatic injury** has been described during the mobilization of the superior pole and is of no consequence if recognized and repaired. In laparoscopic splenectomies, it may be more difficult to recognize the injury given the pneumoperitoneum, but a high index of suspicion can help to minimize its occurrence. The pleural space should be evacuated under positive pressure ventilation prior to closure of the defect to minimize the pneumothorax.
II. **Early postoperative complications**
   A. **Pulmonary complications** develop in nearly 10% of patients after open splenectomy, and these range from atelectasis to pneumonia and pleural effusion. Pulmonary complications are significantly less common with the laparoscopic approach and occur in only 3% to 4% of patients who undergo a laparoscopic splenectomy.
   B. **Subphrenic abscess** occurs in 2% to 3% of patients after open splenectomy but is distinctly uncommon after laparoscopic splenectomy (0.7%). Treatment usually consists of percutaneous drainage and the intravenous administration of antibiotics.

C. **Wound problems** such as hematomas, seromas, and wound infections occur commonly after open splenectomy because of the underlying hematologic disorders, in 4% to 5% of patients. Wound complications after laparoscopic splenectomy are usually minor and occur less frequently (1.5%).

D. **Thrombocytosis and thrombotic complications** can occur after either open or laparoscopic splenectomy. The presumed causes of thrombosis after splenectomy relate to the normal occurrence of thrombocytosis, alterations in platelet function, and a low-flow stasis phenomenon in the ligated splenic vein. Symptomatic portal vein thrombosis occurs more commonly than expected (8% to 10%) and can result in extensive mesenteric thrombosis if not recognized promptly and treated expeditiously. Massive splenomegaly and myelofibrosis are the two main risk factors for portal vein thrombosis (*Am J Surg* 2002;184:631).

E. **Ileus** can occur after open splenectomy, as with any open intra-abdominal operation, but a prolonged postoperative ileus should prompt the surgeon to search for other concomitant problems such as a subphrenic abscess or portal vein thrombosis.

III. **Late postoperative complications**

A. **Overwhelming postsplenectomy infection (OPSI)** is a late complication that may occur at any point in a patient's lifetime. Patients present with non-specific flu-like symptoms rapidly progressing to fulminant sepsis, consumptive coagulopathy, bacteremia, and ultimately death within 12 to 48 hours in asplenic or hyposplenic individuals. The majority of cases occur within the first 2 years following splenectomy. Encapsulated bacteria, especially *Streptococcus pneumoniae*, *H. influenzae* type B, and *Neisseria meningitidis*, are the most commonly involved organisms. The loss of splenic reticuloendothelial cells (which have the unique ability to clear particulate antigen in the absence of antibody), loss of opsonin synthesis, and change in lymphocyte subpopulations limit the ability of asplenic patients to respond appropriately to infection. Successful treatment of OPSI requires prompt recognition and is generally supportive. Initial treatment is high-dose third-generation cephalosporins. Daily prophylactic antibiotics have been recommended after operation in all children younger than 5 years and in immunocompromised patients because these patients are unlikely to produce adequate antibody in response to pneumococcal vaccination. All patients who have had splenectomy should be educated about the risk of OPSI and the need for early physician consultation in the event that fever or other prodromal symptoms should occur.

B. **Splenosis** is the presence of disseminated intra-abdominal splenic tissue, which usually occurs after splenic rupture. Splenosis does not appear to be more common after laparoscopic splenectomy, but care should be taken during splenic morcellation to avoid bag rupture and spillage of splenic tissue.

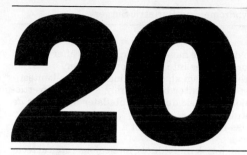

Fistulas, Short-Bowel Syndrome, and Bariatric Surgery

Valerie J. Halpin and
J. Christopher Eagon

GASTROENTEROLOGIC DISORDERS

I. A **fistula** is a communication between two epithelialized surfaces. Fistulas may be categorized according to anatomy, output, or etiology.
   A. **Anatomy**
      1. **External fistulas** are the most common fistulas and connect an internal organ system with the skin (e.g., enterocutaneous fistula).
      2. **Internal fistulas** connect two hollow structures of the same or different organ systems without external communication (e.g., colovesical fistula). In some cases, these are created intentionally (e.g., gastroenterostomy, choledochojejunostomy).
      3. **Proximal fistulas** are located in the upper gastrointestinal (GI) tract. They are usually associated with high outputs (3 L per day or more) and severe symptoms and sequelae, and they often have a poor prognosis.
      4. **Distal fistulas** arise in the distal ileum, colon, or rectum. They are often associated with fewer complications than are proximal fistulas, and they often close with nonoperative treatment.
      5. **Simple fistulas** have a single tract, whereas complicated fistulas have multiple and varied tracts connecting one or more organs.
   B. **Output**
      1. **High-output fistulas** drain more than 500 mL per day.
      2. **Low-output fistulas** drain less than 500 mL per day.
   C. **Etiology**
      1. **Abdominal surgical procedures** are the leading cause of fistula formation, accounting for 67% to 80% of cases. The risk is greatest for operations performed for inflammatory bowel disease, ischemia, malignancy, or extensive intestinal adhesions. Dissection of diseased bowel may result in unrecognized bowel perforation, devascularization, and serosal disruption. Anastomotic disruption, leak, and perianastomotic abscess also are common causes. Malnutrition significantly increases the risk of fistula formation.
      2. **Inflammatory bowel disease.** Fistulas typically occur where the inflammatory disease is worse, usually in the lower GI tract. Internal fistulization is especially common with Crohn's enteritis.
      3. **Diverticular disease** causes fistulas when localized abscesses drain into adjacent organs. Common examples include colovesical and colovaginal fistulas. Internal fistulas should be suspected in patients with diverticular disease who exhibit persistent and recurrent sepsis.
      4. **Malignancy.** Fistulas form as cancers perforate or invade adjacent structures. Healing does not occur if cancer is present, and surgical resection is the only means of cure.
      5. **Radiation enteritis** predisposes to fistula formation after surgery, regardless of the timing of exposure.
      6. **Trauma.** Fistula formation occurs more frequently after penetrating trauma than after blunt trauma. Unrecognized enterotomies as well as injuries that are repaired amid contamination may be prone to fistula formation. Viscus rupture caused by blunt trauma may go unrecognized, and subsequent abscess formation and drainage into adjacent structures

may result in fistula formation. This most commonly occurs after rupture of the duodenum, colon, or pancreas into the retroperitoneum.
   7. **Congenital fistulas.** Tracheoesophageal, rectovaginal, and vitellointestinal duct fistulas manifest shortly after birth. Rarely, a Meckel diverticulum or a patent omphalomesenteric duct presents later in life as a *de novo* enterocutaneous fistula.
   8. **Other causes of GI fistulas** include presence of a foreign body, vascular insufficiency, and amebiasis.
D. Prevention. Identification of high-risk individuals, meticulous surgical technique, and proper use of perioperative antibiotics are important. Thorough preoperative bowel preparation significantly reduces the risk of fistula formation.
E. Pathophysiology. Fistula-associated complications may be life-threatening and require rapid intervention to avoid morbidity and mortality. The overall mortality for all fistulas is 5% to 20%.
   1. **Loss of GI contents**
      a. **Hypovolemia.** High-output fistulas may discharge large volumes of fluid, which cannot be adequately replaced by enteral means, leading to dehydration and intravascular volume depletion.
      b. **Acid-base and electrolyte abnormalities.** Loss of large fluid volumes and associated electrolytes results in metabolic derangements. Severity is directly correlated with the quantity of fistula output.
   2. **Malnutrition** is caused by caloric intake insufficient to meet increased metabolic demands associated with fistula formation, such as the demands related to sepsis. Additionally, substantial portions of the GI tract may be functionally excluded from contact with enteric contents. The ensuing malabsorption leads to alterations in carbohydrate, fat, and protein metabolism; hypovitaminosis; and mineral deficiency.
   3. **Sepsis** is the main determinant of mortality from a fistula. Sepsis accompanies a large percentage of fistulas and is caused by seeding of the fistula tract by organisms indigenous to the bowel. A septic focus diminishes the potential for healing.
F. Initial management
   1. **Fluid resuscitation** to correct hypovolemia and ensure adequate tissue perfusion is a priority. Once the fluid deficit is corrected, accurate measurement of ongoing fluid losses and prompt replacement are essential to maintain euvolemia. Intravenous fluid administration is typically necessary because attempts at enteral replacement result in increased fluid loss from the fistula. Serum electrolytes and acid-base status must be followed closely and abnormalities corrected. Fluid replacement composition depends on the site of the fistula in the GI tract and the quantity of fluid loss, and content must be tailored to meet the specific replacement demands (see Table 4-1). High-output gastric fistulas occasionally may require the addition of hydrochloric acid. Biliary and pancreatic fistula effluent is hypertonic and associated with large bicarbonate and sodium losses.
   2. **Complete bowel rest** is instituted in the initial management of patients with fistulas. This may reduce fistula drainage and may simplify the evaluation and stabilization of the patient. Nasogastric suction has not proved beneficial except in the presence of distal obstruction.
      Nutritional support should be instituted within 24 hours of diagnosis. Early, aggressive parenteral nutritional therapy has dramatically decreased mortality from fistulas from 58% to 16% (*Am J Surg* 1964;108:157).
      a. **Enteral feeding,** if possible, is the primary method of choice for providing nutrients. Patients with colocutaneous and ileal low-output fistulas, including the terminal ileum or cecum, may be safely treated with enteral feeding. Adequate nutrient absorption requires at least 4 feet of functional intestinal tract. Standard enteral formulas are

sufficient in most cases; however, if the available bowel is short, elemental feeding may maximize absorption. In cases of proximal fistula, such as esophageal, gastric, duodenal, and proximal jejunal sites, enteral feeding can be given below the fistula if distal enteral access is available (i.e., feeding jejunostomy tube).

b. **Parenteral nutrition** is the secondary modality available to provide adequate calories and nutrients along with complete bowel rest. Indications include intolerance to enteral nutrition, jejunal and ileal high-output fistulas, and proximal fistulas if distal enteral access is not possible. The benefit of GI tract absorption is lost. However, providing adequate nutrition parenterally is vital when the GI tract cannot be used.

3. **Sepsis must be controlled early.**

a. **Intra-abdominal abscess** should be excluded in each patient with a GI fistula by abdominopelvic computed tomographic (CT) scan. Abscess drainage, whether percutaneous or open, is a therapeutic priority.

b. **Intravenous antibiotics** are indicated when infection is present. Antimicrobial therapy is directed at bowel flora and should consist of treatment against Gram-negative bacteria and anaerobes. Continuous bacterial seeding from the GI tract promotes persistent and recurrent sepsis, which is an indication for operation if uncontrolled with appropriate antimicrobial therapy.

c. **Infected wounds** are adequately opened and packed to allow complete drainage, débridement, and healing by secondary intention. Frequent dressing changes may be required.

4. **Fistula drainage** is controlled by wound management and pharmacotherapy.

a. **Dressings** may be used for low-output fistulas to absorb drainage fluid. However, prolonged contact of enteric contents with a surrounding wound or the skin may impede healing and cause skin breakdown. Intubation of matured fistula tracts may be beneficial. A suction or sump drainage system for high-output fistulas is preferred.

b. **Pharmacologic management** with somatostatin analogs has demonstrated mixed results. Some studies have shown decreased fistula output (*Lancet* 1987;2:672) and decreased time to closure; however, these results have not been uniformly replicated. In addition, H_2-receptor antagonists reduce gastric and duodenal fistula output and provide stress ulceration prophylaxis; however, their efficacy in reducing time to fistula closure has not been proven.

5. **Skin protection must be instituted promptly.** Irritation and excoriation of skin surrounding the site of fistula drainage are common and can be very painful, complicate wound management, and become secondarily infected. Skin surrounding a fistula is protected with a barrier device or powder [e.g., DuoDERM (ConvaTec, Princeton, NJ)]. The skin should be examined and cleansed frequently. An enterostomal therapist is helpful in managing complex wounds. A vacuum-assisted wound closure device may help in controlling skin irritation and fistula closure.

G. **Fistula assessment.** In the initial 4 to 6 weeks, 50% to 70% of fistulas close. The frequency of closure is not necessarily related to the quantity of initial fistula output. The difficult decision on how long to wait for spontaneous closure depends on individual circumstances and the complexity of the underlying illness. There has been a trend toward allowing longer periods for fistula closure because of improved home intravenous therapy, parenteral nutrition, and use of somatostatin analogue. If spontaneous closure does not appear likely, surgical therapy is indicated. The anatomy of the fistula is defined to assist planning of the appropriate surgical procedure.

1. **Contrast radiography** is most commonly used. Fistulography may be performed in mature fistula tracts (usually after 7 to 10 days) and typically provides good visualization of all tracts and sites of communication with

the GI tract. If the fistula tract is not mature, fistulography may be contraindicated. Oral contrast studies can demonstrate contrast extravasation through the fistula and are most valuable for assessing internal fistulas and distal obstruction. Contrast enema is the study of choice for rectal or colonic fistulas. Pyelography and cystography may be used in cases that involve the urinary tract.

2. **Endoscopy** (i.e., esophagogastroduodenoscopy, colonoscopy, or cystoscopy) aids in the assessment of coexistent disease in the organ from which the fistula arises, such as peptic ulceration, inflammatory bowel disease, and cancer. Fistula openings may be difficult to identify by endoscopy.

3. **Abdominopelvic CT scan** is the study of choice for evaluating for abscess. Its value is limited in the absence of abscess.

H. **Surgical treatment** is indicated when fistulas fail to heal with nonoperative measures and when sepsis cannot be controlled. Common conditions under which fistulas fail to close include malignancy, radiation, obstruction distal to the fistula, inflammation, presence of a foreign body, and epithelialization of the fistula tract. The goals of surgery are to eradicate the fistula tract and to restore the epithelial continuity of the associated organ systems.

1. **Gastric fistulas.** High-output gastric fistulas arise from anastomotic breakdown or ulcer perforation and require surgical repair. Most low-output gastric fistulas close spontaneously (e.g., gastrostomy closure after removal of gastrostomy tubes). In cases that do not close, primary repair or serosal patch placement usually is successful.

2. **Duodenal fistulas** are caused by breakdown of an anastomosis, trauma, or, less commonly, peptic ulceration. The high enzyme content of the effluent can cause severe skin excoriation. Most duodenal fistulas close spontaneously with conservative measures. If the fistula is secondary to inflammatory bowel disease, spontaneous closure is unlikely. When surgical intervention is required, primary closure of small duodenal wall disruptions may be performed, but duodenal stricture is associated with primary closure of large defects. Close proximity of the defect to the ampulla may also prevent primary closure. In these cases, duodenal wall integrity may be restored by serosal patch using another portion of bowel. Alternatively, a Roux-en-Y duodenoenterostomy may be performed to divert duodenal output into the bowel.

3. **Biliary and pancreatic fistulas** almost always close with nonsurgical therapeutic measures, which may include percutaneous interventional or endoscopic drainage techniques. Octreotide therapy may be beneficial.

4. **Small-bowel fistulas** are typically cured with bowel resection and primary reanastomosis. In rare severe cases, a temporary diverting enterostomy may be necessary. For internal fistulas, if the openings are in close proximity, the involved region can be resected in continuity.

5. **Large-bowel fistulas** generally are associated with high spontaneous closure rates. Fluid and electrolyte abnormalities are rare because outputs tend to be low. However, sepsis rates may be greater. If surgical closure is required, an adequate mechanical bowel preparation is important. Primary closure, as opposed to resection with primary reanastomosis, depends on associated conditions, the nutritional status of the patient, and the location and complexity of the lesion.

6. **Gastrostomy or enterostomy feeding tubes** placed at the time of definitive repair may facilitate postoperative management. Antibiotic therapy and nutritional support should continue into the postoperative period.

II. **Short-bowel syndrome**

A. **Etiology and pathophysiology.** Short-bowel syndrome is characterized by dehydration, electrolyte derangements, acidic diarrhea, steatorrhea, malnutrition, and weight loss. Congenital anomalies leading to short-bowel syndrome include intestinal atresia, midgut volvulus with intestinal necrosis, and necrotizing enterocolitis. In middle-aged adults, inflammatory bowel disease and trauma are the leading causes of massive intestinal resection. In the elderly, prominent causes include mesenteric ischemia, strangulated hernia, and extensive resection for malignancy.

B. In the adult, the length of the small bowel varies from 300 to 600 cm and correlates directly with body surface area. Several factors determine the severity of short-bowel syndrome, including the extent of resection, the part of the GI tract removed, the type of disease necessitating the resection, the presence of coexistent disease in the remaining bowel, and the adaptability of the remaining bowel. Generally, resection resulting in less than 120 cm of intact bowel leads to short-bowel syndrome. Resection of up to 50% of the small bowel in adults can be tolerated without serious complications, and resection of up to 70% can be tolerated if the terminal ileum and cecum are preserved. Infants may survive after resection of up to 85% of bowel owing to the enhanced ability of the bowel to adapt and grow with the child. Loss of the ileocecal valve results in rapid emptying of enteral contents into the colon and reflux of colonic bacterial flora into the small bowel. Because of its specialized absorptive function, resection of the ileum is also not well tolerated. However, the entire jejunum can be resected without serious adverse nutritional sequelae.

C. Adaptation. The distal small intestine has the greatest adaptive potential and can assume many of the absorptive properties of the proximal GI tract. Cellular hyperplasia and bowel hypertrophy occur over a 2- to 3-year period, increasing the absorptive surface area. Fat absorption is the metabolic process most likely to be permanently impaired; other functions adjust and normalize fairly well. Bowel motility also changes, with the more proximal intestine developing motility patterns similar to those of the normal ileum.

D. Fluid and electrolyte response. Of the 8 to 10 L of chyme presented daily to the small intestine, only 1 to 2 L are delivered into the colon. Significant quantities of electrolytes are absorbed in this process. With short-bowel syndrome, this physiology is altered. Strict intake and output records as well as close monitoring of serum electrolytes are critical in the early management of patients with short-bowel syndrome. The pH of enteric drainage should be monitored, whether from fistulas, stomata, or feces.

E. Malabsorption and malnutrition

1. **Gastric hypersecretion,** seen in the early postoperative period, can persist for prolonged periods. Increased acid load may injure distal bowel mucosa, leading to hypermotility and impaired absorption. The severity of hypersecretion correlates directly with the extent of bowel resection. This generally is more pronounced after jejunal resection than after ileal resection. Loss of an intestinal inhibitory hormone has been implicated.

2. **Cholelithiasis.** Altered bilirubin metabolism after ileal resection increases the risk of pigment gallstones secondary to a decreased bile salt pool, which causes a shift in the cholesterol saturation index. Chronic total parenteral nutrition (TPN) also predisposes to increased risk of cholelithiasis.

3. **Hyperoxaluria and nephrolithiasis.** Excessive fatty acids within the colonic lumen bind intraluminal calcium. Unbound oxalate, normally made insoluble by calcium binding and excreted in the feces, thus is absorbed readily, resulting in hyperoxaluria and calcium oxalate urinary stone formation.

4. **Diarrhea and steatorrhea** are caused by rapid intestinal transit, presence of hyperosmolar enteric contents in the distal bowel, disruption of the enterohepatic bile acid circulation, and bacterial overgrowth. Fat absorption is most severely impaired by ileal resection. The delivery of bile acids into the colon produces a reactive watery diarrhea that may be severe. Unabsorbed fats in the colon further inhibit absorption and stimulate secretion of water and electrolytes.

5. Intestinal microflora. Loss of the ileocecal valve permits reflux of colonic bacteria into the small bowel. Intestinal dysmotility further promotes bacterial colonization. Bacterial overgrowth and change in the indigenous microbial population result in pH alteration and deconjugation of bile salts, with resultant malabsorption, fluid loss, and decreased vitamin B_{12} absorption. Infectious diarrhea, bacterial or viral, is a major cause of morbidity.

F. Effects on intestinal motility. Normal motility depends on the quantity and concentration of enteric contents in the bowel lumen. Trophic factors also play a role. In short-bowel syndrome, these parameters are altered. Because the ileum has the greatest capacity for absorption of fluid and electrolytes and for postresection adaptation, short-bowel syndrome symptoms are most likely to occur after ileal resection.

G. Early postoperative management

1. **Fluids and electrolytes.** The primary goal is to stabilize the metabolic, respiratory, and cardiovascular parameters related to the fluid shift and sepsis that frequently accompany massive small-bowel resection. All fluid losses should be strictly accounted for and replaced.

2. **Ileus** may be prolonged because of deranged motility patterns and changes in intraluminal milieu. Parenteral nutrition should be provided until GI tract function resumes. If ileus persists for an unduly prolonged period, mechanical obstruction or sepsis should be ruled out. Short-bowel syndrome ileus generally resolves more quickly in children than in adults.

3. **Gastric hypersecretion.** H_2-receptor antagonists or proton pump inhibitors reduce the hypersecretion response and protect against peptic ulceration. Antacids neutralize acid on contact and should be administered for nasogastric aspirate pH of less than 5.

4. **Nutritional support** should be instituted early to maintain positive nitrogen balance and to promote wound healing and adaptation of the remaining bowel. Enteral nutrition has a positive trophic effect on the bowel mucosa and should be started as soon as possible. Feeding tubes placed at laparotomy can be very helpful. Even if caloric goals are not met, enteral formula stimulates the remaining intestine and facilitates adaptation. Feeds should initially be low volume, low fat, and isosmotic and then be advanced as tolerated. Elemental feeding may be required in severe cases of short-bowel syndrome.

H. Long-term management

1. **Diarrhea** has many causes in short-bowel syndrome. Frequently, dietary modification improves symptoms. H_2-receptor antagonists reduce acid production and the volume of enteric contents. Chelating resins, such as cholestyramine, reduce intraluminal bile salts and subsequent diarrhea but affect the available systemic bile salt pools. Antisecretory medications, such as loperamide and somatostatin analogue, may be beneficial. Low-dose oral narcotics, such as diphenoxylate hydrochloride and atropine (Lomotil) or codeine, are efficacious but addictive. Bacterial overgrowth should be evaluated by stool culture, and prophylactic antimicrobials, such as metronidazole, should be administered as needed.

2. **Nutritional support.** Vitamins, trace elements and minerals, and essential fatty acids should be parenterally administered until adequate enteral absorption is established. If the patient is unable to assume an oral dietary regimen, parenteral vitamin and mineral supplementation is warranted. The absorption of fat-soluble vitamins A, D, E, and K is especially likely to be compromised. Vitamin B_{12} and calcium absorption are also affected by altered fat absorption and should be supplemented. Chronic TPN can be administered nightly to permit normal daily life.

3. **Late complications,** mostly secondary to metabolic derangements, are common. Anastomotic leak, fistula, stricture, and obstruction can occur well beyond the early postoperative period. Massive bowel resection typically is undertaken in the presence of soiling, necrosis, and abscess. Late

obstruction (partial or complete) is fairly common, and reoperative rates are high. Other problems include nephrolithiasis, cholelithiasis, nutritional deficiency (e.g., anemia, bone disease, coagulopathy), liver dysfunction, TPN-related complications, and central venous catheter–related problems (e.g., sepsis, thrombosis).

I. **Surgical therapy.** Various surgical procedures have been described for the management of short-bowel syndrome, although they have not been widely adopted. Most applications are in the pediatric age group. Most important is the prevention of complications by minimizing the extent of initial bowel resection.

1. **Slowing of intestinal transit.** If intestinal transit times are slowed, enteric contents have a greater opportunity to be absorbed.

   a. An **antiperistaltic segment** is created by reversing a segment of the intestinal tract; counterpulsation then acts to slow transit time. The antiperistaltic effect, however, has been shown to decrease with time.

   b. The **recirculating loop** has poor results because of a high incidence of stasis enteritis.

   c. **Colonic interposition** provides a slower intrinsic rate of motility and a larger luminal diameter. Results are limited.

   d. **Intestinal pacing** in the distal GI tract produces retrograde peristalsis, thereby slowing transit times. This procedure is experimental.

   e. **Increased intestinal surface area.** A tapering and lengthening procedure (tapering enteroplasty) may double bowel length (*J Pediatr Surg* 1980;15:145). It is technically difficult to perform, however, especially when extensive adhesions or mesenteric thickening is present. Results have been moderate.

   f. **Intestinal transplantation.** Future advances in immunosuppression and preservation techniques may make isolated bowel transplantation, which is still somewhat controversial, a more attractive alternative in some patients, especially those with massive resection and virtually no remaining bowel.

III. **Radiation enteritis**

A. **Etiology and pathophysiology.** Approximately 2% to 5% of patients who undergo abdominopelvic external beam radiation, typically for the treatment of malignancies, have radiation-induced bowel damage. Toxicity depends on dose. Small bowel is most susceptible, followed by colon and, lastly, rectum. Radiation-induced injury causes an obliterative endarteritis, resulting in chronic tissue ischemia, followed later by ischemic fibrosis and vascular and lymphatic ectasia. The presence of preexisting vascular disease (diabetes, hypertension, and cardiovascular disease) increases risk. Risk is also greater in thin patients; during concomitant chemotherapy, with damage to replicating mucosa; and when prior abdominal surgery has left fixed loops of bowel in the pelvis.

B. **Acute radiation injury,** seen within hours or days of radiation delivery, causes depletion of actively proliferating cells in the bowel mucosa. A leukocytic infiltrate, with crypt abscess formation, follows. Symptoms include periumbilical abdominal pain, diarrhea, nausea, and vomiting. Contrast and endoscopic studies reveal edematous bowel mucosa. Therapy revolves around treatment of symptoms and avoidance of further injury. A 10% reduction in radiation dose usually prevents further episodes of acute radiation enteritis.

C. **Chronic radiation injury** may be observed decades after radiation exposure. Bowel wall thickening, neovascularization, and telangiectasia may progress slowly. Fibrous bands and strictures form secondary to mesenchymal injury. More commonly, preexisting radiation damage impairs the ability of the bowel to heal after some other primary insult, such as inflammation, malignancy, or surgical manipulation.

D. **Clinical presentation** is highly variable and depends on the bowel segment involved.

1. **Small-bowel enteritis symptoms** range from nausea, vomiting, and abdominal pain to obstruction, perforation, and fistula formation. Oral contrast studies delineate the extent of disease. Findings include bowel wall thickening, decreased peristalsis, and stricture.

2. **The colon and rectum** are more resistant to radiation injury. Nonetheless, radiation therapy commonly is targeted in these areas by external beam or endocavitary delivery. **Symptoms** include rectal bleeding, diarrhea, tenesmus, abdominal pain, and constipation. Proctosigmoidoscopy reveals edematous, inflamed, and friable mucosa. Barium enema can rule out fistula or stricture.

E. **Medical management** is aimed at controlling symptoms by dietary modification and medication. Low-fat, low-residue, and lactose-free diets are recommended. In severe cases, bowel rest and TPN may be indicated. Agents that reduce bowel motility may help in mild cases. Antispasmodic and bile salt chelating agents also are used. Prostaglandin synthesis inhibition with aspirin has been shown to reduce symptoms in a prospective, randomized trial (*Lancet* 1975;2:942). Corticosteroids, in combination with TPN, are believed to reduce the inflammatory reaction, thereby alleviating symptoms. Radiation coloproctitis is treated with sitz baths, steroid retention enemas, and stool-bulking agents. If ulcerative lesions are identified, biopsy should be performed to rule out new or recurrent malignancy.

F. **Surgical therapy** is indicated for partial or complete obstruction, bowel perforation, fistula, and bleeding. Those without an identified lesion do not benefit from surgery. Poor healing associated with irradiated intestine must be taken into account. A thorough history of the original malignancy and the timing and total dose of radiation received guide surgical management. A careful GI workup identifies the location and extent of disease. TPN should be provided if nutritional status is poor. Preoperative ureteral stent placement is often desirable.

1. **Intraoperative efforts** are individualized and revolve around the pathologic lesion. Adhesions should be anticipated and lysis avoided except where absolutely necessary. Enteral bypass may be a better alternative than resection in rare cases. Adequate blood supply to the anastomotic margin must be ensured. Frozen section of this area has been advocated to ensure absence of disease. If there is any doubt, the bowel should be resected to briskly bleeding edges. A feeding enterostomy tube can usually be placed in the distal GI tract to aid in postoperative management. Postoperative gastric decompression is important, and oral intake should proceed cautiously.

2. **Surgical indications** for colonic disease include perforation, obstruction, fistula, and radiation proctitis. Bleeding is usually secondary to mucosal telangiectasia, and noninvasive local control should be attempted. Colonic or abdominoperineal resection with diversion may be necessary. Diversion of the GI tract as a primary treatment modality does provide symptomatic relief, but it has not been shown to alter the course of radiation-induced injury to the colon and rectum, nor does it stop bleeding. Early diversion with later definitive repair is the therapeutic standard in severe cases.

IV. **Bariatric surgery**
A. **Obesity,** a disease of modernization, is a major health epidemic and is common in the United States. The primary cause of obesity is related to dietary factors, but genetic predisposition is important. Rarely, endocrine dysfunction is the cause. **Morbid obesity** is defined as a body mass index (BMI; weight in kilograms divided by square of height in meters) greater than 40, or roughly 100 pounds greater than ideal body weight.

B. **Complications of morbid obesity are significant.** Morbidly obese young men have 12 times the mortality risk than the matched general population. Of the many medical sequelae associated with obesity, nearly all are reversible on resolution of the obese state.

1. **Cardiopulmonary effects.** Systemic hypertension is the most common complication associated with morbid obesity. Coronary atherosclerosis is 10 times more prevalent in obese populations than in those matched for age, gender, and other risk factors. Patients are also 10 times more likely to experience sleep apnea than are the nonobese. Decreased chest wall compliance results in hypoventilation or pickwickian syndrome, with resultant hypoxia and acidosis, leading to pulmonary hypertension and eventual right-sided heart failure.
2. **Non-insulin-dependent diabetes mellitus (NIDDM)** is secondary to increased peripheral resistance to insulin. On reversal of the obese state, diabetes resolves in two-thirds of patients. Diabetic microvascular disease leads to cardiac, renal, and ocular problems.
3. **Degenerative joint disease** from mechanical overbearing of the joint synovial surface results in degeneration, inflammation, and disabling pain.
4. **Hiatal hernia and gastroesophageal reflux** are secondary to increased intra-abdominal pressure.
5. **Cholelithiasis** is three times more common than in the general population.
6. **Thromboembolic disorders** arise from venous insufficiency, leading to stasis and thrombosis. Thrombophlebitis is very common, and the risk of pulmonary embolism is high.
7. **Endocrine dysfunction.** Obese females often develop amenorrhea and menometrorrhagia, with associated hirsutism and breast atrophy, whereas obese males sometimes have feminization syndromes caused by excessive estrogen production by adipocytes.
8. **Psychosocial problems.** Low self-esteem and depression make recovery from the obese condition very difficult.
9. **Other complications** include nonalcoholic fatty liver disease, pseudotumor cerebri (benign intracranial hypertension), complications of pregnancy, and gout.
C. **Medical treatment**
   1. **Medical therapy** can consist of low-calorie diets, behavior modification, exercise, and pharmacotherapy. These therapies may produce temporary reductions in weight, but medical management is difficult, with extremely high relapse rates after 1 to 2 years. Newer medications that suppress appetite and promote weight loss may be used in conjunction.
   2. **Psychological assessment** is necessary to treat underlying depression and low self-esteem as well as to prepare patients for surgical therapy.
D. **Bariatric surgery** was first performed in the 1950s. Weight loss results with jejunoileal bypass were good, but unacceptable long-term complication rates and the poor long-term weight loss results of horizontal gastroplasties caused interest to wane after 1980. The development and improved success of newer surgical procedures led to a National Institutes of Health Consensus Development Conference on morbid obesity (*Am J Clin Nutr* 1992;55:615S) and renewed enthusiasm. Interest has further increased with the application of minimally invasive techniques in bariatric surgery in the late 1990s.
   1. **Indications.** Patients who have failed intensive efforts at weight control using medical means are candidates for bariatric surgery if they have a body mass index greater than 40 or greater than 35 with associated comorbidities, including diabetes, hypertension, and sleep apnea syndrome.
   2. **Benefits** of surgery are related to the reversal of the disease processes associated with severe obesity. Hypertension resolves in 50% of patients and improves in another 25%. NIDDM is reversed in two-thirds of cases, and the incidence of new-onset diabetes is decreased by a factor of 30 compared with untreated controls. Frequently, sleep apnea and gastroesophageal reflux disease are improved or resolve. The quality of life is markedly better.

3. **Preoperative medical evaluation** includes input from the primary care physician, dietitian, physical therapist, and psychiatrist or psychologist, with special attention to the patient's weight history, dietary habits, motivation, social history, and comorbid medical conditions.

4. **Bariatric surgical procedures** rely on one or more of several effects on GI motor function. Gastric restriction produces a small gastric reservoir, thereby producing early satiety and so reducing oral intake. Malabsorption of varying degrees is induced by bypass of selected portions of the proximal small bowel.

    a. **Adjustable silicon gastric banding** was approved for use in the United States in 2001. This is a purely restrictive procedure. The band consists of an inflatable balloon placed around the angle of His. It is connected to a reservoir that is implanted over the rectus sheath. The patient undergoes serial adjustments to inflate the band and create a small proximal gastric pouch. Most complications are related to band slippage or problems with the port. Excess weight loss is approximately 50% at one year. Advantages are adjustability and reversability.

    b. **Vertical banded gastroplasty** is associated with a low incidence of metabolic derangement because it maintains GI tract continuity. An end-to-end anastomosis (EEA) stapler is used to create a window in the midbody of the stomach. A vertical staple line then is placed from the angle of His to the window in order to partition the stomach, leaving a small reservoir. Then, through the hole, a mesh band is positioned around the lesser curve to restrict the size of the passage for enteric content. Complications, though rare, include breakdown of the suture line and erosion of the mesh band into the gastric wall, resulting in **perforation.** Metabolic complications and malnutrition are less frequent than with procedures that include a malabsorptive component. Mortality is less than 1%. Weight loss is approximately 45% of excess body weight at 1 year.

    c. **Roux-en-Y gastric bypass (RYGBP)** is currently the most popular procedure. A 30-mL proximal gastric pouch is created either by transection or by occlusion using a stapling device. A 1-cm diameter anastomosis is then performed between the pouch and a Roux-en-Y limb of small bowel. This results in a small reservoir, a small passage for pouch emptying, and bypass of the distal stomach, duodenum, and proximal jejunum. The length of the Roux limb directly correlates with the degree of postoperative weight loss. Mortality is 1%, most commonly secondary to pulmonary embolism, myocardial infarction, or a leak at the gastrojejunostomy, which occurs in 2% to 4% of patients. Late complications include incisional hernia, stomal stenosis, and ulcer. Nutritional complications include folate, vitamin B_{12}, iron, and calcium deficiency. Weight loss is 70% of excess weight at 1 year. Reversal of NIDDM occurs rapidly, often within 2 weeks. Dumping syndrome occurs in most patients but is desirable and reinforces dietary behavior modification to avoid sweets and high-calorie foods.

    d. **Biliopancreatic diversion (BPD)** and **biliopancreatic diversion with duodenal switch (BPD-DS)** are two additional procedures for patients with a high BMI. BPD requires antrectomy with formation of a 200-cm alimentary channel and a 50- to 75-cm common channel. BPD-DS includes a sleeve gastrectomy, preservation of the pylorus, a 150-cm alimentary channel and a 75- to 100-cm common channel. These procedures are done at select centers for the superobese. Long-term outcomes indicate excess weight loss of 75% at 1 year, but nutritional deficiencies are more common than for RYGBP. The applicability of these procedures to the obese population remains to be determined.

    e. **Jejunoileal bypass** is a purely malabsorptive procedure. At one time the most frequently performed weight reduction procedure, it has a high rate of long-term complications, including diarrhea, bypass or stasis enteritis (characterized by abdominal pain and distention), excessive flatulence, electrolyte abnormalities, cholelithiasis, hepatic dysfunction, and nephrolithiasis secondary to hyperoxaluria. The long-term mortality rate is 10%. As a result, this procedure is no longer performed for obesity, and those with severe sequelae should be reversed and converted to a gastric bypass.

E. Laparoscopic bariatric surgery

1. **Indications** for laparoscopic bariatric surgery are the same as those for open procedures.

2. **Contraindications** to laparoscopic bariatric surgery vary by institution. A BMI of greater than 60, previous upper abdominal surgery, evidence of an excessively large liver, and the presence of a large ventral hernia are relative contraindications.

3. RYGBP and adjustable gastric banding are procedures amenable to a laparoscopic approach. RYGBP appears to be most beneficial in terms of producing long-term weight loss. BPD-DS can be performed laparoscopically in selected centers, although it is technically more difficult and may be done in a two-stage manner, with sleeve gastrectomy as the initial stage.

4. **Laparoscopic RYGBP** is a technically challenging operation. The patient is initially positioned supine in reverse Trendelenburg with the left lateral section of the liver retracted superiorly, thereby exposing the gastroesophageal junction. Dissection is carried out between the left gastric artery and the lesser curvature 4 cm distal to the gastroesophageal junction and on the greater curve at the angle of His to create windows into the lesser sac. A Baker tube is inserted into the stomach and the balloon inflated with 15 mL of saline to size the proximal gastric pouch. A gastrotomy is created directly over the balloon. The anvil of a 21-mm EEA stapler is passed into the gastric lumen via a second gastrotomy created in the distal stomach. The post of the anvil is passed through the upper gastrotomy and secured in place with a purse string suture. The stomach is then transected distal to the anvil, and the lower gastrotomy is oversewn. The jejunum is then measured 30 cm distal to the ligament of Treitz and transected. Seventy-five to 150 cm of distal jejunum is used for the Roux limb and a functional end-to-side jejunojejunostomy is created. The Roux limb is passed into the lesser sac through a defect created in the transverse mesocolon. After the creation of an enterotomy in the proximal Roux limb, the base of the EEA stapler is inserted in an antegrade fashion. The spike of the stapler is passed through the antimesenteric border of the Roux limb, mated to the post of the anvil, and fired. The Roux limb enterotomy is stapled closed, and the gastrojejunostomy is tested for leakage by instillation of 40 mL of methylene blue via a Baker tube.

F. Complications in the immediate postoperative period are similar for laparoscopic and open gastric bypass and include wound infection, bleeding, deep venous thrombosis, pulmonary embolism, anastomotic leakage, myocardial infarction, and a 1% to 2% mortality. The laparoscopic approach decreases the incidence of wound-related complications such as infection, seroma, and hernia. The laparoscopic approach may also result in less postoperative impairment of the respiratory, immune, and GI systems.

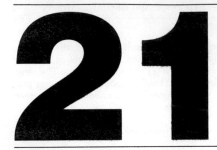

Occlusive Arterial Disease

Douglas W. Green and Gregorio A. Sicard

Stenosis or occlusion of branches of the arterial tree can generate a variety of clinical syndromes. The specific symptoms and severity depend on the downstream organ(s), the degree of stenosis, the chronicity of obstruction, and the extent of collateral circulation. The vast majority of occlusive disease is secondary to atherosclerotic change of the arterial intima. This is, in general, a progressive disorder, influenced to a degree by genetic predisposition. However, the evolution of the disease for most individuals can be modified by changes in environmental factors, particularly diet and exercise. Atherosclerotic disease is a systemic illness, and although symptomatic disease may predominate in one organ, subclinical disease, particularly of the coronary arteries, is generally present. In fact, 50% of the mortality associated with peripheral arterial reconstructions for atherosclerotic disease is cardiac in nature. Other less common causes of occlusive disease include fibromuscular dysplasia, radiation-induced vascular injury, and the vasculitides (e.g., Takayasu arteritis and Buerger disease).

ACUTE ARTERIAL OCCLUSION OF THE EXTREMITY

Symptoms of acute arterial insufficiency occur abruptly. The presentation generally includes the **five Ps** of acute ischemia: **pain, pallor, pulselessness, paresthesias, and paralysis;** some add poikilothermy, the inability to thermoregulate, to this list. The level of occlusion may be localized by the absence of pulses and the level of coolness of the limb. If adequate collateral circulation is not present, irreversible changes may appear as early as 4 to 6 hours after onset. Therefore, priority must be given to restoration of blood flow within this time period. Once the occlusive process has begun, regardless of its cause, vasospasm and propagation of thrombus distal to the site of initial occlusion can contribute to further ischemia.

I. **Etiology**
   A. The most common cause of acute arterial insufficiency is **embolization.**
      1. **Cardiac sources** account for more than 70% of emboli and usually are the result of mural thrombi that develop due to cardiac aneurysms following myocardial infarction or arrhythmias such as atrial fibrillation. Other cardiac causes of emboli include valvular heart disease, prosthetic heart valves, bacterial endocarditis, and atrial myxoma.
      2. **Arterial-arterial emboli** can result from ulcerated atheroma or aneurysms, although embolization from abdominal aortic aneurysms is distinctly rare. The blue toe syndrome occurs in patients with microemboli from unstable proximal arterial plaques and is characterized by the presence of intact pulses and painful ischemic lesions in the distal extremity. Atheroemboli in the lower extremity secondary to plaque disruption by catheters can occur. The severely diseased distal aorta in some of these patients is evident on CT scan and arteriography and has been termed *shaggy aorta.*
      3. **Venous-arterial emboli** (paradoxical emboli) can result from an intracardiac shunt (e.g., patent foramen ovale) or intrapulmonary arteriovenous malformations (e.g., Osler-Weber-Rendu syndrome).
      4. Occasionally, it is difficult to discern whether a person with advanced atherosclerotic disease has had an embolus or whether an already compromised vessel has undergone acute thrombosis. This is particularly true in patients without arrhythmias or prior myocardial infarction. The

presence of contralateral pulses and no past history of claudication may help in making this differentiation.

B. **Direct arterial trauma** is frequently obvious but may initially be occult and may result in arterial stenosis or occlusion only after an intimal flap or arterial wall hematoma progresses sufficiently to cause symptoms. Careful initial examination may help avoid this pitfall. Arterial compromise can also occur in the setting of compression by joint dislocations (e.g., knee), bone fragments (e.g., tibial plateau fracture), or compartment syndrome.

C. Other causes of acute ischemia include arterial thrombosis, aortic dissection, venous outflow occlusion, and low-flow state.

II. Diagnosis and evaluation

A. If history and physical examination demonstrate clear evidence of embolization, **definitive therapy** should not be delayed. If there is a concern that the occlusive process may be thrombotic, however, **arteriography** may be indicated. Angiographically, embolic occlusions can be distinguished from thrombotic occlusions by their occurrence just distal to vascular bifurcations and by the concave shadow formed at the interface with the contrast. In select cases, thrombolysis may be a useful adjunct for defining underlying occlusive disease. In general, patients with acute ischemia unrelated to trauma should be considered to have coexistent cardiac disease. All patients should have an electrocardiogram and chest x-ray performed. After limb revascularization, a transesophageal echocardiogram can be useful in diagnosing a cardiac source. Laboratory determinations usually are of little benefit in the early assessment but are important in the later management of the patient.

B. Patients who present with penetrating **trauma,** long bone fractures, or joint dislocations may have vascular injuries. **Hard signs** of arterial injury include diminished or absent pulses distal to an injury, ischemia distal to an injury, visible arterial bleeding from a wound, a bruit at or distal to the site of injury, and the presence of a large, expanding, or pulsatile hematoma. Patients with penetrating injuries who display clear signs of arterial injury need urgent surgical intervention without preoperative angiography. **Soft signs** of injury include the anatomic proximity of a wound to a major vessel, injury to an anatomically related nerve, unexplained hemorrhagic shock, or a moderately sized hematoma. In those with only soft signs, a careful documentation of pulses by **Doppler pressures** distal to the injury should be undertaken, along with comparison with the contralateral limb. A difference of greater than 10% to 20% suggests the need for arteriography or exploration. In certain situations, duplex scan of the injured area can be useful in the diagnosis of intimal flap, pseudoaneurysm, or arterial or venous thrombi.

III. Management

A. Once a diagnosis of acute arterial ischemia due to emboli or thrombi is made, **heparin** should be administered immediately. An intravenous bolus of 80 units/kg followed by an intravenous infusion of 18 units/kg per hour is usually satisfactory. Partial thromboplastin time (PTT) should be maintained between 60 and 80 seconds.

1. **Surgical therapy,** such as embolectomy, should be performed urgently in patients with an obvious embolus and acute ischemia. Embolectomy can be done under local anesthesia if the patient cannot tolerate general anesthesia. Once the artery is isolated, a Fogarty catheter is passed proximally and distally to extract the embolus and associated thrombus. In some cases, intraoperative thrombolysis may be necessary, as distal vessels may be thrombosed beyond the reach of the Fogarty catheter. Distal patency can be proved, if necessary, with an intraoperative arteriogram, depending on the status of distal vessels and pulses after embolectomy. In the leg, if adequate distal perfusion is not established and an angiogram demonstrates distal thrombus, the distal popliteal artery may be explored, with selective passage of the embolectomy catheter into the anterior tibial, posterior tibial, and peroneal arteries. The arteriotomy can be closed with a patch graft if there is arterial narrowing. Bypass grafting may also be required if significant preexisting arterial disease in the affected segment is discovered.

2. **High-dose heparinization** (20,000-unit initial bolus followed by 2,000 to 4,000 units per hour) may be used in patients who are at extremely high risk for surgery and who have advanced ischemia with a nonviable extremity. The goal is to preserve as much tissue as possible by limiting progressive thrombosis.

3. **Thrombolytic therapy** may be useful in patients with clearly viable extremities in whom thrombosis is the likely underlying cause of their acute ischemia. In general, the fresher the thrombus, the more successful thrombolysis can be. Thrombolysis and follow-up angiography frequently identify an underlying stenosis, which may be treated by balloon angioplasty/stent or by surgical means.

   a. **Urokinase** was the agent of choice until 1999, when the U.S. Food and Drug Administration withdrew the drug from the market because of production concerns. It has recently been reinstated and is in limited use. Urokinase is instilled through an intra-arterial catheter placed as close to the thrombus as possible. Dosing varies from 60,000 to 120,000 units/hour, with an optional loading dose of approximately 200,000 units. Full-dose intravenous heparinization is undertaken concurrently to achieve a PTT of 60 to 80. Reteplase (0.5 to 0.75 units/hour) and alteplase (0.5 to 1.0 mg/hour) are also in use and are administered with subtherapeutic heparin (approximately 400 units/hour intravenously). Complication rates of less than 10% have been reported for thrombolysis. Repeat arteriography is performed 6 to 18 hours after initiation of treatment to gauge the results. Duration of therapy is generally between 4 and 16 hours but may extend for as long as 30 hours.

   b. **Glycoprotein IIb/IIIa inhibitors** may also play a role in combination with a thrombolytic agent. Trials using 0.25 mg/kg abciximab intra-arterially in combination with reteplase have been performed. Significant bleeding occurred in approximately 10% of cases.

   c. During thrombolysis, the patient is usually monitored in the **intensive care unit (ICU).** Thrombin time, fibrinogen level, fibrin degradation product level, PTT, and complete blood count are followed closely to limit the risk of hemorrhage. In general, the likelihood of serious hemorrhagic complications increases when fibrinogen levels drop below 100 mg/dL and the PTT rises above three to five times normal. Once the artery is open, the patient can be managed either with systemic anticoagulation or with surgical intervention (i.e., operative arterial reconstruction, balloon angioplasty).

4. Percutaneous aspiration thromboembolectomy is an investigative technique and may prove useful as an adjunct to thrombolysis by decreasing clot volume. Various devices are currently undergoing clinical trials.

B. In the setting of **trauma**, operative exploration should be performed in any limb that is ischemic or if arteriography demonstrates a significant intimal flap or other pathology. In the presence of coexistent neurologic or orthopedic injuries, it is essential to reestablish arterial flow first, either by direct repair or bypass grafting. At the conclusion of the orthopedic repair, the arterial repair should be reexamined to ensure that it has not been disrupted and has been correctly fashioned to the final bone length. In cases of joint dislocation, reduction of the dislocation should be accomplished first because this may alleviate the need for arterial reconstruction.

1. Intraoperatively it is essential to **obtain proximal and distal control** of the injured artery before exploring the hematoma or wound. When repairing an artery, an end-to-end anastomosis is preferable. A few centimeters of the artery can usually be mobilized proximally and distally to accomplish

reapproximation. However, the uninjured leg or other potential vein harvest site should be prepared in case a conduit is required. It is preferable to use autologous tissue in this setting. If concomitant venous injuries are identified, these should be repaired as well. If injuries to the great vessels are suspected, the patient's chest should be prepared, as a median sternotomy or thoracotomy may be required. A completion arteriography can help to document distal flow. This is especially important if significant spasm is present and distal pulses are not readily palpable.

2. In general, injuries to the subclavian, axillary, brachial, femoral, superficial femoral, profunda femoral, and popliteal arteries should be repaired. The radial or ulnar artery may be ligated if the other vessel is intact and functioning. Similarly, isolated injuries to the tibial arteries may be ligated if one or more of the tibial arteries is intact.

IV. **Complications**
A. **Reperfusion injury** occurs after reestablishment of arterial flow to an ischemic tissue bed, which can lead to further tissue death. It results from the formation of oxygen-free radicals, which directly damage the tissue and cause white blood cell accumulation and sequestration in the microcirculatory system. This process tends to prolong the ischemic interval because it impairs adequate nutrient flow to the tissue despite the restoration of axial blood flow. Currently, there is no proven therapy that limits reperfusion injury.

B. **Rhabdomyolysis** following reperfusion releases the by-products of ischemic muscle, including potassium, lactic acid, myoglobin, and creatinine phosphokinase, into the systemic circulation. The electrolyte and pH changes that occur can trigger dangerous arrhythmias, and precipitation of myoglobin in the renal tubules can cause pigment nephropathy and ultimately acute renal failure. The likelihood that a patient will develop these complications relates to the duration of ischemia and the muscle mass at risk. In an attempt to ameliorate this, some surgeons clamp the femoral vein prior to revascularization and perform a transverse venotomy after lower-extremity arterial inflow is reestablished. The first 250 to 500 mL of blood are discarded or aspirated to an autotransfusion system, thereby removing the hyperkalemic and acidotic plasma. Aggressive hydration, diuresis promotion with mannitol (25 g intravenously), and intravenous infusion of bicarbonate to alkalinize the urine are also accepted methods.

C. **Compartment syndrome** results when prolonged ischemia causes cell membrane damage and leakage of fluid into the interstitium. The edema can result in extremely high intracompartmental pressures, particularly in the lower extremity. When these intracompartmental pressures exceed capillary perfusion pressure, further muscle and nerve necrosis ensues. A four-compartment fasciotomy should be performed when there is concern about the possible development of leg compartment syndrome. Fasciotomy should be routine in any patient with more than 6 hours of lower-extremity ischemia or in the presence of combined arterial and venous injuries. Leg fasciotomies usually are performed through two incisions, one anterolateral and another posteromedial. The skin is left open, to be closed either secondarily or by skin graft at a later time.

D. **Catheter-related complications** can occur early or late. Early complications result from arterial wall trauma and include arterial perforation and rupture, intimal dissection, and pseudoaneurysm formation. A late catheter-related complication is the development of accelerated atherosclerosis in the embolectomized vessel, probably due to endothelial denudation and medial injury.

V. Follow-up care usually is directed at treating the underlying cause of the obstruction. Patients with mural thrombi or arrhythmias require long-term anticoagulation. The in-hospital mortality rate associated with embolectomy is as high as 20% to 30%, mostly due to coexistent cardiac disease.

CHRONIC ARTERIAL OCCLUSIVE DISEASE OF THE EXTREMITY

The lower extremities are most frequently affected by chronic occlusive disease, although upper-extremity disease can occur. The principal early symptom of arterial occlusive disease is claudication, which is usually described as a cramping pain or heaviness in the affected extremity that occurs after physical exertion. Claudication is relieved by rest but recurs predictably with exercise. Lower-extremity occlusive disease is subdivided into three anatomic sections based on symptoms and treatment options. Aortoiliac occlusive disease, or "inflow disease," affects the infrarenal aorta and the common and external iliac arteries. Femoral-popliteal occlusive disease, or "outflow disease," affects the common femoral, superficial femoral, and popliteal arteries. Finally, tibial-peroneal disease, or "runoff disease," affects the vessels distal to the popliteal artery.

I. **Clinical presentation**

A. **Aortoiliac disease** presents with **symptoms of lower-extremity claudication,** usually of the **hip, thigh, or buttock.** It may coexist with femoral-popliteal disease, contributing to more distal symptoms as well. The symptoms usually develop gradually, although sudden worsening of symptoms may suggest the acute thrombosis of a diseased vessel. These patients ultimately develop incapacitating claudication but not rest pain unless distal disease is present as well. Leriche syndrome is a constellation of symptoms in men that results from the gradual occlusion of the terminal aorta. Symptoms include sexual impotence, buttock and leg claudication, leg musculature atrophy, trophic changes of the feet, and leg pallor. In contrast to the male predominance in chronic peripheral vascular disease (PVD), isolated aortoiliac disease affects women and men equally.

B. Patients with **femoral-popliteal** and **tibial disease** present with claudication of the lower extremity, usually most prominent in the **calves.** More severe impairment of arterial flow can present as rest pain. Rest pain is a burning pain in the distal foot, usually worse at night or when the leg is elevated, and is relieved by placing the leg in a dependent position. Examination of the chronically ischemic extremity reveals decreased or absent distal pulses and trophic changes that include thickening of the nails, loss of leg hair, shiny skin, and ulceration at the tips of the toes.

C. Symptomatic arterial occlusive disease of the **upper extremity** is relatively rare.

1. The proximal subclavian artery is most commonly affected by **atherosclerotic disease,** followed by axillary and brachial arteries. These patients typically present with arm claudication or finger-hand ischemia or necrosis. Occasionally, ulcerated plaques of the innominate or subclavian arteries can be a source of embolization to the hand.

2. **Vertebral steal** can result when an occlusive subclavian artery lesion is located proximal to the origin of the vertebral artery. The arm's demand for blood is supplied by reversed flow in the ipsilateral vertebral artery, which shunts blood from the posterior cerebral circulation. Most patients with proximal subclavian lesions are completely asymptomatic. Others may present with arm ischemia or posterior circulation symptoms, such as drop attacks, ataxia, sensory loss, or diplopia occurring after exercise of the affected limb.

II. **Diagnosis**

A. The diagnosis of chronic arterial occlusive disease is concerned with determining the presence of **significant flow-limiting lesions** and distinguishing the disease from those that may mimic it, such as arthritis, gout, and neuromuscular disorders. The degree of arterial flow limitation and the impact of reduced tissue perfusion determine the appropriate therapy.

B. For patients presenting with **lower-extremity symptoms,** it is essential to examine the femoral and distal pulses at rest and after exercise. The absence of femoral pulses is indicative of aortoiliac disease, although some patients with aortoiliac disease have palpable pulses at rest that are lost after exercise. Bruits may also be appreciated over the lower abdomen or femoral vessels.

C. Noninvasive testing can quantify flow through larger vessels and tissue perfusion.

1. **Segmental arterial Doppler** readings with waveforms should be performed in all patients with suspected symptomatic arterial disease. The **ankle-arm index (AAI;** the ratio of the blood pressure in the leg to that in the arm) allows one to quantify the degree of ischemia. Patients without vascular disease have an AAI of more than 1.0, patients with claudication have an AAI of less than 0.6, and patients with rest pain and severe ischemia have an AAI of less than 0.4. Waveform changes help localize the site of significant disease.

2. Transcutaneous measurement of **local tissue oxygenation** has been developed to attempt to quantify the physiologic derangements of ischemia. However, the usefulness of this test in the general vascular patient has not been validated.

D. Digital subtraction arteriography is the **gold standard** for evaluating the arterial tree before planned revascularization. Typical digital subtraction arteriography of the lower extremities includes images of the infrarenal aorta and the renal, iliac, femoral, tibial, and pedal vessels. **MRA** is an excellent imaging modality for these areas as well and is especially useful in patients with renal insufficiency. It is in widespread use currently.

III. Management

A. Intermittent claudication by itself is not an indication for surgical intervention because it has a benign course in most patients. In patients presenting with claudication alone, 70% to 80% remain stable or improve and 10% to 20% worsen. Only 5% to 10% of patients develop gangrene and are at risk for limb loss. Therefore, first-line treatment for patients with claudication should be medical therapy, with a stress on risk factor modification. Essentially, there are three **indications for surgical intervention.**

1. **Limb salvage** is the goal of surgery in patients with ischemic rest pain or tissue loss, including frank distal gangrene. Multilevel femoral-popliteal-tibial disease is the typical distribution in these patients. When significant aortoiliac disease and distal disease are jointly present in a patient with a threatened limb, however, an inflow (aortoiliac) procedure should be performed first.

2. **Peripheral atheroembolization** from aortoiliac ulcerated plaques, even if there is little or no history of claudication, is an indication for exclusion and bypass or endarterectomy of the aortoiliac system.

3. **Incapacitating claudication** that jeopardizes a patient's livelihood or influences his or her quality of life indicates disease likely to respond well to treatment. These patients should adhere to a program of risk factor reduction as well.

B. Medical therapy is available for those patients with symptoms who are not candidates for surgical intervention. However, no medical therapy is available to significantly halt the progression or reverse the changes of advanced atherosclerotic disease.

1. **Risk factor modification** is the single most important intervention for reducing the impact of advanced atherosclerotic disease. Control of hypertension and serum glucose, cessation of smoking, management of lipid disorders, attainment of ideal body weight, and regular exercise should be the goals.

2. Evidence is now accumulating that **aspirin** alone or combined with dipyridamole may have an impact on the natural progression of claudication due to atherosclerotic disease. Further, because many of these patients have concomitant coronary artery or cerebrovascular disease, lifelong therapy with 81- or 325-mg aspirin daily may reduce the risk of myocardial infarction or stroke.

3. **Clopidogrel** and **ticlopidine** are chemically related **antiplatelet agents** that have been shown to reduce vascular death and the need for revascularization in some recent studies in patients with intermittent claudication. However, the evidence suggests they are no better than aspirin.
4. **Pentoxifylline** is a **rheologic agent** thought to reduce blood viscosity and allow for improved flow through small arterioles and stenotic arteries. Although the drug is frequently prescribed, its benefit is unpredictable and generally small. It may be best suited for patients with severe disease not amenable to reconstruction.
5. **Cilostazol** is a type III **phosphodiesterase inhibitor** and the newest agent available for treatment of claudication. Cilostazol acts to inhibit platelet aggregation and cause vasodilation. Given at 50 mg or 100 mg twice a day, it increases walking distances when compared with placebo and pentoxifylline. Early studies suggest that the drug is safe in most patients, although its use is contraindicated in those with class III or IV heart failure due to the toxicity of phosphodiesterase inhibitors in patients with congestive heart failure.

C. **Preoperative care** of patients with PVD includes a complete arterial evaluation. In addition to angiographic evaluation of the symptomatic arterial tree, patients generally undergo screening for associated cardiac, renal, cerebrovascular, and pulmonary disease so that any correctable lesions can be addressed. Myocardial complications account for the majority of early and late deaths; therefore, patients with questionable myocardial function may require more extensive cardiac evaluation. Screening for carotid disease should also be performed and include a history of stroke or transient ischemic attack (TIA) and carotid auscultation. On the day before surgery involving the abdominal aorta, patients are kept on a liquid diet, hydrated well, and given a mechanical bowel preparation. Parenteral antibiotics are started 1 to 2 hours preoperatively and are continued for 24 hours after surgery.

D. **Endovascular surgical therapy.** See Chapter 23.

E. **Open surgical therapy**
1. **Aortoiliac occlusive disease**
a. **Aortobifemoral grafting** is the treatment of choice in low-risk patients. This procedure may be performed through a transperitoneal or a retroperitoneal approach. Results at our institution suggest that the retroperitoneal approach reduces postoperative complications, especially ileus. Although a number of grafts are available for use as replacement conduit, the knitted polyethylene terephthalate (Dacron) prosthesis is the most commonly used. A distal endarterectomy may be performed in conjunction with a bypass to improve outflow. Similarly, if significant renal artery disease is identified preoperatively, renal revascularization by endarterectomy or bypass grafting can be performed at the time of aortic reconstruction. Results are excellent, with reported patency rates of up to 95% at 5 years.
b. **Femorofemoral, ilioiliac, or iliofemoral bypasses** are alternatives in high-risk patients with unilateral iliac disease. The patency rates are lower than those achieved with aortobifemoral grafts.
c. **Axillobifemoral bypass** is an adequate alternative for high-risk patients who need revascularization. This bypass avoids an intraabdominal procedure and the need for cross-clamping the aorta. The patency rates are significantly worse than those achieved with aortobifemoral bypass, although for patients with a short life expectancy (<5 years), it may be a reasonable alternative.
d. **Aortoiliac endarterectomy** may be considered for patients who have disease localized to the distal aorta and common iliac vessels. Advantages include the avoidance of prosthetic material and better flow into the hypogastric arteries. This procedure should not be done in patients with aneurysmal changes of the aorta, a completely occluded aorta to

the level of the renal arteries, or extension of disease into the external iliac vessels.

2. **Femoral, popliteal, and tibial occlusive disease**
   a. In patients with above-knee occlusion, an **above-knee femoral-popliteal bypass** is indicated. In patients who have disease below the knee, a more distal bypass may be performed to the below-knee popliteal, posterior tibial, anterior tibial, or peroneal arteries. In extreme cases, if all tibial vessels are occluded, pedal vessels may serve as suitable outflow vessels. These grafts usually originate from the common femoral artery, although a more distal vessel may be used if the inflow into that vessel is adequate.
   b. The best results are obtained with the use of **autologous vein** as a conduit. The greater saphenous is the vein of choice. The lesser saphenous vein or the arm veins may provide good alternatives. These autologous grafts can be used either *in situ* or reversed. The advantages of the *in situ* bypass are that (1) the vein's nutrient supply is left intact and (2) the vein orientation allows for a better size match (the large end of the vein is sewn to the large common femoral artery, and the small end is sewn to the distal vessel). The advantage of the reversed-vein bypass is that endothelial trauma is minimized because valve lysis is not necessary.
   c. When autologous vein is not available, **cryopreserved vein grafts** can be used. Comparable patency rates have also been achieved using polytetrafluoroethylene for above-knee grafts. In extreme cases, prosthetic grafts can be bypassed to the tibial vessels, but the results are inferior. An alternative is to combine the prosthetic graft with a vein graft as a composite or to use a small cuff of vein (Miller cuff) or patch angioplasty (Taylor patch) just at the distal anastomosis. These modifications are believed to improve prosthetic graft patency by improving compliance match at the distal anastomosis.
   d. **Endarterectomy** as the sole procedure in an extremity is rarely performed except in cases of isolated short-segment stenosis of the superficial femoral artery. Endarterectomy may have a role in patients with limited vein availability or in the presence of an infected field. In these patients, a superficial femoral artery endarterectomy may obviate the need for a prosthetic graft.
   e. **Sympathectomy** sometimes is used as an adjunct to vascular reconstructions and involves division of the sympathetic chain and L3-5 ganglia. With the development of percutaneous alcohol ablation of the sympathetic ganglia, this procedure is becoming more popular. Although it does not increase blood supply to the muscles, it does result in maximal dilation of small arterioles and collaterals, providing increased blood flow to the skin and subcutaneous tissues. The effect is short lived, lasting only 4 to 6 weeks, but occasionally sympathectomy relieves rest pain and helps in the healing of small ulcerations.
   f. **Amputation** is reserved for patients with gangrene or persistent painful ischemia not amenable to vascular reconstruction. These patients often have severe coexistent vascular and cardiovascular disease, and the survival rate for patients undergoing major amputations is approximately 50% at 3 years and 30% at 5 years.
      (1) The **level of amputation** is determined clinically. Important factors include the level necessary to remove all the infected tissue and the adequacy of the blood supply to heal the amputation at a given level. A general principle is to preserve as much length of the extremity as safely possible, as this improves the patient's opportunity for rehabilitation. In some cases, revascularization before amputation enables a more distal amputation to heal adequately.
      (2) **Digital amputations** are performed commonly in diabetic patients who develop osteomyelitis or severe foot infections.

(3) **Transmetatarsal amputations** usually are performed when several toes are involved in the ischemic process or after previous single-digit amputations.

(4) **Syme amputation** involves the removal of the entire foot and calcaneus while preserving the entire tibia. It is rarely appropriate for PVD.

(5) **Below-knee amputation (BKA)** is the most common type of amputation performed for patients with severe occlusive disease.

(6) **Above-knee amputation (AKA)** heals more easily than BKA and is useful in older patients who do not ambulate.

(7) **Hip disarticulation** rarely is performed for PVD.

3. **Upper-extremity occlusive disease**

   a. For proximal subclavian disease, the **choice of bypass procedure** depends primarily on the patency of the ipsilateral common carotid artery.

   b. If the ipsilateral common carotid artery is patent, **carotid-subclavian bypass** is performed through a supraclavicular approach using a prosthetic graft (vein grafts are to be avoided). Subclavian artery transposition to ipsilateral carotid artery is another good alternative if anatomically feasible, and it avoids the use of a bypass conduit.

   c. If the ipsilateral carotid artery is occluded, **subclavian-subclavian bypass** may be performed. This is an extra-anatomic approach using a longer-segment prosthetic graft, and the patency is thereby diminished somewhat.

4. **Intraoperative anticoagulation** is employed during most vascular reconstructions. Generally, unfractionated heparin (100 to 150 units/kg) is administered intravenously shortly before cross-clamping and supplemented as necessary with 50 units/kg until the cross-clamps are removed. Anticoagualtion can be monitored intraoperatively by following activated clotting time (ACT) levels. Reversal with protamine administration is generally done to reduce bleeding complications.

F. **Postoperative care**

   1. For open aortic procedures, early postoperative care is usually administered in the ICU, where frequent hemodynamic and hematologic measurements are performed. Assessment of distal pulses should be done intraoperatively, immediately after reconstruction and regularly thereafter. In uncomplicated cases, the patients usually are extubated the day of surgery or on postoperative day 1. Patients are kept well hydrated for the first 2 postoperative days, after which third-space fluid begins to mobilize and diuresis ensues. Fluid management may be guided by Swan-Ganz catheter pressure monitoring. Antibiotics are continued for 24 hours postoperatively. A nasogastric tube is kept in place until return of bowel function. Patients are instructed not to sit with the hips flexed at greater than 60 degrees for the first 72 hours after graft placement, although ambulation as early as possible is encouraged.

   2. For distal bypass grafts, **pulses should be assessed frequently** for the first 24 hours and then several times a day. Antibiotics are continued for 48 hours postoperatively or longer if infected ulcers warrant such treatment. Ambulation as early as possible is encouraged in patients without tissue necrosis. In patients who are unable to ambulate immediately, physical therapy can help increase strength in the limb and prevent contracture. Sitting with the hips flexed to 90 degrees is discouraged in any patient with a femoral anastomosis. Patients should be discharged with instructions to keep their legs elevated to help resolve the edema that develops in the revascularized extremity. Staples are left in place for 2 to 3 weeks because these patients frequently have delayed wound healing.

   3. **Perioperative antithrombotic therapy** should include aspirin (81 to 325 mg per day) for all prosthetic infrainguinal reconstructions. Also, any bypass distal to the knee should likely include aspirin. Dipyridamole

(75 mg 3 times daily) may be added, although the increment of additional benefit is unknown. In patients sensitive to aspirin, clopidogrel (75 mg per day) may be substituted.

4. Postoperative oral anticoagulation has a more limited role. Owing in part to the increased risk of hemorrhage, anticoagulation with warfarin (international normalized ratio 2.0 to 3.0) is generally limited to grafts considered to be at a high risk for thrombosis. There may be some benefit to be gained from the administration of dextran 40 (0.5 mL/kg per hour intravenously) for up to 72 hours postoperatively in high-risk grafts.

5. For amputations, weightbearing is delayed for 4 to 6 weeks. Some advocate the use of compressive wraps to aid in the maturation of the stump. In all cases, early consultation with a physical therapist is recommended. Physical therapy is essential for maintaining strength in the limb, preventing contracture, and rehabilitating the patient once a prosthesis is fitted. In addition, as soon as the patient is ready, he or she should be fitted for a prosthesis, and ambulation training should begin. Rehabilitation rates (ability to walk without assistance) for patients undergoing major amputation are 60% and 30%, respectively, for patients with a unilateral BKA or AKA. For those with bilateral amputations, rehabilitation rates drop to 40% for patients with bilateral BKA and 10% for patients with bilateral AKA.

6. **Long-term follow-up** for distal bypass grafts should consist of arterial Doppler examinations every 3 months for the first 18 months, then every 6 months for a year, and then yearly. Less frequent follow-up is necessary for aortoiliac bypasses. Significant reduction in the AAI or flow velocities predicts pending graft failure, and such grafts should be studied further by arteriography. Intervention to repair or revise stenosed grafts results in much higher long-term patency than repairing or replacing occluded grafts.

G. **Complications**
1. Early complications occur in approximately 5% to 10% of patients after aortic surgery and frequently relate to preoperative comorbid disease. Myocardial infarction, congestive heart failure, pulmonary insufficiency, and renal insufficiency are most common. Complications related directly to the aortic reconstruction include hemorrhage, embolization or thrombosis of the distal arterial tree, microembolization, ischemic colitis, ureteral injuries, impotence, paraplegia, and wound infection. Late complications include anastomotic pseudoaneurysm or graft dilatation, graft limb occlusion, aortoenteric erosion or fistula, and graft infections.

2. In distal revascularizations, most of the early complications are also related to comorbid conditions. Early graft thrombosis (within 30 days of surgery) most often results from technical errors, hypercoagulability, inadequate distal runoff, and postoperative hypotension. Technical errors are responsible for more than 50% of early graft failures and include graft kinks, retained valve leaflets, valvulotome trauma, intimal flaps, significant residual arteriovenous fistulas, and the use of an inadequate conduit (i.e., small vein).

EXTRACRANIAL CEREBROVASCULAR DISEASE

Atherosclerotic occlusive disease of the extracranial carotid artery is a major risk factor for stroke. Stroke is a primary cause of disability and the third most common cause of death in the United States, with more than 160 new strokes per 100,000 people occurring each year. The initial mortality from stroke is between 20% and 30%. Of patients who survive the initial event, one-third function normally, one-third recover with mild deficits, and one-third recover with significant deficits. A smaller percentage of patients require total custodial care. Of patients who survive, approximately 50% die of recurrent stroke within 5 years.

I. Presentation

 A. The clinical presentation of patients with symptomatic occlusive disease is a **neurologic deficit.** Extracranial vascular occlusive disease can result in lateralizing and global symptoms. However, many patients may have an asymptomatic stenosis that is identified by a health care provider based on auscultation of carotid bruits or screening Doppler study.

 B. **Lateralizing ischemic events** can result in aphasia (expressive or receptive), combined sensory and motor deficits, and various visual disturbances. Deficits such as these are usually associated with the anterior cerebral circulation (i.e., the internal carotid artery and its branches).

  1. **TIAs** are transient hemispheric neurologic deficits that may last from several seconds to hours but fewer than 24 hours. TIAs that occur in rapid succession, interspersed with complete recovery but with progressively smaller intervals between attacks (crescendo TIAs), carry a high risk of progression to a permanent neurologic deficit and must be evaluated emergently.

  2. **Amaurosis fugax,** or temporary monocular blindness, described as a shade coming down over the eye, results from emboli lodging in the ophthalmic artery. Funduscopic examination can demonstrate these cholesterol plaques, commonly known as Hollenhorst plaques.

  3. A **reversible ischemic neurologic deficit** is a longer-lasting neurologic deficit that can last for up to 7 days but ultimately resolves completely.

  4. If the neurologic deficit is fixed and persists beyond 7 days, it is considered a **completed stroke.** In addition, some patients may present with a neurologic deficit that fluctuates, gradually worsening over a period of hours or days while the patient is under observation. This situation is considered a stroke in evolution and, like crescendo TIAs, needs prompt treatment.

 C. **Global ischemic events** are manifested by symptoms such as vertigo, dizziness, perioral numbness, ataxia, or drop attacks. These usually are associated with interruption of the brainstem or posterior circulation (i.e., the vertebrobasilar system).

II. Pathophysiology and epidemiology. Ischemic events in patients with extracranial vascular disease can be the result of emboli or a low-flow state. Although it can be clinically significant, disease of the vertebral arteries often remains asymptomatic. On the other hand, even asymptomatic significant occlusive carotid arterial disease carries with it a doubling of baseline stroke risk. Once a significant carotid lesion results in an ipsilateral lateralizing cerebral event, the risk of stroke may be as high as 26% over 2 years.

III. Diagnosis. A careful neurologic examination is performed before obtaining any diagnostic studies. Imaging of the carotid arterial system attempts to classify the degree of stenosis because of the prognostic implications. Due to methodologic differences in calculating the percentage of stenosis encountered in different studies, there is some disagreement about exact cutoff percentages. However, in general, there are essentially four levels of stenosis (with approximate percentages): mild (<50%), moderate (50% to 69%), severe (70% to 99%), and occluded (100%).

 A. A variety of noninvasive and invasive diagnostic studies are available. **Color-flow duplex scanning** uses real-time B-mode ultrasound and color-enhanced pulsed Doppler flow measurements to determine the extent of the carotid stenosis. This is the initial screening test for carotid disease. The reliability of this study depends in large part on the abilities of the vascular technicians; if adequate, validated vascular laboratory studies are preformed, treatment of most carotid lesions can be instituted based on ultrasound or duplex scanning alone.

 B. **Arteriography** remains the gold standard for the diagnosis of cerebrovascular disease. Unlike duplex scanning, however, arteriography remains an invasive procedure with inherent risks, such as contrast allergy, renal toxicity, and stroke (2% to 4% of patients). Because of these risks and improvements

in duplex ultrasonography, carotid arteriography is generally limited to patients with technically inadequate duplex ultrasonography or for verification of carotid occlusion.
  C. Although **MR angiography** is a highly sensitive technique for the evaluation of patients for symptomatic cerebrovascular disease, its precision remains inferior to that of conventional angiography. Recently CT angiography has been introduced as an alternative to arteriography.
IV. **Management**
  A. **Medical therapy.** It is important to make every effort to modify risk factors to prevent progression of carotid occlusive disease. Control of hypertension, cessation of smoking, management of lipid disorders, attainment of ideal body weight, and regular exercise should be undertaken. No drug therapy has been shown to reduce the risk of stroke in patients with asymptomatic carotid disease. Medical management in symptomatic patients is focused primarily on the use of antiplatelet agents, specifically aspirin. Aspirin is effective in reducing stroke and stroke-related deaths as well as myocardial infarctions. Low doses (81 mg per day) are as efficacious as higher doses (1,200 mg per day). Other antiplatelet agents, such as dipyridamole and ticlopidine (250 mg orally twice a day), are no better than aspirin alone. Anticoagulation with heparin sodium is beneficial in patients who have cardiac emboli. In evolving strokes, heparin may be useful in preventing progression of thrombus. The major contraindication to heparinization is a recent hemorrhagic brain infarct; therefore, a computed tomographic (CT) scan of the brain should be obtained before heparin is given.
  B. **Surgical therapy.** Surgical management is the treatment of choice for extracranial cerebrovascular disease and has been documented to reduce stroke. However, it should be performed only in centers of excellence in which the combined stroke and mortality rate is less than 3%.
    1. **Indications**
       a. **Asymptomatic patients with greater than 70% stenosis**
       b. **Symptomatic patients with greater than 50% stenosis**
       c. **Symptomatic patients with greater than 50% stenosis** who have an **ulcerated lesion** or whose **symptoms persist** while they are on **aspirin**
       d. **Selected patients with stroke in evolution.** Operation is performed to restore normal blood flow to allow recovery of ischemic brain tissue that is nonfunctional yet metabolically alive. Surgical candidates have mild to moderate neurologic defects and no evidence of hemorrhage on CT scan. The timing of surgery in these cases is controversial.
       e. **Selected patients with completed strokes.** Operation is performed in the hope of reducing stroke recurrence, which is 7% to 8% per year with nonsurgical therapy. Patients with a mild deficit and greater than 70% stenosis or with greater than 50% stenosis and an ulcer are candidates for surgery. So are patients with a moderate deficit, a lesion greater than 70%, and a contralateral occluded carotid artery. The timing of surgery in these cases is debatable. A prudent approach is to wait 4 to 6 weeks to minimize the risk of postoperative hemorrhage.
       f. Rarely, endarterectomy is performed on patients with **completely occluded carotid arteries.** Candidates for surgery include patients who have undergone endarterectomy and develop immediate postoperative thrombosis or symptoms, patients who are asymptomatic and have had a bruit disappear while under observation, patients who have had a recent occlusion and have fluctuating or progressive symptoms, and patients who are symptomatic and have a new internal carotid occlusion that can be operated on within 2 to 4 hours of the onset of symptoms.
    2. **Carotid endarterectomy** has been performed for more than 40 years and is the most commonly performed vascular operation. A beneficial outcome depends on meticulous technique. The use of such technique can keep the perioperative adverse event rate (stroke and death) below 3%.

    a. Anesthesia for carotid endarterectomy can be general endotracheal anesthesia, regional cervical block, or local anesthesia. The choice of anesthesia depends on a combination of patient factors and surgeon expertise. No single method of anesthesia has proved superior.

    b. During **dissection and mobilization** of the common carotid artery and its branches, it is important to proceed with gentle dissection and minimal manipulation of the carotid bulb to prevent embolization from the atherosclerotic plaque.

    c. After **systemic heparinization** of the patient, the carotid artery is occluded, and a longitudinal arteriotomy is made from just proximal to the plaque in the common carotid artery to just beyond the distal extent of the plaque in the internal carotid artery.

    d. Placement of tubing to **shunt** blood from the common carotid artery around the operative field to the internal carotid artery during endarterectomy is a controversial practice. Although some surgeons "always shunt" and a few "never shunt," most surgeons "selectively shunt" based on preoperative patient factors (e.g., the presence of contralateral internal carotid artery occlusion) or intraoperative neurologic assessment.

        (1) For patients undergoing anesthesia for carotid endarterectomy with local or regional anesthesia, **intraoperative neurologic assessment** can be as simple as having the patient squeeze a noise toy in the contralateral hand after carotid occlusion and answering a few simple questions.

        (2) For patients under general anesthesia, several different methods have been used to **assess cerebral perfusion or neurologic function** after clamping of the carotid artery. These include transcranial Doppler measurements and intraoperative electroencephalogram (EEG) monitoring.

    e. The **plaque** is carefully separated from the media and removed. The carotid endarterectomy is closed using a running suture, and if the internal carotid artery is small, a patch angioplasty can be performed.

3. Postoperative care

    a. Immediately after endarterectomy, **neurologic function and blood pressure (BP) alterations** should be monitored. Hypertension and hypotension are common after endarterectomy and may cause neurologic complications. The extremes of BP should be treated with either sodium nitroprusside or phenylephrine (Neo-Synephrine) to keep the systolic BP between 140 and 160 mm Hg (slightly higher in chronically hypertensive patients). The wound should be examined for hematoma formation. Aspirin is resumed in the immediate postoperative period. In patients with reactive platelets, dextran 40 (up to 20 mL/kg per 24 hours for up to 72 hours) may be started intraoperatively and continued into the early postoperative period. Anaphylaxis can occur with dextran use; therefore, a hapten (Promit, 15% dextran 1) may be given before the start of infusion to bind antibodies to dextran.

    b. Patient follow-up. A baseline duplex scan is obtained 2 to 3 weeks after the procedure and again at 6 months. After that, patients can be followed yearly. Patients who can tolerate aspirin are given 325 mg per day.

4. Complications

    a. Stroke rates must be low (3%) to make operative management of cerebrovascular disease reasonable, especially in asymptomatic patients.

    b. Myocardial infarction remains the most common cause of death in the early postoperative period. As many as 25% of patients who undergo endarterectomy have severe, correctable coronary artery lesions.

    c. Cranial nerve injuries occur in 5% to 10% of patients who undergo carotid endarterectomy. The most commonly injured nerve is by far

the marginal mandibular, followed by the recurrent laryngeal, superior laryngeal, and hypoglossal nerves.
d. **Recurrent carotid stenosis** has been reported to occur in 5% to 10% of cases, although symptoms are present in fewer than 3%. Two types of lesions have been characterized. A myofibroblastic lesion that occurs early (within 3 years) results from uncontrolled proliferation of the medial smooth-muscle cells and extracellular matrix. Recurrent atherosclerosis can also cause restenosis. The presence of symptoms is an indication for treatment of a recurrent lesion. Frequently, these lesions do not lend themselves to endarterectomy and are best treated by vein patching or excision and saphenous vein bypass grafting.

RENOVASCULAR DISEASE

Stenosis or occlusion of the renal arteries may result in hypertension, ischemic nephropathy, or both. Renovascular hypertension is the most common form of surgically correctable secondary hypertension. However, because of the predominance of primary hypertension and difficulties in clinical diagnosis of renovascular hypertension, its exact prevalence is difficult to assess.
  I. **Clinical presentation**
     A. A high index of suspicion is necessary to distinguish patients with potentially correctable renovascular hypertension from the majority of patients with primary hypertension. There are several clinical features that may be used to identify patients with potential renovascular hypertension.
        1. The presence of **severe hypertension** in a child or young adult or an adult older than age 50 years
        2. The **sudden development** or **worsening** of hypertension at any age
        3. **Hypertension and unexplained impairment of renal function**
        4. Hypertension that is **refractory** to appropriate three-drug therapy
        5. **Hypertension** in a patient with **extensive coronary disease, cerebral vascular disease, or PVD**
        6. **Worsening of renal function**
     B. On **physical examination,** these patients may have an epigastric, subcostal, or flank bruit. The finding of a unilateral small kidney by any clinical study is a possible indicator.
     C. **Deterioration of renal function in the elderly** may also be a clinical clue, as up to 15% of elderly patients hospitalized for the treatment of renal failure are ultimately diagnosed with ischemic nephropathy.
 II. **Pathophysiology**
     A. Renal arterial stenosis is perceived by the ipsilateral kidney as a hypovolemic state and as such activates the **renin-angiotensin-aldosterone system**. Typical renovascular hypertension results from unilateral renal artery stenosis (renin-dependent hypertension): renin release by the affected kidney remains high, as the resulting increase in intravascular volume is eliminated by the unaffected contralateral kidney. Bilateral renal artery stenosis (volume-dependent hypertension) results in an initial rise in renin; once the intravascular volume increases, however, feedback mechanisms return renin levels to near normal.
     B. Even in the **absence of hypertension,** a significant renal artery stenosis may be present and may lead to renal failure.
        1. In **acute renal failure,** renal arterial stenosis should be considered in the differential diagnosis if the urinary sediment is unremarkable and there are no signs of acute tubular necrosis, glomerulonephritis, or interstitial nephritis. Acute ischemic nephropathy may occur within 2 weeks of starting an angiotensin-converting enzyme (ACE) inhibitor or other antihypertensive or diuretic.
        2. Renal artery stenoses may account for up to 20% of **unexplained chronic renal failure** in patients older than 50 years of age. The diagnosis is more

likely in those with generalized atherosclerosis or uncontrolled hypertension.

3. Isolated unilateral renal artery stenosis generally does not cause an increase in the serum creatinine concentration to greater than 2.0 mg/dL.

C. Atherosclerosis causes approximately two-thirds of all renovascular lesions in adults and usually affects the ostia and proximal 2 cm of the renal artery. Associated extrarenal atherosclerosis occurs in 15% to 20% of patients.

D. The second most common renovascular lesion is **fibromuscular dysplasia,** most commonly medial fibroplasia. These lesions are multifocal, have a characteristic string-of-beads appearance on angiography, and typically occur in young and middle-aged women.

III. **Diagnosis**

A. Testing for clinically significant renal artery disease must evaluate the **anatomic and physiologic changes.** Anatomic lesions of the renal arteries by themselves correlate poorly with physiologic effect. More important, they correlate poorly with treatment response.

B. **Arteriography** remains the best test for making the diagnosis of anatomic renal artery stenosis. However, the usual caveats regarding the risks of arteriography, especially the nephrotoxic effects of the contrast agent, are important to consider.

C. In patients with a relative contraindication to arteriography, **duplex scanning** is useful for screening. However, this procedure is highly technician dependent.

D. **MR angiography** with gadolinium-based intravenous contrast is an excellent test for evaluating kidney and main renal artery morphology without nephrotoxins. It may also be useful for evaluating the functional significance of renal artery stenoses. Limitations include imaging of distal renal artery stenoses and patients with implanted devices, morbid obesity, or claustrophobia.

E. The two most commonly used tests to determine the functional significance of a renal artery lesion are **captopril renal scintigraphy** and **selective renal vein renin measurement.** These tests can be complicated to perform and interpret, especially in patients with bilateral disease or in those taking ACE inhibitors or beta-blockers.

IV. **Management of fibromuscular disease**

A. Renal artery stenoses resulting from fibromuscular dysplasia rarely cause renal failure, and endovascular treatment of the lesions is frequently successful in treating the hypertension.

B. Failure of endovascular treatment (see Chapter 23). Surgical therapy may be employed, including *ex vivo* repair for complex disease as described in Section V.C.2.d.

V. **Management of atherosclerotic disease**

A. **Therapy for renal artery stenosis** due to atherosclerotic disease has a dual purpose: to control target organ damage from hypertension and to avoid progressive ischemic renal failure. However, even with functional studies, response to therapy is difficult to predict because the hypertension may be primarily essential and the renal failure due to hypertensive glomerulosclerosis. No careful studies have been done comparing best medical therapy to surgical or endovascular intervention.

B. **Medical therapy** with antihypertensive drugs is often successful in the management of patients with renovascular hypertension. A combination of beta-blockers and a calcium channel blocker, an ACE inhibitor, or an angiotensin II receptor inhibitor is commonly used as first-line therapy. ACE inhibitors are often effective, but they should be used cautiously when the entire renal parenchymal mass is at risk, as occurs in renovascular hypertensive patients who have bilateral disease or a solitary kidney. Diuretics should be reserved for second-line therapy.

C. Surgical therapy
1. The **indications** for intervention are evolving. Classically, surgery usually has been reserved for patients with uncontrollable hypertension refractory to maximal medical therapy. Evidence is accumulating that revascularization may be more important as a means of maintaining renal mass. Consideration should also be given to renal revascularization in patients undergoing aortic bypass for aneurysmal or occlusive disease and concomitant renal stenoses.
2. **Procedures**
   a. **Aortorenal bypass** is the classic open treatment for renal revascularization. The stenotic renal artery is isolated with a segment of infrarenal aorta, and bypass is accomplished using saphenous vein, autologous hypogastric artery, or prosthetic graft.
   b. **Renal endarterectomy** is also an excellent choice for renal revascularization and is the treatment of choice for bilateral orificial lesions. Most commonly, a transverse arteriotomy is made over the orifices of both renal arteries. Distal endpoints and adequacy of endarterectomy can be assessed intraoperatively using duplex scanning.
   c. **Alternative bypass procedures** are available for patients who are not good candidates for aortorenal bypass due to prior aortic surgery, the presence of severe aortic disease, or unfavorable anatomy. Grafts can be taken from the supraceliac aorta or the superior mesenteric, common hepatic, gastroduodenal, splenic, or iliac arteries. Results for these procedures are comparable to those for direct aortic reconstruction but with significantly less morbidity and mortality.
   d. *Ex vivo* **renal artery reconstruction** with renal autotransplantation is useful in patients with complex lesions that require microvascular techniques and for which exposure *in situ* is inadequate. These procedures are time consuming, and adequate hypothermic protection from ischemic renal injury may be difficult with the kidney *in situ*. In general, operations requiring more than two branch artery reconstructions or anastomoses should be considered for *ex vivo* repair. Once repair is accomplished, the kidney can be transplanted orthotopically or heterotopically to the ipsilateral iliac fossa.
   e. **Endovascular techniques** (see Chapter 23)
   f. **Nephrectomy** may be required in patients who have renal infarction, severe nephrosclerosis, severe renal atrophy, noncorrectable renal vascular lesions, failed revascularizations, or a normal contralateral kidney and who are high-risk surgical candidates.
3. **Postoperative care**
   a. **Immediately after operation,** patients should be kept well hydrated to maintain adequate urine output. Concern about the patency of the reconstruction may be addressed by a renal scan or duplex scan.
   b. **Patient follow-up** should consist of routine BP monitoring, a renal scan, and creatinine determination at 3 months, 12 months, and then yearly. Any recurrence of hypertension or deterioration in renal function should prompt arteriography. Duplex scanning is also a useful test for following these reconstructions.
4. **Complications** of renal revascularization include persistent hypertension, acute renal failure, renal artery restenosis, thrombosis, aneurysm formation, and distal embolization.

MESENTERIC ISCHEMIA

Diagnosing mesenteric vascular disease can be difficult. Most patients are asymptomatic until late in the disease process. Although considerable advances have been made in perioperative care as well as in the diagnosis and treatment of intestinal ischemia, mortality remains as high as 70% to 80% due to delays in diagnosis.

I. Acute occlusion

A. Clinical presentation

1. Patients with emboli to the gastrointestinal tract usually have acute abdominal pain in the presence of significant cardiac disease (frequently atrial fibrillation). Patients who experience arterial thrombosis usually have associated severe atherosclerotic disease and may have a history consistent with chronic intestinal ischemia. Patients with mesenteric thrombosis usually are older and may recently have had a low–cardiac-output event.

2. Because of previous underlying vascular disease, the time until frank bowel infarction may be delayed by collateral circulation. In either case, the pain usually is sudden in onset and intermittent at first, progressing to continuous severe pain, often described as pain out of proportion to the degree of abdominal tenderness. These patients may also have bloody diarrhea before or after the onset of pain.

3. Patients develop abdominal tenderness when the bowel wall inflammation or necrosis becomes transmural.

4. **Mesenteric venous thrombosis** presents with varying manifestations, ranging from an asymptomatic state to catastrophic illness. Patients usually complain of prolonged, generalized abdominal pain that develops somewhat less rapidly than with acute mesenteric arterial occlusion. These patients may have occult gastrointestinal bleeding but no frank hemorrhage.

B. Pathophysiology. The cause may be either an embolus to or thrombosis of the superior mesenteric artery. Bowel ischemia also can result from portomesenteric venous thrombosis.

C. Diagnosis

1. The mainstay of diagnosis is **angiography** of the mesenteric circulation, including lateral views of the celiac axis and superior mesenteric artery.

2. Other **laboratory findings** can include an elevated white blood cell count with a left shift, persistent metabolic acidosis, and an unexplained elevated serum potassium level.

3. After acute arterial occlusion, the abdominal plain x-ray appears relatively normal. After venous thrombosis, x-rays may show small-bowel wall thickening or air in the portal venous system. If mesenteric venous thrombosis is suspected, a CT scan may be useful in making the diagnosis.

D. Surgical therapy

1. If an embolus or thrombosis is demonstrated, an **emergent embolectomy** should be performed. If a proximal stenosis is present in the superior mesenteric artery, aortomesenteric bypass should be performed using autologous graft.

   a. **Assessment of bowel viability** at laparotomy is made based on the gross characteristics of the bowel. The bowel is likely viable if it appears pink and if arterial pulsations are present. A number of other techniques have been described, including the use of fluorescein dye, Doppler studies, and tissue oximetry, but these are not substitutes for experienced clinical judgment.

   b. **Second-look procedures** are prudent when bowel viability is questionable. Whether to perform a second operation 24 to 48 hours after initial exploration is decided at the time of initial laparotomy, and that decision should not be changed even if the patient's condition improves. This approach is especially important in patients who have extensive bowel involvement and in whom resection of all questionable areas would result in the loss of most of the bowel.

2. For **venous occlusion**, surgical intervention rarely is helpful, although anecdotal reports suggest that portomesenteric venous thrombectomy may be beneficial. Similarly, the role of lytic therapy in the treatment of this disorder is unclear. It is imperative to begin systemic anticoagulation as soon as the diagnosis is made to limit the thrombotic process.

Frequently, the diagnosis is made at laparotomy. If the diagnosis is made before exploration, however, operation should be reserved until evidence of bowel infarction exists.

E. **Perioperative care** usually requires maximal medical support; these patients frequently are hemodynamically unstable and develop multiple organ system failure. Admission to the ICU, prolonged endotracheal intubation, parenteral nutrition, and broad-spectrum antibiotic therapy are typical.

II. **Chronic intestinal ischemia**

A. **Clinical presentation.** Patients with chronic intestinal ischemia present with **intestinal angina,** which is pain related to eating, usually beginning within an hour after eating and abating within 4 hours. Such patients experience significant weight loss related to the decreased ability to absorb food and decreased intake secondary to recurrent pain. The diagnosis usually is made from history alone because the only physical finding may be the presence of an abdominal bruit. In patients with a low-cardiac-output state and chronic intestinal angina, persistent shock may represent acute thrombosis and intestinal necrosis. This can occur in the absence of major vessel thrombosis on angiography, and the mortality associated with it is as high as 90%.

B. **Surgical therapy.** Elective revascularization of the superior mesenteric and celiac arteries via an autologous graft from the aorta or aortic endarterectomy is the treatment of choice. The orificial nature of most of these lesions has contributed to the poor success of balloon angioplasty.

C. **Perioperative care.** These patients often are malnourished. Some advocate parenteral nutrition for 1 to 2 weeks before surgery, which is continued postoperatively. Some patients develop a revascularization syndrome consisting of abdominal pain, tachycardia, leukocytosis, and intestinal edema. Concern about the adequacy of revascularization should prompt angiography.

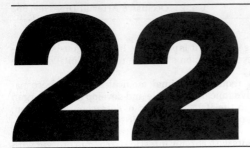

Aneurysmal Arterial Disease

Ravi K. Veeraswamy and Robert W. Thompson

The arterial wall is composed of the intima, media, and adventitia. The intima is composed of endothelium. The media contains layers of smooth muscle cells and an extracellular matrix (ECM) of elastin, collagen, and proteoglycans. The adventitia is made of loose connective tissue and fibroblasts. An arterial aneurysm is a weakness of the arterial wall resulting in a permanent localized dilatation >50% of the normal vessel diameter. All three layers are dilated with the majority of degeneration occurring in the media layer.

I. **Abdominal aortic aneurysms**
   A. **Incidence.** Abdominal aortic aneurysms (AAAs) are the most common type of arterial aneurysm, occurring in 3% to 10% of people older than 50 years of age in the United States. They are five times more common in men than in women and three and one-half times more common in Caucasians than in African Americans.
   B. **Pathophysiology.** Ninety percent of AAAs are believed to be degenerative in origin; 5% are inflammatory. Matrix metalloproteinases (MMPs) have been documented to have increased activity in aneurysmal tissues. Infection and possible autoimmune processes may play a role in AAA formation. Chlamydia pneumonia, B lymphocytes, plasma cells, and large amounts of immunoglobulin have been found in the walls of AAAs. Familial clustering of AAAs has been noted in 15% to 25% of patients undergoing surgery for AAAs. The risk of rupture correlates with wall tension in accordance with Laplace's law, such that the risk of aneurysm rupture correlates directly with aneurysm diameter (Fig. 22-1). Ninety-five percent of AAAs are infrarenal, 25% involve the iliac arteries, and 2% involve the renal or other visceral arteries. Four percent are associated with peripheral (e.g., femoral or popliteal) aneurysms. The major complications of AAA are ruptures, of which 20% are intraperitoneal and have a high mortality rate.
   C. **Diagnosis**
      1. **Clinical manifestations.** Seventy-five percent of AAAs are asymptomatic and are found incidentally. Aneurysm expansion or rupture may cause severe back, flank, or abdominal pain and varying degrees of shock. Distal embolization, thrombosis, and duodenal or ureteral compression can produce symptoms. Fifty percent of AAAs are identified on physical examination as a pulsatile mass at or above the umbilicus. The differential diagnosis includes a tortuous aorta or an abdominal mass lying adjacent to the normal aorta that might transmit aortic pulsations (e.g., lymphoma, pancreatic pseudocysts or carcinoma, mesenteric masses). AAA rupture may mimic renal colic, peritonitis, duodenal perforation, pancreatitis, degenerative spine disease, acute disk herniation, or myocardial infarction. Given its immediately life-threatening nature and potential for surgical repair, AAA must be considered first in symptomatic patients.
      2. **Radiologic evaluation**
         Abdominal cross-table lateral films. In 75% of patients with an AAA, arterial wall calcification permits estimation of aneurysm diameter. **Ultrasonography and computed tomography (CT) scanning** demonstrate AAAs with an accuracy of 95% and 100%, respectively, and are useful for serial examinations of small aneurysms. **Magnetic resonance (MR) scan** is comparable to CT but avoids radiation exposure and is useful

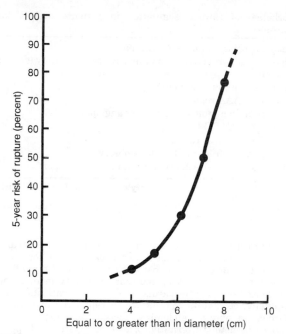

Figure 22-1. The 5-year risk of rupture is plotted against aneurysm size, showing the sharp increase in risk of rupture beyond a diameter of 6 cm. (Reprinted with permission from Hollier L, Rutherford RB. Infrarenal aortic aneurysms. In: Rutherford RB, ed. *Vascular Surgery.* 3rd ed. Philadelphia: WB Saunders, 1989:912.)

in patients with intravenous contrast contraindications. **Aortography** is **not** sensitive for the diagnosis of AAA because it may underestimate the aneurysm size or fail to reveal the aneurysm owing to the presence of mural thrombus. However, aortography is indicated to evaluate suspected renal or mesenteric artery stenosis and lower-extremity occlusive disease.

D. **Elective management of abdominal aortic aneurysm.** The risk of aneurysm rupture correlates best with aneurysm size (Fig. 22-1). However, even small aneurysms can rupture.

   1. **Medical management.** Patients with small aneurysms without risk factors for rupture can be followed using ultrasound or CT scan every 6 months, with larger ones followed more frequently. Smoking cessation and control of hypertension are very important. Doxycycline is being investigated as an agent that may retard aneurysm growth, based on its MMP-inhibiting properties.

   2. **Surgical management.** Indications for repair include symptomatic aneurysms of any size, aneurysms exceeding 5 cm, those increasing in diameter by more than 0.5 cm per year, and saccular aneurysms (usually infected). Relative indications for repair of smaller AAAs include poorly controlled hypertension [diastolic blood pressure (BP) ≥ 100 mm Hg] and significant chronic obstructive pulmonary disease (1-second forced expiratory volume $<50\%$ of predicted value). Relative contraindications to elective repair include recent myocardial infarction, intractable congestive heart failure, unreconstructible coronary artery disease, life expectancy of <2 years, and incapacitating neurologic deficits after a stroke. Operative mortality ranges from $<2\%$ for uncomplicated AAA to $>50\%$

Table 22-1. Schemes of cardiac evaluation in patients with abdominal aortic aneurysms (AAAs)

I Asymptomatic cardiac status → AAA repair
II Mild, stable cardiac symptoms → noninvasive cardiac study (dobutamine echocardiogram or dipyridamole-thallium stress test)
   Study positive → coronary angioplasty
   Study negative → AAA repair
III Significant cardiac symptoms → coronary angioplasty
   Significant CAD → CABG
   Insignificant CAD → AAA repair
IV Very elderly, LVEF <20%, small AAA → observe
   Unreconstructible CAD → AAA repair with cardiac support

CABG, coronary artery bypass grafting; CAD, coronary artery disease; LVEF, left ventricular ejection fraction.
Reprinted with permission from Hollier L, Rutherford RB. Infrarenal aortic aneurysms. In: Rutherford RB, ed. *Vascular Surgery*. 3rd ed. Philadelphia: WB Saunders, 1989:915.

for ruptured AAA. Five-year survival after elective repair of AAA is no different from that for age-matched patients without AAA. Associated cardiovascular disease, hypertension, decreased renal function, chronic obstructive lung disease, and morbid obesity increase operative risk. Table 22-1 outlines the cardiac evaluation of patients with an AAA.

3. **Operative technique.** In the standard repair, the aneurysm is approached through a midline abdominal incision and exposed by incising the retroperitoneum. Alternatively, a left retroperitoneal approach is advantageous in obese patients or those with previous intraabdominal surgery. In addition, proximal control of the aorta at or above the celiac axis is more easily achieved via this approach. Next, the duodenum and left renal vein are dissected off the aorta. After heparinization, the aorta is cross-clamped first distal and then proximal to the aneurysm. Aortotomy is then made and extended longitudinally to the aneurysm "neck," where the aorta is either transected or cut in a T fashion. The aneurysm is opened, thrombus is removed, and bleeding lumbar arteries are suture ligated. Using a tube or bifurcation graft, the proximal anastomosis is performed to nonaneurysmal aorta. The distal anastomosis is completed at the aortic bifurcation (tube graft) or at the iliac or femoral arteries (bifurcation graft), as the disease dictates. Cross-clamping can be safely performed for at least 60 minutes. After the clamps have been removed and hemostasis is ensured, the aneurysm wall is closed over the graft.

E. **Management of ruptured abdominal aortic aneurysm**
   1. **Preoperative management.** Unstable patients are resuscitated with fluids (crystalloid, colloid, or blood) and transferred immediately to the operating room for laparotomy. Stable patients may undergo emergency ultrasonography or CT scanning to confirm the diagnosis.
   2. **Operative management** is aimed at rapidly controlling the aorta. Anesthetic induction is delayed until the surgeon is ready to make the abdominal incision. Through a midline incision, the aorta is cross-clamped or compressed at the diaphragmatic hiatus. The retroperitoneal hematoma is opened, and the aneurysm is identified. After obtaining distal control of the iliac and collateral arteries, the proximal clamp is placed immediately above the aneurysm to allow perfusion of the visceral and renal arteries. Subsequent management is similar to repair of an elective AAA. Bifurcation grafts should be avoided in favor of the more expeditious tube graft techniques. Heparin should also be avoided.
F. **Endovascular management of abdominal aortic aneurysm.** Endovascular management of AAA is discussed in Chapter 23.

G. Complications

1. **Arrhythmia, myocardial ischemia, or infarction** may occur.

2. **Intraoperative hemorrhage** can be reduced by clamping the aorta proximal to the aneurysm and the iliac arteries distally. Once the aneurysm is opened, retrograde bleeding from lumbar arteries must be controlled rapidly with transfixing ligatures. Blood should be salvaged in the operating room and autotransfused to the patient.

3. **Aortic cross-clamping shock,** which may occur on release of the aortic cross-clamp, may be obviated by adequate hydration and slow release of the aortic cross-clamp.

4. **Renal insufficiency** may be related to intravenous contrast, inadequate hydration, hypotension, a period of aortic clamping above the renal arteries, or embolization of the renal arteries.

5. **Lower-extremity ischemia** may result from embolism or thrombosis, especially in emergency operations for which heparin might not be used. Embolism to the lower extremities can be prevented by minimizing manipulation of the aneurysm prior to clamping and by perfusing the hypogastric arteries before perfusing the external iliac arteries at the time of unclamping. Use of a Fogarty catheter to remove a clot from lower-extremity vessels is indicated when leg ischemia is identified in the operating room.

6. **Microemboli** arising from atherosclerotic debris can cause cutaneous ischemia ("trash foot"), which should be treated expectantly. Amputation may be required if significant necrosis results.

7. **Gastrointestinal complications** may consist of prolonged paralytic ileus, anorexia, periodic constipation, or diarrhea. This problem is diminished by using the left retroperitoneal approach. A more serious complication, ischemic colitis of the sigmoid colon, is related to ligation of the inferior mesenteric artery in the absence of adequate collateral circulation. Symptoms include leukocytosis, significant fluid requirement in the first 8 to 12 postoperative hours, fever, and peritoneal irritation. Diagnosis is made by sigmoidoscopy to 20 cm above the anal verge. Necrosis that is limited to the mucosa may be treated expectantly. Necrosis of the muscularis causes segmental strictures, which may require delayed segmental resection. Transmural necrosis requires immediate resection of necrotic colon and construction of an end colostomy.

8. **Paraplegia** may occur after repair of a ruptured AAA when the aorta is clamped near the diaphragm, due to spinal cord ischemia. Paraplegia is rare following elective infrarenal AAA repair. Obliteration or embolization of important spinal artery collateral flow via the internal iliac arteries or an abnormally low origin of the accessory spinal artery (artery of Adamkiewicz) can result in paraplegia.

9. **Sexual dysfunction** and retrograde ejaculation result from damage to the sympathetic plexus during dissection near the aortic bifurcation, especially the proximal left common iliac artery.

II. Thoracic aortic aneurysms

A. **Incidence.** This is primarily a disease of the elderly. Ascending and transverse arch aneurysms each comprise 25% of thoracic aortic aneurysms (TAAs). The remaining 50% occur in the descending aorta (thoracic or thoracoabdominal). Most descending TAAs begin just distal to the left subclavian artery

B. **Pathophysiology.** TAAs are divided into five main types: ascending, transverse, descending, thoracoabdominal, and traumatic. Ascending aortic aneurysms are usually caused by medial degeneration. Transverse, descending, and thoracoabdominal aortic aneurysms are related to atherosclerosis. Hypertension contributes to expansion.

C. **Diagnosis**

1. **Clinical manifestations** are usually absent; most nontraumatic TAAs are detected as incidental findings on chest films obtained for other purposes.

A minority of patients may present with chest discomfort or pain that intensifies with aneurysm expansion or rupture, aortic valvular regurgitation, congestive heart failure, compression of adjacent structures (recurrent laryngeal nerve, left main-stem bronchus, esophagus, superior vena cava, porta hepatis), or erosion into adjacent structures (esophagus, lung, airway).

2. **Radiologic evaluation. Chest films** may reveal a widened mediastinum or an enlarged calcific aortic shadow. Traumatic aneurysms may be associated with skeletal fractures. **MR or CT scanning** with intravenous contrast provides precise estimation of the size and extent of these aneurysms and facilitates the planning of surgical therapy. **Echocardiography** is useful in evaluating aneurysms involving the aortic arch. **Aortography** demonstrates the proximal and distal extent of the aneurysm and the vessels arising from it.

D. **Surgical management.** Surgical management depends on the type and location of the TAA. Repair of proximal arch aneurysms requires cardiopulmonary bypass and circulatory arrest. Preclotted woven polyethylene terephthalate (Dacron) is the graft of choice. The ascending and transverse arches are repaired through a median sternotomy incision. The descending and thoracoabdominal aortas are approached through a left posterolateral thoracotomy incision. Intraoperative management of patients undergoing thoracotomy is facilitated by selective ventilation of the right lung using a double-lumen endobronchial tube. Cerebrospinal fluid drainage during and after surgery can lower the incidence of postoperative paraplegia.

1. **Ascending aortic arch aneurysms**
   a. **Indications** for surgical repair include symptomatic or rapidly expanding aneurysms, aneurysms >7 cm in diameter, ascending aortic dissections, mycotic aneurysms, and asymptomatic aneurysms >5.5 cm in diameter in patients with Marfan's syndrome.
   b. **Operative management.** An aneurysm arising distal to the coronary ostia is replaced with an interposition graft. A proximal aneurysm resulting in aortic valve incompetency is replaced with a composite valved conduit (Bentall procedure) or a supracoronary graft with separate aortic valve replacement. Ascending arch aneurysms due to Marfan's syndrome or cystic medial necrosis are repaired with aortic valve replacement owing to the high incidence of valvular incompetence associated with aneurysmal dilation of the native aortic root. When a composite graft is used, the coronary arteries are anastomosed directly to the conduit.

2. **Transverse aortic arch aneurysms**
   a. **Indications** for repair include aneurysms >6 cm in diameter, aortic arch dissections, and ascending arch aneurysms that extend into the transverse arch.
   b. **Operative management.** After opening the aorta under hypothermic circulatory arrest, the distal anastomosis is performed using a beveled graft, followed by anastomosis of an island of the brachiocephalic vessels to the superior aspect of the graft. The proximal anastomosis is constructed to the supracoronary aorta (if the aortic valve is not involved) or to a segment of composite valved conduit interposed to complete the arch reconstruction. Involvement of the transverse arch and its branch vessels requires interposition grafting to the involved vessels.

3. **Descending thoracic aortic aneurysms**
   a. **Indications** for repair include symptomatic aneurysms and asymptomatic aneurysms >6 cm in diameter.
   b. **Operative management.** Before cross-clamping, the anesthesiologist pharmacologically controls proximal BP with sodium nitroprusside. After the distal clamp is applied, a proximal clamp is placed just distal to the left subclavian artery or between the left common carotid and

left subclavian arteries. Selected intercostal branches are reattached to the aortic interposition graft. Use of left heart partial bypass is a valuable adjunct, and catheter-based drainage of cerebrospinal fluid may reduce the incidence of postoperative paraplegia.

4. **Thoracoabdominal aneurysms**
   a. **Indications** for repair include symptomatic aneurysms and aneurysms >6 cm in diameter.
   b. **Operative management** consists of tube graft replacement, along with anastomosis of major branches to the graft. Aneurysms involving the thoracic and proximal abdominal aortic segments may be approached through a left posterolateral thoracotomy extended to the umbilicus. Left heart partial bypass (atriofemoral) is often used, both to protect the heart from overdistention and to provide distal blood flow while the aorta is clamped. Sodium nitroprusside may be given before cross-clamping to reduce proximal BP, and cerebrospinal fluid drainage may decrease the incidence of postoperative paraplegia. The aneurysm is opened, and the orifices of all major aortic branches are occluded with balloon catheters or suture ligatures. The proximal anastomosis is performed, followed by end-to-side anastomosis of significant aortic branches to the graft, especially the celiac axis and superior mesenteric artery, and the renal arteries. The distal anastomosis is made either to the uninvolved aorta or to the iliac arteries.

5. **Traumatic aortic aneurysms**
   a. **Indications** for repair. Urgent repair is indicated, except when precluded by more compelling life-threatening injuries or major central nervous system trauma.
   b. **Operative management.** Using proximal and distal control, these aneurysms may be repaired by primary aortorrhaphy, aneurysmectomy and end-to-end reanastomosis, or by interposition grafting.

E. **Complications.** Possible complications of thoracic aortic surgery include arrhythmia, myocardial infarction, intraoperative hemorrhage, stroke, aortic cross-clamp shock, renal insufficiency, lower-extremity ischemia, microemboli, and disseminated intravascular coagulopathy. The incidence of paraplegia may be as high as 10% to 30% with some types of TAAs. This risk can be reduced by multimodal therapies implemented to prevent or minimize spinal cord ischemia: distal aortic perfusion, intercostal and lumbar artery reimplantation, preoperative or intraoperative localization of spinal blood supply, hypothermia, cerebrospinal fluid drainage, or pharmacotherapy.

III. **Peripheral arterial aneurysms.** Popliteal and femoral artery aneurysms account for more than 90% of all peripheral aneurysms and are often associated with aneurysms in other locations. The male–female ratio is >30:1. Nearly all are degenerative and associated with atherosclerosis. These aneurysms have a propensity to thrombose and cause embolic occlusion of distal vessels. Rupture, compression of adjacent structures, or distal embolization can also occur.

A. **Popliteal aneurysms**
   1. **Incidence.** Popliteal aneurysms account for nearly 70% of peripheral aneurysms. Fifty percent to 70% are bilateral, 40% to 50% are associated with AAAs, and nearly 40% of patients have a concurrent femoral artery aneurysm.
   2. **Pathophysiology.** Atherosclerosis, trauma, wall stress due to vibrations and turbulence proximal to a branching point, sex-linked genetic abnormalities, ECM breakdown, and infection (e.g., syphilis) contribute to aneurysm formation.
   3. **Diagnosis**
      a. **Clinical manifestations** related to thromboembolism include claudication, rest pain, ulceration, and neuropathy. Mass effect may produce a pulsatile mass or venous obstruction. Approximately 45% are asymptomatic.

      b. Physical examination may reveal a pulsatile mass in the popliteal fossa if the aneurysm is patent. Conversely, a thrombosed popliteal aneurysm may feel firm but not pulsatile.

      c. Radiologic evaluation. Lower-extremity plain films may demonstrate calcified aneurysms. **Ultrasonography, CT scanning** with intravenous contrast, or **MR scanning** confirms the diagnosis and is used to rule out bilateral aneurysms or an associated AAA. **Arteriography** is useful in evaluating distal runoff and in planning reconstruction.

    4. Operative management is aimed at preventing thromboembolic complications and restoring adequate blood flow to the distal extremity. The procedure most often used is bypass of the aneurysm, preferably using an autologous conduit and ligation of the artery proximal and distal to the aneurysm to exclude it from circulation. Alternatively, popliteal aneurysms that cause local symptoms may be repaired with aneurysmectomy and interposition of autologous vein or prosthetic graft. For thrombosed aneurysms, preoperative thrombolysis lyses thrombosed runoff vessels for potential bypass outflow and improves limb salvage. An intraoperative arteriogram after repair is recommended to confirm adequacy of outflow. Amputation is required in 10% to 20% of patients who present with acute thrombosis and limb-threatening ischemia.

B. Femoral artery aneurysms

    1. Incidence. Femoral artery aneurysms are the second most common peripheral aneurysm. Seventy percent are bilateral, 80% are associated with AAA, and 40% are associated with popliteal aneurysms.

    2. Pathophysiology. Fifty percent of these aneurysms occur proximal to the femoral bifurcation (type I); the other 50% involve the profunda femoris (type II). Atherosclerosis is a major etiology, although degeneration of the ECM and connective tissue disorders also plays a role.

    3. Diagnosis

      a. Clinical manifestations are often limited to a pulsatile groin mass. Approximately 40% are asymptomatic at the time of diagnosis. Symptomatic patients may present with local pain, mass effect with nerve or vein compression, or lower-extremity ischemia. **Differential diagnosis** includes pseudoaneurysms due to percutaneous catheterization, anastomotic leaks, trauma, or intravenous drug abuse misadventures.

      b. Radiologic evaluation. Ultrasonography, CT, or MR scan can confirm the diagnosis and is useful in evaluating the infrarenal aorta and popliteal regions. **Angiography** is useful in demonstrating involvement of the profunda femoris ostium and in evaluating distal runoff.

    4. Operative management consists of aneurysmectomy and end-to-end graft replacement using autologous vein or prosthetic graft repair. In type II aneurysms, a separate graft can be used to connect the profunda femoris to the main graft. Preservation of the profunda femoris is necessary for limb salvage.

C. Proximal subclavian artery aneurysms

    1. Incidence. The presence of such an aneurysm is associated with a 30% to 50% incidence of aortoiliac or peripheral artery aneurysms and should therefore provoke an evaluation to identify synchronous aneurysmal disease.

    2. Pathophysiology. Proximal subclavian artery aneurysms arise most commonly from atherosclerosis.

    3. Diagnosis

      a. Clinical manifestations. Acute expansion or rupture may cause pain in the patient's neck, chest, or shoulder. **Local compression** of adjacent structures, such as the brachial plexus, recurrent laryngeal nerve, or trachea, may cause corresponding symptoms of upper-extremity neuropathies, hoarseness, or respiratory distress, respectively. **Ischemia** can occur due to thromboembolism to the brain or the upper extremity.

b. **Physical examination** may reveal a pulsatile supraclavicular mass or bruit, absent or diminished upper-extremity pulses, "blue finger syndrome," sensory and motor deficits in the ipsilateral upper extremity, vocal cord paralysis, or Horner's syndrome.

c. **Radiology.** Complete aortic arch and upper-extremity angiography. This imaging test defines the aneurysm, assesses for distal occlusive disease, and evaluates the contralateral vertebral system, especially when the ipsilateral vertebral artery arises from the aneurysm.

4. **Operative treatment** of proximal subclavian artery aneurysms requires resection with either primary anastomosis or interposition grafting using prosthetic or autologous grafts. A lesion on the right is generally approached through a median sternotomy, whereas a left-sided aneurysm can be treated through a left thoracotomy.

D. **Distal subclavian artery aneurysms**

1. **Pathophysiology.** These are also called *subclavian-axillary artery aneurysms.* They arise secondary to compression of the artery by a cervical rib or band of fibrous and muscular tissue as part of thoracic outlet syndrome. Poststenotic dilatation progresses to aneurysmal changes in the arterial wall over time. Once the arterial wall is aneurysmal, symptoms of ischemia or local compression develop as with proximal subclavian aneurysms.

2. **Diagnosis** is established with angiography as previously described (see Section III.C.3).

3. **Operative treatment** includes complete resection of the cervical rib and scalenus anterior. Aneurysm resection is indicated for asymptomatic patients with aneurysms larger than twice the normal vessel diameter or those with thromboembolic complications. Catheter embolectomy is mandatory for recently occluded distal arteries. Reconstruction of the subclavian artery is similar to that for proximal lesions (see Section III.C.4).

E. **Ulnar artery aneurysm (hypothenar hammer syndrome)**

1. **Incidence.** Ulnar artery aneurysms are most commonly seen in men younger than 50 years of age and in people who use the palms of their hands for pushing, pounding, or twisting.

2. **Pathophysiology.** Repetitive trauma to the ulnar artery is the most common cause.

3. **Diagnosis**

a. **Clinical manifestations.** Many patients have a severe lacerating pain over the hypothenar eminence at the time of injury followed by a chronic, dull aching pain. Ischemic symptoms, most commonly of the fourth and fifth fingers or any digit except the thumb, develop weeks or months later.

b. **Physical examination** reveals the ischemic changes of the fingers, tenderness, and/or pulsatile mass over the hypothenar eminence. An abnormal Allen's test is present in the majority of patients.

c. **Radiologic evaluation. Digital plethysmography and duplex ultrasonography** are helpful in making the diagnosis. **Angiography** is mandatory.

4. **Treatments** include cervicodorsal sympathectomy, excision of the ulnar artery aneurysm with ligation of the ulnar artery, and aneurysmectomy with microsurgical reconstruction of the ulnar artery by reanastomosis or interposition vein graft. Preoperative thrombolytic therapy plays an important role in patients with ulnar aneurysm thrombosis. Medical therapies including calcium channel blockers, smoking cessation, and avoiding further hand trauma can also be helpful.

IV. Splanchnic aneurysms. Splanchnic artery aneurysms are uncommon. The arteries most often involved are the splenic (60%), hepatic (20%), superior mesenteric (5.5%), celiac (4%), gastric and gastroepiploic (4%), and intestinal (3%) arteries. Most of these aneurysms are caused by atherosclerosis. The risk of rupture is >50% in hepatic, celiac, and superior mesenteric aneurysms.

A. Splenic artery aneurysms

1. **Incidence.** These aneurysms occur in 0.02% to 0.16% of the U.S. population, with a 4:1 female predominance in women of childbearing age. Incidence correlates with multiparity.

2. **Pathophysiology** is related to systemic arterial fibrodysplasia, portal hypertension, and increased splenic blood flow during pregnancy. Most splenic artery aneurysms occur at the bifurcation of the distal splenic artery. Twenty percent are multiple. Rupture most often occurs into the lesser sac and can progress to free intraperitoneal hemorrhage via the foramen of Winslow. The overall risk of rupture is 5% to 10%; however, 95% of ruptures occur during pregnancy.

3. **Diagnosis**

   a. **Clinical manifestations.** Most are asymptomatic. Vague left upper quadrant or epigastric pain may occur with acute aneurysm enlargement. Gastrointestinal bleeding occurs with rupture into the stomach or pancreatic duct. **Differential diagnosis** for ruptured splenic aneurysms in pregnant women includes placental abruption, uterine rupture, and amniotic fluid embolization. A ruptured hepatic adenoma should also be ruled out. Splenic artery pseudoaneurysms secondary to pancreatitis can present in a manner similar to that of true splenic artery aneurysms.

   b. **Radiologic evaluation. Abdominal plain films** reveal a signet ring–like calcification in the left upper quadrant in 70% of patients. Often, **CT or MR scan** can visualize the aneurysm and confirm any leak from it. **Aortography** confirms the diagnosis.

4. **Operative management** is indicated in symptomatic aneurysms, pregnant patients, and women who anticipate future pregnancy. Proximal aneurysms are approached through the lesser sac and are treated with aneurysmectomy or ligation without arterial reconstruction. Midsplenic artery aneurysms can be ligated from within the aneurysm sac. Distal aneurysms may be resected with a distal pancreatectomy. Splenic hilar aneurysms are treated with splenectomy, suture ligation, or aneurysmorrhaphy. Transcatheter embolization may be performed in high-risk patients. After aneurysm rupture, operative maternal and fetal mortality is 70% and 95%, respectively.

B. Hepatic artery aneurysms

1. **Incidence.** Hepatic artery aneurysms are the second most common splanchnic artery aneurysms, occurring most often in the elderly, with a male–female ratio of 2:1.

2. **Pathophysiology** is related to atherosclerosis (32%), medial degeneration (24%), trauma (22%), and mycotic infection (10%). The vast majority is extrahepatic and involves the common hepatic (63%), right hepatic (29%), left hepatic (5%), or right and left hepatic (4%) arteries. Rupture and compression of the hepatobiliary tree are the most frequent complications. Fifty percent of ruptures are intraperitoneal; the other 50% are into the hepatobiliary tree.

3. **Diagnosis**

   a. **Clinical manifestations** are usually absent but may include persistent right upper quadrant or epigastric pain. Severe pain or radiation to the patient's back suggests an expanding aneurysm. Rupture into the hepatobiliary tree produces hematemesis, biliary colic, and jaundice. **Differential diagnosis** includes AAA, cholecystitis, pancreatitis, and perforated duodenal ulcer.

    b. Physical examination may reveal an abdominal bruit, a pulsatile right upper quadrant, or an epigastric mass (uncommon).

    c. Laboratory tests may reveal elevated serum bilirubin, alkaline phosphatase, or liver enzymes in the presence of hepatobiliary obstruction.

    d. Radiologic evaluation. Arteriography is the diagnostic tool of choice and is recommended for planning surgical therapy. Many aneurysms are identified first on a CT scan.

  4. Operative management is usually indicated owing to the high mortality (>35%) associated with rupture. Common hepatic artery aneurysms can be treated with aneurysmectomy, aneurysmorrhaphy, or aneurysm exclusion with or without arterial reconstruction, depending on the adequacy of collateral flow. Aneurysms of the proper hepatic artery are treated with aneurysmorrhaphy, aneurysmectomy with primary artery repair (small aneurysms), or bypass. Intrahepatic aneurysms can be treated with liver resection, proximal artery ligation, or percutaneous transcatheter embolization (in high-risk patients).

V. Other arterial aneurysms

  A. Renal artery aneurysms

    1. Incidence. Renal artery aneurysms occur in 1% to 10% of the population and constitute approximately 1% of all aneurysms.

    2. Pathophysiology. These aneurysms may be either extrarenal (85%) or intrarenal (15%) in location. Extrarenal renal artery aneurysms are subdivided into saccular (most common), fusiform, and dissecting. Saccular aneurysms classically occur near the bifurcation of the renal artery. Fusiform aneurysms are poststenotic dilatations associated with renal artery stenosis. Renal artery dissections are associated with renal artery fibroplasias. Intrarenal aneurysms may be congenital, traumatic, or related to collagen vascular disease.

    3. Diagnosis

      a. Clinical manifestations are usually absent until complications arise. Rupture and dissection may produce flank pain or hematuria (intrarenal aneurysms).

      b. Physical examination commonly reveals hypertension and an abdominal bruit. A palpable mass occurs in fewer than 10% of cases.

      c. Laboratory tests may reveal anemia or hematuria.

      d. Radiologic evaluation. Abdominal films may demonstrate ring-shaped calcifications in the renal hilum in patients with calcific saccular aneurysms. **CT scan** may reveal an incidental renal artery aneurysm. **Arteriography** confirms the diagnosis and details the anatomy of the renal branches.

    4. Operative management. Treatment is indicated for aneurysms that rupture, are associated with dissection, or produce renal artery stenosis leading to hypertension. Saccular aneurysms are repaired in pregnant women owing to an increased risk of rupture. Small aneurysms at the bifurcation can be treated with aneurysmectomy and reconstruction of the bifurcation. Aneurysmectomy with aortorenal or splenorenal bypass is advised for large aneurysms or stenotic lesions. Polar renal artery aneurysms can be excised with end-to-end arterial reanastomosis. Ruptured renal artery aneurysms are treated with nephrectomy.

  B. Infected aneurysms

    1. Incidence. The incidence of infected arterial aneurysms has risen with the increased prevalence of immunocompromised patients, invasive transarterial procedures, and drug addiction.

    2. Pathophysiology. Infected aneurysms can be divided into four types: mycotic aneurysm, microbial arteritis with aneurysm, infected preexisting aneurysm, and posttraumatic infected false aneurysm. The clinical characteristics of each type are summarized in Table 22-2. *Staphylococcus aureus* is the most common pathogen. *Salmonella* species (arteritis),

Table 22-2. Clinical characteristics of infected aneurysm

	Mycotic aneurysm	Microbial arteritis	Infection of existing aneurysms	Posttraumatic infected false aneurysm
Etiology	Endocarditis	Bacteremia	Bacteremia	Narcotic addiction; trauma
Age (yr)	30–50	>50	>50	<30
Incidence	Rare	Common	Unusual	Very common
Location	Aorta; visceral; intracranial; peripheral	Atherosclerosis; aortoiliac; intimal defects	Infrarenal aorta	Femoral; carotid; injection sites
Bacteriology	Gram-positive cocci	*Salmonella* spp.; others	*Staphylococcus* spp.; *Escherichia coli*; others	*Staphylococcus aureus*; polymicrobial
Mortality (%)	25	75	90	5

Reprinted with permission from Wilson SE, Van Wagenen P, Passaro E Jr. Arterial infection. *Curr Probl Surg* 1978;15:11.

Streptococcus species, and Staphylococcus epidermidis (preexisting aneurysms) also predominate. The risk of rupture for Gram-negative infections exceeds that for Gram-positive infections.
3. **Diagnosis**
   a. **Clinical manifestations** may be absent or include fever, tenderness, or sepsis.
   b. **Physical examination** may demonstrate a tender, warm, palpable mass in an extremity aneurysm.
   c. **Laboratory tests** may reveal leukocytosis. Aerobic and anaerobic blood cultures should be obtained, but only 50% of cultures are positive.
   d. **Radiologic evaluation**
      Abdominal plain films. Aneurysms associated with vertebral body erosion suggest infection. **MR or CT scanning** can demonstrate an aneurysm and verify its rupture. **Angiography** delineates the characteristics of the aneurysm. Aneurysms that are saccular, multilobed, or eccentric with a narrow neck are more likely a result of infection.
4. **Management**
   a. **Preoperative management.** Broad-spectrum antibiotics should be administered intravenously after aerobic and anaerobic blood cultures have been obtained.
   b. **Operative management** includes (1) controlling hemorrhage; (2) obtaining arterial specimens for Gram's stain, aerobic and anaerobic cultures, and drug sensitivities; (3) resecting the aneurysm with wide debridement and drainage; and (4) reconstructing major arteries through uninfected tissue planes. Extra-anatomic bypass may be necessary to avoid contamination of the graft.
   c. **Postoperative management** requires adequate drainage of the aneurysm cavity and long-term antibiotic therapy.

23

Endovascular Surgery

**Toby J. Dunn and
Luis A. Sanchez**

Endovascular approaches to the treatment of peripheral vascular disease are rapidly evolving and favorably competing with many established vascular reconstruction techniques. They allow treatment with less invasive techniques to avoid major vascular reconstructions and their associated morbidity and costs. The endovascular approach also provides a favorable treatment alternative to individuals at high risk for complications with traditional vascular reconstructions. Because of the ongoing evolution of devices and endovascular techniques, there are limited long-term clinical outcomes data for most procedures, and guidelines for the application of endovascular techniques continue to evolve.

TECHNIQUES AND INDICATIONS FOR ENDOVASCULAR SURGERY

I. **Techniques and devices**
   A. **Angioscopy.** Satisfactory endovascular visualization requires a small, flexible fiberoptic scope and sufficient irrigation to avoid opacification by blood.
      1. **General indications.** Angioscopy is of limited utility but has been used to assess various interventions, including thromboembolectomy, endarterectomy, venous valvulotomy, and venous bypass side branch occlusion. Angioscopy has been found to be most useful in infrainguinal bypass graft procedures (with *in situ* vein bypass and with revision of failed bypass grafts).
      2. **Complications.** Adequate visualization may require vigorous irrigation. This may lead to fluid overload or air embolization. Passage of the angioscope may also injure the vessel wall or venous conduit.
   B. **Intravascular ultrasound (IVUS)** allows evaluation of vessel wall morphology and intraluminal pathology.
      1. **General indications**
         a. **Allows diagnosis of complex arterial pathology**
         b. **Provides guidance in maneuvering intravascular instruments**
         c. **Evaluates results of endovascular interventions**
         d. Limits the use of nephrotoxic contrast agents in **patients with renal insufficiency**
      2. **Complications** include vessel wall injury from passage of the ultrasound probe.
   C. **Balloon angioplasty**
      1. **General indications.** Best results are obtained with short-segment (<10 cm) stenoses within large, high-flow vessels (e.g., iliac artery).
      2. **Results.** Patency rates for balloon angioplasty of occlusive lesions are generally inferior to those of open surgical bypass except at the aortoiliac level. Unsuccessful angioplasty usually occurs because of inability to cross the lesion, elastic recoil, severe arterial calcification, and vessel wall dissection. However, angioplasty failures and restenoses are often amenable to repeat endovascular intervention, with variable results.
      3. **Complications.** Balloon angioplasty causes luminal dilation by fracturing the occlusive atherosclerotic plaque. This may expose the bloodstream to thrombogenic material, which may lead to vessel occlusion. Balloon

dilation also may create an intimal flap, leading to medial dissection and luminal narrowing or occlusion.
D. **Intravascular stenting.** Two general types of intravascular stents are available: balloon expandable (e.g., Palmaz stent) and self-expanding (e.g., Wallstent). Important characteristics of balloon-expandable stents include significant rigidity, radial strength, and minimal stent shortening with deployment. By contrast, self-expanding stents are more flexible, they have less radial strength, and some shorten with expansion, making precise stent placement more difficult. A rapidly growing variety of balloon expandable and self-expanding stents are becoming commercially available. Newer drug-eluting stents that inhibit neo-intimal hyperplasia (NIH) may replace current peripheral stents, but these are only currently approved for the coronary circulation.
   1. **General indications.** Intravascular stents have been used to address occlusive arterial lesions in a variety of locations. Stent placement was generally reserved for cases of early and late angioplasty failure (i.e., unsuccessful angioplasty and restenosis after prior angioplasty). However, at this time, stents are often used primarily in lesions known to have decreased patency with angioplasty alone. Their role in the treatment of infrainguinal disease is limited but continues to grow.
   2. **Results.** Restenosis rates after intravascular stent deployment have been shown to be similar to results with balloon angioplasty treatment alone in infrainguinal vessels but to be better in more proximal vessels (i.e., iliac, renal, mesenteric, aortic arch branches, carotid). Antiplatelet agents (e.g., aspirin, clopidogrel) are typically administered to decrease the incidence of stent thrombosis and to decrease the risk of NIH.
   3. **Complications.** In addition to complications associated with device introduction (embolization, dissection, vessel rupture, thrombosis, pseudoaneurysm formation at the arteriotomy site), stent migration or inappropriate stent deployment may occur. Pseudoaneurysms may also occur at the site of stent deployment.
E. **Endovascular grafts**
   1. **General indications.** Intravascular stents covered with prosthetic graft material [polytetrafluoroethylene (PTFE) or Dacron] have been developed for treatment of aneurysmal, occlusive, and traumatic arterial lesions. Most of the current designs include full-length stent support to prevent rotation or kinking of the unsupported graft.
   2. **Results.** Experience with endovascular grafting continues to increase. The short- and midterm results have been encouraging in the treatment of aneurysms, selected occlusive lesions, and traumatic arterial lesions. These devices are currently approved for the treatment of infrarenal abdominal aortic aneurysms and are likely to be approved for the treatment of thoracic aneurysms and other lesions in the near future.
   3. **Complications** are similar to those with intravascular stents.
F. **Atherectomy devices.** Various devices have been developed to mechanically debulk arterial occlusive lesions.
   1. **General indications.** The indications for use of atherectomy devices are very narrow in patients with peripheral vascular disease: instances in which balloon angioplasty (with or without stent placement) is unsuccessful or contraindicated. Bulky arterial lesions or stenoses associated with NIH may be amenable to treatment with atherectomy devices. New lower profile and user-friendly devices may broaden their application.
   2. **Results and complications.** Early devices were associated with significant complications and early thrombosis. In addition, none of these devices prevented restenosis, and their long-term results are no better than those for balloon angioplasty with or without stents. Newer devices have lower complication rates but their role and results are still unclear.

II. Specific indications for endovascular surgery
A. Aneurysms
1. **Abdominal aortic aneurysm (AAA)**
   a. **Indications.** The indications for endovascular treatment of AAA are no different than for traditional open operative repair. Generally, any AAA that is symptomatic, has a diameter greater than 5.0 cm, or has been growing >5 mm per year warrants consideration for surgical intervention.
   b. **Selection criteria.** The most important selection criteria for endovascular treatment of an AAA is aortoiliac anatomy. Assessment of the proximal neck of the AAA includes the following factors: length and diameter of nondilated and healthy infrarenal aorta, the angle between the neck and aneurysm, the presence of intraluminal thrombus, and the shape of the aortic neck. Most devices require a proximal neck that is 1.5 cm long, and some devices allow suprarenal attachment with an open stent segment. Current endograft dimensions at the proximal end are up to 32 mm in diameter. Significant angulation between the neck and adjacent aneurysm (>45 degrees) makes proximal graft deployment technically difficult and is associated with a higher risk of treatment failure. Significant mural thrombus or atheroma in the proximal neck can prevent adequate sealing of an endograft and therefore represents a contraindication for endovascular treatment. The proximal neck segment geometry is also important in that a cone-shaped neck or reverse taper (i.e., widens more distally) precludes adequate apposition of the endograft to the aortic wall. The distal neck of the AAA is important only for placement of straight aortic endografts, which are now rarely used. The vast majority of aortic endografts placed today are bifurcated and extend to the iliac arteries. The anatomy of the iliac arteries also has a significant influence on whether an aortic endograft can be placed successfully. Iliac artery tortuosity, calcification, and luminal narrowing, in combination with the profile of the delivery system, are critical for successful endograft delivery and deployment without complication. Patent aortic branches may influence the decision as to whether to proceed with endograft placement. A renal artery or accessory renal artery arising from the proximal neck or aneurysm or the presence of a horseshoe kidney with multiple renal arteries is often a contraindication for endograft placement. Patent lumbar arteries arising from the aneurysm do not preclude endograft placement. A patent inferior mesenteric artery (IMA) associated with large mesenteric collaterals (e.g., meandering mesenteric artery) or a large patent IMA suggests abnormal mesenteric blood supply and risk of large-bowel ischemia with endograft coverage of the IMA orifice. Therefore, these vascular patterns are contraindications to endograft placement.
   c. **Imaging studies.** Spiral computed tomographic (CT) scans with three-dimensional reconstruction are usually obtained to assess anatomic feasibility of endovascular stent graft deployment. Calibrated conventional angiography can also be obtained to assess aneurysm length and luminal dimensions for selection of the most appropriate endovascular graft.
   d. **Technique.** All current aortic endovascular grafts are usually introduced through direct femoral artery exposure. Percutaneous techniques for graft deployment are currently being developed. Most endovascular grafts are bifurcated, and many devices are modular (consisting of two or more components). Endografts typically have a full-length stent skeleton that prevents graft kinking. The deployment is mostly by unsheathing of self-expanding stents. Oversized stent grafts (by 10% to 15%) are selected based on preoperative assessment

of arterial diameter to ensure adequate graft apposition to the aortic wall. If necessary, graft length can be tailored by means of overlapping extension segments in modular devices. Positioning of the iliac limbs in bifurcated unibody aortic stent grafts is performed using guidewires and pullwires placed across the aortic bifurcation. Modular aortic stent grafts include a bifurcated portion with short and long limbs. After deployment of the main graft and long limb, a separate wire is placed through the short graft limb in a retrograde fashion from the contralateral femoral artery to guide deployment of an appropriate limb extension. The hypogastric artery is identified by intraoperative angiography, and the distal attachment site of the stent graft is positioned proximal to the hypogastric artery.

e. **Complications.** Early complications of endograft placement include distal embolization, graft thrombosis, and arterial injury (especially external iliac artery avulsion at the common iliac bifurcation in patients with tortuous diseased iliac arteries). These complications may require emergent conversion to open repair. Arterial dissection may occur with device introduction, but this may not require additional treatment if the endograft spans the segment of dissection. As with open surgical AAA repair, bowel ischemia may occur postoperatively secondary to embolization or hypoperfusion. Renal dysfunction may occur because of the nephrotoxicity of the contrast agent used for intraoperative angiography or because of direct injury due to embolization or renal artery occlusion. Late complications include graft migration and endoleak. Graft migration can typically be treated with secondary endovascular procedures. Endoleak, a unique complication of endovascular repair, is defined as failure to exclude the aneurysmal sac fully from arterial blood flow, potentially predisposing to rupture of the aneurysm sac. Management strategies for endoleaks discovered on follow-up imaging studies are evolving. In general, endoleaks from the proximal or distal attachment sites (type I) warrant intervention, because these are frequently associated with increasing aneurysm sac size. Type II endoleaks are due to collateral flow (IMA, lumbar arteries) and are generally closely observed. Type III endoleaks are usually due to component separation, and they should be corrected as soon as they are diagnosed. Type IV endoleaks are due to porosity of the graft material and are usually self-limiting. For any endoleak that is associated with aneurysm sac enlargement, intervention is required. Endoleaks are usually corrected by endovascular means but may require conversion to open surgical repair. Proximal endoleaks may be sealed with angioplasty or placement of a stent graft segment. Collateral bleeding may be treated with embolization through collateral vessels (via the hypogastric artery for lumbar branch bleeding, via the superior mesenteric artery for IMA bleeding) or directly through the aneurysm sac via a translumbar approach, which is usually the most successful strategy.

f. **Results.** Relative to open surgical repair, endovascular treatment of AAA is associated with a reduction in perioperative morbidity and a shorter duration of hospitalization. Recent studies from statewide databases also suggest a reduction of perioperative mortality. The short- and midterm results are encouraging and are similar to results seen with open repair, but long-term results are not yet available. Close follow-up with CT scanning every 6 months initially and yearly after the first year is essential to understand the behavior of these devices. Future fenestrated and branch devices may allow treatment of pararenal and other more complex AAAs.

2. **Thoracic aortic aneurysm (TAA)**
   a. **Indications and technique.** Because of the considerable morbidity and mortality associated with surgical repair of descending TAAs, the

endovascular approach to aneurysm exclusion is particularly attractive. The decision to proceed with endovascular graft placement is based on similar anatomic considerations as for AAA: adequate length (2 cm) and diameter (20 to 40 mm) of the proximal and distal aneurysm necks, cylindrical shape of aneurysm neck, absence of significant mural thrombus within the neck, and aortic and iliofemoral anatomy amenable to device introduction. In situations in which the proximal neck length is too short, seating of the proximal graft end over the origin of the left subclavian artery has been performed successfully with or without an adjunctive left carotid–left subclavian transposition or bypass. These devices are frequently used outside of the United States for the treatment of thoracic aortic lesions. None is currently approved for use in the United States.

   b. **Results and complications.** Early results for the use of commercial devices are encouraging. Various studies have suggested low morbidity and mortality and high rates of aneurysm exclusion. Future fenestrated and branched devices may allow endovascular treatment of more complex arch and thoracoabdominal aneurysms, but this technology is very early in its development.

3. **Aortic dissection.** In descending aortic dissections (type B, Stanford classification), organ ischemia may occur in two situations: (1) the dissection proceeds into branch vessels without a reentry lesion, causing narrowing of the true lumen, or (2) the intimal flap of a dissection reentry point occludes the lumen of an aortic branch. In both of these situations, stent placement in the involved aortic branch vessels may restore adequate perfusion. Endovascular strategies to promote increased blood flow in the true aortic lumen include stent graft coverage of the intimal tear and intimal flap balloon fenestration to create a communication between the true and false lumens. These interventions increase true lumen blood flow and help to prevent true lumen collapse and end-organ ischemia.

4. **Peripheral aneurysms**

   a. **Iliac aneurysms.** Most iliac artery aneurysms occur in association with AAA, and isolated iliac artery aneurysms are rare. Unilateral common iliac aneurysms can be treated by stent graft placement, with preservation of hypogastric artery flow if possible. When the unilateral common iliac aneurysm is located close to the iliac bifurcation, there are two options: (1) proximal embolization of the hypogastric artery to maintain pelvic collateral flow and stent graft placement across the common iliac aneurysm, or (2) open bypass for preservation of hypogastric artery blood flow. Internal iliac (hypogastric) artery aneurysms can be treated with embolization of the aneurysm distally (and proximally if possible) and endovascular graft occlusion of the internal iliac artery orifice to ensure exclusion. Patients should be monitored closely for the development of pelvic ischemia in the postoperative period, especially if both hypogastrics are occluded.

   b. **Popliteal aneurysms.** Treatment of popliteal artery aneurysms with stent grafts is technically feasible, but experience is limited. The incidence of popliteal aneurysm stent graft thrombosis is unacceptably high. Based on the known inferior patency rates of prosthetic grafts in this position, open surgical bypass with vein graft and aneurysm ligation is to date the preferred treatment. Endovascular treatment should be limited to patients who are in poor medical condition and unable to tolerate open reconstruction. Patency of endovascular devices is more likely in patients with good runoff and large superficial femoral and distal popliteal arteries for graft attachment.

   c. **Subclavian and axillary aneurysms.** These aneurysms can be readily excluded by endovascular means with very limited morbidity and mortality when no major branches need to be sacrificed (e.g., vertebral, carotid, or internal mammary in a patient with a coronary bypass graft). The durability of these devices in the thoracic outlet has been in question due to the compression forces at the site. Nevertheless, endovascular grafts have been successfully used to exclude true and false aneurysms in this location, with good short-term results.

B. Occlusive disease

  1. Aortoiliac occlusive disease

    a. Indications. Balloon angioplasty and intravascular stent placement across aortoiliac occlusive lesions have been demonstrated to be technically feasible and have excellent results. These procedures are indicated for symptomatic stenotic lesions (i.e., emboligenic lesions or lesions causing hypoperfusion) and in cases of distal bypass graft construction to improve graft inflow. Short-segment (<10 cm) concentric stenotic lesions have the highest long-term patency rates when treated with angioplasty alone or with stent placement. Angioplasty failure (residual luminal diameter reduction of 30% or more, 5 to 10 mm Hg or greater mean blood pressure gradient across the lesion, intimal flap, and medial dissection) is an indication for arterial stenting. Other indications for iliac stenting include eccentric stenotic lesions, recanalized iliac occlusions, restenosis after previous angioplasty, and ulcerated emboligenic lesions.

    b. Technique. Intra-arterial access for iliac artery angioplasty and stenting is generally via the femoral artery. For balloon angioplasty, the angioplasty balloon is positioned across the stenosis over a guidewire under fluoroscopy. When the occlusive lesion is in the distal aorta or proximal common iliac artery close to the aortic bifurcation, angioplasty should be performed using two balloons, one in each iliac artery and both partially projecting into the distal aorta ("kissing balloons"). The rationale for this is that lesions in proximity to the aortic bifurcation typically involve the distal aorta and both common iliac arteries. Unilateral balloon dilatation may cause plaque fracture and dissection and narrowing of the contralateral vessel. Balloon inflation to 6 to 10 atmospheres of pressure is maintained for 30 to 90 seconds, after which a second inflation is performed to check for residual stenosis (as seen by a deformed balloon profile). In cases of residual stenosis, repeat dilation with higher pressure may be attempted. If this is unsuccessful, stenting may produce a more favorable result. Finally, completion angiography is performed. Intra-arterial pressures also may be recorded across the dilated region to assess for hemodynamically significant residual stenosis. Pullback pressures can be obtained after pharmacologic vasodilation (nitroglycerin or papaverine) of the distal vascular bed. A resting gradient of 5 to 10 mm Hg and a vasodilated gradient of 10 to 20 mm Hg are considered hemodynamically significant. Balloon-expandable stents are generally dilated 10% to 15% more than the adjacent normal artery to ensure satisfactory stent apposition to the vessel wall. Balloon angioplasty is also commonly performed after deployment of self-expanding stents.

    c. Complications include arterial wall dissection, vessel occlusion (either from thrombosis or dissection), arterial rupture, and distal embolization.

    d. Results. Early balloon angioplasty failure can result from elastic recoil of atherosclerotic plaque or arterial wall dissection. These complications are potentially amenable to stent placement. Cases of late failure are due to intimal hyperplasia or progressive atherosclerosis. Iliac artery balloon angioplasty 2-year patency rates of between 60% and 70% have been reported. Reports on iliac artery stenting demonstrate 4-year patency rates as high as 85%. The results in general are better for common iliac artery lesions than for external iliac artery lesions and better for short-segment disease than for long-segment disease. Poor distal runoff is also associated with decreased patency.

2. **Infrainguinal occlusive disease**
   a. **Indications.** To date, balloon angioplasty and stenting of infrainguinal occlusive lesions have had poorer results than surgical bypass procedures. Nevertheless, endovascular treatment of these lesions may be appropriate in certain circumstances. In cases of limb-threatening ischemia in patients without sufficient autologous conduit or in patients at high operative risk, angioplasty and stenting may allow limb salvage despite poor long-term patency. There is no evidence to support primary stenting of femoral-popliteal stenotic lesions at this time. Stenting may be useful in cases of unsuccessful angioplasty (residual stenosis, intimal flap, dissection) or recurrent stenosis after previous angioplasty. Balloon angioplasty has been proposed for treatment of focal (<1.5 cm) infrainguinal vein bypass graft stenoses. Although surgical revision has been the treatment of choice, endovascular treatment is reasonable for certain high-risk patients in whom reoperation is deemed difficult, risky, or both. Up to 80% of patients who initially undergo percutaneous attempts at limb salvage will require standard operative intervention at some point.
   b. **Results.** The results of femoral-popliteal artery angioplasty and stenting are rapidly improving. Early data suggest that stent placement in the femoropopliteal area is associated with a 30% to 50% primary patency rate at 2 years. Stent placement in infrageniculate vessels is associated with a 20% patency rate at 2 years. The most important factor associated with early success is the type of lesion (stenosis better than occlusion); late success is most dependent on the runoff status. In addition, long-segment lesions (>10 cm) are associated with poor long-term results. Two-year patency rates as high as 66% have been reported after balloon angioplasty of favorable vein graft stenotic lesions. Newer techniques and devices (cryoplasty balloons, atherectomy catheters, recanalization devices) may lead to improved outcomes in the future.
3. **Renal artery stenosis**
   a. **Indications.** Clinically significant renal artery stenosis typically manifests as hypertension or ischemic nephropathy. Indications for interventional therapy of clinically significant renal artery stenosis include poorly controlled hypertension and worsening renal function. Balloon angioplasty is the treatment of choice for clinically significant fibromuscular dysplastic lesions of the renal artery. Angioplasty of renal artery atherosclerotic lesions has less favorable results but entails significantly less procedure-related morbidity than surgical bypass or endarterectomy. When indications exist for open aortic surgery (e.g., AAA repair), renal artery bypass or endarterectomy can be performed at the same time. Surgical therapy also may be preferable in cases of long-segment disease or occlusions or when atherosclerosis is severe and widespread (i.e., to avoid the risk of atheroembolic complications with intra-arterial instrumentation). Therefore, indications for angioplasty of renal artery stenosis include the failure of medical management of renovascular hypertension in the absence of any clear indications for open aortic surgery. Renal artery stents are routinely used for restenosis after previous angioplasty, treatment of procedural complications (e.g., dissection), and the treatment of atherosclerotic ostial lesions.
   b. **Technique.** Intravascular access to the renal artery may be obtained from the femoral, brachial, or axillary arteries (access from the upper extremity may be preferable in cases of caudally angled renal arteries). In patients at high risk for renal failure (e.g., type II diabetes, preexisting renal insufficiency), nephrotoxic contrast may be avoided and angiography can be performed using gadolinium or carbon dioxide. Technical success for renal artery angioplasty is defined as a less

than 30% residual stenosis and a pressure gradient across the lesion of less than 5 to 10 mm Hg.

c. Results. Patients with fibromuscular dysplasia respond favorably to percutaneous transluminal angioplasty, with cure rates of greater than 50%. Patients with atherosclerotic disease respond less favorably in the long-term, although immediate technical success is seen in up to 99% of patients. Improvements in blood pressure are seen in approximately two-thirds of patients; however, only 15% of patients with renal insufficiency demonstrate improved excretory renal function. Additionally, up to 15% of patients exhibit decreased renal excretory function following intervention. Angiographic restenosis occurs in 15% to 20% of patients within 1 year of treatment, most commonly in small renal arteries (<4mm). Based on this data, percutaneous angioplasty with stenting of atherosclerotic disease of the renal artery yields blood pressure, renal function, and anatomic results that are slightly inferior but comparable to contemporary surgical results. Percutaneous intervention is, however, associated with lower morbidity and mortality rates than open surgical intervention.

4. Carotid occlusive disease
   a. Indications. The indications for surgical treatment of carotid occlusive disease are based on several large prospective studies [e.g., Asymptomatic Carotid Atherosclerosis Study (ACAS) and North American Symptomatic Carotid Endarterectomy Trial (NASCET)], and standard carotid endarterectomy is performed with minimal morbidity and mortality. Indications for endovascular treatment of these lesions, therefore, require a large-scale prospective study [e.g., Carotid Revascularization Endarterectomy versus Stent Trial (CREST), Endarterectomy versus Angioplasty in Patients with Severe Symptomatic Carotid Stenosis Study (EVA-3S)] to demonstrate that angioplasty and stenting can be performed with equivalent or less morbidity and mortality than traditional endarterectomy. The lesions most suitable for this approach may be those for which endarterectomy would be difficult and risky, for example, lesions in a reoperative neck, cervical fibrosis from irradiation, high internal carotid lesions, and lesions in patients with severe comorbidities.

   b. Technique. Vascular access to carotid occlusive lesions is usually from the femoral artery. Several different cerebral protection devices have been developed to minimize cerebral embolic events caused by intravascular instrumentation. Two types of protection devices are currently being evaluated: occlusive balloons and filter devices. With the balloon devices, a subset of patients with insufficient collateral flow do not tolerate internal carotid artery (ICA) balloon occlusion during stent deployment and require temporary shunt placement. The advantage of filter devices is that they allow the maintenance of antegrade carotid flow (and better angiographic visualization) during stent placement and deployment. After localization of the stenotic lesion, balloon angioplasty is performed, followed by stent deployment.

   c. Results. The short-term results of carotid artery stenting are approaching those of open endarterectomy, but long-term results are lacking. Conversion to endarterectomy is occasionally required due to various technical problems, such as inability to cross the occlusive lesion, thrombus within the stent, and ICA kink. Several small studies have reported few (2% to 5%) periprocedural neurologic complications after internal carotid artery angioplasty and stenting using cerebral protection devices. This compares favorably with the 7% to 10% neurologic complication rates reported before the development of cerebral protection devices and lower-profile stents. Early data suggest that the perioperative myocardial infarction, stroke, and death rates in "high-risk" patients are lower when they are treated with carotid artery stenting than with surgical endarterectomy. Long-term data from current studies should clarify the role of stenting in the management of carotid artery stenosis.

5. Supra-aortic trunk occlusive disease

  a. Indications. The indications for endovascular treatment of occlusive lesions of aortic arch branches are the same as those for open surgical treatment. For proximal subclavian artery lesions, the indications are arm claudication, digital embolization, symptoms of vertebrobasilar insufficiency, and preparation for coronary artery bypass using the internal mammary artery. For innominate and common carotid lesions, indications include stenosis of greater than 75% and referable symptoms such as transient ischemic attack, amaurosis fugax, or ipsilateral nondisabling stroke.

  b. Technique. Access to the occlusive lesion is either from the femoral, brachial, or common carotid arteries. Early results with angioplasty alone were notable for poor short- and midterm patency rates. Therefore, current endovascular treatment of these lesions is with stent deployment. The majority of devices currently used are balloon-expandable stents for orificial lesions because of their increased radial force. Self-expanding, more flexible stents are used for more tortuous areas.

  c. Results. Short- and midterm follow-up of patients undergoing angioplasty with stenting of supra-aortic trunk occlusive lesions shows a 3-year patency rate of up to 85%. Long-term results of endovascular treatment of these lesions are not yet available. Nevertheless, endovascular treatment of these lesions is significantly less morbid than open operative approaches that require thoracotomy, sternotomy, or claviculectomy.

C. Venous disease. Endovascular techniques have been used successfully in the treatment of venous disease.

  1. Deep venous thromboses (DVTs) of the ileofemoral system have been treated with catheter-based techniques involving local administration of thrombolytics. This approach may result in earlier thrombus resolution and a reduced incidence of postthrombotic syndrome than systemic anticoagulation. Bleeding complications can occur.

  2. Vena cava interruption can be performed percutaneously, usually via a femoral or internal jugular approach. Indications include patients with DVT and contraindications to anticoagulation, patients with pulmonary embolism while therapeutically anticoagulated, and patients felt to be at high risk for the development of DVT and subsequent pulmonary embolism (e.g., patients with spinal cord injury). Pulmonary embolism can occur in up to 4% of patients treated with vena caval filters. Complications include filter migration, caval thrombosis, and local insertion site complications.

  3. Transvenous pulmonary embolectomy has been performed percutaneously in select patients, avoiding the risks of general anesthesia and sternotomy or bleeding complications associated with systemic lytic use.

D. Vascular trauma Experience with endovascular treatment of traumatic arterial injuries has largely been limited to arteriovenous fistulas and pseudoaneurysms in the hemodynamically stable patient. Successful stent graft treatment of arteriovenous fistulas and pseudoaneurysms at various locations has been reported. However, the overall experience has been limited, and besides demonstrating technical feasibility, no guidelines have been determined regarding appropriate indications for endovascular treatment. In patients with multiple injuries, endovascular treatment of severe arterial lesions is potentially very attractive despite the limited long-term results available.

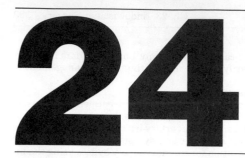

24

Venous Disease, Thromboembolism, and Lymphedema

Jason Lee and
Brian Rubin

VENOUS ANATOMY

Venous anatomy is divided into the superficial, deep, and perforator components. In the lower extremity, the major superficial veins are the greater saphenous vein (located anterior to the medial malleolus and traveling medially to the fossa ovalis in the groin), the lesser saphenous vein (posterior to the lateral malleolus, coursing posterolaterally to the popliteal fossa), and the posterior arch vein, also called *Leonardo's vein* (beginning in the medial ankle and joining the greater saphenous vein below the knee). The deep veins in the leg are named according to their paired arteries. The deep veins of the calf typically are duplicated as venae comitantes with numerous communicating branches. The posterior tibial and peroneal veins also communicate with the soleal sinusoids. In the thigh, the deep venous system includes the superficial and deep femoral veins that join about 4 cm below the inguinal ligament. The superficial and deep systems are connected by perforating veins (direct and indirect). Most blood flows from the superficial to the deep system via the direct perforators, but indirect perforators (small superficial veins draining into muscles that connect to the deep system via intramuscular veins) are also important. Blood is propelled toward the heart by compression of the deep veins by calf muscle contractions during walking, and flow is unidirectional due to a series of one-way valves. Of surgical interest are five groups of direct medial calf perforators joining either the greater saphenous vein or the posterior arch vein to the posterior tibial vein (*J Vasc Surg* 1996;24:800). They are named **Cockett** or **paratibial perforators**, depending on their anatomic location, which can be variable. The saphenous nerve travels medially, close to the saphenous vein near the ankle, making it susceptible to injury during stripping of the lower saphenous vein.

CHRONIC VENOUS INSUFFICIENCY

Chronic venous disease spans a broad clinical spectrum, which includes cosmetically undesirable telangiectases, varicose veins, and venous ulceration. Advances in noninvasive imaging techniques (duplex scanning) and minimally invasive surgical techniques are being used to tailor medical and surgical therapies, resulting in marked improvement in clinical outcomes and patient satisfaction.

   I. **Pathophysiology**
      A. **Reflux disease** from venous valvular incompetence accounts for most (>80%) chronic venous disease. Valve malfunction can be inherited or acquired through sclerosis or elongation of valve cusps; it also can result from dilation of the valve annulus despite normal valve cusps. Varicose veins may represent superficial venous insufficiency in the presence of competent deep and perforator systems, or they may be a manifestation of perforator or deep disease. Valvular disease below the knee appears to be more critical in the pathophysiology of severe disease than does deep valvular disease above the knee. The perforator veins are frequently implicated when venous ulcers exist, but any component of the venous system, either alone or in combination, may be incompetent. Therefore, all components need evaluation in the workup of chronic venous insufficiency (CVI) (*Am J Surg* 1995;169:572).

B. Obstructive physiology is a less common cause of venous pathology, with reflux often being present simultaneously.

II. **Etiology.** Venous disease can be congenital (although it may present later in life), primary (cause undetermined), or secondary (postthrombotic, posttraumatic, or other). Deep venous thrombosis (DVT) accounts for most secondary cases and may be responsible for a significant number of other cases because many deep vein thrombi are asymptomatic. Other contributing factors include pregnancy, hormone therapy, and obstruction in a proximal segment (e.g., from adenopathy, arterial compression, or pregnancy).

III. **Diagnosis** is made by history, physical examination, and noninvasive studies.

   A. **History.** A history of any DVT or trauma should be sought, as well as any family history of varicose veins or CVI. Patients may complain of lower-extremity edema, aching, skin irritation, or varicose veins. Leg pain is described as a dull ache, worsening at the end of the day, and often relieved with exercise or elevation. In severe cases, individuals can experience acute, bursting pain with ambulation (**venous claudication**). Prolonged rest and leg elevation (20 minutes) are needed to obtain relief.

   B. **Physical examination** can reveal ankle edema, subcutaneous fibrosis, hyperpigmentation (brownish discoloration secondary to hemosiderin deposition), lipodermatosclerosis, venous eczema, and dilatation of subcutaneous veins, including telangiectases (0.1 to 1.0 mm), reticular veins (1 to 4 mm), and varicose veins (>4 mm). Ultimately, ulcers develop, typically proximal to the medial malleolus. Any signs of infection should be noted. Arterial pulses should be examined and are usually adequate.

   C. **Noninvasive studies**

   1. **Duplex scanning** (B-mode ultrasound imaging combined with Doppler frequency shift display) has become invaluable in assessing valvular incompetence and obstruction. For evaluation of patients with valvular incompetence, a modified duplex study is performed. With the individual standing, cuffs are placed on the thigh, calf, and foot and inflated; then the cuffs are rapidly deflated in an attempt to create retrograde venous blood flow in segments of valvular incompetence. Competent valves generally take no more than 0.5 to 1.0 seconds to close. Detailed mapping of valve competence of each segment of the venous system is possible, including the common femoral, superficial femoral, greater saphenous, lesser saphenous, popliteal, posterior tibial, and perforator veins. In one report, this method was found to have a predictive value of 77% for diagnosing reflux leading to severe symptoms, compared with a predictive value of 44% for descending phlebography, previously considered the gold standard (*J Vasc Surg* 1992;16:687). Descending phlebography is limited by its inability to study valves distal to a competent proximal valve.

   2. **Continuous-wave Doppler** examination is easily performed in the office using a handheld probe. The study is helpful for screening for reflux at the saphenofemoral and saphenopopliteal junctions. Its use is limited owing to its inability to quantitate reflux and to provide precise anatomic information.

   3. **Trendelenburg test** is easy to perform but has been largely replaced by the much more accurate duplex imaging studies. First, the patient's leg is elevated to drain venous blood. An elastic tourniquet is applied at the saphenofemoral junction, and the patient then stands. Rapid filling (<30 seconds) of the saphenous system from the deep system indicates perforator valve incompetence. When the tourniquet is released, additional filling of the saphenous system occurs if the saphenofemoral valve is also incompetent.

IV. **Differential diagnosis.** Lower-extremity venous disease must be differentiated from arterial occlusive disease, chronic lymphedema, squamous cell carcinoma, trauma, arteriovenous malformations, and orthostatic edema. Ischemic

Table 24-1. Classification of chronic lower-extremity venous disease

Classification	Definition
C	Clinical signs (grade 0–6),* supplemented by (A) for asymptomatic or (S) for symptomatic presentation
E	Etiologic classification (congenital, primary, or secondary)
A	Anatomic distribution (superficial, deep, or perforator; alone or in combination)
P	Pathophysiologic dysfunction (reflux or obstruction; alone or in combination)

*See Table 24-2.
Reprinted with permission from Porter JM, Moneta GL. Reporting standards in venous disease: an update. International Consensus Committee on Chronic Venous Disease. *J Vasc Surg* 1995;21:635.

ulcers from arterial disease are more likely to be on the patient's foot, with discrete edges and pale bases; they are more painful than venous ulcers. Other signs or symptoms of arterial disease may be present, such as poor pulses, dependent rubor, pallor with elevation, and claudication. Lymphedema typically causes pitting edema without pigmentation and ulceration. Lymphedema is less responsive to elevation, usually requiring several days to improve.

V. **Nomenclature.** Based on the conclusions of an international consensus committee, a standardized nomenclature of chronic venous disease has been established (*J Vasc Surg* 1995;21:635). Disease is classified according to a **CEAP** system: **c**linical signs, **e**tiology, **a**natomic distribution, and **p**athophysiology (Tables 24-1 and 24-2).

VI. **Nonsurgical treatment**
    A. **Infected ulcers** necessitate treatment of the infection first. *Staphylococcus aureus*, *Streptococcus pyogenes*, and *Pseudomonas* species are responsible for most infections and can usually be treated with local wound care, wet-to-dry dressings, and oral antibiotics. Topical antiseptics should be avoided. Severe infections require intravenous antibiotics.
    B. **Leg elevation** can temporarily decrease edema and should be instituted when swelling occurs. This should be done before a patient is fitted for stockings or boots.
    C. **Compression therapy** is the primary treatment for CVI.
        1. **Elastic compression stockings** are fitted to provide a compression gradient from 30 to 40 mm Hg, with the greatest compression at the ankle. They should be donned on arising from bed and removed at bedtime. Stockings are effective in healing ulcers but can take months to obtain good results. In a study of 113 patients treated with initial bedrest, local wound care, and elastic compression stockings, there was a 93% ulcer

Table 24-2. Clinical classification of chronic lower-extremity venous disease

Grade	Characteristics
0	No visible or palpable signs of venous disease
1	Telangiectases, reticular veins, or malleolar flare
2	Varicose veins
3	Edema without skin changes
4	Skin changes ascribed to venous disease (e.g., pigmentation, venous eczema, or lipodermatosclerosis)
5	Skin changes as defined above and healed ulceration
6	Skin changes as defined above and active ulceration

Adapted with permission from Porter JM, Moneta GL. Reporting standards in venous disease: an update. International Consensus Committee on Chronic Venous Disease. *J Vasc Surg* 1995;21:635.

healing rate in a mean of 5.3 months (*Surgery* 1991;109:575). Because stockings do not correct the abnormal venous hemodynamics, they must be worn after the ulcer has healed to prevent recurrence. Their principal drawback is patient compliance. Recurrence for compliant patients in the same study was 16% at a mean follow-up of 30 months.

2. **Unna boots** are paste gauze compression dressings that contain zinc oxide, calamine, and glycerin and are used to help prevent further skin breakdown. They essentially provide nonelastic compression therapy. Typically, medical personnel apply the dressing and change it once or twice a week. Healing time for ulcers is less than that of elastic compression alone, with 70% of ulcers healed by 7 versus 11 weeks (*J Am Acad Dermatol* 1985;12:90).

3. **Pneumatic compression devices** provide dynamic sequential compression. They are used primarily in the prevention of deep vein thrombi in hospitalized patients, but they have also been used successfully to treat venous insufficiency. In a prospective study comparing local wound care and gradient compression stockings with or without sequential pneumatic compression for 4 hours a day, there was an ulcer healing rate of 2.1% of the ulcer area per week without dynamic compression compared with 19.8% with dynamic compression (*Surgery* 1990;108:871).

D. **Topical medications** for venous stasis ulcers have largely been ineffective. Topical therapy is directed at absorbing wound drainage and avoiding desiccation of the wound. Antiseptics can be counterproductive. Hydrogen peroxide, povidone-iodine, acetic acid, and sodium hypochlorite are toxic to cultured fibroblasts and should be used for the shortest duration necessary to control ulcer infection.

E. **Sclerotherapy** can be effective in treating telangiectases, reticular varicosities, and small varicose veins. If saphenous reflux is present, it should be corrected first. Contraindications include arterial occlusive disease, immobility, acute thrombophlebitis, and hypersensitivity to the drug. Sclerosing agents include 1% or 3% sodium tetradecyl sulfate, sodium morrhuate (rarely used because of anaphylactic reactions), hypertonic saline, and polidocanol (not currently approved in the United States). Varices are marked while the patient is standing. A 25-gauge needle is used to inject 0.25 to 0.50 mL sclerosant slowly into the lumen of larger veins. A 30-gauge needle is used for sclerosing reticular veins and telangiectases in supine patients. Compression stockings are applied at the end of the procedure and are worn for several days to 6 weeks. Patients should walk for 30 minutes after the procedure. Complications include cutaneous necrosis, hyperpigmentation, telangiectatic matting (new, fine, red telangiectases), thrombophlebitis, anaphylaxis, and allergic reaction (*Dermatol Surg* 1995;21:19).

VII. **Surgical therapy** is indicated for severe disease refractory to medical treatment and for patients who cannot comply with the lifelong regimen of compression therapy. Surgical therapy includes skin grafting, saphenous vein stripping, endovenous obliteration of the saphenous vein, varicose vein stab avulsion, subfascial endoscopic perforator ligation, and valvuloplasty.

A. **Preoperative evaluation** consists primarily of duplex imaging in a reliable vascular laboratory. All components of the venous system should be studied and the precise location of pathology noted. Surgical therapy is directed at the component or components found to have pathology. For valve reconstruction, ascending or descending phlebography may be useful.

B. **Skin grafting** is occasionally used to speed healing of large ulcers. The ulcer bed should be dry and free of infection. A fenestrated split-thickness skin graft is preferred to allow for serous drainage. Bedrest is recommended until the ulcer has healed completely. Recurrence is common unless the underlying venous pathology is corrected or conservative support (elastic compression) is initiated and maintained after skin grafting.

C. **Stripping the greater saphenous vein** has been one of the classic treatments for varicose veins. The vein should be stripped only in the regions where pathology occurs. If the entire vein is involved, one incision is made anterior to the medial malleolus and another just below the inguinal crease. A stripper is inserted into the vein lumen at one site and run through the lumen to the other site. High ligation of the vein is done at the saphenofemoral junction, including all tributaries. Reconnection of the saphenous to the femoral system via multiple tributaries near the saphenofemoral junction is thought to be the major cause of recurrent varices. The vein is then stripped from one site to the other. Compressive bandages are applied to reduce hematoma formation, and compression stockings are worn for several weeks. Complications include ecchymosis, DVT, and saphenous nerve injury. Stripping only the thigh portion is probably the most important aspect of the procedure (*Lancet* 1996;348:210). Not stripping the calf eliminates much of the risk to the saphenous nerve because this nerve is closely associated with the saphenous vein from the knee to the ankle; it also allows the portion of the vein below the knee to be used for arterial bypass if needed in the future. The same technique can be applied to the lesser saphenous vein.

D. **Endovenous radiofrequency or laser obliteration** of the greater saphenous vein has been shown to effectively treat saphenous reflux and associated varicose veins with less morbidity than saphenectomy (*J Vasc Surg* 2003;38:207). A probe is inserted into the greater saphenous vein under ultrasound guidance. The probe emits either laser or radiofrequency energy, which coagulates and coapts the vein walls, causing complete obliteration of the lumen. Potential complications of this technique include skin burns, deep venous thrombosis, pulmonary thromboembolism, vein perforation and hematoma, paresthesias, and phlebitis. Reported outcomes achieved with endovenous radiofrequency and laser obliteration are comparable to those resulting from saphenectomy (*J Vasc Surg* 2002;35:1190; *J Vasc Interv Radiol* 2003;14:991). Incomplete obliteration and recanalization occurs in a small percentage of patients. One contraindication to endovenous obliteration is saphenous vein thrombosis.

E. The **stab avulsion technique** allows a cosmetically acceptable surgical approach to varicose veins. Preoperatively, the patient's varicose veins are carefully marked with indelible ink while the patient is standing. Some authors consider this the most important technical step in the procedure (*Am J Surg* 1996;172:278). An incision (2 to 3 mm) is made next to the markings. The vein is pulled out of the incision with a small vein hook, and the two arms of the vein are pulled taut and avulsed. This can be repeated many times to remove large clusters of veins. The small incisions can be closed with Steri-Strips. The patient's leg is covered with compression stockings for several days to weeks. This technique is often used in conjunction with saphenous stripping to provide optimal results. Alternatively, the greater saphenous vein can be removed by sequential avulsion instead of stripping. This has been shown prospectively to decrease pain and bruising (*Br J Surg* 1996;83:1559).

F. For most severe CVI, **more extensive surgery** is required, usually directed at correction of saphenous reflux and ligation of incompetent medial calf perforators. Even in the presence of combined superficial and deep incompetence, treatment of only the superficial and perforator incompetence can significantly improve clinical symptoms and hemodynamics (*J Vasc Surg* 1996;124:711) by disrupting continued transmission of high deep venous pressure to the skin. Traditionally, treatment of perforator reflux has been accomplished via an **open surgical subfascial ligation** (the Linton procedure), which requires an incision through diseased skin and extensive subcutaneous dissection. Wound complications have limited the acceptance of this procedure. **Subfascial endoscopic perforator surgery** is becoming increasingly popular because of its decreased morbidity. This procedure is performed by making small port incisions in unaffected skin in the calf and fascia of the posterior superficial compartment. Various types of endoscopes (laparoscopic, arthroplastic, or bronchoscopic) may be used for visualization. Carbon dioxide insufflation in the subfascial space may or may not be used. A balloon expander can expand the subfascial space to improve visualization. Typically, two to six perforators are identified and ligated. Most patients are discharged within 24 hours of surgery. Preliminary results indicate an ulcer-healing rate of 88% at a mean follow-up of 5 months (*J Vasc Surg* 1997;25:94). Pain, edema, pigmentation, and lipodermatosclerosis have all been shown to improve. Complications include wound infection, superficial thrombophlebitis, cellulitis, and saphenous neuralgia, but the overall morbidity is less than that resulting from the open technique. A newer technique, "mini-incision" ligation of perforators, has had good results and produces fewer wound complications. In this method, perforators are first identified in the vascular laboratory, and their location is marked on the skin. Small purse-string sutures are then placed at these marks to ligate the vessels (*J Vasc Surg* 1997;25:437).

G. **Direct venous valve reconstruction** can be performed to restore competence to floppy or redundant valves. Generally, this excludes patients with venous reflux secondary to DVT because the inflammatory thrombotic process tends to fibrose and shorten the valve cusps. Valvuloplasty can be done using an open or closed technique (*J Vasc Surg* 199;16:694). For the open procedure, a venotomy is made above the valve, and the cusps are sutured until competence is achieved. Alternatively, an angioscope can be inserted through a tributary, and repair of the valve can be viewed directly without a venotomy. To correct an incompetent superficial femoral vein, transfer of a valved vein segment is performed using end-to-end anastomosis either to the proximal saphenous vein or to the deep femoral vein, thus providing a competent proximal valve. Autotransplantation of a segment of axillary or brachial vein into the proximal popliteal vein has also been used with variable success.

VENOUS THROMBOEMBOLISM

I. **Epidemiology.** Venous thromboembolism, which includes DVT and pulmonary embolism (PE), is a common cause of death. The true incidence of DVT is difficult to determine because its clinical diagnosis can be inaccurate and it often occurs in the setting of other critical illnesses. One population-based study in Worcester, Massachusetts, reported 48 cases of DVT per 100,000 population (*Arch Intern Med* 1991;151:5). This figure was based on hospital discharge diagnoses and is likely to underrepresent the true incidence. Extrapolation of the Worcester data leads to the estimate that there are approximately 260,000 cases of DVT diagnosed in acute care hospitals annually.

II. **Pathophysiology.** DVT starts as a platelet nidus, usually in the venous valves of the calf. The thrombogenic nature of the nidus activates the clotting cascade, leading to a thrombus that grows by accumulating more platelets and fibrin. The fibrinolytic system is also activated, and thrombogenesis and thrombolysis compete for dominance. The thrombus grows if thrombogenesis predominates. A thrombus can detach from the endothelium and migrate into the pulmonary system, becoming a PE. A thrombus can also organize and grow into the endothelium, resulting in venous valve incompetency and phlebitis. Thrombi localized to the calf have less tendency to embolize than thrombi that extend to the thigh veins (*Am Rev Respir Dis* 1990;141:1). Approximately 20% of cases of calf DVT propagate to the thigh, and 50% of cases of thigh or proximal DVT embolize. Significant PE results in increased right ventricular afterload, which may lead to right ventricular dysfunction, decreased cardiac output, or arrhythmias. Remodeling or fibrinolytic dissolution of the embolus also occurs, although few patients have complete normalization of pulmonary arterial pressures after PE. Most patients survive the first hour after a PE, although many of these occurrences are not detected. If not diagnosed, recurrent episodes of PE pose a greater risk of mortality. Among patients correctly diagnosed and treated, the recurrence rate of clinically detected PE is 8.3%, and the early fatality rate is approximately 2.5% (*N Engl J Med* 1992;326:19). PE usually recurs within 1 week, and the early fatalities occur within 2 weeks of the initial episode. One year after PE, approximately 24% of patients die from underlying cardiovascular disease, pulmonary disease, or malignancy.

III. **Risk factors for venous thromboembolism**

A. **Malignancy.** Trousseau was the first to suggest an association between malignancy and a hypercoagulable state when he observed episodic migratory thrombophlebitis in his cancer patients. Several pathogenic mechanisms have been described for this association. Tumor cell activation of the clotting cascade can occur directly through interactions with factors VIIa and X and tissue factor (TF). Indirect clotting activation can occur through stimulation of mononuclear cells to produce TF or factor X activators and stimulation of macrophages to produce TF activators.

B. **Endothelial injury.** Another mechanism for the association of malignancy and thrombus formation is endothelial injury. Adhesion of tumor cells to endothelium can lead to disruption of endothelial intracellular junctions and expose the highly thrombogenic subendothelial surface. Chemotherapeutic drugs, such as bleomycin, carmustine, vincristine, and doxorubicin (Adriamycin), can also cause vascular endothelial cell damage.

C. **Reactive thrombocytosis** can occur in patients with malignancy, especially those with advanced disease of the lung, colon, stomach, or breast. Thrombocytosis may be caused by spontaneous clumping of platelets or increased levels of thrombopoietin, a glycoprotein that regulates the maturation of megakaryocytes.

D. **Venous stasis** can be caused by immobility, venous obstruction, increased venous pressure, and increased blood viscosity. Venous stasis promotes thrombus formation by reducing clearance of activated coagulation factors and by causing endothelial hypoxia, leading to reduced levels of surface-bound thrombomodulin and increased expression of TF. Two very common causes of immobility leading to DVT formation are surgery and critical illness. Major chest surgery, abdominal/pelvic surgery, and lower-extremity surgery have all been associated with increased risk of DVT development. Similarly, a prolonged nonambulatory state, such as fracture of the hip, pelvis, or leg; multisystem trauma; neurologic injury; or other critical injury requiring bedrest can increase DVT risk.

E. The use of **oral contraceptives (OCPs)** and **estrogen hormone replacement therapy** have been linked to increased risk of venous thrombus formation. Many studies have found an odds ratio of 3.0 to 5.0 for risk of DVT in patients taking OCPs compared to non-OCP-using patients. This increased risk is still found with patients using third-generation OCPs containing new progestins. In a matched-control study from Oxford, the authors found a 3.7-fold increase in the risk of venous thrombus in older women undergoing hormone replacement therapy. The mechanism causing the increased risk is still unknown, especially because the estrogens used in hormone replacement therapy are different from those used in OCPs.

F. **Hypercoagulable states** can also lead to DVT formation. Primary hypercoagulable states are inherited conditions that can lead to abnormal endothelial cell thromboregulation (e.g., decreased thrombomodulin-dependent activation of protein C, impaired heparin binding of antithrombin III, down-regulation of membrane-associated plasmin production) or decreased thrombogenic inhibitors (e.g., antithrombin III, protein C, protein S). Secondary hypercoagulable states are states in which endothelial activation by cytokines leads to an inflammatory thrombogenic vessel wall. Antiphospholipid syndrome, heparin-induced thrombopathy, myeloproliferative syndromes, and cancer are among the more common syndromes leading to secondary hypercoagulable states. Some chemotherapy agents, such as cyclophosphamide, methotrexate, and 5-fluorouracil, can cause a decrease in the plasma levels of proteins C and S.

IV. **Diagnosis of venous thromboembolism.** Approximately 75% of patients with
suspected DVT or PE turn out not to have these conditions. Nevertheless, objective studies are indicated when suspicion is high because clinical diagnosis
alone is inaccurate and undetected or untreated DVT or PE can have a fatal
outcome.
  A. The **initial evaluation** for suspected venous thromboembolism in a patient
begins with an assessment of the risk factors mentioned earlier in this chapter. The clinical presentation of a patient with DVT includes pain of the extremity, increased circumference of that extremity with respect to the contralateral extremity, dilation of superficial veins of the suspected extremity
only, and calf pain on dorsiflexion of the ankle. A more severe presentation
of DVT is phlegmasia cerulea dolens, in which limb pain and swelling are
accompanied by cyanosis, a sign of arterial ischemia.
  B. **PE** can have many clinical presentations, most of which are nonspecific; they
include tachycardia, fever, hypoxia, and cardiac arrhythmia. Myocardial ischemia, cardiogenic shock, and sepsis share common signs with PE and often
need to be ruled out at the time of presentation. Venous thromboembolism
may occur without clear clinical signs.
  C. For **suspected DVT,** compression ultrasonography of the femoral, popliteal,
and calf trifurcation veins is highly sensitive (>90%) in detecting thrombosis of the proximal veins (femoral and popliteal) but less sensitive (50%) in
detecting calf vein thrombosis. Ultrasonography is the preferred diagnostic
modality because it is less invasive than the reference standard of venography and more sensitive than impedance plethysmography. Approximately
2% of patients with initial normal ultrasound results have positive results
on repeat tests performed 7 days later. This delayed detection rate is attributed to extension of calf vein thrombi or small, nonocclusive proximal
vein thrombi.
  D. For detecting PE in cases where it is suspected, **contrast-enhanced spiral
computed tomography (CT)** has sensitivity (70% to 90%) comparable to that
of pulmonary angiography. Spiral CT is preferable to angiography because
it is less invasive and less expensive. Its sensitivity is limited to subsegmen-
tal pulmonary artery occlusion. Chest CT can be combined with CT angiography of pelvic and deep thigh veins to detect DVT as well as PE. Patients
with significant contrast allergy or renal insufficiency are not candidates for
CT scanning.
  E. Radionucleotide ventilation and perfusion lung imaging (VQ scan) has been
replaced by chest CT as the initial imaging test for suspected PE. VQ scanning can be used in situations where CT scanning is not feasible. A VQ scan
result of "high probability" strongly suggests the presence of PE. However,
more than 50% of patients have "intermediate probability" results. Because
approximately 25% of these patients have PE, further evaluation or initiation of empiric treatment must be considered.
  F. **Pulmonary angiography,** the reference test, is reserved for patients whose
diagnosis is still uncertain.
V. **Prevention and treatment of venous thromboembolism.** The prevention of
venous thromboembolism depends on knowledge of risk factors in individual
patients. As detailed previously in this chapter, prolonged immobility, cancer,
estrogen use, and hypercoagulable states are well-known risk factors. Other
risk factors include age greater than 40, prior DVT, obesity, varicose veins,
congestive heart failure, myocardial infarction, and stroke. The rationale for
venous thromboembolism prophylaxis is that the disease is of a silent nature.
DVT and PE may manifest few clinical symptoms, and the diagnosis is sometimes uncertain. Although treatment of detected venous thromboembolism is
effective, many patients who die from PE do so in the first 30 minutes of the
event, too soon for anticoagulation to have full effect. In the absence of prophylaxis, the frequency of fatal postoperative PE ranges from 0.1% to 0.8%
in patients who are undergoing elective general surgery, 0.3% to 1.7% in patients undergoing elective hip surgery, and 4% to 7% in patients undergoing

emergency hip surgery (*Haemostasis and Thrombosis: Basic Principles and Clinical Practice.* 3rd ed. Philadelphia: JB Lippincott Co., 1994). Prophylaxis is achieved by either altering the blood coagulation state, preventing venous stasis, or preventing embolization.

A. **Low-dose unfractionated heparin** is given subcutaneously at 5,000 units 2 hours before surgery and every 8 or 12 hours postoperatively. Low-dose heparin reduces the risk of venous thromboembolism by 50% to 70% (*N Engl J Med* 1988;318:18) and does not require laboratory monitoring. Because of the potential for minor bleeding, it should not be used for patients undergoing cerebral, ocular, or spinal surgery. **Graduated compression stockings** are effective in preventing DVT formation by reducing venous stasis. However, this efficacy has been shown just for calf DVT, and insufficient data exist to conclude that they aid in the prevention of proximal DVT or PE. In surgery patients, the combination of graduated compression stockings and low-dose heparin is significantly more effective than low-dose heparin alone (*Br J Surg* 1985;72:7). Graduated compression stockings are relatively inexpensive and should be considered for all high-risk patients, even when other forms of prophylaxis are used.

B. **Intermittent pneumatic compression of the extremities** enhances blood flow in the deep veins and increases blood fibrinolytic activity. For patients with significant bleeding risk with anticoagulation, pneumatic compression is an effective alternative. Compression devices should not be placed on an extremity with known DVT. In the case of known bilateral lower-extremity DVT, the compression device can be placed on the upper extremity. Pedal compression devices are also effective in patients whose body habitus does not allow conventionally sized devices to fit around their thighs or calves.

C. **Low–molecular-weight heparins (LMWHs)** have several advantages over unfractionated heparin. They have longer half-lives, the dose response is more predictable, and in laboratory animals they cause fewer bleeding complications with equivalent anticoagulation effects. In large randomized trials of patients with DVT, outpatient treatment with a LMWH was as safe and effective as inpatient treatment with intravenous unfractionated heparin. LMWHs seem to be slightly better than low-dose heparin for prophylaxis against DVT formation because LMWHs cause fewer wound hematomas and are more convenient to dose.

D. **Caval interruption with intracaval filters** has been available since the 1960s as a method of preventing PE. However, unfractionated heparin followed by warfarin therapy for 3 months is 95% effective in preventing PE in patients with known DVT. Thus, filter placement was restricted in patients with DVT who also had contraindications to anticoagulation or had failure of anticoagulation therapy. With the development of percutaneous methods of filter placement (which have low complication rates), indications for filter use have widened. According to recent estimates from industry manufacturers, 30,000 to 40,000 filters are inserted in the United States annually.

E. The **choice of prophylaxis method** depends on the risk of venous thromboembolism compared with the risk of anticoagulation. See Chapter 1, Section II.A.2, for a detailed description.

F. **Catheter-directed thrombolysis** of acute DVT with or without mechanical thrombectomy devices has been advocated in order to avoid sequelae of DVT. The goals are to restore venous flow, preserve venous valve function, and eliminate the possibility of thromboembolism. Technical success and early clinical benefit have been reported, but long-term data is unavailable.

LYMPHEDEMA

I. **Pathophysiology**
A. **Primary lymphedema** is the result of congenital aplasia, hypoplasia, or hyperplasia of lymphatic vessels and nodes that causes the accumulation of a protein-rich fluid in the interstitial space. Swelling of the patient's leg

initially produces pitting edema, which progresses to a nonpitting form and may lead to dermal fibrosis and disfigurement. Primary lymphedema is classified according to age at presentation as congenital (present at birth), praecox (early in life), or tarda (late in life). Congenital lymphedema (10% to 15% of cases) can be hereditary (Milroy disease) or nonhereditary. Praecox lymphedema (70% to 80% of cases) is seen in female patients 80% to 90% of the time and presents during adolescence. Lymphedema tarda (10% to 15% of cases) is seen equally in men and women and presents after the third or fourth decade.

B. Secondary lymphedema results from impaired lymphatic drainage secondary to a known cause. Surgical or traumatic interruption of lymphatic vessels (often from an axillary or groin lymph node dissection), carcinoma, infection, venous thrombosis, and radiation are causes of secondary lymphedema.

II. Lymphedema is diagnosed by history, physical examination, and exclusion of other causes of a swollen extremity. Imaging studies, especially lymphoscintigraphy, can aid in the diagnosis. Typically, however, imaging studies are directed at ruling out venous thrombosis or extrinsic venous compression as the cause of leg swelling.

A. Clinical presentation

1. Symptoms. Early lymphedema is characterized by unilateral or bilateral arm or pedal swelling that resolves overnight. With disease progression, the swelling increases and extends up the extremity, producing discomfort and thickened skin. With more advanced disease, swelling is not relieved overnight. Significant pain is unusual. With secondary lymphedema, symptoms related to the principal disease are present. Patients commonly present with repeated episodes of cellulitis secondary to high interstitial protein content.

2. Physical examination reveals edema of the affected extremity. When the lower extremity is involved, the toes are often spared. With advanced disease, the extremity becomes tense with nonpitting edema. Dermal fibrosis results in skin thickening, hair loss, and generalized keratosis.

B. Imaging studies

1. Lymphoscintigraphy is the injection of radiolabeled (technetium-99m) colloid into the web space between the patient's second and third toes or fingers. The patient's limb is exercised periodically, and images are taken of the involved extremity and the whole body. Lymphedema is seen as an abnormal accumulation of tracer or as slow tracer clearance along with the presence of collaterals. For the diagnosis of lymphedema, the study has a sensitivity and specificity of 92% and 100%, respectively (*J Vasc Surg* 1989;9:683).

2. CT and MR scan are able to exclude any mass obstructing the lymphatic system. MR scan has been able to differentiate lymphedema from chronic venous edema and lipedema (excessive subcutaneous fat and fluid).

3. Lymphangiography involves catheter placement and injection of radiopaque dye directly into lymphatic channels; it has largely been replaced by lymphoscintigraphy and CT. A decreased total number of lymphatic channels and structural abnormalities can be seen. Lymphangiography can demonstrate the site of a lymphatic leak in postsurgical or traumatic situations. Complications include lymphangitis and hypersensitivity reaction to the dye.

III. Differential diagnosis includes all other causes of a swollen extremity, including trauma, infection, arterial disease, venous disease, lipedema, neoplasm, radiation effects, and other systemic diseases, such as right ventricular failure, myxedema, nephrosis, nephritis, and protein deficiency. These causes must be excluded before invasive study.

IV. Treatment

A. Medical management is limited by the physiologic and anatomic nature of the disease. The use of diuretics to remove fluid is not effective because of the high interstitial protein concentration. Development of fibrosis and irreversible changes in the subcutaneous tissue further limit options. The objectives of conservative treatment are to control edema, maintain healthy skin, and avoid cellulitis and lymphangitis.

1. **Combination of physical therapies (CPT)** is the primary approach recommended in a consensus document by the International Society of Lymphology Executive Committee (*Lymphology* 1995;28:113). CPT involves gentle manual manipulation of tissues to direct lymph flow, physical therapy exercises, and compression bandages. It is followed by the wearing of custom-made compression garments. In a study of 119 patients with 3-year follow-up, CPT reduced lymphedema by 63% (*Oncology* 11:99, 1997).

2. **Sequential pneumatic compression** has been shown to improve lymphedema. Several designs have been used with various degrees of success. Elastic stockings or sleeves should be fitted and worn afterward to maintain results. Extremity elevation may also help.

3. **Skin care and good hygiene** are important. Topical hydrocortisone cream may be needed for eczema.

4. **Benzopyrones** (such as warfarin) have been effective in reducing lymphedema due to filariasis. Their action is believed to derive from enhanced macrophage activity and extralymphatic absorption of interstitial proteins.

5. **Cellulitis and lymphangitis** should be suspected when sudden onset of pain, swelling, or erythema of the leg occurs. Intravenous antibiotics should be initiated to cover staphylococci and β-hemolytic streptococci. Broad-spectrum penicillins, cephalosporins, or vancomycin usually are adequate. Limb elevation and immobilization should be initiated, and warm compresses can be used for symptomatic relief. Topical antifungal cream may be needed for chronic infections.

B. **Surgical options** include excision with skin grafting, closure of disrupted lymphatic channels, omental transposition, lymphatic transposition, and microsurgical lymphovenous anastomosis. Only 10% of patients with lymphedema are surgical candidates, and surgery is directed at reducing limb size. Indications for operation are related to function because cosmetic deformities persist postoperatively. Results are best when surgery is performed for severely impaired movement and recurrent cellulitis.

1. **Total subcutaneous excision** is performed for extensive swelling and skin changes. Circumferential excision of the skin and subcutaneous tissue from the tibial tuberosity to the malleoli is performed. The defect is closed with a split- or full-thickness skin graft from the resected specimen or a split-thickness skin graft from an uninvolved site. Good functional results can be expected in 60% to 100% of patients (*Plast Reconstr Surg* 1977;60:589). Recurrent lymphedema and hyperpigmentation occur more frequently when split-thickness skin grafts are used. Lymphatic reconstruction includes direct (lymphovenous bypass, lymphatic grafting) and indirect (mesenteric bridge, omental flap) procedures.

2. **Lymphovenous anastomoses** bypass the obstructed lymphatic system in patients with chronic lymphedema. With improved microvascular techniques, patency rates of 50% to 70% can be expected months after surgery (*J Vasc Surg* 1986;4:148). Lymphatic grafting is performed for upper-extremity or unilateral lower-extremity lymphedema. Good results have been reported in 80% of patients (*Plast Reconstr Surg* 1990;85:64). A mesenteric bridge is formed by suturing a segment of mucosa-stripped ileum with intact blood supply to transected distal iliac or inguinal nodes. An omental flap placed in a swollen limb is believed to improve lymphatic drainage through spontaneous lympholymphatic anastomoses. Due to their complexity and associated complications, indirect procedures are not widely used.

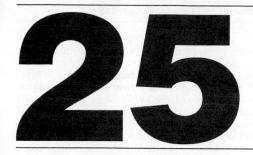

Hereditary Tumor Syndromes and Genetic Counseling

Mark S. Cohen and Jeffrey F. Moley

TUMORS AND GENETICS

I. **Introduction.** Cancer is a genetic disease in that the cause of malignant transformation lies in genetic alterations that take place within cells. While not all cancers are hereditary, there are many families that are affected by a predisposition to certain tumors and malignant syndromes. The ability to diagnose carriers of these hereditary tumors using modern genetic testing has improved the way many of these disorders are treated, and preventative strategies have been instituted for some disorders. Although the science of genetic testing has answered many questions, it has also raised new ones, including ethical and moral concerns that affect not only the patients and their families but also the society in which they live and work. Genetic testing is an important component of the multidisciplinary approach to cancer care. Genetic counselors are vital members of this team, translating complicated medical information to familes in a nonbiased way to allow them to consider their options and make informed treatment decisions.

II. **Tumor syndromes**

A. **Breast cancer.** Inherited breast cancer accounts for approximately 5% to 10% of all breast cancers, amounting to almost 20,000 cases per year in the United States alone.

1. **Diagnosis and screening.** A detailed family history should be taken in any individual with breast cancer and should include paternal as well as maternal information. *BRCA1* **and** *BRCA2* **genes** account for 45% and 35% of hereditary breast cancer, respectively. It is an autosomal dominant genetic disorder with high penetrance. The *BRCA1* gene was cloned from the long arm of chromosome 17 and spans approximately 100,000 nucleic acids, with more than 1,600 different mutations reported. Over 100 different mutations have been reported for *BRCA2*, an even larger gene. Risk of breast cancer among disease gene carriers varies, depending on the clinical setting. In high-risk families, patients with a mutated *BRCA1* gene have an 87% lifetime risk of breast cancer, and patients with a mutated *BRCA2* gene have an 80% risk. In the Ashkenazi Jewish population, *BRCA1* and *BRCA2* mutations confer a risk of 56% by age 70. Different types of mutations are associated with varying risks of breast cancer. Carriers of *BRCA* mutations also have a higher risk for other cancers. *BRCA* patients have a lifetime risk of 40% to 60% for developing ovarian cancer (*Am J Hum Genet* 1995;56:265). Ovarian cancer in these patients appears to have a better prognosis than sporadic ovarian cancer (*N Engl J Med* 1996;335:1413). Men who are *BRCA2* mutation carriers have a higher risk of breast cancer, although not as high as women. Commercial tests to detect mutations in the *BRCA1* and *BRCA2* genes are available but still relatively costly. Genetic testing may identify a mutation of unknown significance. Genetic counseling is essential and highly encouraged before any test is administered.

2. **Treatment.** For *BRCA* mutation carriers, treatment includes close surveillance, chemoprevention, and prophylactic surgery. Therapy options should be tailored to individuals based on their desires and the perceived risk. Women should have yearly mammograms starting in their

midtwenties, compared with 40 years of age for women who are not gene carriers. Tamoxifen has been shown to reduce the risk of cancer in the contralateral breast after an initial diagnosis of cancer. A review of high-risk women found a 90% reduction in breast cancer after bilateral prophylactic mastectomies (*N Engl J Med* 1999;340:77). A prospective study found a significant reduction in breast cancer in women with *BRCA1* or *BRCA2* mutations who elected to have prophylactic mastectomies (*N Engl J Med* 2001;345:159). If bilateral mastectomies are performed, the patient should continue to have close surveillance yearly for changes in the remaining breast tissue.

B. Li-Fraumeni syndrome (LFS). LFS is a rare autosomal dominant disorder characterized by an inherited predisposition to breast cancer and at least five childhood cancers, including soft-tissue sarcoma, osteosarcoma, leukemia, brain tumor, and adrenocortical carcinoma. Approximately 50% of LFS families have been found to have germline mutations in the gene for tumor protein p53 (*TP53*) (*Am J Hum Genet* 1995;56:608). Because a significant number of LFS kindreds do not have a *TP53* germline mutation, genetic heterogeneity is likely. The protein product of the gene functions as a transcription factor, preventing DNA synthesis when damage has occurred to the cell's DNA. While other tumors have been reported with LFS, breast cancer is the most common, and almost 90% of carriers develop it by age 50. LFS accounts for 1% of all breast cancers, and approximately 50% of carriers develop some type of invasive breast cancer by age 30. These patients also have an increased sensitivity to radiation effects.

C. Cowden disease (multiple hamartoma syndrome). Cowden disease is an autosomal dominant syndrome characterized by multiple facial trichilemmomas, oral papillomas, "cobblestoning" of the tongue, acral keratoses, bilateral breast cancer, gastrointestinal polyposis, and thyroid tumors. Lipomas, hemangiomas, macrocephaly, and brain tumors have also been reported. Breast cancer develops in 30% to 50% of patients by age 50. Germline mutations in the *PTEN* gene (also known as *MMAC1*) are responsible for the syndrome (*Nat Genet* 1997;15:307). The protein product is a tyrosine phosphatase. Currently genetic testing for *PTEN* mutations is available only in select centers, and genetic counseling is primarily based on clinical judgement and family pedigrees.

D. Ataxia-telangiectasia (AT). AT is an autosomal recessive disease with a varied phenotype, including progressive cerebellar ataxia, oculocutaneous telangiectasias, progeric skin changes, immune dysfunction, and increased cancer susceptibility. The hallmark of ataxia-telangiectasia is cerebellar ataxia, often seen at a young age. Most patients are unable to walk by age 10. The responsible gene (*ATM*) is required for transcription of p53 in response to radiation damage. These individuals are extremely sensitive to ionizing radiation. Carriers are prone to a variety of cancers, particularly leukemia and lymphoma, but also breast, pancreatic, stomach, bladder, and ovarian cancer. Heterozygote carriers of AT are reported to have an increased risk of breast cancer and to account for up to 5% to 7% of breast cancers (*Cancer Genet Cytogenet* 1996; 92:130), but this number may be an overestimate.

E. Colorectal cancer. Inherited cancers may account for up to 15% of the 150,000 new cases of colorectal cancer diagnosed annually in the United States.

1. Familial adenomatous polyposis (FAP). FAP is an inherited autosomal dominant syndrome characterized by florid colonic polyposis and caused by mutations in the *APC* tumor-suppressor gene on chromosome 5q21. The gene encodes a 300-kd protein, which can bind microtubules and β-catenin. The location of a mutation within the gene can produce different phenotypes. For example, congenital hypertrophy of the retinal pigment epithelium, once thought to be a signature of the disease, occurs when the mutation resides between codons 463 and 1387. Virtually

100% of affected individuals develop colorectal cancer if not treated. Carriers typically develop hundreds to thousands of adenomatous polyps that carpet the large intestine during the second or third decades of life. The polyps are indistinguishable from sporadic polyps; however, because of their enormous numbers and the early age at which they develop, the likelihood of one of them progressing to malignancy is close to 100%. The median age of cancer diagnosis for untreated individuals is 39 years, almost 30 years earlier than for sporadic colorectal cancer. Affected individuals are also prone to development of duodenal, gastric, and ileal polyps and are at risk for developing duodenal, stomach, periampullary, thyroid, and other cancers as well. Upper gastrointestinal cancers, usually duodenal tumors, pose the greatest risk of mortality once the risk of colorectal cancer is eliminated. Upper endoscopic surveillance should be performed every 3 years. Polypectomy, if possible, is thought to be adequate treatment for most polyps, followed by annual screening.

   a. **FAP variants.** There are several phenotypic variations of FAP that were previously thought to be distinct syndromes:

      (1) **Gardner syndrome,** associated with mutations in codons 1403 to 1578, is characterized by gastrointestinal polyposis, desmoid tumors, osteomas of the mandible or skull, and sebaceous cysts. Desmoid tumors also appear as a phenotypic characteristic in 10% to 20% of FAP patients. Although not malignant, they can be locally aggressive and a significant cause of mortality. Desmoids often arise in surgical scars or small-bowel mesentery after abdominal surgery. Diffuse fibrosis may lead to ureteral, vascular, or gastrointestinal obstruction. Further surgical resection may not be possible, and even when resection is initially successful, desmoids often recur.

      (2) **Turcot syndrome** is associated with malignant central nervous system tumors, gastrointestinal polyposis, and colorectal cancer.

      (3) **Somatic mutations** in the *APC* gene also occur in more than 80% of sporadic cases of colorectal cancer as well as in early sporadic adenomas.

   b. **Screening.** Any at-risk individual whose family has never been tested should have the entire *APC* gene sequenced to detect a mutation. Several centers across the United States perform linkage analysis for *APC* gene mutation carriers. The protein truncation test detects more than 95% of mutations but should only be performed as a screening test once a mutation that causes truncation has been established in the family. Screening for affected children should begin in their preteen years via lower endoscopy and should continue annually. Affected individuals should undergo lifelong surveillance of their upper gastrointestinal tract for a secondary malignancy.

   c. **Surgery.** Operative therapy is performed when polyposis is detected, usually in the late teen years or early twenties. In younger patients, two options exist for removing the colon: either a total proctocolectomy with an ileal pouch–anal anastomosis (IPAA) or a total colectomy with an ileorectal anastomosis. An ileorectal anastomosis is usually better tolerated than an IPAA, even with a variety of pouch configurations, mainly due to morbidities of sphincter dysfunction and impotence in men following IPAA. Leaving behind rectal mucosa, however, carries a significant risk for developing rectal cancer over time, and close surveillance of this mucosa is paramount for patients with an ileorectal anastomosis. The rate of rectal cancer after ileorectal anastomosis has been reported to range from 12% to 20% at 20 years (*Semin Surg Oncol* 1995;11:423), and high rectal polyp density as well as rectal stumps greater than 7 cm in length were found to correlate with an increased risk of cancer. Multiple factors should be considered when

deciding on the appropriate surgical procedure, including extent of
rectal disease, location of any cancer, sphincter function, extracolonic
disease, surgeon experience, and patient follow-up.

2. **Hereditary nonpolyposis colorectal cancer syndrome (HNPCC or Lynch
syndrome).** HNPCC is an autosomal dominant disease caused by inacti-
vation of one of at least five DNA mismatch repair genes, which produces
DNA microsatellite instability and replication errors. HNPCC accounts
for approximately 5% of all colorectal cancers. The lifetime risk of colorectal cancer is approximately 70% to 80%, and the median age of cancer development is 44 years. These patients do not develop polyposis, but
the polyps that do develop have an accelerated rate of tumor progression.
The cancers tend to be right-sided (70% proximal to the splenic flexure).
In addition, synchronous and metachronous colorectal cancers are seen
in 25% to 30% of cases. These patients do better, stage for stage, than
their sporadic counterparts. Extracolonic malignancies are also seen, especially endometrial cancer, as well as ovarian, small-bowel, stomach,
pancreas, urologic tract, bladder, and, occasionally, breast cancer. Patients who develop extracolonic malignancies have sometimes been described as belonging to Lynch type II kindreds, whereas patients with
colorectal malignancies alone are considered Lynch I.

   a. **The Amsterdam criteria clinically define HNPCC.** The criteria are as
   follows: (1) The family includes at least three relatives with proven
   colorectal cancer, and one of them is a primary relative of the other
   two; (2) at least two generations are affected; and (3) one individual
   was diagnosed before age 50. To enhance the diagnostic accuracy of the
   Amsterdam criteria, some groups have also suggested the inclusion of
   replication error status (*Cancer* 1996;77:265).

   b. **Mismatch repair genes.** *MSH2, MLH1, MSH6, PMS1,* and *PMS2* are
   the DNA mismatch repair genes responsible for most cases of HN-
   PCC when inactivated. *MSH2* and *MLH1* account for two-thirds of
   HNPCC. If these genes are inactivated, the cell cannot repair errors
   made by DNA polymerase during DNA replication, leading to genome
   wide mutations. Microsatellite instability (additions or deletions in
   the number of dinucleotide DNA repeats) characterizes the DNA of
   these individuals and is the basis for genetic testing. Genetic testing
   for *MSH2* and *MLH1* is now available at many centers in the United
   States but is time consuming and costly. High-risk individuals should
   be screened with colonoscopy every 2 years beginning at age 20 to 25
   and annually after age 30. Women should undergo endometrial surface sampling annually beginning at age 30. Surveillance for ovarian
   cancer is limited, but transvaginal ultrasound and CA-125 should be
   considered.

   c. **Treatment** for HNPCC kindreds has not been well defined. If a
   germline mutation is detected, prophylactic surgery should be considered. The general principles of treatment are the same as for FAP,
   but a colectomy with an ileorectal anastomosis may be a more reasonable alternative, because these tumors have a proximal predilection.
   Alternatively, nonoperative management with screening colonoscopy
   every 1 to 2 years in known gene carriers is an option. Prophylactic
   total abdominal hysterectomy and bilateral salpingo-oophorectomy is
   an option for women who do not want more children. Again, genetic
   counseling is strongly advised prior to surgical therapy.

3. **Muir-Torre syndrome (MTS).** MTS is a rare autosomal dominant hereditary cancer syndrome characterized by the presence of at least one sebaceous gland tumor and a visceral cancer. The sebaceous gland tumors
often appear as yellow facial papules and are a hallmark of this disease.
The most common internal malignancy is colorectal cancer, but other tumors occur, especially genitourinary tumors. Clinical similarities with
HNPCC include a tendency for proximal colon cancers and for better

survival than for sporadic cancers. Microsatellite instability is found in tumors in about half of affected individuals. Germline mutations have been found in the *MSH2* and the *MLH1* genes in different kindreds (*Am J Hum Genet* 1996;59:736).

4. **Peutz-Jeghers syndrome.** Peutz-Jeghers syndrome is a rare autosomal dominant disease characterized by gastrointestinal hamartomatous polyposis and mucocutaneous pigmentation. The melanin pigmentations usually appear in childhood and may occur on the lips, oral mucosa, hands, feet, and perianal and umbilical areas. Hamartomas occur throughout the gastrointestinal tract, with the small intestine being the most frequent location. The polyps have an uncertain malignant potential but can cause obstruction, intussusception, and bleeding. Both malignancies of the gastrointestinal tract, including pancreatic cancer, and extraintestinal cancers occur with increased frequency. These patients should have a baseline upper endoscopy and colonoscopy at approximately 20 years of age, with frequent surveillance thereafter. Some have advocated a subtotal colectomy if the polyps are too numerous to follow. Diagnostic and predictive genetic testing is now possible in many families due to the recent identification of causative mutations in the serine/threonine kinase *STK11* gene (also known as the *LKB1* gene) (*Expert Rev Anticancer Ther* 2003;3:518).

5. **Familial juvenile polyposis (FJP).** FJP is another rare autosomal dominant disease characterized by hamartomatous polyposis. The polyps, usually numbering 50 to 200, primarily occur in the colon and rectum but can also be found in the duodenum and stomach. The lifetime risk for developing colorectal cancer is estimated to be 25% to 50%, and the cancer develops mostly at an early age. There is also an increased risk for upper gastrointestinal tumors. Typically, children first present with diarrhea or rectal bleeding. Associated congenital abnormalities include cerebral and pulmonary arteriovenous malformations, cardiac anomalies, polydactyly, malrotation, and cranial malformations. Colonoscopic surveillance should begin by age 12. The *SMAD4* gene has recently been linked to some of the kindreds with this syndrome (*Science* 1998;15:1086). The recommended treatment for FJP is subtotal colectomy with ileorectal anastomosis; however, rectal recurrence is possible with any retained rectal mucosa, and some authors advocate a restorative proctocolectomy with IPAA and pouch surveillance.

F. **Endocrine tumors**
1. **Multiple endocrine neoplasia syndromes (MEN)**
   a. **Multiple endocrine neoplasia type 1 (MEN-1).** MEN-1 is an autosomal dominant syndrome characterized by tumors of the parathyroid glands, pancreatic islet cells, and pituitary gland. Hyperparathyroidism (HPT) occurs in virtually all patients. Clinical evidence of pancreatic islet cell and pituitary tumors develops in 50% and 25% of patients, respectively. Lipomas, thymic or bronchial carcinoid tumors, and tumors of the thyroid, adrenal cortex, and central nervous system (CNS) may also develop. The gene responsible for MEN 1, *MENIN*, is located on chromosome 11q13 and appears to act through transcription factors (*Science* 1997;276:404). Genetic testing is available in many centers, but if it is not available, screening of family members should begin in their early teens, including yearly determinations of plasma calcium, glucose, gastrin, fasting insulin, vasoactive intestinal polypeptide, pancreatic polypeptide, prolactin, growth hormone, and β-human gonadotropin hormone.

      (1) **Hyperparathyroidism.** Since HPT is frequently the first detectable abnormality in patients with MEN-1, yearly calcium screening of asymptomatic kindred members is recommended. Patients with HPT and MEN-1 usually have generalized (four-gland) parathyroid enlargement. Surgery should consist of $3\frac{1}{2}$-gland

parathyroidectomy or a total parathyroidectomy with autotransplantation of parathyroid tissue to the forearm. This method achieves cure in more than 90% of cases and results in hypoparathyroidism in less than 5%. Graft-dependent recurrent HPT, however, is seen in up to 50% of cases. It is managed by resecting a portion of the autografted material (*Ann Surg* 1980;192:451).

(2) **Pituitary tumors** occur in up to 40% of MEN-1 patients and most commonly are benign prolactin-producing adenomas. Growthhormone, adrenocorticotropic hormone–producing, and nonfunctioning tumors are also seen. Patients may present with headache, diplopia, or symptoms referable to hormone overproduction. Bromocriptine inhibits prolactin production and may reduce tumor bulk and obviate the need for surgical intervention. Transsphenoidal hypophysectomy may be necessary if medical treatment fails.

(3) **Pancreatic islet cell tumors** pose the most difficult clinical challenge and account for most of the morbidity and mortality of the syndrome. Gastrinomas (Zollinger-Ellison syndrome) are most common, but vasoactive intestinal polypeptide–secreting tumors, insulinomas, glucagonomas, and somatostatinomas are also encountered. The pancreas is usually diffusely involved, with islet cell hyperplasia and multifocal tumors. Tumors may be found in the proximal duodenum and peripancreatic areas (gastrinoma triangle), and these are virtually always malignant. The treatment goal is relief of symptoms related to excessive hormone production and cure or palliation of the malignant process. Patients frequently require medical and surgical therapy. Before surgical exploration, the patient should be evaluated for an adrenal tumor by measuring urinary excretion rates of glucocorticoids, mineralocorticoids, sex hormones, and plasma metanephrines.

2. **MEN-2 syndrome.** MEN-2 is characterized by medullary thyroid carcinoma (MTC) and includes MEN-2A, MEN-2B, and familial, non-MEN MTC [familial MTC (FMTC)]. These autosomal dominant syndromes are caused by gain-of-function mutations in the *RET* proto-oncogene, which encodes a transmembrane tyrosine kinase receptor. Mutations in *RET* lead to constitutive activation (tyrosine phosphorylation) of the RET protein, which drives tumorigenesis. Genetic testing should be performed on all suspected individuals. In more than 50% of patients with medullary thyroid carcinoma, the cancer will recur after primary surgical resection. While reoperation is advocated for local recurrence, there is no accepted adjuvant regimen to effectively treat metastatic disease. Investigational therapies and clinical trials with targeted inhibitors of RET tyrosine kinase activity are currently being evaluated (*Surgery* 2002;132:960)

a. **MEN-2A.** All patients with MEN-2A will develop MTC, whereas pheochromocytomas arise in approximately 40% to 50% of patients, and hyperplasia of the parathyroid glands (HPT) arises in approximately 25% to 35%. Patients with MEN-2A also develop gastrointestinal manifestions, including abdominal pain, distention, and constipation as well as Hirschsprung disease (*Ann Surg* 2002;235:648). On genetic analysis, patients with MEN-2A and Hirschsprung disease (MEN2A-HD) share common mutations in either codon 609, 618, or 620 of exon 10 of the *RET* proto-oncogene.

(1) **MTC** develops at an early age on a background of C-cell hyperplasia and is multifocal. Treatment is total thyroidectomy with central lymph node neck dissection, which entails removal of all nodes and fatty tissue between the carotid sheaths and the innominate artery. Many authors also recommend ipsilateral or bilateral functional neck dissections to remove lateral cervical lymph nodes, which are found in up to 80% of patients at time of presentation. Parathyroidectomy with autotransplantation of parathyroid

tissue into the forearm (MEN-2A) or sternocleidomastoid (MEN-2B, FMTC) can be performed. Patients should be screened for pheochromocytomas before undergoing surgery. MTC cells produce the hormone calcitonin, which can be measured in screening and follow-up examinations, especially for residual or recurrent disease. Infusing the secretagogues calcium gluconate and pentagastrin before measuring calcitonin provides more reliable results than following basal calcitonin levels. Patients who are found to have a known *RET* mutation based on genetic testing should undergo preventative thyroidectomy before age 6 for MEN-2A and FMTC and in infancy for MEN-2B. Genetic counseling for parents of affected children is crucial prior to prophylatic surgery.

(2) **Pheochromocytomas** in MEN-2A and MEN-2B are generally not metastatic or extra-adrenal, but 10% may be bilateral and up to 10% are malignant. Screening, which should be done at the same time as screening for MTC, consists of plasma or 24-hour urinary measurements of catecholamines, vanillylmandelic acid (VMA), and urine metanephrines. Operatively, most tumors can be approached laparoscopically, with the likely exception of extremely large tumors or malignant tumors. Preoperative preparation with alpha blockade and hydration is necessary.

b. **MEN-2B** is a variant of MEN-2 in which patients develop MTC and pheochromocytomas but not hyperparathyroidism. Patients also develop ganglioneuromatosis and a characteristic physical appearance, with hypergnathism of the midface, marfanoid body habitus, and multiple mucosal neuromas. MTC is particularly aggressive in these patients. MEN-2B patients also demonstrate multiple gastrointestinal symptoms and megacolon.

c. **FMTC** is characterized only by the hereditary development of MTC without other endocinopathies. MTC is generally more indolent in these patients.

G. **Sarcomas.** Soft tissue sarcomas have been identified in several familial cancer syndromes, including LFS (Section II.B), hereditary retinoblastoma, and neurofibromatosis types 1 and 2. The prognosis is highly dependent on the tumor grade.

H. **Neurofibromatosis type 1 (NF1).** H. NF1 is a common autosomal dominant disorder that affects more than 80,000 people in the United States and is caused by mutations in the *NF1* gene. The three hallmarks of the disease are multiple neurofibromas, café au lait spots, and Lisch nodules (benign iris hamartomas). Neurofibromas may be removed for pain, functional impairment, or cosmetic reasons. In the gastrointestinal tract, neurofibromas may result in bleeding, obstruction, or intussusception. NF1 patients have a much greater likelihood of developing neurofibrosarcomas and are also at risk for pheochromocytomas, CNS tumors, and leukemias. An enlarging mass, localized pain, or neuropathy should be considered a neurofibrosarcoma until proved otherwise. These tumors are generally resistant to chemoradiation.

I. **Neurofibromatosis type 2 (NF2)** is a much rarer autosomal dominant disorder characterized by the defining feature of bilateral vestibular schwannomas and caused by the *NF2* gene (merlin or schwannomin on chromosome 22q11-13). The syndrome is also characterized by skin neurofibromas, café au lait spots, cataracts, and other CNS tumors, including gliomas, meningiomas, schwannomas, and neurofibromas.

J. **Retinoblastoma (RB).** Familial retinoblastoma is an autosomal dominant syndrome with 90% penetrance due to mutations in the *RB* gene on chromosome 13q14, and it is characterized by bilateral retinoblastomas in infants and children. Most familial cases occur *de novo,* and early screening, which can decrease mortality by 55%, includes ophthalmologic exams every 3 months to age 2 years, then every 6 months to age 10 years.

K. **Von Hippel-Lindau syndrome (VHL).** VHL is an autosomal dominant syndrome in which benign and malignant tumors may develop in the kidneys, brain, spine, eyes, adrenals, pancreas, inner ear, and epididymis. Mean age of diagnosis is around 26 years. Retinal hemangioblastomas are the most common presentation, with a mean age of diagnosis of 25 years. Renal cell carcinomas are less common, with a mean age of diagnois of 44 years. Multiple bilateral renal cysts (>100) are common, with up to 75% of patients developing cysts, tumors, or both. VHL protein appears to regulate the transcription of DNA to mRNA by RNA polymerase II. VHL has also been proposed to regulate vascularization by altering the stability of vascular endothelial growth factor (VEGF). VHL is broken into 3 types based on genetic phenotype. Type I patients do not develop pheochromocytomas. Type 2A patients develop pheochromocytomas but not renal cell carcinomas. Finally, Type 2B patients manifest both pheochromocytomas and renal cell carcinomas. Nephron-sparing surgery is the treatment of choice to preserve as much kidney function as possible; however, recurrence occurs in 40% to 50% of patients, necessitating close follow-up. Renal transplantation has been used successfully for extensive disease. Pheochromocytomas should be resected when found.

L. **Hereditary renal carcinoma (HRC).** Hereditary renal carcinoma may be either clear cell (HCRC) or papillary (HPRC) in nature. HCRC carcinomas are bilateral and multifocal. HCRC patients have a translocation of part of chromosome 3p, and the disease is due to gain-of-function mutations in the MET proto-oncogene, encoding a tyrosine kinase receptor on chromosome 7q31-34. The median age of survival for patients with HCRC is 52 years.

M. **Wilm tumor (nephroblastoma).** Nephroblastoma is the most common intra-abdominal solid tumor in children, with a peak incidence at 3 to 4 years of age. Only 1% are inherited, and the rest are obtained sporadically. Three syndromes are associated with a genetic predisposition to Wilm tumors: **WAGR syndrome,** characterized by Wilm tumors, aniridia, genitourinary malformations, and mental retardation; **Denys-Drash syndrome (DDS),** characterized by Wilm tumors, mesangial sclerosis leading to renal failure, and ambiguous genitalia; and **Beckwith-Wiedemann syndrome (BWS),** characterized by overgrowth, omphalocele, and predisposition to embryonic malignancies such as Wilm tumors. Wilm tumors may also be familial and without association with other syndromes. The best surveillance method for patients at risk for developing Wilm tumor is intra-abdominal ultrasound every 3 months until age 7 (*Hematol Oncol Clin North Am* 1995;9:1253). A baseline abdominal CT should also be obtained to evaluate for other malignancies. Treatment consists of surgical resection and chemotherapy, with the addition of radiation for advanced disease. Wilm tumors carry an 80% cure rate.

N. **Melanoma.** Melanoma is familial in approximately 10% of cases, and in these cases it is often associated with multiple atypical moles. **Familial atypical multiple-mole melanoma syndrome (FAMMM)** has also been called *dysplastic nevus syndrome, B-K syndrome,* and *large atypical nevus syndrome.* A National Institutes of Health Consensus Conference defined FAMMM using these criteria: (1) the occurrence of malignant melanoma in one or more first- or second-degree relatives; (2) a large number of melanocytic nevi, usually more than 50, some of which are atypical and variable in size; and (3) melanocytic nevi that have certain histopathologic features, including an architectural disorder with asymmetry, subepidermal fibroplasia, and lentiginous melanocytic hyperplasia with spindle or epithelial melanocyte nests. The lesions predominantly occur on the trunk but are also found on the buttocks, scalp, and lower extremities. The relative risk for developing melanoma when multiple atypical moles are present ranges from 5 to 11 based on multiple studies. The median age for melanoma diagnosis is 34. *CDKN2*, a cell cycle protein gene, has been found to contain germline mutations in some kindreds with familial melanoma (*Nat Genet* 1994;8:15).

Other malignancies have been related to mutations in the *CDKN2* gene, especially pancreatic cancer. There may be other genes contributing to FAMMM. **Screening** for FAMMM begins at around puberty and consists of yearly physical examinations, including a total body skin examination. For patients who have a large number of moles, baseline photographs or computerized scanning are helpful. Patients should examine their own skin regularly. Suspicious lesions should undergo biopsy. Sun exposure should be avoided. Regular ophthalmologic examinations should be performed due to the increased risk of ocular nevi and ocular melanoma.

III. **Genetic testing and counseling.** A detailed family history should be taken on all patients with cancer. An inherited cancer syndrome should be suspected if the same cancer affects several close relatives, if the cancer occurs at an earlier age than sporadic cases, or if the cancer is bilateral. A family pedigree helps identify potential gene carriers and guides counseling and testing. Genetic counselors complement surgeons in the discussion of test results and can aid in reviewing limitations, confidentiality, and therapeutic options in a nonbiased manner. In an evaluation of the use of the commercial *APC* gene test, more than 30% of physicians misinterpreted the test results (*N Engl J Med* 1997;336:823). Genetic counselors should be consulted about any patient who has undergone genetic testing. In order for patients to make informed decisions regarding their care and therapy, the oncology team, including genetic counselors, must address not only the medical and therapeutic goals of treatment but also the social and ethical concerns of the patient, which in many circumstances is a more challenging task.

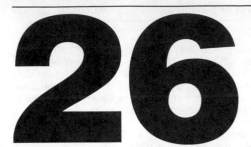

Endocrine Surgery

Alliric I. Willis and
Bruce L. Hall

THYROID

The thyroid gland develops from the endoderm of the primitive foregut, arises in the ventral pharynx in the region of the base of the tongue, and descends into the neck. This course of descent of the thyroid is the embryological reason for the pyramidal lobe and findings such as thyroglossal duct cysts and undescended thyroid at the base of the tongue. The parafollicular cells, or C cells, are derived from the neural crest and migrate to the thyroid. The thyroid is stimulated to release thyroid hormone in response to thyroid-stimulating hormone (TSH) from the anterior pituitary gland, which is stimulated by thyrotropin-releasing hormone (TRH) from the hypothalamus. Thyroid hormone synthesis begins when dietary iodide is ingested, actively transported into the thyroid gland, and then oxidized by thyroid peroxidase into iodine. Iodinization of tyrosine results in monoiodotyrosine (MIT) and diiodotyrosine (DIT). Iodine coupling of MIT and DIT results in the formation of T_3 and T_4, which are bound to thyroglobulin while in the thyroid. Upon release into plasma, the majority of T_3 and T_4 are bound to thyroid-binding globulin (TBG). Only the unbound or "free" hormones are active (i.e., available to tissues).

I. **Evaluation of thyroid disorders**
A. **Clinical features of hyperthyroidism** reflect increased catabolism and excessive sympathetic activity caused by excess circulating thyroid hormones. Symptoms of hyperthyroidism include weight loss despite normal or increased appetite, heat intolerance, excessive perspiration, anxiety, irritability, palpitations, fatigue, muscle weakness, and oligomenorrhea. Signs of hyperthyroidism include goiter, sinus tachycardia or atrial fibrillation, tremor, hyperreflexia, fine or thinning hair, thyroid bruit, and muscle wasting. The presentation of hyperthyroidism can vary considerably with age: Young patients usually present with hypermetabolism, whereas older patients may present primarily with tachyarrhythmias or cardiac failure. Rarely, elderly patients experience only wasting, apathy, confusion, or depression (apathetic hyperthyroidism). **Clinical features of hypothyroidism** include cold intolerance, weight gain, constipation, edema (especially of the eyelids, hands, and feet), dry skin, dry and thinning hair, weakness, somnolence, and menorrhagia.
B. **Biochemical thyroid function testing** confirms clinically suspected abnormalities in thyroid function; however, test results must be interpreted in the context of clinical findings. The introduction of sensitive thyrotropin assays has transformed thyroid function testing from strategies based on thyroxine (T_4) to strategies based on thyroid-stimulating hormone (TSH) (*Mayo Clin Proc* 1994;69:469). Currently, measurement of serum TSH level and free T_4 (FT_4) is the best and most efficient combination of blood tests for diagnosis of most patients with thyroid disorders.
1. Measurement of **TSH** (0.3 to 5.0 mIU/L) by a second-generation sensitive TSH (sTSH) test is the single most useful biochemical test in the diagnosis of thyroid illness. **In most ambulatory and hospitalized patients without pituitary disease, increased TSH signifies hypothyroidism, suppressed TSH suggests hyperthyroidism, and normal TSH reflects a euthyroid state.** Of note, critically ill, hospitalized patients, especially those receiving drugs such as dopamine or glucocorticoids,

may have transient changes in TSH (usually elevated) without true abnormalities in thyroid function.

2. Assessment of T_4 concentration corroborates identified abnormalities in TSH and provides an index of severity of thyroid dysfunction. **Total T_4** (3 to 12 μg/dL) measurements quantify bound and unbound hormone and do not directly reflect the small "free" or active T_4 fractions. Factors that increase the thyroxine-binding globulin (TBG) concentration (estrogens, pregnancy, liver disease) may elevate the total T_4 or triiodothyronine (T_3) despite a normal free hormone concentration and a euthyroid state. Androgens, severe hypoproteinemia, chronic liver disease, and acromegaly result in decreased TBG.

3. **The FT_4 index** [FT_4I = total T_4 × RT_3U (RT_3U is the resin T_3 uptake)] (0.85 to 3.50) correlates more closely with the level of FT_4, eliminates ambiguity introduced by altered thyroglobulin levels, and is the preferred test for estimating FT_4.

4. **The resin T_3 uptake (RT_3U)** (20% to 40%) test measures unoccupied thyroid hormone–binding sites on TBG by allowing radiolabeled T_3 to compete for binding between TBG and a resin. This assay provides an indirect measure of FT_4. In patients with hyperthyroidism, the resin uptake is elevated because most of the sites on TBG are occupied by T_4 so that more radioactive T_3 binds to the resin. The RT_3U is directly related to the FT_4 fraction and inversely related to the TBG binding sites.

5. **Measurement of T_3** (80 to 200 ng/dL) is unreliable as a test for hypothyroidism. This test is useful in the occasional patient with suspected hyperthyroidism, suppressed sTSH, and normal FT_4I (T_3 thyrotoxicosis).

6. **Antithyroid microsomal antibodies** are found in the serum of patients with autoimmune thyroiditis (Hashimoto thyroiditis), and measurement of these antibodies is helpful for diagnosing this common cause of hypothyroidism. **Anti-TSH receptor antibodies**, which stimulate the TSH receptor, are detectable in more than 90% of patients with autoimmune hyperthyroidism (Graves disease); however, their measurement is not often needed in the diagnosis of this disease.

7. A useful **thyroid function test algorithm** (*Clin Lab Med* 1993;13:673) includes TSH assay as the initial test. If this is normal, no further tests are needed. If TSH is elevated, FT_4I and microsomal antibodies are measured to confirm hypothyroidism, which is often autoimmune. If TSH is suppressed, FT_4I is measured to confirm primary hyperthyroidism. If TSH is low and FT_4I is normal, T_3 is measured to diagnose T_3 thyrotoxicosis.

C. **Thyroid imaging** is most often accomplished with radionuclide scanning or ultrasound; other imaging modes, including computed tomography (CT) and MR scan, are useful in special circumstances.

1. **Technetium thyroid scanning** 20 minutes after the intravenous injection of technetium-99m (^{99m}Tc) is useful in determining the size of the thyroid and in differentiating solitary functioning nodules from multinodular goiter or Graves disease. Hypofunctioning areas (cyst, neoplasm, or suppressed tissue adjacent to autonomous nodules) are "cold" whereas areas of increased synthesis are "hot." Thyroid scans cannot differentiate benign from malignant thyroid nodules. Cold nodules have a 15% to 20% risk of malignancy; hence, most should be removed. Hot nodules are almost never malignant. ^{99m}Tc thyroid scans are most useful as adjunctive tests to assess risk of malignancy in patients with indeterminate thyroid nodule cytology discovered by fine-needle aspiration (FNA) or in hyperthyroid patients suspected of having a hyperfunctioning thyroid adenoma. Thyroid scanning 4 to 24 hours after administration of oral iodine-131 (^{131}I) is useful for identifying metastatic

differentiated thyroid tumors and for both confirming a diagnosis of Graves disease and predicting a response to ^{131}I radioablation.

2. **Thyroid ultrasonography** with high-frequency (7.5 to 10.0 MHz) transducers accurately determines gland volume as well as the number and character of thyroid nodules (*Am J Med* 1995;99:642). Although not completely reliable, features suggestive of malignancy on ultrasound include hypoechoic pattern, incomplete peripheral halo, irregular margins, and microcalcifications. Ultrasound is useful for guiding FNA biopsy and cyst aspiration. Cysts seen on ultrasound, especially those larger than 3 cm, are malignant in up to 14% of cases. Ultrasound followed by FNA of abnormalities larger than 1 cm is the most common imaging and diagnostic algorithm.

3. **CT scanning and MR scan** of the thyroid are costly and generally are reserved for assessing substernal or retrosternal masses suspected to be goiters.

II. **Specific thyroid disorders**

A. Autoimmune diffuse toxic goiter (**Graves disease**) is the most common cause of hyperthyroidism and may be caused by stimulating immunoglobulins directed against the TSH receptor. Graves disease may be treated with antithyroid drugs, ablation with radioactive iodine (RAI), or surgery, depending on the clinical situation.

1. **Ablation with RAI is the treatment of choice for most patients with Graves disease.** A dose of 5 to 10 mCi of ^{131}I is given orally and is 75% effective after 4 to 12 weeks. In the 25% of patients with persistent thyrotoxicosis after 12 weeks, double the initial dose is repeated. After treatment, there is a high incidence (70%) of eventual permanent hypothyroidism, which is managed easily by replacement therapy. There are virtually no other long-term side effects of RAI (i.e., no significantly increased risk of thyroid cancer, leukemia, or teratogenicity). Contraindications to radiotherapy include pregnant women, newborns, patients who refuse, or patients with low RAI uptake (<20%) in the thyroid. Treatment of children or young adults (<30 years) with RAI is controversial because of presumed long-term oncogenic risks.

2. Thionamide drugs, such as **propylthiouracil (PTU) or methimazole,** are used for antithyroid drug therapy. PTU (100 to 300 mg orally 3 times daily) is given for 4 to 6 weeks until the patient becomes euthyroid; then the dosage usually is decreased (100 mg orally 3 times daily). The patient is then treated empirically for 6 to 18 months, at which time the drugs are withdrawn. Clinical features that favor remission include small gland size and mild hypothyroidism. However, overall, long-term remission is achieved in less than 20% to 30% of patients. Antithyroid drugs also are used to prepare thyrotoxic patients for surgery or ablative therapy. PTU may be given during pregnancy at reduced doses, especially if thyroidectomy is necessary in the second trimester. Minor adverse reactions occur infrequently and include rash, hepatitis, arthralgias, and a lupuslike syndrome. Agranulocytosis is a rare (0.5%) but serious side effect of thionamide therapy.

3. **Thyroidectomy for Graves disease** may be indicated for children and adolescents, pregnant women (late second or early third trimester), patients unresponsive to or noncompliant with medical therapy, and patients who refuse RAI. One surgical option is bilateral subtotal thyroidectomy, performed with the goal of leaving a 1- to 2-g vascularized cuff of thyroid on each side. However, some centers advocate total thyroidectomy as primary treatment to decrease the recurrence rate of goitrous disease. Risks of surgery are extremely small (<1%) in experienced hands but include hypoparathyroidism and injury to the recurrent laryngeal nerve. Surgery usually results in hypothyroidism. The long-term incidence of recurrent hyperthyroidism after surgery is

approximately 10% but depends on amount of tissue left behind. Patients with recurrent hyperthyroidism after thyroidectomy should be considered for treatment with RAI, since reoperation carries a somewhat higher risk of complication.

B. In **multinodular goiter,** a large goiter or retrosternal extension can compress the trachea. Subtotal or total thyroidectomy is the treatment of choice if there are symptoms of compression, suspicion of malignancy, or questionable nodules or if the gland is cosmetically bothersome.

C. Toxic adenoma is an autonomously functioning thyroid nodule that produces hyperthyroidism and is treated by surgical excision (thyroid lobectomy) or RAI.

D. Rare causes of hyperthyroidism include self-administration of excessive thyroid hormone (factitious hyperthyroidism), iodine-induced hyperthyroidism, pituitary TSH-secreting adenoma, trophoblastic tumors secreting chorionic gonadotropin (which has TSH-like activity), struma ovarii, and thyroiditis.

III. Hypothyroidism is almost always caused by primary hypofunction of the thyroid gland. Clinically, hypothyroid patients should be separated into those without goiter (primary atrophy), those with goitrous hypothyroidism (i.e., Hashimoto thyroiditis, drug-induced hypothyroidism, iodine deficiency, and congenital causes of dyshormonogenesis), and those with postablative hypothyroidism (after thyroidectomy or treatment with RAI). Postablative hypothyroidism and Hashimoto thyroiditis are the most important causes of hypothyroidism encountered by the surgeon. Diagnosis rests on the characteristic clinical features and laboratory findings of an elevated TSH (usually >15 units/mL) and a decreased FT_4 level. A low TSH in association with low T_4 suggests pituitary or hypothalamic failure.

IV. Thyroiditis represents a diverse group of autoimmune and inflammatory disorders characterized by infiltration of the thyroid with inflammatory cells and subsequent fibrosis of the gland.

A. Hashimoto thyroiditis is a chronic autoimmune disorder characterized by destructive lymphocytic infiltration of the thyroid. The disease is 15 times more common in women, and more than 90% of patients have circulating antibodies directed against thyroid microsomes and thyroglobulin. Although patients initially are euthyroid, hypothyroidism may occur later. A firm symmetric or asymmetric goiter is palpable and usually (but not always) nontender. Cervical lymphadenopathy is uncommon. Euthyroid patients may not require treatment. Thyroid hormone is given to hypothyroid patients both as replacement therapy and to suppress TSH. Thyroidectomy is indicated for compressive symptoms, for a dominant nodule suspicious for malignancy, or for cosmetic preference.

B. Acute suppurative thyroiditis is rare and is caused by infection with *Streptococcus* or *Staphylococcus* species. Treatment consists of appropriate antibiotic therapy and surgical drainage of abscesses.

C. Subacute (de Quervain) thyroiditis is a rare condition that occurs in young women, often after a viral upper respiratory tract infection. Symptoms of fatigue, weakness, and painful thyroid enlargement radiating to the patient's jaw or ear are treated with nonsteroidal anti-inflammatory drugs or with steroids. The condition almost always remits spontaneously within a few weeks. Thyroidectomy may be indicated in rare cases of persistent thyroiditis after months of unsuccessful steroid treatment.

D. Riedel thyroiditis is a rare, progressive inflammatory condition of the entire thyroid gland, strap muscles, and other neck structures. Its cause is unknown, and it can be associated with other fibrotic processes, including retroperitoneal fibrosis, sclerosing cholangitis, and fibrosing mediastinitis. The lymphocytic infiltrate and dense fibrous tissue reaction in the thyroid result in a firm, nontender goiter with a woody texture. Riedel's thyroiditis may require surgical excision to exclude malignancy or relieve compressive symptoms.

V. **A solitary thyroid nodule** commonly occurs (4% to 7% of adults) and is usually a benign lesion. Such nodules may be associated with a multinodular goiter or with an otherwise normal thyroid. The malignant potential of the newly discovered thyroid nodule is of justifiable concern to both physician and patient, and the goal of diagnostic testing is to separate the relatively few patients with thyroid malignancy from the larger group of patients with benign thyroid nodules. Surgical intervention is appropriate for all malignant or suspicious thyroid nodules. The frequency of cancer in surgically excised nodules is 8% to 17% (*N Engl J Med* 1993;328:553).

A. **History and physical examination** are invaluable in the management of the thyroid nodule. Nodules in the very young and very old (especially men) are more likely to be malignant. Exposure to ionizing radiation increases the incidence of both benign and malignant thyroid nodules and is a well-recognized risk factor for the development of thyroid carcinoma. A family history of thyroid malignancy, familial polyposis, or other endocrine disease also increases the risk of cancer. Rapid nodule growth, pain, compressive symptoms, or hoarseness of voice increase the likelihood of malignancy but are nonspecific. Physical findings of a solitary nodule with firm or irregular texture or with fixation to surrounding structures suggest malignancy. Similarly, the presence of enlarged cervical lymph nodes is extremely important because this finding is highly indicative of thyroid cancer. Malignancy is uncommon in hyperfunctioning nodules, and all patients should have a serum TSH measured to exclude clinical or subclinical thyrotoxicosis.

B. **FNA** is the initial diagnostic test of choice for the euthyroid patient with a solitary thyroid nodule. This procedure is safe, inexpensive, and easy to perform, and it allows better selection of patients for operation than does any other technique (*Ann Intern Med* 1993;118:282).

1. **The technique of FNA** involves palpation of the nodule, aspiration of sufficient material, and adequate preparation and staining of a smear of the aspirated cells. The equipment required includes a 25-gauge hypodermic needle, a 10-mL syringe, and a syringe holder (e.g., Cameco Ltd., London), which allows operation with a single hand. The thyroid gland is palpated with the patient supine and his or her neck slightly extended. The operator stands on the side opposite the lobe to be aspirated and immobilizes the nodule between the index and middle fingers of his or her nondominant hand. The overlying skin is cleansed with povidone-iodine or alcohol. No local anesthetic is required. The needle is introduced into the nodule, then either the piston of the syringe is retracted to create suction or material is allowed to pass into the syringe by passive action to minimize blood in the specimen. The needle tip can be gently angled in multiple directions within the nodule, again in an attempt to avoid excess trauma and bloody specimen. Before removing the needle, the suction is released to prevent aspiration of the needle contents into the syringe. Then the needle is detached, and air is introduced into the syringe before aspirated cells are expressed onto a slide. The smear is air-dried and stained using the May-Grünwald-Giemsa method, or it is alcohol-fixed and stained using the Papanicolaou method. Usually, two or three passes are made to limit sampling error. Ultrasound-guided FNA is useful when lesions are small or difficult to palpate.

2. Cytologic **results of FNA** can be benign, malignant, or indeterminate, provided that an adequate specimen is obtained (an adequate specimen has at least 10 groups of well-preserved follicular cells, with 10 cells per group, obtained from two separate needle passes). The accuracy of the results ranges from 70% to 90% and is highly dependent on the skill and experience of the cytopathologist. The false-negative rate of FNA is low (<6%), and patients with negative (i.e., not cancerous or indeterminate) cytology can be followed safely (*Surgery* 1989;106:980). Indeterminate aspirations pose difficult management decisions because carcinoma

occurs in 10% to 30% of these cases. Follicular and Hürthle cell neoplasms and the follicular variant of papillary cancer account for many indeterminate results, whereas papillary, medullary, and undifferentiated thyroid carcinomas usually have distinctive cytopathologic features. Diagnostic thyroid lobectomy is indicated for all FNA-indeterminate and FNA-positive thyroid nodules and for all nodules, regardless of FNA result, in patients with a history of radiation exposure. An inadequate FNA biopsy is obtained in up to 20% of cases; half of these can be diagnosed with repeated aspiration. The management of nodules with persistently inadequate FNA should be guided by clinical criteria.

C. **Radionuclide thyroid scans** detect areas of active or decreased thyroid hormone synthesis but do not provide information that allows clear separation of benign and malignant nodules. Approximately 20% of nodules that are hypofunctioning ("cold") on thyroid scintiscan are malignant, but the majority are benign. Hyperfunctioning ("hot") nodules carry a low risk of malignancy, but exceptions occur. Thyroid scanning may be useful in patients with indeterminate FNA cytology because, in such patients, hyperfunctioning nodules almost always are benign.

D. **Ultrasonography** is a sensitive method for determining whether a lesion is solid or cystic, but it cannot distinguish reliably between benign and malignant nodules. Although thyroid cysts have a lower likelihood of being malignant, larger carcinomas can undergo cystic degeneration. Cysts may disappear after FNA, but those that persist, recur, or yield insufficient material for interpretation should be excised.

E. **Thyroid lobectomy** is indicated for (1) nodules with malignant or indeterminate aspiration cytology, (2) nodules in children, (3) nodules in patients with either a history of neck irradiation or a family history of thyroid cancer, and (4) symptomatic or cosmetically bothersome nodules.

VI. **Thyroid neoplasms**

A. **Differentiated (papillary and follicular) thyroid cancer** is among the most curable of human cancers (*N Engl J Med* 1998;338:297). These cancers are rare in children and increase in frequency with age; the female to male ratio is approximately 2.5:1.0. The cause of these cancers is unknown, but childhood exposure to radiation (10 to 1,500 cGy) is the best-known etiologic factor. Approximately 30% of exposed children develop thyroid nodules, and of these, an estimated 30% are malignant. The appropriate initial procedure for a solitary thyroid nodule suspected of being malignant is a total lobectomy and isthmectomy. Controversy exists about the extent of surgery (lobectomy versus total thyroidectomy) that should be performed for patients with proven differentiated thyroid cancer, principally because these patients have a good prognosis irrespective of the surgical treatment. The prognosis depends mostly on the patient's age as well as the extent and histologic subtype of the disease. Several prognostic index systems have been developed, including the MACIS (*m*etastasis, *a*ge, completeness of resection, *i*nvasion, and *s*ize) and the tumor, node, metastasis classification adjusted for patient age. In all, 85% to 90% of patients fall into a low-risk category with favorable prognosis.

1. **Papillary thyroid carcinoma (PTC)** represents 85% of thyroid carcinomas and occurs in any age group, especially children and women younger than 40 years. PTC is often multifocal and frequently metastasizes to cervical lymph nodes. Occult, clinically insignificant foci of microscopic PTC are found in 4% to 28% of autopsies or in thyroidectomy specimens for benign diseases. A young age at diagnosis is a favorable prognostic factor, and even involvement of cervical nodes does not affect the prognosis adversely. Total thyroidectomy is appropriate for patients with gross evidence of bilateral disease, multifocal PTC, or a history of neck irradiation. Total thyroidectomy is arguably the treatment of choice for unilateral tumors larger than 1.0 to 1.5 cm. Advantages of

total thyroidectomy include the ability to treat extrathyroidal metastases or recurrences with RAI and to use serum thyroglobulin to monitor therapy. Retrospective studies also show a decreased risk of recurrence or death. Complications of total thyroidectomy include hypoparathyroidism and recurrent laryngeal nerve (RLN) injury, which occur in less than 1% of cases. Prophylactic neck dissection is not indicated for PTC, but a modified ipsilateral, central neck dissection is indicated for patients with palpable metastases in cervical nodes. Studies have been reported on the successful use of sentinel lymph node biopsy in patients with papillary thyroid cancer to guide regional lymph node dissection, and these demonstrate very high levels of concordance between sentinel node status and final regional node status as well as between intraoperative frozen section diagnosis and permanent section diagnosis (*Cancer* 2001;92:2868–2874). Radioablation of residual thyroid tissue or metastatic or residual cancer is performed with 75 to 100 mCi of ^{131}I 4 weeks after total thyroidectomy while the patient is hypothyroid (i.e., **TSH >30 μlU/mL** on no replacement of T_4). As demonstrated in a published study from our institution, radioablation therapy may be further streamlined since TSH >30 can be achieved in most patients 1 to 3 weeks after discontinuing thyroxine (*J Nucl Med* 2004;45:567–570). Thyroid replacement may be resumed for 3 to 6 months and then discontinued for 1 month before obtaining a second ^{131}I scintiscan to test for remaining functional thyroid tissue. Ablation may be repeated at higher doses if the scan is positive. Long-term suppression therapy with T_4 decreases recurrences and may improve survival.

2. **Follicular thyroid carcinoma** (10% of thyroid carcinomas) is rare before age 30 years and has a slightly worse prognosis than PTC. Unlike PTC, follicular thyroid cancer spreads hematogenously to bone, lung, or liver, either at the time of diagnosis or years after resection. Small (<1.0 cm), unilateral follicular carcinomas with limited invasion of the tumor capsule or limited spread along blood vessels may be treated with thyroid lobectomy, whereas larger tumors (>1.0 cm), multicentric tumors, and tumors with more extensive invasion or distant metastases are treated with total thyroidectomy. Radioablation is indicated after total thyroidectomy, followed by lifelong thyroid hormone suppression.

B. **Medullary thyroid carcinoma (MTC)** arises from the thyroid C cells that derive from the neural crest and secrete calcitonin. MTC may occur sporadically or may be inherited, either alone or as a component of multiple endocrine neoplasia (MEN) types 2A or 2B. Sporadic MTC usually is detected as a firm, palpable, unilateral nodule with or without involved cervical lymph nodes. Patients with hereditary MTC develop bilateral, multifocal tumors and often are diagnosed on the basis of family screening. MTC should be suspected if tumor calcification is noted on plain x-rays or if the patient has profuse diarrhea and episodic flushing (caused by excess calcitonin release). MTC spreads early to cervical lymph nodes and may metastasize to liver, lungs, or bone. All patients with suspected or known MTC should have a careful family history taken, be tested biochemically for pheochromocytoma before thyroidectomy, and be genetically tested for DNA mutations in the tyrosine kinase receptor *RET* proto-oncogene (*Hum Mol Genet* 1993;2:851).

1. **The biochemical diagnosis** of MTC is made by demonstration of an elevated plasma calcitonin level after the intravenous administration of calcium and pentagastrin. The patient should fast overnight. A peripheral 21-gauge "butterfly" intravenous line connected to a three-way stopcock is started to provide a simple and rapid way to administer medicines and draw blood samples. Blood is drawn before and at 1, 2, 3, and 5 minutes after the intravenous administration of calcium gluconate (2 mg/kg over 1 minute) and pentagastrin (0.5 μg/kg over 5 seconds). Plasma calcitonin is measured by radioimmunoassay.

Stimulated calcitonin testing is also a sensitive way to detect residual or recurrent MTC postoperatively.

2. **Treatment** of MTC is total thyroidectomy with removal of the lymph nodes in the central zone of the patient's neck (from the sternal notch to the hyoid bone and laterally to the carotid sheaths). A modified neck dissection is indicated for clinically involved ipsilateral cervical lymph nodes. Of patients with persistently elevated calcitonin levels after initial thyroidectomy, 28% had normalized early postoperative calcitonin levels after a subsequent meticulous bilateral microdissection of cervical lymph nodes (*Surgery* 1993;114:1090). There are no proven systemic chemotherapy options for MTC; however, *in vitro* research has demonstrated inhibition of MTC cell growth and RET tyrosine kinase activity resulting from treatment with tyrosine kinase inhibitors (*Surgery* 2004:132:960–966).

C. **Undifferentiated or anaplastic thyroid carcinoma** (1% to 2% of thyroid carcinomas) carries an extremely poor prognosis; usually presents as a fixed, sometimes painful goiter; and usually occurs in patients older than 50 years. Invasion of local structures, with resultant dysphagia, respiratory compromise, or hoarseness due to recurrent laryngeal nerve involvement, can preclude curative resection. External irradiation or chemotherapy may provide limited palliation.

D. **Primary malignant lymphoma of the thyroid** often is associated with Hashimoto thyroiditis. Radiotherapy is the treatment of choice for disease confined to the patient's neck, and radical surgical resection is not indicated once a diagnosis is made. Compressive symptoms usually respond rapidly to radiotherapy.

VII. **Postoperative thyroid hormone replacement** is necessary after total or near total thyroidectomy or ablation with radioiodine. Oral levothyroxine is begun before discharge at an average dose of 100 μg per day (0.8 μg/lb per day). Adequacy of thyroid hormone replacement is assessed by measuring T_4 and TSH at 6 to 12 weeks after surgery. Adjustments to the dose should not be more frequent than monthly in the absence of symptoms and should be cautious (12.5- to 25.0-μg increments).

VIII. **Management of complications after thyroidectomy**
A. **Hemorrhage** is a rare but serious complication of thyroidectomy that usually occurs within 6 hours of surgery. Management can require control of the airway by endotracheal intubation and, rarely, can require urgent opening of incision and evacuation of hematoma before return to the operating room for wound irrigation and ligation of the bleeding point.

B. **Transient hypocalcemia** commonly occurs 24 to 48 hours after thyroidectomy but infrequently requires treatment. Patients who are markedly symptomatic or who have serum calcium below 7 mg/dL are given 1 to 2 ampules (10 to 20 mL) of 10% calcium gluconate intravenously over 1 to 2 minutes, followed by temporary oral calcium carbonate (500 mg orally 3 times a day). More prolonged intravenous replacement is achieved by mixing 6 ampules of 10% calcium gluconate (540 mg elemental calcium) in D5W, 500 mL, for infusion at 1 mL/kg per hour. Permanent hypoparathyroidism is uncommon after total thyroidectomy. Normal parathyroid tissue removed or devascularized at the time of total thyroidectomy may be autotransplanted into sternocleidomastoid muscle to prevent postoperative hypocalcemia (*Ann Surg* 1996;223:472).

C. **Recurrent laryngeal nerve (RLN) injury** is a devastating complication of thyroidectomy that should occur rarely (<1%). Unilateral RLN injury causes hoarseness, and bilateral injury compromises the airway, necessitating tracheostomy. Repeat neck exploration, thyroidectomy for extensive goiter or Graves disease, and thyroidectomy for fixed, locally invasive cancers are procedures particularly prone to RLN injury. Intentional (as with locally invasive cancer) or inadvertent transection of the RLN can be repaired primarily or with a nerve graft, although the efficacy of these repairs is not known. Temporary RLN palsies can occur during thyroidectomy, and these usually resolve over a period of 4 to 6 weeks. The **external branch of the superior laryngeal nerve** may be injured if not identified during ligation of the superior thyroid pole vascular bundle. This injury results in weakness of the patient's voice at high pitch. The best prevention of these injuries is a thorough understanding of the anatomy of these nerves.

PARATHYROID

I. **Hyperparathyroidism (HPT)** refers to hypercalcemia caused by inappropriate parathyroid hormone (PTH) release from the parathyroid glands. Primary HPT results from autonomous release of PTH from parathyroid adenoma or hyperplastic parathyroid glands. Secondary HPT results from a defect in mineral homeostasis (e.g., renal failure), with a compensatory increase in parathyroid function. Tertiary HPT results from the development of autonomous, calcium-insensitive parathyroids after prolonged secondary stimulation (e.g., prolonged renal failure).

A. **Primary HPT**

1. **Incidence.** Primary HPT has an incidence of 0.25 to 1.00 per 1,000 population in the United States and is especially common in postmenopausal women. It most often occurs sporadically, but it can be inherited alone or as a component of familial endocrinopathies, including MEN types 1 and 2A.

2. The more common **clinical findings associated with HPT** include nephrolithiasis, osteoporosis, hypertension, and emotional disturbances. The widespread use of the multichannel autoanalyzer has led to more patients being diagnosed with **"asymptomatic" hypercalcemia** or with earlier symptoms, such as muscle weakness, polyuria, anorexia, and nausea. When they are carefully questioned, many patients with HPT turn out to be symptomatic.

3. **Differential diagnosis of hypercalcemia** includes HPT, malignancy, granulomatous disease (e.g., sarcoidosis), immobility, hyperthyroidism, milk-alkali syndrome, and familial hypocalciuric hypercalcemia (FHH). Patients with hypercalcemia and suspected HPT at a minimum should have their serum calcium, phosphate, creatinine, and PTH measured. The diagnosis of HPT is biochemical and requires demonstration of hypercalcemia (serum calcium >10.5 mg/dL) and an elevated PTH level. Currently, the assay of choice for PTH is the highly sensitive and specific intact PTH level radioimmunoassay. Free calcium level (ionized calcium) is a more sensitive test of physiologically active calcium and is the test of choice for hypercalcemia. Hypercalcemia without an elevated PTH can be due to a variety of causes (especially malignancy, Paget disease, sarcoidosis, and milk-alkali syndrome) that must be excluded. Serum alkaline phosphatase is elevated in 10% to 40% of patients with HPT, and serum phosphate is decreased in 50% of patients with HPT if renal function is normal. Elevated PTH promotes bicarbonate excretion, causing hyperchloremic metabolic acidosis; the chloride-phosphate ratio exceeds 33 in 96% of patients with HPT (*Ann Intern Med* 1974;80:200). Radiographic features of HPT are seen in advanced cases and include decreased bone density, osteitis fibrosa cystica, and the pathognomonic sign of subperiosteal bone resorption on the radial aspect of the phalanges of the second or third digits of the hand.

4. **Preoperative localization** of parathyroid adenomas is generally not necessary before a careful neck exploration by an experienced endocrine surgeon, as stated by the 1991 National Institutes of Health consensus conference. However, current practice makes use of several techniques to facilitate limited neck exploration to ensure a high success rate and optimal cosmesis in the outpatient setting. These techniques

include radio- and/or image-guided exploration (sestamibi- or ultrasound-guided), videoscopic exploration, and intraoperative intact PTH level monitoring (*Surgery* 1997;122:1107). The most frequently applied approach is preoperative sestamibi scanning, followed by direct excision of the scan-identified gland and confirmation of cure by intraoperative PTH measurement. This intraoperative test requires the availability of a rapid assay of intact PTH, which confirms the success of the surgery immediately if the PTH level falls more than 50% 10 minutes after the apparent source of PTH has been removed. If the preoperative localization scan is not informative, then the standard full neck exploration is appropriate.

5. **Parathyroidectomy is indicated** for all patients with symptomatic HPT. Nephrolithiasis, bone disease, and neuromuscular symptoms are improved more often than renal insufficiency, hypertension, and psychiatric symptoms. Parathyroidectomy for asymptomatic IIPT is somewhat controversial. A recent large prospective study of patients with asymptomatic HPT found that 27% developed symptoms of hypercalcemia with 10-year follow-up (*N Engl J Med* 1999;341:1249). Accepted indications include markedly elevated serum calcium, hypercalcemic crisis, reduced creatinine clearance, asymptomatic kidney stones, markedly elevated urinary calcium excretion, and advanced osteoporosis. Close observation is required for patients not treated surgically.

6. **Neck exploration and parathyroidectomy** for HPT result in normocalcemia in more than 95% of patients when performed by an experienced surgeon without any preoperative or intraoperative localization studies. The neck is exposed through a transverse cervical incision. The patient is typically under general anesthesia, although current localization techniques increasingly allow the use of local or regional anesthesia. A thorough, orderly search and identification of all four parathyroid glands are the cornerstones of the standard surgical management of HPT. Parathyroid glands are red-brown to yellow and flat or oval, with a characteristic vascular architecture; however, it may be difficult to distinguish them from fat or lymphoid tissue. Superior parathyroid glands develop from the fourth pharyngeal pouch and most commonly are located dorsally along the middle or upper thyroid lobe, near the intersection of the inferior thyroid artery and recurrent laryngeal nerve, dorsal to the nerve. Ectopic superior glands usually are found posteriorly in the tracheoesophageal groove or cranial to the superior thyroid pole, or rarely in the posterior mediastinum. Inferior parathyroid glands develop in conjunction with the thymus from the third pharyngeal pouch, are more variable in position than are the superior glands, and usually are located ventral to the recurrent laryngeal nerve at the inferior pole of the thyroid lobe within the thyrothymic ligament. Ectopic inferior glands are most likely found embedded in the thymus in the anterior mediastinum. The parathyroid gland is normally about 3 mm by 6 mm and weighs 25 to 40 mg. Determination that a parathyroid gland is abnormally enlarged is best made by the surgeon at the time of operation and not by hypercellularity or other features on histologic examination. Most often, a single adenomatous gland is found; the other, normal parathyroid glands should be left in place. Routine biopsy of normal parathyroid glands is expensive, risks devascularization of the glands, and is not routinely necessary. Occasionally, multiple parathyroid adenomas are found, which should be removed, leaving at least one normal parathyroid behind. Management of four-gland parathyroid hyperplasia is controversial and may include total parathyroidectomy and parathyroid autotransplantation or 3.5-gland parathyroidectomy. **The dictation of a clear, factual operative note detailing the identification and position of each parathyroid gland is essential.** This information is invaluable in the unlikely event of reoperation for persistent or recurrent HPT.

7. **Familial primary HPT** may occur alone or as a component of MEN type 1 and type 2A. HPT in these syndromes is primarily chief cell hyperplasia and variable enlargement of all four glands. These patients have a higher incidence of recurrent or persistent hypercalcemia after parathyroidectomy. Familial benign hypocalciuric hypercalcemia (FHH) is an autosomal dominant form of HPT in which affected family members have mild hypercalcemia, hypocalciuria (urinary excretion of <100 mg of calcium daily), and hypomagnesemia and rarely develop renal or bone complications (*J Pediatr* 1972;17:1060). Parathyroidectomy is ineffective for FHH.

B. Hypercalcemia from **secondary and tertiary HPT** is treated initially with dietary phosphate restriction, phosphate binders, and vitamin D supplementation. Patients with medically unresponsive, symptomatic HPT (e.g., bone pain and osteopenia, ectopic calcification, or pruritus) may be surgically treated with total parathyroidectomy and heterotopic autotransplantation.

II. **Reoperative parathyroid surgery** may be necessary for persistent or recurrent HPT. In all cases, HPT must be reconfirmed biochemically, and 24-hour urinary calcium should be obtained to exclude FHH. Preoperative localization is mandatory and includes careful review of the operative note from the initial surgery and concordant noninvasive studies. Approximately 70% to 80% of patients undergoing reexploration after an initial failed operation have a missed gland that is accessible through a cervical incision. Reoperative parathyroid surgery carries a substantially higher risk of injury to the recurrent laryngeal nerve and of hypocalcemia due to postoperative scarring and disruption of normal tissue planes.

A. **Preoperative localization** of the hyperfunctioning parathyroid should be attempted in nearly all reoperative cases by ^{99m}Tc-sestamibi scintigraphy and ultrasound or CT scanning. These noninvasive studies are successful in localizing the missed gland in 25% to 75% of cases (*Radiology* 1987;162:133). With combined use of CT scan, ultrasonography, and scintigraphy, at least one imaging study identifies the tumor in more than 75% of patients. Noninvasive localizing studies must be interpreted in the context of the operative note. Invasive imaging tests, including angiography, are associated with greater morbidity and measurable mortality; they should be reserved for complex cases with negative or equivocal noninvasive studies. The success of these tests in localizing the concealed tumor is highly dependent on the skill and experience of the radiologist (*Radiology* 1987;162:138). Invasive studies are most helpful for identifying rare glands located outside the patient's neck (e.g., mediastinum).

B. **Operative strategy.** The goal of reexploration is to perform an orderly search based on the information gained from the initial operation and from localization studies.

1. **Missed parathyroid glands** are found either in the usual position or in ectopic sites, as determined by the embryology of parathyroid development. Rarely, a parathyroid gland is intrathyroidal (especially in patients with multinodular goiter), and intraoperative thyroid ultrasound followed by thyroid lobectomy can be performed if an exhaustive search fails to identify the parathyroid adenoma. If four normal glands have been located, the adenoma is likely to represent a supernumerary (fifth) gland. Intraoperative ultrasound is an effective tool for localizing parathyroid glands.

2. **Mediastinal adenomas** within the thymus are managed by resecting the cranial portion of the thymus by gentle traction on the thyrothymic ligament or by a complete transcervical thymectomy using a specialized substernal retractor (*Ann Surg* 1991;214:555). Median sternotomy carries a higher morbidity and increased postoperative pain, and the possibility of these should be discussed with the patient preoperatively.

III. **Parathyroid autotransplantation**

A. Indications for **total parathyroidectomy and heterotopic parathyroid autotransplantation** include HPT in patients with renal failure, in patients with four-gland parathyroid hyperplasia, and in patients undergoing neck reexploration in which the adenoma is the only remaining parathyroid tissue. The site of parathyroid autotransplantation may be the sternocleidomastoid muscle or the brachioradialis muscle of the patient's nondominant forearm. Parathyroid grafting into the patient's forearm is advantageous if recurrent HPT is possible (e.g., MEN type 1 or 2A). If HPT recurs, the hyperplastic parathyroid tissue may be partially excised from the patient's forearm under local anesthesia.

   B. Technique. Freshly removed parathyroid gland tissue is cut into fine pieces approximately 1 mm by 1 mm by 2 mm and placed in sterile iced saline. An incision is made in the patient's nondominant forearm, and separate intramuscular beds are created by spreading the fibers of the brachioradialis with a fine forceps. Approximately four to five pieces are placed in each site, and a total of approximately 100 mg of parathyroid tissue are transplanted. The beds are closed with a silk suture to mark the site of the transplanted tissue. Transplanted parathyroid tissue begins to function within 14 to 21 days of surgery.

   C. Cryopreservation of parathyroid glands is performed in MEN patients and all patients who may become aparathyroid after repeat exploration. Cryopreservation may be performed by freezing approximately 200 mg of finely cut parathyroid tissue in vials containing 10% dimethyl sulfoxide, 10% autologous serum, and 80% Waymouth medium. Cryopreserved parathyroid tissue can be used for autotransplantation in patients who become aparathyroid or in patients with failure of the initial grafted parathyroid tissue.

IV. Postoperative hypocalcemia

   A. Transient hypocalcemia commonly occurs after total thyroidectomy or parathyroidectomy and requires treatment if it is severe (total serum calcium <7.5 mg/dL) or if the patient is symptomatic. Chvostek sign (twitching of the facial muscles when the examiner percusses over the facial nerve anterior to the patient's ear) is a sign of relative hypocalcemia but is present in up to 15% of the normal population. This sign is not necessarily an indication for calcium replacement.

   B. Patients with **persistent hypocalcemia** after total thyroidectomy or after parathyroid autotransplantation can require continued supplementation for 6 to 8 weeks postoperatively. Usually, patients are given calcium carbonate, 500 to 1,000 mg orally 3 times per day, and 1,25-dihydroxyvitamin D_3, 0.25 μg orally per day.

   C. Hypocalcemic tetany is a medical emergency that is treated with rapid intravenous administration of 10% calcium gluconate or calcium chloride until the patient recovers. Specifically, 1 to 2 ampules (10 to 20 mL) of 10% calcium gluconate are given intravenously over 10 minutes, and the dose may be repeated every 15 to 20 minutes, as required. Subsequently, a continuous infusion of 10% calcium gluconate (90 mg elemental calcium/10 mL), 60 mL in 500 mL D5W (1 mg/mL), is initiated at 0.5 to 2.0 mg/kg per hour to maintain the serum calcium at 8 to 9 mg/dL. Patients with severe hypocalcemia also must have correction of hypomagnesemia.

V. Parathyroid carcinoma is rare and accounts for less than 1% of patients with HPT. Approximately 50% of these patients have a palpable neck mass, and serum calcium levels may exceed 15 mg/dL.

   A. Diagnosis is made by the histologic finding of vascular or capsular invasion, lymph node or distant metastases, or gross invasion of local structures.

   B. Surgical treatment is radical local excision of the tumor, surrounding soft tissue, lymph nodes, and ipsilateral thyroid lobe when the disease is recognized preoperatively or intraoperatively. Reoperation is indicated for local recurrence in an attempt to control malignant hypercalcemia.

   C. Patients with parathyroid carcinoma and some patients with benign HPT may develop **hyperparathyroid crisis.** Symptoms of this acute, sometimes fatal, illness include profound muscular weakness, nausea and vomiting, drowsiness, and confusion. Hypercalcemia (16 to 20 mg/dL) and azotemia are usually present. Ultimate treatment of "parathyroid crisis" is parathyroidectomy; however, hypercalcemia and volume and electrolyte abnormalities should be addressed first. Treatment is warranted for symptoms or a serum calcium level greater than 12 mg/dL. First-line therapy is infusion of 300 to 500 mL per hour of 0.9% sodium chloride (5 to 10 L per day intravenously) to restore intravascular volume and to promote renal excretion of calcium. After urinary output exceeds 100 mL per hour, furosemide (80 to 100 mg intravenously every 2 to 6 hours) may be given to promote further renal sodium and calcium excretion. Thiazide diuretics impair calcium excretion and should be avoided. Hypokalemia and hypomagnesemia are complications of forced saline diuresis and should be corrected. If diuresis alone is unsuccessful in lowering the serum calcium, other calcium-lowering agents may be used. These include the **bisphosphonates** pamidronate (60 to 90 mg in 1 L 0.9% saline infused over 24 hours) and etidronate (7.5 mg/kg intravenously over 2 to 4 hours daily for 3 days); **mithramycin** [25 μg/kg intravenously over 4 to 6 hours daily for 3 to 4 days (malignant hypercalcemia only)]; and salmon **calcitonin** (initial dose, 4 IU/kg subcutaneously or intramuscularly every 12 hours, increasing as necessary to a maximum dose of 8 IU/kg subcutaneously or intramuscularly every 6 hours). Orthophosphate, gallium nitrate, and glucocorticoids also have calcium-lowering effects.

ENDOCRINE PANCREAS

Pancreatic islet cell tumors are rare tumors that produce clinical syndromes related to the specific hormone secreted. Insulinomas are the most common of these tumors, followed by gastrinoma, then the rarer VIPoma (vasoactive intestinal polypeptide–secreting tumor), glucagonoma, and somatostatinoma. Recognition of **characteristic syndromes** is key to the diagnosis, which **must be confirmed biochemically.** Islet cell tumors are often occult, and their localization may be difficult, especially for small, multifocal, or extrapancreatic tumors. Islet cell tumors may occur sporadically or as a component of MEN type 1 or von Hippel-Lindau disease (nearly always multifocal). Islet cell tumors may be benign or malignant, although prediction may be based on the hormone produced rather than the tumor size.

  I. **Insulinoma**
   A. **Clinical features.** Patients with insulinoma develop profound hypoglycemia during fasting or after exercise. The clinical picture includes the signs and symptoms of neuroglycopenia (anxiety, tremor, confusion, and obtundation) and the sympathetic response to hypoglycemia (hunger, sweating, and tachycardia). These bizarre complaints initially may be attributed to malingering or a psychosomatic etiology unless the association with fasting is recognized. Many patients eat excessively to avoid symptoms, causing significant weight gain. **Whipple triad** refers to the clinical criteria for the diagnosis of insulinoma: (1) hypoglycemic symptoms during monitored fasting, (2) blood glucose levels less than 50 mg/dL, and (3) relief of symptoms after administration of intravenous glucose. Factitious hypoglycemia (excess exogenous insulin administration) and postprandial reactive hypoglycemia must be excluded.
   B. A supervised, in-hospital **72-hour fast** is required to diagnose insulinoma. Patients are observed for hypoglycemic episodes and have 6-hour measurement of plasma glucose, insulin, proinsulin, and C peptide. During the fast, the patient is allowed noncaloric beverages, and the fast is terminated when symptoms of neuroglycopenia develop. Nearly all patients with insulinoma develop neuroglycopenic symptoms and have inappropriately elevated plasma insulin (>5 μU/mL) associated with hypoglycemia (glucose <50 mg/dL). Elevated levels of C peptide and proinsulin usually are present as well (*Curr Probl Surg* 1994;31:79).
   C. **Localization.** Insulinomas typically are small (<2 cm), solitary, benign tumors that may occur anywhere in the pancreas. Rarely, an insulinoma may develop in extrapancreatic rests of pancreatic tissue. Dynamic CT scanning at 5-mm intervals with oral and intravenous contrast is the initial

localizing test for insulinoma, with success in 35% to 85% of cases. Endoscopic ultrasound is also effective but is operator dependent (*N Engl J Med* 1992;326:1721). The effectiveness of indium-111 (^{111}In)–octreotide scintigraphy for localizing insulinoma (approximately 50%) is less than for other islet cell tumors because insulinomas typically have few somatostatin receptors. Selective arteriography with observation of a tumor "blush" is the single best diagnostic study for the primary tumor and hepatic metastases. If a tumor is still not identified, regional localization to the head, body, or tail of the pancreas can be accomplished by portal venous sampling for insulin or by calcium angiography. Calcium angiography involves injection of calcium into selectively catheterized pancreatic arteries and measurement of plasma insulin through a catheter positioned in a hepatic vein.

D. Treatment of Insulinoma is surgical in nearly all cases. Surgical management of insulinomas consists of localization of the tumor by careful inspection and palpation of the gland after mobilization of the duodenum and the inferior border of the pancreas. Use of intraoperative ultrasonography greatly facilitates identification of small tumors, especially those located in the pancreatic head or uncinate process. Most insulinomas can be enucleated from surrounding pancreas, although those in the body or tail may require resection. In general, blind pancreatectomy should not be performed when the tumor cannot be identified. Approximately 5% of insulinomas are malignant, and 10% are multiple (usually in association with MEN type 1). Medical treatment for insulinoma with diazoxide, verapamil, or octreotide has limited effectiveness but may be used in preparation for surgery or for patients unfit for surgery.

II. Gastrinoma

A. Patients with **gastrinoma and the Zollinger-Ellison syndrome** (ZES) have severe peptic ulcer disease (PUD) due to gastrin-mediated gastric acid hypersecretion. Most patients present with epigastric pain, and 80% have active duodenal ulceration at the time of diagnosis. Diarrhea and weight loss are common (40% of patients). ZES is uncommon (0.1% to 1.0% of PUD cases), and most patients present with typical duodenal ulcer. Gastrinoma and ZES should be considered in any patient with (1) PUD refractory to treatment for *Helicobacter pylori* and conventional doses of H_2 blockers or omeprazole; (2) recurrent, multiple, or atypically located (e.g., distal duodenum or jejunum) peptic ulcers; (3) complications of PUD (i.e., bleeding, perforation, or obstruction); (4) PUD with significant diarrhea; and (5) PUD with HPT, nephrolithiasis, or familial endocrinopathy. All patients considered for elective surgery for PUD should have ZES excluded preoperatively.

B. Diagnosis of ZES requires demonstration of fasting hypergastrinemia and basal gastric acid hypersecretion. A fasting serum gastrin level of 100 pg/mL or greater and a basal gastric acid output (BAO) of 15 mEq per hour or more (>5 mEq per hour in patients with previous ulcer surgery) secure the diagnosis of ZES in nearly all cases. Fasting hypergastrinemia without elevated basal gastric acid output is seen in atrophic gastritis, in renal failure, and in patients taking H_2-receptor antagonists or omeprazole. Fasting hypergastrinemia with elevated basal gastric acid output is seen in retained gastric antrum syndrome, gastric outlet obstruction, and antral G-cell hyperplasia. A **secretin stimulation test** is used to distinguish ZES from these conditions. This test is performed by measuring fasting serum gastrin levels before and 2, 5, 10, and 15 minutes after the intravenous administration of secretin (2 units/kg). Eighty-five percent of patients with ZES have an increase in gastrin levels (>200 pg/mL over baseline) in response to a secretin stimulation test, whereas patients with other conditions do not. This test is most useful when ZES is suspected in patients who have had prior gastric surgery and in patients with moderately increased fasting gastrin levels (100 to 1,000 pg/mL).

C. Localization of gastrinoma should be performed in all patients considered for surgery. Approximately 80% of gastrinomas are located within the "gastrinoma triangle," which includes the duodenum and head of the pancreas. Gastrinomas are often malignant, with spread to lymph nodes or liver occurring in up to 60% of cases. Approximately 20% of patients with ZES have familial MEN type 1; these patients often have multiple, concurrent islet cell tumors. Dynamic CT scanning, ^{111}In-octreotide scintigraphy, endoscopic ultrasound, and MR scan are useful noninvasive tests for localizing gastrinoma; however, preoperative localization is unsuccessful up to 50% of the time. Selective angiography with or without secretin injection of the gastroduodenal, superior mesenteric, and splenic arteries and measurement of hepatic vein gastrin can localize occult gastrinoma in up to 70% to 90% of cases.

D. In cases of ZES, **medical treatment** of gastric hyperacidity with H_2 histamine receptor antagonists and omeprazole is highly effective. These medications are indicated preoperatively in patients undergoing operation for cure and in patients with unresectable or metastatic gastrinoma. Increased doses of oral histamine receptor antagonists can be required and often are given at 6-hour intervals. Starting doses (cimetidine, 300 mg orally every 6 hours; ranitidine, 150 mg orally every 6 hours; famotidine, 20 mg orally every 6 hours) are increased until the gastric acid secretion is less than 10 mEq per hour before the next dose. Alternatively, a continuous intravenous infusion can be initiated (e.g., ranitidine, 0.5 mg/kg per hour) and increased until control of gastric acid secretion is achieved. Omeprazole is given by mouth or nasogastric tube at 20 mg per day or twice a day.

E. **Surgical management of ZES** is indicated in all fit patients with nonmetastatic, sporadic gastrinoma. Goals of surgery include precise localization and curative resection of the tumor. Resection of primary gastrinoma alters the malignant progression of tumor and decreases hepatic metastases in patients with ZES. Intraoperative localization of gastrinomas is facilitated by extended duodenotomy and palpation, intraoperative ultrasonography, or endoscopic duodenal transillumination. Gastrinomas within the duodenum, pancreatic head, or uncinate process are treated by enucleation, whereas tumors in the body or tail of the pancreas can be removed by distal or subtotal pancreatectomy. Immediate cure rates are 40% to 90% for resections by experienced surgeons; however, half of patients initially cured according to biochemical tests experience recurrence within five years. **Gastric acid hypersecretion is controllable with H_2 blockers or omeprazole in most patients with ZES, rendering gastrectomy unnecessary.** If a gastrinoma cannot be localized intraoperatively, a parietal cell vagotomy may be performed. Surgical debulking of metastatic or unresectable primary gastrinoma facilitates medical treatment and prolongs life expectancy in select patients. Patients with ZES and MEN 1 most often cannot be cured surgically and usually are treated medically.

III. **Unusual islet cell tumors**

A. **VIPomas** secrete vasoactive intestinal peptide and cause profuse secretory diarrhea (fasting stool output of >1 L per day), hypokalemia, and either achlorhydria or hypochlorhydria (watery diarrhea, hypokalemia, and achlorhydria are the symptoms of Verner-Morrison syndrome). Hyperglycemia, hypercalcemia, and cutaneous flushing may be seen. Other, more common causes of diarrhea and malabsorption must be excluded. A diagnosis of VIPoma is established by the finding of elevated fasting serum vasoactive intestinal peptide levels (>190 pg/mL) and secretory diarrhea in association with an islet cell tumor. Octreotide (150 g subcutaneously every 8 hours) is highly effective as a means of controlling the diarrhea and correcting electrolyte abnormalities before resection. Most VIPomas occur in the distal pancreas and are amenable to distal pancreatectomy. Metastatic disease is commonly encountered (50%); nevertheless, surgical debulking is indicated to alleviate symptoms.

B. **Glucagonomas** secrete excess glucagon and result in type II diabetes, hypoaminoacidemia, anemia, weight loss, and a characteristic skin rash, necrolytic migratory erythema. Diagnosis is suggested by symptoms and by biopsy of the skin rash but is confirmed by elevated plasma glucagon levels (usually >1,000 pg/mL). Tumors are large and are readily seen on CT scan. Resection is indicated in fit patients after nutritional support, even if metastases are present.

C. **Somatostatinomas** are the rarest of the islet cell tumors and cause a syndrome of diabetes, steatorrhea, and cholelithiasis. These tumors are frequently located in the head of the pancreas and are often metastatic at the time of presentation.

D. **Other rare islet cell tumors** include pancreatic polypeptide-secreting, neurotensin-secreting, and adrenocorticotropic hormone (ACTH)–secreting tumors as well as nonfunctioning islet cell tumors. These tumors usually are large and often malignant. Treatment is surgical resection.

CARCINOID TUMORS

Carcinoid tumors are classified according to their embryologic origin: foregut (bronchial, thymic, gastroduodenal, and pancreatic), midgut (jejunal, ileal, appendiceal, right colic), and hindgut (distal colic, rectal). Depending on the site of origin, carcinoids secrete hormones differently and have different clinical features. Carcinoid tumors most frequently occur in the gastrointestinal tract. Bronchial and thymic carcinoids occur less commonly. In general, the diagnosis of carcinoid rests on the finding of elevated circulating serotonin or urinary metabolites [5-hydroxyindoleacetic acid (5-HIAA)] and localizing studies. The single best biochemical test is an elevated urinary 5-HIAA (normal, 2 to 8 mg per 24 hours). Rectal or jejunoileal tumors may be visualized by contrast studies, whereas bronchial carcinoids can be identified on chest x-rays, CT scans, or bronchoscopy. Abdominal or hepatic metastases are best identified by CT scanning, ultrasonography, or angiography. As with other neuroendocrine tumors, some carcinoids can be detected with metaiodobenzylguanidine ([131]I- MIBG) scanning, and most are detectable by ^{111}In-octreotide scintigraphy.

I. **Carcinoid of the appendix** is by far the most common carcinoid tumor and is found in up to 1 in 300 appendectomies. The risk of lymph node metastases and the prognosis of appendiceal carcinoids depend on the size: Tumors less than 1 cm never metastasize, tumors 1 to 2 cm have a 1% risk of metastasis, and tumors larger than 2 cm have a 30% risk of metastasis (*World J Surg* 1996;20:183). Extent of surgery for appendiceal carcinoid is based on size: simple appendectomy for tumors less than 1 cm, right hemicolectomy for tumors larger than 2 cm, and selective right hemicolectomy for tumors 1 to 2 cm. Prognosis for completely resected appendiceal carcinoid is favorable, with 5-year survival of 90% to 100%.

II. **Small-intestinal carcinoid tumors** usually present with vague abdominal symptoms that uncommonly lead to preoperative diagnosis. Most patients are operated on for intestinal obstruction, which is caused by a desmoplastic reaction in the mesentery around the tumor rather than by the tumor itself. Extended resection, including the mesentery and lymph nodes, is required, even for small tumors. Meticulous examination of the remaining bowel is mandatory because tumors are multicentric in 20% to 40% of cases, and synchronous adenocarcinomas are found in up to 10% of cases. An almost linear relationship exists between size of tumor and risk of nodal metastases, with a risk of up to 85% for tumors larger than 2 cm. Prognosis depends on the size and extent of disease; overall survival is 50% to 60%, which is substantially decreased if liver metastases are present. Small-bowel carcinoids have the highest propensity to metastasize to liver and produce the carcinoid syndrome.

III. **Rectal carcinoids** are typically small, submucosal nodules that are often asymptomatic or produce one or more of the nonspecific symptoms of bleeding, constipation, and tenesmus. These tumors are hormonally inactive and almost never produce the carcinoid syndrome, even when spread to the liver occurs. Treatment of small (<1 cm) rectal carcinoids is endoscopic removal.

Transmural excision of tumors 1 to 2 cm can be done locally. Treatment of 2-cm and larger tumors or invasive tumors is controversial but may include anterior or abdominoperineal resection for fit patients without metastases.

IV. Foregut carcinoids include gastroduodenal, bronchial, and thymic carcinoids. These are a heterogeneous group of tumors with variable prognosis. They do not release serotonin and may produce atypical symptoms (e.g., violaceous flushing of the skin) related to release of histamine. Gastroduodenal carcinoids may produce gastrin and cause ZES. Resection is advocated for localized disease.

The **carcinoid syndrome** occurs in less than 10% of patients with a carcinoid and develops when venous drainage from the tumor gains access to the systemic circulation, as with hepatic metastases. The classic syndrome consists of flushing, diarrhea, bronchospasm, and right-sided cardiac valvular fibrosis. Symptoms are paroxysmal and may be provoked by alcohol, cheese, chocolate, or red wine. Diagnosis is made by 24-hour measurement of urinary 5-HIAA or of whole blood 5-hydroxytryptamine. Surgical cure usually is not possible with extensive abdominal or hepatic metastases; however, debulking of the tumor may alleviate symptoms and improve survival, when it can be performed safely. Hepatic metastases also have been treated with chemoembolization using doxorubicin, 5-fluorouracil, and cisplatin. **Carcinoid crisis** with severe bronchospasm and hemodynamic collapse may occur perioperatively in patients with an undiagnosed carcinoid. Prompt recognition is crucial, as administration of octreotide (100 μg intravenously) can be lifesaving.

ADRENAL-PITUITARY AXIS

I. **Adrenal cortex**
   A. **Cushing syndrome** results from exogenous steroid administration or excess endogenous cortisol secretion. The clinical manifestations of Cushing syndrome include hypertension, edema, muscle weakness, glucose intolerance, osteoporosis, easy bruising, cutaneous striae, and truncal obesity (buffalo hump, moon facies). Women may develop acne, hirsutism, and amenorrhea as a result of adrenal androgen excess.
      1. **Pathophysiology**
         a. The most common cause of Cushing syndrome is **iatrogenic,** namely, the administration of exogenous glucocorticoids or ACTH.
         b. Hypersecretion of ACTH from the anterior pituitary gland (**Cushing disease**) is the most common pathologic cause (65% to 70% of cases) of endogenous hypercortisolism. The adrenal glands respond normally to the elevated ACTH, and the result is bilateral adrenal hyperplasia. Excessive release of corticotropin-releasing factor by the hypothalamus is a rare cause of hypercortisolism.
         c. Abnormal secretion of cortisol from a primary adrenal adenoma or carcinoma is the cause of hypercortisolism in 10% to 20% of cases. **Primary adrenal neoplasms** secrete corticosteroids independently of ACTH and usually result in suppressed plasma ACTH levels and atrophy of the adjacent and contralateral adrenocortical tissue.
         d. In approximately 15% of cases, Cushing syndrome is caused by **ectopic secretion of ACTH** or an ACTH-like substance from a small-cell bronchogenic carcinoma, carcinoid tumor, pancreatic carcinoma, thymic carcinoma, medullary thyroid cancer, or other neuroendocrine neoplasm. Patients with ectopic ACTH-secreting neoplasms can present primarily with hypokalemia, glucose intolerance, and hyperpigmentation but with few other chronic signs of Cushing syndrome.
      2. **Diagnosis** of Cushing syndrome is biochemical. The goals are to first establish hypercortisolism and then identify the source. However, all of the available tests are complicated by a lack of specificity and an overlap in the biochemical responses of patients with the different disease states.

a. Establishing the presence of hypercortisolism

(1) The best **screening test for hypercortisolism** is a 24-hour measurement of the urinary excretion of free cortisol. Urinary excretion of more than 100 μg per day of free cortisol in two independent collections is virtually diagnostic of Cushing syndrome. Measurement of plasma cortisol level alone is not a reliable method of diagnosing Cushing syndrome due to overlap of the levels in normal and abnormal patients.

(2) An **overnight dexamethasone suppression test** (dexamethasone, 1 mg orally at 11 PM, and measurement of plasma cortisol at 8 AM) is used to confirm Cushing syndrome, especially in obese or depressed patients who may have marginally elevated urinary cortisol. Patients with true hypercortisolism have lost normal adrenal-pituitary feedback and usually fail to suppress the morning plasma cortisol level to less than 5 μg/dL.

b. Localization of the cause of hypercortisolism

(1) **Determination of basal ACTH by immunoradiometric assay** is the best method of determining the cause of hypercortisolism. Suppression of the absolute level of ACTH below 5 pg/mL is nearly diagnostic of adrenocortical neoplasms. ACTH levels in Cushing disease may range from the upper limits of normal (15 pg/mL) to 500 pg/mL. The highest plasma levels of ACTH (>1,000 pg/mL) have been observed in patients with ectopic ACTH syndrome.

(2) Standard **high-dose dexamethasone suppression testing** is used to distinguish a pituitary from an ectopic source of ACTH. Normal individuals and most patients with a pituitary ACTH-producing neoplasm respond to a high-dose dexamethasone suppression test (2 mg orally every 6 hours for 48 hours) with a reduction of urinary free cortisol and urinary 17-hydroxysteroids to less than 50% of basal values. Most patients with a primary adrenal tumor or an ectopic source of ACTH production fail to suppress to this level. However, this test does not separate clearly pituitary and ectopic ACTH hypersecretion because 25% of patients with the ectopic ACTH syndrome also have suppressible tumors.

(3) Additional tests that may be useful include the **metyrapone test** (an inhibitor of the final step of cortisol synthesis) and the **corticotropin-releasing factor infusion test.** Patients with pituitary hypersecretion of ACTH respond to these tests with a compensatory rise in ACTH and urinary 17-hydroxysteroids, whereas patients with a suppressed hypothalamic-pituitary axis (primary adrenal tumor, ectopic ACTH syndrome) usually do not have a compensatory rise.

3. **Imaging tests** are useful for identifying lesions suspected on the basis of biochemical testing. Reliance on radiologic studies to diagnose the cause of Cushing syndrome should be discouraged.

a. Patients with ACTH-independent hypercortisolism require thin-section **CT scan or MRI scan of the adrenal gland,** both of which identify adrenal abnormalities with more than 95% sensitivity. Patients with ACTH-dependent hypercortisolism and either markedly elevated ACTH or a negative pituitary MRI scan should have **CT scan of the chest** to identify a tumor producing ectopic ACTH.

b. Gadolinium-enhanced MRI scan of the sella turcica is the best imaging test for pituitary adenomas suspected of causing ACTH-dependent hypercortisolism.

c. Bilateral **inferior petrosal sinus sampling** can delineate unclear cases of Cushing disease from other causes of hypercortisolism. Simultaneous bilateral petrosal sinus and peripheral blood samples are obtained before and after peripheral intravenous injection of 1 μg/kg corticotropin-releasing hormone. A ratio of inferior petrosal sinus to peripheral plasma ACTH of 2.0 at basal or of 3.0 after corticotropin-releasing hormone administration is 100% sensitive and specific for pituitary adenoma.

4. **Surgical treatment of Cushing syndrome** involves removing the cause of cortisol excess (a primary adrenal lesion or pituitary or ectopic tumors secreting excessive ACTH). Transsphenoidal resection of an ACTH-producing pituitary tumor is successful in 80% or more of cases of Cushing disease. Treatment of ectopic ACTH syndrome involves resection of the primary lesion, if possible. Primary adrenal causes of Cushing syndrome are treated by removal of the adrenal gland containing the tumor. All patients who undergo adrenalectomy for primary adrenal causes of Cushing syndrome require perioperative and postoperative glucocorticoid replacement because the pituitary-adrenal axis is suppressed.

B. **Primary aldosteronism** (Conn syndrome) is a syndrome of hypertension and hypokalemia caused by hypersecretion of the mineralocorticoid aldosterone. This uncommon syndrome accounts for less than 1% of unselected patients with hypertension. An aldosterone-producing adrenal adenoma (APA) is the cause of primary aldosteronism in two-thirds of cases and is one of the few surgically correctable causes of hypertension. Idiopathic bilateral adrenal hyperplasia (IHA) causes 30% to 40% of cases of primary aldosteronism. Adrenocortical carcinoma and autosomal dominant glucocorticoid-suppressible aldosteronism are rare causes of primary aldosteronism. **Secondary aldosteronism** is a physiologic response of the renin-angiotensin system to renal artery stenosis, cirrhosis, congestive heart failure, and normal pregnancy. In these conditions, the adrenal gland functions normally.

1. **Diagnosis.** Aldosterone-mediated retention of sodium and excretion of potassium and hydrogen ion by the kidney causes **hypokalemia and moderate diastolic hypertension.** Edema is characteristically absent. Laboratory diagnosis of primary aldosteronism requires demonstration of hypokalemia (<3.5 mEq/L), inappropriate kaliuresis (>30 mEq per day), and elevated aldosterone (>15 ng/dL) with normal cortisol. Upright plasma renin activity (PRA) of less than 3 ng/mL per hour corroborates the diagnosis. A ratio of plasma aldosterone (ng/dL) to PRA (ng/mL per hour) of greater than 20 to 25 further suggests primary hyperaldosteronism. Confirmation of primary aldosteronism involves determination of serum potassium and PRA and a 24-hour urine collection for sodium, cortisol, and aldosterone after 5 days of a high-sodium diet. Patients with primary hyperaldosteronism do not demonstrate aldosterone suppressibility (>14 μg per 24 hours) after salt loading. Alternatively, plasma aldosterone and PRA can be measured before and 2 hours after oral administration of 25 mg of captopril. Failure to suppress plasma aldosterone to less than 15 ng/dL is a positive test. Before biochemical studies, all diuretics and antihypertensives are discontinued for 2 to 4 weeks, and a daily sodium intake of at least 100 mEq is provided. **Differentiation between adrenal adenoma and IHA is important because unilateral adenomas are treated by surgical excision whereas bilateral hyperplasia is treated medically.** Because suppression of the renin-angiotensin system is more complete in APA than in IHA, these two disorders can be distinguished imperfectly (with approximately 85% accuracy) by measuring plasma aldosterone and PRA after overnight recumbency and then after 4 hours of upright posture. Patients with IHA usually have an increase in PRA and aldosterone in response to upright posture, but patients with adenoma usually show continued suppression of PRA, and their level of aldosterone does not change or falls paradoxically. In practice, this test usually is not necessary because, after a biochemical diagnosis of primary hyperaldosteronism, sensitive imaging tests are used to localize the lesion or lesions.

2. **Localization.** High-resolution adrenal CT scan should be the initial step in localization of an adrenal tumor. CT scanning localizes an adrenal

adenoma in 90% of cases overall, and the presence of a unilateral adenoma larger than 1 cm on CT scan and supportive biochemical evidence of an aldosteronoma are generally all that is needed to make the diagnosis of Conn syndrome. Uncertainty regarding APA versus IHA after biochemical testing and noninvasive localization may be definitively resolved by bilateral adrenal venous sampling for aldosterone and cortisol. Simultaneous adrenal vein blood samples for aldosterone and cortisol are taken: the ratio of aldosterone to cortisol is greater than 4:1 for a diagnosis of aldosteronoma and less than 4:1 for a diagnosis of IHA.

3. **Treatment.** Surgical removal of an APA through a posterior or laparoscopic approach results in immediate cure or substantial improvement of hypertension and hyperkalemia in more than 90% of patients with Conn syndrome. The patient should be treated with spironolactone (200 to 400 mg per day) preoperatively for 2 to 3 weeks to control blood pressure and to correct hypokalemia. Patients with IHA should be treated medically with spironolactone (200 to 400 mg per day). A potassium-sparing diuretic, such as amiloride (5 to 20 mg per day), and calcium channel blockers have also been used. Surgical excision rarely cures bilateral hyperplasia.

C. **Acute adrenal insufficiency** is an emergency and should be suspected in stressed patients with a history of either adrenal insufficiency or exogenous steroid use. Adrenocortical insufficiency is most often caused by acute withdrawal of chronic corticosteroid therapy but can result from autoimmune destruction of the adrenal cortex, from adrenal hemorrhage (Waterhouse-Friderichsen syndrome), or rarely from infiltration with metastatic carcinoma. Recently, adrenal insufficiency in acutely ill patients has been elucidated as being multifactorial and difficult to diagnose clinically. However, the diagnosis and prompt treatment of it can be of significant benefit in acutely ill patients (*N Engl J Med* 2003;20;348:727–734).

   1. **Signs and symptoms** include fever, nausea, vomiting, severe hypotension, and lethargy. Characteristic laboratory findings of adrenal insufficiency include hyponatremia, hyperkalemia, azotemia, and fasting or reactive hypoglycemia.

   2. **Diagnosis:** A rapid ACTH stimulation test is used to test for adrenal insufficiency. Corticotropin (250 μg), synthetic ACTH, is administered intravenously, and plasma cortisol levels are measured upon completion of the administration then 30 and 60 minutes later. Normal peak cortisol response should exceed 20 μg/dL. The most benefit from adrenocortical hormone replacement in critically ill septic patients is reported in those whose cortisol levels rose <9 μg/dL from baseline in response to corticotropin stimulation (*N Engl J Med* 2003;20;348:727–734).

   3. **Treatment of adrenal crisis must be immediate, based on clinical suspicion,** before laboratory confirmation is available. Intravenous volume replacement with normal or hypertonic saline and dextrose is essential, as is immediate intravenous steroid replacement therapy with **4 mg dexamethasone.** Thereafter, 100 mg of hydrocortisone is administered intravenously every 6 to 8 hours and is tapered to standard replacement doses as the patient's condition stabilizes. Subsequent recognition and treatment of the underlying cause, particularly if it is infectious, usually resolves the crisis. Mineralocorticoid replacement is not required until intravenous fluids are discontinued and oral intake resumes.

   4. **Prevention.** Patients who have known adrenal insufficiency or have received supraphysiologic doses of steroid for at least 1 week in the year preceding surgery should receive 100 mg of hydrocortisone the evening before and the morning of major surgery, followed by 100 mg of hydrocortisone every 8 hours during the first postoperative 24 hours.

II. **Adrenal medulla: pheochromocytoma**

A. **Pathophysiology.** Pheochromocytomas are neoplasms derived from the chromaffin cells of the sympathoadrenal system that result in unregulated,

episodic oversecretion of catecholamines. Most pheochromocytomas secrete predominantly norepinephrine and smaller amounts of epinephrine. Rarely, epinephrine is secreted predominantly or exclusively.
  B. **Clinical features.** Approximately 80% to 85% of pheochromocytomas in adults arise in the adrenal medulla, whereas 10% to 15% arise in the extra-adrenal chromaffin tissue, including the paravertebral ganglia, posterior mediastinum, organ of Zuckerkandl, and urinary bladder. Symptoms of pheochromocytoma are related to excess sympathetic stimulation from catecholamines and include paroxysms of pounding frontal headache, diaphoresis, palpitations, flushing, or anxiety. The most common sign is episodic or sustained hypertension, but pheochromocytoma accounts for only 0.1% to 0.2% of patients with sustained diastolic hypertension. Uncommonly, patients present with complications of prolonged uncontrolled hypertension (e.g., myocardial infarction, cerebrovascular accident, or renal disease). Pheochromocytomas can occur in association with several hereditary syndromes, including MEN types 2A and 2B and von Hippel-Lindau syndrome. Tumors that arise in familial settings frequently are bilateral.
  C. The **biochemical diagnosis** of pheochromocytoma is made by demonstrating elevated 24-hour urinary excretion of catecholamines and their metabolites (metanephrines, vanillylmandelic acid). If possible, antihypertensive medications (especially monoamine oxidase inhibitors) should be discontinued before the 24-hour urine collection, and creatinine excretion should be measured simultaneously to assess the adequacy of the sample. Plasma catecholamines also are elevated during the paroxysms of hypertension, but they are more difficult to measure and interpret and therefore have limited clinical application.
  D. **Radiographic tests** are used to demonstrate the presence of an adrenal mass.
    1. **CT scanning** is the imaging test of choice and identifies 90% to 95% of pheochromocytomas larger than 1 cm. MR scan can also be useful because T2-weighted images have a characteristic high intensity in patients with pheochromocytoma and metastatic tumor compared with adenomas.
    2. **Scintigraphic scanning** after the administration of ^{131}I-MIBG provides a functional and anatomic test of hyperfunctioning chromaffin tissue. MIBG scanning is very specific for both intra- and extra-adrenal pheochromocytomas.
  E. **The treatment of benign and malignant pheochromocytomas is surgical excision.**
    1. **Preoperative preparation** includes administration of an alpha-adrenergic blocker to control hypertension and to permit reexpansion of intravascular volume. Phenoxybenzamine, 10 mg orally twice a day, is initiated and increased to 20 to 40 mg orally twice a day until the desired effect or prohibitive side effects are encountered. Postural hypertension is expected and is the desired endpoint. β-Adrenergic blockade (e.g., propranolol) may be added if tachycardia or arrhythmias develop but only **after complete** α-**adrenergic blockade.** Patients with cardiopulmonary dysfunction may require a pulmonary artery (Swan-Ganz) catheter perioperatively, and all patients should be monitored in the surgical intensive care unit in the immediate postoperative period.
    2. **The classic operative approach** for familial pheochromocytomas is exploration of both adrenal glands, the preaortic and paravertebral areas, and the organ of Zuckerkandl through a midline or bilateral subcostal incision. In patients with MEN type 2A or 2B and a unilateral pheochromocytoma, it is acceptable policy to remove only the involved gland (*Ann Surg* 1993;217:595). In patients with a sporadic, unilateral pheochromocytoma localized by preoperative imaging studies, adrenalectomy may be performed by an anterior or posterior approach or (increasingly) by laparoscopic adrenalectomy. Intraoperative labile hypertension can occur during resection of pheochromocytoma. This can be prevented by

minimal manipulation of the tumor but can be controlled most effectively with intravenous sodium nitroprusside (0.5 to 10.0 μg/kg per minute) or phentolamine (5 mg).

III. **Adrenocortical carcinoma** is a rare but aggressive malignancy; most patients with this cancer present with locally advanced disease. Syndromes of adrenal hormone overproduction may include rapidly progressive hypercortisolism, hyperaldosteronism, or virilization. Large (>6 cm) adrenal masses that extend to nearby structures on CT scanning likely represent carcinoma. **Complete surgical resection of locally confined tumor is the only chance for cure of adrenocortical carcinoma.** Definitive diagnosis of adrenocortical carcinoma requires operative and pathologic demonstration of nodal or distant metastases. Any adrenal neoplasm weighing more than 50 g should be considered malignant. Often, patients with adrenocortical carcinoma present with metastatic disease, most often involving the lung, lymph nodes, liver, or bone. Palliative surgical debulking of locally advanced or metastatic adrenocortical carcinoma may provide these patients with symptomatic relief from some slow-growing, hormone-producing cancers. Chemotherapy with mitotane may be somewhat effective. Overall, the prognosis for patients with adrenocortical carcinoma is poor.

IV. **Incidental adrenal masses** are detected in 0.6% to 1.5% of abdominal CT scans obtained for other reasons. Most incidentally discovered adrenal masses are benign, nonfunctioning cortical adenomas of no clinical significance. The **NIH consensus state-of-the-science statement** from 2002 on adrenal incidentalomas recommends that patients with an incidentaloma should have a 1-mg dexamethasone suppression test and a measurement of plasma-free metanephrines. Patients with coexisting hypertension should also be evaluated for primary aldosteronism. Surgery should be considered in all patients with clinically apparent functional adrenal cortical tumors and pheochromocytomas. Tumors greater than 6 cm should be surgically removed. Tumors less than 4 cm should be monitored clinically and radiologically. Either open or laparoscopic adrenalectomy is acceptable. Laparoscopic adrenalectomy has been associated with shorter hospitalization and faster recovery. Its use is generally limited to malignant lesions less than 5 cm in diameter and benign-appearing lesions up to 8 to 10 cm in diameter.

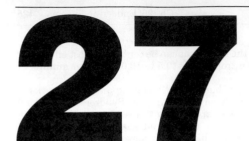

Trauma Surgery

**Aalok Sahai and
Douglas Schuerer**

Injury remains a leading cause of death and disability around the world. This chapter outlines an overall approach to trauma care, provides a framework for therapy, highlights critical aspects of decision making, and focuses on selected key diagnoses and interventions. These points illustrate the four main features of effective trauma care: (1) Therapy should be comprehensive, extending from the initial field evaluation through the completion of rehabilitation; (2) it should be multidisciplinary, involving the coordination of a dedicated team of health professionals; (3) it should be systematic so as to provide a framework for the timely and accurate identification of all injuries and comorbidities; and (4) it should be rapid, which means that the injuries and the interventions required to treat them need to be identified and properly prioritized as quickly as possible.

TRAUMA CARE

I. **Prehospital care** of the trauma patient is provided by a wide range of emergency medical service (EMS) personnel with varying levels of skills training (first responders, emergency medical technicians, and paramedics). These field professionals are responsible for performing the three major functions of prehospital care: (1) assessment of the injury scene, (2) stabilization and monitoring of injured patients, and (3) safe and rapid transportation of critically ill patients to the appropriate trauma center. The observations and interventions performed are important in guiding the resuscitation of an injured patient. The MVIT (*m*echanism, *v*ital signs, *i*njury inventory, *t*reatment) system of reporting is one method of communicating data to the trauma team in an efficient, fast, and organized manner.

A. The **mechanism of a trauma** partially determines the pattern and severity of injuries sustained in the event. The pattern of injury can often be predicted based on the type of trauma. Front-end car collisions can cause direct contact between the driver's knees and the dashboard. Such trauma can result in combination patellar fracture, posterior knee dislocation (with popliteal artery injury), femoral shaft fracture, and posterior rim fracture of the acetabulum. Feet-first falls from significant heights cause axial loading and a possible combination of calcaneal fracture, lower extremity long bone fracture, acetabular injury, and lumbar spine compression fracture. Adult pedestrians struck by motor vehicles often have a pattern of three distinct injuries: (1) injury to the tibia and fibula from striking the bumper, (2) injury to the head from striking the windshield or hood after being swept from the ground, and (3) injury to the upper extremity from falling to the pavement. In young children struck by a motor vehicle, the constellation of injuries is known as the Waddell triad: (1) femur fracture from striking the bumper, (2) abdominal solid organ injury (liver or spleen) from striking the fender, and (3) opposite side head injury from landing on the pavement.

B. **Vital signs**, including level of consciousness and voluntary movement, give insight into the clinical trajectory of the patient and are a key element in leveling trauma. EMS providers typically measure and report these values, often in less than ideal conditions. Deterioration of vital signs en route to the trauma center suggests the existence of life threats requiring immediate intervention. Improvement in vital signs *en route* may reflect transient compensatory responses by the patient. They may, however, only reflect human error in obtaining data in difficult circumstances.

C. The **injury inventory** consists of the description of injuries as observed by the EMS personnel. The inventory should be considered a minimal list, and every aspect of the report must be confirmed or excluded by the trauma team. Important prehospital observations include whether the patient was trapped in a vehicle, was crushed under a heavy object, or suffered significant exposure secondary to prolonged extrication. Such findings alert the trauma team to critical secondary injuries, including rhabdomyolysis, traumatic asphyxia, and hypothermia, that can have a profound impact on outcome.

D. **Prehospital treatment** is aimed at stabilization of the injured patient and involves securing an airway, providing adequate ventilation, assessing and supporting circulation, and stabilizing the spine. EMS caregivers fulfill these goals through various therapies that include (but are not limited to) administration of oxygen and intravenous fluids, prevention of heat loss, and immobilization of the spine with a backboard and properly fitting hard cervical collar. Any patient suspected of having injuries to the cervical spine must be placed in a rigid collar. All such interventions need to be taken into acount during the initial evaluation, including immediate confirmation of any prehospital airway.

E. **Initial hospital care.** Trauma deaths have a **trimodal distribution**: (1) immediate death occurring at the time of injury due to devastating wounds; (2) early death occurring within the first few hours of injury due to major intracranial, thoracic, abdominal, pelvic, and extremity injuries; and (3) late death occurring days to weeks after the initial injury due to secondary complications (sepsis, acute respiratory distress syndrome, systemic inflammatory response syndrome, or multiple organ dysfunction and failure). Initial hospital care usually takes place in the emergency department and has two main components: the primary and secondary surveys. The goal of the **primary survey** is to identify and treat those injuries that can result in early death within the first few minutes of injury. The goal of the **secondary survey** is to initiate and maintain the resuscitation of physiologic functions, catalogue all injuries sustained, and institute appropriate therapy or supportive measures.

II. **Primary survey.** The primary survey is a systematic, rapid evaluation of the injured patient following the **mnemonic ABCDE (*a*irway, *b*reathing, *c*irculation, *d*isability, *e*xposure).** On completion of the survey, the patient should have an established airway with cervical spine control, adequate ventilation and oxygenation, and proper intravenous access and control of hemorrhage; an inventory of the patient's neurologic status and disability should have been done; and the patient should have undergone complete exposure with environmental control. During the survey, a rudimentary history is obtained (if possible). This history follows the acronym **AMPLE** (*a*llergies, *m*edications, *p*ast medical history, *l*ast oral intake, *e*vents surrounding the injury).

A. **Airway.** Establishing a patent airway is the highest priority in the care of a trauma patient because without one irreversible brain damage can occur within minutes. Because the status of the cervical spine in an injured patient is often unknown, the airway should always be secured under cervical spine control. Engaging the patient in conversation on arrival at the emergency department allows for immediate evaluation of the airway. A patient who is able to respond verbally has a patent airway. A patient who cannot respond verbally must be assumed to have an obstructed airway until proven otherwise. The causes of airway obstruction in the trauma patient can be myriad, and the means of establishing an airway vary from simple maneuvers to emergent surgical procedures. Every trauma patient initially should have oxygen administered (via nasal cannula or bag valve facemask) and an oxygen saturation monitor (i.e., pulse oximeter) placed. An oximeter device is helpful, but it is important to remember that its output readings can be misleading in certain clinical situations (e.g., patients with severe anemia, insufficient pulse pressure, hypothermia, or burns with inhalation injury).

1. **Basic maneuvers.** A frequent cause of airway loss in the trauma patient is mechanical obstruction caused by vomitus, phlegm, or other debris in the oropharynx. Simple suctioning can remove such blockage. In the semiconscious or unconscious patient, the tongue itself can occlude the airway. The jaw-thrust maneuver can successfully displace the tongue anteriorly from the pharyngeal inlet, relieving the obstruction. In the unconscious patient, the placement of an oropharyngeal airway (or, in the absence of head trauma, a nasopharyngeal airway) can mechanically displace the tongue anteriorly, securing patency. In the semiconscious patient, the nasopharyngeal airway can be used in certain circumstances to ensure an open airway. Both devices, however, can cause significant irritation of the upper aerodigestive tract, with resultant vomiting, and thus should not be used on fully conscious patients. Even though the basic maneuvers just mentioned can be lifesaving by providing temporary airway function, tracheal intubation is the definitive means of securing an airway in the trauma patient.

2. **Tracheal intubation** is indicated in any patient in whom concern for airway integrity exists (unconscious or semiconscious patients, patients with mechanical obstruction secondary to facial trauma or debris, combative and hypoxic patients). The emergent tracheal intubation of an uncooperative trauma patient is a high-risk undertaking. The most skilled operator available should secure the airway by the most expeditious means possible. The preferred method of intubation is via the orotracheal route using **rapid sequence induction (RSI).** Nasotracheal intubation should be discouraged. Rapid sequence intubation follows a systematic protocol to ensure successful provision of an airway. The patient is first **spontaneously ventilated with 100% oxygen.** During this time, a team member provides in-line cervical spine stabilization to prevent unintentional manipulation as the hard cervical collar is removed anteriorly. Another team member provides anterior pressure on the cricoid cartilage to occlude the esophagus (Sellick maneuver). This pressure prevents aspiration during intubation. Following preoxygenation, a **short-acting sedative or hypnotic medication is administered** via a functioning intravenous line with a stopcock. The choice of medication depends on the clinical situation. In general, etomidate, 0.3 mg/kg intravenously, or a short-acting benzodiazepine, such as midazolam, 1.0 to 2.5 mg intravenously, is used because these medications tend to have minimal effects on the cardiovascular status of the patient. In addition, midazolam provides anterograde amnesia. Opiates, such as fentanyl citrate, 2 μg/kg intravenously, should be used only in patients who are adequately perfused because their mild cardiac depressant activity can cause unexpected cardiovascular decompensation in hypoxic, hypoperfused patients. Sodium thiopental, 2 to 5 mg/kg intravenously, is exclusively reserved for the well-perfused patient with a seemingly isolated head injury because it diminishes the transient elevation in intracranial pressure (ICP) associated with tracheal intubation. A **paralytic agent is administered immediately after the sedative.** Succinylcholine, 1.00 to 1.25 mg/kg intravenously, is the paralytic of choice because, as a depolarizing muscle relaxant, it has a rapid onset (fasciculations within seconds) and a short half-life (recovery within 1 to 2 minutes). Contraindications in the acute trauma setting are limited to patients with known pseudocholinesterase deficiency or previous spinal injury. Succinylcholine can be used safely in patients with acute burns or spinal trauma. Rocuronium, 0.60 to 0.85 mg/kg intravenously, is an alternative paralytic, but as a nondepolarizing relaxant, it has a slower onset (up to 90 seconds) and a longer half-life (recovery after 40 minutes) than succinylcholine. **After onset of paralysis, the**

endotracheal tube (the largest for patient size and airway) is inserted through the vocal cords under direct vision with the assistance of a laryngoscope and with the balloon inflated. The tube position is usually around 21 cm from the incisors in women and 23 cm from the incisors in men. Proper positioning of the tube in the trachea should be confirmed by exhalation of carbon dioxide over several breaths (using a litmus paper device or capnometer). **Adequacy of ventilation** should be verified by bilateral auscultation in each axilla. A chest x-ray should be taken within the next few minutes and checked to ensure proper endotracheal tube position. Tracheal intubation should secure an airway within 90 to 120 seconds (about three attempts). If it is unsuccessful, an airway placed directly through the cricoid membrane is often necessary.

3. **Cricothyrotomy** is the method of choice for establishing a surgical airway in adults in instances where orotracheal intubation is not possible (unsuccessful orotracheal attempts or massive facial trauma). The cricoid membrane is easily palpated between the cricoid cartilage and the larynx. Being both superficial and relatively avascular, it provides rapid, easy access to the trachea. After identification of the membrane, a 1.5-cm transverse skin incision is made over it (no skin preparation is necessary). A scalpel is used to poke a hole through the membrane. Care is taken to avoid exiting through the trachea posteriorly, thereby injuring the esophagus. Next, the scalpel handle, a tracheal spreader, or a similar surgical instrument is used to expand the hole. Finally, a 6.0-mm endotracheal or tracheostomy tube is inserted into the trachea through the cricothyrotomy, the balloon is inflated, and the tube sutured into place. Historically, a cricothyrotomy would eventually require revision to a tracheostomy to decrease the risk of tracheal stenosis, but this has been challenged, and many institutions will now use the cricothyrotomy site as a tracheostomy site. Cricothyrotomy is contraindicated in children younger than 12 years of age because of the anatomic difficulty in performing the procedure. In this situation, percutaneous transtracheal ventilation is an alternative.

4. **Percutaneous transtracheal ventilation** can provide a temporary airway until a formal surgical airway can be supplied, especially in young children in whom cricothyrotomy is not possible. A small cannula (usually a 14-gauge intravenous catheter) is placed through the cricoid membrane. The cannula is connected to oxygen tubing containing a precut side hole. Temporary occlusion of the side hole provides passage of oxygen into the lungs via the cannula. Exhalation occurs passively through the vocal cords. Through this means, alveolar oxygen concentrations are transiently maintained for approximately 30 to 45 minutes.

B. **Breathing.** Once an airway is established, attention is directed at assessing the patient's breathing (i.e., the oxygenation and ventilation of the lungs). A patent airway does not ensure adequate breathing because the trachea can be ventilated without successfully ventilating the alveoli. Through the secured airway, 100% oxygen is administered. The chest is then examined, and the axillae are auscultated to assess gas delivery to the peripheral lung. Any abnormal sounds suggest potentially life-threatening conditions. The chest wall motion is observed, and the position of the trachea is noted. The use of accessory muscles of respiration is sought (this is often a sign of severe respiratory compromise and impending cardiovascular collapse). In this manner, important life-threatening abnormalities involving the thorax can be identified and treated. The following are potentially fatal conditions that require immediate attention and treatment. (See Chapter 42, Section II.B, for a description of the **technique of tube thoracostomy.**)

1. **Tension pneumothorax.** Signs of a tension pneumothorax include the absence of breath sounds, hyperresonance in the lung field, tracheal deviation away from the side of the abnormality, and associated hypotension due to decreased venous return. Immediate decompressive therapy is indicated (a chest x-ray should not delay treatment). Decompression

involves placement of a 14-gauge intravenous catheter in the second intercostal space in the midclavicular line. A tube thoracostomy should promptly follow decompression. A chest x-ray should be obtained only after the chest tube placement is complete.

2. **Pneumothorax or hemothorax.** Absent or decreased breath sounds in a lung field without tracheal deviation usually indicate a simple pneumothorax or hemothorax on the affected side. A chest x-ray can usually confirm these conditions. Treatment consists of tube thoracostomy (28 Fr. or larger). The chest tube should be connected to an underwater seal-suction device adjusted to −20 cm water suction.

3. **Flail chest.** Paradoxical chest wall motion with spontaneous respirations indicates a flail chest (three or more ribs with two or more fractures per rib). Pulmonary contusion often accompanies such an injury. Chest x-ray often reveals the extent of fractures and underlying lung injury. Treatment involves adequate pain control (often with epidural analgesia), aggressive pulmonary toilet, and respiratory support. Many of these patients will require early mechanical ventilatory support. Intensive care monitoring is recommended for elderly or debilitated patients.

4. **Open pneumothorax.** Any chest wound communicating with the pleural space that is greater than two-thirds the diameter of the trachea will preferentially draw air into the thorax ("sucking chest wound"). Open chest wounds therefore must be covered with a partially occlusive bandage secured on three sides (securing all four sides can result in a tension pneumothorax and should be avoided). In this manner, air is prevented from entering the thorax through the wound but can exit via the wound if necessary. Prompt tube thoracostomy should follow placement of the partially occlusive dressing.

5. **Tracheobronchial disruption.** Severe subcutaneous emphysema with respiratory compromise can suggest tracheobronchial disruption. The tube thoracostomy placed on the affected side will reveal a large air leak, and the collapsed lung may fail to reexpand. Bronchoscopy is diagnostic. Treatment involves intubation of the unaffected bronchus followed by operative repair (see Section V.D.2).

C. **Circulation.** After evaluation of both the airway and breathing, circulation is assessed. The goal of this portion of the primary survey is to identify and treat the presence of shock. Initially, all active external hemorrhage is controlled with direct pressure, and obvious fractures are stabilized. The pulse is characterized, and a blood pressure (BP) is obtained. The skin perfusion is determined by noting skin temperature and evaluating capillary refill. Over time, end-organ perfusion during a trauma resuscitation is estimated using mental status and urine flow as markers. Shock is defined as the inadequate delivery of oxygen and nutrients to tissue. The etiologies of shock can be divided into three broad categories: hypovolemic, cardiogenic, and distributive. The trauma team must be familiar with the manifestations and therapy of each category of shock because any of the three may be encountered in the injured patient.

1. **Hypovolemic shock.** The most common type of shock encountered in the trauma patient is a form of hypovolemic shock known as hemorrhagic shock. It occurs as a result of decreased intravascular volume secondary to blood loss and can be divided into four classes (Table 27-1). In its severe form, it can manifest as a rapid pulse, decreased pulse pressure, diminished capillary refill, and cool, clammy skin. Therapy involves restoring the intravascular volume. As a result, the patient should have **two large-bore intravenous lines placed (14- or 16-gauge). The antecubital veins are the preferred sites.** If a peripheral intravenous catheter cannot be placed secondary to venous collapse, an 8.5 Fr. cannula (Cordis catheter) should be placed via the Seldinger technique into the **femoral vein.** The subclavian and internal jugular veins should be reserved for those patients in whom major venous intra-abdominal injury or pelvic fractures

Table 27-1. Estimated blood loss by initial hemodynamic variables

	Class I	Class II	Class III	Class IV
Blood loss (mL)	Up to 750	750–1,500	1,500–2,000	>2,000
Blood loss (% blood volume)	Up to 15%	15–30%	30–40%	>40%
Pulse rate	<100	>100	>120	>140
Blood pressure (mm Hg)	Normal	Normal	Decreased	Decreased
Pulse pressure (mm Hg)	Normal or increased	Decreased	Decreased	Decreased
Urinary output (mL/hr)	>30	20–30	5–15	Negligible

would prevent intravascular repletion. Short, wide intravenous catheters are used to maximize the flow of resuscitation fluids into the circulation (the rate of fluid flow is proportional to the cross-sectional area of a conduit and inversely proportional to the fourth power of its radius). A blood specimen should be simultaneously obtained for cross-matching and for any other pertinent labs. Resuscitation should consist of an **initial bolus of 2 L of crystalloid solution** (children should receive an initial bolus of 20 mL/kg). All fluids administered should be warmed to prevent hypothermia. Whole blood should be administered if further resuscitation is required. If time has not allowed proper cross-matching (as is frequently the case), type O blood should be used. Premenopausal women should receive Rh– blood. Men and postmenopausal women can receive either Rh– or Rh+ blood. In the setting of penetrating torso injury involving a large blood vessel, less aggressive resuscitation (keeping BP around 90 mm Hg) until formal surgical control of the bleeding site is obtained has been shown to have some benefit in diminishing blood loss (*N Engl J Med* 1994;331:1105). Emergency department thoracotomy (EDT) is sometimes indicated for severe cardiopulmonary collapse (see Section VI.A.1).

2. **Cardiogenic shock** occurs when the heart is unable to provide adequate cardiac output to perfuse the peripheral tissues. In the trauma setting, such shock can occur in one of two ways: **(1) extrinsic compression** of the heart leading to decreased venous return and cardiac output or **(2) myocardial injury** causing inadequate myocardial contraction and decreased cardiac output. Patients in cardiogenic shock secondary to extrinsic compression of the heart usually present with cool, pale skin; decreased BP; and distended jugular veins. They often respond transiently to an initial fluid bolus, but more definite therapy is always needed. Tension pneumothorax is the most common etiology. Cardiac tamponade is a less common cause. It usually occurs in the setting of a penetrating injury near the heart. Rapid diagnosis can be obtained with the use of ultrasound. Therapy consists of pericardial drainage and repair of the injury, usually a proximal great vessel or cardiac wound (see Sections V.D.5.a and V.D.6.a). EDT may be required. Patients in cardiogenic shock secondary to myocardial injury can also present with cool skin, decreased BP, and distended jugular veins. Acute myocardial infarction can manifest in this way. Often, it is responsible for the traumatic event, but it can also occur as a result of the stress following an injury. Diagnosis of a myocardial infarction is via electrocardiogram (ECG) and troponin levels. Therapy should follow Advanced Cardiac Life Support guidelines, keeping in mind that anticoagulants may need to be avoided early on until active bleeding related to the trauma has been excluded. Severe blunt cardiac injury is another manifestation. It usually occurs in the setting of high-speed motor vehicle crashes. An ECG and possibly an echocardiogram are essential. Therapy ranges from close monitoring with

pharmacologic support in an intensive care unit to operative repair (see
Section V.D.6.b).

3. **Distributive shock** occurs as a result of an increase in venous capacitance leading to decreased venous return. Neurogenic shock secondary
to acute quadriplegia or paraplegia is one type. Loss of peripheral sympathetic tone is responsible for the increased venous capacitance and
decreased venous return. These patients present with warm skin, absent rectal tone, and inappropriate bradycardia. They often respond to
an initial fluid bolus but will eventually require pharmacologic support
to help restore sympathetic tone. Phenylephrine is the drug of choice. It
is administered via a central venous catheter at an initial rate of 30 to
60 μg per minute and titrated to effect (using BP as a guide). Of note,
the leading cause of shock in a trauma patient is hypovolemia, and thus
neurogenic shock is usually a diagnosis of exclusion.

D. **Disability.** The goal of this phase of the primary survey is to identify and
treat life-threatening neurologic injuries, and priority is given to evaluating
level of consciousness and looking for lateralizing neurologic signs. The level
of consciousness is quickly assessed using the **AVPU system** (ascertaining
whether the patient is **a**wake, opens eyes to **v**oice, opens eyes to **p**ainful
stimulus, or is **u**narousable). The pupils are examined, and their size, symmetry, and responsiveness to light are noted. Focal neurologic deficits are
noted. Signs of significant neurologic impairment include inability to follow
simple commands, asymmetry of pupils or their response to light, and gross
asymmetry of limb movement to painful stimuli. Severe neurologic injuries
require urgent evaluation and are either intracranial or spinal in origin.

1. **Intracranial injuries.** Head injury remains a leading cause of trauma fatality in the United States. **Herniation (either uncal or cerebellar) is often
the final common pathway leading to death.** Vigilance on the part of the
trauma team can sometimes trigger interventions before such an event
becomes irreversible. For example, uncal herniation is often associated
with a "blown" (fixed, dilated) pupil on the side of herniation secondary
to compression of either the constrictor (Edinger-Westphal) nucleus of
the pupil or its outgoing fibers in the third cranial nerve. As this compression begins, the pupil assumes an ovoid shape. Such a finding can
alert the trauma team to impending herniation and the need for immediate intervention. Acute therapy of severe intracranial injuries focuses on
maximizing cerebral perfusion pressure (CPP) to provide an adequate
supply of glucose and oxygen to the injured tissue. *CPP* is defined as
the difference between mean arterial pressure (MAP) and ICP: CPP =
MAP − ICP. Maximization of CPP therefore involves manipulating both
MAP and ICP, and this is achieved when the BP is adequate (MAP >70 to
80 mm Hg) and the ICP is normal (<10 to 15 mm Hg in adults). A CPP
of more than 60 to 70 mm Hg is the goal.

   a. **Mean arterial pressure (MAP).** Maintaining an adequate MAP is very
   important in the patient with head trauma because hypotension is
   a major risk factor for poor outcome. The patient should be kept euvolemic or hypervolemic. In addition, pharmacologic support should
   be used as necessary to maintain an adequate BP. Extreme hypertension should be avoided. Hypoxia is especially detrimental in traumatic
   head injuries, and all efforts to maintain adequate oxygenation should
   be made during trauma resuscitations.

   b. **Intracranial pressure (ICP)** is defined according to the modified Monro-
   Kellie hypothesis. This hypothesis is that the intracranial contents are
   contained in a rigid sphere (skull) in which the total volume occupied
   by the three major constituents—brain, blood, and cerebrospinal fluid
   (CSF)—is constant and in which the pressure is evenly distributed.
   An increase in the volume occupied by one constituent therefore must
   be accompanied by a decrease in the volume occupied by one of the
   remaining constituents or there will be a rise in pressure. In the

trauma setting, early and rapid delineation of intracranial injuries by computed tomography (CT) scan is important, as it allows decisions regarding the need for ICP monitoring to be made early. Although usually reserved for the intensive care unit or operating room, ICP monitoring is usually accomplished via the placement of a **subarachnoid pressure monitor ("bolt")**. An **intraventricular catheter** placed in the nondominant lateral ventricle can also be used. This placement has the advantage of providing a means of draining CSF when necessary. General measures used to prevent an increase in the ICP include elevating the head of the bed to 30 to 45 degrees and maintaining the patient's head in the midline position to prevent obstruction of jugular venous outflow. If ICP remains elevated, pharmacologic diuretic therapy to reduce the volume of both the CSF and the brain can be used. **Mannitol, 0.25 to 1.00 g/kg,** is the preferred agent. Sedation and therapeutic paralysis can acutely lower ICP, but they have the disadvantage of obscuring ongoing clinical neurologic examination. Although once advocated as an initial means of lowering ICP, hyperventilation is no longer recommended as a first- line therapy because of its adverse ischemic effects (it decreases ICP by causing intracranial vasoconstriction secondary to inducing hypocarbic alkalosis). It may be used in an acute setting with impending herniation until pharmacologic agents are available, and if it is used, the P_{CO_2} should be closely monitored and kept at a level of 30 to 35 mm Hg. The effective reduction in ICP secondary to hyperventilation lasts no more than 24 to 48 hours because of renal compensation for the respiratory alkalosis. Another second-line modality for decreasing ICP is barbiturate-induced coma (pentobarbital or thiopental), which decreases cerebral blood flow by reducing the metabolic needs of the central nervous system (CNS). It should not be used in the acute setting due to the severe vasomotor instability that may be associated with barbiturate administration, and it should be used only after consultation with a neurosurgeon.

  2. **Spinal cord injuries.** Acute injury to the spinal cord can result in neurogenic shock, which should be treated appropriately (see Section II.C.3). In addition, spinal cord trauma produces debilitating neurologic loss of function. The appropriate acute management of such deficits remains somewhat controversial. A multicenter trial showed that **high-dose infusion of methylprednisolone immediately after blunt injuries** to the spinal cord (complete or incomplete) resulted in modest but statistically significant functional preservation (*N Engl J Med* 1990;322:1405). This study has been followed by several other prospective trials. Currently, most trauma centers administer an intravenous bolus dose of methylprednisolone at 30 mg/kg over 1 hour, followed by a 23-hour infusion of the same drug at a rate of 5.4 mg/kg per hour, in all patients presenting with blunt spinal trauma within 8 hours of injury. Patients presenting with penetrating spinal trauma or being treated more than 8 hours after blunt spinal trauma should not receive any regimen.
  3. **Neurosurgical consultation.** A neurosurgeon should be consulted immediately in all patients with severe neurologic injuries. Early radiologic evaluation of the CNS to exclude evacuable intracranial mass lesions is also critical (see section III.D.3).
E. **Exposure.** The last component of the primary survey is exposure with environmental control. Its purpose is to allow for complete visual inspection of the injured patient while preventing excessive heat loss. The patient is first completely disrobed, with clothing cut away so as not to disturb occult injuries. The patient then undergoes visual inspection, including logrolling to examine the back, splaying of the legs to examine the perineum, and elevation of the arms to inspect the axillae. The nude patient loses heat rapidly to the environment unless specific countermeasures are undertaken. The

resuscitation room should be kept as warm as possible. Any cold metal backboard should be removed as quickly as possible, and all soggy clothing or bedclothes should be taken off expeditiously. All resuscitation fluid should be warmed. Finally, the patient should be covered with warm blankets or a "hot air" heating blanket.

III. **Completion of the primary survey.** The completion of the primary survey should be followed by a brief assessment of the adequacy of the initial resuscitation efforts.

A. **Monitoring.** Appropriate monitoring is essential to determine the clinical trajectory of the injured patient. If not already in place, **ECG leads and a pulse oximeter** should be applied. An **automatic cuff** should be placed for serial BP measurements, although it should be kept in mind that such measurements can be inaccurate in a patient with a systolic blood pressure <90. Finally, an **indwelling urinary catheter** should be placed. Before insertion of the catheter, however, the urethral meatus should be inspected and found free of blood (the labia and scrotum should not harbor a hematoma). In addition, all male patients require palpation of the prostate to ensure that it is in the normal position, not displaced superiorly ("high riding"). If any genitourinary structures are abnormal, a retrograde urethrogram is necessary. If it is normal, the catheter may be passed. If urethral injuries are present, immediate consultation with an urologist is required before attempting to pass the catheter.

B. **Laboratory values.** After placement of two intravenous catheters (see Section II.C.1), blood should be sent for laboratory studies. The most important test to obtain is the cross-match. Other studies include blood chemistries, hematologic analysis, coagulation profile, blood gas with base deficit, toxicologic analysis (with ethanol level), urinalysis, and β-human chorionic gonadotropin level if the patient is a woman of childbearing age. The hematocrit value is the most commonly misinterpreted measure because it is not immediately altered with acute hemorrhage. It should not, therefore, be considered an indicator of circulating blood volume in the trauma patient. (Serial hematocrit values, however, may give an indication of ongoing blood loss.)

C. **Adequacy of resuscitation.** The adequacy of resuscitation can best be determined using urine output and blood pH. Resuscitation, therefore, should strive for a blood pH of 7.4 and a urinary output of 0.5 to 1.0 mL/kg per hour in adults (1 to 2 mL/kg per hour in children). Base deficit and lactic acid levels are also used as markers of adequate resuscitation and have been shown to have prognostic value.

D. **Radiographic investigations.** Essential radiographic investigations are ordered during this period. These tests can provide critical data regarding injuries sustained in a trauma, but their performance should not get in the way of ongoing physical examinations and interventions.

1. **Plain radiography**
   a. **Blunt trauma.** Patients who have sustained blunt trauma with major energy transfer require **chest and pelvic radiographs.** If time permits and the patient is stable, a formal three-view cervical spine series (lateral, anteroposterior, and odontoid) should be obtained. If there is not any evidence of spinal or pelvic injury, an upright chest x-ray should be obtained because it provides crucial information with regard to hemothorax, pneumothorax, mediastinal widening, and subdiaphragmatic gas that sometimes cannot be gleaned from a supine film. Finally, plain radiographs should be obtained of any area of localized blunt trauma, especially if fractures are suspected on the basis of physical exam.
   b. **Penetrating trauma.** Patients who have sustained penetrating injuries require regional plane radiographs to localize foreign bodies and exclude perforation of gas-filled organs (e.g., intestines, lungs). When these films are being obtained, all entrance and exit sites should

be identified with a radiopaque marker. This technique gives insight into the trajectory of the penetrating object and the potential organs injured.

2. **Trauma ultrasonography.** Many trauma centers now employ **focused abdominal sonography for trauma (FAST)** as an initial radiographic screening evaluation for all trauma following the primary survey. As the name implies, it is a focused examination designed to identify free intraperitoneal fluid and/or pericardial fluid. An ultrasound machine is used to take multiple views of six standard areas on the torso: **(1) right paracolic gutter, (2) Morison pouch, (3) pericardium, (4) perisplenic region, (5) left paracolic gutter, and (6) suprapubic region.** Free fluid in the abdomen and within the pericardium appears anechoic. FAST has many advantages: it is portable, rapid, inexpensive, accurate, noninvasive, and repeatable. Its disadvantages include operator variability as well as difficulty of use in morbidly obese patients or those with large amounts of subcutaneous fat. It is most useful in evaluating patients with blunt abdominal trauma, especially those who are hypotensive. It may not be as useful in evaluating children or patients with penetrating trauma. It is important to note that if a FAST exam is negative, it does not exclude major intra-abdominal injury. Finally, some trauma centers are using sonography to evaluate the thorax for traumatic effusions and pneumothoraces.

3. **Computed tomography (CT).** Occasionally, a severely injured patient may require immediate CT evaluation before completion of the secondary survey. For example, patients with severe head injury in whom a compressive intracranial lesion is suspected should undergo emergent CT evaluation to rule out an operable (and potentially lifesaving) condition (e.g., epidural or subdural hematoma). In general, however, the use of CT scan for evaluation of the abdomen or pelvis has become a standard of care, and the availability of more rapid scanners has allowed for the development of protocols in some centers that call for the scanning of trauma patients with a complete body scan (i.e., head, cervical spine, chest, abdomen, and pelvis). Radiology investigation protocols for the trauma setting continue to evolve but usually remain dependent on the availability of equipment and skilled technicians or radiologists in any particular institution.

IV. **Secondary Survey.** The secondary survey follows the primary survey. It is a complete head-to-toe examination of the patient designed to inventory all injuries sustained in the trauma. Thoroughness is the key to finding all injuries, and a systematic approach is required. Only limited diagnostic evaluation is necessary for making decisions about subsequent interventions or evaluations. A review of important aspects of the secondary survey according to anatomic region follows. This review emphasizes only highlights and is not to be considered exhaustive.

A. **Head.** The patient should be evaluated for best motor and verbal responses to graded stimuli so that a **Glasgow Coma Score (GCS)** can be calculated. The GCS is highly reproducible and exhibits little interobserver variability. Severity of head trauma can be stratified according to the score obtained. Any patient with a GCS of 8 or below is considered to have severe neurologic depression and should be intubated to protect the airway (see Chapter 38 and Table 38-1). Inspection and palpation of the head are used to identify obvious lacerations and bony irregularities. All wounds require specific evaluation for evidence of depressed skull fractures or devitalized bone. Signs suggestive of basal skull fractures should be sought. These include periorbital hematomas ("raccoon eyes"), mastoid hematomas ("battle sign"), hemotympanum, and CSF rhinorrhea and otorrhea.

B. **The face** should be inspected for lacerations, hematomas, asymmetry, and deformities. The cranial nerves should be evaluated. The bones should be palpated in a systematic fashion to search for evidence of tenderness, crepitus, or bony discontinuity. In particular, the presence of a midfacial fracture should be sought by grasping the maxilla and attempting to move it. If a fracture is present, it should be classified according to the LeFort criteria. The nares should be examined for evidence of a septal hematoma. The oral cavity should be illuminated and inspected for evidence of mucosal violation (commonly seen in mandibular fractures). All dentures and/or displaced teeth should be removed to prevent airway occlusion. The conscious patient should be asked to bite down to determine if abnormal dental occlusion is present (highly suggestive of a maxillary or mandibular fracture). The eyes should be examined for signs of orbital entrapment and the pupils reexamined. Finally, a nasogastric tube (contraindicated if there is a question of trauma to the midface) or orogastric tube (in patients who have midfacial fractures or are comatose) should be placed to decompress the stomach.

C. **The neck** should be inspected and palpated to exclude cervical spine, vascular, or aerodigestive tract injury.
   1. **Cervical spine evaluation.** Assessing the status of the cervical spine is an important aspect of the secondary survey. Signs of cervical spine injury include midline cervical spine tenderness or vertebral step-off on palpation. Excluding the presence of a cervical injury can often be challenging. The proper algorithm is often dictated by the overall condition of the patient.
      a. **Awake, unimpaired patient.** In the awake, unimpaired, neurologically intact patient, the cervical spine should be palpated for signs of injury (e.g., midline cervical spine tenderness, vertebral step-off). If positive findings are present, the stabilizing cervical collar should remain in place, and a formal three-view cervical spine x-ray series should be obtained. If the physical examination is normal, the patient may be allowed, under supervision, to move the neck through the full range of motion. If there is not any cervical spine pain during this movement, the likelihood of a cervical spine injury is very low, and the stabilizing cervical collar can be removed. If any cervical spine pain is elicited during this movement, the stabilizing cervical collar should remain in place, and a formal cervical spine x-ray series should be obtained. If these x-rays are interpreted as normal, then the possibility of ligamentous injury should be entertained, and the patient should undergo supervised flexion-extension radiographs of the neck. If these films are interpreted as normal, the likelihood of cervical spine injury is low, and the stabilizing cervical collar can be removed (a soft collar may be placed for comfort). If the patient is unable to undergo the 30 degrees of excursion, the collar should be replaced and repeat films obtained at a later time.
      b. **Unconscious or impaired patient.** In the unconscious or impaired (e.g., acutely intoxicated) patient, the cervical spine should be considered unstable until a reliable clinical examination can be performed because significant ligamentous instability can exist with a normal three-view cervical spine x-ray series. The stabilizing cervical collar, therefore, should remain in place until the patient is fully awake and unimpaired. The patient then can be evaluated as previously described [see Section IV.C.1.a]. A CT or MR scan of the cervical spine is a useful adjunct in patients who are unlikely to regain consciousness for extended periods of time.
   2. **Vascular/aerodigestive evaluation.** In addition to evaluating the cervical spine, the neck should be inspected for active hemorrhage and palpated for local tenderness, hematomas, and evidence of subcutaneous air. Wounds should be classified according to their depth and their location. A wound is considered superficial if it does not penetrate the platysma; it is considered deep if the platysma is penetrated. The neck

is divided anatomically into three zones: **zone I** covers the thoracic inlet (manubrium to cricoid cartilage), **zone II** encompasses the midneck (cricoid cartilage to angle of the mandible), and **zone III** spans the upper neck (angle of mandible to base of skull).

D. Thorax. Significant pulmonary, cardiac, or great vessel injury may result from both penetrating and blunt trauma. In all cases, examination of the thorax includes inspection, palpation, percussion, and auscultation. Particular attention should be directed at observing the position of the trachea, checking for symmetric excursion of the chest, palpating for fractures and subcutaneous emphysema, and auscultating the quality and location of breath sounds. Two points bear further comment. First, thoracic extra-anatomic air (subcutaneous air, pneumomediastinum, or pneumopericardium) is frequently noted on physical examination or chest radiography in trauma patients (*Surg Clin North Am* 1996;76:725). Such a finding should alert the trauma team to four potential etiologies: (1) pulmonary parenchymal injury with occult pneumothorax (most common cause), (2) tracheobronchial injury, (3) esophageal perforation, and (4) cervicofacial trauma (usually self-limiting). Second, symmetric breath sounds are not a guarantee of adequate ventilation and oxygenation. End-tidal carbon dioxide, oxygen saturation, and arterial blood gas values must be monitored to ensure that breathing is intact.

E. The abdomen extends from the diaphragm to the pelvic floor, corresponding to the space **between the nipples and the inguinal creases** on the anterior aspect of the torso. When examining the abdomen during the secondary survey, the primary goal is to determine the presence of an intra-abdominal injury rather than to characterize its exact nature. Detecting those patients with occult injuries of the abdomen requiring operative intervention remains a diagnostic challenge. The mechanism of injury, however, often provides important clues.

    1. Penetrating trauma. Stab wounds to the abdomen can be divided into thirds: one-third do not penetrate the peritoneal cavity, one-third penetrate the peritoneal cavity but do not cause any significant intraabdominal injury, and one-third penetrate the peritoneal cavity and do cause significant intra-abdominal damage. As a result, the ability to exclude penetration of the peritoneal cavity in the patient with a stab wound to the abdomen has important therapeutic implications. In the stable patient without obvious signs of intra-abdominal injury (e.g., peritonitis), **local wound exploration** remains a viable screening option. It is a well-defined procedure that entails preparing and draping the area of the wound, infiltrating the wound with local anesthetic, and extending the wound as necessary to follow its track. If the track terminates without entering the peritoneum (as occurs in approximately half of the patients who undergo the procedure), the injury can be managed as a deep laceration. Otherwise, penetration of the peritoneum is assumed, and significant injury must be excluded by further diagnostic evaluation. Options include laparoscopy or celiotomy, CT, FAST, diagnostic peritoneal lavage (DPL, with a lowered red blood cell count of >10,000 as the positive cutoff value), and admission and observation. Gunshot wounds within the surface markings of the abdomen have a high probability of causing a significant intra-abdominal injury and have therefore been taken to require immediate celiotomy, but this imperative has recently been challenged for those patients with stable hemodynamics and no peritoneal signs on physical examination. In a large retrospective study of patients with abdominal gunshot wounds, selective nonoperative management was reported to result in a significant decrease in the percentage of unnecessary laparatomies (*Ann Surg* 2001;234:395). This probably should only be considered in institutions with adequte resources and personnel so that the patient can be closely monitored and undergo frequent abdominal exams. Furthermore, it would be prudent to proceed with

CT scan investigations to delineate the trajectory of the bullet and to exclude any significant injuries.

2. **Blunt trauma.** In the patient sustaining blunt abdominal trauma, physical signs of significant organ involvement are often lacking. As a result, a number of algorithms have been proposed to exclude the presence of serious intra-abdominal injury.

   a. **In the awake, unimpaired patient** without abdominal complaints, combining hospital admission and serial abdominal examinations is a cost-effective strategy for excluding serious abdominal injury as long as the patient is not scheduled to undergo an anesthetic that would interfere with observation. However, such patients are rare in the trauma setting.

   b. **Unstable patient with abdominal injury.** An unstable patient with injuries confined to the abdomen requires immediate celiotomy.

   c. **Unstable patient with multiple injuries.** If an unstable patient has multiple injuries and there is uncertainty whether the abdomen is the source of shock, a FAST exam may be useful. If a patient is fairly stable and access to CT is readily available, head and abdomen/pelvis CT scans can be obtained. DPL may be useful in patients with head injuries requiring immediate operative therapy. In many large centers, a CT scan can be obtained as readily as the performance of a DPL.

   d. **Stable patient with multiple injuries.** If a stable patient has multiple injuries and the abdomen may harbor occult organ involvement that is not immediately life-threatening, a CT evaluation is necessary (see Section VI.C.2). In addition to identifying the presence of intra-abdominal injury, CT scanning can provide information helpful for determining the probability that a celiotomy will be therapeutic. Laparoscopy has also been proposed as an adjunct in this situation.

F. **The pelvis** should be assessed for stability by palpating the iliac wings. Signs of fracture include scrotal hematoma, unequal leg length, and iliac wing hematomas. Careful inspection for lacerations (and possible open fracture) is undertaken.

G. **The back** should be inspected for wounds and hematomas, and the spine should be palpated for vertebral step-off or tenderness. If there are positive signs of spinal injury, anteroposterior and lateral radiographs of the appropriate region (i.e., thoracic, lumbar, sacral) should be obtained.

H. **The genitalia and perineum** should be inspected closely for blood, hematoma, and lacerations. In particular, signs of urethral injury should be sought (see Section III.A). A rectal examination is mandatory to assess rectal tone and to look for the presence of gross blood in the rectum.

I. **The extremities** should be inspected and palpated to exclude the presence of soft tissue and orthopedic, vascular, or neurologic injury. Inspection should look for gross deformity of the limb, active bleeding, open wounds, expanding hematomas, and evidence of ischemia. Obvious dislocations or displaced fractures should be reduced as soon as possible. All wounds should be examined for continuity with joint spaces or bone fractures. The limb should be palpated for subcutaneous air, hematomas, and the presence and character of peripheral pulses. A thorough neurologic examination should be undertaken to determine the presence of peripheral nerve deficits. Radiographs of suspected fracture sites should be obtained, and ankle-brachial indices (ABIs) should be measured in the setting of possible vascular injury even if pulses are normal.

J. **General.** During the secondary survey (and throughout the initial evaluation of the injured patient), any rapid decompensation by the patient should initiate a return to the primary survey in an attempt to identify the cause. Finally, in any penetrating trauma, all entrance and exit wounds must be accounted for during the secondary survey to avoid missing injuries.

V. **Definitive Hospital Care.** With the completion of the primary and secondary surveys, definitive hospital care is undertaken. During this phase of care for the trauma patient, extensive diagnostic evaluations are completed and therapeutic interventions performed. In this section, important therapeutic principles are discussed according to the anatomic location of the injury.

A. Head injuries
1. **Lacerations.** Active bleeding from scalp wounds can result in significant blood loss. Initial therapy involves application of direct pressure and inspection of the wound to exclude bone involvement (i.e., depressed skull fracture). If significant bone injury has been excluded, the wound may be irrigated and débrided. A snug mass closure incorporating all the layers of the scalp will effectively control any hemorrhage and should be done as soon as possible (i.e., before CT evaluations).
2. **Intracranial lesions.** Traumatic intracranial lesions are myriad. They include extraparenchymal lesions, such as epidural hematomas, subdural hematomas, and subarachnoid hemorrhages, as well as intraparenchymal injuries, such as contusions and hematomas. CT is the diagnostic modality of choice. Acute therapy to control ICP and maximize CPP has been discussed previously (see Section II.D.1). A neurosurgeon should be consulted early because emergent surgical intervention can be required.

B. Maxillofacial injuries
1. **Lacerations.** All lacerations of the face should be meticulously irrigated, débrided, and closed primarily with fine nonabsorbable sutures. Alignment of anatomic landmarks is essential. Wounds involving the eyes, lips, ears, nose, and oral cavity may require consultation with a qualified specialist. Given the highly vascular nature of the face, primary closure can be performed up to 24 hours after an injury (except a bite wound) as long as it is accompanied by adequate irrigation and débridement. Any deep laceration in the region of the parotid or lacrimal ducts should be examined for ductal involvement. If either parotid or lacrimal ductal injury is present, consultation with the appropriate specialist should be undertaken. Any patients with mucosal violation require appropriate antibiotic bacterial coverage of oral flora (i.e., penicillin or clindamycin).
2. **Fractures.** Patients with significant craniofacial soft-tissue injury or clinical signs of facial fractures require radiographic evaluation to determine bony integrity. Facial CT (with both axial and coronal 3-mm views) has supplanted most facial plain films other than the Panorex view (obtained for mandible fractures) and is often required in complex midface fractures to define fracture fragments in detail. Therapy is predicated on the type of fracture present.
   a. **Frontal sinus fractures.** Therapy for frontal sinus fractures varies depending on the severity of injury. Nondisplaced anterior table fractures are treated with broad-spectrum antibiotics and observation. Displaced anterior table fractures and posterior table fractures require operative intervention by a specialist.
   b. **Nasal fractures** are one of the most common maxillofacial fractures encountered in the injured patient. Displaced fractures can usually be reduced nonoperatively, with subsequent packing of the nasal cavity for stability. The presence of a septal hematoma requires immediate incision and drainage to prevent avascular necrosis and resultant saddle-nose deformity.
   c. **Maxillary fractures** are classified according to the LeFort system. These fractures often require complex open reduction and fixation. A surgical specialist experienced in these complicated repairs is essential.
   d. **Mandibular fractures.** Fractures of the mandible typically occur in areas of relative weakness, including the parasymphyseal region, angle, and condyle. These injuries can often be treated by a surgical specialist with maxillomandibular fixation, but such therapy requires a 4- to 6-week interval. Rigid fixation using plates is another option. Patients with open fractures should receive antibiotics covering mouth flora.

C. Neck injuries
1. **Penetrating neck wounds.** The diagnostic evaluation of penetrating neck trauma depends on both the depth and location of the wound. Lacerations superficial to the platysma should be irrigated, débrided, and closed primarily. Lacerations longer than 7 cm should be evaluated and closed in the operating room to decrease the risk of infection. Wounds deep to the platysma require evaluation based on the anatomic zone of the injury.
   a. **Zone I injuries.** Thoracic inlet injuries commonly involve the great vessels. Routine four-vessel arteriography has been advocated by many surgeons owing to difficulty in the clinical evaluation and operative exposure of this region. In two prospective studies (*Br J Surg* 1993;80:1534; *World J Surg* 1997;21:41), only 5% of zone I injuries required operation for vascular trauma. Furthermore, routine arteriography did not identify any clinically significant vascular injuries that did not already possess "hard" evidence of vascular trauma (severe active hemorrhage, shock unresponsive to volume expansion, absent ipsilateral upper extremity pulse, neurologic deficit) or "soft" evidence (bruit, widened mediastinum, hematoma, decreased upper-extremity pulse, shock responsive to volume expansion). Additionally, patients who lacked clinical evidence of vascular trauma and were managed conservatively did not have any morbidity or mortality as a result of missed vascular injuries. A recent retrospective analysis supported such observations (*J Trauma* 2000;48:208). Evaluation of the aerodigestive tract can also be approached selectively. Patients with clinical evidence of aerodigestive tract injury (hemoptysis, hoarseness, odynophagia, subcutaneous emphysema, hematemesis) should undergo dual evaluation with bronchoscopy and meglumine diatrizoate (Gastrografin) or thin barium swallow. Esophagoscopy may be substituted for obtunded patients or patients otherwise unable to participate in the swallow study. Finally, CT arteriography has recently been shown to be a good alternative for evaluating vascular and aerodigestive injuries.
   b. **Zone II injuries.** The proper diagnostic algorithm for midneck injuries is somewhat controversial. Little disagreement exists as to the need for immediate operative exploration in the patient with evidence of obvious vascular or aerodigestive tract injury. In stable patients without such signs, multiple selective approaches have been advocated. These approaches have ranged from routine arteriography with panendoscopy to observation alone (*J Vasc Surg* 2000;32:483). Several studies have suggested that contrast-enhanced CT can be useful by demonstrating the trajectory of the missile to vital structures and thus can aid in decision-making regarding further invasive studies or surgical exploration (*Arch Surg* 2001;136:1231; *Trauma* 2001;51:315). Furthermore, studies have shown CT angiography to be useful and comparable to conventional angiography in evaluating for possible vascular injury (*Radiology* 2000;216:356; 2002;224:336). Finally, some authors continue to recommend traditional ipsilateral cervical exploration despite the increased incidence of negative explorations and the associated increased hospital costs. None of these algorithms for management of penetrating zone II injuries has shown superiority over the others, and management is probably best dictated by the manpower and imaging services available to the surgeon.
   c. **Zone III injuries.** Upper neck injuries with clinical evidence of vascular involvement require prompt CT angiography owing to the difficulty of gaining exposure and control of vessels in this region. Embolotherapy can be used for temporary or definitive management, except for the internal carotid artery. An injury without clinical evidence of vascular trauma may be managed selectively, with further evaluation by CT. Direct pharyngoscopy suffices to exclude aerodigestive trauma. In

neck vascular injuries, endovascular stenting and/or embolization, especially in zones I and III, may be beneficial and should be considered if available.

   d. **Operative therapy.** Regardless of the location of the cervical injury, common operative principles apply once surgical exploration is undertaken. Adequate exposure, including proximal and distal control of vascular structures, is essential. The most common approach is through an incision along the anterior border of the sternocleidomastoid muscle. A collar incision is reserved for repair of isolated aerodigestive injuries or for bilateral explorations (e.g., transcervical injuries). The track of the wound must be followed to its termination. Arterial injuries are repaired primarily if possible. Otherwise, prosthetic vascular grafts can be used. Veins can be ligated, except in the case of bilateral internal jugular injury. Tracheal and esophageal injuries should be repaired primarily using synthetic absorbable sutures. If these injuries occur in tandem, a well-vascularized flap of muscle or fascia should be interposed between the repairs to decrease the incidence of posttraumatic tracheoesophageal fistula. Unexpected laryngeal injuries should be evaluated with endoscopy. A drain may be placed if there is any suspicion of aerodigestive tract violation. This maneuver will allow for controlled cutaneous drainage of any leak, thereby preventing lethal mediastinitis. In the case of combined aerodigestive and vascular injuries, the aerodigestive repair should be drained to the contralateral neck to prevent breakdown of the vascular repair from gastrointestinal (GI) secretions should the aerodigestive repair leak.

2. **Blunt neck trauma.** Severe blunt neck trauma can result in significant laryngeal and vascular injuries. In the patient with a stable airway, CT is the best modality for evaluation of a suspected laryngeal injury because it can help determine the need for operative intervention. Minor laryngeal injuries can be treated expectantly with airway protection, head-of-bed elevation, and corticosteroids. Major laryngeal injuries require operative exploration and repair. Blunt vascular trauma usually involves the internal or common carotid artery, but there may also be injury to the vertebral vessels without symptomatology. These injuries can be devastating because they often are not diagnosed until the onset of neurologic deficits. Four-vessel arteriography and CT angiography are the preferred diagnostic modalities, but color flow Doppler has also been suggested. Because the severity of the deficit and the time to diagnosis are strongly associated with outcome, a high index of suspicion is needed. Some authors have even advocated selective arteriography in asymptomatic patients with injury patterns or mechanisms suggestive of a blunt carotid or vertebral artery injury (i.e., severe hyperextension or flexion with rotation of the neck; direct blow to the neck; significant anterior neck soft-tissue injury; cervical spine fracture; displaced midface fractures or mandibular fractures; basilar skull fracture involving the sphenoid, mastoid, petrous, or foramen lacerum) (*Ann Surg* 1998;228:462). The current recommendation is for operative repair of surgically accessible lesions. Systemic anticoagulation (unless contraindicated) with heparin appears to improve neurologic outcome, and it is therefore recommended for surgically inaccessible lesions.

D. **Thoracic injuries.** Rapid diagnosis and treatment of thoracic injuries are often necessary to prevent devastating complications.

1. **Chest wall injuries.** Lacerations of the chest without pleural space involvement require simple irrigation, débridement, and closure. A chest wound communicating with the pleural space constitutes an open pneumothorax and should be treated accordingly (see Section II.B.4). Significant soft-tissue loss may occasionally be encountered and can be initially repaired with polytetrafluoroethylene (PTFE) mesh. Complex

myocutaneous flap or prosthetic closure, however, is often required for
definitive treatment. Rib fractures are common, especially in blunt
trauma. They are readily identified on chest x-ray. Any rib fracture can
trigger a progression of pain, splinting, atelectasis, and hypoxemia. Preventing this cascade through the use of adequate analgesia and pulmonary toilet is essential. Parenteral narcotics are often required. In the
case of multiple rib fractures, intercostal regional blockade using local
anesthetics or epidural analgesia using either narcotics or local anesthetics may be useful. Flail chest often results in significant respiratory
embarrassment and must be treated aggressively (see Section II.B.3).
Finally, the location of rib fractures can provide insight into possible associated injuries (e.g., thoracic aortic injuries are associate with first and
second rib fractures, and hepatic or splenic injuries are associated with
lower rib fractures).

2. **Tracheobronchial injuries** often present with massive subcutaneous emphysema. Prompt diagnosis and initial stabilization are essential. The operative approach is dictated by the location of the injury. Upper tracheal
injuries require a median sternotomy. Distal tracheal or right bronchial
injuries are repaired via a right thoracotomy. Left bronchial injuries mandate a left thoracotomy. Penetrating injuries can be débrided and repaired
primarily using synthetic absorbable suture. Transections resulting from
blunt injuries usually require débridement of the tracheobronchial segment with reanastomosis. Tracheal defects involving up to two rings can
usually be repaired primarily through adequate mobilization. Complex
bronchoplastic procedures or pulmonary resections are rarely required.

3. **Esophageal injuries** are most commonly encountered after penetrating
trauma, and they can pose difficult diagnostic and therapeutic challenges.
These injuries require prompt recognition because delay in diagnosis is
often lethal (mortality can increase threefold when repair is delayed by
24 hours). CT can be helpful for delineating the trajectory of the missile
and possible esophageal injury. Esophagoscopy combined with meglumine diatrizoate (Gastrografin) swallow can detect virtually all injuries,
but either modality is probably adequate for evaluating the thoracic
esophagus. Such evaluations must be performed expeditiously, however,
because their use can cause delays that impact the morbidity of an
esophageal injury repair (*J Trauma* 2001;50:289). As in the case of tracheobronchial injuries, the operative approach is determined by the location of the injury. A right thoracotomy provides excellent exposure for
most thoracic esophageal injuries, particularly those in the midesopha-
gus. A left thoracotomy is recommended for distal esophageal injuries.
Primary repair should be undertaken whenever possible and consists
of closure using an absorbable synthetic suture. The repair can be buttressed with a vascularized flap (i.e., pleural or pericardial) or fundoplication (for distal injuries). Drain placement near (but not adjacent to) the
repair is recommended. Treatment options in late recognized esophageal
injuries include esophageal repair and wide pleural drainage, diversion
with injury exclusion, complex flap closure, and esophageal resection
(reserved for the esophagus with underlying pathology). Morbidity and
mortality are high in this situation.

4. **Pulmonary injuries.** All pulmonary injuries can potentially have an associated pneumothorax (simple or tension). Prompt diagnosis and treatment can be lifesaving (see Section II.B).

   a. **Pulmonary contusion** can be associated with both blunt and penetrating thoracic trauma. These lesions often have adequate perfusion but decreased ventilation. The consequent ventilation-perfusion
mismatch results in severe hypoxemia. Diagnosis is often made by
chest x-ray. Therapy consists of aggressive pulmonary toilet and respiratory support. Occasionally, positioning the patient with the uninjured side in the dependent position will promote perfusion to the

better-ventilated lung, although bleeding into this lung is a concern. Severe contusions often require intubation and mechanical ventilatory support. The management of such patients is extremely challenging because unusual modes of ventilation (e.g., pressure-controlled, inverse-ratio ventilation) may be needed. Consultation with a critical care specialist is often essential.

b. **Hemothorax** is typically diagnosed as opacification on chest x-ray, and it commonly arises from penetrating chest injuries. In the majority of cases, tube thoracostomy is sufficient therapy. A chest x-ray obtained after placement of the tube should be inspected for both tube placement and adequacy of drainage of the hemothorax. A persistent hemothorax with a properly placed thoracostomy tube should raise the possibility of persistent hemorrhage within the hemithorax. Operative intervention is often based on the amount of initial sanguinous drainage and ongoing hemorrhage from the tube. Guidelines vary according to institution and should be individualized to the clinical situation. In general, patients who drain *more than 1.5 L of blood at tube insertion or who have an ongoing blood loss greater than 200 mL per hour over 6 hours* should undergo operative thoracotomy for control of hemorrhage. Significant intrathoracic bleeding can result from pulmonary hilar or great vessel injury (see Section V.D.5). Pulmonary parenchymal hemorrhage can often be controlled with pulmonary tractotomy and oversewing of bleeding intrapulmonary vasculature. Pulmonary resection (lobectomy or pneumonectomy) may be considered for intractable pulmonary hemorrhage (usually from a hilar injury). Morbidity and mortality after pulmonary resection in the trauma setting, however, are significant, and it should therefore be considered a last resort. Air embolism can develop in the setting of significant pulmonary parenchymal injury, especially in the patient on positive-pressure mechanical ventilation. It usually presents as sudden cardiovascular collapse, and therapy consists of placing the patient in steep Trendelenburg, aspirating air from the right ventricle, and providing cardiovascular support. Chest wall intrathoracic hemorrhage usually originates from an intercostal or internal mammary artery and is best treated by ligation.

5. **Great vessel injury**
   a. **Penetrating trauma.** Thoracic great vessel injury most commonly occurs secondary to penetrating trauma. These patients often present in profound shock with an associated hemothorax. Occasionally, they present with pericardial tamponade due to a proximal aortic or vena caval injury. Often, diagnostic investigations are not performed because immediate operative intervention is indicated (e.g., massive hemothorax, pericardial tamponade). In certain circumstances, however, diagnostic evaluation is possible and can be rather extensive. For example, the stable patient suffering from a transmediastinal gunshot injury requires evaluation of the thoracic great vessels, esophagus, trachea, and heart unless the trajectory of the missile clearly avoids those structures. Aortography, endoscopy with radiographic swallow study, echocardiography, and CT may be needed, therefore, to exclude significant injury. CT angiography of the chest to delineate the trajectory of the bullet missile and arterial injury has been used in some centers to determine the need for ancillary studies or surgical interventions. This strategy may provide a more directed approach and avoid potential complications related to the use of diagnostic or operative procedures. The operative approach depends on the vessel involved. Median sternotomy is ideal for access to the proximal aorta, superior vena cava, right subclavian artery, and carotid artery. A left infraclavicular extension ("trapdoor") to the median sternotomy provides exposure to the left subclavian artery, but a high left anterolateral thoracotomy

is probably a better approach. Finally, rapid median sternotomy with either right or left infraclavicular extensions is most appropriate in the patient who has undergone EDT before arrival in the operating room. Whenever possible, primary repair should be performed for arterial and vena caval injuries. Prosthetic grafting may be necessary for complex reconstructions. Brachiocephalic and innominate venous injuries can be ligated. Endovascular approaches may be helpful but remain experimental.

   b. Blunt trauma associated with rapid deceleration (e.g., motor vehicle crashes, falls) can result in thoracic great vessel injury. The descending thoracic aorta just below the origin of the left subclavian artery is particularly prone to rupture from rapid deceleration because it is tethered by the ligamentum arteriosum. Often such a trauma results in complete transection of the aorta and immediate death from exsanguination. In some patients, however, only partial disruption of the aorta occurs, and there is tamponade of the hemorrhage. These patients can arrive at the trauma center alive. If their injury goes unrecognized, however, mortality is near universal. All patients presenting with blunt trauma associated with rapid deceleration therefore must be screened with a chest x-ray, preferably upright. Those patients with positive findings on chest x-ray (widened mediastinum, obscured aortic knob, deviation of the left main-stem bronchus or nasogastric tube, and opacification of the aortopulmonary window) require further evaluation. Helical (spiral) CT is then undertaken, and if it is interpreted as normal, the likelihood of a blunt aortic injury is near zero. If the helical CT is interpreted as indeterminate for aortic injury, immediate four-vessel arteriography is necessary. Arteriographic evidence of an aortic injury mandates prompt operative intervention. In some institutions, direct helical CT evidence of an aortic injury is sufficient to mandate operative repair, whereas in other institutions, it is followed by arteriography. Transesophageal echocardiography is an appropriate diagnostic modality in patients who are unable to undergo helical CT or arteriography. When a blunt aortic injury is present, operative repair should be undertaken as quickly as possible. A left anterolateral thoracotomy is the preferred approach to this portion of the aorta. Often, a prosthetic interposition graft is inserted at the level of the injury, but primary repair can also be performed. Whether to use partial cardiopulmonary bypass as a circulatory adjunct or the "clamp-and-sew" technique remains controversial. Currently, definitive studies demonstrating the superiority of one method of the other in terms of morbidity and mortality do not exist. Sufficient prospective data do exist, however, to recommend delaying operative repair in patients requiring other emergent interventions (e.g., laparotomy or craniotomy) for more immediately life-threatening injuries or in patients who are poor operative candidates due to age or comorbidities (*J Trauma* 2000;48:1128). These patients require close pharmacologic control of their BP until surgical repair can be accomplished. As in penetrating injury, the use of endovascular stents in this setting remains experimental at this time but offers another potential management strategy.

  6. Cardiac injury

    a. Penetrating trauma. Cardiac injury is usually associated with penetrating anterior chest trauma between the midclavicular lines, but it can occur in the setting of penetrating trauma outside these anatomic landmarks. The presentation of a penetrating cardiac injury can range from hemodynamic stability to complete cardiovascular collapse. Pericardial tamponade should be suspected in the patient presenting in shock with distended neck veins and diminished heart sounds **(Beck triad)**. Tension pneumothorax must be excluded, however, by auscultating the lung fields. Additionally, patients with pericardial tamponade can present with jugular venous distention on inspiration (Kussmaul sign). In the hemodynamically stable patient with suspicion for an occult penetrating cardiac injury, echocardiography is the diagnostic modality of choice. Transesophageal examination is preferred. The presence of pericardial fluid warrants emergent operative exploration. Another diagnostic modality is immediate subxiphoid pericardial exploration, especially in the setting of multiple injuries requiring emergent interventions. This procedure is performed in the operating room under general anesthesia. The pericardium is exposed via a subxiphoid approach, and a 1-cm longitudinal incision is made along it. The presence of straw-colored fluid within the pericardium constitutes a negative examination. Blood within the pericardium mandates definitive exploration and cardiorrhaphy. In the hemodynamically unstable patient, EDT is often the means of diagnosis. The preferred operative approach to the repair of penetrating cardiac injuries is via median sternotomy. Atrial and ventricular cardiac wounds are repaired primarily using interrupted or running monofilament sutures. Skin staples may also be used (especially in the setting of EDT). A foley may also be placed into the cardiac wound and the balloon inflated as a temporary measure until definitive management can be performed in the operating room. Care must be taken to avoid injury to coronary arteries during the repair. Wounds adjacent to major branches of the coronary circulation therefore require horizontal mattress sutures placed beneath the artery. Distal coronary artery branches may be ligated. Early consultation with a cardiothoracic surgeon is essential, especially in cases involving complex repairs or cardiopulmonary bypass.

  b. **Blunt trauma.** Blunt cardiac injury (BCI) should be suspected in all patients presenting with the appropriate mechanism of injury (e.g., motor vehicle crash with chest trauma) or in those manifesting an inappropriate cardiovascular response to the injury sustained (*J Trauma* 1998;44:941, 1998). Presentations range from unexplained sinus tachycardia to cardiogenic shock with cardiovascular collapse. Studies suggest that cardiac enzymes have little to no *clinical* value in the diagnosis or treatment of BCI. ECG is the screening modality of choice. A normal ECG excludes significant BCI while the presence of an ECG abnormality (i.e., arrhythmia, ST changes, ischemia, heart block, unexplained sinus tachycardia) in the stable patient warrants admission for 24-hour continuous cardiac monitoring. In the unstable patient, a transthoracic echocardiogram should be performed to identify any dyskinetic/akinetic myocardium or valvular damage. If the transthoracic evaluation is suboptimal, a transesophageal study is mandatory [Eastern Association for the Surgery of Trauma (EAST) guidelines, 1998]. Therapy is dictated by the echocardiogram findings. Patients with frank myocardial or valvular rupture require emergent operative repair. Otherwise, supportive therapy with continuous monitoring and appropriate pharmacologic support (i.e., inotropes and vasopressors) in an intensive care setting is warranted. Any arrhythmias are managed according to standard Advanced Cardiac Life Support protocols. Rarely, invasive mechanical cardiac support is necessary. Aneurysmal degeneration can be a long-term complication of blunt cardiac injury.

E. **Abdominal injuries.** The management of abdominal injuries must often be individualized to meet the needs of each patient, but certain guidelines do apply. All patients undergoing laparotomy for trauma should be prepared and draped from the sternal notch to the knees anteriorly and from each posterior axillary line laterally to have access to the thorax if needed and to the saphenous vein for any potential vascular reconstruction.

1. **Diaphragmatic injuries** occur most commonly as a result of penetrating thoracic or abdominal trauma. Blunt trauma, however, can produce rupture secondary to rapid elevation of intra-abdominal pressure. Frequently, diagnosis is made during celiotomy, but injury can occasionally be recognized on radiographic studies (e.g., chest x-ray or CT). Therapy entails primary repair using monofilament synthetic sutures in a horizontal mattress fashion. In certain circumstances, PTFE mesh closure may be required to cover large defects. Immediate repair prevents the long-term complications associated with diaphragmatic hernias.

2. **Abdominal esophageal injuries** are managed much like thoracic esophageal wounds (see Section V.D.3). In addition to primary repair and drain placement, the fundus of the stomach can be used to buttress the site via a 360-degree (Nissen) wrap. Exposure of this portion of the esophagus can be difficult. Often, the left lobe of the liver must be mobilized and the crus of the diaphragm partially divided. Finally, placement of a feeding jejunostomy should be considered to allow for enteral nutrition in the postoperative period.

3. **Gastric injuries.** Injuries to the stomach occur most often in the setting of penetrating trauma. Sanguineous drainage from a nasogastric (or orogastric) tube should raise the possibility of gastric injury. Diagnosis is usually made at laparotomy. Simple lacerations can be repaired in one layer using synthetic absorbable suture. Alternatively, a full-thickness closure can be reinforced with Lembert stitches. Massive devitalization may require formal resection with restoration of GI continuity via gastroenterostomy. In such cases, vagotomy is helpful in reducing the risk of marginal ulcer.

4. **Hepatic injuries.** The use of CT in blunt trauma has increased the diagnosis of occult liver injuries, making the liver the most commonly injured abdominal solid organ.

   a. **Penetrating trauma.** The diagnosis of penetrating hepatic injury is usually made at exploratory laparotomy, although CT has been used to identify injuries. Hemorrhage in the setting of hepatic trauma can be massive, and familiarity with maneuvers to gain temporary and definitive control of such bleeding is essential.

      (1) **Initial hemostasis.** Rapid mobilization of the injured lobe with bimanual compression can often provide initial hemostasis. Perihepatic packing with laparotomy pads placed over the bleeding site and on the anterior and superior aspects of the liver to compress the wound is an extremely effective alternative. Temporary occlusion of the contents of the hepatoduodenal ligament (Pringle maneuver) with a vascular clamp decreases hepatic vascular inflow and is successful in controlling most intraparenchymal bleeding. It is often employed to allow further mobilization of the liver and exposure and repair of injuries. Occlusion times should not exceed 30 to 60 minutes because longer intervals of warm ischemia are poorly tolerated by the liver. Failure of the Pringle maneuver to significantly decrease bleeding suggests major hepatic venous involvement, including juxtahepatic and retrohepatic inferior vena caval injuries. Prompt recognition and temporary vascular control of such injuries via the placement of an atrial-caval shunt (Schrock shunt) can be lifesaving. Another option in this setting is total hepatic vascular isolation achieved by placing vascular clamps on the hepatoduodenal ligament (if not already done), the descending aorta at the level of the diaphragm, and the suprahepatic and suprarenal vena cava. Finally, bleeding from deep penetrating injuries (e.g., transhepatic gunshot wounds) can sometimes be temporarily controlled through placement of an occluding intrahepatic balloon catheter.

(2) Definitive hemostasis is attained via multiple techniques. Raw surface oozing can be controlled by electrocautery, argon beam coagulation, or parenchymal sutures [horizontal mattress stitches placed in a plane parallel to the injury using large absorbable (No. 2 chromic) sutures on a wide-sweep, blunt-tip needle]. Topical hemostatic agents are also useful (i.e., microcrystalline collagen, thrombin, oxidized cellulose). Deeper wounds are usually managed by hepatotomy and with selective ligation of bleeding vessels. A finger-fracture technique is employed to separate overlying liver parenchyma within a wound until the injured vessel is identified, isolated, and controlled. Major venous injuries should be repaired primarily. Omental packing of open injuries can provide buttressing. Resectional débridement is limited to frankly devitalized tissue. Hepatic artery ligation is reserved for deep lobar arterial injuries where hepatotomy may result in significant blood loss. Formal anatomic resection should be avoided because of its high associated morbidity and mortality. Finally, closed suction drains should be placed near the wound to help identify and control biliary leaks.

(3) Damage control principles are frequently applied to complex hepatic injuries. Perihepatic packing with intensive care admission and resuscitation, followed by return to the operating room in 24 to 48 hours, is common. On occasion, an intrahepatic balloon catheter is used. Liberal use of this algorithm can decrease mortality.

b. **Blunt trauma.** The management of blunt hepatic trauma has undergone a dramatic change over the last decade, largely due to improvement in CT imaging. Currently, CT is the recommended diagnostic modality for evaluation of the stable patient suspected of having blunt hepatic trauma because it can reliably identify and characterize the degree of an injury. Oral and intravenous contrast is necessary to help exclude concomitant hollow viscus injury. In the presence of hepatic trauma, therapy should be predicated on the hemodynamic status of the patient. The unstable patient requires operative exploration and control of hemorrhage as described (see Section V.E.4.a). The stable patient without an alternate indication for celiotomy should be admitted for close hemodynamic monitoring (preferably in an intensive care setting) and serial hematocrit determinations. Operative intervention should be promptly undertaken for hemodynamic instability. Evidence of ongoing blood loss in the hemodynamically stable patient warrants angiographic evaluation and embolization of the bleeding source. Transfusions are administered as indicated. The frequency of follow-up CT evaluation of the lesion should be dictated by the clinical status of the patient. Resumption of normal activity should be based on evidence of healing of the injury. Stable patients therefore do not require strict bed rest. Complications of blunt hepatic trauma include biliary leak and abscess formation, both of which are readily amenable to endoscopic and percutaneous therapy. Delayed hemorrhage is rare, but pseudoaneurysm formation can occur with hemorrhage or hemobilia, requiring angiography and embolization. Nonoperative management is successful in the vast majority of blunt hepatic injuries and has even been reported in certain cases of penetrating hepatic wounds.

5. **Gallbladder injuries.** Injury to the gallbladder frequently coexists with hepatic, portal triad, and pancreaticoduodenal trauma. Treatment consists of cholecystectomy. The gallbladder also provides an effective means of assessing biliary tree integrity via cholangiography.

6. **Common bile duct injuries.** Penetrating trauma is most often responsible for common bile duct injuries. Like gallbladder injuries, they often occur in association with other right upper quadrant organ trauma. Most often, diagnosis is apparent at the time of laparotomy, but occult injuries can occur. Intraoperative cholangiography, therefore, is warranted when biliary involvement is suspected. Primary repair of the injured duct over a T tube is the preferred management, but Roux-en-Y choledochojejunostomy is sometimes required (i.e., when significant segmental loss of the duct is present). Choledochoduodenostomy and cholecystojejunostomy are poor options and should be avoided.
7. **Duodenal injuries** frequently coexist with devastating GI and abdominal vascular trauma and, as a result, can represent a diagnostic and therapeutic challenge. The type and severity of duodenal injury determine management.
   a. **Duodenal hematoma.** Intramural duodenal hematomas usually occur after blunt trauma to the upper abdomen. Patients present with abdominal pain, nausea, and vomiting. Diagnosis is made with CT or upper GI fluoroscopy using meglumine diatrizoate (Gastrografin). Therapy consists of long-term nasogastric decompression and nutritional support (parenteral or enteral distal to the level of injury). The majority of duodenal hematomas are effectively treated in this manner, but operative evacuation may be indicated if obstruction persists for more than 14 days and CT reimaging confirms persistent hematoma.
   b. **Duodenal perforation** can be difficult to diagnose. Patients often complain only of vague back or flank pain, and symptoms can evolve slowly. Plane radiographic signs suggestive of perforation include evidence of retroperitoneal gas, blurring of the right psoas muscle, and leftward scoliosis. Upper GI fluoroscopy using water-soluble contrast (meglumine diatrizoate) may also show evidence of a leak. The diagnostic modality of choice, however, is CT using oral and intravenous contrast, with the oral contrast administered in the trauma room. Operative therapy depends on the degree of injury, but complete mobilization of the duodenum (Kocher maneuver) is essential for proper visualization and repair. Most defects (approximately 80%) can be repaired primarily in two layers, with a transverse closure to avoid luminal narrowing. Closed suction drainage placed around the repair is strongly recommended to control any anastomotic leak. Nasoduodenal decompression should be instigated. Alternatively, antegrade or retrograde (preferred) tube duodenostomy can be performed in conjunction with tube gastrostomy and feeding jejunostomy, the so-called triple tube drainage (*J Trauma* 1979;19:334).
   c. **Complex duodenal injuries** are an operative challenge, and management remains controversial, especially in the presence of tissue devitalization. Whenever possible, débridement with primary repair should be performed. The repair should be protected via triple-tube drainage or pyloric exclusion with diverting gastrojejunostomy. For large defects not amenable to primary closure, a retrocolic Roux-en-Y duodenojejunostomy is an option. Finally, pancreaticoduodenectomy (Whipple procedure) should be reserved only for the most complex injuries, including duodenal devascularization or severe combined injuries involving the pancreatic head and bile duct. This procedure has a very high morbidity and mortality in the trauma setting.
8. **Pancreatic injuries.** Injury to the pancreas often occurs as a result of penetrating trauma, although a significant number of cases do involve blunt mechanisms. Associated morbidity and mortality remain significant and increase with the number of associated injuries. However, isolated pancreatic trauma is rare. Typically, the liver or stomach is also involved, but concomitant duodenal-pancreatic or biliary-pancreatic

injuries do happen. Currently, CT is the best diagnostic imaging modality available, but occasionally endoscopic retrograde cholangiopancreatography or MR cholangiopancreatography studies should be used to help clarify the presence or absence of pancreatic duct injury. *Pancreatic enzymes are not helpful in the diagnosis.* Treatment focuses on determining the presence and location of major ductal involvement. Commonly, such information is obtained during operative inspection of the gland, but occasionally intraoperative pancreatography (endoscopic or transduodenal) may be necessary. Adequate exploration entails performing a Kocher maneuver (to visualize the head of the pancreas) as well as transecting the gastrohepatic and gastrocolic ligaments (to inspect the body and tail of the pancreas). If necessary, the retroperitoneal attachments along the inferior border are divided (to view the posterior aspect of the pancreas) (*Curr Probl Surg* 1999;36:325). When the pancreatic duct is intact, injuries (e.g., contusions, lacerations) are often treated with débridement and closed drainage. Pancreatorrhaphy is employed when indicated. Transection of the pancreatic duct requires more extensive procedures. For ductal injuries occurring to the right of the superior mesenteric vessels, treatment consists of closing the proximal end of the duct with a stapler or suture and draining the distal end via a Roux-en-Y pancreaticojejunostomy. Distal pancreatectomy (with or without splenectomy) should be used for transections occurring to the left of the superior mesenteric vessels. Additionally, it is an option for more proximal injuries in which resection would preserve greater than 10% of the pancreas. Whatever the procedure, the proximal end of the duct should be closed, and the pancreatic bed should be extensively drained. The liberal use of closed suction drainage helps decrease morbidity by controlling pancreatic leaks. Finally, severe injury to the head of the pancreas, especially in conjunction with duodenal and biliary trauma, may require pancreaticoduodenectomy but usually not during the initial operation.

9. **Splenic injuries.** The spleen is the second most common solid organ injured in abdominal trauma. Like hepatic trauma, the management of splenic injuries has undergone an evolution over the past decade.

   a. **Penetrating trauma.** In general, penetrating splenic injuries are diagnosed at laparotomy, although they are sometimes identified on CT imaging. Management depends on complete mobilization of the spleen. Initial hemostasis is possible through manual compression. Minor injuries contained within the splenic capsule do not require any intervention. Bleeding from small capsular lacerations can be controlled with direct pressure or topical hemostatic agents. More complex injuries are treated according to the hemodynamic status of the patient. In the stable patient, splenorrhaphy can be employed in an attempt to preserve immune function (requiring salvage of 40% of the splenic mass). Devitalized tissue should be débrided and the wound closed with absorbable horizontal mattress sutures (usually 2-0 chromic). Alternatively, the spleen can be wrapped in absorbable mesh. Partial resection is indicated for isolated superior or inferior pole injuries. In unstable patients or in patients in whom splenic salvage fails, splenectomy should be performed in an expeditious manner. Drainage of the splenic bed is not necessary unless pancreatic injury is suspected. All patients who undergo emergent splenectomy are at risk for overwhelming postsplenectomy sepsis infection. Although this complication is rare (maximum risk is 0.5% in prepubertal children), the mortality is up to 50%. Therefore, all patients undergoing emergent splenectomy require postoperative immunization against *Streptococcus pneumoniae, Haemophilus influenzae,* and *Neisseria meningitidis.* Some authors even recommend penicillin prophylaxis for children because they are at highest risk. Yearly

viral influenza vaccines are also recommended for postsplenectomy patients.
  b. **Blunt trauma.** Today, most blunt splenic injuries are initially treated with nonoperative observation. CT remains the diagnostic modality of choice. All hemodynamically stable patients without an alternate indication for laparotomy should undergo close observation with continuous monitoring of vital signs, initial bed rest, nasogastric decompression (unless contraindicated), and serial hematocrit determinations. Patients with CT evidence of a contrast "blush" or evidence of continuing blood loss who remain stable should undergo transfusion and selective angiographic embolization. Patients who are hemodynamically unstable or are failing nonoperative management (e.g., require continuing transfusion) should undergo operative exploration and therapy as described (see Section V.E.9.a). Most often, splenectomy is performed. CT reimaging should be performed as clinical status indicates.
 10. **Small-bowel injuries.** Given its large volume and anatomy (tethering at the duodenojejunal flexure), the small bowel is prone to both penetrating (e.g., gunshot) and blunt (e.g., lap belt) trauma. Diagnosis is made at laparotomy or via radiographic imaging (plane radiograph or CT). Treatment consists of primary repair or segmental resection with anastomosis. Mesenteric defects should be closed.
 11. **Large-bowel injuries.** The management of large-bowel injuries is currently undergoing revision. Colonic injuries typically occur secondary to penetrating trauma and are diagnosed at the time of laparotomy. Traditional management emphasized débridement and two-layer primary closure for stab wounds or low-velocity gunshot wounds. Excision, diverting colostomy creation, and Hartmann pouch formation was advocated in patients with multiple injuries, prolonged shock, or large wounds requiring resection and in cases of significant fecal contamination. Recently, however, a prospective multicenter study demonstrated that the surgical management (primary repair versus diversion) of penetrating colonic injuries did not affect the incidence of abdominal complications regardless of associated risk factors (*J Trauma* 2001;50:765). The only independent risk factors for such complications were severe fecal contamination, large transfusion requirement (greater than four units) in the first 24 hours, and single-agent antibiotic prophylaxis. *Primary repair, therefore, should be considered in all penetrating colonic injuries.*
 12. **Rectal injuries.** Penetrating trauma is also responsible for most rectal injuries. They often occur in association with genitourinary or pelvic vascular trauma, and they can be diagnosed via proctoscopy or CT or at laparotomy. Traditional management advocated rectal washout (débridement), diverting sigmoid colostomy creation, and presacral drain placement (the so-called three *D*s). A prospective, randomized trial, however, demonstrated that omission of presacral drains in the management of low-velocity penetrating rectal injuries did not increase infectious complications (*J Trauma* 1998;45:656). Débridement (with primary repair of rectal wounds when possible) and diverting colostomy formation therefore seem sufficient management. Distal stump mucous fistula construction can simplify subsequent reconstruction because it obviates the need to search for a Hartmann pouch in the pelvis. Reversal can be undertaken after 6 weeks if barium enema reveals healing of the rectum and the patient is medically stable.
  F. **Retroperitoneal vascular injuries.** Injuries to the major retroperitoneal vessels or their abdominal branches can be life-threatening. These wounds usually present with frank intra-abdominal hemorrhage or retroperitoneal hematoma formation. Management is based on both mechanism of trauma and location of injury.

1. **Penetrating trauma.** The majority of retroperitoneal vascular injuries are the result of penetrating trauma. By definition, any hematoma formed by a penetrating mechanism is uncontained and requires prompt exploration.
   a. **Initial access and hemostasis.** At times, vascular injuries present with massive intra-abdominal bleeding, and familiarity with techniques to control such hemorrhage expeditiously and to obtain access to vessels efficiently can be lifesaving. Packing the site of injury with laparotomy pads is always a reliable temporizing option. Often, initial control requires occluding the supraceliac aorta at the level of the diaphragmatic hiatus using a vascular clamp, a T-bar, or direct pressure. Division of the gastrohepatic ligament and mobilization of the stomach and esophagus can provide access to this section of the aorta. Occasionally, division of the diaphragmatic crus is necessary for more proximal control. Once the proximal aorta has been occluded, definitive identification and repair of vascular injuries require adequate exposure of the involved vessels. A left medial visceral rotation (Mattox maneuver) provides excellent access to the aorta, celiac axis, superior mesenteric artery (SMA), left renal artery, and iliac arteries. A right medial visceral rotation (Catell maneuver) readily exposes the vena cava (with a combined Kocher maneuver), right renal vessels, and iliac veins. The infrarenal aorta may also be approached via a transperitoneal incision at the base of the mesocolon.
   b. **Repair of vascular injuries.** Most aortic and iliac arterial injuries can be repaired directly by lateral arteriorrhaphy. On occasion, reconstruction with graft prosthesis or autologous venous graft is necessary for significant circumferential or segmental defects. If enteric contamination is extensive, extra-anatomic bypass with oversewing of the proximal stump is mandatory. Injuries to the celiac root or certain of its branches (left gastric or splenic arteries) can often be ligated without adverse outcome, especially in young patients. Splenectomy must follow splenic artery ligation. Common hepatic artery injuries should be repaired when possible (via lateral arteriorrhaphy, resection and reanastomosis, or graft), but ligation can be tolerated at times. SMA defects must be repaired. Vena caval and iliac venous injuries are repaired by lateral venorrhaphy. Injuries to the superior mesenteric vein (SMV) and portal vein should undergo repair, but cases of successful outcome after ligation have been reported. Because of the risk of postoperative thrombosis leading to portal hypertension or superior mesenteric infarction, SMV and portal venous reconstructions must be closely followed, and anticoagulation is often administered. Finally, major renal arterial and venous injuries require primary repair, whereas partial nephrectomy is recommended for segmental vessel involvement. Endovascular treatment has an expanding role in the treatment of all vascular trauma and may be beneficial.
2. **Blunt trauma** can cause retroperitoneal vascular injury with resultant hematoma formation. Often, these hematomas are discovered at operative exploration, but they are sometimes seen on preoperative imaging. The character and location of the hematoma determine management.
   a. **Central abdominal hematomas (zone I).** All central abdominal hematomas caused by blunt trauma require operative exploration. Supramesocolic hematomas are usually due to injuries to the suprarenal aorta, celiac axis, proximal SMA, or proximal renal artery. They should be approached via a left medial visceral rotation. Inframesocolic hematomas are secondary to infrarenal aortic or inferior vena caval injuries and are best exposed by a transperitoneal incision at the base of the mesocolon. As with any vascular repair, proximal and distal control of the involved vessel should be obtained prior to exploration if possible.

b. **Flank hematomas (zone II).** Flank hematomas are suggestive of renal artery, renal vein, or kidney parenchymal injury. Unless they are rapidly expanding, pulsatile, or ruptured, they should not be explored if discovered at the time of celiotomy. Radiographic evaluation of the ipsilateral kidney is necessary in this situation to assess its function, usually by means of CT imaging. Evidence of nonfunction should prompt arteriography of the renal artery because blunt abdominal trauma often causes intimal tears, with resulting thrombosis of the artery. If it is discovered within 6 hours of the injury, revascularization is performed, although the success rate is only 20%. Otherwise, nonoperative management is preferred. Nephrectomy is sometimes indicated when laparotomy is performed for associated injuries in a stable patient. In this setting, removal of the nonfunctioning kidney will decrease long-term renal complications (e.g., urinoma, hypertension, delayed bleeding). When operative exploration of a flank hematoma is required, vascular control should be obtained outside the Gerota fascia. Total or partial (to preserve renal mass) nephrectomy may be necessary for a shattered kidney.

c. **Pelvic hematomas.** Central pelvic hematomas in the setting of blunt trauma are usually due to pelvic fractures. If discovered at celiotomy, they should not be explored unless iliac vessel injury is suspected (loss of ipsilateral groin pulse, rapidly expanding hematoma, pulsatile hematoma) or rupture has occurred. Bleeding from pelvic fractures can be massive, and management should focus on nonoperative control. Unstable pelvic fractures in association with hypotension should undergo some form of external stabilization. In extreme circumstances, temporary control of hemorrhage can be achieved by wrapping a sheet tightly around the pelvis. Formal external fixation should follow as soon as possible. It should also be considered in those patients with unstable pelvic fractures who require celiotomy or who are hemodynamically stable but have a need for continued resuscitation. Pelvic angiography with selective embolization is the preferred intervention for patients in whom major pelvic fractures are the suspected source of ongoing bleeding. It should also be considered in patients with major pelvic fractures when CT imaging reveals evidence of arterial extravasation in the pelvis or when bleeding in the pelvis cannot be controlled at laparotomy.

G. **Genitourinary injuries.** Injuries to the genitourinary tract are discussed in detail in Chapter 40. Three points, however, warrant discussion in the context of trauma. Urethral injuries complicate the placement of an indwelling catheter. Their diagnosis and management have been discussed (Section III.A). In blunt abdominal trauma, **gross hematuria *or* microscopic hematuria in the setting of hemodynamic instability** mandates urologic evaluation. The absence of hematuria, however, does not always exclude an injury to the urinary tract, especially in the setting of penetrating torso trauma. CT is the best imaging modality for demonstrating urologic injury in the trauma patient who does not require laparotomy for other reasons, and it provides information regarding kidney perfusion. Although once commonly used, excretory urography (IVP) in the trauma patient is often unsatisfactory and is now rarely used. In patients with suspected bladder rupture, especially those with gross *hematuria or pelvic fluid on CT in the presence of pelvic fractures,* cystography should be performed. **CT cystography** has been demonstrated to be equivalent to conventional cystography in assessing bladder injury (EAST guidelines, 2003).

H. **Orthopedic injuries** are discussed in detail in Chapter 39, but three important considerations bear mentioning.

1. **Blood loss.** Fractures can produce large blood losses. A broken rib can be associated with a 125-mL blood loss, a forearm fracture with a 250-mL blood loss, a broken humerus with a 500-mL blood loss, a femur fracture

with a 1,000-mL blood loss, and a complex pelvic fracture with a blood loss of 2,000 mL or more. Stabilization of fractures can minimize the amount of bleeding. Although the MAST trouser (pneumatic antishock device) has been largely discredited as a device for raising BP, it may afford transient pneumatic stabilization to lower-extremity and pelvis fractures, thereby attenuating further blood loss while the patient is being prepared for more specific interventions (e.g., traction, fixation, or arteriography and embolization).

2. **Spinal fractures.** Fractures of the spine are multiple in 10% of cases. Complete radiographic evaluation of the spine is necessary, therefore, when a single fracture is discovered.

3. **Joint involvement.** Two joints overlie single-access arteries: the elbow and the knee. Fractures or dislocations of either of these joints increase the risk of ischemic complications of the involved distal limb. The integrity of the underlying artery therefore must be confirmed by ABIs, serial evaluation, or, in some cases, arteriography.

I. **Extremity injuries.** Extremity trauma can result in devastating injuries requiring the coordination of multiple specialists to perform complex reconstructions. The goal of management is limb preservation and restoration of function, and it should focus on ensuring vascular continuity, maintaining skeletal integrity, and providing adequate soft-tissue coverage.

1. **Penetrating trauma.** Penetrating extremity trauma typically occurs in males younger than 40 years old. Multiple injuries can occur in association with such trauma, and a high index of suspicion is necessary for diagnosing and repairing them expeditiously.

2. **Vascular injuries.** A wounded extremity can tolerate approximately 6 hours of ischemia before the onset of irreversible loss of function. Quickly identifying and repairing vascular injuries, therefore, is essential in any extremity trauma. Immediate operative exploration is indicated for obvious (hard) signs of vascular involvement (pulse deficit, pulsatile bleeding, bruit, thrill, expanding hematoma) in gunshot or stab wounds without associated skeletal injury. Arteriography should be employed for those patients with hard vascular signs in the setting of associated skeletal injury (fracture, dislocation) or shotgun trauma. Patients with possible (soft) signs of vascular injury (nerve deficit, nonexpanding hematoma, associated fracture, significant soft-tissue injury, history of bleeding or hypotension) require evaluation of vascular integrity. A useful algorithm is to check the ABI initially. If the ABI for the affected limb is greater than 0.9, no further radiographic evaluation is necessary. If it is less than 0.9, noninvasive Doppler ultrasonography should follow to exclude vascular injury. If ultrasonography is equivocal, arteriography is indicated; if it is positive, either operative exploration or arteriography can follow (depending on the institution). Patients without hard or soft signs do not require arteriography to exclude vascular involvement. Occult vascular injuries can be managed nonoperatively, with subsequent repair as indicated, without an increase in morbidity. Arterial injuries should be repaired within 6 hours to maximize limb salvage rates. The operative approach is similar to elective vascular procedures and endovascular therapy may be feasible if available. Proximal and distal control of the involved vessel is essential. Primary repair using monofilament suture should be performed for limited arterial lacerations. For complex injuries (large segmental or circumferential defects), resection with reanastomosis, patch angioplasty, or interposition grafting is preferred. Whenever possible, autologous vein should be used instead of PTFE for patching or grafting because of its higher patency rates. Ligation of single-artery forearm and calf injuries is possible in the presence of normal counterparts. Restoration of blood flow (via temporary shunt or formal repair) should precede any skeletal reconstruction in cases of combined injuries. Completion arteriography should

be performed after any arterial repair. Venous injuries should undergo lateral venorrhaphy or resection with end-to-end reanastomosis if the patient is hemodynamically stable. Ligation with postoperative leg elevation and compression stocking placement (to reduce edema) is indicated in all other cases. Multiple compartment fasciotomies should be liberally used, especially after prolonged ischemia or in the presence of associated injuries.

3. **Skeletal injuries** are diagnosed with plane radiography. Restoration of skeletal integrity is attained by means of either internal or external fixation. Temporary vascular shunting should be performed before stabilization of an unstable fracture in the setting of combined injuries. External fixation is preferred in the presence of gross contamination or tissue loss (see Chapter 39 for further details).

4. **Soft-tissue injuries.** Definitive closure of large soft-tissue defects rarely occurs at the initial operation for extremity trauma. Complex wounds are often thoroughly irrigated and débrided, dressed, and reviewed daily in the operating room. Delayed closure is then undertaken and may require advanced soft-tissue flaps (pedicle or free). On rare occasions, a so-called mangled extremity may require primary amputation if there are severe soft-tissue defects, major bone injury, or unreconstructable peripheral nerve injury and loss of limb function.

5. **Blunt trauma.** Blunt extremity trauma can result in debilitating crush or near-avulsion injuries. Diagnosis and management are the same as in penetrating trauma, but limb salvage and preservation of function tend to be worse due to the extent of injury. These wounds often require the coordinated involvement of multiple specialists.

6. **Extremity compartment syndromes.** Compartment syndromes are common in distal extremity trauma. They typically occur in association with prolonged limb ischemia or external pressure, fractures, crush or vascular injuries (especially combined arterial and venous injuries), and burns. **Increased tissue pressure (>30 mm Hg)** within the inelastic fascial compartment leads to occlusion of capillary flow and ischemia. Signs and symptoms of compartment syndrome include **pain (especially on passive motion), pressure, paralysis, paresthesia, pulselessness, and pallor (the so-called six *Ps*).** A high index of suspicion is necessary for early diagnosis because signs often occur late in the process, especially the loss of pulses. Serial compartment pressure measurements should therefore be undertaken in any patient with risk factors. Fasciotomy of all involved compartments is necessary when pressures are 30 to 40 mm Hg (or lower if evidence of ischemia exists). Additionally, fasciotomy should be performed if pressures cannot be obtained.

J. **Damage control surgery.** Over the last decade, the concept of damage control has gained increasing support among trauma surgeons as a valuable adjunct in the surgical care of severely injured patients (*Surg Clin North Am* 1997;77:753). Evolving in response to changing patterns of injury in urban American settings, the damage control philosophy centers on coordinating staged operative interventions with periods of aggressive resuscitation to salvage trauma patients sustaining major injuries. These patients are often at the limits of their physiologic reserve when they present to the operating room, and persistent operative effort results in exacerbation of their underlying **hypothermia, coagulopathy, and acidosis,** initiating a vicious cycle that culminates in death. In these situations, abrupt termination of the procedure after control of surgical hemorrhage and contamination, followed by intensive care resuscitation and staged reconstruction, can be lifesaving. Although often discussed in the context of abdominal trauma, the practice of damage control can be applied to all organ systems. It is divided into three phases: initial exploration, secondary resuscitation, and definitive operation.

1. **Phase I (initial exploration).** The first phase in the damage control algorithm consists of performing an initial operative exploration to attain rapid control of active hemorrhage and contamination. The decision to revert to a damage control approach should occur early in the course of such an exploration. In the setting of abdominal trauma, the patient is prepared and draped as previously described (see Section V.E), and the abdomen is entered via a midline incision. Any clot or debris present on entering the abdomen is promptly removed. If exsanguinating hemorrhage is encountered, four-quadrant packing should be performed. The packing is then removed sequentially, and all surgical hemorrhage within a particular quadrant is controlled before proceeding. Following control of bleeding, attention is directed at containment of any enteric spillage. Any violations of the GI tract should be treated with suture closure or segmental stapled resection. Anastomosis and stoma formation should be deferred until later definitive reconstruction, and any stapled ends of the bowel should be returned to the abdomen. External drains are placed to control any major pancreatic or biliary injuries. Laparotomy packs are then reinserted, especially in the presence of coagulopathic bleeding. Often, primary abdominal fascial closure is not possible secondary to edematous bowel or hemodynamic instability. Alternative methods of closing the abdomen include skin closure via towel clips or running suture, Bogota bag placement, prosthetic mesh insertion, or abdominal wall zipper creation. Of all these techniques, the Bogota bag is the most commonly used. It is fashioned by opening the seams of a 3-L sterile urologic irrigation bag and suturing it to the skin edges. Closed suction drains covered with a sterile adhesive dressing eases wound care in the ICU. Throughout the initial operative exploration, communication between the surgeons, anesthesia team, and nursing staff is essential for optimal outcome.

2. **Phase II (secondary resuscitation).** The second phase in the damage control approach focuses on secondary resuscitation to correct hypothermia, coagulopathy, and acidosis. Following completion of the initial exploration, the critically ill patient is rapidly transferred to the ICU. Invasive monitoring and complete ventilatory support are often needed. Rewarming is initiated by elevating the room temperature, placing warming blankets, and heating ventilator circuits. All intravenous fluids, blood, and blood products are prewarmed. As body temperature normalizes, coagulopathy improves, but rapid infusion of clotting factors (fresh frozen plasma, cryoprecipitate, and platelets) is often still required. Circulating blood volume is restored with aggressive fluid and blood product resuscitation, improving end-organ perfusion and correcting acidosis. With these interventions, hemodynamic stability returns, urinary output increases, invasive monitoring parameters improve, and serum lactate levels and blood pH analysis improve. In the setting of abdominal trauma, a potentially lethal complication that can occur during this phase is abdominal compartment syndrome. It is a form of intra-abdominal vascular insufficiency secondary to increased intra-abdominal pressure. Presentation includes abdominal distention, low urinary output, ventilatory insufficiency in association with high peak inspiratory pressures, and low cardiac output secondary to decreased venous return (preload). Diagnosis is made via measurement of urinary bladder pressure (>25 cm H_2O). When present, prompt operative reexploration is mandated to relieve the increased pressure. If surgical bleeding is found to be the cause of the intra-abdominal hypertension, it should be controlled and the abdomen closed. If severe edema of the intra-abdominal contents is the source of the compartment syndrome, the abdomen should be closed using a Bogota bag to reduce intra-abdominal pressure. Following correction of the problem, phase II resuscitation is continued.

3. **Phase III (definitive operation).** The third phase of damage control consists of planned reexploration and definitive repair of injuries. This phase typically occurs 48 to 72 hours following the initial operation and after successful secondary resuscitation. In the setting of abdominal trauma, all complex injuries are repaired, with precedence going to those involving the vasculature. Conservative principles should be applied. Risky GI anastomoses or complex GI reconstructions should be avoided. The abdomen should be closed primarily if possible. Otherwise, biologic mesh or simple skin closure and staged repair of the resulting ventral hernia should be performed. Even though the damage control approach allows for salvage of many severely injured patients, it is still associated with substantial morbidity and mortality. Outcome is often determined by providing excellent supportive care (ventilation, nutrition, appropriate antibiotics, and physical therapy with rehabilitation services).

VI. **Miscellaneous aspects of general trauma care**
   A. **Emergency department thoracotomy (EDT)** is performed in a final attempt to salvage a certain subset of patients presenting in extremis to the emergency department. The goals are to control intrathoracic hemorrhage, relieve cardiac tamponade, cross-clamp the thoracic aorta, and restore cardiac output.
      1. **Indications.** The indications for EDT have been refined over time. Currently, it should be used in the management of penetrating chest trauma associated with significant hemodynamic deterioration (systolic BP of <60 mm Hg) or cardiopulmonary arrest occurring within the emergency department or shortly before arrival (<10 to 12 minutes). Additionally, it can be used in certain cases of penetrating abdominal trauma fulfilling the same criteria. Current thinking is that it is contraindicated in blunt chest or abdominal trauma resulting in cardiopulmonary arrest because survival after such an intervention almost never occurs.
      2. **Technique.** EDT is performed via an anterolateral left thoracotomy in the fifth or sixth intercostal space. The skin, subcutaneous tissues, and intercostal musculature are opened sharply. A Finochietto retractor is placed to spread the ribs and aid in exposure. First, the pericardium is identified and incised vertically anterior to the phrenic nerve. Any clot or debris is removed from around the heart. Specific cardiac injury is then sought, and repair is undertaken as previously described (see Section V.D.6.a). After cardiorrhaphy, air is evacuated from the heart by needle aspiration, and the adequacy of cardiac filling is assessed to determine intravascular volume status. In the absence of associated pulmonary vascular or great vessel injury, vigorous volume resuscitation is undertaken. If peripheral vascular access is insufficient, direct infusion into the right atrial appendage can be performed. In severely hypovolemic patients, the descending thoracic aorta may be exposed and cross-clamped to maintain coronary and cerebral perfusion. The aorta should also be clamped if any intra-abdominal hemorrhage is suspected. During volume resuscitation, open cardiac massage is employed to provide adequate circulation. After restoration of adequate circulatory volume, the underlying cardiac rhythm is assessed, and internal cardioversion is used when appropriate. The patient should be transported to the operating room for definitive injury management and wound closure after a successful resuscitation.
      3. **Complications of EDT** are many. They include lung injury while gaining access to the heart, transection of the phrenic nerve while performing pericardotomy, injury to the coronary vessels during cardiorrhaphy, and esophageal trauma while clamping the descending thoracic aorta. Therefore, care must be taken during each step of the procedure to avoid causing additional injuries.
   B. **Diagnostic peritoneal lavage (DPL).** Since the advent of FAST and rapid helical CT imaging, DPL is now rarely used in the evaluation of patients with

suspected intra-abdominal injuries. It remains, however, a useful diagnostic modality in certain situations.

1. **Indications.** DPL is useful in excluding the presence of significant intra-abdominal organ injury in the presence of blunt trauma or a stab wound to the abdomen. It should be employed when less invasive techniques (e.g., serial abdominal examinations, CT, or FAST) are unavailable or if the patient develops unexplained hemodynamic instability while in the operating room for another injury. The only absolute contraindication to DPL is a planned celiotomy. Pelvic fracture, pregnancy, and prior abdominal surgery often mandate a change in indication and technique. All patients undergoing DPL require prior evacuation of the stomach via a gastric tube as well as drainage of the bladder by indwelling catheter.

2. **Technique.** Aspiration of 10 mL of gross blood or any enteric contents is considered a positive DPL. Additionally, the microscopic presence of 100,000 red blood cells/μL or 500 white blood cells/μL in the setting of blunt abdominal trauma and the presence of 10,000 red blood cells/μL or 50 white blood cells/μL in the setting of penetrating abdominal trauma is considered a positive finding on DPL.

3. **Complications.** DPL can produce false-positive results due to bleeding near the incision or from pelvic fractures hemorrhaging into the anterior preperitoneal space of Retzius. False-negative findings can occur from improper placement of the catheter and infusion of fluid into the space of Retzius. Puncture of viscera is also possible, especially in the setting of pregnancy or adhesions from prior abdominal operations. An open technique is essential in such circumstances. Although it is associated with certain complications, DPL is a safe, simple, reliable procedure for detecting intra-abdominal injuries with excellent sensitivity (>95%).

C. **CT imaging in trauma care.** CT imaging has emerged as a powerful tool in the evaluation of the trauma patient. Since its inception, its role has expanded from assessing intracranial injuries (its use in the 1970s) to whole body imaging. Although it is an extremely useful modality, three points must be kept in mind when deciding to perform a CT scan in the trauma setting.

1. **Patient status.** The overall status of the trauma patient is crucial in determining whether CT is the proper modality to use. Even though a CT facility may be located adjacent to a resuscitation area, a patient is often inaccessible while centered in the CT torus for an examination. Unstable patients therefore should not undergo CT imaging. Instead, they should have specific interventions performed to stabilize vital functions and then proceed to the CT facility and/or the operating room.

2. **Appropriateness of CT evaluation.** CT imaging may be an inappropriate modality early in the course of treatment for a trauma patient. For example, a patient with evidence of free air on plane radiography requires emergent celiotomy for treatment of a ruptured hollow viscus, not an immediate CT evaluation of the abdomen unless other injuries are suspected. Furthermore, a high-resolution CT of a facial fracture should not delay treatment of more immediate life threats. CT would be an appropriate modality, however, for determining major organ system injuries in a patient without significant external evidence of trauma. It is also particularly effective in recreating the trajectory of a penetrating missile and its relationship to major vascular or aerodigestive structures. Soft-tissue hemorrhage and edema, bone and missile fragments, foreign bodies, and soft-tissue gas can be followed through successive CT panels to determine the course of the missile through the body and its relationship to important structures.

3. **Order and timing of CT evaluations.** Often, trauma patients will require multiple CT examinations as part of their diagnostic evaluation. Determining the proper order of such imaging is important. Head CT should take precedence over all other CT studies because emergent craniotomy

may be necessary to drain a mass lesion. Chest CT should follow the head CT when suspicion of a mediastinal hematoma (i.e., great vessel injury) exists. Abdominal CT usually follows the head and chest CTs. The patient should receive enteral contrast before arriving at the CT scanner, especially if duodenal hematoma is suspected. It is not, however, absolutely required. Intravenous contrast should be administered for chest and abdominal CTs unless contraindicated. Use of dynamic and spiral protocols improves the resolution and speed of abdominal imaging and the information gained from it. CT evaluation of bony structures (e.g., face, spine, pelvis) often requires multiple, tightly spaced images that take time to obtain. Such studies can be obtained immediately if the patient is stable.

D. Antibiotics in trauma care. Many injuries violate natural barriers to infection. Contamination of wounds with microorganisms is therefore common, and antibiotic therapy is used to help reduce bacterial counts to allow effective immune system response. The selection of antibiotics is based on the nature of the barrier violation and the organisms most likely to be involved.

  1. **Skin injuries.** Traumatic violation of the skin is not an indication for antibiotic therapy in and of itself. Débridement and irrigation of the wound usually reduce bacterial counts to levels at which healing can occur without infection. Antibiotic therapy is indicated when the patient is at high risk for infection due to age or intercurrent disease (e.g., immunosuppression). It should also be used when the potential contaminating organisms are particularly virulent (e.g., those found in pond water, human saliva, or soil). Rarely, antibiotics are given because local wound care is inadequate. A first-generation cephalosporin, such as cefazolin, should be used to cover endogenous skin flora. Clindamycin is a safe alternative when hypersensitivity to β-lactams exists. When covering virulent organisms, specific coverage should be tailored to those most likely to contaminate the wound. Finally, with any skin wound, tetanus prophylaxis should be given when indicated.

  2. **GI injuries.** Traumatic violation of the GI tract releases anaerobes and Gram-negative organisms. These bacteria usually can be treated with a second-generation cephalosporin or cephamycin, such as cefotetan or cefoxitin. Use of combination therapy, such as clindamycin with gentamicin or aztreonam, is usually reserved for patients with documented β-lactam hypersensitivity. All patients undergoing celiotomy for abdominal trauma should receive a single preoperative dose of a broad-spectrum antibiotic with aerobic and anaerobic coverage as prophylaxis. In the setting of penetrating trauma with hollow viscus injury, the antibiotic need only be continued for 24 hours after the operation. Adjusted doses are needed for hemodynamically unstable patients.

  3. **Orthopedic injuries.** Open fractures are prone to infection. Although débridement and irrigation are the mainstays of therapy, adjunctive antibiotics are indicated. Because the most common contaminants are skin flora, a first-generation cephalosporin is often selected. An aminoglycoside is sometimes added for complex wounds. Simple open fractures require 24 hours of therapy. Complex fractures require no more than 72 hours of antibiotics after wound closure.

  4. **CNS injuries.** A traumatic violation of the dura exposes the meninges, CSF, and neural tissue, predisposing them to infection. Although controversy exists regarding the necessity of antibiotic therapy, most neurosurgeons routinely prescribe a β-lactam (e.g., oxacillin) that easily crosses the blood-brain barrier. Planned placement of an ICP monitoring catheter in a trauma patient does not require antibiotic therapy.

E. Deep venous thrombosis with pulmonary embolus is the leading cause of preventable morbidity and mortality in trauma patients. Some form of prophylaxis is required in all such patients. When neural injuries (i.e., CNS or spinal cord injuries) are absent, subcutaneous heparin should be administered. When lower-extremity injuries do not preclude their use, sequential pneumatic compression devices are beneficial. Therapy combining compression devices with subcutaneous heparin is thought to be synergistic. Low–molecular-weight heparin solutions are also being used in many centers as the primary form of deep venous thrombosis prophylaxis. When the preceding techniques are contraindicated, serious consideration should be given to early placement of a vena caval filter. Although such a filter does not prevent thrombosis, it substantially decreases the risk of a deadly pulmonary embolus.

F. Nutrition in trauma care. Nutritional support remains a cornerstone in the care of trauma patients. In general, the passage of 5 days without protein-calorie support renders most injured patients deeply catabolic, potentially compromising their immune system. Nutrition should be started quickly, therefore, especially if a prolonged hospital course is anticipated. The GI tract is the preferred route of administration, and placement of a feeding enterostomy should be considered at the end of every celiotomy for trauma. Enteral nutrition helps maintain the immune function and integrity of the GI tract, thereby preventing bacterial translocation. Glutamine is the fuel of the enterocyte and functions as an essential amino acid in the setting of trauma. In patients without a functional GI tract, parenteral nutrition should be used. It requires central venous access for its administration and therapeutic complications (e.g., line sepsis, vein thrombosis) tend to be greater.

G. Gastroduodenal ulceration. Injured patients remain at risk for stress gastroduodenal ulceration and concomitant hemorrhage. Prophylaxis is therefore recommended. Enteral feeding remains the most effective method. When such feeding is not possible, a topical agent such as sucralfate can be used as a safe, inexpensive alternative. Parenteral histamine-receptor blockers also prevent posttraumatic GI bleeding in ventilated or coagulopathic patients. Finally, newer intravenous proton pump inhibitors may find a role in prophylaxis, but their expense may prove prohibitive.

H. Analgesia in trauma care. Providing adequate analgesia for trauma patients continues to remain a therapeutic challenge. When properly administered, analgesia can control sympathetic hyperactivity and allow a patient to maintain ventilation and mobility. In general, the best techniques are those that address the injured parts directly (e.g., neuraxis and locoregional analgesia). They often, however, require time, normal coagulation parameters, and patient cooperation. When these criteria are not met, patient-controlled intravenous opiate administration is the best alternative. Most commonly, morphine sulfate is given by means of a patient-controlled analgesic device. Intermittent intravenous opiate therapy is a less optimal option. Intramuscular opiate injection is an ineffective and inefficient means of analgesic control and should be avoided.

I. Neuropsychiatric disorders. Neuropsychiatric disorders are common in trauma patients. They can include substance withdrawal, anxiety, depression, or underlying psychosis. The onset of posttraumatic delirium should always trigger a search for a toxic, metabolic, or structural cause. Failure to identify such an etiology should suggest the possibility of a treatable psychiatric disturbance. A mental health history from the patient or family obtained at admission can provide important insight into the cause of the delirium. Additionally, a high index of suspicion for substance withdrawal is needed because certain types can be fatal (e.g., alcohol). Patients undergoing withdrawal from a drug typically present with signs and symptoms in opposition to the typical effects of the substance abused. Treatment is tailored to the withdrawal syndrome encountered.

J. Rehabilitation in trauma care. Rehabilitation is a crucial aspect of trauma care, and its planning should begin at the time of admission. Contractures and pressure sores can begin within hours of injury, and as a result standardized prevention must be initiated promptly on the arrival of the patient on the ward. Regular turning of the patient, placement of air mattresses, and elevation of distal extremities (especially the heel) off the bed can decrease the formation of debilitating pressure sores. Specially designed orthotic splints, braces, and stockings prevent joint and scar contractures that can inhibit return of function. Finally, early physical and occupational therapy initiates the recovery process and prepares the patient for the often difficult rehabilitation to daily activity.

CONCLUSION

A chapter of this nature is brief by necessity, but a comprehensive strategy for the care of patients who have been involved with traumatic events will clearly improve outcomes. This care should be coordinated by dedicated general surgeons with an interest or special training in trauma and should ideally use surgical specialty services staffed by individuals with trauma expertise. Although all institutions will not be able to have dedicated trauma-oriented surgeons on staff, the development of statewide trauma systems facilitates the care of patients by directing care of these patients toward those institutions with appropriate resources. For these statewide trauma systems to survive and for the hospitals within the systems to remain financially intact, there needs to be ongoing governmental financial support for the care of trauma victims. Trauma is a serious public health concern that requires comprehensive public health and governmental strategies for managing the complicated issues surrounding the trauma care.

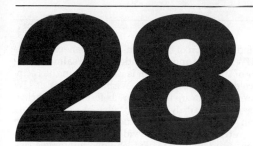

Transplantation

Jeremy Goodman,
Jeffrey A. Lowell, and
Daniel C. Brennan

TRANSPLANT ORGAN PROCUREMENT

I. **Donor selection.** The greatest obstacle to organ transplantation today is the lack of suitable donor organs. Live donation has provided an important source of organs, with annual living kidney donors recently surpassing deceased donors. Less frequently, live donation is being utilized in liver and lung transplantation. The patients waiting for organs still outnumber the available organs, and the waiting list for organ transplants grows each year. In the United States, more than 80,000 people await a solid-organ transplant (http://www.unos.org).

II. **Deceased donors.** This group of donors was formerly known as *brain-dead* or *cadaveric donors.* The causes of death in deceased donors are most frequently intracerebral hemorrhage or trauma. Strict criteria for establishing brain death include the presence of irreversible coma and the absence of brainstem reflexes (i.e., pupillary, corneal, vestibulo-ocular, or gag reflexes). Other useful diagnostic tests include blood flow scan, arteriography, and an apnea test. **Consent** is required from the family, and inquiries into the donor's medical history are made. Ideally, the donor should have stable hemodynamics, although the use of vasopressors is common. The fact that a potential donor required cardiopulmonary resuscitation may not preclude donation, particularly in a witnessed arrest with prompt institution of resuscitation and recovery of vital signs. The criteria for donor organ acceptance and use are not absolute; therefore, all patients meeting brain death criteria should be considered as potential donors. Contraindications for organ donation include a history of intravenous drug abuse or the presence of a malignancy (with the exception of a primary brain tumor). **Exclusion criteria** for specific organs also exist. Potential kidney donors ideally have normal renal function before brain death. Acute tubular necrosis (ATN) in the donor, underlying medical disease (e.g., diabetes, hypertension), or prolonged cold ischemia time may preclude the use of a donor kidney. Selection of a donor liver for a given recipient takes into account donor size, ABO blood type, age, liver function studies, hospital course, hemodynamics, and prior medical and social history. "Expanded-criteria" donors, those not meeting traditional inclusion criteria, have been used for recipients whose wait-list time is considered prohibitive.

III. **Donation following cardiac death (DCD)** refers to those who do not meet strict brain death criteria but who are otherwise considered to have nonsurvival neurologic insults. Life support is discontinued in the operating room, and organ procurement is initiated after a specified interval following cardiac asystole.

IV. **Deceased-donor organ recovery.** The initial dissection identifies hepatic hilar structures, including the common bile duct, portal vein, hepatic artery, and any aberrant arterial blood supply, such as a left hepatic artery branch arising from the left gastric artery or a right hepatic artery from the superior mesenteric artery (SMA). After this dissection, the liver is flushed and cooled with University of Wisconsin (UW) preservation solution (a cold-storage solution containing a high concentration of potassium, lactobionate, hydroxyethyl starch, and other antioxidants) via cannulae placed in the portal vein and the aorta proximal to the iliac artery. A clamp is applied to the supraceliac aorta. The donor liver is removed with its diaphragmatic attachments, a cuff of aorta surrounding

461

the celiac axis and the SMA, and a portion of the supra- and infrahepatic vena cava. The liver is packaged in UW solution and surrounded by iced saline during transportation. The remainder of the liver dissection is performed in the recipient's operating room under cold-storage conditions. With the advent of UW solution, donor livers can be preserved for up to 12 hours before revascularization, with only a low incidence of allograft dysfunction. Ideally, cold ischemia time is minimized to less than 8 hours. The donor kidneys are removed *en bloc* and then separated. The ureters are dissected widely to minimize devascularization and are divided near the bladder. This technique minimizes risk of injury to the arteries and allows identification of multiple renal arteries, if present. The pancreas may also be removed for transplantation in a suitable donor. The pancreas and duodenum are removed *en bloc*. The blood supply for the pancreas allograft comes from the donor splenic and superior mesenteric arteries, and outflow is via the portal vein. The mesentery below the pancreas is divided with a stapling device.

V. **Histocompatibility.** Antibodies to human leukocyte antigen (HLA) do not occur naturally but are produced in response to exposure to foreign histocompatibility antigens that may occur after pregnancy, blood transfusions, or previous transplants. The traditional test used for detecting specific sensitization against donor histocompatibility antigens is termed a **cross-match** or **complement-dependent lymphocytotoxicity assay.** Several methods are available for performing the cross-match, each involving the addition of recipient serum, donor cells (T cells, B cells, or monocytes), and complement. If specific antidonor antibodies are present, antibody binding results in complement fixation and lysis of the donor lymphocytes. Flow cytometry also can be used for cross-matching. This method permits the detection of noncytotoxic antibodies and the definition of cell specificity or antibody binding. Polymerase chain reaction (PCR) and enzyme-linked immunosorbent assay technology are being used increasingly for HLA typing, particularly for the major histocompatibility (MHC) class II HLA antigens. HLA matching is of practical significance only in renal and pancreatic transplantation.

IMMUNOSUPPRESSION

A variety of immunosuppressive medications are used in transplant patients to prevent rejection. The protocols outlined in the following sections are the ones currently in use at Washington University and are intended to serve as guidelines. Variations on these protocols are used at other transplantation centers. Most protocols rely on the use of several drugs owing to the different mechanisms and synergies of these medications.

I. **Immunosuppressive medications**

A. **Prednisone or methylprednisolone sodium succinate (Solu-Medrol).** Steroids are part of most multiple-drug immunosuppressive regimens and are the first-line drug in the treatment of rejection. Steroids modify antigen processing and presentation, inhibit lymphocyte proliferation, and inhibit cytokine and prostaglandin production. After surgery, patients are placed on a steroid taper and maintained on a low dose of prednisone or eventually withdrawn from the drug altogether. Late steroid withdrawal is inadvisable, but steroid avoidance protocols have had good short-term results. The long-term results are unknown. The acute and chronic side effects of steroid therapy include diabetes mellitus, infections, cataracts, hypertension, weight gain, and bone disease.

B. **Cyclosporine (Sandimmune, Neoral, Gengraf).** Cyclosporine's development and use has been one of the most significant advances in transplantation. It is a small fungal cyclic peptide that blocks T-cell activation, inhibiting T-lymphocyte proliferation, interleukin-2 (IL-2) production, IL-2 receptor expression, and interferon-γ release. Two-hour peaks, 12-hour troughs, or both, are monitored and adjusted based on time from transplant, HLA match, and so forth. Side effects include nephrotoxicity, hypertension, tremors, seizures, hyperkalemia, hyperuricemia, hypercholesterolemia, gingival hyperplasia, and hirsutism. Cyclosporine is metabolized by the liver. Common medications that may increase cyclosporine levels include diltiazem, verapamil, erythromycin, fluconazole, ketoconazole, tetracycline, metoclopramide, and cimetidine. Medications that decrease levels include intravenous Bactrim, isoniazid, rifampin, phenytoin, phenobarbital, carbamazepine, and omeprazole.

C. **Tacrolimus (Prograf, FK506)** is a macrolide that has a mechanism of action similar to that of cyclosporine but is approximately 100 times more potent. Tacrolimus doses are adjusted to maintain 12-hour trough levels between 5 and 10 ng/mL (FPIA assay). The side effect profile is similar to that of cyclosporine but does not include hirsutism and gingival hyperplasia. Alopecia and posttransplant diabetes mellitus (PTDM) are more common with tacrolimus.

D. **Sirolimus (Rapamycin, Rapammum)** is a newer anti-T cell agent that has a mechanism of action similar to cyclosporine and tacrolimus as well as unique inhibitory properties derived from the mTOR molecule, which blocks T-cell signal transduction. It is increasingly being utilized as first-line therapy following transplantation. Side effects include thrombocytopenia, hyperlipidemia, mouth ulcers, anemia, and impairment of wound healing.

E. **Azathioprine (Imuran)** is an antimetabolite that is a thioguanine derivative of mercaptopurine. This purine analogue alters the function or synthesis of DNA and RNA, inhibiting T- and B-lymphocyte proliferation. One of the major side effects of this drug is bone marrow suppression, manifested as leukopenia and thrombocytopenia. An important drug interaction occurs with allopurinol, which blocks the metabolism of azathioprine and increases the degree of bone marrow suppression.

F. **Mycophenolate mofetil (CellCept)** is a relatively selective inhibitor of T- and B-cell proliferation, cytotoxic T-cell generation, and antibody formation. It is used as an alternative to azathioprine, and is the antimetabolite of choice in 90% of transplant programs. Major toxicities include gastrointestinal disturbances and increased cytomegalovirus infection.

G. **Polyclonal antithymocyte antibodies.** Polyclonal antibodies are immunologic products with antibodies to a wide variety of T cell antigens, adhesion molecules, costimulatory molecules, cytokines, the T-cell receptor, and class I and II MHC molecules. These agents are used as induction therapy in the perioperative period or as rescue therapy following acute rejection. The two preparations available in the United States are **Thymoglobulin** and **Atgam**. Thymoglobulin, a rabbit-derived product, is more potent than Atgam, a horse-derived product. Common side effects of both include fever, leukopenia, and thrombocytopenia.

H. **Monoclonal antibodies. OKT3** is a murine monoclonal antibody that recognizes the T-cell receptor and blocks antigen recognition, hindering T-cell effector functions and potentiating T-cell lysis. OKT3 usually is administered to patients with steroid-resistant, severe rejection. Immediate side effects can include fever, chills, hypotension, respiratory distress, and pulmonary edema, all of which are secondary to the **cytokine release syndrome. Daclizumab (Zenapax)** and **basiliximab (Simulect)**, which are IL-2 receptor–specific monoclonal antibodies increasingly being used as induction therapy, are begun immediately prior to transplantation and continued in the immediate postoperative period.

I. **Other antibodies** against costimulatory molecules, including leukocyte function–associated antigen 1, intercellular adhesion molecule 1, CD40, and CD52 (Campath-1H), are currently being tested for their potential efficacy in the treatment of rejection.

II. **Complications of immunosuppression**

A. **Bacterial infections.** Infectious complications after transplantation characteristically are caused by opportunistic organisms. Routine bacterial infections, such as pneumonia or urinary tract infections, can also occur.

Table 28-1. Prophylaxis and treatment of infections in immunosuppressed patients

Herpes simplex virus (HSV)
  Prophylaxis
    Acyclovir 200 mg p.o. b.i.d. for 3 mo (only if CMV D$^-$/R$^-$; otherwise CMV
      treatment will also cover HSV)
    For liver transplant patients, for 3–6 mo or until prednisone is <10 mg per day
  Treatment
    Decrease immunosuppression
    Acyclovir, 5–10 mg i.v. for 7–10 days
CMV
  Prophylaxis
    Ganciclovir, 1,000 mg p.o. t.i.d. (1 year for D$^+$/R$^-$, 6 mo for D$^+$/R$^+$, 3 mo for
      D$^-$/R$^+$), or
    Valganciclovir, 450 mg p.o. b.i.d. (must reduce dose for renal insufficiency)
  Treatment
    Ganciclovir, 5 mg/kg i.v. q. 12 h for 3 wk, or
    Valganciclovir, 450 mg p.o. b.i.d. for 3 wk, in the absence of invasive disease
    Consider unselected IgG, 500 mg/kg i.v. q.i.d. for 5 days for pneumonitis or
      colitis, or
    Hyperimmune CMV IgG, 100 mg/kg i.v. q.i.d. for 5 doses for pneumonitis or
      colitis
Epstein-Barr virus
  Prophylaxis
    Acyclovir, 200 mg p.o. b.i.d. for life (D$^+$/R$^-$)
  Treatment
    Consider reduction or withdrawal of immunosuppression
    Consider ganciclovir, 5 mg/kg i.v. q. 12 h for 3 wk
    Consider chemotherapy for patients with lymphoproliferative disorders
Candida
  Prophylaxis of oral candidiasis
    Nystatin, 5 mL (500,000 units) swish and swallow q.i.d. for 3 mo, or
    Miconazole, troche suck and swallow q.i.d. for 3 mo, or
    Fluconazole, 100 mg q. wk for 3 mo
  Treatment of esophageal candidiasis
    Fluconazole, 100 mg p.o. b.i.d., or
    Voriconazole, 200 mg p.o. b.i.d.
Pneumocystis carinii pneumonia
  Prophylaxis (for life)
    Bactrim, 1 double-strength tablet p.o. q.d. for serum creatinine <3 mg/dL, or
    Bactrim, 1 single-strength tablet p.o. q.d. for serum creatinine >3 mg/dL, or
    Dapsone, 50 mg p.o. q.d. for sulfa allergy, or
    Pentamidine, 300 mg per nebulizer q. month for sulfa allergy and G6PD
      deficiency

D, donor; R, recipient.

      B. Viral infections. The most common viral infections after transplantation in-
clude **cytomegalovirus (CMV), Epstein-Barr virus (EBV), herpes simplex
virus (HSV),** and **BK virus.** See Table 28-1 for a summary of prophylaxis and
treatment for common viral and fungal infections.
         1. CMV infection can occur at any time after transplantation but is most com-
monly seen 1 to 4 months posttransplant. CMV may infrequently infect
the recipient's liver, lungs, or gastrointestinal tract. Signs and symptoms
of CMV infection include fever, chills, malaise, anorexia, nausea, vomiting,

cough, abdominal pain, hypoxia, leukopenia, and elevation in liver transaminases. CMV antibody titers (IgG, IgM) and peripheral blood PCR are the most common tools for diagnosing CMV infection. CMV can be associated with significant morbidity and even mortality, but it typically responds well to early diagnosis and treatment. There is also evidence that CMV contributes to allograft injury.

Prophylactic administration of ganciclovir (1,000 mg orally three times a day) or valganciclovir (900 mg orally per day) may be useful in any patient who receives a CMV-positive allograft because many of these patients develop a significant CMV infection if left untreated. Treatment consists of decreasing immunosuppression and administering ganciclovir (5 mg/kg intravenously every 12 hours for 3 weeks), which inhibits DNA synthesis. Valganciclovir, intravenous ganciclovir, and, to a lesser extent, oral ganciclovir dosing must be adjusted for renal dysfunction. The most common side effects of valganciclovir and ganciclovir are anemia, neutropenia, and thrombocytopenia.

2. **EBV** can infect B cells at any time after transplantation and may be associated with the development of a lymphoproliferative disorder (lymphoma), usually of B-cell origin. Infiltration of the hematopoietic system, CNS, lungs, or other solid organs may occur. The patient usually presents with fever, chills, sweats, enlarged lymph nodes, and elevated uric acid. Diagnosis is made by physical examination; EBV serology; CT scan of the head, chest, and abdomen (to look for lymph nodes or masses); and biopsy of potential sites or lesions. Treatment consists of reducing or withdrawing immunosuppression. Intravenous ganciclovir inhibits EBV-associated DNA polymerase and may be added but is not of proven benefit. Acyclovir prophylaxis for life (200 mg twice a day) may be considered in EBV donor+/recipient- patients. Additionally, standard chemotherapy should be considered for advanced disease or polyclonal tumors that have not responded to other measures.

3. **HSV** causes characteristic ulcers on the oral mucosa, in the genital region, and in the esophagus. Renal transplant patients are given prophylactic acyclovir at a dosage of 200 mg orally twice a day for 3 months. Active HSV infections are treated by decreasing the patient's immunosuppression and instituting acyclovir therapy (5 to 10 mg/kg intravenously every 8 hours for 7 to 10 days). Side effects of acyclovir are rare but include nephrotoxicity, phlebitis, bone marrow suppression, and CNS toxicity.

4. **BK virus** is a member of the polyoma virus family. Approximately 90% of individuals are seropositive. BK viruria detected by "decoy cell" shedding or PCR develops in 30% of kidney transplant recipients and progresses to viremia in 15% of recipients within the first year. Persistent BK viremia leads to BK nephropathy, which occurs in up to 10% of kidney transplant recipients during the first year. There is no known effective treatment, though low-dose cidofovir (0.25 mg/kg intravenously every 2 weeks) has been tried. Early graft loss occurs in 50% of patients with BK nephropathy, and the other 50% are left with chronic allograft dysfunction.

C. **Fungal infections** can range from mild asymptomatic colonization to lethal invasive infections. Oral **candidiasis** can be prevented and treated with oral nystatin (Mycostatin, 500,000 units orally four times a day for 3 months). Esophageal candidiasis can be treated with a short course of intravenous amphotericin B or fluconazole (100 mg orally twice a day). Serious fungal infections are treated with intravenous amphotericin B.

D. **Other opportunistic infections.** *Pneumocystis carinii* **pneumonia** is a potentially lethal pneumonia that occurs in 5% to 10% of renal transplant patients receiving no prophylactic treatment. Patients typically present with fever, dyspnea, nonproductive cough, hypoxia, and pulmonary infiltrates. The diagnosis is made by bronchoalveolar lavage or a lung biopsy. It can be prevented by low-dose Bactrim or inhaled pentamidine. Treatment of pneumonia involves much higher doses of these agents, with a concomitant decrease in immunosuppression.

E. **Malignancies.** Some of the cancers that occur at a higher frequency in transplant recipients than in the general population are squamous cell carcinoma, basal cell carcinoma, Kaposi sarcoma, lymphomas, hepatobiliary carcinoma, and cervical carcinoma. Other common cancers do not have a higher incidence among transplant recipients.

DIALYSIS

Acute renal failure (ARF) is defined by a rise in the serum creatinine of more than 0.5 mg/dL (0.04 mmol/L) when the baseline serum creatinine is less than 3.0 mg/dL (0.27 mmol/L) or by a rise of more than 1.0 mg/dL (0.09 mmol/L) when the serum creatinine baseline is 3.0 mg/dL (0.27 mmol/L) or above. **End-stage renal disease (ESRD)** results when the functioning renal mass deteriorates to less than 10% to 20% of normal. ESRD may affect multiple organ systems, resulting in altered fluid and electrolyte homeostasis, accumulation of metabolic waste products, anemia, hypertension, and metabolic bone disease.

I. **Treatment of renal failure**
   A. **Conservative treatment** of renal failure begins with dietary restrictions. Fluid intake is limited to urine output plus insensible losses, usually 1.5 to 2.0 L per day. Protein is restricted to 0.7 to 1.2 g/kg per day to minimize the rise in blood urea nitrogen (BUN). Sodium chloride is restricted to 2 g per day (sodium, 35 mEq per day), potassium chloride is restricted to 2 g per day (potassium, 25 mEq per day), and phosphorus, magnesium, and aluminum are avoided as much as possible. Control of serum phosphorus can be accomplished through the use of calcium carbonate (500 to 2,500 mg orally within 30 minutes of meals and at bedtime). Sodium bicarbonate (650 mg orally 2 to three times a day) is used to control acidosis when the serum bicarbonate is less than 20 mg/dL (20 mmol/L). Loop diuretics in combination with thiazide or thiazide-like diuretics are useful adjuncts for maintaining fluid homeostasis. Typically, chlorthalidone (500 mg intravenously twice a day) or metolazone (5 mg orally twice a day), followed by furosemide (80 to 200 mg intravenously twice a day), is given. The thiazide prevents distal tubule adaptation and salt reclamation, which occurs after administration of furosemide. When conservative therapy is inadequate, death ensues without either dialysis or transplantation.
   B. **Dialysis** removes fluids and wastes and adjusts acid-base and electrolyte disturbances by diffusion and osmosis across a semipermeable membrane. This is accomplished in hemodialysis (HD) by the semipermeable membrane of an artificial kidney or in peritoneal dialysis (PD) by the semipermeable peritoneal membrane. Both methods may be used either acutely or chronically.
   C. **Transplantation** is the treatment of choice for many patients with ESRD.
   D. **Mortality** for ARF is as high as 50% for patients admitted to the intensive care unit with ARF, despite the availability of dialysis. This high mortality is generally due to the patient's underlying disease processes and associated comorbidities.

II. **Indications for acute dialysis** can be remembered by the mnemonic **AEIOU-PP (acidosis, electrolyte disturbances, intoxicants, overload, uremia, and pericarditis and polyneuropathy).**
   A. **Acidosis.** Dialysis for acidosis should be considered when the serum bicarbonate is less than 10 mEq/L (10 mmol/L) and administration of further alkali is contraindicated.
   B. **Electrolyte disturbances.** A serum potassium acutely greater than 6 mEq/dL (6 mmol/L) is the most common indication for dialysis. Sodium, calcium, and magnesium also can be corrected with dialysis.
   C. **Intoxicants.** Common dialyzable intoxicants include lithium, ethylene glycol, methanol, salicylates, and theophylline.

D. Fluid **overload** unresponsive to diuretics is another common indication for dialysis.

E. Uremia is a syndrome characterized by vomiting, anorexia, nausea, itching, listlessness, and asterixis associated with renal failure. A patient's symptoms may not correlate directly with the degree of azotemia because many uremic toxins are not yet identified. Furthermore, in ARF no survival advantage is conferred by early dialysis for patients with azotemic symptoms.

F. Pericarditis and **polyneuropathy** are two absolute indications for dialysis caused by uremia. Pericarditis due to uremia may not necessarily present with elevated ST segments on electrocardiography. Pericardial friction rubs often are ephemeral and may require repeated examinations to detect. Polyneuropathy most commonly manifests as a wrist or foot drop. Without early dialysis, these symptoms may become irreversible.

III. Hemodialysis (HD)

A. Types of HD

1. Chronic intermittent maintenance HD usually requires dialysis three times a week for 3 to 4 hours per treatment. Determination of dialysis adequacy uses clearance of BUN as a marker for treatment of uremia. For HD, a urea reduction ratio (predialysis BUN − postdialysis BUN/predialysis BUN) of more than 70% or a **KT/V** of more than 1.3 [where K is the clearance of the dialyzer (in mL per minute), T is the duration of dialysis in minutes, and V is the volume of distribution of urea (in mL)] confers a survival advantage in chronic renal failure.

2. Continuous arteriovenous hemofiltration (CAVH). This method of HD and **continuous venovenous hemofiltration (CVVH)**, also known as *slow continuous ultrafiltration*, are the methods of HD used most frequently in critically ill patients with hemodynamic instability and volume overload. Because the patient's arterial BP provides the ultrafiltration pressure, a systolic pressure of 80 mm Hg is required to support CAVH. The access for CAVH is obtained by placing a 7 Fr. single-lumen catheter into a femoral artery and a large central vein. CVVH is accomplished with a double-lumen venous cannula. The ultrafiltrate is essentially plasma, and its rate of collection may exceed 1,000 mL per hour.

B. Complications of HD

1. Hypotension commonly occurs with HD and may occur even without ultrafiltration. Measures to prevent it include the use of bicarbonate (rather than acetate) dialysis fluid; low-temperature (35°C) dialysate; infusion of a saline, blood, or albumin prime at the beginning of dialysis or during the dialysis run; high-sodium dialysate; or ultrafiltration without HD during the first hour.

2. Dyspnea. The effect of complement and adhesion molecules on circulating leukocytes and endothelium results in leukocyte pooling in the pulmonary circulation and dyspnea. Use of biocompatible cellulose acetate or synthetic membranes helps to prevent dyspnea.

3. Bleeding occurs secondary to dysfunctional platelets associated with uremia or the use of heparin. Bleeding can be minimized by performing dialysis with low-dose or no heparin or by preventing clotting with the use of citrate or frequent flushes with saline.

4. Disequilibrium syndrome is characterized by mental status deterioration associated with dialysis and is due to the rapid removal of metabolic waste products or fluid and electrolyte shifts. It may be prevented by limiting the percent reduction in urea to 25% with the first dialysis session.

IV. Peritoneal dialysis (PD)

A. Technique. Access is gained through an intraperitoneal soft silicone (Tenckhoff) catheter. Continuous ambulatory PD requires 4 to 5 exchanges of 2 to 3 L of dialysis fluid daily. The dialysis fluid is composed of dextrose at various concentrations (1.5%, 2.5%, or 4.0%) and electrolytes. Each exchange dwells in the peritoneum for 2 to 4 hours, with the last exchange of the day remaining overnight. A typical exchange takes 20 to 40 minutes.

Some patients are able to perform continuous cycler–assisted PD. This form of PD uses a machine to warm, infuse, and drain 10 to 16 L of dialysis fluid overnight while the patient sleeps. For PD, a weekly total *KT/V* of 2.0 per week and total creatinine clearance of 60 L per week per 1.73 m² is considered minimally adequate dialysis. Acute PD is used when acute HD cannot be performed, most often owing to hemodynamic instability.

B. **Complications of PD**

1. **Peritonitis.** Despite improvements in equipment and techniques (e.g., Y-system, bagless system, and ultraviolet light box disinfectant bag spiker), one-third of patients on PD develop peritonitis each year. The diagnosis is suggested by a fever, abdominal pain, cloudy dialysate fluid, more than 100 polymorphonuclear cells per mL of PD fluid, bacteremia, or a positive peritoneal fluid Gram stain or culture. The infection is usually caused by Gram-positive organisms. Less frequent causes include Gram-negative bacteria, yeast, and mycobacteria or atypical mycobacteria. Treatment usually is empiric, with antibiotics added to the dialysate. Fungal peritonitis and pseudomonal peritonitis are difficult to eradicate and often require removal of the PD catheter.

2. **Access.** Catheter malposition, obstruction, leakage, and (rarely) bowel perforation are complications associated with PD catheters. Exit-site infections occur commonly and can often be treated locally. A tunnel infection is more difficult to eradicate and often leads to peritonitis.

3. **Obesity.** Dextrose is the osmotic agent used in PD and provides 200 to 500 calories per exchange. With normal serum glucose, 80% of the dextrose is absorbed. This caloric intake must be considered relative to the patient's needs.

4. **Membrane failure** occurs eventually and more frequently after episodes of peritonitis. After 1 year, only one-half of the patients who start PD are able to remain on it.

5. **Other.** Abdominal wall hernias, low back pain, and protein loss are also potential complications of PD.

KIDNEY TRANSPLANTATION

I. **Indications** for renal transplantation include the presence of ESRD with an irreversible glomerular filtration rate of less than 20 mL per minute. Excellent short- and long-term results can be achieved regardless of the cause of renal failure (Table 28-2). Renal failure secondary to diabetes mellitus, once thought to be a contraindication to transplantation, is now the single most common disease process in the United States requiring renal transplantation, comprising as many as 25% of all cases.

Table 28-2. Causes of renal failure requiring renal transplantation

Type	Characteristics
Congenital	Aplasia, obstructive uropathy
Hereditary	Alport syndrome (hereditary nephritis), polycystic disease, tuberous sclerosis
Neoplastic	Renal cell carcinoma, Wilms tumor
Progressive	Diabetic nephropathy, chronic pyelonephritis, Goodpasture syndrome (anti–glomerular basement membrane disease), hypertension, chronic glomerulonephritis, lupus nephritis, nephrotic syndrome, obstructive uropathy, scleroderma, amyloidosis
Traumatic	Vascular occlusion, parenchymal destruction

II. Contraindications. Although the indications for transplantation are broad, some conditions must be considered contraindications.

   A. Recent or metastatic malignancy. Immunosuppressive drugs may unfavorably influence the natural history of the malignancy, and aggressive local and metastatic recurrence is more likely. In general, most transplantation centers require a significant (2- to 5-year) disease-free interval after the treatment of a malignant tumor. Exceptions include early stage skin cancers and *in situ* cancers.

   B. Chronic infection. The presence of any active, life-threatening infection precludes transplantation and the use of immunosuppressive therapy. If the infection can be treated either medically or surgically, the patient should be reconsidered for transplantation after therapy. Infection with the human immunodeficiency virus (HIV) is a strong contraindication to renal transplantation at most centers.

   C. Severe extrarenal disease may preclude transplantation in certain circumstances, either because the patient is not an operative candidate or because the transplantation and associated immunosuppression may accelerate disease progression (i.e., chronic liver disease, chronic lung disease, and advanced uncorrectable heart disease). Severe peripheral vascular disease may also be a contraindication.

   D. Noncompliance. Any patient with a history of repeated noncompliance with medical therapy should be considered high risk. A period of compliance before being placed on the waiting list is generally advised. This is especially true of adolescent patients.

   E. Psychiatric Illness. Organic mental syndromes, psychosis, and mental retardation that impairs the patient's capacity to understand the transplantation procedure and its complications are contraindications to transplantation. Patients with alcohol or other drug addiction must enter and successfully complete a rehabilitation program before being offered transplantation.

III. Preoperative workup and evaluation. Patients referred to a transplantation center are seen by a transplantation surgeon, nephrologist, social worker, and a transplantation coordinator. Evaluation of a potential recipient is outlined in Table 28-3. The evaluation identifies coexisting problems or disease entities that must be addressed to improve the outcome of the transplantation. Family history is important because it may provide information about the patient's kidney disease and allows a discussion about potential living donors. When the evaluation is complete, the patient is presented at a multidisciplinary evaluation committee meeting, where a decision is made as to whether to accept the patient as a potential recipient. Allocation of a given organ to a specific patient is done using a computer-generated algorithm run by the United Network for Organ Sharing (UNOS) and is based on specific criteria, which are different for each organ [e.g., blood type, HLA matching, waiting time, prior sensitization (i.e., high panel reactive antibodies [PRA] rating), and medical urgency for kidney allocation]. Once a patient is active on the waiting list, blood is sent monthly to the tissue-typing laboratory for cross-matching and to determine the PRA.

The **PRA (panel reactive antibodies)** helps predict the likelihood that a patient will have a positive cross-match. It is determined by testing the potential recipient's serum against a panel of cells of various HLA specificities in a manner similar to the cross-match. The percentage of specificities in the panel that the patient's sera react with is the PRA. Most normal individuals do not have preformed anti-HLA antibodies and thus have a low PRA (0% to 5%). Patients who have been exposed to other HLAs through blood transfusions, previous transplantations, or pregnancies or who have autoimmune diseases with antibodies recognizing HLAs may have a high PRA. These patients are more likely to have a positive cross-match.

   A. Special considerations. The lower urinary tract should be sterile, continent, and compliant before transplantation. In patients with a history of

Table 28-3. Pretransplantation evaluation of renal transplant recipients

Initial workup
   History and physical examination
   Laboratory analyses: complete blood cell count; partial thromboplastin time;
      prothrombin time; serum electrolytes; total protein, albumin, cholesterol,
      glucose, calcium, magnesium, and phosphorus; liver function tests; intact
      parathyroid hormone; prostate-specific antigen for men >40 yr; viral
      serologies (including herpes simplex; Epstein-Barr virus; varicella-zoster
      virus; cytomegalovirus; hepatitis A, B, and C; and human immunodeficiency
      virus); urinalysis and urine culture; purified protein derivative; panel-reactive
      antibody; ABO and human leukocyte antigen typing; serum for frozen storage
   Electrocardiography
   Chest x-ray
Routine examinations
   Dental
   Stool guaiac (Hemoccult)
   Pap smear
   Mammogram (women >35 yr)
   Ophthalmologic (diabetic patients)
   Psychosocial
Secondary workup (based on preliminary findings)
   Cardiac: exercise stress electrocardiography, dobutamine stress
      echocardiography, coronary angiography
   Gastrointestinal tract: upper and lower endoscopy, right upper quadrant
      ultrasonography
   Genitourinary: voiding cystourethrography, cystoscopy, retrograde ureterography
   Pulmonary: arterial blood gases, pulmonary function tests

---

bladder dysfunction, diabetes mellitus, and recurrent urinary tract infections, a voiding cystourethrogram may be obtained before transplantation.
Transplant ureter implantation into the native bladder is preferred and
usually can be achieved, even in small bladders and those that have been
diverted previously.

B. Pretransplantation native nephrectomy has been avoided secondary to the
anemia that develops following removal of the kidneys and their endogenous erythropietin production. It is only performed in patients with chronic
renal parenchymal infection, infected renal calculi, heavy proteinuria, intractable hypertension, massive polycystic kidney disease with pain or
bleeding, renal cystic disease that is suspicious for carcinoma, and infected
reflux nephropathy. Erythropoietin renders pretransplantation nephrectomy more acceptable, especially in patients with intractable hypertension whose posttransplantation management can be difficult without
nephrectomy.

C. Living donors. Living kidney donation has become an important part of renal transplant practice. Parent-child or sibling combinations are the most
common, although biologically unrelated donors are increasingly being
used. Advantages of living-donor transplantation include improved short-
and long-term graft survival (1-year survival >95%); improved immediate
allograft function, planned operative timing to allow for optimization of the
recipient's medical condition (and, in many cases, avoidance of dialysis),
fewer rejection and infection episodes, and shorter hospital stays. Although
expanded-criteria deceased donors (who tend to be older) have increased
the donor pool, a living donor, if available, is preferred to a deceased donor.
   The primary goal in evaluating a potential living donor is to ensure the
donor's well-being and safety. The donor must be in excellent health and

must not have any illnesses, such as hypertension or diabetes, that may threaten his or her own renal function in the future. The donor anatomy is evaluated preoperatively with arteriography or CT/MR angiography. Donor kidneys are now commonly removed using laparoscopic or mininephrectomy techniques to minimize donor morbidity.

IV. **Preoperative considerations.** When a kidney becomes available, the recipient is admitted to the hospital, and the surgeon, nephrologist, and anesthesiologist perform a final preoperative evaluation. Routine laboratory studies and a final cross-match are performed. The need for preoperative dialysis depends on the patient's volume status and serum potassium. Generally, a patient with evidence of volume overload or a serum potassium greater than 5.6 mEq/L (5.6 mmol/L) requires preoperative hemodialysis. Induction therapy with a polyclonal antibody preparation is begun intraoperatively.

V. **Operative considerations**

A. **Technique.** In the operating room, a Foley catheter is inserted, and the patient's bladder is irrigated with antibiotic-containing solution. A central venous pressure (CVP) line is inserted, and a first-generation cephalosporin is administered. The renal vein and artery typically are anastomosed to the external iliac vein and artery, respectively. A heparin bolus of 3,000 units is administered before venous clamping. Before reperfusion of the kidney, mannitol (25 g) and furosemide (100 mg) are administered intravenously, and the patient's systolic BP is maintained above 120 mm Hg, with a CVP of at least 10 mm Hg to ensure optimal perfusion of the transplanted kidney. The ureter can be anastomosed to either the recipient bladder or the ipsilateral ureter, although the bladder is the preferred location. Establishing an antireflux mechanism is essential for preventing posttransplantation reflux pyelonephritis. This is accomplished by performing an extravesical ureteroneocystostomy (Litch).

B. **Intraoperative fluid management.** The newly transplanted kidney is sensitive to volume contraction, and adequate perfusion is essential for immediate postoperative diuresis and acute tubular necrosis (ATN) prevention. Volume contraction should not occur, and volume status is constantly monitored by checking the patient's cardiac function, CVP, and BP. The initial posttransplantation urine outputs can vary dramatically based on many factors. It is imperative to know the patient's native urine volume to assess the contribution of the native and the transplanted kidney to posttransplantation urine output. Dopamine may be administered at a level of 2 to 5 μg/kg per minute intravenously to promote renal blood flow and support systemic blood pressure.

VI. **Postoperative considerations**

A. **General care.** Many aspects of postoperative care are the same as those for any other general surgical patient. Early ambulation is encouraged, and the need for good pulmonary toilet and wound care is the same. Due to immunosuppression, sutures and skin staples are left in place for 2 to 3 weeks to allow for slower wound healing. The bladder catheter is left in place for 3 to 7 days. Meperidine is avoided because its metabolites are excreted renally and can rise to toxic levels in the patient whose allograft is not functioning immediately after transplantation.

B. **Intravenous fluid replacement.** In general, the patient should be kept euvolemic or mildly hypervolemic in the early posttransplantation period. Hourly urine output is replaced with one-half normal saline on a milliliter-for-milliliter basis because the sodium concentration of the urine from a newly transplanted kidney is 60 to 80 mEq/L (60 to 80 mmol/L). Insensible fluid losses during this period typically are 30 to 60 mL per hour and essentially are losses of water that can be replaced by a solution of 5% dextrose in 0.45% normal saline at 30 mL per hour. Therefore, during the early posttransplantation period, the patient's intravenous fluid consists of one-half normal saline administered at a rate equal to the previous hour's urine output plus 30 mL of 5% dextrose in 0.45% normal saline. This formula requires the patient's volume status to be assessed repeatedly. If the post-transplantation urine output is low and the patient is thought to be hy-povolemic (based on clinical and hemodynamic evaluation), isotonic saline boluses are given. Potassium chloride replacement usually is not required unless the urine output is very high, and even then it should be given with great care. Potassium chloride especially should be avoided in the oliguric posttransplantation patient.

C. GI tract. Gastritis and peptic ulcer disease occur secondary to steroid ther-apy in the transplantation patient. Therefore, patients are prophylactically treated with famotidine (20 mg per day orally or intravenously). If severe gastroesophageal reflux, leukopenia, or mental status changes occur while the patient is receiving famotidine, lansoprazole may be given (30 mg per day orally).

D. Renal allograft function or nonfunction. If the patient's urine output is low in the early postoperative period (<50 mL per hour), volume status must be addressed first. If the patient is hypovolemic, 250 to 500 mL iso-tonic saline should be given in bolus fashion and repeated once, if needed. If the patient is euvolemic, the bladder catheter should be irrigated to en-sure patency. If clots are encountered, a larger catheter and/or continuous bladder irrigation may be needed. If the catheter is patent and the patient is euvolemic or hypervolemic, furosemide (100 to 200 mg intravenously for recipients of deceased-donor transplants, 20 to 40 mg intravenously for those with living-donor transplants) should be given. If diuresis follows these maneuvers, urine output is again replaced milliliter for milliliter with one-half normal saline. Early nonfunction of a transplanted kidney is most commonly due to reversible ATN. Ischemia of the kidney is the most frequent cause; it is due to hypotension in the donor, warm ischemia during procurement, prolonged cold ischemia, or excessive warm ischemia during the transplantation procedure. Immunologic injury and reperfusion injury also may play some role in the mechanism of injury leading to ATN. Before the diagnosis of ATN can be made, however, noninvasive studies (renal Doppler ultrasonography or technetium-99m renal scan) demon-strating vascular patency and good renal blood flow in the absence of hy-dronephrosis or urinary leak (renal ultrasonography) must be obtained. If flow is confirmed, dialysis can be continued until the transplanted kidney recovers.

E. Immunosuppression. A variety of immunosuppressive protocols exist. The protocol currently in use at Washington University is outlined here. In-duction therapy with Thymoglobulin (1.5 mg/kg intravenously) is given intraoperatively and then daily during the first three posttransplantation days. On posttransplantation days 1 to 30, patients receive cyclosporine (4 mg/kg orally twice a day) to maintain a trough level of 250 to 300 ng/mL (FPIA) or tacrolimus (0.05 mg/kg orally twice a day); azathio-prine (2.5 mg/kg orally per day) or mycophenolate mofetil (1,000 mg orally twice a day for 5 days, reduced to 500 mg orally twice a day thereafter); and prednisone (1 mg/kg orally per day for days 1 to 3, 0.5 mg/kg orally per day for days 4 to 14, then 25 mg orally per day, decreasing by 2.5 to 5 mg each week to a goal of 5 mg per day by week 13). Methylprednisolone (7 mg/kg intravenously) is given in the operating room.

VII. Rejection. An allografted kidney is a foreign body that is capable of eliciting an immune response and thus can be rejected. There are several different types of rejection; some are preventable, whereas others can be treated with varying degrees of success.

A. Hyperacute rejection occurs when preformed anti-HLA antibodies bind the endothelium of the allograft and initiate a cascade of events culminat-ing in vascular thrombosis and ischemic necrosis of the graft. Hyperacute rejection usually can be prevented by cross-matching donor lymphocytes with recipient serum. Hyperacute rejection usually occurs within minutes of cross-clamp release and is irreversible. Viability of the allograft can be

assessed by intraoperative biopsy. The only therapeutic option is to remove the allograft immediately.
B. **Accelerated** rejection also appears to be antibody-mediated and usually occurs 12 to 72 hours after transplantation. The patient usually is anuric or oliguric and has fever and graft tenderness. Although treatment for this form of rejection is not well defined, administration of an antilymphocyte preparation may salvage the graft. Accelerated rejection can lead to an immunologically mediated ATN from which good renal function recovery can occur.
C. **Acute** rejection is cell mediated and involves T lymphocytes and soluble mediators called lymphokines. It happens in 20% to 40% of patients and typically occurs 1 to 6 weeks after transplantation. The development of a rising creatinine level should prompt the consideration of rejection. Technetium-99m renal scan demonstrates decreased but persistent perfusion. Diagnosis is confirmed by percutaneous needle biopsy. There are two basic treatment modalities (Table 28-4): high-dose methylprednisolone or an antilymphocyte preparation. The latter generally is reserved for steroid-resistant rejection, although antilymphocyte therapy may be used as first-line therapy for moderate or severe rejections with arteritis. Maintenance immunosuppression may also be switched (i.e., from cyclosporine to tacrolimus). More than 90% of acute rejection episodes can be treated successfully.
D. **Chronic** rejection is a poorly understood phenomenon that can occur weeks to years after transplantation. Eventually, kidney function deteriorates to the point that either retransplantation or dialysis is required. Emerging evidence suggests that the humoral immune response is an important contributor to chronic rejection. Detection of anti-donor specific antibodies, an elevated posttransplant PRA, or C4d staining on a biopsy are supportive of humoral or antibody-mediated rejection.
VIII. **Surgical complications of renal transplantation.** Wound seromas, hematomas, and infections are treated according to usual surgical principles. Other complications require special consideration.
A. **Lymphoceles** are collections of lymph that occur because of lymphatic leaks in the retroperitoneum. They present 1 week to several weeks after transplantation and are best diagnosed by ultrasonography. They may produce ureteral obstruction, deep venous thrombosis, leg swelling, or incontinence secondary to bladder compression. Most lymphoceles arise from leakage of lymph from the donor kidney. Treatment consists of percutaneous drainage. Open or laparoscopic internal drainage by marsupialization into the peritoneal cavity may be necessary, as repeated percutaneous drainage is not advised and seldom leads to resolution of the lymphocele.
B. **Renal artery and vein thrombosis.** Arterial and venous thrombosis most often occur in the first 2 to 3 days after transplantation. If the kidney had been functioning but a sudden cessation of urine output occurs, graft thrombosis should be suspected. A rapid rise in serum creatinine, graft swelling, and local pain ensue. If the allograft had not been functioning or if the native kidneys make a large amount of urine, there may be no signs of graft thrombosis. The transplanted kidney has no collateral circulation and has a low tolerance for warm ischemia. The diagnosis is made by technetium-99m renal scan or Doppler ultrasonography. Unless the problem is diagnosed quickly and repair performed immediately, the graft will be lost, and transplantation nephrectomy will be required.
C. **Urine leak.** The etiology is usually anastomotic leak or ureteral sloughing secondary to ureteral blood supply disruption. Urine leaks present with pain, rising creatinine, and possibly urine draining from the wound. Diagnosis is made by locating the fluid collection with ultrasonography and then aspirating the fluid and comparing its creatinine level to the serum creatinine level. A renal scan demonstrates radioisotope outside the urinary tract, and a cystogram shows leakage of contrast outside the bladder.

Table 28-4. Treatment of rejection

Azathioprine
    Consider increasing dose if white blood cell count >3,000
    Azathioprine will not treat rejection but may prevent relapse
Steroids
    Intravenous pulse, methylprednisolone
        7 mg/kg q.d. for 3 days
        Use if patient is unreliable or on n.p.o. status
        Consider if rejection is early (<3 mo) or mild
    Oral pulse (prednisone)
        3 mg/kg q.d. in 2–4 divided doses for 3–5 days
        After pulse, restart steroids at previous dose
        Use if patient reliable and rejection early or mild
Cyclosporine
    Increase dose to achieve trough level >300 ng/mL for 1 month
Antilymphocyte preparations
    Thymoglobulin
        Use if poor OKT3 response or positive anti-OKT3 antibodies
        1.5 mg/kg i.v. q.d. for 7–10 days
    OKT3
        5 mg/d i.v. for 7–14 days
        Use immediately for vascular/humoral rejection and moderate rejection with
            arteritis
        Monitor CD3 and CD5 counts the day after the first dose
        If the patient has had prior OKT3, check anti-mouse antibodies; if titer
            >1:1000, OKT3 will probably be ineffective
        Premedicate with diphenhydramine (Benadryl), acetaminophen (Tylenol), and
            methylprednisolone on days 1 & 2
    Atgam
        Use if poor OKT3 response or positive anti-OKT3 antibodies
        15–30 mg/kg i.v. q.d. for 7–14 days
    IVIgG
        Use if BK$^+$ virus in urine or blood
        500 mg/kg i.v. q.d. for 3 days
Mycophenolate mofetil
    1,000 mg p.o. b.i.d.
    1,500 mg p.o. b.i.d. for rejection while on mycophenolate mofetil or refractory
        rejection
    Use for early moderate or vascular rejection on azathioprine and chronic
        rejection with creatinine <4 mg/dL
Tacrolimus
    5 mg p.o. b.i.d., target level 5–15 ng/mL
    Use for refractory rejection despite maximal cyclosporine
    Stop cyclosporine when using tacrolimus
Rapamycin
    10 mg p.o. load, then 4 mg p.o. q.d., target level 8–20 ng/mL
Leflunomide
    20 mg p.o. q.d.
    Reduce to 10 mg p.o. q.d. or 20 mg p.o. M/W/F for GI intolerance
    Consider if concomitant viral infection
Plasmapheresis
    Consider for severe vascular rejection
Local irradiation
    150 rads q.d. for 5–7 days
    Consider for refractory rejection or infected patient

Table 28-5. Long-term maintenance immunosuppression for renal transplantation

Azathioprine
  2.5 mg/kg p.o. q.d. in evening
  Decrease or hold for leukopenia (WBC count <3,000/mm^3) or thrombocytopenia
    (plt <50,000–75,000/mm^3)
Mycophenolate mofetil
  1,000 mg p.o. b.i.d.
  Reduce to 500 mg p.o. b.i.d. for WBC count <5,000/mm^3, diarrhea, 1st week
    posttransplant
Prednisone (p.o.)
  1 mg/kg q.d. for days 1–3
  0.5 mg/kg q.d. for days 4–14
  25 mg q.d. for week 3
  20 mg q.d. for week 4
  15 mg q.d. for week 5
  12.5 mg q.d. for week 6
  10 mg q.d. for week 7
  7.5 mg q.d. for week 8
  then 5 mg q.d.
  >12 mo, consider steroids every other day or withdrawal if no rejection for 6 mo
Cyclosporine
  8 mg/kg q.d. for first month, level 250–300 ng/mL (FPIA)
  7 mg/kg q.d. for months 2–3, level 250–300 ng/mL
  6 mg/kg q.d. for months 3–6, level 150–250 ng/mL
  5 mg/kg q.d. >6 mo, level 100–200 ng/mL
  Trough levels >400 ng/mL are considered toxic; however, peak (2-hr) levels may
    be more relevant than trough levels
  Peak 800–1,200 ng/mL at <1 mo, 600–1,000 at 1–3mo, 400–600 at >3 mo
Tacrolimus
  5 mg p.o. b.i.d., level 5–10 ng/mL (FPIA)
  Levels >20 ng/mL are considered toxic

Urine leaks are treated by placing a bladder catheter to reduce intravesical pressure and subsequent surgical exploration. The type of repair depends on the level of the leak. If an anastomotic leak is found, the distal ureter can be resected and reimplanted. If the transplantation ureter is nonviable or of inadequate length, ureteroureterostomy over a double-J stent using the ipsilateral native ureter can be performed. The stent can be removed via cystoscopy several weeks later.

IX. **Long-term follow-up.** Immunosuppression (Table 28-5) and infection prophylaxis (Table 28-1) should be tapered with time. After the initial 3-month period, when acute rejection becomes less of a risk, cyclosporine and steroid dosages are tapered. Chronic long-term immunosuppression can be maintained at lower levels than those required for induction. However, immunosuppression can almost never be discontinued completely. Specific metabolic consequences of cyclosporine administration include hypertension, nephrotoxicity, hypercholesterolemia, and hyperuricemia. Gradual dose reduction can be helpful, but often specific therapy is needed to correct these side effects. Weight gain is the predominant side effect of steroid therapy. Dietary manipulation and gradual dosage reduction are important. Long-term complications of steroids include joint deterioration with avascular necrosis, osteoporosis, cataract formation, and diabetes mellitus (10% of patients). The incidence of these problems can be minimized by using as low a dose of prednisone as

Table 28-6. Most common indications for orthotopic liver transplantation

Adults
  Chronic hepatitis C
  Alcoholic liver disease
  Chronic hepatitis B
  Primary biliary cirrhosis
  Primary sclerosing cholangitis
  Autoimmune hepatitis
Children
  Extrahepatic biliary atresia
  α-1-Antitrypsin deficiency

possible. Antibiotic prophylaxis should be used before any surgical or dental procedure.

LIVER TRANSPLANTATION

I. **Indications for hepatic transplantation** are complications attributable to end-stage liver disease (ESLD). In the absence of other medical contraindications, virtually any disease resulting in ESLD is amenable to transplantation. The most common diseases for which orthotopic liver transplantation (OLT) is performed are listed in Table 28-6. Common indications for OLT in patients with ESLD include variceal hemorrhage, intractable ascites, encephalopathy, intractable pruritus, and poor synthetic function. Stage I or II hepatocellular carcinoma in a cirrhotic liver is an increasingly common indication for transplantation. Single lesions less than 5 cm or three lesions less than 3 cm may be treated in this way.

II. **Contraindications.** There are a few absolute contraindications to liver transplantation: multisystem organ failure, extrahepatic malignancy, poor cardiac or pulmonary reserve, severe infection, and ongoing substance abuse. Renal insufficiency, either chronic or acute, increases the morbidity of hepatic transplantation but is not a contraindication. Renal transplantation can be performed at the time of liver transplantation for patients with ESRD. Some degree of preoperative renal insufficiency is often reversible after successful liver transplantation.

III. **Preoperative evaluation.** Referrals to transplantation centers are made on an elective or urgent basis. The evaluation determines the need and urgency for OLT as well as its technical feasibility.

  A. **Elective transplantation.** Under elective conditions, the potential candidate is presented to a multidisciplinary committee for evaluation. The patient's evaluation is based on history, physical examination, laboratory evaluation, results of endoscopic procedures, cardiac and pulmonary evaluation, and radiologic examination (Table 28-7). Active infection should be treated promptly, and transplantation should be postponed until the infection resolves. Patients with a recent history of alcohol or other substance abuse should also be evaluated by a specialist prior to transplantation.

  B. **Urgent transplantation.** Acceptable results with OLT also can be achieved in selected patients with acute liver failure. The pretransplantation evaluation is performed in a manner similar to that outlined for the elective patient; however, timing, neurologic status, and hemodynamic stability may limit the number of tests obtained.

  A careful neurologic examination must be done in this setting, and the grade of coma should be determined. Patients in grade IV (unresponsive) coma have been shown in some studies to benefit from continuous

Table 28-7. Pretransplantation evaluation of liver transplant recipients

Initial workup

History

  Etiology of liver disease

  Duration of liver disease

  Complications of liver disease

  Previous surgical procedures

  Additional medical problems

  Access to transplant center

  Social support

Physical examination

  Stigmata of chronic liver disease

  Jaundice

  Fluid retention

  Nutritional status

  Abdominal mass

  Asterixis or encephalopathy

  Growth and development (pediatric age group)

Laboratory analyses

  ABO blood type; complete blood cell count; prothrombin time; partial thromboplastin time; serum electrolytes; urinary electrolytes; total protein, albumin, glucose, calcium, magnesium, and phosphorus; total and direct bilirubin; aspartate aminotransferase; alanine aminotransferase; alkaline phosphatase; γ-glutamyl transpeptidase; cholesterol; serum ammonia; viral serologies (including human immunodeficiency virus; hepatitis A, B, and C; cytomegalovirus; Epstein-Barr virus; and herpes simplex virus); urinalysis and urine culture; cell count; and culture of ascitic fluid and purified protein derivative

Electrocardiogram

Chest x-ray

Arterial blood gas

Dobutamine stress echocardiography

Pulmonary function tests

CT or MR scan of the abdomen with liver volume

Esophagogastroduodenoscopy

Doppler ultrasonography

Psychosocial evaluation

Optional examinations

  CT scan of chest and bone scan for patient with malignancy

  Visceral angiogram

  Cardiac catheterization

  Endoscopic retrograde cholangiogram or percutaneous transhepatic cholangiography with brush biopsy for patients with sclerosing cholangitis (10% coincidence of cholangiocarcinoma in these patients)

  Colonoscopy for patients with inflammatory bowel disease, sclerosing cholangitis, Hemoccult-positive stools, family history of colon cancer, previous history of colonic polyps

CT, computed tomography; MR, magnetic resonance.

perioperative monitoring of intracranial pressure (ICP) because untreated severe elevations in ICP can result in permanent brain injury and death. An attempt is made to keep cerebral perfusion pressure (mean arterial BP minus ICP) above 60 mm Hg. Low mean arterial BP is treated with vasopressors after volume resuscitation. Elevation in ICP is treated with hyperventilation, mannitol, and elevation of the head of the bed more than 45 degrees. ICP monitor placement may be complicated by severe coagulopathy and thrombocytopenia, which is common in these patients.

Patients with acute hepatic failure may develop ARF as well, which can require hemofiltration or HD. Sepsis also is seen in acute hepatic failure and requires broad-spectrum antibiotics and antifungals. Pulmonary insufficiency is a common accompaniment of acute liver failure and may require intubation, high-concentration oxygen, and positive end-expiratory pressure.

IV. **Organ allocation.** Livers are now allocated based on the **Model for End-Stage Liver Disease (MELD)** scoring system. The MELD score is derived from the values for bilirubin, serum creatinine, and the international normalized ratio (INR) and ranges from 6 to 40. Livers are allocated to appropriate patients with the highest MELD scores. Special exception points may be granted, such as in cases of hepatocellular carcinoma. Children are graded based on the Pediatric End-Stage Liver Disease (PELD) score.

V. **Donor selection.** Selection of an appropriate donor liver takes into account donor size, ABO blood type, age, presence of infection, history of malignancy, liver function studies, hospital course, hemodynamic stability, and prior alcohol or drug use. Absolute contraindications to the use of a donor liver include the presence of extrahepatic malignancy and HIV. The use of expanded donor criteria allows transplantation of organs from older patients, patients with fatty livers, and patients with positive hepatitis B or C serologies.

VI. **Hepatic transplantation procedure**
   A. **Whole-organ liver transplantation.** Conceptually, transplantation of the liver can be thought of as comprising three distinct sequential phases. The **first phase** involves the dissection of the recipient's diseased liver. The **second phase**, known as the **anhepatic phase**, refers to the period starting with devascularization of the recipient's liver and ending with revascularization of the newly implanted liver. During the anhepatic phase, venovenous bypass (VVB) may be used. VVB shunts blood from the portal vein and infrahepatic inferior vena cava (IVC) to the axillary, subclavian, or jugular veins. Maintenance of venous return from the kidneys and lower extremities during the anhepatic phase results in a smoother hemodynamic course, allows time for a more deliberate approach to hemostasis, reduces visceral edema and splanchnic venous pooling, and lowers the incidence of postoperative renal dysfunction. The liver allograft is implanted by anastomosing first the suprahepatic vena cava and then the infrahepatic IVC. The portal vein anastomosis is performed, and blood flow to the liver is reestablished. Finally, the hepatic arterial anastomosis is performed. If the recipient hepatic artery is not suitable for anastomosis, a donor iliac arterial graft can be used as a conduit from the infra- or suprarenal aorta. The **third phase** includes biliary reconstruction and abdominal closure. Biliary continuity is established via a duct-to-duct anastomosis over a T tube or a choledochojejunostomy. A duct-to-duct anastomosis is preferable, but it may not be possible when there is a donor-recipient bile duct size discrepancy or a diseased recipient bile duct (e.g., with primary sclerosing cholangitis, biliary atresia, and secondary biliary cirrhosis).

   In a modification of the above technique, the recipient's retrohepatic IVC is preserved, and the donor suprahepatic IVC is anastomosed to the confluence of the recipient's right, middle, and left hepatic veins. The donor infrahepatic IVC is then oversewn. A temporary end-to-side portacaval shunt is also created at the beginning of the hepatectomy. This technique has all the advantages of VVB without its associated risks and costs.

B. Reduced and split-liver transplantation was developed to support the needs of pediatric patients awaiting appropriately sized transplants. Benefits include the ability to better match the size of the donor liver to the recipient and the option of using a single liver to provide grafts for multiple patients. These benefits have translated to the adult population as well. The liver has a remarkable capacity for regeneration. It can be divided based on the anatomic segments of Couinaud into a left lateral section (segments 2 and 3), a left lobe graft (segments 2 to 4), or a right lobe graft (segments 5 to 8). The left lateral section is most commonly used in children. Comparison of the size of the donor and the recipient is used to determine the appropriate-sized graft. The mortality of pediatric recipients on the waiting list for a liver transplant has been reduced by the use of split-liver transplantation.

C. Living-donor liver transplantation has been developed as a result of the success of reduced liver transplantation. The left lateral section or left lobe of the liver is usually used as the donor graft for adult-to-child transplantation. Advantages similar to those observed with living related kidney donors have also been observed, such as reduced ischemic time and the inherent benefits of an elective operation. Adult-to-adult living-donor liver transplantation necessitates the use of the larger right hepatic lobe. An amount of liver approximately equal to 0.1% of patient weight (e.g., 700 g for a 70-kg recipient) is required.

VII. Postoperative care

A. Hemodynamic. Intravascular volume resuscitation usually is required in the immediate postoperative period secondary to third-space losses, increased body temperature, and vasodilatation. Adequate perfusion is assessed by left and right heart filling pressures, cardiac output, urine output, and the absence of metabolic acidosis. Hypertension is common and should be aggressively treated.

B. Pulmonary. Ventilatory support is required postoperatively until the patient is awake and alert, is able to follow commands and protect the airway, and is able to maintain adequate oxygenation and ventilation.

C. Hepatic allograft function. Monitoring of hepatic allograft function begins intraoperatively after revascularization. Signs of satisfactory graft function include hemodynamic stability and normalization of acid-base status, body temperature, coagulation studies, maintenance of glucose metabolism, and bile production. Reassessment of hepatic allograft function continues postoperatively, initially occurring every 6 hours. Satisfactory hepatic allograft function is indicated by an improving coagulation profile, decreasing transaminase levels, normal blood glucose, hemodynamic stability, adequate urine output, bile production, and clearance of anesthesia. Early elevations of bilirubin and transaminase levels may be indicators of preservation injury. The peak levels of serum glutamic-oxaloacetic transaminase and serum glutamate pyruvate transaminase usually are less than 2,000 units/L and should decrease rapidly over the first 24 to 48 hours postoperatively. After the patient leaves the intensive care unit, liver function tests are obtained daily. Bile is inspected daily, a T-tube cholangiogram may be obtained to ensure adequate biliary drainage and to rule out extravasation. If hepatic dysfunction becomes evident at any time, prompt evaluation must be undertaken and treatment must be initiated. It is important to correctly diagnose the cause of liver dysfunction, because each cause has its own unique treatment.

1. Primary nonfunction and initial poor function. The use of UW solution for organ preservation has decreased the incidence of primary nonfunction. For poorly understood reasons, however, 1% to 9% of transplanted livers fail immediately after the surgery. Primary nonfunction is characterized by hemodynamic instability, poor quantity and quality of bile, renal dysfunction, failure to regain consciousness, increasing coagulopathy, persistent hypothermia, and lactic acidosis in the face of patent vascular anastomosis (as demonstrated by Doppler ultrasonography). Without retransplantation, death ensues.

2. **Rejection.** Acute rejection is relatively common after liver transplantation, with 60% of recipients experiencing at least one cell-mediated or acute rejection episode. However, rejection is an extremely uncommon cause of graft loss. The most common causes of early graft loss include primary nonfunction and hepatic artery thrombosis.

3. **Technical complications.** A variety of technical problems can lead to liver allograft dysfunction, including hepatic artery stenosis or thrombosis, portal vein stenosis or thrombosis, biliary tract obstruction, bile duct leak, and hepatic vein or vena caval thrombosis. **Hepatic artery thrombosis** that occurs in the early posttransplantation period may lead to fever, hemodynamic instability, and rapid deterioration of the patient, with a marked elevation of the transaminases. An associated bile leak may be noted soon after liver transplantation due to the loss of the bile ducts' main vascular supply. Acute hepatic artery thrombosis may be treated by attempted thrombectomy. If this is unsuccessful, retransplantation is needed. Hepatic artery thrombosis that occurs long after liver transplantation may produce intra- and extrahepatic bile duct strictures and may be an indication for elective retransplantation. Occasionally, hepatic artery thrombosis is completely asymptomatic.

   Portal vein stenosis or thrombosis is rare. When it occurs, the patient's condition may deteriorate rapidly, with profound hepatic dysfunction, massive ascites, renal failure, and hemodynamic instability. Although surgical thrombectomy may be successful, urgent retransplantation is often necessary. Late portal vein thrombosis may allow normal liver function but usually results in variceal bleeding and ascites.

   Bile duct obstruction is diagnosed by cholangiography. A single short bile duct stricture may be treated by either percutaneous or retrograde balloon dilation. A long stricture, ampullary dysfunction, or failed dilation necessitates revision of the biliary tract anastomosis. Fever and abdominal pain in the early posttransplantation period should raise the possibility of biliary anastomotic disruption, which requires urgent surgical revision.

4. **Recurrent infection and neoplasm.** CMV can cause hepatic allograft dysfunction and usually occurs within 8 weeks of transplantation. Diagnosis is made by liver biopsy, with CMV inclusion bodies being found with light microscopy or by PCR in peripheral blood. Treatment consists of decreasing baseline immunosuppression and administering ganciclovir (5 mg/kg every 12 hours via central venous access for 3 weeks).

   Viral hepatitis and malignancy (e.g., hepatoma, cholangiocarcinoma, neuroendocrine tumors) can recur in the hepatic allograft but are uncommon in the early posttransplantation period. The clinical presentation includes elevations on liver function tests. The diagnosis is made by liver biopsy. Imaging studies (e.g., CT scan, liver ultrasonography) are important for following patients transplanted for neoplasms. Patients transplanted for hepatocellular carcinoma also should have surveillance with CT scan and tumor markers at regular intervals.

D. **Electrolytes and glucose.** The use of diuretics may result in hypokalemia, whereas cyclosporine or tacrolimus toxicity may cause hyperkalemia. Magnesium levels are maintained above 2 mg/dL (0.82 mmol/L) because the seizure threshold is lowered by the combination of hypomagnesemia and cyclosporine or tacrolimus. Calcium should be measured as free ionized calcium and kept above 4.4 mg/dL (1.1 mmol/L). Phosphorus levels should be maintained above 2.5 mg/dL (0.81 mmol/L) to avoid respiratory muscle weakness and altered oxygen hemoglobin dissociation. Glucose homeostasis is necessary because steroid administration may result in hyperglycemia, which is best managed with intravenous insulin because it is short acting and easily absorbed. Cyclosporine and tacrolimus are diabetogenic immunosuppressants and may alter glucose homeostasis. Hypoglycemia is a complication of liver failure, and in the presence of liver dysfunction, glucose administration may be necessary.

E. GI tract. H_2 blockade, proton pump inhibition, and/or antacids are used to prevent stress ulcers. Endoscopy is performed liberally for any GI bleeding to determine the etiology. Nystatin and GI tract decontamination solution containing gentamicin and polymyxin B are used in the perioperative period to prevent esophageal candidiasis and translocation of bacterial pathogens.

F. Nutrition. Patients who are severely malnourished should be placed on nutritional supplementation as soon as stable fluid and electrolyte status and adequate graft function have been reached. Patients with adequate preoperative nutrition can be maintained on routine intravenous fluids until GI tract function returns (usually 3 to 5 days). Enteral nutrition is used as soon as the postoperative ileus resolves. Total parenteral nutrition (TPN) is indicated when the GI tract is nonfunctional.

G. Infection surveillance. The most common causes of bacterial infection after liver transplantation include line sepsis, urinary tract infection, infected ascites, cholangitis, pneumonia, biliary anastomotic leak, and intraabdominal abscess. Prophylactic antibiotics covering biliary pathogens are administered for the first 48 hours after liver transplantation. If a fever develops in the liver transplant recipient, a thorough examination should be performed. A chest x-ray and cultures of blood, urine, indwelling lines, and bile also are necessary. A T-tube cholangiogram and Doppler ultrasonography of the liver can be performed to rule out perihepatic fluid collection and to evaluate hepatic vasculature.

Hepatitis B or C recurs in the liver allograft following transplantation. Therefore, protocols are currently under investigation using different combinations of hepatitis B Ig, hepatitis B vaccines, lamivudine, retroviral agents, and monoclonal antibodies. The diagnosis is suspected if the level of liver transaminases increases, and it is confirmed by biopsy. Recurrent disease may be severe enough to lead to life-threatening hepatitis and cirrhosis. Strategies to prevent hepatitis B recurrence include the use of lamivudine before transplant to arrest viral replication and high-dose hepatitis B Ig and lamivudine after transplant. Hepatitis C recurrence after transplant, although it is ubiquitous, does not commonly lead to significant problems for many years and is associated with mild transaminitis. Occasionally, hepatitis C recurrence can be early, aggressive, and severe. Antiviral therapy has been used to treat hepatitis C recurrence but with very limited success.

H. Posttransplantation immunosuppression. Currently, the immunosuppressive agents used to prevent rejection include corticosteroids and cyclosporine or tacrolimus. Occasionally, azathioprine or mycophenolate mofetil may be added to reduce cyclosporine or tacrolimus doses in patients with renal disease or autoimmune liver disease.

VIII. Rejection. Many liver transplant recipients experience at least one acute rejection episode, and it commonly occurs between the 4th and 21st day postoperatively. Rejection is characterized by fever; increased ascites; decreased bile quality and quantity; and elevation of total white blood cell and eosinophil count, bilirubin, and transaminase levels. Liver transplant rejection is diagnosed by percutaneous liver biopsy. In the early posttransplantation period, technical causes of hepatic dysfunction are ruled out by Doppler ultrasonography to ensure vascular patency, and T-tube cholangiography is obtained to rule out a bile duct obstruction or leak. Typical biopsy findings consistent with acute rejection include the triad consisting of portal lymphocytes, endothelialitis (subendothelial deposits of mononuclear cells), and bile duct infiltration and damage. The first-line treatment for acute rejection is a bolus of corticosteroids (methylprednisolone, 1 g intravenously). If the rejection responds appropriately, the patient undergoes steroid recycling (methylprednisolone, 50 mg intravenously four times a day for four doses; 40 mg intravenously four times a day for four doses; 30 mg intravenously four times a day for four doses; 20 mg intravenously four times a day for four doses; 20 mg intravenously twice a day for two doses; and finally prednisone, 20 mg per day orally) and optimizing of the immunosuppressive regimen (which may include the addition of azathioprine or mycophenolate mofetil).

PANCREAS TRANSPLANTATION

I. **Indications.** Diabetes mellitus (DM) affects 6.3% of Americans and is the sixth leading cause of death. It is the leading cause of renal failure and blindness in adults. Other long-term complications caused by diabetes include myocardial infarction, stroke, amputation, and neuropathy. Invasive methods for maintaining euglycemia and preventing the long-term complications of DM include the use of autoregulating insulin pumps, pancreatic islet cell transplants, and whole organ pancreatic transplantation.

Pancreas transplantation is commonly performed in the setting of kidney transplantation (either simultaneously or afterwards) for diabetes complicated by end-stage renal disease. A limited number of simple pancreas transplants are also performed.

II. **Contraindications** to pancreas transplantation are the same as those for kidney transplantation, including disabilities secondary to DM, such as peripheral gangrene, intractable cardiac decompensation, and incapacitating peripheral neuropathy. Continued tobacco use also is considered a relatively strong contraindication to pancreas transplantation.

III. **Preoperative workup and evaluation.** Workup of the potential pancreas transplantation patient is similar to that of the kidney recipient and identifies co-existing diseases, as outlined in Table 28-3. To allow identification of beneficial effects of pancreas transplantation on the complications of DM, a careful preoperative evaluation of the patient's neurologic and ophthalmologic status should be performed.

IV. **Donor pancreas procurement** occurs as part of a multiorgan retrieval. Contraindications to pancreas donation include the presence of diabetes, pancreatitis, trauma to the pancreas, or significant intra-abdominal contamination. Although the liver and pancreas may share blood supply, combined retrieval can be performed safely without compromising either organ. During the organ retrieval procedure, it is important to identify accessory or replaced hepatic arteries that may arise from the left gastric artery or the SMA. The abdominal viscera are flushed with UW solution, and the liver, pancreas, duodenum, and spleen are removed *en bloc* and separated under cold-storage conditions. The splenic artery is divided from the celiac, and the SMA is divided at its origin or distal to a replaced right hepatic artery, if present. The mesentery of the small intestine is either oversewn or stapled.

V. **Deceased-donor pancreas transplantation operation**
A. **Forms of pancreatic transplantation**
1. **Isolated pancreas transplantation.** The most widely accepted technique of pancreatic transplantation in the United States uses whole organ pancreas with venous drainage into the systemic circulation and enteric exocrine drainage. Some centers advocate portal venous drainage, which may be associated with fewer episodes of acute rejection.

Under cold-storage conditions, the portal vein is isolated. If it is too short to allow for a tension-free anastomosis, an extension autograft is placed using donor iliac vein. The SMA and splenic artery then are reconstructed with a donor iliac artery Y-bifurcation autograft. Only the second portion of the duodenum is retained with the pancreas. Then the portal vein is anastomosed to the iliac vein or the superior mesenteric vein, and the donor common iliac artery graft is anastomosed to the recipient's external iliac artery. The duodenal segment of the transplant is then opened, and a duodenocystostomy is created. Alternatively, the duodenal segment can be anastomosed to a Roux-en-Y limb for enteric drainage. The pancreas transplant is left in the right paracolic gutter, and if kidney transplantation is to be performed, it is done on the left side.

2. **Simultaneous kidney-pancreas transplantation** may be considered in insulin-dependent diabetic patients who are dialysis dependent or imminent and have a creatinine clearance of less than 30 mL per minute. Some of the advantages of combined transplantation include the ability to monitor rejection of the pancreas by monitoring renal rejection and the fact that the patient is exposed to only one set of donor antigens.

3. **Pancreatic islet cell transplantation** is still investigational and has not yet received widespread acceptance. Pancreatic islet cells are isolated and injected into the portal vein for engraftment in the liver. The major problems encountered have been obtaining enough islet cells to attain glucose homeostasis and failure in achieving long-term insulin independence. New immunosuppressive protocols and improved isolation techniques, however, promise to raise the historically low success rate (*N Engl J Med* 2000;343:230), and a number of clinical trials are currently underway.

B. **Exocrine drainage**

1. **Enteric drainage.** Most programs now use enteric drainage, which avoids the acidosis, volume depletion, and urologic complications associated with bladder drainage. Enteric drainage can be performed by anastomosing the duodenal segment to small bowel in a side-to-side fashion or via a Roux-en-Y limb. Disadvantages of enteric drainage include the inability to monitor exocrine secretions and a higher rate of technical failure.

2. **Bladder drainage.** Advantages of this technique include the ability to measure urinary amylase, which can facilitate the early diagnosis of rejection. Cystoscopic transduodenal needle biopsy can also be performed in the diagnosis of rejection. The major disadvantages of bladder drainage are fluid and electrolyte disturbances and urologic complications (including hematuria, urinary tract infections, urethral strictures, and reflux pancreatitis) caused by the drainage of fluid, bicarbonate, and enzymes into the bladder.

VI. **Postoperative management and monitoring**

A. **Immunosuppression** consists of quadruple therapy with antibody induction, tacrolimus, prednisone, and mycophenolate mofetil.

B. **Serum glucose** is followed during and after the transplantation. Intravenous insulin infusions are stopped within the first few hours after pancreas transplantation.

C. **Rejection** of the pancreas transplant is suggested by a rise in serum amylase or a fall in urinary amylase. Rejection of pancreas and kidney transplants usually occurs in parallel but at times may be discordant. The diagnosis of kidney rejection is suggested by a rise in creatinine, which is then confirmed by biopsy. Biopsy of the pancreas transplant is performed percutaneously or via cystoscopy. Rejection is treated with corticosteroids or antilymphocyte preparations.

D. **Graft-related complications.** Besides rejection, complications of pancreas transplantation include metabolic acidosis and dehydration. These are due to the loss of sodium and bicarbonate into the urine from the transplanted duodenum, and they are avoided with enteric drainage. Other common complications include pancreatitis, urinary tract infections, urethritis, and anastomotic leak from the duodenocystostomy. Infections with CMV also may occur.

Table 28-8. Causes of intestinal failure

Superior mesenteric artery thrombosis	Crohn disease
Superior mesenteric artery embolization	Trauma
Necrotizing enterocolitis	Radiation
Volvulus	Tumor (desmoid, polyposis)
Gastroschisis	Pseudo-obstruction
Intestinal atresia	

VII. **Effect on secondary complications of diabetes.** The full effect of pancreatic transplantation on secondary complications of diabetes is still unknown. Pancreatic transplantation may prevent the development of diabetic nephropathy in the transplanted kidney. It also may stabilize diabetic retinopathy and improve diabetic neuropathy.

INTESTINAL TRANSPLANTATION

Intestinal failure occurs when the functioning GI tract mucosal surface area has been reduced below the minimal amount necessary for adequate digestion and absorption of food. This may be caused by intestinal loss or intestinal disease (Table 28-8). The development of TPN has led to the possibility of long-term survival for infants and adults with intestinal failure. However, TPN has limitations and its own associated morbidity.

I. **Indications.** Adults and children who have documented intestinal failure without the potential for long-term survival on TPN are candidates for intestinal transplantation. **Intestinal failure** is said to occur when any child younger than 1 year requires more than 50% of his or her caloric needs from TPN after neonatal small-bowel resection or when a child older than 4 years requires more than 30% of calories from TPN. Older children and adults receiving more than 50% of their nutritional requirements from TPN for more than 1 year also should be considered for intestinal transplantation. Other considerations include venous access, recurrent infectious complications related to central venous catheters, prolonged hospitalizations, growth retardation, and hepatobiliary dysfunction secondary to prolonged TPN.

II. **Donor intestinal procurement generally** uses multiorgan recovery techniques. The liver, stomach, duodenum, pancreas, and small intestine are removed *en bloc* and separated under cold-storage conditions. Alternatively, the intestine may be recovered alone or with the liver.

III. **Intestinal transplantation operation.** Patients who receive isolated intestinal allografts have vascular anastomoses created between the donor superior mesenteric vein and the recipient portal vein and between the donor SMA and the recipient aorta. Vascular reconstruction for patients who receive combined liver-intestinal grafts parallels that for patients undergoing a standard OLT. Supra- and infrahepatic vena caval anastomoses are completed, and arterial inflow is accomplished after the portal vein anastomosis by using a patch of aorta that contains the SMA and celiac.

IV. **Postoperative management**

    A. **Immunosuppression and infectious prophylaxis.** Posttransplantation immunosuppression uses tacrolimus and prednisone. Monitoring for graft rejection is done through frequent endoscopic biopsies. Watery diarrhea may be a sign of either rejection or superinfection. With the return of intestinal function, feedings are begun with an elemental diet and then advanced as tolerated. Viral and fungal infection prophylaxis includes ganciclovir, oral antibiotic bowel preparation, and low-dose amphotericin B.

    B. **Potential complications.** Inherent risks with intestinal transplantation include up to 50% graft failure (rejection) at 3 years. Combined liver-intestine transplantation carries all the additional risks inherent in liver transplantation. Risks that are increased in intestinal transplant recipients include the development of graft-versus-host disease and posttransplantation lymphoproliferative disease. Complications related to tacrolimus-based immunosuppression include diabetes mellitus, headaches, CNS neurotoxicity, peripheral neurotoxicity, and nephrotoxicity. As with any effective immunosuppressant, there is an increased risk of infection and malignancy.

REFERENCE

Norman DJ, Turka LA, eds. *Primer on Transplantation.* 2nd ed. Thorofare, NJ: American Society of Transplant Physicians; 2001.

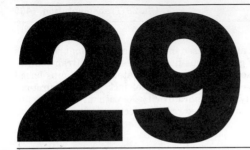

Burns

Jack Oak and
J. Perren Cobb

Burns are tissue injuries resulting from direct contact with hot liquids, gases, or surfaces; caustic chemicals; electricity; or radiation. Most commonly, the skin is injured, which compromises its function as a barrier to injury and infection and as a regulator of body temperature, fluid loss, and sensation. More than 2 million individuals in the United States sustain burns each year, of whom more than 50,000 are hospitalized. Seventy-five percent of those hospitalized have burns covering <10% of their body-surface area (BSA) (*N Engl J Med* 1996;335:1581). Advances in burn care management continue to reduce mortality and improve the quality of life for burn victims.

ASSESSMENT AND MANAGEMENT OF BURN INJURIES

I. **Assessment**
   A. **The mechanism of injury** identified by the patient or witnesses helps to direct the assessment. Burns sustained in a closed environment, such as a structure fire, often produce inhalation injury in addition to thermal trauma. Explosions can cause barometric injury to the lungs and may cause blunt trauma. Burn source, duration of exposure, time of injury, and environment are documented carefully.
   B. **Associated injuries** may be present in the burn patient and can result from explosions, falls, or jumping in escape attempts. Fractures, abdominal organ injury, pulmonary contusion, and pneumothorax sometimes occur.
   C. **Patient age** has a major effect on outcome, with infants and elderly patients being at highest risk. Inpatient, outpatient, or burn unit management decisions also are influenced by patient age. Burns are a common form of child abuse and should be suspected when the mechanism of injury appears to be incongruent with the injury pattern. Elderly patients often have diminished organ system reserve and comorbid medical problems that place them at increased risk.
   D. **State of health.** Preexisting medical problems affecting management should be noted, including allergies, medications, hypertension, and diabetes mellitus. A careful review of systems should be obtained, with particular attention paid to cardiac, renal, pulmonary, and gastrointestinal systems.
   E. **Prehospital treatment** is ascertained and recorded, including care provided by the patient and by the emergency response team. Administered fluids are documented carefully and subtracted from estimated fluid requirements for the first 24 hours of injury.
   F. **Physical examination**
      1. **Airway** assessment and support have the highest priority. Supraglottic tissue edema progresses over the first 12 hours and can obstruct the airway rapidly. The larynx protects subglottic tissue from direct thermal injury but not from injury due to inhaled toxic gases. Inhalation injury should be suspected if the patient was burned in an enclosed structure or explosion. Physical signs include hoarseness, stridor, facial burns, singed facial hair, expectoration of carbonaceous sputum, or presence of carbon in the oropharynx. Direct laryngoscopy is useful in equivocal cases but should not delay expeditious endotracheal intubation with a large-bore tube based on clinical indications. Bronchoscopy is particularly helpful in diagnosing inhalation injury in patients with clinically silent airway

injuries, in facilitating difficult intubations, and in predicting the onset of adult respiratory distress syndrome (*J Trauma* 1994;36:59).

2. **Breathing** is evaluated for effort, depth of respiration, and auscultation of breath sounds. Wheezing or rales suggest either inhalation injury or aspiration of gastric contents. Circumferential deep burn of the thorax can restrict inspiration, necessitating escharotomies in the anterior axillary lines bilaterally. Carboxyhemoglobin levels >10% indicate inhalation injury (in nonsmokers). Levels >30% are associated with mental status changes, and those >60% are not compatible with survival.

3. **Circulation** is assessed for the presence of shock (rapid, weak, or absent pulse) and tissue perfusion. Signs of impairment in central perfusion include cyanosis, agitation, and reduced mentation. Intravascular volume shifts to the interstitial compartment, coupled with exudative and evaporative water loss from the burn injury, can reduce circulating blood volume rapidly. Full-thickness circumferential extremity or neck burns require escharotomy if circulation distal to the injury is impaired. Escharotomies are rarely needed within the first 6 hours of injury.

4. **Remove all clothing** to halt continued burn from melted synthetic compounds or chemicals and to assess the full extent of body-surface involvement in the initial examination. Irrigate injuries with water or saline to remove harmful residues. **Remove jewelry** (particularly rings) to prevent injury resulting from increasing tissue edema.

G. **Depth of burn** (Table 29-1)
1. **First-degree burns** are limited to the epidermis. The skin is painful and red. There are no blisters. These burns should heal spontaneously in 3 to 4 days.
2. **Second-degree burns**, which are subdivided into **superficial or deep partial-thickness**, are limited to the dermal layers of the skin. **Superficial** partial-thickness burns involve the papillary dermis. They appear red, warm, edematous, and blistered, often with denuded, moist, mottled red or pink epithelium. The injured tissue is very painful, especially when exposed to air. Such burns frequently arise from brief contact with hot surfaces, liquids, flames, or chemicals. **Deep** second-degree burns involve the reticular dermis and thus can damage some dermal appendages (e.g., nerves, sweat glands, or hair follicles). Hence, such burns can be less sensitive, or hairs may be easily plucked out of areas with deep partial-thickness burns. Still, the only definitive method of differentiating superficial and deep partial-thickness burns is by length of time to heal. Superficial burns heal in <2 weeks; deep ones require at least 3 weeks. Further, any partial-thickness burn can convert to full-thickness injury over time, especially if early fluid resuscitation is inadequate.
3. **Full-thickness** (third- or fourth-degree) burns involve all layers of the skin and some subcutaneous tissue. In **third-degree** burns, all the skin appendages, including hair follicles and sweat and sebaceous glands, and sensory fibers for touch, pain, temperature, and pressure are destroyed. This results in an initially painless, insensate dry surface that may appear either white and leathery or charred and cracked, with exposure of underlying fat. **Fourth-degree** burns also involve fascia, muscle, and bone. They often result from prolonged contact with thermal sources or high electrical current. All full-thickness burns are managed surgically, and immediate burn expertise should be sought.

H. **Percentage of BSA estimation**
1. **Small areas: palm of patient's hand equals 1% of BSA.**
2. **Large areas: rule of nines.** Regions of the body approximating 9% BSA or multiples thereof are shown in Table 29-2. Note that infants and babies have a proportionally greater percentage of BSA in the head and neck region and less in the lower extremities compared with adults.

Table 29-1. Treatment algorithm for the three clinically important burn depths[a]

Burn depth[b]	Level of injury	Clinical features	Treatment	Usual result
Superficial partial-thickness	Papillary dermis	Blisters Erythema Capillary refill Intact pain sensation	Tetanus prophy-laxis Cleaning (e.g., with chlorhexi-dine gluconate) Topical agent (e.g., 1% silver sulfadiazine) Sterile gauze dressing[c] Physical therapy Splints as neces-sary	Epithelializa-tion in 7–21 days Hypertrophic scar rare Return of full function
Deep partial-thick-ness	Reticular dermis	Blisters Pale white or yellow color Absent pain sensation	As for superficial partial-thick-ness burns Early surgical excision and skin grafting an option	Epithelializa-tion in 21–60 days in the absence of surgery Hypertrophic scar common Earlier return of function with surgi-cal therapy
Full thick-ness	Subcutane-ous fat, fascia, muscle, or bone	Blisters may be absent Leathery, in classic, wrinkled appearance over bony prominences No capillary refill Thrombosed subcutaneous vessels may be visible Absent pain sen-sation	As for superficial partial-thick-ness burns Wound excision and grafting at earliest feasi-ble time	Functional limitation more fre-quent Hypertrophic scar mainly at graft margins

[a]Epidermal (first-degree) burns present clinically with cutaneous erythema, pain, and tenderness; they resolve rapidly and generally require only symptomatic treatment.
[b]No clinically useful objective method of measuring burn depth exists; classification depends on clinical judgment.
[c]Sterile gauze dressings are frequently omitted on the face and neck.
Reprinted with permission from Monafo WW. Initial management of burns. *N Engl J Med* 1996;335:1581.

Table 29-2. Rule of nines estimation of percentage of body surface area

	Head and neck	Trunk		Extremity		Genital
		Anterior	Posterior	Upper	Lower	
Adult	9	18	18	9	18	1
Infant	18	128	18	9	14	—

II. Management
A. Emergency room
1. **Resuscitation.** A surgical consultation is initiated for all patients with major injury (*N Engl J Med* 1996;335:1581).
   a. **Oxygen** should be provided to patients with all but the most minor injuries. A 100% oxygen high-humidity face mask for those with possible inhalation injury assists the patient's expectoration from dry airways and treats carbon monoxide poisoning. Others can benefit from 2 to 6 L oxygen via nasal cannula.
   b. **Intravenous access.** All patients with ≥20% BSA burns require intravenous fluids. A 16-gauge or larger peripheral venous access should be started immediately to provide circulatory volume support. Peripheral access in the upper extremities is preferred over central venous access because of the risk of catheter-related infection. An intravenous catheter may be placed through the burn if other suitable sites are unavailable. Avoid lower-extremity catheters, if possible, to prevent phlebitic complications.
   c. **Fluid** is administered intravenously to all patients with ≥20% BSA burns. Increased capillary permeability in injured tissue results in edema and evaporative losses. Evaporative cooling results in heat loss, and hypothermia may result. Acute metabolic acidosis usually is secondary to inadequate fluid resuscitation. Persistent metabolic acidosis also can result from anaerobic metabolism secondary to carbon monoxide binding to cellular cytochrome.
      (1) **Modified Parkland formula.** The estimated crystalloid requirement for the first 24 hours after injury is calculated based on patient weight and BSA burn percentage. **Lactated Ringer solution volume in the first 24 hours = 4 mL × % BSA** (second-, third-, and fourth-degree burns only) × **body weight (kg).** One-half of the calculated volume is given in the first 8 hours after injury, and the remaining volume is infused over the next 16 hours. Fluid resuscitation calculations are based on the time of injury, not the time when the patient is evaluated. Prehospital intravenous hydration is subtracted from the total volume estimate. It should be emphasized that formulas are only estimates, and more or less fluid may be required to maintain adequate tissue perfusion as measured by rate of urine output. Patients with inhalational injury, associated mechanical trauma, electrical injury, escharotomies, or delayed resuscitation require more fluid than that based on the formula alone. Further, for children weighing ≤30 kg, 5% dextrose (D5) in ¼ normal saline maintenance fluids should supplement the Parkland formula to compensate for ongoing evaporative losses. Patient **body weight** is determined early after the burn as a baseline measurement for fluid calculations and as a daily reference for fluid management.
      (2) **Colloid-containing** solutions are best held for intravenous therapy until after the first 24 hours postburn. The role of albumin therapy in resuscitation has been reviewed recently, and one conclusion is that it should be used with great caution (*BMJ* 1998;317:235; *Evid Based Med* 1999;4:19; *ACP J Club* 1999;130:6). If given to patients with inhalation injury early in resuscitation, albumin may move into the interstitium and may increase pulmonary complications. By 24 hours, capillary leak diminishes. For patients with >30% BSA burn, a one-time bolus of 5% albumin solution (0.3 to 0.5 mL/kg per 1% of BSA) should be infused to restore plasma oncotic pressure. Otherwise, replace insensible losses with D5W in adults or D5 in ¼ normal saline in children weighing ≤30 kg. Such fluids replace evaporative

losses and mitigate the hypernatremia after resuscitation (*Shock* 1996;5:4).

d. A Foley catheter is used to monitor hourly urine production as an index of adequate tissue perfusion. In the absence of underlying renal disease, a minimum urine production rate of 1 mL/kg per hour in children (weighing ≤30 kg) and 0.5 mL/kg per hour in adults is the guideline for adequate intravenous infusion. To minimize edema, consider reducing intravenous hydration if urine output exceeds 1.5 mL/kg per hour in adult patients.

e. Nasogastric tube insertion with low intermittent suction is performed if patients are intubated or develop nausea, vomiting, and abdominal distention consistent with adynamic ileus. Virtually all patients with >25% BSA burns have an adynamic ileus.

f. Escharotomy may be necessary in full-thickness circumferential burns of the neck, torso, or extremities when increasing tissue edema impairs peripheral circulation or when chest involvement restricts respiratory efforts. Full-thickness incisions through (but no deeper than) the insensate burn eschar provide immediate relief. Longitudinal escharotomies are performed on the lateral or medial aspect of the extremities and the anterior axillary lines of the chest, where indicated (Fig. 29-1). Usually, they are done at the bedside and require no anesthesia. However, if the digits were burned so severely that desiccation results, midlateral escharotomies have minimal benefit. Escharotomies are rarely required within the first 6 hours after injury. Indications for escharotomy rest on clinical grounds. Traditionally, to aid in assessing peripheral circulation, the documentation

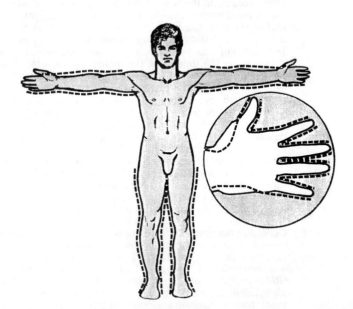

Figure 29-1. Placement of escharotomies. Midaxial escharotomies should be performed if vascular compromise occurs. Incisions should be performed through the dermis and subcutaneous tissue to allow maximal expansion of the underlying fascia. (Reprinted with permission from Eichelberger M. *Pediatric Trauma.* St. Louis: Mosby, 1993.)

of palpable peripheral pulse or the presence of a Doppler signal has been used. However, studies have indicated that correlation of intramuscular pressure with signs and symptoms of extremity compression, including Doppler pulse, was poor (*Am J Surg* 1980;140:825–831). Infrared photoplethysmograph (PPG or pulse oximetry) has been a useful adjunct in assessing the need of escharotomies. PPG has been correlated with blood flow and direct measurement of compartment pressure. In one study of 55 extremity injuries, there were clinical signs suggesting the use of escharotomy in 6 of 29 patients. However, normal PPG signals were present, and conservative management resulted in no long-term morbidity (*J Hand Surg* 1984;9:314–319).

2. **Monitors.** Continuous pulse oximetry to measure oxygen saturation is useful. One caveat is that falsely elevated levels can be observed in carbon monoxide poisoning.

3. **Laboratory examination** includes a baseline complete blood cell count, type and cross-match, electrolytes and renal indices, β-human chorionic gonadotropin (in women), arterial carboxyhemoglobin, arterial blood gas, and urinalysis. A toxicology screen and an alcohol level are obtained when suggested by history or mental status examination. A chest x-ray is obtained with the understanding that it rarely reflects early inhalation injury. Additional chest films are obtained should endotracheal intubation or central line placement become necessary. An electrocardiogram is useful initially, particularly in elderly patients or those with electrical burns. Fluid and electrolyte fluxes during resuscitation and later mobilization of third-space edema can result in arrhythmias and interval electrocardiographic changes.

4. **Moist dressings** applied to partial-thickness burns provide pain relief from air exposure. Cool water applied to small partial-thickness burns can provide relief but must be avoided in patients with major burns (>25% BSA) and especially in infants—groups that are at high risk for hypothermia. Cold water also can cause vasoconstriction and can extend the depth and surface area of injury.

5. **Analgesia** is given intravenously every 1 to 2 hours to manage pain but in small doses to guard against hypotension, oversedation, and respiratory depression.

6. **Photographs or diagrams** of the BSA involvement and thickness of burns are useful in documenting the injury. They also can facilitate communication between the various members of the team caring for the patient and serve medicolegal purposes in the case of assault or child abuse.

7. **Early irrigation and débridement** are performed using normal saline and sterile instruments to remove all loose epidermal skin layers, followed by the application of topical antimicrobial agents and sterile dressings. In general, it is safe to leave blisters intact because they permit healing in a sterile environment and offer some protection to the underlying dermis. Once they are ruptured, or if the bullae are large (>2 cm) and thin-walled, débridement is indicated to prevent infection. If the burns resulted from liquid chemical exposure, they are irrigated continuously for 20 to 30 minutes. Dry chemicals are removed from the skin before irrigation to prevent them from dissolving into solution and causing further injury. Corneal burns of the eye require continuous irrigation for several hours and immediate ophthalmologic consultation.

8. **Topical antimicrobial agents** are the mainstay of burn management. The most common organisms complicating the burn injury are *Staphylococcus aureus*, *Pseudomonas aeruginosa*, *Enterococcus* species, Enterobacteriaceae, group A streptococci, and *Candida albicans*. Systemic antibiotics are not administered prophylactically but are reserved for documented infection. Bacterial proliferation may occur underneath the

eschar at the viable-nonviable interface, resulting in subeschar suppuration and separation of the eschar. Microorganisms can invade the underlying tissue, producing invasive burn wound sepsis. The risk of invasive infection is higher in patients with multiorgan failure or burns >30% BSA to total BSA. When the identity of the specific organism is established, antibiotic therapy is targeted to that organism. It may be useful on occasion to diagnose invasive infection. The technique requires a 500-mg biopsy of suspicious eschar and underlying unburned tissue. The presence of microorganisms in viable tissue confirms the diagnosis. The number of microorganisms in viable tissue correlates with mortality. Treatment requires infected eschar excision and appropriate topical/systemic antibiotic therapy (*World J Surg* 1998;22:135).

  a. Silver sulfadiazine (e.g., Silvadene) is the most commonly used agent because it is not irritating and has the fewest adverse side effects, the worst being a transient leukopenia in the first 1 to 3 days. It is formulated as a cream, which helps to minimize evaporative water and heat loss and thus diminishes caloric requirements. It is **contraindicated** in patients with glucose 6-phosphatase deficiency.

  b. Mafenide acetate (Sulfamylon) is **bacteriostatic** and has better Gram-negative (particularly against *P. aeruginosa*) and anaerobic coverage as well as deeper eschar penetration. Further, burns over avascular cartilage, such as the ear, are ideal for mafenide acetate therapy. However, it is painful and readily absorbed systemically; it can also lead to metabolic **hyperchloremic** acidosis by inhibiting carbonic anhydrase.

  c. Polymyxin B sulfate (Polysporin) is tolerated well on facial burns and does not discolor skin, as silver sulfadiazine sometimes can.

  d. Silver nitrate has lost favor because of the severe electrolyte abnormalities resulting from Na^+, K^+, and Cl^- leaching from the wound and because it readily stains skin and clothing. However, for patients with a sulfa allergy, it is a reasonable choice, provided that electrolytes are closely monitored.

  e. Acticoat (Westaim Biomedical, Exeter, NH) has recently gained acceptance. This dressing comes as an easy-to-apply sheet, slowly releases silver ions, has good antimicrobial activity, and can be left in place for 3 days. However, its expense may prove prohibitive for some types of injury.

9. **Tetanus prophylaxis** should be administered as tetanus toxoid, 0.5 mL intramuscularly, if the last booster dose was more than 5 years before the injury. If immunization status is unknown, human tetanus immunoglobulin (Hyper-Tet), 250 to 500 units, should be administered intramuscularly using a syringe and injection site different from those used for tetanus toxoid administration.

10. **Critical care issues with burns.** Such issues include burn wound infection, pneumonia, sepsis, ileus, Curling ulcer (gastroduodenal), acalculous cholecystitis, and superior mesenteric artery syndrome.

  a. Stress ulcer prophylaxis (e.g., H_2 blockers, antacids, or omeprazole) should be provided for patients who have major burns and can receive nothing by mouth, especially those with coagulopathy.

  b. Deep venous thrombosis and thromboembolic complications were considered to be rare in burn patients, even when their protracted immobility, hypercoagulability, and common need for femoral central venous access were taken into account. There is currently no consensus on the advisability of routine prophylaxis, but some type is increasingly being prescribed for adult burn patients during prolonged critical illness.

  c. Glucose monitoring is also of paramount importance. Glucose control has been associated with a reduced incidence of infectious complications and enhanced survival.

  d. Sepsis. Recent studies are now available suggesting that recombinant activated protein C (r-APC) may have some benefit in select patients with systemic sepsis and sudden organ failure. Its judicious use is mandated for the potential of bleeding complications and the cost of the therapy. Data for burn patients are mostly anecdotal, but r-APC may not be useful in burn patients who have relatively chronic organ dysfunction and large wounds.

B. Outpatient. Only minor first-degree or partial-thickness injuries should be considered for outpatient management. Whether to use outpatient management depends on many factors, including patient reliability, opportunity for follow-up, and accessibility to health professionals. Surgical consultation is recommended at the time of initial evaluation in all but the most minor injuries.

  1. Dressings are often managed by the patient when the injury is easily accessible. Home health nursing is a useful adjunct when self-application is suboptimal or wounds are in early healing stages, requiring close follow-up. Silver sulfadiazine is often applied as a light coating, followed by sterile dressings once or twice daily.

  2. Antibiotics are not prescribed prophylactically because they allow resistant organisms to multiply. Their use is limited to documented infection of the wounds.

  3. Follow-up usually occurs once or twice a week during the initial healing of partial-thickness burns and split-thickness skin grafts until epithelialization is complete. Thereafter, patients are followed at 1- to 3-month intervals to evaluate and treat scar hypertrophy (application of foam tape or Jobst garments), hyperpigmentation (avoidance of direct sunlight, use of sunscreen), dry skin (unscented lotion massage), pruritus (antihistamines), and rehabilitation potential and therapy (physical, occupational, social, and psychological).

C. Inpatient

  1. Transfer to a burn center should follow the guidelines of the American Burn Association. These criteria reflect multiple studies showing that age and BSA burn percentage remain the two most important prognostic factors.

   a. Patients younger than 10 years or older than 50 years sustaining partial- or full-thickness burns to >10% BSA

   b. Partial- or full-thickness burns to >20% BSA in other age groups

   c. Specialized regions, including joints, hands, feet, perineum, genitalia, face, eyes, or ears

   d. Full-thickness burns to >5% BSA

   e. Significant inhalation, chemical, or electrical injury

   f. Burns in combination with significant associated mechanical trauma or preexisting medical problems

   g. Patients requiring specialized rehabilitation, psychological support, or social services (including suspected neglect or child abuse)

  2. Nutrition. The daily estimated metabolic requirement (EMR) can be calculated from the Curreri formula: EMR = [25 kcal × body weight (kg)] + (40 kcal ×% BSA). Protein losses from metabolism and burn wound extravasation are replaced by supplying 1.5 to 2.0 g/kg per day. Therapeutic strategies should target prevention of body weight loss of more than 10% of the patient's baseline weight. Losses of more than 10% of lean body mass may lead to impaired immune function and delayed wound healing. Losses of more than 40% lead to imminent mortality (*Shock* 1998;10:155–160).

   a. Enteral feedings are the preferred route when tolerated and can be administered through an enteral feeding tube positioned in the duodenum. For severe burns, early feeding within the first 24 hours has been shown to improve a number of outcome measures, including length of hospital stay (*Burns* 1997;23(suppl 1):519). Overfeeding may become an issue in patients with a prolonged recovery course. Overfeeding results in hyperglycemia, which has a negative influence on the outcome of septic and critically ill patients (*J Trauma* 2001;51:540–544). Furthermore, the high caloric enteral diet may lead to an impairment of the splanchnic oxygen balance in burned septic patients (*Burns* 2002;28:60–64). The use of the Curreri formula has not been validated in patients with more than 40% BSA burns. Thus, some have encouraged the use of CO_2 gap as a parameter for splanchnic oxygen balance.

   b. Total parenteral nutrition should be initiated after fluid resuscitation only if the patient is unable to tolerate enteral feeding.

   c. Daily vitamin supplementation in adults should include 1.5 g ascorbic acid, 500 mg nicotinamide, 50 mg riboflavin, 50 mg thiamine, and 220 mg zinc. Patients with large burns may remain hypermetabolic for weeks to months after the burn wound is closed; early tapering of nutritional intake in these patients should be avoided.

3. Wound care

   a. Analgesia and sedation for dressing changes are necessary for major burns. Valium (0.1 mg/kg intramuscularly) plus ketamine (0.5 mg/kg intramuscularly) is one sedative regimen that has been used. Alternatively, in patients with a secure airway (typically intubated), intravenous propofol has the desired effects of ease of titration and quick onset and offset of action. Either of these sedative regimens in concert with narcotic analgesia is well tolerated.

   b. Daily dressing changes. While the wounds are exposed, the surgeon can properly assess the continued demarcation and healing of the injury. Physical therapy with **active range of motion** is performed at this time, before reapplying splints and dressings.

   c. Débridement of all nonviable tissue should take place using sterile technique and instruments when demarcation occurs. Soft eschar can be abraded lightly, using wet gauze. Enzymatic treatments (i.e., Travase, sutilains ointment) can be useful in dissolving eschar to develop granulation tissue for tissue grafting.

   d. Temporary dressings for massive burns with limited donor sites

   (1) Biologic. Fresh or cryopreserved cadaver allografts have been the gold standard. Recently, however, our center has had success using porcine xenografts. This alternative provides the advantages of ease of acquisition and application while providing barrier protection and a biologic bed under which dermis can granulate.

   After several days, the allograft can be removed, and a meshed autograft may be replaced for definitive coverage. The use of cultured autologous epithelium, cultured allogeneic epidermis, and allograft dermis has had encouraging results in some burn centers but remains largely investigational. (*Surg Clin North Am* 1993;73:363).

   (2) Using a **synthetic** membrane (e.g., Integra artificial skin, Dermagraft-TC) is an attractive alternative. Integra consists of an epidermal analogue, Silastic film, and a dermal analogue, a collagen matrix with chondroitin 6-sulfate. The patient's dermal fibroblasts can grow into this matrix. Once adequate vascularization is seen through the Silastic film, the film is removed, and an ultrathin autograft is placed onto the artificial dermis. The autograft is thin so that donor sites can be reharvested more quickly. This technique has been reported to give results similar to those obtained using allografts (*J Trauma* 2001;50:358). Dermagraft-TC has had similar success. This bilaminate skin substitute consists of a dermal matrix impregnated with human neonatal fibroblasts and a silicone epidermal analogue. After a few days, the bilaminate artificial skin comes off easily and can be replaced with autograft (*J Burn Care Rehabil* 1997;18:52).

4. **Operative management**
   a. **Early tangential excision** of burn eschar to the level of bleeding capillaries should follow the resuscitation phase. Debate persists as to the optimal timing of burn wound excision (range is 1 to 10 days). Excision can be performed using a Goulian or Humbly knife for small surfaces and a power- or gas-driven dermatome for larger surfaces. For each trip to the operating theater, consider limiting burn excision to <20% BSA or 2 hours operating time. Even within such limits, aggressive débridement frequently produces profound blood loss and hypothermia.
   b. **Split-thickness skin grafts** are harvested at a thickness of 12 to 15 thousandths of an inch with a meshed expansion ratio from 1.5:1 to 3.0:1. The graft is immobilized with absorbable sutures or staples. For very large wounds, 4:1 autograft can be overlaid with meshed allograft skin (Fig. 29-2). However, cosmesis is poor, and graft take may be less; thus, this technique is used on the back, flanks, or other less visible areas. Nonadherent dressings and bolsters are applied to minimize shear forces on the fresh grafts. **Splints or pins** may be required to improve graft survival at joints and to prevent contracture. **Ideal point positions** are extension in the neck, knee, elbow, wrist, and interphalangeal joints; **15-degree flexion** at metacarpophalangeal joints; and **abduction** at the shoulder.
   c. **For large burns that cannot be completely covered with available autograft**, allograft or xenograft can be used to cover the remaining wound temporarily. Currently, porcine xenograft, or processed porcine dermis, is the only xenograft in common use. In 3 to 5 days, the temporary grafts can be removed, and autograft should take well on the granulating dermis.

D. **Follow-up**
   1. **Wound healing**
      a. **Infection** is minimized by using topical antimicrobial agents.
      b. **Granulation** tissue that fails to epithelialize at skin graft sites can be cauterized using an applicator stick tipped with silver nitrate.

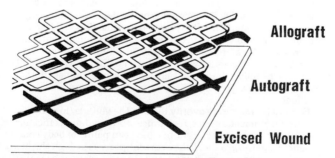

Allograft

Autograft

Excised Wound

Figure 29-2. Combined skin graft to cover burn wounds too extensive for other methods. The widely meshed autograft would allow continued fluid fluxes during the more extended time required for epithelialization. A more narrowly meshed allograft placed superficial to the autograft can accelerate the process by providing temporary coverage while the autograft fills in. (Reprinted with permission from Eichelberger M. *Pediatric Trauma*. St. Louis: Mosby, 1993.)

  c. **Hyperpigmentation** is best prevented by avoiding direct sunlight exposure for up to 1 year. When exposure to sunlight is unavoidable, a topical sunblock agent should be used.

  d. **Scar hypertrophy** is minimized by local tissue compression, tailored Jobst garments, foam sponge, foam tape, silicone gel sheets, and massage regimens. Hypertrophic scarring can be described with a rating system such as the Vancouver Scar Scale (VSS). This scale is based on four factors: pigmentation, vascularity, pliability, and height.

  e. **Contractures** are best prevented by using active range of motion. When present, release (Z-plasty) or excision and skin grafting may be necessary.

  f. **Pruritus** can be palliated with antihistamines. Recently, doxepin, an antidepressant with strong antihistamine properties, has been approved for topical use.

  g. **Rehabilitation** with ongoing evaluation is provided by occupational and physical therapists.

III. Burn mechanisms: special considerations

 A. Inhalational. Thermal injury to the airway generally is limited to the oropharynx or glottis. The glottis generally protects the subglottic airway from heat, unless the patient has been exposed to superheated steam. Edema formation can compromise the patency of the upper airway, mandating early assessment and constant reevaluation of the airway (*J Trauma* 1994;36:59). **Gases** containing substances that have undergone incomplete combustion (particularly aldehydes), toxic fumes (hydrogen cyanide), and carbon monoxide can cause tracheobronchitis, pneumonitis, and edema. Further, mortality may be increased by as much as 20%. **Carbon monoxide** exposure is suggested by a history of exposure in a confined space with symptoms of nausea, vomiting, headache, mental status changes, and cherry-red lips. Carbon monoxide binds to hemoglobin with an affinity 249 times greater than that of oxygen, resulting in extremely slow dissociation (250-minute half-life with room air) unless the patient is administered supplemental oxygen (40-minute half-life with 100% oxygen via nonrebreathing mask). The arterial **carboxyhemoglobin** level is obtained as a baseline, and if it is elevated (>5% in nonsmokers or >10% in smokers), oxygen therapy should continue until normal levels are achieved. Inhaled chemical products of combustion may include acids, phosgene, and cyanide derived from burning polyvinylchloride and polyurethane. The increased ventilation-perfusion gradient and the reduction in peak airway flow in distal airways and alveoli can be evaluated using a xenon-133 ventilation-perfusion lung scan. **Management** of minor inhalation injury is by delivery of humidified oxygen. Major injuries require endotracheal intubation with a large-bore tube (7.5 to 8.0 mm) to facilitate pulmonary toilet of viscous secretions and mechanical ventilation with positive pressure. Numerous studies indicate that low-volume ventilation has shown benefit in patients with respiratory failure. Hypoxic intubated patients may benefit from oscillation-type mechanical ventilation (*Crit Care Med* 1997;25:937).

 B. Electrical

  1. **Factors influencing severity** include the voltage (high is >1,000 V), current, duration of contact, resistance, and grounding efficiency. Electrical current passes in a straight line between points of body contact with the source and the ground. When current passes through the heart or brain, cardiopulmonary arrest can result. In most cases, these injuries respond to resuscitation and usually do not cause permanent damage. **Severity of injury frequently is underestimated** when only the entrance and exit wounds are considered.

   a. **Tissue resistance.** Heat and subsequent injury from thermal necrosis is directly proportional to resistance to current flow. Tissues are listed here from lowest to highest resistance: nerve, blood vessels, muscle, skin, tendon, fat, and bone. In addition to direct tissue injury, thrombosis can occur with distal soft-tissue ischemia. Peripheral perfusion should be monitored closely because fasciotomy may become necessary to treat compartment syndrome. Fluid resuscitation requirements often are higher than calculated by published formulas.

   b. Current

   (1) Alternating current (household, power lines) produces severe muscle contraction with each cycle and can result in fractures in addition to the thermal injury at skin entrance and exit points. High-voltage injury, which is commonly seen in workers operating near power lines, can present with full-thickness, charred skin at the entrance and exit wounds, with full arrest, and with fractures sustained while current passed through the body or during a fall.

   (2) Direct current emanates from batteries and lightning. With a voltage of at least 100 million volts and a current of 200,000 amps, lightning kills 150 to 300 people in the United States every year. Injury can result from direct strikes or side flashes. Current can travel on the surface of the body rather than through it, producing a "splashed-on" pattern of skin burn.

2. **Complications** include **cardiopulmonary arrest** (more common with alternating current), **thrombosis, associated fractures** related to fall or severe muscle contraction, **spinal cord injury**, and **cataracts. Rhabdomyolysis** may occur and result in myoglobin release from injured cells. Precipitation of protein in the renal tubules can cause acute renal failure. Dark urine is the first clinical indication of myoglobinuria, and intravenous lactated Ringer solution should be administered to maintain a urine output >100 mL per hour. Alternatively, 3 ampules of sodium bicarbonate (~135 mEq sodium) in 1 L D5W provide an isotonic solution to alkalinize the urine more effectively and minimize nephrotoxicity from the myoglobinuria.

C. Chemical injury may result from contact with alkali, acid, or petroleum compounds. Removal of the offending agent is the cornerstone of treatment. Dry chemicals should be brushed off or aspirated into a closed suction container before irrigating with copious amounts of water for at least 20 to 30 minutes. Alkali burns, which penetrate more deeply than acid burns, require longer periods of irrigation. Neutralizing the chemicals is no longer recommended because the resulting reaction generates more heat, which can exacerbate the injury. Eye injury from alkali burns mandates 8 hours of continuous irrigation after injury. **Tar** can cause ongoing burn if not removed. Cool the tar with cold water. Then, use an adhesive remover to remove any remaining tar.

D. Cold injury

1. **Classification of hypothermia** is based on core temperature (usually approximated with a rectal or esophageal thermometer): mild, 32°C to 35°C; moderate, 30°C to 32°C; and severe, <30°C. The elderly and children are particularly susceptible, and contributing factors include drug or alcohol ingestion, hypothyroidism, immobilization, moisture, sepsis, diabetes mellitus, and cerebral ischemia. Signs include reduced levels of consciousness, and patients may appear cold, gray, cyanotic, or asystolic. Rewarming is accomplished by a warm-water bath, endotracheal intubation, ventilation with warm gases, and/or central venous infusion of warm lactated Ringer solution. More invasive methods include peritoneal lavage, thoracic-pleural lavage, hemodialysis, and cardiopulmonary bypass. Serial arterial blood gases are obtained during rewarming to monitor the development of systemic acidosis as tissue beds reperfuse. Care is taken to avoid overstimulation, which can lead to ventricular dysrhythmias. The heart becomes increasingly irritable at core temperatures below 34°C. Asystole may occur below 28°C, and cardiopulmonary resuscitation should be started and maintained until the patient reaches 36°C.

2. **Frostbite** results from the formation of intracellular ice crystals and microvascular occlusion. Factors affecting severity are temperature, duration of exposure, and environmental conditions promoting rapid heat loss, such as wind velocity, moisture, immobilization, and open wounds. The fingers, toes, and ears are most commonly injured, particularly when reduced tissue perfusion has resulted from other causes, such as shock.

   a. **Classification**

      (1) **First-degree:** hyperemia and edema, without skin necrosis

      (2) **Second-degree:** superficial vesicle formation containing clear or milky fluid surrounded by hyperemia, edema, and partial-thickness necrosis

      (3) **Third-degree:** hemorrhagic bullae and full-thickness necrosis

      (4) **Fourth-degree:** gangrene with full-thickness involvement of skin, muscle, and bone

   b. **Treatment** is rapid rewarming using 40°C water until the tissue perfusion returns. Because mechanical pressure or friction can injure the tissue further, massage and weightbearing are discouraged. Rewarming can be painful, and therefore intravenous analgesia should be provided. Dry dressings are applied, and the injured area is kept warm and elevated to reduce edema formation. Tetanus prophylaxis is administered, and follow-up over several weeks is recommended to allow for demarcation of full-thickness injury. Escharotomy may be required for severe injury. Early amputation is not recommended because improvement in tissue viability can occur weeks after injury.

IV. **Future burn care management.** Burn mortality has dramatically improved. At the U.S. Army Institute of Surgical Research, the LA50, the size of a burn that kills half of patients, is 75.6% SBA in adults and 90% SBA in children younger than 15 years of age (*J Burn Care Rehabil* 1997;18:S2). With aggressive early tangential excision, early coverage, alternative dressings, and better understanding of aggressive wound infection, clinicians have an augmented arsenal to combat morbidity and mortality. Earlier detection of bacterial infections of wounds may lead to earlier intervention before serious illness or further wound damage occurs. Molecular diagnostic approaches such as the use of the polymerase chain reaction (PCR) have been used to identify strains of MRSA within 2 hours, as compared with the days typically required for culture using conventional microbiological procedures. Ongoing immunologic and clinical studies on burn-induced immunosuppression, cytokines, and artificial bilaminate skin may provide the next advances in burn care. The biggest challenge, however, may still be prevention education.

Soft-Tissue and Skin Tumors

Keith D. Amos,
Jeffrey F. Moley, and
Timothy J. Eberlein

DIAGNOSIS OF SKIN LESIONS AND SOFT-TISSUE MASSES

Most patients present with a visible or palpable lesion or mass. Physical examination is a key to diagnosis. Biopsy is often performed to confirm or establish the diagnosis. For large or deep soft-tissue tumors, radiologic evaluation often precedes biopsy.

I. **Skin lesions**
   A. **History.** Pigmented lesions with a change in size, borders, and coloration are important. The presence of itching, bleeding, or ulceration should be noted.
   B. **Physical examination.** Color, size, shape, borders, elevation, location, firmness, and surface characteristics should be recorded for each skin lesion. In general, uniformly colored, small, round, circumscribed lesions are benign. Irregularly colored, larger, asymmetric lesions with indistinct borders and ulceration are more likely to be malignant.
   C. **Biopsy.** Lesions that change over a period of observation should have a tissue diagnosis. Any lesion that needs a full thickness of tissue, particularly suspected melanomas, should receive a punch biopsy or excisional biopsy. In general, shave biopsies should be avoided. A punch biopsy involves using a cylindrical blade to remove a small core of skin. Excisional biopsy is the same as for soft-tissue masses, discussed in Section II.D.

II. **Soft-tissue masses**
   A. **History.** An enlarging, painless mass is the most common presentation. There is a frequently perceived association with antecedent trauma. Pain is a late symptom. Any symptom or enlargement is important. Lesions often are misdiagnosed as hematomas or pulled muscles.
   B. **Physical examination.** The key factors to note on physical examination are size, extent of anatomic relationships with surrounding structures, borders, and mobility. A neurovascular examination of the affected area should be performed.
   C. **Radiologic evaluation**
      1. **MR scan** is the best choice for imaging soft-tissue masses. However, it can be difficult to distinguish tissue edema surrounding tumor from tumor itself. The combination of T2-weighted image and gadolinium enhancement is very good at distinguishing tumor from surrounding normal tissue.
      2. **Computed tomography (CT)** is used for larger, deeper tumors to assess the character and extent of the tumor and involvement of other structures, as well as to help determine surgical access to the tumor. CT-guided core-needle biopsy can be attempted for deep tumors with difficult surgical access. A CT scan of the chest should be performed on all patients with soft-tissue sarcomas (STSs), and CT may be helpful in evaluating the pelvis and retroperitoneum.
   D. **Biopsy.** Ideally, the oncologic surgeon who will perform the definitive resection should perform the biopsy.
      1. **Incisional biopsy** is the gold standard. It is usually performed in the operating room under appropriate anesthesia. A small incision should be made so that it can be excised for a possible subsequent operation. The incision should be oriented along the long axis of the extremity. Incisional biopsy rather than excisional biopsy should be performed for a tumor >3 cm

(or >5 cm if it is consistent with a lipoma), because if the tumor is a sarcoma, the subsequent total excision will be complicated by the potential contamination of a broad area by the initial excision. Drains should be avoided; meticulous hemostasis to prevent hemorrhage from spreading tumor is critical. If drains are needed, drain sites should be in line with the incision, to be excised in any subsequent operation.

2. **Core-needle biopsy** provides a section of intact tissue for histologic analysis and can be performed in the clinic; it has the potential to provide the same information as that rendered by incisional biopsy if a good core of tissue is obtained. A very small incision is made to allow easy entrance of the needle through the skin. Most indeterminate or negative results should be confirmed with either incisional or excisional biopsy.

3. **Excisional biopsy** is performed for tumors that are probably benign or <3 cm in diameter. The usual procedure is an elliptical incision around the tumor along the skin lines of minimal tension, with anticipation of primary closure. The tumor should be excised completely with a thin envelope of normal tissue.

4. **Fine-needle aspiration** is the least invasive but also the least informative form of tissue diagnosis. As the needle enters the mass, multiple passes are made through the mass in various directions; the plunger is released before removing the needle from the mass. The specimen is then fixed and sent for cytopathologic evaluation. Fine-needle aspiration usually cannot give the grade but often can determine the presence of malignancy and the histologic type of tumor. Indeterminate results should be followed by further evaluation.

BENIGN LESIONS

I. **Seborrheic keratoses** are benign skin growths that originate in the epidermis. They appear in older people as multiple, raised, irregularly rounded lesions with a verrucous, friable, waxy surface and variable pigmentation from yellowish to brownish black. They are often found on the face, neck, and trunk. If removal is desired, treatment may consist of excision or curettage followed by electrodesiccation, as well as topical agents, such as trichloroacetic acid, or cryotherapy with liquid nitrogen.

II. **Actinic keratoses** are caused by sun exposure and are found predominantly in elderly, fair-skinned patients. They are small, usually multiple, flat to slightly elevated lesions with a rough or scaly surface ranging from red to yellowish brown to black and are found in areas of chronic sun exposure. Unlike seborrheic keratoses, these lesions have malignant potential: 15% to 20% of lesions become squamous cell carcinoma. Metastases are rare under these circumstances. Benign appearing actinic keratoses can be observed. When indicated, treatment consists of topical application of 5-fluorouracil twice a day for 2 to 6 weeks.

III. **Nevi.** Junctional nevus cells actually are located in the epidermis and at the dermal-epidermal junction. These nevi are small (<6 mm), well-circumscribed, light brown or black macules found on any area of the body. They rarely develop in people older than 40 years, and any new lesion in someone older than 40 should be considered a possible early melanoma.

IV. **Epidermal inclusion cysts** are lined by epidermal cells containing lipid and keratinous material. Asymptomatic cysts may be removed for diagnosis, prevention of infection, or cosmesis. Excision of the cyst should include the entire cyst lining, preferably without interruption of the lining, to prevent recurrence and should include any skin tract or drainage site.

V. **Neurofibromas** are benign tumors that arise from Schwann cells and are seen most frequently in the setting of neurofibromatosis (von Recklinghausen disease). Neurofibromas are soft, pendulous, sometimes lobulated subcutaneous masses that vary widely in size. The overwhelming majority of these tumors do not require excision. These tumors are removed for symptoms of pain, for an observed increase in size, or for cosmetic reasons.

VI. **Ganglion cysts** are subcutaneous cysts attached to the joint capsule or tendon sheath of the hands and wrists; they are most commonly seen in young and middle-aged women. They present as firm, round masses often seen on the dorsum of the wrist, but they also can be found on the radial volar wrist, along the flexor tendon sheaths of the hand, or in the dorsum of the distal interphalangeal joint. They have an extremely low recurrence rate if treated by surgical excision; in addition to the cyst, the capsular attachment and a small portion of the joint capsule should be removed to prevent recurrence.

VII. **Lipomas** are benign tumors consisting of lobules of fat and are perhaps the most common human neoplasms. There is very little potential for malignancy; sarcomatous elements occur in fewer than 1% of cases. They are soft, fatty, subcutaneous masses and vary widely in size. Asymptomatic small tumors can be followed clinically, but rapidly growing tumors should be removed. Large tumors (>5 cm) should be evaluated by incisional biopsy to make certain they are not malignant. Lipomas are enucleated easily from the surrounding normal fat.

MALIGNANT LESIONS

I. **Dermatofibrosarcoma protuberans** is a locally aggressive tumor that does not metastasize. Margins of 2 to 5 cm should be achieved if possible. Alternatively, Mohs micrographic surgery involves serial excisions of the tumor, with microscopic examination for areas of positive margins that have been mapped and are then reexcised, one section at a time, until a negative margin is reached. Although time consuming and expensive, this surgery has been advocated in the management of dermatofibrosarcoma protuberans for improved tissue conservation, cosmetic advantages, and low recurrence rates.

II. **Desmoid tumors** are nonmetastasizing but locally aggressive tumors that arise from connective tissue. Wide excision with a margin of normal tissue should be performed if possible, but limb function should be spared. Local recurrences are common, and reexcision is often required. Tamoxifen, nonsteroidal anti-inflammatory drugs (e.g., sulindac), or a combination has been used with only anecdotal success and may be attempted as a conservative alternative to surgery. These drug regimens have been advocated in recurrent or unresectable cases as well. Recommendations as to future pregnancies are conflicting and unclear. Patients with a desmoid tumor should undergo colonoscopy to exclude the diagnosis of familial adenomatous polyposis.

III. **Melanoma.** The incidence of malignant melanoma is increasing at a rate faster than any other cancer. The annual incidence in the United States is approximately 55,000, with approximately 7,900 deaths expected in the year 2004.

   A. Lesions. Most pigmented lesions are benign, but approximately one-third of all melanomas arise from pigmented nevi. It is essential to differentiate between benign, premalignant, and malignant lesions.

      1. Premalignant lesions

         a. Dysplastic nevi have variegated color (tan to brown on a pink base); are large (5 to 12 mm); appear indistinct, with irregular edges; and have macular and papular components. There is a familial association between dysplastic nevi and a high incidence of melanoma. Melanomas may develop *de novo* or from preexisting dysplastic nevi.

         b. Congenital nevi are notable for their presence since birth and are commonly referred to as "birthmarks." They can be premalignant; there is an increased risk of melanoma developing from these lesions, particularly if the nevus is larger than 20 cm.

      2. Malignant lesions

         a. Superficial spreading melanoma is the most common form of melanoma (80%), with approximately one-half arising from a preexisting mole. The lesions usually are slow growing and brown, with small discrete nodules of various differing colors. They tend to spread laterally but usually are slightly elevated. They are found most commonly on the back in men and women and on the lower extremities of women.

   b. **Nodular melanoma** is the most aggressive form, rapidly becoming a palpable, elevated, firm nodule that may be dense black or reddish blue-black. A distinct convex nodular development indicates deep dermal invasion. Nodular melanomas arise from the epidermal-dermal junction and invade deeply into the dermis and subcutaneous tissue. Approximately 5% are amelanotic (flesh colored).

   c. **Lentigo maligna melanoma** usually is found on older patients as a large melanotic freckle on the temple or malar region known as **Hutchinson freckle**. It usually is slow growing but becomes large, often reaching 5 to 6 cm in diameter. Initially, it is flat, but it becomes raised and thicker, with discrete brown to black nodules and irregular edges.

   d. **Acral lentiginous melanoma** occurs on the palms, soles, and nail beds; occurs primarily in darker-skinned people; and metastasizes more frequently than do other melanomas.

   e. **In-transit metastases** and **satellites** both signify a poor prognosis with a high risk of local recurrence and distant metastasis. In-transit metastases are lesions in the skin more than 2 cm from the primary lesion; they arise from tumor cells in intradermal lymphatics. Satellites are metastatic lesions in the skin within 2 cm of the primary tumor.

B. **History and risk factors.** A history of melanoma should include an assessment of risk factors and family history for melanoma.

   1. **Risk factors.** Each of the risk factors listed below are considered to carry a more than threefold increase in risk for melanoma; the presence of three or more risk factors carries approximately 20 times the risk.

      a. **Family or personal history of melanoma**
      b. **Blond or red hair**
      c. **Freckling of the upper back**
      d. **Three or more blistering sunburns before age 20 years**
      e. **Presence of actinic keratosis**
      f. **Blue, green, or gray eyes**

C. **Clinical features.** Early melanoma and dysplastic lesions can be recognized by the features highlighted in the mnemonic **ABCD:** *a*symmetry, *b*order irregularity, *c*olor variegation, and *d*iameter >6 mm. Advanced lesions are more readily apparent and may be nodular or ulcerated.

D. **Staging and prognosis.** Tumor thickness is the most important factor in staging the tumor. Tumors <1 mm thick have a cure rate >95%, whereas 10-year survival for lesions more than 4 mm thick is 46%. Thickness also has been correlated with the risk of regional node and distant metastasis. The Breslow scale for thickness is helpful in classifying melanoma depth (Table 30-1). The anatomic level of invasion, known as *Clark's level* (Table 30-2), is also still occasionally used, but the revised American Joint Committee on Cancer (AJCC) system of TNM (tumor, node, metastasis) classification for melanoma (Tables 30-3 and 30-4) is preferred over both these systems. The AJCC staging system for melanoma was revised in 2002 to provide more accurate and precise information regarding patient prognosis. Older age, male gender, satellitosis, ulceration, and location on the *b*ack, posterolateral

Table 30-1. Breslow's classification (thickness) of melanoma

<0.75 mm
0.76–1.50 mm
1.51–4.0 mm
>4.0 mm

Table 30-2. Clark's classification (level of invasion) of melanoma

Level I	Lesions involving only the epidermis (*in situ* melanoma); not an invasive lesion
Level II	Invasion of the papillary dermis but does not reach the papillary-reticular dermal interface
Level III	Invasion fills and expands the papillary dermis but does not penetrate the reticular dermis
Level IV	Invasion into the reticular dermis but not into the subcutaneous tissue
Level V	Invasion through the reticular dermis into the subcutaneous tissue

arm, neck, or scalp (the BANS region) all carry a worse prognosis. The presence of regional node metastasis severely worsens prognosis (10-year survival, 25% to 30%). Distant metastases have a dismal prognosis (median survival, 2 to 11 months).

E. Treatment

1. Surgery

    a. Wide local excision of the lesion is the primary definitive treatment for most melanomas and premalignant lesions. The size of the surgical margins depends on the tumor thickness: thin melanomas

Table 30-3. Revised AJCC TNM (tumor, node, metastasis) definitions of melanoma

T Classification

T1	≤1.0 mm	a. without ulceration
		b. with ulceration or level IV or V
T2	1.01–2.0 mm	a. without ulceration
		b. with ulceration
T3	2.01–4.0 mm	a. without ulceration
		b. with ulceration
T4	>4.0 mm	a. without ulceration
		b. with ulceration

Regional lymph nodes (N)

N1	One lymph node	a. micrometastasis[a]
		b. macrometastasis[b]
N2	2–3 lymph nodes	a. micrometastasis[a]
		b. macrometastasis[b]
		c. in-transit met(s)/satellite(s) without metastatic lymph node(s)
N3	4 or > metastatic lymph nodes, matted lymph nodes, or combinations of in-transit met(s)/satellite(s) and metastatic lymph node(s)	

Distant metastasis (M)

M1	Distant skin, subcutaneous, or lymph node mets	Normal LDH
M2	Lung mets	Normal LDH
M3	All other visceral or any distant mets	Normal LDH
		Elevated LDH

[a]Micrometastases are diagnosed after sentinel or elective lymphadenectomy.
[b]Macrometastases are defined as clinically detectable lymph node metastases confirmed by therapeutic lymphadenectomy or when any lymph node metastasis exhibits gross extracapsular extension. mets, metastases.
Modified from Balch CM, Buzaid AC, Soong SJ, et al., New TNM melanoma staging system: Linking Biology and Natural History to Clinical Outcomes. *Semin. Surg. Oncol.* 2003;21:43–52.

Table 30-4. AJCC stage groupings for cutaneous melanoma

	Clinical Staging[a]	Pathologic Staging[b]
0	Tis N0 M0	Tis N0 M0
IA	T1a N0 M0	T1a N0 M0
IB	T1b N0 M0	T1b N0 M0
	T2a N0 M0	T2a N0 M0
IIA	T2b N0 M0	T2b N0 M0
	T3a N0 M0	T3a N0 M0
IIB	T3b N0 M0	T3b N0 M0
	T4a N0 M0	T4a N0 M0
IIC	T4b N0 M0	T4b N0 M0
III[c]	Any T N1 M0	
	N2	
	N3	
IIIA		T1–4a N1a M0
		T1–4a N2a M0
IIIB		T1–4b N1a M0
		T1–4b N2a M0
		T1–4a N1b M0
		T1–4a N2b M0
		T1–4a/b N2c M0
IIIC		T1–4b N1b M0
		T1–4b N2b M0
		Any T N3 M0
IV	Any T Any N Any M1	Any T Any N Any M1

[a]Clinical staging includes microstaging of the primary melanoma and clinical/radiologic evaluation for metastases. By convention, it should be used after complete excision of the primary melanoma with clinical assessment for regional and distant metastases.
[b]Pathologic staging includes microstaging of the primary melanoma and pathologic information about the regional lymph nodes after partial or complete lymphadenectomy, except for pathologic stage 0 or stage Ia patients, who do not need pathologic evaluation of their lymph nodes.
[c]There are no stage III subgroups for clinical staging.
Modified from Balch CM, Buzaid AC, Soong SJ, et al., New TNM melanoma staging system: Linking Biology and Natural History to Clinical Outcomes. *Semin. Surg. Oncol.* 2003;21:43–52.

(<1 mm) should have a margin of 1 cm; lesions between 1 and 2 mm and all scalp lesions should have a margin of 2 cm; lesions >2 mm should have margins of 2 to 3 cm (*Ann Surg Oncol* 2000;7:87). In general, the wounds should be closed primarily, with flaps or skin grafts reserved for large defects if needed. Mohs micrographic surgery has been advocated by some groups for areas where wide and deep excisions are difficult. Further trials using this technique for melanoma are ongoing.

b. **Elective lymph node dissection** is still a controversial issue. Several large trials, such as the World Health Organization trial number 1, World Health Organization trial number 14, the Mayo Clinical Surgical Trial, and the Intergroup Melanoma Surgical Trial, have attempted to address this topic. The Intergroup Trial showed that elective lymph node dissection in patients with intermediate-thickness tumors (1 to 4 mm) improves survival, especially in those under the age of 60. Elective lymph node dissection has not been shown to benefit other subgroups (*Ann Surg* 1996;224:255).

c. **Sentinel lymph node (SLN) biopsy.** The efficacy of intraoperative lymphatic mapping and selective lymphadenectomy has been established for melanoma. This technique is based on the documented pattern of lymphatic drainage of melanomas to a specific lymph node, termed the *sentinel lymph node*, before further spread. The histology of SLN should reflect that of the rest of the nodal basin. If the SLN is negative for metastases, a more radical and morbid lymph node dissection can be avoided. This procedure requires expertise and a multidisciplinary approach, including the participation of nuclear medicine, pathology, and radiology. The SLN can be accurately identified 96% of the time using dyes and radiolymphoscintigraphy. Currently, it appears that SLN is most beneficial for intermediate-thickness melanomas (1 to 4 mm) (*Ann Surg* 2001;233:250).

The presence of disease in the SLN identifies patients who may benefit from a complete lymph node dissection or adjuvant therapy. Recently, submicroscopic disease in the SLN has been diagnosed based on genetic changes detectable by the polymerase chain reaction. Initial studies indicate improved prediction of disease recurrence and improved survival over histologic evaluation alone.

- **d. Therapeutic lymph node dissection** should be performed for involved axillary and superficial inguinal lymph nodes unless unresectable distant metastases are present. Deep inguinal node dissection should be reserved for patients whose survival is thought to justify the potential morbidity of the procedure.
- **e. Resection of metastases.** Satellites can be treated by including them in the excision of the primary tumor. Distant metastases that are few and accessible may be resected for palliation and (in rare cases) for cure.

2. **Isolated limb perfusion** is used for recurrent limb melanoma that is locally advanced and cannot be resected by simple surgical means. Isolated limb perfusion delivers high-dose regional chemotherapy and establishes a hyperthermic environment to an extremity while its circulation has been isolated from the rest of the body. Melphalan is commonly used as a chemotherapeutic agent for this procedure. Overall response rates with isolated limb perfusion are between 80% and 90%. Patients who are elderly or who have medical comorbidities or systemic metastases are generally not suitable for this procedure.

3. **Adjuvant therapy.** Chemotherapeutic approaches to treating melanoma have been disappointing. No single agent has a greater than 25% response rate, and dacarbazine is the only agent approved by the U.S. Food and Drug Administration for treatment of melanoma. Interferon-alpha 2b is the only adjuvant therapy that has been shown to improve disease-free survival and overall survival (in patients with stage IIB–III disease). Other biologic response modifiers, such as interferon-gamma and interleukin-2, have been investigated. Extensive research into immune-based therapies is under way. Several melanoma tumor antigens have recently been identified, and vaccines using these antigens with dendritic cells have shown initial success. Larger trials and newer treatment approaches are currently being planned.

OTHER MALIGNANT SKIN TUMORS

I. **Basal cell carcinoma** is the most common malignant neoplasm of the skin; it derives from the basal cells of the epidermis and adnexal structures. They are slow growing and very rarely metastasize (<0.1%) but can be locally aggressive. Sun exposure is the most significant epidemiologic factor; consequently, this neoplasm is found most commonly on the skin of the head and neck (85%) in fair-skinned patients older than 40 years.

- **A. Lesions.** It is particularly important to identify the morpheaform carcinoma because it is more aggressive, with a tendency toward deep infiltration and local recurrence. These carcinomas are flat, indurated lesions with a smooth, whitish, waxy surface and indistinct borders. The noduloulcerative form is the most common and is characterized by shiny, translucent nodules with a central umbilication that often becomes ulcerated, with pearly, rolled, telangiectatic edges.

B. Treatment

1. **Excisional biopsy** is adequate treatment for small tumors, with intraoperative frozen-section analysis (to confirm negative margins) and primary closure. Larger tumors may be diagnosed by incisional or punch biopsy followed by removal, with closure using a flap or skin graft if necessary. A margin of 2 to 4 mm on all sides of visible tumor should be obtained, and positive margins on frozen-section analysis should be reexcised. Margins of dysplasia or actinic changes need not be reexcised because local recurrence generally does not occur in these cases. The patient should be warned about possible pigmentation persistence.

2. **Mohs micrographic surgery** may be useful for recurrent tumors or in situations in which tissue conservation is important.

3. **Curettage with electrodesiccation** can be performed for small superficial tumors, with little risk of recurrence.

4. **Liquid nitrogen** can be used for tumors of <1 cm in diameter.

5. **Radiation therapy** can be used in certain situations for structures difficult to reconstruct, such as the eyelids. It also can be used for palliation in patients who have large tumors and who might refuse an extensive operation, especially the elderly. Although reexcision is indicated for recurrences or positive margins, radiation therapy can be used in individual circumstances.

II. **Squamous cell carcinoma** is the second most common skin cancer in fair-skinned people and is the most common cancer in darkly pigmented people. As with the other skin malignancies, sunlight is the major etiology, with the greatest risk in elderly men who have a history of chronic sun exposure. The mean age of presentation is 68 years, and men predominate two to one. Squamous cell carcinoma can be found on any sun-exposed area, including mucous membranes. It also is known to develop from draining sinuses, radiation, chronic ulcers, and scars (particularly burn scars, in which case it is called a *Marjolin ulcer*).

A. **Lesions.** Squamous cell carcinoma presents as small, firm, erythematous plaques with a smooth or verrucous surface and indistinct margins. As they grow, the lesions become raised, fixed, and ulcerated. Ulceration tends to occur earlier in aggressive lesions. Most lesions are preceded by actinic keratosis, which results in a slow-growing, locally invasive lesion without metastases. If not preceded by actinic keratosis, the cancer tends to be more aggressive, with more rapid growth, invasion, and metastatic spread. Perineural invasion has a poorer prognosis and higher recurrence rate.

B. **Treatment** is similar to that for basal cell carcinoma. Tumor-free margins of 5 mm for tumors of <1 cm and tumor-free margins of 1 to 2 cm for tumors of more than 2 cm in diameter should be obtained. Curettage with electrodesiccation and laser vaporization have been used for small, superficial squamous carcinomas, but there is no way to assess margins of treatment. Solitary metastases should be resected if possible, because there is a relatively high cure rate compared with other cancers.

SOFT-TISSUE SARCOMAS (STSs)

STSs derive from mesodermal tissues and are rare, constituting approximately 1% of adult malignant neoplasms and causing 3,100 deaths annually. Most of these tumors arise *de novo*, rarely from premalignant tumors. In a minority of cases, STSs are associated with cancer predisposition syndromes such as von Recklinghausen disease, Werner syndrome, or Li-Fraumeni syndrome. Lymphedema and radiation have been shown to be etiologic factors in certain rare sarcomas.

I. **Lesions.** Sarcomas are classified by histologic cell type of origin and grade. The most common subtype is malignant fibrous histiocytoma (40%), followed by liposarcoma (25%). Patients typically present with an asymptomatic lump or mass that has grown to be visible or palpable. Retroperitoneal tumor can reach massive proportions before increased abdominal girth and vague symptoms bring it to the physician's attention. Tumors also may grow unnoticed to large sizes in the thigh or trunk.

II. **Diagnosis.** Biopsy (usually core or incisional) is necessary for diagnosis. Care is needed to orient incisions to aid in the definitive operation. Even small, apparently benign lesions should be biopsied or excised. Adequate tissue must be provided to pathology for histologic assessment.

III. **Staging and prognosis** (Table 30-5). The AJCC staging system is based on tumor size, nodal status, histologic grade, and metastasis. Of these, size and grade are the most important.

   A. **Grade.** The grade of the tumor is the major prognostic factor. Grade is obtained from histopathologic analysis of biopsy tissue and is generally based on the number mitotic index, nuclear morphology, and degree of anaplasia. However, many centers have varying criteria, and rates of discordance between even expert pathologists of up to 40% have been observed.

Table 30-5. Soft-tissue sarcoma staging

Tumor grade (G)	Stage IA[a]
GX: Grade cannot be assessed	G1, T1a, N0, M0
G1: Well differentiated	G1, T1b, N0, M0
G2: Moderately differentiated	G2, T1a, N0, M0
G3: Poorly differentiated	G2, T1b, N0, M0
G4: Undifferentiated	Stage IB[b]
Primary tumor (T)	G1, T2a, N0, M0
TX: Primary tumor cannot be assessed	G2, T2a, N0, M0
T0: No evidence of primary tumor	Stage IIA[c]
T1: Tumor 5 cm or less in greatest dimension	G1, T2b, N0, M0
T1a: Superficial tumor[d]	G2, T2b, N0, M0
T1b: Deep tumor[d]	Stage IIB[e]
T2: Tumor more than 5 cm in greatest dimension	G3, T1a, N0, M0
T2a: Superficial tumor[d]	G3, T1b, N0, M0
T2b: Deep tumor[d]	G4, T1a, N0, M0
Regional lymph nodes (N)	G4, T1b, N0, M0
NX: Regional lymph nodes cannot be assessed	Stage IIC[f]
N0: No regional lymph node metastasis	G3, T2a, N0, M0
N1: Regional lymph node metastasis	G4, T2a, N0, M0
Distant metastasis (M)	Stage III[g]
MX: Distant metastasis cannot be assessed	G3, T2b, N0, M0
M0: No distant metastasis	G4, T2b, N0, M0
M1: Distant metastasis	Stage IV[h]
	Any G, any T, N1, M0
	Any G, any T, N0, M1

[a]Stage IA tumor is defined as low grade, small, superficial, and deep.
[b]Stage IB tumor is defined as low grade, large, and superficial.
[c]Stage IIA tumor is defined as low grade, large, and deep.
[d]Superficial tumor is located exclusively above the superficial fascia without invasion of the fascia; deep tumor either is located exclusively beneath the superficial fascia or superficial to the fascia with invasion of or through the fascia or is located superficial and beneath the fascia. Retroperitoneal, mediastinal, and pelvic sarcomas are classified as deep tumors.
[e]Stage IIB tumor is defined as high grade, small, superficial, and deep.
[f]Stage IIC tumor is defined as high grade, large, and superficial.
[g]Stage III tumor is defined as high grade, large, and deep.
[h]Stage IV tumor is defined as any metastasis to lymph nodes or distant sites.
M, metastasis; N, node; T, tumor.

B. Staging for STS includes physical examination and CT or MR scan to assess the size and extent of tumor. Because metastases most commonly are found in the lungs, CT scan of the lungs is a required study for grade II and III lesions. Abdominal CT scan is required for evaluation of retroperitoneal sarcomas, not only to evaluate the tumor but also to assess for hepatic metastases, which are more common for this site. In general, retroperitoneal and truncal STSs have worse prognoses than extremity STSs.

C. Prognosis. Almost 80% of metastases are to the lungs and occur within 2 to 3 years of diagnosis. If the pulmonary disease is resectable, 30% survival at 3 years can be expected. In addition, tumor size, grade, margins after resection, and anatomic location all have an impact on various outcome measures such as local recurrence, overall survival, and tumor-free survival. Local recurrence should be resected aggressively, and long-term follow-up is required, as late recurrences may occur.

IV. Surgical treatment

A. Resection. Smaller, grade I tumors can be excised with a minimum 1-cm margin, usually without adjuvant radiation. Larger tumors may benefit from a larger margin or radiation to prevent recurrence. Grade II and III tumors, in general, require radiation therapy in addition to excision to avoid more radical surgery. Depending on the size and grade of tumor, compartment resection may be indicated.

B. Limb-sparing resection combined with radiation therapy offers survival equivalent to that achieved with amputation (*Ann Surg* 1982;196:305). Limb-sparing procedures have a distinct psychological as well as functional advantage and are the procedures of choice for most tumors. The tumor should be removed with an envelope of normal tissue surrounding it, if possible. The resection should include the area of previous incision and biopsy and any drain sites. The resection field should be marked with clips to guide radiation therapy.

C. Gastrointestinal stromal tumors (GISTs) are sarcomatous tumors of the gastrointestinal tract. These tumors are rare and most commonly arise from the stomach. GISTs can present with acute or subacute gastrointestinal bleeding, vague abdominal pain, a palpable abdominal mass, or as an incidental mass found on CT scan of the abdomen. These tumors are distinguished from other tumors of the GI tract by expression of c-kit (CD117). Surgical resection with microscopically negative margins is standard treatment. Gleevec (imatinib mesylate) has been approved to treat patients with unresectable or metastatic GISTs.

D. Retroperitoneal sarcomas are considerably more difficult to treat because the tumors often involve vital structures, but the general therapeutic principles remain the same (i.e., resection of as much tumor as possible with as wide a margin as possible). Organs associated with the tumor should be resected *en bloc* to completely remove the tumor. Radiation therapy may be used in some cases but is associated with relatively high morbidity. Wide margins as a rule are not achievable in the retroperitoneum and limit the effectiveness of therapy. For tumor recurrences, surgical resection is the therapy of choice.

V. Other adjuvant therapy

A. Interstitial perioperative radiation therapy (brachytherapy) involves the use of catheters or implants placed at the time of surgery to provide radiation directly to the tumor bed. Afterloading involves loading of the radiation source through catheters postoperatively to deliver localized high-dose radiation to the tumor bed. Brachytherapy has at least two advantages: it requires a short course of in-hospital treatment rather than 5 to 6 weeks of outpatient external-beam radiation therapy, and it may provide dose control near sensitive areas, such as joints and blood vessels. There is evidence that it is effective at decreasing local recurrence for high-grade tumors when combined with surgery.

B. Chemotherapy. Several randomized prospective trials failed to show any improvement in survival with adjuvant chemotherapy for adult grade II or III sarcomas. The two drugs with the greatest efficacy are doxorubicin and ifosfamide; however, even these have at best a 40% to 60% response rate. The use of various chemotherapeutic agents, their patterns of delivery, and their combination with cytokine administration continue to be evaluated and are currently being studied in randomized trials.

C. Isolated limb perfusion provides increased delivery of therapy (e.g., hyperthermic therapy and chemotherapy) to an extremity sarcoma while reducing systemic toxicity. There is some suggestion of decreased local recurrence with definite downstaging of the tumor, but there is no improvement in survival. Although systemic toxicity may be reduced, local toxicity can be severe. This approach would benefit from a randomized prospective trial comparing it with wide excision (compartment) and external-beam radiation therapy.

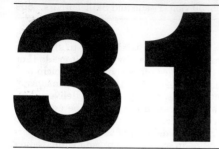

Hernias

**Felix G. Fernandez and
L. Michael Brunt**

I. Inguinal hernias

A. Incidence. The true incidence and prevalence of inguinal hernia are unknown. In the United States, 756,000 inguinal hernia repairs were performed in 1996, of which 176,000 were bilateral. Laparoscopic studies have reported rates of contralateral defects as high as 22%, with 28% of these going on to become symptomatic during short-term follow-up. The male-female ratio is greater than 10:1. Lifetime prevalence is 25% in men and 2% in women. Two-thirds of inguinal hernias are indirect. Nearly two-thirds of recurrent hernias are direct. Inguinal hernias have an approximate incidence of incarceration of 10%, and a portion of these may become strangulated. Recurrence rates are <1% in children and vary in adults according to the method of hernia repair.

B. Terminology

1. **Direct hernias** are those in which viscera protrude through a weakness in the posterior inguinal wall. The base of the hernia sac is medial to the inferior epigastric vessels through the Hesselbach triangle, which is limited by the inferior epigastric artery, the lateral edge of the rectus sheath, and the inguinal ligament.

2. **Indirect hernia sacs** pass through the internal inguinal ring lateral to the inferior epigastric vessels and lie within the spermatic cord. The sac is covered by cremaster muscle fibers.

3. **In combined (pantaloon) hernias,** direct and indirect hernias coexist.

4. A **sliding hernia** (usually indirect inguinal in location) is a hernia in which a part of the wall of the hernia sac is formed by an intra-abdominal viscus (usually colon, sometimes bladder). In a Richter hernia, part (rather than the entire circumference) of the bowel wall is trapped. A Littré hernia is one that contains a Meckel diverticulum.

5. **Incarcerated hernias** cannot be reduced into the abdominal cavity, whereas strangulated hernias have incarcerated contents with vascular compromise. Frequently, intense pain is caused by ischemia of the incarcerated segment.

C. Diagnosis

1. **Clinical presentation**

   a. **Most inguinal hernias** present as an intermittent bulge that appears in the groin, usually related to exertion or long periods of standing. The patient may complain of unilateral discomfort without noting a mass. Often, a purposeful Valsalva maneuver can reproduce the symptoms. In infants and children, a groin bulge often is noted by caregivers during episodes of crying or defecation. Rarely, patients present with bowel obstruction without noting a groin abnormality. All patients with a small-bowel obstruction must be questioned carefully and examined for hernias.

   b. **Physical examination.** The main diagnostic maneuver for inguinal hernias is palpation of the inguinal region. The patient is best examined while standing and straining (cough or Valsalva). Hernias manifest themselves as bulges with smooth, rounded surfaces that become more evident with straining. The hernia sac can also be examined more clearly by invaginating the hemiscrotum to introduce an index finger through the external inguinal ring. This may become uncomfortable for the patient and is unnecessary if an obvious bulge is present. Incarcerated inguinal hernias present with abdominal distention, nausea, and vomiting due to intestinal obstruction.

2. **Radiographic evaluation.** x-ray studies are rarely indicated. Ultrasonography or CT scanning may occasionally be used to diagnose an occult groin hernia, particularly in the obese patient. Plain abdominal x-rays may verify intestinal obstruction in cases of incarceration.

D. **Differential diagnosis.** Inguinal hernias should be distinguished from femoral hernias, which protrude below the inguinal ligament. Inguinal adenopathy, lipomas, dilatation of the saphenous vein, epididymitis, testicular torsion, and groin abscess all should be considered in appropriate situations.

E. **Treatment**
1. **Preoperative evaluation and preparation.** Most patients with hernias should be treated surgically, although "watchful waiting" may be appropriate for elderly individuals with small asymptomatic hernias. Associated abnormalities that can increase intra-abdominal pressure (such as chronic cough, constipation, or bladder outlet obstruction) should be evaluated and remedied to the extent possible before elective herniorrhaphy. In cases of intestinal obstruction and possible strangulation, broadspectrum antibiotics and nasogastric suction may be indicated. Correction of volume status and electrolyte abnormalities is important when there is an associated small-bowel obstruction.

2. **Reduction.** Temporary management includes manual reduction. In uncomplicated cases, the hernia reduces with palpation over the inguinal canal with the patient supine. If this does not occur, the physician applies gentle pressure over the hernia with the concavity of the palm of his or her hand and fingers. The palm of the physician's hand exerts a steady but gentle pressure and also maintains the direction to be followed: craniad and lateral for direct hernias, craniad and posterior for femoral hernias. If the herniated viscera do not reduce, gentle traction over the mass with compression may allow bowel gas to leave the herniated segment, making the mass reducible. Sedation and the Trendelenburg position may be required for reduction of an incarcerated hernia, but the difficulty of distinguishing between acute incarceration and strangulation should be noted: the inguinal canal can become quite tender with or without ischemic contents. When an incarcerated hernia is reduced nonsurgically, the patient should be observed for the potential development of peritonitis caused by perforation of a loop of strangulated bowel. If there is strong suspicion of strangulation, no attempt should be made to reduce the hernia because of the potential for *en masse* reduction of a gangrenous segment of bowel.

3. **Surgical treatment**
a. **Choice of anesthetic.** Local anesthesia, which has several advantages over general or regional (spinal or epidural) anesthesia, is the preferred anesthetic for elective open repair. Local anesthesia results in better postoperative analgesia, a shorter recovery room stay, and a negligible rate of postoperative urinary retention; it is the lowest-risk anesthetic for patients with underlying cardiopulmonary disorders. Commonly, a mixture of a short-acting agent (lidocaine 1%) and longer-acting agent (bupivacaine 0.25% to 0.50%) is used. The dose limits for local anesthesia are 300 mg plain lidocaine or 500 mg lidocaine with epinephrine and 175 mg plain bupivacaine or 225 mg bupivacaine with epinephrine. Use of local anesthesia for herniorrhaphy in our hospital is routinely supplemented by monitored anesthesia care and administration of intravenous midazolam and propofol. Virtually all patients who undergo hernia repair under local anesthesia can be managed as outpatients unless associated medical conditions or extenuating social circumstances necessitate overnight observation in the hospital.

Laparoscopic hernia repair has been carried out under local or regional anesthesia but is more commonly done under general anesthesia.
   b. Treatment of the hernia sac. In indirect hernias, the sac is dissected free from the cord structures and cremasteric fibers. The sac should be opened away from any herniated contents. The contents are then reduced, and the sac is ligated deep to the internal ring with an absorbable suture. Alternatively, the hernia sac may be invaginated back into the abdomen without ligation. Large, indirect sacs that extend into the scrotum should not be dissected beyond the pubic tubercle because of an increased risk of ischemic orchitis. Similarly, one should avoid translocating the testicle into the inguinal canal during hernia repair owing to the risk of ischemia. Cord lipomas are frequently encountered during repair and should be excised to avoid future confusion with a recurrent hernia. Sliding hernia sacs can usually be managed by reducing the sac and attached viscera. Direct sacs are usually too broadly based for ligation and should not be opened but instead are simply freed from attenuated transversalis fibers and inverted. In preperitoneal repairs, the sac is usually reduced but not ligated because the repair is insinuated between the peritoneum and abdominal wall.
   c. Inguinal floor reconstruction. Some method of reconstruction of the inguinal floor is necessary in all adult hernia repairs to prevent recurrence. Various techniques for inguinal floor repair are available, and factors that influence the choice of repair include the type of hernia as well as the surgeon's preference and expertise. Three broad categories of repairs are available: primary tissue repairs, anterior tension-free mesh repairs, and preperitoneal repairs, including the laparoscopic approach.
      (1) Primary tissue repairs. Primary repairs without mesh were the mainstay of hernia surgery for decades. The advantages of these repairs are simplicity of the repair and the absence of any foreign body in the groin. Disadvantages include higher recurrence rates (5% to 10% for primary repairs and 15% to 30% for repair of recurrent hernias) due to tension on the repair and a slower return to unrestricted physical activity. Consequently, the vast majority of hernia repairs performed today in the United States use some form of tension-free mesh technique. The principal features of the more commonly performed tissue repairs are the following:
         (a) Bassini repair. The inferior arch of the transversalis fascia or conjoint tendon is approximated to the shelving portion of the inguinal ligament with interrupted, nonabsorbable sutures (Fig. 31-1). The Bassini repair has been used for simple, indirect hernias, including inguinal hernias in women (Fig 31-2).
         (b) McVay repair. The transversalis fascia is sutured to the Cooper ligament medial to the femoral vein and the inguinal ligament at the level of, and lateral to, the femoral vein. This operation usually requires placement of a relaxing incision medially to avoid undue tension on the repair. The McVay repair closes the femoral space and therefore, unlike the Bassini repair, is effective for femoral hernias.
         (c) Shouldice repair. In this repair, the transversalis fascia is incised (and partially excised if weakened) and reapproximated. The overlying tissues (the conjoint tendon, iliopubic tract, and inguinal ligament) are approximated in multiple, imbricated layers of running nonabsorbable suture. The experience of the Shouldice Clinic with this repair has been excellent, with recurrence rates of <1%, but higher recurrence rates have been reported in nonspecialized centers.
      (2) Open tension-free repairs. The most common mesh inguinal hernia repairs performed today are the tension-free mesh hernioplasty

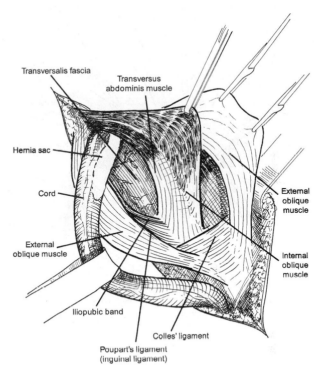

Transversalis fascia

Transversus
abdominis muscle

Hernia sac

Cord

External
oblique
muscle

External
oblique muscle

Internal
oblique
muscle

Iliopubic band

Colles' ligament

Poupart's ligament
(inguinal ligament)

Figure 31-1. Exposure of the right inguinal region for repair of an indirect hernia.

(Lichtenstein repair) and the patch-and-plug technique. In the Lichtenstein repair, a piece of polypropylene mesh approximately 5 × 3 in. is used to reconstruct the inguinal floor. The mesh is sutured to the fascia overlying the pubic tubercle inferiorly, the transversalis fascia and conjoint tendon medially, and the inguinal ligament laterally (Fig. 31-3). The mesh is slit at the level of the internal ring, and the two limbs are crossed around the spermatic cord and then tacked to the inguinal ligament, effectively creating a new internal ring of mesh. This repair avoids the approximation of attenuated tissues under tension, and recurrence rates with this technique have been consistently 1% or less. Moreover, because the repair is without tension, patients are allowed to return to unrestricted physical activity in 2 weeks or less. The mesh plug technique entails placement of a preformed plug of mesh in the hernia defect (e.g., internal ring) that is sutured to the rings of the fascial opening. An onlay piece of mesh is then placed over the inguinal floor, which may or may not be sutured to the fascia. Mesh plugs may be ideally suited for the repair of small, tight defects, such as femoral hernias. Another technique involves the use of a bilayer mesh in which the posterior leaflet is placed in the preperitoneal space and the anterior leaflet is sutured to the same layers as with the Lichtenstein repair.

(3) **Laparoscopic and preperitoneal repairs.** Approximately 15% of hernia repairs in the United States are now carried out using a laparoscopic preperitoneal approach. The anatomy of the

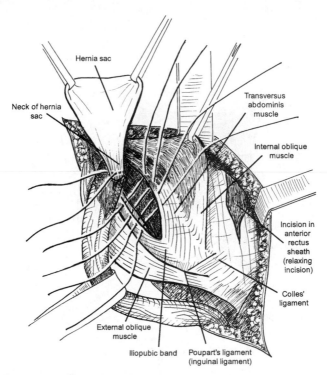

Figure 31-2. Stitch placement for high ligation of the hernia sac, once separated from the cord structures, and the Bassini (iliopubic tract) rapair.

preperitoneal space is shown in Figure 31-4. The laparoscopic hernia repair is based on the technique of Stoppa, who used an open preperitoneal approach to reduce the hernia and placed a large piece of mesh to cover the entire inguinal floor and myopectineal orifice. Preperitoneal hernia repairs may also be performed without mesh, an approach that is rarely used today for routine hernia repair but that can be a good option in patients with strangulated hernias. Advantages of the preperitoneal approach in this setting are that it may facilitate reduction of the incarcerated or strangulated hernia contents and that, if gangrenous bowel is found, resection can be carried out through the preperitoneal incision, whereas this is difficult to accomplish through a standard groin incision.

In **laparoscopic hernia repair,** the preperitoneal space is reached by either transabdominal laparoscopy [the transabdominal preperitoneal (TAPP) procedure] or by a totally extraperitoneal repair (TEP). With the TAPP repair, the peritoneal space is entered by conventional laparoscopy at the umbilicus, and the peritoneum overlying the inguinal floor is dissected away as a flap. With the TEP repair, the preperitoneal space is developed with a balloon inserted between the posterior rectus sheath and the peritoneum. The balloon is then inflated to dissect the peritoneal flap away from the posterior abdominal wall and the direct and indirect spaces, and the other ports are inserted into this preperitoneal space without ever entering the peritoneal cavity. The advantages

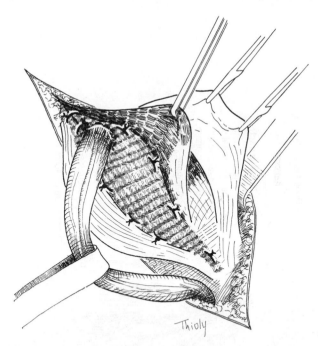

Figure 31-3. Placement of mesh to effect a tension-free conjoint tendon–to–iliopubic tract repair.

of the TAPP approach are that there is a large working space, familiar anatomic landmarks are visible, and the contralateral groin can be examined for an occult hernia. The advantages of the TEP repair are that the abdominal cavity is not violated, the peritoneum is not opened, much of the dissection is done by balloon, and the procedure can be performed under regional or even local anesthesia (with sedation).

After laparoscopic dissection and reduction of the hernia sac, a large piece of mesh (6 × 4 in.) is placed over the inguinal floor. This is stapled superiorly to the posterior abdominal wall fascia on either side of the inferior epigastric vessels, medially to the Cooper ligament and the midline, and superolateral to the fascia above the internal ring. Staples must not be placed in or posterior to the iliopubic tract or lateral to the iliac crest because of the risk of neurovascular injuries to the ilioinguinal, genitofemoral, lateral femoral cutaneous, and femoral nerves as well as the external iliac vessels. Comparative studies of laparoscopic and open hernia repair have shown that laparoscopic repairs are associated with less postoperative pain and faster recovery than open repairs, but hospital costs have been higher for the laparoscopic technique. Operative times, complications, and recurrence rates (<3% for laparoscopic repair) have been similar. Laparoscopic hernia repair is at this time still used selectively for patients with a unilateral inguinal hernia. Special circumstances in which laparoscopic repair may be favored include (1) recurrent hernias to avoid the scar tissue in the inguinal canal; (2) bilateral hernias, because both sides of the groin can be repaired with the same three small incisions used

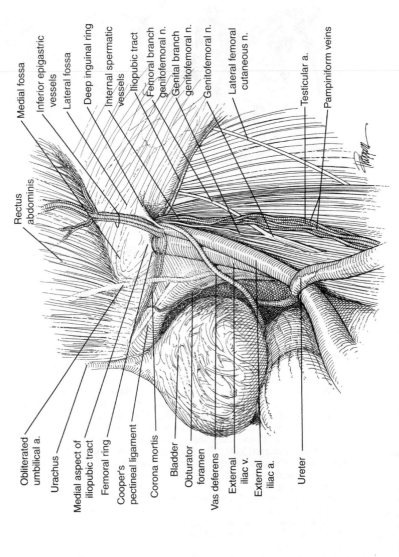

Labels (clockwise from top): Medial fossa, Inferior epigastric vessels, Lateral fossa, Deep inguinal ring, Internal spermatic vessels, Iliopubic tract, Femoral branch genitofemoral n., Genital branch genitofemoral n., Genitofemoral n., Lateral femoral cutaneous n., Testicular a., Pampiniform veins, Rectus abdominis, Obliterated umbilical a., Urachus, Medial aspect of iliopubic tract, Femoral ring, Cooper's pectineal ligament, Corona mortis, Bladder, Obturator foramen, Vas deferens, External iliac v., External iliac a., Ureter

Figure 31-4. Anatomy of the preperitoneal space from the laparoscopic perspective. (Reprinted with permission from Fitzgibbons RJ, Filipi, CJ. The transabdominal preperitoneal laparoscopic herniorrhaphy. In: RJ Fitzgibbons and AG Greenburg, eds. *Nyhus and Condon's Hernia.* 5th ed. Philadelphia: Lippincott Williams & Wilkins; 2002).

for the unilateral repair; (3) individuals with a unilateral hernia for whom a rapid recovery is critical (e.g., athletes and laborers); and (4) obese patients. Laparoscopic hernia repair is contraindicated in patients who have large scrotal hernias or who have undergone prior extensive lower abdominal surgery.

The **Kugel repair** is a preperitoneal repair in which a preformed polypropylene patch with a stiff ring around the edges is placed in the preperitoneal space through an open incision. The preperitoneal space is accessed through an oblique skin incision about 2 to 3 cm above the inguinal ring halfway between the anterior superior iliac spine and the pubic tubercle. After the preperitoneal space is entered, the peritoneum is dissected free by blunt dissection, and the hernia sac is gently reduced. The mesh patch is then placed into the preperitoneal space to cover the hernia defect. The Kugel technique is a preperitoneal alternative to the laparoscopic repair that can be performed under local anesthesia.

d. **Complications.** Surgical complications include wound hematoma, infection, nerve injury (ilioinguinal, iliohypogastric, genital branch of the genitofemoral, lateral femoral cutaneous, femoral), vascular injury (femoral vessels, testicular artery, pampiniform venous plexus), vas deferens injury, ischemic orchitis, and testicular atrophy. Recurrence rates after tension-free mesh repairs for primary hernias are 1% to 2% or less.

e. **Recurrent inguinal hernias** are more difficult to repair because the scar makes dissection difficult and the disease process has continued. Recurrence within 1 year of initial repair suggests an inadequate initial attempt, such as overlooking an indirect hernia sac. Recurrence after 2 or more years suggests progression of the disease process that caused the initial hernia (e.g., increased intra-abdominal pressure, degeneration of tissues). Recurrences should be repaired because the defect usually is small with fixed edges that are prone to complications, such as incarceration or strangulation. Repair can be done by an anterior approach through the old operative field or by a posterior (open preperitoneal or laparoscopic) approach. Prosthetic mesh is almost always used to reinforce attenuated tissues unless the operative field is contaminated.

II. **Femoral hernias**
A. **Incidence.** Femoral hernias constitute up to 2% to 4% of all groin hernias; 70% occur in women. Approximately 25% of femoral hernias become incarcerated or strangulated, and a similar number are missed or diagnosed late.
B. **Anatomy.** The abdominal viscera and peritoneum protrude through the femoral canal into the upper thigh. The boundaries of the femoral canal are the lacunar ligament medially, the femoral vein laterally, the iliopubic tract anteriorly, and the Cooper ligament posteriorly.
C. **Diagnosis**
1. **Clinical presentation**
a. **Symptoms.** Patients may complain of an intermittent groin bulge or a groin mass that may be tender. Because femoral hernias have a high incidence of incarceration, small-bowel obstruction may be the presenting feature in some patients. Elderly patients, in whom femoral hernias occur most commonly, may not complain of groin pain, even in the setting of incarceration. Therefore, an occult femoral hernia should be considered in the differential diagnosis of any patient with small-bowel obstruction, especially if there is no history of previous abdominal surgery.
b. **Physical examination.** The characteristic finding is a small, rounded bulge that appears in the upper thigh just below the inguinal ligament. An incarcerated femoral hernia usually presents as a firm, tender mass. The differential diagnosis is the same as for inguinal hernia.

    c. Radiographic evaluation. Radiographic studies are rarely indicated. Occasionally, a femoral hernia is found on a CT scan or gastrointestinal contrast study performed to evaluate a small-bowel obstruction.

D. Treatment. The surgical approach can be inguinal, preperitoneal, or femoral.

    1. Inguinal approach. A Cooper ligament repair (McVay) using the inguinal canal approach allows reduction of the hernia sac with visualization from above the inguinal ligament and closure of the femoral space. Occasionally, it may be necessary to divide the inguinal ligament to reduce the hernia. The repair can be performed with or without mesh.

    2. Preperitoneal approach. A transverse suprainguinal incision permits access to the extraperitoneal spaces of Bogros and Retzius. The hernia is reduced from inside the femoral space, and the hernia defect is repaired preperitoneally, usually with mesh, but can be repaired primarily. This approach is especially useful for incarcerated or strangulated femoral hernias. Uncomplicated femoral hernias can also be repaired laparoscopically.

    3. Femoral approach. A horizontal incision is made over the hernia, inferior and parallel to the inguinal ligament. After the hernia sac is dissected free, it can be resected or invaginated. The femoral canal is closed by placing interrupted stitches to approximate the Cooper ligament to the inguinal ligament or by using a plug of prosthetic material.

    4. Complications. Complications are similar to those for inguinal hernia repair. The femoral vein may be especially susceptible to injury because it forms the lateral border of the femoral canal.

III. Internal hernias

A. Incidence. Of patients who present with acute intestinal obstruction, fewer than 5% have an internal hernia. When internal hernias are complicated by intestinal volvulus, there is an 80% incidence of strangulation or gangrene.

B. Etiology. Internal hernias occur within the abdominal cavity owing to congenital or acquired causes. Congenital causes include abnormal intestinal rotation (paraduodenal hernias) and openings in the ileocecal mesentery (transmesenteric hernias). Other, less frequent types are pericecal hernias, hernias through the sigmoid mesocolon, and hernias through defects in the transverse mesocolon, gastrocolic ligament, gastrohepatic ligament, or greater omentum. Acquired causes include hernias through mesenteric defects created by bowel resections or ostomy formation. The small bowel may also herniate beneath an adhesion from previous surgery.

C. Diagnosis

    1. Clinical presentation. These hernias usually are diagnosed because an intestinal segment becomes incarcerated within the internal defect, resulting in small-bowel obstruction. Patients with congenital causes usually have not had prior abdominal surgery. The reported mortality in acute intestinal obstruction secondary to internal hernias is 10% to 16%.

        a. Symptoms usually are of intestinal obstruction (see Chapter 13, Section IV.C.1) without evidence of an external hernia. When there is intestinal obstruction or intestinal strangulation, the diagnosis is based on clinical rather than on laboratory findings.

        b. Physical examination (see Chapter 13, Section IV.C.2)

    2. Radiographic studies. Plain abdominal films may show small-bowel obstruction. An abdominal CT scan can sometimes establish the diagnosis of an internal hernia preoperatively. Contrast studies may also sometimes be useful.

D. Differential diagnosis includes other causes of intestinal obstruction, such as adhesions, external hernia, malignancy, gallstone ileus, and intussusception (see Chapter 13, section IV.D).

E. Surgical treatment. The diagnosis of internal hernia is often made at laparotomy for small-bowel obstruction. Intestinal loops proximal to the obstruction are dilated, friable, and edematous above the obstruction and collapsed distal to it. Once the hernia is reduced, intestinal viability is assessed, and nonviable intestine is removed. If a large percentage of bowel is of questionable viability, a limited bowel resection followed by a second-look laparotomy in 24 to 48 hours may preserve small-bowel length. The hernia defect should be closed primarily with nonabsorbable suture.

IV. Abdominal wall hernias
  A. Incidence and etiology
    1. Incisional hernias occur at sites of previous incisions at which there has been dehiscence of the abdominal wall. The causes are multiple and include obesity, wound infections, malnutrition, and technical wound closure factors. Hernias occur in up to 20% of patients undergoing abdominal operations and are most commonly seen with midline incisions. Most incisional hernias are now repaired with a mesh technique either open or laparoscopically.
    2. Umbilical hernias are congenital defects. They are more frequent in African Americans than in Caucasians. Most newborn umbilical hernias close spontaneously by the second year of life. However, umbilical hernias are also common in adults. Patients with ascites have a high incidence of umbilical hernias. When large, the hernias may cause gastrointestinal tract symptoms. When small, they rarely cause symptoms and may go unnoticed. Umbilical hernias have a fairly high rate of incarceration, usually with preperitoneal fat or omentum.
    3. Epigastric hernias are hernias of the linea alba above the umbilicus. They occur more frequently in athletically active young men. When small or in obese individuals, epigastric hernias may be hard to palpate, making the diagnosis difficult as well. Usually, they produce epigastric pain that may be falsely attributed to other abdominal diagnoses. The diagnosis is made by palpation of a subcutaneous epigastric mass; most such hernias occur within a few centimeters of the umbilicus and are associated with a small (1 to 2 cm) fascial defect.
    4. Spigelian hernias protrude through the spigelian fascia, near the termination of the transversus abdominis muscle along the lateral edge of the rectus abdominis near the junction of the linea semilunaris and linea semicircularis. Because the herniated visceral contents are intraparietal (between the abdominal wall muscles), these hernias can be difficult to diagnose and therefore are included in the differential diagnosis of obscure abdominal pain. Ultrasonography, CT scan, or laparoscopy can be useful confirmatory tools in patients with focal symptoms in the appropriate region.
    5. The **most common type of lumbar hernia** is an incisional hernia from a previous retroperitoneal or flank incision. Lumbar hernias may also occur in two different triangles: the Petit triangle and the Grynfeltt triangle. Lower lumbar hernias of the Petit triangle are located in a weak area limited posteriorly by the latissimus dorsi, anteriorly by the external oblique muscle, and inferiorly by the iliac crest. Grynfeltt hernias are upper lumbar in location, below the lowest rib.
    6. Obturator hernias are very rare hernias that occur predominantly in thin, older women and are difficult to diagnose. Patients classically present with bowel obstruction and focal tenderness on rectal examination. Pain along the medial aspect of the thigh with medial thigh rotation, known as the *Howship-Romberg sign*, results from obturator nerve compression and, when present, may aid in the clinical diagnosis of an obturator hernia.
  B. Treatment and operative management. Small epigastric, umbilical, obturator, and spigelian hernias may be repaired primarily. Most incisional hernias and lumbar and obturator hernias require the use of prosthetic mesh because of their size, the often poor quality of surrounding tissue, and high recurrence rates after primary repair.

1. **Open repairs.** The principles for ventral hernia repair include dissection and identification of all defects and repair with nonabsorbable sutures placed in healthy tissue. Most sizable incisional hernias are now repaired with some type of mesh prosthesis that should be anchored by nonabsorbable sutures placed in healthy fascial tissue several centimeters beyond the margins of the defect. The mesh should be durable and well tolerated by the patient, with a low risk for infection. A variety of mesh products are available for repair, including polypropylene, polytetrafluoroethylene (PTFE, Gore-Tex), and a composite mesh of polypropylene and PTFE. A newer mesh product is Parietex Composite (Sofradim Inc., France), which is a polyester mesh coated with a resorbable hydrophobic film to minimize tissue attachment. Nonsynthetic products available for closure of defects in contaminated fields include AlloDerm (Lifecell Corporation, Branchberg, NJ), which is a decellularized human skin preparation that acts as a matrix for tissue ingrowth, and Surgisis (Cook Surgical, Bloomington, Ind), which is a porcine small intestine submucosa product that also promotes tissue ingrowth. One should try to avoid placing polypropylene mesh in direct contact with the intestine because of the risk of adhesion formation and fistulization. Rarely, in patients with massive incisional defects and loss of domain of intestinal contents, preoperative pneumoperitoneum can be used to stretch the abdominal wall to provide sufficient autogenous tissue for repair. Peritoneal insufflation of air (500 to 1,000 mL per day for 5 to 10 days) may allow primary closure when not otherwise possible and may obviate the need for a prosthetic graft.

2. **Laparoscopic repairs.** The laparoscopic approach is an increasingly used alternative method for repair of incisional hernias. The repair generally is performed intra-abdominally and involves placement of an intraperitoneal mesh prosthesis to cover the hernia defect. The contents of the hernia should be reduced, but the sac itself is not removed. There should be a 3- to 5-cm margin of mesh lateral to the hernia defect. The mesh should then be anchored in place with sutures and staples. Early results show that the techniques are safe, simple and effective, with results that are equivalent to, if not better than, the results of open repair. Early recurrence rates are reported at 1% to 10% and complication rates at 10% to 25%. Length of hospital stay and pain medication requirements are less than with open repair. Contraindications to laparoscopic ventral hernia repair include inability to establish pneumoperitoneum safely, an acute abdomen with strangulated or infarcted bowel, or the presence of peritonitis.

32

Breast Surgery

Keith D. Amos and
Jill R. Dietz

DIAGNOSIS AND EVALUATION

I. **Patients seek medical attention** most commonly for an abnormal mammogram, a new breast mass, pain and tenderness without a mass, nipple discharge, or skin changes. **Patient history** should include questions regarding the duration of the symptoms or mass, change in size, associated pain or skin changes, relationship to pregnancy or the menstrual cycle, and previous trauma. Nipple discharge should be characterized according to its color and whether it is spontaneous, unilateral, or emanating from a single duct. Any skin changes in the nipple or areola should be noted. The hormonal history includes age of menarche, date of last menstrual period, regularity of menstrual cycle, number of pregnancies, age at first-term pregnancy, lactational history, and age at menopause or surgical menopause (note if oophorectomy performed). A history of previous breast biopsies, breast cancer, or cyst aspiration should be ascertained, including any known pathology results and treatment regimens. A history of previous oral contraceptive use and hormonal replacement therapy should be elicited. The patient should provide dates of previous mammograms and location of the films. A detailed family history of breast and gynecologic cancer should be recorded, including the age at diagnosis and the location. This history should include at least two generations as well as any associated cancers, such as ovary, colon, or prostate (in men).

II. **Physical examination**
   A. **Inspect the breasts** with the patient in the upright position, initially with the arms and pectoral muscles relaxed, then with the pectoral muscles contracted, and, finally, with the arms raised. Look for symmetry; deformity; skin changes, such as erythema or edema; and prior biopsy scars. Skin retraction may be more obvious with the patient's arms raised. The nipples are inspected for retraction, discoloration, inversion, ulceration, and eczematous changes.
   B. The **regional nodes should be palpated** with the patient in the upright position, pectoral muscles relaxed. Axillary and supraclavicular nodal regions are evaluated. Size, number, and fixation of nodes should be noted. The patient's breasts should be palpated in the upright and supine positions. In the supine position, the patient's breast is examined with the ipsilateral arm raised above and behind the head. The flat surface of the examiner's fingers should be used to palpate the entire breast systematically. The examination should extend to the clavicle, sternum, lower rib cage, and midaxillary line. If a dominant mass is palpated, its size, shape, texture, tenderness, fixation to skin or deep tissues, location, and relationship to the areola should be noted. A diagram in the chart noting these features is helpful. Examine for nipple discharge by palpating around the areola and noting where pressure elicits discharge. It is important to note whether the discharge is from a single duct, its appearance (e.g., serous, sanguineous), and whether it is associated with a mass. A Hemoccult test should be performed to evaluate for the presence of blood.

III. **Breast imaging**
   A. **Mammography**
      1. A **screening mammogram** is performed in the asymptomatic patient and consists of two standard views, mediolateral and craniocaudal. Studies

have shown that screening mammography reduces mortality by 24% to 44%, depending on the age group. The current recommendation from the National Cancer Institute and American College of Surgeons is annual screening mammography for women aged 40 years and older. In the presence of hereditary breast cancer with known BRCA mutations, annual mammograms should begin at age 25 to 30 years, along with semiannual physical examinations. In patients with a strong family history of undocumented genetic mutation, annual mammograms and semiannual physical examinations should begin 10 years earlier than the age of the youngest affected relative and no later than age 40 years.

The American College of Radiology has described categories for grading breast lesions, along with a scale ranging from 1 to 5, where 1 = negative; 2 = benign-appearing lesion; 3 = probably benign lesion, 6-month follow-up recommended; 4 = findings suspicious for breast cancer, biopsy recommended; and 5 = highly suspicious for breast cancer. Any suspicious lesion should undergo further evaluation.

2. **Diagnostic mammograms** are performed in the symptomatic patient or to follow up on an abnormality noted on a screening mammogram. Patients are usually examined by a mammographer, and the films are interpreted immediately. Additional views, such as spot-compression views or magnification views, are performed to further characterize any lesions noted. The false-negative and false-positive rates are both approximately 10%. A normal mammogram in the presence of a palpable mass does not exclude malignancy, and either further workup with a different imaging modality (ultrasound) or a biopsy should be performed. Mammography is not generally performed in lactating women or patients younger than age 30 years unless the degree of clinical suspicion is high. In the augmented breast, displacement views should be ordered to maximize the amount of parenchyma that can be visualized.

3. **Benign mammographic findings**
   a. **Radial scar.** The finding of a radial scar on mammography is an indication for biopsy. This variant of fibrocystic breast condition (FBC) is associated with proliferative epithelium in the center of the fibrotic area in approximately one-third of cases.
   b. **Fat necrosis** can occur after local trauma to the breast, such as a seatbelt injury. The patient may not recall any history of trauma. Fat necrosis may resemble carcinoma on palpation and on mammography. Tissue diagnosis should be obtained to exclude carcinoma. The fat may liquefy instead of scarring, which results in a characteristic oil cyst.
   c. **Milk of calcium** is associated with FBC and is caused by calcified debris in the base of the acini. Characteristic microcalcifications appear discoid on craniocaudal view and sickle-shaped on mediolateral view. These changes are benign and do not require biopsy.
   d. **Cysts** may feel like smooth, mobile, well-defined masses on palpation. If a cyst is tense with fluid, its texture may be firm, resembling a malignant mass. Solid masses cannot be distinguished from cysts by mammography. Aspiration can quickly determine the nature of the mass. Cyst fluid may vary in color from clear to straw-colored to dark green. Cytology is not routinely necessary. If the aspirate is bloody or a mass remains after drainage, excisional biopsy is indicated. If no palpable mass is present after drainage, the patient should be evaluated in 3 to 4 weeks. If the cyst recurs, it can be reaspirated; however, repeated recurrence is an indication for excisional biopsy to exclude intracystic tumor (*Arch Surg* 1989;124:253).

4. **Mammographic findings** suggestive of **malignancy** are new or spiculated masses, clustered microcalcifications in linear or branching arrays, and architectural distortion.

B. **Ultrasonography** is used to further characterize a lesion identified by either physical examination or mammography. Ultrasound can be used to determine whether a lesion is solid or cystic or to better define its size, contour, or internal texture. Although not a useful screening modality by itself due to significant false-positive and false-negative rates, when used as an adjunct with mammography, ultrasonography may improve diagnostic sensitivity of benign findings to >90%, especially among younger patients, for whom mammographic sensitivity is lower.

C. Other imaging modalities. MR scan of the breast is still considered experimental. It has been shown to be useful as an adjunct to mammography in detecting multicentric disease and in evaluating the dense distorted breast. It is also the most sensitive modality for evaluating the integrity of implants. Limitations of MR include an inability to identify microcalcifications or differentiate between inflammatory breast cancer and abscesses.

IV. Breast biopsy
  A. Palpable masses
    1. Fine-needle aspiration biopsy (FNAB) is a reliable and accurate office technique with sensitivity greater than 90%. A 22- to 25-gauge needle on a 10-mL syringe is advanced into the mass, and suction is applied. The needle is moved back and forth within the tumor with quick short strokes in nearly the same line as the original puncture. Cells are collected in the hub of the needle. The suction is released and the needle withdrawn. The contents of the needle are expelled onto a glass slide. A second glass slide is inverted over the first, and the two are pulled apart. One slide is fixed immediately, and the second is allowed to air dry. Two to three passes are performed for a total of four to six slides. False-negative findings are caused by inadequate sampling or improper specimen processing. FNAB results should be concordant with clinical impression and mammographic findings of the lesion (triple diagnostic test). Fine-needle aspiration diagnoses the presence of malignant cells; however, it does not give information on tumor grade or the presence of invasion. Fewer than 5% of malignant masses are comprised of ductal carcinoma *in situ* (DCIS). Nondiagnostic or indeterminate aspirates do not exclude malignancy and require a surgical biopsy (*Am J Surg* 1997;174:372). Estrogen and progesterone receptors can be determined by immunohistochemistry on malignant FNAB specimens.
    2. Core biopsy, with either a Tru-Cut or spring-loaded Monopty device, can be used to obtain more tissue. The skin is infiltrated with lidocaine and a nick made in the skin. The needle is inserted into the mass and fired. Three to five cores are taken and placed in formalin. Invasion, grade, and receptor status can be determined. For indeterminate specimens, an open surgical biopsy is necessary.
    3. Excisional biopsy is performed in the operating room using local anesthesia and intravenous sedation. Incisions should be oriented along Langer lines for optimal cosmesis (curvilinear, parallel to the areola). All incisions should be planned so that they can be incorporated into a mastectomy incision. Masses should be excised as a single specimen, the specimen should be oriented so that a short suture is placed superiorly and a long suture laterally, and the margins should be inked. Improper specimen handling may obscure margin status.
    4. Incisional biopsy removes a wedge of tissue from a palpable breast mass. It is indicated for the evaluation of a large breast mass suspicious for malignancy but for which a definitive diagnosis cannot be made by FNAB or core biopsy.
  B. Nonpalpable lesions
    1. Stereotactic core biopsy is a minimally invasive method of obtaining core samples of nonpalpable, mammographically suspicious lesions under radiographic control. This technique is ideally suited to establish tissue diagnoses of several foci in disparate quadrants of the breast. Using a computer-driven stereotactic unit, two mammographic images, each at

a 15-degree angle from the center, are taken to triangulate the position of the site to be biopsied in three-dimensional space. A computer determines the depth of the lesion and the alignment of the needle, which can be positioned within 1 mm of the intended target. Biopsies are taken, and postfire images are obtained of the breast and specimen. **Contraindications** include lesions close to the chest wall or in the axillary tail and thin or ptotic breasts that would allow needle strike-through. Radial scars should undergo needle-localized biopsy (NLB) because the entire lesion must be evaluated for definitive diagnosis. A diagnosis of atypical ductal hyperplasia (ADH) mandates NLB to exclude the presence of coexistent DCIS or invasive cancer, which can be missed by core needle biopsy. Core needle biopsy may underestimate the degree of pathology in lesions that contain ADH and DCIS. As many as 50% of women found to have ADH and 20% of women found to have DCIS on core biopsy were determined to have DCIS or invasive cancer, respectively, at the time of surgical excision. For indeterminate specimens, an open surgical biopsy is necessary. Nondiagnostic and insufficient specimens should also undergo NLB.

2. **Vacuum-assisted biopsy,** with either the Mammotome (Ethicon Endo-Surgery, Cincinnati, Ohio) or the Minimally Invasive Breast Biopsy device (US Surgical, Norwalk, Conn), has been developed as a response to the difficulties that FNAB and core biopsy have with evaluating microcalcifications and DCIS. The Mammotome uses an 11-gauge biopsy probe to contiguously acquire tissue, which is pulled into the probe by vacuum suction. The advantage of this tool is that it can pull back several larger volume samples of tissue into the probe while the device remains in the breast. This technique allows removal of all of the tissue around a cluster of calcifications during a single insertion of the probe. This device also has the ability to place a marking clip through the probe to allow for future identification of the biopsy site. These modalities have fewer underestimates of ADH and DCIS pathology than does FNAB or core biopsy and have become the most commonly used tissue acquisition instruments for the percutaneous biopsy of DCIS lesions (*J Am Coll Surg* 2001; 192:197).

3. **Needle localization biopsy** is performed by placing a needle and hookwire into the patient's breast adjacent to the lesion under mammographic guidance. The patient is then brought to the operating room. With the localization mammograms as a map, an excisional biopsy is performed, encompassing the tissue around the wire and lesion. The specimen is oriented and a radiograph obtained to confirm the presence of the lesion in the specimen. It is not necessary to remove skin around the needle insertion site.

4. **Emerging techniques.** Iodine-125 seed localization biopsy is a new technique that avoids needle placement for localization and allows for greater flexibility in operative planning. A titanium seed containing 0.05 to 0.3 mCi^{125}I is inserted into the breast lesion or area of microcalcifications by the nuclear medicine radiologist under radiographic guidance, and a skin marker is placed. The titanium seed is localized by dissection with the aid of a handheld gamma detector, and the tissue around the seed is excised. The remaining cavity can be probed for residual activity to ensure adequate circumferential dissection, and the biopsy specimen is examined radiographically to confirm removal of the seed and the lesion. Seeds can be inserted the day before a scheduled biopsy to allow for more flexibility in operative planning.

V. **Assessment of breast cancer risk**
   A. Breast cancer is the most common malignancy among women worldwide (*Int J Cancer* 1999;80:827). **Genetics, hormonal exposure, or pathologic factors** may be correlated to a risk for breast cancer. A family history of

breast cancer in a first-degree relative is associated with an approximate doubling of risk. If two first-degree relatives have a history of breast cancer (e.g., a mother and a sister have had breast cancer), the risk is even higher. These familial effects are enhanced if the relative had either early-onset cancer or bilateral disease. Factors that increase a patient's risk by 1.5- to 4.0-fold include increased exposure to estrogen or progesterone due to early menarche (before age 12 years) and late menopause (age >55 years), high body-mass index after menopause, presence of hyperplastic breast tissue with atypia, and exposure to ionizing radiation. A late age at first full-term pregnancy is an important determinant of breast cancer risk. Women with a first birth after age 30 years were shown to have twice the risk of those with a first birth before age 18 years. Breast-feeding may exert a protective effect against the development of breast cancer. Lifetime and 5-year breast cancer risk can be estimated using the Gail model, which is based on age, onset of menses, onset of menopause, age at first birth, and prior breast biopsies. This model is used for entering women in chemopreventive trials.

B. Certain pathologic features observed on breast biopsy are associated with increased breast cancer risk. No increased risk is associated with adenosis, cysts, duct ectasia, or apocrine metaplasia. There is a slightly increased risk with moderate or florid hyperplasia, papillomatosis, and complex fibroadenomas. Atypical ductal or lobular hyperplasia carries a 4- to 5-fold increased risk of developing cancer; the risk increases to 10-fold if there is a positive family history. Patients with increased risk should be counseled appropriately. Those with atypia or lobular carcinoma *in situ* (LCIS) should be followed with semiannual physical examinations and yearly mammograms.

C. *BRCA*. *BRCA1* and *BRCA2* are breast cancer susceptibility genes associated with 80% of hereditary breast cancers, and they account for approximately 5% to 10% of all breast cancers. Women with *BRCA1* mutations have an estimated risk of 85% for breast cancer by age 70 years, a 50% chance of developing a second primary breast cancer, and a 20% chance of developing ovarian cancer. *BRCA2* mutations carry a lower risk for breast cancer and account for 4% to 6% of all male breast cancers. Surveillance should include a monthly breast self-examination, semiannual clinical examination, and annual mammography beginning at age 25 to 35 years. Screening for *BRCA1* and *BRCA2* gene mutations should be reserved for women who have a strong family history and have undergone a multidisciplinary evaluation, including genetic counseling. Prophylactic bilateral mastectomy provides a cancer risk reduction of 90% to 100% and is an option for some patients. Preliminary studies show a significantly reduced risk of breast cancer after prophylactic oophorectomy in patients with *BRCA* mutations; however, no large randomized prospective trials have been completed to date.

D. ErbB2 (*Her2/neu*) oncogene overexpression is seen in approximately 30% of breast adenocarcinomas, and its presence in a tumor specimen is a negative prognostic factor. Current research is investigating methods of targeting this oncogene for future therapies.

E. Chemoprevention. The first large chemopreventive trial was conducted by the National Surgical Breast and Bowel Project (NSABP). P-1 was a large randomized, prospective trial begun in 1992 to evaluate the use of tamoxifen, an estrogen antagonist, as a cancer prevention drug in women at risk for developing breast cancer. Women taking tamoxifen achieved an overall reduction in the risk of developing invasive breast carcinoma of 49% and a reduction in the risk of developing noninvasive breast cancer of 50%. In subgroups of women with a history of LCIS and with a history of atypical hyperplasia, tamoxifen reduced the risk of developing invasive breast cancer by 65% and 86%, respectively. Tamoxifen also provided a significant reduction in hip fractures in women over 50 years of age. There was no difference noted in the incidence of ischemic heart disease for women taking tamoxifen. The NSABP B-24 trial looked at the benefit of tamoxifen in women with DCIS as adjuvant therapy after lumpectomy and radiation. After a median follow-up of 74 months, tamoxifen provided a 37% overall risk reduction for all breast cancers (invasive and noninvasive). The toxicities of this drug entail an increased risk of endometrial cancer and thrombotic vascular events. Women on tamoxifen also reported increases in vasomotor symptoms (hot flashes) and vaginal discharge. Tamoxifen has been approved by the U.S. Food and Drug Administration for (1) the treatment of metastatic breast cancer, (2) adjuvant treatment of breast cancer, and (3) chemoprevention of invasive or contralateral breast cancer in high-risk women. The dosage approved for chemoprevention is 20 mg per day for 5 years. It is estimated that chemoprevention could prevent as many as 500,000 invasive and 200,000 noninvasive breast cancers over 5 years in the United States alone. Current clinical trials are evaluating newer selective estrogen-receptor modulators as well as retinoids, peroxisome proliferator–activated receptor-gamma ligands, and cyclooxygenase-2 inhibitors.

NONMALIGNANT BREAST CONDITIONS

I.   **Fibrocystic breast change (FBC)** is a descriptive term encompassing several of the following pathologic features: stromal fibrosis, macro- and microcysts, apocrine metaplasia, hyperplasia, and adenosis, which may be sclerosing, blunt-duct, or florid. FBC is common and may present as breast pain, a breast mass, nipple discharge, or abnormalities on mammography. The patient presenting with a breast mass or thickening and suspected FBC should be reexamined on day 10 of the menstrual cycle, when the hormonal influence is at its nadir. Often, the mass will have diminished in size. A persistent dominant mass must undergo further evaluation, biopsy, or both to exclude carcinoma.

II. **Breast cysts** frequently present as a tender mass or as a smooth, well-defined mass on palpation. Symptomatic cysts should be aspirated. Cysts discovered by mammography are confirmed as simple cysts by ultrasound and, if asymptomatic, are usually observed. Cysts that are associated with a solid mass and recur after aspiration or have a bloody aspirate should be excised.

III. **Fibroadenoma** is the most common discrete mass in women younger than 30 years. Fibroadenomas enlarge during pregnancy and involute after menopause. They present as smooth, firm mobile masses. On mammography and ultrasound, they have well-circumscribed borders. These masses may be managed conservatively if clinical and radiographic appearance is consistent with a fibroadenoma. If, however, the mass enlarges or is greater than 2 cm, it should be excised.

IV. **Breast pain.** Most women experience some form of breast pain or discomfort during their lifetime. The pain may be cyclic or not, focal or diffuse. Benign disease is the etiology in the majority of cases. However, pain may be associated with cancer in up to 10% of patients. Features that raise the suspicion of cancer are noncyclic pain in a focal area, pain associated with a mass, or bloody nipple discharge. Once cancer has been excluded, most patients can be managed successfully with reassurance. In 15% of patients, however, the pain may be so disabling that it interferes with activities of daily living.
     A. **Cyclic breast pain** is often described as a heaviness or tenderness. It may be maximal in the upper outer quadrant and radiate to the inner surface of the upper arm. Many patients experience symptomatic relief by reducing the caffeine content of their diet or by ingesting vitamin E (400 to 800 units per day), although there is no scientific proof that these methods are valuable.
        1. **Evening primrose oil** (1,000 mg three times a day) is the first-line treatment. It contains the essential fatty acids linoleic and linolenic acid.

Evening primrose oil is thought to act by increasing the synthesis of prostaglandin E_1, which inhibits the action of prolactin peripherally. After 2 to 4 months of ingestion, more than 50% of women experience improvement, with few adverse reactions. Evening primrose oil can be purchased over the counter at health food stores.

2. **Danazol** (a derivative of testosterone) is reserved for severe breast pain that fails to respond to other measures. The initial dosage is 100 mg per day for 2 months to induce remission; this is decreased to 100 mg per day from days 14 to 28 of the menstrual cycle. The dosage is reduced progressively thereafter. Adverse reactions include hirsutism, voice changes, acne, amenorrhea, and abnormal liver function. Treatment should start on the first day of the menstrual cycle to exclude pregnancy.

B. **Noncyclic breast pain** occurs in premenopausal and in postmenopausal women. It is described as burning, stabbing, or drawing and frequently occurs in the subareolar area or medial aspect of the breast. Evening primrose oil is the first-line treatment, followed by danazol for severe pain. An injection of lidocaine and prednisolone into the tender spot is helpful in some patients. Excision of the trigger spot via breast biopsy has a response rate of 50%.

C. **Tietze syndrome or costochondritis** may be confused with breast pain. It may be unilateral or bilateral and involve the second to fourth costal cartilages. Patients are locally tender in the parasternal area. Treatment is with nonsteroidal anti-inflammatory agents.

D. **Superficial thrombophlebitis** of the veins overlying the breast and occasionally the upper abdomen is referred to as *Mondor disease*. It may present with breast pain. A cord can be palpated corresponding to the thrombosed vein. It is a self-limiting condition and usually resolves over several weeks. Nonsteroidal anti-inflammatory agents may be helpful. Hot compresses may provide symptomatic relief.

E. **Breast pain in pregnancy and lactation** can occur from several other sources, including engorgement, clogged ducts, trauma to the areola and nipple from pumping or nursing, or any of the above-mentioned sources. Clogged ducts are usually treated with warm compresses, soaks, and massage.

F. **Cervical radiculopathy** can also cause referred pain to the breast.

V. **Nipple discharge**

A. **Lactation** is the most common physiologic cause of nipple discharge and may continue for up to 2 years after cessation of breast-feeding. In parous nonlactating women, a small amount of milk may be expressed from multiple ducts bilaterally. This requires no treatment.

B. **Galactorrhea** is milky discharge unrelated to breast-feeding. Physiologic galactorrhea is the continued production of milk after lactation has ceased and menses resumed. Often, it is caused by continued mechanical stimulation of the nipples.

1. **Drug-related galactorrhea** is caused by medications that affect the hypothalamic-pituitary axis by depleting dopamine (tricyclic antidepressants, reserpine, methyldopa, cimetidine, and benzodiazepines), blocking the dopamine receptor (phenothiazine, metoclopramide, and haloperidol), or having an estrogenic effect (digitalis). Discharge is generally bilateral and nonbloody.

2. **Spontaneous galactorrhea in a nonlactating patient** may be due to a pituitary adenoma or to a microadenoma producing prolactin. Amenorrhea may be an associated feature. The diagnosis is established by measuring the serum prolactin level and performing a computed tomographic (CT) or MR scan of the pituitary gland. Treatment is administration of bromocriptine or surgical removal.

C. **Pathologic nipple discharge** is spontaneous and unilateral, originates from a single duct, and is either serous, serosanguineous, bloody, or watery.

The presence of blood can be confirmed with a Hemoccult test. Cytologic evaluation of the discharge is not generally useful. In the absence of detectable abnormality by either physical examination or mammography, the most likely etiologies are benign intraductal papilloma, duct ectasia, or fibrocystic changes; however, malignancy is the underlying cause in 10% of patients. In lactating women, serosanguineous or bloody discharge can also be associated with duct trauma, infection, or epithelial proliferation associated with breast enlargement. A solitary papilloma with a fibrovascular core places the patient at marginally increased risk for the development of breast cancer. Patients with persistent spontaneous discharge from a single duct require a surgical microdochectomy, ductoscopy, or major duct excision.

1. **Microdochectomy** involves excision of the involved duct and associated lobule. This procedure is performed with local anesthesia and often with intravenous sedation. Immediately before surgery, the involved duct is cannulated, and radiopaque or methylene blue contrast is injected. The ductogram identifies the location of the lesions as filling defects and serves as a guide to excision. After the ductogram is obtained, the patient is taken to the operating room. Through a circumareolar incision, the duct is identified and excised, along with the associated lobule.

2. **Ductoscopy** is a minimally invasive surgical technique that utilizes a 1-mm rigid videoscope to perform an internal exploration of the major ducts of the breast. Saline is irrigated through the scope to fully distend the ductal system. Once a ductal mass is identified, this single duct can be excised.

3. **Major duct excision** is performed through a circumareolar incision. An areolar flap is raised to reach the major ducts. All the retroareolar ducts are transected and excised, along with a cone of tissue extending up to several centimeters posterior to the patient's nipple. A preoperative ductogram is obtained to identify the location of the lesion. Major duct excisions are rarely indicated because the lesions should be identified on ductogram. Major duct excision may be used for women with bloody nipple discharge from multiple ducts or in postmenopausal women with bloody nipple discharge.

VI. **Breast infections**
 A. **Lactational mastitis** may occur either sporadically or in epidemics. The most common causative organism is *Staphylococcus aureus*. The patient's breast is swollen, erythematous, and tender. Purulent discharge from the nipple is uncommon. In the cellulitic phase, it is treated with oral or intravenous antibiotics. If it occurs in the early stages of infection, the frequency of nursing or pumping should be increased. Approximately 25% of cases progress to abscess formation. Breast abscesses often are not fluctuant, and therefore the diagnosis is made by failure to improve on antibiotics, abscess cavity seen on ultrasound, or aspiration of pus. Treatment is cessation of nursing, surgical drainage, and wound packing.
 B. **Nonpuerperal abscess** occurs as a result of duct ectasia with periductal mastitis, infected cysts, infected hematoma, or hematogenous spread from another source. If the abscess is subareolar, anaerobes are the most common causative agent. Treatment is administration of the appropriate antibiotic or surgical drainage for an abscess. These abscesses have a high recurrence rate. For women who experience recurrence, treatment is a central duct excision. Recurrent or unresolved infection requires biopsy of the abscess cavity to exclude cancer.
 C. **Duct ectasia, periductal mastitis, or mammary fistula.** The causes of duct ectasia and periductal mastitis are unclear. These conditions may present as subareolar abscess, periareolar cellulitis, and thick discharge from the nipple or as a fistula. Patients often have a chronic relapsing course with multiple infections requiring surgical drainage. Both anaerobic and aerobic organisms can be cultured from the ectatic ducts. Antibiotic treatment

should cover both types of organisms. Repeated infections can result in a chronically draining periareolar lesion or a mammary fistula, which is lined with squamous epithelium. These are treated by duct excision along with excision of the fistula once the acute infection resolves. The patient should be advised that the condition can recur, even after surgery.

VII. Gynecomastia is defined as hypertrophy of breast tissue in men. Pubertal hypertrophy occurs in young adolescent boys, is usually bilateral, and resolves spontaneously in 6 to 12 months. Senescent gynecomastia is commonly seen after age 70 years, as testosterone levels decrease. Drugs or excessive hormone production may cause gynecomastia in adults. Drugs associated with gynecomastia are similar to those that cause galactorrhea in women and include digoxin, spironolactone, methyldopa, cimetidine, tricyclic antidepressants, phenothiazine, reserpine, and marijuana. Excess hormonal secretion of estrogens may be due to such tumors as testicular teratomas and seminomas, bronchogenic carcinomas, and adrenal tumors. Tumors of the pituitary and hypothalamus may also cause breast enlargement. Gynecomastia may be a manifestation of such systemic diseases as hepatic cirrhosis, renal failure, and malnutrition. Carcinoma should be excluded by mammography and biopsy. Excision of breast tissue via a periareolar incision is performed if workup fails to reveal a medically treatable cause or if the enlargement fails to regress or is cosmetically unacceptable.

VIII. Breast conditions during pregnancy. Bloody nipple discharge may occur in the second or third trimester. It is the result of epithelial proliferation under hormonal influences and usually resolves by 2 months postpartum. Breast masses occurring during pregnancy include galactoceles, lactating adenoma, simple cysts, breast infarcts, and carcinoma. Fibroadenomas may grow during pregnancy due to hormonal stimulation. Masses should be carefully evaluated by ultrasound, and a biopsy should be performed for any suspicious lesion. Ultrasound distinguishes between a solid mass and cysts. FNAB, vacuum-assisted biopsy, and core biopsy can be safely performed. Mammography can be performed with uterine shielding but is rarely helpful due to the increased density of the patient's breast. If a breast lesion is diagnosed as malignant, the patient should be given the same treatment options stage for stage as a nonpregnant woman, and the treatment should not be delayed because of the pregnancy.

MALIGNANCY OF THE BREAST

Management of breast cancer is multidisciplinary, involving cooperation between the surgeon, radiation oncologist, and medical oncologist. Current staging of breast cancer is based on the TNM (tumor, node, metastasis) staging system (Tables 32-1 and 32-2). Patients should be assigned a clinical stage based on physical examination, which may be modified when the final pathology report is available.

I. Preoperative staging in breast cancer (stages I and II). Before definitive surgery is undertaken, preoperative workup should include a complete blood cell count, complete metabolic panel, and chest x-ray. A bone scan should be obtained if the alkaline phosphatase or calcium level is elevated. Alterations in liver function tests are indications for CT scan of the liver. If metastatic disease is detected, local treatment is no longer a priority, and the patient should undergo chemotherapy, hormonal therapy, or both.

II. Noninvasive breast pathology is confined to the mammary ducts or lobules and is classified as either DCIS or LCIS, respectively.

A. DCIS, or intraductal carcinoma, is treated as a malignancy. These lesions comprise malignant cells that have not penetrated the basement membrane. Mammographic screening has significantly increased the diagnosis of DCIS; because of this, DCIS is currently the subtype of breast cancer most rapidly increasing in incidence, with over 55,000 new cases in the United States in 2003 (approximately 20% of all new breast cancers). The most common mammographic findings are clustered pleomorphic

Table 32-1. American Joint Committee on Cancer TNM (tumor, node, metastasis) staging for breast cancer

Stage	Description
Tumor	
TX	Primary tumor not assessable
T0	No evidence of primary tumor
Tis	Carcinoma *in situ*
T1	Tumor ≤ 2 cm in greatest dimension
T1 mic	Microinvasion ≤ 0.1 cm in greatest dimension
T1a	Tumor >0.1 cm but not >0.5 cm
T1b	Tumor >0.5 cm but not >1 cm
T1c	Tumor >1 cm but not >2 cm
T2	Tumor >2 cm but <5 cm in greatest dimension
T3	Tumor >5 cm in greatest dimension
T4	Tumor of any size with direct extension into the chest wall or skin
T4a	Extension to chest wall (ribs, intercostals, or serratus anterior)
T4b	*Peau d'orange,* ulceration, or satellite skin nodules
T4c	T4a + b
T4d	Inflammatory breast cancer
Regional lymph nodes	
NX	Regional lymph nodes not assessable
N0	No regional lymph node involvement
N1	Metastasis to movable ipsilateral axillary lymph nodes
N2	Metastases to ipsilateral axillary lymph nodes fixed to one another or to other structures
N3	Metastases to ipsilateral internal mammary lymph node with or without axillary lymph node involvement, or in clinically apparent in that clavicular lymph nodes.
Distant metastases	
MX	Presence of distant metastases not assessable
M0	No distant metastases
M1	Existent distant metastases (including ipsilateral supraclavicular nodes)

Reprinted with permission from Fleming ID, Cooper JS, Henson DE, et al., eds. *AJCC cancer staging manual*. 5th ed. Philadelphia: Lippincott Williams & Wilkins; 1998.

calcifications. The physical examination is normal in the majority of patients. Impalpable, mammographically detected lesions require either NLB, stereotactic core biopsy, or vacuum-assisted biopsy to obtain material for histology.

1. Several **classification systems** have been proposed for DCIS. A DCIS pathology consensus conference in 1997 failed to agree on a unified classification system; however, factors such as margin status, tumor size, nuclear grade, cell polarization, and architecture should be recorded on specimens. Although there are five architectural subtypes (papillary, micropapillary, solid, cribriform, and comedo), specimens are mainly grouped as comedo versus noncomedo. The comedo or high-grade subtype is more often associated with microinvasion, a higher proliferation rate, aneuploidy, *Her2/neu* gene amplification, and a higher local recurrence rate. DCIS may advance in a segmental manner, with gaps between disease areas. Lesions can be multifocal (two or more lesions >5 mm apart within the same index quadrant) or multicentric (in different quadrants).

Table 32-2. American Joint Committee on Cancer classification for breast cancer based on TNM (tumor, node, metastasis) criteria

Stage	Tumor	Nodes	Metastases
0	Tis	N0	M0
I	T1	N0	M0
IIA	T0, 1	N1	M0
	T2	N0	M0
IIB	T2	N1	M0
	T3	N0	M0
IIIA	T0, 1, 2	N2	M0
	T3	N1, 2	M0
IIIB	T4	Any N	M0
	Any T	N3	M0
IV	Any T	Any N	M1

Reprinted with permission from Fleming ID, Cooper JS, Henson DE, et al., eds. *AJCC cancer staging manual*, 5th ed. Philadelphia: Lippincott Williams & Wilkins; 1998.

2. Although complete **excision** should be curative, excision alone is associated with a reported local recurrence rate of up to 40% at 5 years, with one-half the recurrences presenting as invasive ductal carcinoma. Margin status is an important factor in predicting risk of local recurrence, as patients with free margins >10 mm have a 10% to 15% likelihood of recurrent disease (after additional radiation therapy). Traditionally, these patients were treated with mastectomy, which carries a 0% to 2% recurrence rate; however, based on recent clinical trials, breast conservation surgery is as effective as mastectomy in overall survival. Therefore, therapeutic options range from simple excision to total mastectomy or skin-sparing mastectomy with reconstruction, depending on the size, grade, margin status, multicentricity of disease, and age of the patient. Although the NSABP B-17 trial demonstrated that adjuvant radiation therapy was effective in decreasing the rate of recurrence in patients with DCIS, it may not be necessary for all patients with DCIS. Current clinical trials are evaluating which patients may benefit the most from radiation therapy. The addition of adjuvant radiation has not been shown to affect breast cancer mortality. However, it should be given to patients with DCIS who wish breast conservation. This is especially true for younger women with close margins or large tumors. Adjuvant tamoxifen may further reduce the risk of recurrence in these patients.

3. Axillary dissection is not performed for pure DCIS. For patients with extensive DCIS lesions treated with mastectomy, a **sentinel lymph node biopsy (SLNB)** can be performed at the time of mastectomy to evaluate the axilla. The sentinel lymph node should be evaluated by hematoxylin and eosin staining, followed by immunohistochemistry for cytokeratin if negative. A positive sentinel node indicates invasive breast cancer, changing the stage of the disease and possibly the treatment as well. For pure DCIS, there is no added benefit from chemotherapy, because this disease is confined to the ducts of the breast; however, adjuvant tamoxifen has been shown to reduce the risk of breast cancer recurrence by 37% over 5 years as well as to decrease the risk of developing cancer in the contralateral breast (NSABP B-24 trial). The Van Nuys Prognostic Index (Table 32-3) is a numerical algorithm used by many surgeons to stratify patients into three groups to determine who is at greatest risk of developing recurrent disease and would therefore benefit the most from a more aggressive treatment approach. This index uses several measurable factors (lesion size, margin width, grade,

Table 32-3. Van Nuys scoring system[a]

	Score		
	1	2	3
Size (mm)	d15	>15–40	>40
Margins (mm)	S10	<10 but >1	<1
Histology	Nonhigh grade without necrosis	Nonhigh grade with necrosis	High grade with or without necrosis

[a] A score of 13 points is given for each of the prognostic factors described above, resulting in a total index score ranging from 3 to 9. Scores of 3 and 4 are considered low index values; scores of 5, 6, or 7 are considered intermediate; and scores of 8 or 9 are considered high.
Modified from Silverstein MJ, Lagios MD, Craig PH, et al. A prognostic index for ductal carcinoma *in situ* of the breast. *Cancer* 1996;77:226–227.

and presence of necrosis) to stratify patients into three groups. The low-scoring group is treated with excision alone, as no difference in recurrence rate is demonstrated with the addition of radiation. The intermediate-scoring group has been shown to benefit from adjuvant radiation therapy, and the high-scoring group should undergo mastectomy, as the risk of recurrence with conservative excision is high (*Adv Surg* 2000;34:29).

B. LCIS is an incidental pathologic finding in a breast biopsy specimen. It may be multifocal or bilateral. It is not considered a preinvasive lesion but rather an indicator for increased breast cancer risk of approximately 1% per year or 35% lifetime. The cancer may be either invasive ductal or lobular and may occur in either breast. Two treatment options are currently accepted: lifelong surveillance or possible prophylaxis with tamoxifen in the setting of a clinical trial. Bilateral total mastectomies with immediate reconstruction are reserved for selected women with a strong family history of breast cancer and LCIS, after appropriate counseling. Mastectomy for LCIS is much less frequently performed. If surveillance is chosen, patients should perform monthly self-examination and have annual mammograms and semiannual clinical examinations.

III. Invasive breast cancers are often histologically heterogeneous. Adenocarcinoma of the breast can be divided into five different histologic subtypes: infiltrating ductal (75% to 80%), infiltrating lobular (5% to 10%), medullary (5% to 7%), mucinous (3%), and tubular (1% to 2%). Surgical options for early-stage (I and II) invasive breast cancer include modified radical mastectomy (total mastectomy and axillary dissection) with or without reconstruction or breast conservation therapy (BCT), consisting of lumpectomy and axillary dissection (or SLNB) followed by breast irradiation. Skin-sparing mastectomy with immediate autologous reconstruction is an excellent alternative to mastectomy alone.

A. Axillary lymph node dissection (ALND) or SLNB should be performed in all patients with stage I and II breast cancer for staging purposes, control of the axilla, or both. Axillary staging is a component of modified radical mastectomy and BCT. ALND involves removal of level I lymph nodes (lateral to the pectoralis minor muscle), level II nodes (posterior to the pectoralis minor muscle), and, if grossly involved, possibly level III nodes. An adequate dissection should remove at least eight lymph nodes. Intraoperative complications of axillary dissection include damage to the long thoracic, medial pectoral, thoracodorsal, and intercostobrachial nerves. Postoperatively, the most frequent complications include wound infections and seromas. Several prospective studies have demonstrated a significant decrease in wound infection and seroma rates with the use of one preoperative dose of a cephalosporin and the placement of at least one closed suction drain. Persistent seroma may be treated with repeated aspirations or reinsertion of a drain. One long-term complication of ALND is the increased risk of upper-extremity lymph edema.

For surgeons with adequate experience, **SLNB** has been established as a useful minimally invasive technique for predicting axillary involvement in patients with T1 or T2 tumors. It involves intraoperative lymphatic mapping using **Lymphazurin** blue dye and/or technetium-labeled sulfur colloid to identify the primary draining lymph node(s) in the nodal basin. Twenty percent to 30% of the time, more than one SLN is identified. The histology of the SLN(s) predicts the involvement of the remaining axillary nodes. If the SLN is negative, a more extensive lymph node dissection can be avoided. If the SLN is positive, a standard axillary dissection is performed or radiation therapy is administered to the axilla. The procedure requires a multidisciplinary approach, including nuclear medicine, pathology, and radiology. Experienced surgeons (those who have performed at least 30 SLNBs, with ALNDs for confirmation) can identify the SLN in >90% of patients, accurately predicting the patient's remaining lymph node status in 97% to 99% of cases. Serial sectioning and immunohistochemical staining of SLNB specimens may improve accuracy in detecting micrometastatic disease. Large trials [NSABP B-32, American College of Surgeons Oncology Group (ACOSOG) z-0010 and z-0011] are under way to compare long-term regional control of disease and overall survival in women who undergo SLNB alone versus those who undergo SLNB followed by standard axillary dissection. These trials will help establish what role this modality will play in the care of these breast cancer patients and what is the predictive value of immunohistochemistry detection of micrometastasis.

B. **BCT** comprises complete surgical excision of the cancer followed by radiation therapy, and it may be offered to patients with reasonable tumor-breast ratios. For patients with large tumors who desire BCT, preoperative chemotherapy or hormonal therapy may be offered to reduce the size of the tumor. Adjuvant radiotherapy has been demonstrated to decrease the breast cancer recurrence rate from 30% to less than 7% at 5 years. Radiotherapy is administered daily on an outpatient basis 5 days a week for approximately 6 weeks. After surgery, patients receive 4,500 to 5,000 cGy of radiation to the breast, usually with a boost to the tumor bed.

1. **Contraindications to lumpectomy/quadrantectomy with adjuvant radiation** include two or more primary tumors in separate quadrants of the breast; persistently positive margins after multiple attempts at complete resection; pregnancy (especially in the first or second trimesters); prior radiation to the breast region; collagen vascular disease (e.g., scleroderma); diffuse disease throughout the breast, precluding excision with negative operative margins; and the unavailability of radiation therapy. Extensive intraductal component (i.e., 25% of the primary tumor is intraductal) is not considered a contraindication to BCT, provided that microscopically negative margins can be obtained.

2. **Technique of lumpectomy.** Incisions should be curvilinear and parallel to the nipple-areolar complex. A gross margin of 1 cm should be attempted, and the specimen oriented as already described. A small ellipse of skin is often removed to help orient the specimen, and meticulous hemostasis is achieved. The tumor bed can be marked with radiopaque clips. Use of drains impairs cosmesis. Internal flaps of breast tissue may be used to obliterate the surgical defect, especially if the pectoralis fascia is exposed. The subcutaneous tissue is closed, and the skin is reapproximated with a subcuticular suture. Incisions for lumpectomy and axillary dissection should be separate. Reconstruction is recommended any time that excision or reexcision of a lesion significantly affects the final shape and size of the breast.

3. **Complications of BCT** include infection and bleeding as well as the complications of axillary dissection. Other complications include specific side effects of radiotherapy to the breast, such as early skin

changes (e.g., breast edema, erythema, moist desquamation). Late skin changes include edema, pigmentation changes, and telangiectasias. Radiation to the chest wall may result in interstitial pneumonitis, spontaneous rib fracture, breast fibrosis, pericarditis, pleural effusion, and chest wall myositis (rare). Patients with positive lymph nodes undergo radiation therapy to the axilla, which increases the risk of arm lymph edema to 15%.

4. **Follow-up for BCT** is similar to that for mastectomy. A posttreatment mammogram of the treated side is performed to establish a new baseline mammogram. Mammograms are then performed every 6 to 12 months after the completion of radiotherapy until the surgical changes stabilize, and then annually.

C. **Modified radical mastectomy** is the combination of a total mastectomy and axillary node dissection. It differs from the traditional Halstead radical mastectomy in that the pectoralis major muscle is preserved to enhance cosmesis of the chest wall. Complications include flap necrosis, bleeding, and infection, in addition to the complications of axillary dissection. Follow-up after mastectomy involves physical examination every 3 to 4 months for 2 to 3 years and every 6 months for the next 2 to 3 years. The chest wall should be examined for evidence of recurrence. Mammography of the contralateral breast should continue annually.

D. **Immediate reconstruction** at the time of mastectomy should be offered to eligible patients. Options include latissimus dorsi myocutaneous flaps, transverse rectus abdominis myocutaneous flaps, and inflatable tissue expanders followed by saline implants. A skin-sparing mastectomy may be performed, resulting in improved cosmesis. For this procedure, the nipple-areolar complex, a rim of periareolar breast skin, and the biopsy site are excised. Immediate reconstruction has been shown not to affect patient outcome adversely. The detection of recurrence is not delayed, and the onset of chemotherapy is not changed. Patients who undergo an immediate reconstruction after skin-sparing mastectomy often need additional outpatient procedures for nipple reconstruction or other contour adjustments.

IV. **Locally advanced breast cancer (LABC)** comprises T3 or T4, N1 or greater, and M0 cancers (stages IIIA and IIIB).

A. **Patients with noninflammatory stage IIIB** (chest wall or skin involvement, skin satellites, ulceration, fixed axillary nodes) should receive induction chemotherapy (cyclophosphamide, 5-fluorouracil, and either doxorubicin or methotrexate) as the initial step in treatment, followed by surgery and radiation. The high response rates seen with this approach allow modified radical mastectomy to be carried out, with primary skin closure and possible immediate reconstruction. Treatment includes 3 to 4 cycles of neoadjuvant chemotherapy, followed by modified radical mastectomy with or without reconstruction, radiotherapy to the chest wall axilla and supraclavicular nodes, and further chemotherapy to complete a total of 6 to 12 cycles. Patients with stage IIIA disease receiving neoadjuvant chemotherapy can be converted to BCT candidates with no difference in overall outcome. Approximately 20% of patients with stage III disease present with distant metastases after appropriate staging has been performed.

B. **Inflammatory LABC (T4d).** Inflammatory breast represents 1% to 6% of all breast cancers. It is characterized by erythema, warmth, tenderness, and edema (peau d'orange). An underlying mass is present in 70% of cases. Associated axillary adenopathy occurs in 50% of cases. Delayed diagnosis is common owing to its similarity to mastitis. A breast biopsy that includes a portion of skin confirms the diagnosis. In two-thirds of cases, tumor emboli are seen in dermal lymphatics; 30% of patients have distant metastasis at the time of diagnosis. Inflammatory breast cancer requires aggressive multimodal therapy, as median survival is approximately 2 years, with a 5-year survival of only 5%.

C. **Staging in LABC.** Because of the frequent presence of distant metastasis at the time of presentation, all patients should undergo staging with complete blood cell count, complete metabolic panel, bone scan, and CT scan of chest and abdomen before neoadjuvant chemotherapy.

D. **Follow-up.** Patients with LABC are at higher risk for local and distant recurrence and should be examined every 3 months by all specialists involved in their care.

V. **Treatment of locoregional recurrence.** All patients who present with locoregional recurrence should have a metastatic workup to exclude visceral or bony disease and should be evaluated for systemic chemotherapy or hormonal therapy.

A. **Recurrence in the breast after BCT** requires salvage mastectomy.

B. **Recurrence in the axilla.** Optimal control is obtained with surgical resection followed by radiation to the axilla and consideration of systemic therapy.

C. **Recurrence in the chest wall after mastectomy.** One-third of these patients have distant metastatic disease at the time of recurrence, and more than 50% will have distant disease within 2 years. Excision of the recurrence alone results in poor local control. Therefore, multimodal approaches are necessary. For an isolated local recurrence, excision followed by radiotherapy results in excellent local control. Rarely, patients require radical chest resection with myocutaneous flap closure.

VI. **Adjuvant systemic therapy treatment** is given when all gross tumor has been removed and no measurable tumor remains (Table 32-4).

Table 32-4. Adjuvant systemic treatment based on the St. Gallen Consensus Conference[a]

	Premenopausal	Postmenopausal
Node+		
ER+	**Chemotherapy** ± tamoxifen **Ovarian ablation** ± tamoxifen GnRH analogue **Chemotherapy** ± ovarian ablation ± tamoxifen	**Tamoxifen** ± chemotherapy
ER–	**Chemotherapy**	**Chemotherapy** ± tamoxifen
Node–		
ER+		
Low/minimal risk	No treatment vs. tamoxifen	No treatment vs. tamoxifen
Intermediate risk	**Tamoxifen** ± chemotherapy Ovarian ablation GnRH analogue	**Tamoxifen** ± chemotherapy
High risk	**Chemotherapy** + tamoxifen Ovarian ablation GnRH analogue	**Tamoxifen** + chemotherapy
ER–		
Low risk	Not applicable[b]	Not applicable[b]
Intermediate risk	Not applicable[b]	Not applicable[b]
High risk	**Chemotherapy**	**Chemotherapy** ± tamoxifen

[a]Bold entries are treatments accepted for routine use.
[b]All ER tumors are considered high risk.
ER, estrogen receptor; GnRH, gonadotropin-releasing hormone.
Modified from the Recommendations of the St. Gallen Consensus Panel, St. Gallen, Switzerland, 1998.

A. All **node-positive patients** should receive adjuvant chemotherapy. This treatment is frequently followed with tamoxifen if the tumor is positive for estrogen receptor (ER). Chemotherapeutic regimens comprise four to eight cycles of a combination of cyclophosphamide, 5-fluorouracil and methotrexate or doxorubicin and cyclophosphamide followed by a taxane. In patients with *Her2/neu*-positive tumors, a doxorubicin-based regimen is usually chosen. In postmenopausal women, chemotherapy is frequently used up to age 70. In older patients, chemotherapy is performed less frequently. In ER-positive tumors in postmenopausal women, tamoxifen is the drug of choice.

B. **Node-negative patients** may also benefit from adjuvant therapy in terms of years gained of disease-free survival. Up to 30% of node-negative women die of breast cancer within 10 years if treated with surgery alone. Node-negative patients who are at high risk and benefit the most from adjuvant chemotherapy include those with larger tumors (>1 cm), higher nuclear grade, ER-negative tumors, and lymphovascular invasion. The NSABP B-20 trial and the International Breast Cancer Study Group trial IX were intended to evaluate the effects of tamoxifen alone versus tamoxifen in combination with polychemotherapy in patients with ER-positive and ER-negative tumors. They demonstrate that polychemotherapy in combination with tamoxifen was superior to tamoxifen alone in increasing disease-free and overall survival, especially in ER-negative patients regardless of tumor size. The NSABP B-23 trial looked at two different chemotherapy regimens with or without tamoxifen. Preliminary data showed no significant difference in overall survival between the two chemotherapy regimens regardless of whether tamoxifen was given. The St. Gallen Consensus Panel (1998) suggested that patients who have node-negative disease and whose tumors are small (≤1 cm) and ER-positive may be spared adjuvant chemotherapy but still may benefit from tamoxifen. Ultimately, the decision to use adjuvant therapy should involve an individualized discussion with the patient regarding the risks of recurrence without adjuvant therapy, the cost and toxicities of adjuvant therapy, and the expected benefit in risk reduction and survival from this therapy.

VII. **Indications for postmastectomy radiation** to the chest wall and regional node-bearing areas include T3 and T4 tumors, attachment to the pectoral fascia, positive surgical margins, involved internal mammary nodes, inadequate or no axillary dissection, more than eight positive lymph nodes, and residual tumor on the axillary vein. Randomized, prospective trials have shown a significantly decreased recurrence and improved survival in premenopausal women with these indications treated with chemotherapy and radiation therapy (*N Engl J Med* 1997;337:949, 956).

VIII. **Lymphedema** occurs in approximately 10% of women undergoing axillary dissection, and this fact was the rationale behind the development of SLNB. However, if axillary dissection occurs, the patient should avoid violations of the skin and be advised to avoid blood draws, blood pressure cuffs, and intravenous lines in her affected arm. Infections of the patient's hand or arm should be treated promptly and aggressively because infection can damage lymphatics further. Lymphedema presenting with simultaneous cellulitis should be treated aggressively with antibiotics and arm elevation. Lymphedema can become irreversible after repeated episodes of infection. If lymphedema is treated promptly while it is still reversible, the patient's arm may return to normal size. For persistent lymphedema, the most effective therapy is intense physiomassage treatment. A graded pneumatic compression device has also been used to reduce arm swelling, followed by a professionally fitted compression sleeve. Good results have also been reported for professional massage therapy. With the increasing use of SLNB, this disabling complication may become a rarer event.

IX. **Paget disease of the nipple** is characterized by eczematoid changes of the nipple, which may involve the surrounding areola. Paget disease is almost always accompanied by an underlying malignancy, either invasive ductal carcinoma or DCIS. Burning, pruritus, and hypersensitivity may be prominent symptoms. Palpable masses are present in approximately 60% of patients. Mammography should be performed to identify other areas of involvement. If clinical suspicion is high, a pathologic diagnosis should be obtained by wedge biopsy of the nipple and underlying breast tissue. Treatment is mastectomy or BCT with excision of the nipple-areolar complex, followed by radiation therapy. The prognosis is related to tumor stage.

X. **Breast cancer during pregnancy** may be difficult to diagnose due to the low level of suspicion and breast nodularity and density. It carries an incidence of approximately 1 in 5,000 gestations and accounts for almost 3% of all breast cancers. Mammography and ultrasound may be helpful in characterizing masses. All dominant masses should undergo biopsy. Excisional biopsy can be safely performed under local anesthesia. Therapeutic decisions are influenced by the clinical cancer stage and the trimester of pregnancy and must be individualized. The standard preoperative staging workup is performed. Laboratory values such as alkaline phosphatase may be elevated during pregnancy. For advanced-stage disease, MR scan or ultrasound may be used in lieu of CT scan for staging. Although modified radical mastectomy is the standard treatment for a breast cancer diagnosed during pregnancy, BCT, radiation therapy, and adjuvant chemotherapy may also be applicable as long as the patient understands the risks and teratogenicity of these modalities (*Adv Surg* 2000;34:275, 282). Chemotherapy may be given by the mid-second trimester, and radiation therapy may be given in the latter part of the third trimester.

XI. **Breast cancer in men** accounts for fewer than 1% of male cancers and fewer than 1% of all breast cancers. *BRCA2* mutations are associated with approximately 4% to 6% of these cancers. Patients generally present with a nontender hard mass. This contrasts with unilateral gynecomastia, which is usually firm, central, and tender. Mammography can be helpful in distinguishing gynecomastia from malignancy. Malignant lesions are more likely to be eccentric, with irregular margins, and are often associated with nipple retraction and microcalcification. Biopsy of suspicious lesions is essential. Modified radical mastectomy is the surgical procedure of choice. Eighty-five percent of malignancies are infiltrating ductal carcinoma and are positive for ERs. Adjuvant hormonal and chemotherapy treatment parallels that used in women. Overall survival per stage is comparable to that observed in women.

XII. **Cystosarcoma phyllodes tumors** account for 0.5% to 1.0% of breast cancers. Phyllodes tumor presents as a large, smooth, lobulated mass, and on physical examination, it may be difficult to distinguish from fibroadenoma. These tumors can occur in women of any age but most frequently present between ages 35 and 55. Skin ulcerations may occur secondary to pressure of the underlying mass. FNAB cannot reliably diagnose these tumors. Histologically, stromal overgrowth is the essential characteristic for differentiating phyllodes tumors from fibroadenomas. The biologic behavior of malignant tumors is similar to that of sarcomas. Treatment is wide local excision to tumor-free margins or total mastectomy. Axillary dissection is not indicated unless nodes are clinically positive (which is rare). Currently, there is no role for adjuvant radiation; however, tumors >5 cm in diameter and with evidence of stromal overgrowth may benefit from adjuvant chemotherapy with doxorubicin and ifosfamide (*Cancer* 2000;89:1510). Patients whose tumors were malignant should be followed with semiannual physical examinations and annual mammograms and chest radiographs.

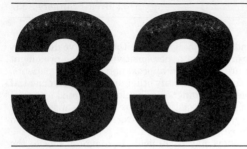

Otolaryngology: Head and Neck Surgery

**Abraham Jacob and
Bruce Haughey**

OTOLARYNGOLOGIC DISORDERS

I. The ear

A. Anatomy and physiology

1. The external ear includes the **auricle** and **external auditory canal.** The auricle is made of cartilage while the **lobule** contains only fibrofatty tissue. The lateral third of the external auditory canal is cartilaginous and contains both sebaceous and ceruminous glands. The medial two-thirds of the ear canal is bony.

2. The **tympanic membrane** that closes the medial end of the external canal is composed of an outer epithelial layer, a middle fibrous layer, and an inner mucosal layer. Its vibratory surface is the **pars tensa,** and the small, flaccid area superior to the neck of the malleus is the **pars flaccida.**

3. The **middle ear** is the space medial to the tympanic membrane and lateral to the otic capsule (inner ear). The **eustachian tube** connects the anterior aspect of the middle ear to the nasopharynx. It protects the middle ear from nasopharyngeal pathogens, aerates the middle ear, and drains fluid into the nasopharynx. Eustachian tube function is dynamic and influenced primarily by the tensor veli palatini muscle. The posterior superior aspect of the middle ear space communicates with the mastoid cavity. The ossicular chain consists of the malleus, incus, and stapes. The manubrium of the malleus is adherent to the tympanic membrane at the umbo. The head of the malleus articulates with the body of the incus while the long process of the incus articulates with the stapes. The stapes footplate transmits vibratory energy to the inner ear via the oval window. Sound energy is conducted and amplified by the pinna, external auditory canal, tympanic membrane, and ossicular chain. The difference in surface area between tympanic membrane and the oval window, along with the lever action of the ossicular chain, leads to a 22-fold amplification in sound energy.

4. The bony **otic capsule** (inner ear) encases the sensory end organs of hearing and balance. These include **the three semicircular canals, the utricle, the saccule, and the cochlea.** The cochlea is a snail-shaped structure with $2\frac{1}{2}$ turns. The three semicircular canals, oriented 90 degrees to each other, are responsible for sensing angular acceleration, while the utricle and saccule detect linear acceleration. The **organ of Corti** in the cochlea, the **cupulae** in the semicircular canals, and the **maculae** in the utricle and saccule convert mechanical energy into neuroelectrical signals that are transmitted centrally via the vestibulocochlear nerve.

5. Cranial nerve VIII, **the vestibulocochlear nerve,** has both a cochlear and vestibular division. It travels through the internal auditory canal and enters the brainstem at the cerebellopontine angle.

6. Cranial nerve VII, **the facial nerve,** courses through the temporal bone. It has a short labyrinthine segment that becomes the tympanic segment after giving off the greater superficial petrosal nerve at the geniculate ganglion (first genu, or turn). The tympanic segment overlies the stapes suprastructure and oval window. At its second genu (turn), the facial nerve enters the mastoid cavity (mastoid segment) and travels vertically

before exiting the temporal bone at the stylomastoid foramen. Before exiting the temporal bone, the facial nerve gives off a motor branch to the stapedius muscle as well as the chorda tympani nerve supplying taste to the anterior two-thirds of the tongue.

B. Hearing loss and tinnitus
1. **Hearing loss** is classified as sensorineural, conductive, or mixed.
   a. **Sensorineural hearing loss (SNHL)** is caused by lesions in the cochlea, cranial nerve VIII, or the central nervous system. The sound conduction apparatus is intact but neuroelectrical impulses are either not generated or not transmitted effectively. Common causes of SNHL include presbycusis (age-related hearing loss), noise exposure, ototoxicity, viral or bacterial infections, autoimmune diseases, temporal bone trauma, CN VIII tumors, and genetic or congenital hearing loss. SNHL is treated with hearing aids. Cochlear implantation is reserved for the profoundly deaf who do not benefit from conventional amplification.
   b. **Conductive hearing loss** is the result of inadequate transmission of sound energy to the inner ear. The problem can arise in the external ear canal, tympanic membrane, or middle ear. Common causes include impacted cerumen, tympanic membrane perforation, otitis media, cholesteatoma, ossicular chain fixation, and ossicular discontinuity. Treatment is often surgical and involves restoring the sound conduction pathway. Those who elect not to have surgery can sometimes be treated with hearing aids.
2. **Tinnitus,** or ringing in the ears, can be objective (heard by the examiner) or subjective (perceived only by the patient). It is usually described as hissing, crickets chirping, whooshing, or ringing. Tinnitus, while often nonspecific or associated with noise exposure, can be the only manifestation of more serious conditions such as eighth nerve tumors or arteriovenous malformations.

C. Evaluation of hearing and balance
1. **Bedside evaluation of hearing** includes the Weber and Rinne tests.
   a. **The Weber test** entails placing a 512-Hz tuning fork on the patient's midline forehead or teeth and asking whether the sound is perceived as louder in one ear or the other. The test is normal if the patient is unable to lateralize the sound to a particular ear. Sound lateralizes to the ear with a conductive hearing loss or contralateralizes to the ear with an SNHL.
   b. **The Rinne test** is performed by placing the tuning fork first lateral to the pinna (air conduction) and then on the mastoid tip (bone conduction). The patient is asked which placement was perceived as louder. Those with normal hearing or those with SNHL perceive air conduction louder than bone conduction. Patients with a conductive hearing loss perceive bone conduction as louder than air conduction.
2. **Formal audiometry** is able to both qualify and quantify hearing loss. The patient's hearing threshold for pure tones (measured in decibels) from 250 to 8,000 Hz, as well as speech audiometry, is tested. Both air and bone conduction thresholds are quantified, and a gap between these thresholds suggests the presence of a conductive component to the hearing loss. Speech audiometry measures speech reception thresholds (decibels) and word recognition scores (percentage correct). A drop in word discrimination out of proportion to the hearing loss by pure tunes suggests the presence of retrocochlear pathology (e.g., acoustic tumors).
   a. **Auditory brainstem response (ABR)** measures EEG waveforms generated in response to sound as neuroelectrical energy is transmitted thru the eighth cranial nerve and brainstem. This test does not require patient cooperation and is useful in testing infants.
   b. **Tympanometry,** or impedance audiometry, measures tympanic membrane compliance, ear canal volume, and the stapedial reflex (seventh/eighth nerve reflex arc). Tympanic membrane perforations,

middle ear mass effect, or ossicular chain abnormalities affect canal volume and eardrum compliance. Conductive hearing losses or retro-cochlear processes impairing neurotransmission along the seventh or eighth cranial nerve alter the stapedial reflex.

3. **Bedside evaluation of the dizzy patient** can be challenging. The physician must first define what it means to the patient to be "dizzy." Patients may use the term to describe lightheadedness, near-syncope, dysequilibrium, or frank vertigo. The differential diagnosis includes cardiovascular or cerebrovascular perfusion abnormalities, central (CNS) pathologies, and inner ear abnormalities. Psychological issues may play into the symptomatology as well. Bedside testing includes orthostatic blood pressure measurements, observation of the patient's gait, cerebellar testing, and maneuvers designed to elicit nystagmus. Types of nystagmus include gaze, positional, positioning, and postheadshake nystagmus. The Dix-Hallpike test, one test of positioning nystagmus, helps in the diagnosis of benign paroxysmal positional nystagmus (BPPV). Saccades and smooth pursuit visual tracking are tasks requiring multisynaptic CNS pathways. Abnormalities in these systems suggest central disease. The constellation of patient symptoms, bedside testing, and formal vestibular testing help to narrow the differential diagnosis.

4. **Formal vestibular testing includes electronystagmography (ENG), dynamic posturography, and rotational chair analysis.** The test most commonly employed is the ENG. One component of this study is **caloric testing**—the application of cold and warm water to the external auditory canal in an effort to stimulate low-frequency horizontal semicircular canal **nystagmus.** Nystagmus is defined by its fast phase. The pneumonic COWS (cold opposite, warm same) can be used as a reminder of the direction of nystagmus induced by caloric testing.

D. **Inflammatory ear disease**
1. **Otitis externa (OE),** commonly referred to as "swimmer's ear," is inflammation of the external auditory canal. A moist ear canal causes changes in the local pH and results in bacterial overgrowth. The most common culprit is *Pseudomonas aeruginosa,* but *Staphylococcus aureus* may also cause otitis externa. Symptoms include severe pain, ear drainage, canal swelling, and a conductive hearing loss. First-line treatment is aural toilet and antibiotic ear drops. If the ear canal is extremely swollen, an ear wick may be placed. This serves as both a stent and facilitates contact between the ear drops and the canal wall. Fungal external otitis (otomycosis) can have both acute and chronic forms. Treatment includes drying and acidifying the ear canal along with use of topical antifungals. Malignant external otitis is essentially skull base osteomyelitis. This tends to be a disease of diabetic or immunocompromised patients and can be rapidly fatal. Aggressive therapy, including systemic antibiotics and surgical débridement, is required.
2. **Eustachian tube dysfunction** refers to inadequate aeration or drainage of the middle ear space by the eustachian tube. The tube is nearly horizontal in infants but elongates and assumes a more vertical alignment with facial growth. Dysfunction results in a negative middle ear pressure and puts patients at risk for otitis media with or without cholesteatoma. Serous otitis media refers to clear or amber-colored fluid behind the tympanic membrane while mucoid otitis media implies a thick mucinous middle ear effusion. Eardrum mobility is restricted, as is evident on pneumatic otoscopy or tympanometry. Eustachian tube dysfunction is treated with antibiotics (if infection is present), insufflation exercises, and myringotomy with tube placement if medical therapy fails. Pressure equalization tubes are generally placed in the anterior pars tensa and tend to remain in place for 6 to 18 months. After extrusion, the tympanic membrane usually heals spontaneously.

3. **Acute otitis media** is predominantly a disease of young children (younger than 5 years old). The most common bacterial pathogens are pneumococci, *Haemophilus influenza*, and *Moraxella catarrhalis*. Symptoms include fever, otalgia, decreased appetite, and irritability, and the diagnosis is made by history and physical examination. The tympanic membrane appears erythematous or dull or may be bulging. Grossly purulent material can sometimes be noted behind the drum, and the drum may perforate spontaneously. Treatment consists of oral antibiotics for 10 to 14 days. Otorrhea can be treated with antibiotic ear drops. Patients with recurrent disease require β-lactamase–inhibiting agents or placement of a pressure equalization tube. Four to 6 episodes of otitis media per year is an indication for tubes. Complications of otitis media include eardrum perforation, mastoiditis, subperiosteal abscess, labyrinthitis, facial nerve palsy, epidural or subdural abscess, meningitis, brain abscess, sigmoid sinus thrombophlebitis, and otitic hydrocephalus.
4. **Chronic suppurative otitis media** describes prolonged infection of the middle ear, and it is often associated with a persistent tympanic membrane perforation. Chronic otorrhea is common. While some cases may be managed medically, most require surgery.
5. A **cholesteatoma** is a keratocyst of the temporal bone further classified as **congenital, primary acquired,** or **secondary acquired.** Congenital cholesteatomas are thought to arise from embryonic rests and present as a white cyst medial to an intact eardrum (often in the anterior-superior quadrant). These patients do not have a history of chronic ear disease. Primary acquired cholesteatomas result from eustachian tube dysfunction and negative pressure in the middle ear. A retraction pocket develops in the pars flaccida and collects squamous debris. Secondary acquired cholesteatomas arise from tympanic membrane perforations with medial migration of squamous epithelium around the edges of the hole. The cholesteatoma matrix is metabolically active and erodes bone by pressure effect and osteoclast activation. Symptoms include a conductive hearing loss, a perilymphatic fistula, SNHL, vertigo, and facial nerve palsy. Treatment requires surgery.
E. **Ear trauma**
   1. Ear trauma is **classified by location.** Trauma to the auricle may result in an auricular hematoma that requires incision and drainage. Failure to do so results in cartilage destruction and a deformed "cauliflower" ear. Tympanic membrane perforations usually heal without intervention. Surgical repair is indicated for chronic perforations. **Temporal bone fractures** are classified as longitudinal (80%) or transverse (20%). While transverse fractures are less common, they are more likely to cause permanent SHNL or facial nerve injury. The decision to pursue surgical intervention is determined by the status of the facial nerve.
   2. **Foreign bodies** in the external canal are common. Care should be used to avoid trauma to the eardrum and ear canal during removal. Organic materials expand when moistened and should not be treated with ear drops. Batteries in the ear canal must be removed immediately, as they can cause severe scarring and stenosis.
F. **Vertigo**
   1. **Vertigo,** from the otolaryngologist's perspective, is a distinct sense of motion in relation to the environment. This is often described as spinning or tumbling, not faintness or lightheadedness. True vertigo usually originates in the inner ear, whereas unsteadiness can be multifactorial. Vertigo resulting from abnormalities in the inner ear does *not* directly cause loss of consciousness.
   2. **Ménière disease** is defined by a symptom complex: episodic vertigo lasting from minutes to hours, fluctuating SNHL, tinnitus, and aural fullness. The histologic correlate is endolymphatic hydrops, defined as an

increase in endolymph volume within the inner ear. Medical management consists of salt restriction, diuretics, and vestibular suppressants. Refractory cases need transtympanic gentamicin, endolymphatic sac surgery, labyrinthectomy, or vestibular nerve section to control the vertigo. Therapy is tailored to the patient's level of disability.

3. **Benign positional vertigo** is a common disorder characterized by transient vertigo that lasts roughly 30 seconds and is precipitated by a sudden upward head tilt toward the affected ear. This disease is thought to be caused by floating calcium carbonate particles in the posterior semicircular canal. Canalith repositioning maneuvers such as the Eppley technique are effective in treatment.

4. **Vestibular neuritis** is thought to result from a viral infection of the inner ear. Vertigo can last days or even weeks, and the patient may be left with persistent dysequilibrium for months. Hearing is generally not affected. Vestibular rehabilitation (physical therapy) is helpful.

G. **The facial nerve.** Central paralysis from a supranuclear lesion (a lesion proximal to the facial nucleus in the pons) spares the ipsilateral forehead because this area receives bilateral cortical innervation. Peripheral lesions (lesions at or distal to the facial nucleus) produce paralysis of the whole face on the ipsilateral side. Bell palsy is the most common cause of facial nerve paralysis and is now thought to be related to the presence of herpes virus in the geniculate ganglion. Treatment is controversial, but most physicians use systemic steroids and oral antivirals. Roughly 15% of patients have a permanent facial palsy from this disease. Surgical decompression of the nerve is considered when patients have >90% denervation as defined by electroneurography (EnoG). Other causes of facial paralysis include trauma; intracranial, intratemporal, and extracranial tumors of the facial nerve or surrounding structures; infections; and autoimmune diseases. Malignancies of the parotid gland damage the nerve in its extratemporal course.

II. **Nose and sinus disorders**

A. **Anatomy and physiology**

1. **The external nose** comprises bone and cartilage. Lined with skin, the nasal vestibule leads into the nasal cavity through the piriform aperture. The nasal septum (cartilage anteriorly and bone posteriorly) divides the nose into a right and left half. Three to 4 mucosa-lined bony prominences, **the inferior, middle, superior, and supreme turbinates,** project from the lateral nasal wall. Just lateral to each turbinate is its corresponding **meatus.** The **olfactory nerve** penetrates the **cribriform plate** and is distributed along the superior aspect of the nasal septum and nasal vault. The nose is lined by a ciliated cuboidal or pseudostratified columnar epithelium and has a submucosa rich in mucous glands, nerves, blood vessels, and inflammatory cells.

2. The paranasal sinuses are paired bony cavities in the forehead, cheeks, nose, and central skull (**the frontal, maxillary, ethmoid, and sphenoid sinuses,** respectively). The mucus produced in these sinuses circulates toward the natural ostium (opening) of each sinus by mucociliary flow and then drains into the nose. The maxillary, frontal, and anterior ethmoid sinuses drain into the middle meatus; and the posterior ethmoids and sphenoid sinus drain into the superior meatus; and the nasolacrimal duct drains into the inferior meatus. The nose opens into the nasopharynx through the posterior **nasal choanae.**

3. The nose and sinuses have **multiple functions.** The nose provides a conduit for air—cleaning, warming, and humidifying it prior to its entry into the lower respiratory tract. Roughly half the resistence to airflow in the respiratory tract occurs at **the nasal valve.** This area is bounded by the nasal septum, upper lateral cartilages, and inferior turbinates. The nose also provides olfaction and helps with taste. The sinuses contribute resonance to the voice, decrease the weight of the skull, and cushion the cranial contents during blunt head trauma. Common symptoms of

sinonasal disorders are nasal congestion, rhinorrhea, nasal obstruction, postnasal drip, facial pressure, altered olfaction, eustachian tube dysfunction, epistaxis, hoarseness, and cough.
B. **Diagnostic tests.** Most sinonasal disorders are diagnosed by a thorough history and a physical examination that includes endoscopic intranasal visualization. Computed tomographic (CT) scans are helpful in delineating sinonasal anatomy for surgical planning and help to rule out mass lesions. Nasal mucus smears may distinguish allergy (characterized by eosinophils) from bacterial or viral infection (characterized by neutrophils and lymphocytes). Skin endpoint titration or radioallergosorbent (RAST) assays confirm sensitivity to particular allergens. **Rhinometry** can provide an objective measure of nasal airflow and nasal volume.
C. **Congenital disorders**
   1. Congenital midline nasal masses in children can be **encephaloceles, gliomas, or dermoid cysts.** These may present intranasally or extranasally as a mass or pit. An MRI should be obtained to rule out intracranial communication, and treatment is surgical excision.
   2. **Posterior nasal choanal atresia** may be unilateral or bilateral. Bilateral choanal atresia presents in the newborn period because infants are obligate nasal breathers. Inability to pass a catheter through the nose into the oropharynx confirms the diagnosis. Those with unilateral atresia present later in life with symptoms similar to rhinosinusitis.
D. **Inflammatory disorders**
   1. **The paranasal sinuses** communicate with the nose via their ostia. Therefore, whereas rhinitis and sinusitis may occur in isolation, the more common scenario is combined **rhinosinusitis.**
   2. **Allergic rhinosinusitis** is characterized by a Gell and Coombs type I reaction. In susceptible patients, inhaled allergens bind to IgE receptors on mast cells, resulting in degranulation and the release of vasoactive mediators such as histamine. Vasodilation and hypersecretion ensue, producing sneezing, nasal congestion, and rhinorrhea. Seasonal allergic rhinitis usually occurs in the spring and fall. Trees and grasses are the allergens in spring, whereas weeds are the usual culprits in the fall. Perennial allergic rhinitis is produced by nonseasonal inhalants such as mold, house dust, and animal dander. Diagnosis is made by history and confirmed by skin tests or radioallergosorbent allergy tests. Treatment includes environmental control, medications, and allergy immunotherapy. The medications utilized include systemic and intranasal antihistamines and steroids, cromolyn nasal spray, and decongestants. Allergy immunotherapy attempts to desensitize the body by inducing the formation of blocking IgG antibodies to each allergen.
   3. **Nonallergic rhinitis** encompasses a variety of other diseases that produce nasal congestion, excessive secretions, and postnasal drip.
      a. **Viral rhinitis** is the typical cold. Viral rhinitis typically occurs in the winter and usually lasts 5 to 10 days. Treatment is supportive and includes humidification, rest, and hydration. Antibiotics are not indicated unless a secondary bacterial infection ensues.
      b. **Rhinitis medicamentosa** is caused by prolonged use of decongestant nasal sprays. Patients using such sprays for more than 5 days experience rebound nasal congestion on withdrawal, which promotes further use and "addiction" to the nasal spray. Treatment consists of discontinuing the offending agent.
      c. **Drug-induced rhinitis** is produced by systemic agents, including alcohol, antithyroid medications, aspirin, estrogen, iodides, and reserpine. Other topical irritants are cocaine, tobacco, and marijuana.
      d. **Vasomotor rhinitis** is characterized by nasal congestion and watery rhinorrhea. The exact etiology is unknown but may be secondary to sinonasal autonomic dysfunction. The nasal mucosa remains in a chronically stimulated state, and the hypersecretion may be worsened

by nonspecific stimulants such as weather changes, stress, and chemical irritants. Treatment consists of antihistamines, decongestants, and nasal steroid sprays. Surgery to reduce the bulk of the turbinates may be indicated in refractory cases. Vidian neurectomy has been largely abandoned as a treatment for this condition.

  e. Atrophic rhinitis is characterized by atrophy of nasal membranes. It typically affects the elderly or those who have undergone excessive resection of the intranasal turbinate architecture during sinus surgery. Often called *ozena*, it results in a foul, malodorous discharge. Therapy includes removal of crusts and use of saline nasal sprays.

  f. Metabolic-endocrine rhinitis typically occurs in pregnancy, during parts of the menstrual cycle, in hypothyroidism, and in patients with diabetes mellitus. The nasal mucosa is boggy and congested. When associated with pregnancy, the condition resolves after birth.

 4. Wegener granulomatosis is an autoimmune vasculitis typically affecting the upper respiratory tract and kidney. In the nose, nasopharynx, and paranasal sinuses, the disease causes erythema and ulceration of the mucosa. Nasal septal cartilage necrosis is highly suspicious for Wegener granulomatosis. It is ultimately diagnosed by history, biopsy, and elevated serum c-ANCA levels.

E. Nasal foreign bodies. Nasal foreign bodies are generally found in children or adults with mental retardation. The history and physical exam is significant for unilateral foul-smelling nasal discharge. Most foreign bodies can be removed in awake patients with topical anesthesia. However, general anesthesia with airway protection may be necessary in some (especially younger or uncooperative children). Organic materials tend to expand and fragment during attempts at removal. Batteries in the nose constitute a medical emergency requiring urgent removal.

F. Nasal septal deviation. A deviated nasal septum may result from nasal trauma or differential growth in septal growth centers during fetal development or childhood. A significantly deviated septum can produce nasal obstruction, interfere with drainage from the sinuses, or cause headaches by contacting turbinate mucosa. Treatment is surgical (septoplasty). The deviated portions of cartilage and bone are removed after elevation of the overlying mucosa.

G. Soft-tissue pathologies

 1. Adenoid hypertrophy. While they are located in the nasopharynx and not the nose, adenoid hypertrophy produces nasal obstruction, mouth breathing, recurrent upper respiratory tract infections, and snoring. Infected adenoid tissue can result in postnasal drip and rhinorrhea simulating sinusitis. The adenoids can obstruct the eustachian tube and cause middle ear effusions. Therapy is surgical (adenoidectomy). The adenoid pad usually atrophies with age.

 2. Inflammatory nasal polyps are pendulous, edematous, hyperplastic regions of nasal mucosa. Their etiology is unknown, but they are commonly associated with allergy or chronic rhinosinusitis. Some patients present with the clinical triad of aspirin sensitivity, asthma, and nasal polyposis. Cystic fibrosis patients tend to form extensive nasal polyps. Inflammatory polyps are usually treated with topical or systemic steroids, antibiotics for associated infections, and surgical debulking. An antrochoanal polyp is a large nasal polyp originating in the maxillary sinus and extending into the nose or even the nasopharynx. Treatment is complete excision.

 3. Neoplasms of the nose and nasopharynx are uncommon.

  a. Papillomas are benign wartlike growths on the septum or lateral nasal wall and are classified as fungiform, inverting, or cylindrical. **Inverting papillomas** tend to occur in the lateral nasal wall and are associated with a 10% incidence of squamous cell carcinoma. Wide local excision is necessary to prevent recurrence.

b. Juvenile nasopharyngeal angiofibroma occurs in adolescent boys and usually presents with nasal obstruction and recurrent epistaxis. Treatment is complete surgical excision. Angiography and embolization of the vascular supply 24 hours prior to resection helps minimize blood loss.

c. The most common sinonasal malignancy is **squamous cell carcinoma.** Carcinoma of the nasopharynx is uncommon in the United States but is very common in Hong Kong and parts of China, where it is associated with the Epstein-Barr virus. There are three histologic types (all considered variants of squamous cell carcinoma): traditional squamous cell carcinoma, nonkeratinizing carcinoma, and undifferentiated carcinoma. Metastasis to the neck is common. Nasopharyngeal carcinoma is treated primarily with radiation, but surgery is required for biopsy and radical resection in isolated cases.

d. Other cancers of the nasopharynx include adenocarcinoma, salivary malignancies, soft-tissue sarcomas, melanoma, lymphoma, and neuroendocrine tumors.

H. Sinus disease

1. **Rhinosinusitis** is a clinical diagnosis based on symptoms (rhinorrhea, postnasal drip, headache, fever, nasal congestion, and facial pressure) and duration of disease (acute, <1month; subacute, 1 to 3 months; chronic, >3 months).

2. **Acute bacterial sinusitis** is characterized by facial pain and pressure, fever, dental pain, nasal congestion, and rhinorrhea. It is usually a short-lived infection often preceded by a nonspecific upper respiratory tract infection. The most common culprits are *Streptococcus pneumoniae, M. catarrhalis,* and *H. influenza.* Treatment consists of antibiotics, decongestants, mucolytic agents, humidification, and hydration. The natural history is resolution within 2 weeks, but clinicians should watch for intraorbital or intracranial complications.

3. **Chronic bacterial sinusitis** is defined as sinonasal infection for >3 months. The predominate symptoms are halitosis, postnasal drip, headache, cough, facial pressure, and nasal airway obstruction. Systemic signs such as fever are usually absent. The disease is a result of obstruction at the **osteomeatal complex** (common drainage pathway in the middle meatus of the frontal, maxillary, and ethmoid sinuses), along with infection. Inhalant allergies, ciliary dysfunction, immune deficiencies, or structural obstruction also contribute. Treatment consists of a 3- to 4-week course of antibiotics, decongestants, nasal and systemic steroids, mucolytic agents, and nasal saline lavages. CT scans even after maximizing medical therapy can demonstrate mucosal thickening, air-fluid levels, or cysts in the sinuses. Endoscopic sinus surgery may be indicated to reestablish the patency of the sinus ostia, ventilate the sinuses, and remove diseased mucosa or polyps.

4. **Fungal sinusitis** is classified as allergic fungal sinusitis, mycetoma (fungus ball), or invasive fungal sinusitis. Invasive fungal sinusitis usually involves *Mucor* organisms and is a disease of debilitated, diabetic, or immunocompromised patients. Treatment includes intravenous antifungals and surgical débridement of nonviable tissue.

I. Nasal-sinus trauma

1. **Nasal fractures** are the result of blunt facial trauma. Nondisplaced fractures without cosmetic deformity require no further intervention. Displaced fractures produce cosmetic changes and nasal obstruction. These require closed or open reduction.

2. **Septal hematomas** may occur with any nasal trauma. Blood collects between the mucoperichondrium and cartilage of the nasal septum. Because the cartilage relies on the overlying tissues for its blood supply, the hematoma causes cartilage necrosis and septal perforation. Treatment is incision and drainage.

3. **Midface fractures** are usually classified according to the **Le Fort system.**
Le Fort I fractures involves the lower midface. The fracture line runs
through the lower maxilla and into the nasal cavity. Le Fort II fractures
pass through the anterior wall of the maxillary sinus, the inferior orbital
rim, and the floor of the orbit and across the nose to the contralateral
side. Fractures of the cribriform plate may occur. Le Fort III (craniofacial
dissociation) fractures involve the zygomatic arch, the lateral orbital wall,
the floor of the orbit, and the nose to the contralateral side. These are often
associated with intracranial injuries. Midface fractures with cosmetic
or functional deformities require open reduction and internal fixation
with commercially available plating systems. Control of the airway is
important in the acute setting. Transnasal intubation or tracheostomy
may be required.

III. **Salivary glands**

A. **Anatomy and physiology**

1. **The major salivary glands** include the parotid, submandibular, and sublingual glands. Hundreds of minor salivary glands exist in the palate,
oral mucosa, and tongue.

a. The **parotid gland** is the largest of the salivary glands. Its secretions
are primarily serous, and it is the dominant producer of saliva during
mastication. It lies anterior to the ear on the surface of the masseter
muscle. The tail of the parotid lies inferior to the angle of the mandible
extending onto the sternocleidomastoid muscle. The parotid is divided
into a superficial and deep lobe by the extracranial branches of the
facial nerve. This is a division of surgical convenience, not an true
anatomic division. The parotid duct (Stensen duct) exits the anterior
portion of the gland running parallel to the buccal branch of the facial
nerve. It crosses the masseter, pierces the buccinator, and enters the
oral cavity adjacent to the second maxillary molar.

b. The **submandibular (submaxillary) gland** lies just inferior and medial
to the mandible. It produces a mixture of mucinous and serous saliva
and produces the majority of baseline saliva when masticating is not
occurring. Its anterior portion wraps around the posterior edge of the
mylohyoid muscle and extends toward the sublingual gland. The submandibular duct (Wharton duct) exits the anterosuperior part of the
gland to enter the floor of mouth just lateral to the frenulum of the
tongue.

c. The **sublingual gland** lies below the floor of the mouth mucosa. Its
multiple ducts enter directly into the floor of the mouth and secrete
primarily mucinous saliva.

2. The paired parotid, submandibular, and sublingual glands supply 1 to 1.5
liters of **saliva** per day. Saliva provides lubrication during mastication,
inhibits bacterial growth, helps maintain dental health, and contains
some digestive enzymes.

B. **Diagnostic tests.** Radiographic studies may be used to evaluate salivary
gland pathology. Plain films can identify salivary calculi. Contrast sialog-
raphy (placing contrast material in the ductal system of the parotid or submandibular gland) has been largely replaced by CT scan with contrast.
Fine-needle biopsies of mass lesions are both sensitive and specific in the
diagnosis salivary neoplasms.

C. **Inflammatory diseases of the salivary glands**

1. **Acute sialadenitis** is defined as acute inflammation of the salivary glands
and usually involves the parotid gland. It typically affects elderly, diabetic, immunocompromised, or dehydrated individuals. Typically of bacterial origin, *S. aureus* is usual culprit. The involved gland is firm and
tender, with purulent exudate emanating from its duct. Pain generally increases with mastication. The treatment includes hydration, antibiotics,
and sialogogues. Abscess formation requires surgical drainage. When
draining parotid abscesses, care must be taken to avoid the facial nerve.

2. **Chronic sialadenitis** is characterized by recurrent episodes of parotid or submandibular swelling. The gland becomes fibrotic and firm, and treatment is surgical removal. Branches of the facial nerve are at increased risk owing to surrounding inflammation and scar.

3. **Mumps** is a childhood viral disease that can involve the parotid glands bilaterally. It produces acute swelling and tenderness but generally resolves with supportive measures. The incubation period is 2 to 3 weeks, and one episode usually results in lifelong immunity.

4. **Obstructive salivary gland disease.** The most frequent cause of salivary gland obstruction is a ductal calculus (**sialolithiasis**). Saliva contains calcium and phosphate salts, which may precipitate to form salivary stones. Sudden swelling and pain of the involved gland is worsened by eating. These stones occur most commonly in the submandibular duct. Most are radiopaque and many can be palpated in the floor of the mouth within the duct. Distal stones may be removed through the mouth, while those closer to the hilum of the gland require removal of the gland itself.

5. **Systemic disease.** Parotid enlargement may occur with starvation, bulimia, cirrhosis of the liver, hypothyroidism, diabetes, menopause, and Cushing disease. Gland enlargement may also occur with ingestion of iodides, lead, copper, and phenothiazines. Cystic parotomegaly is also seen in HIV/AIDS.

D. **Trauma.** Facial lacerations can involve the parotid parenchyma, the Stensen duct, and branches of the facial nerve. Loss of facial function mandates exploration and epineural repair of the nerve. Injury to the parotid duct requires repair of the duct over a stent. **Sialoceles** typically resolve with pressure dressings and intermittent needle aspiration.

E. **Tumors.** Patients presenting with salivary gland mass lesions should be worked up for neoplasms. Workup may require imaging, fine-needle aspiration, or excisional biopsy for diagnosis. It is important to remember that lymphadenopathy may simulate a salivary neoplasm.

1. **Benign tumors.** Approximately 80% of parotid tumors, 50% of submandibular tumors, and 25% of minor salivary gland tumors are benign. **Pleomorphic adenoma** is the most common of all salivary gland tumors, followed by **Warthin tumor** (cystadenoma lymphomatosum). Pleomorphic adenomas grow slowly over many years and are painless. Facial nerve palsy is rare. Histologically, they have a pseudocapsule with microscopic extensions of tumor into the surrounding gland parenchyma. Therapy is a superficial parotidectomy rather than enucleation because the latter is associated with high recurrence rates. Lymphoepithelial cysts may be seen in HIV patients and are typically bilateral. Diagnosis can be made with fine-needle aspiration.

2. **Malignant tumors.** Approximately 20% of parotid tumors, 50% of submandibular tumors, and 75% of minor salivary gland tumors are malignant. **Mucoepidermoid carcinoma** is the most common malignancy of the parotid gland and is the most common salivary gland malignancy overall. Mucoepidermoid carcinomas are classified as low grade (well-differentiated, large mucinous component) or high grade (poorly differentiated, large epidermoid component). Treatment is surgical excision, with postoperative radiation reserved for high-grade lesions. **Adenoid cystic carcinoma** is a high-grade malignancy with a propensity for perineural spread and distant metastases. Treatment is radical resection followed by radiation therapy. Long-term follow-up is required because these tumors often recur years after the initial resection. Other high-grade malignancies include **adenocarcinoma, malignant-mixed tumor,** and **squamous cell carcinoma. Acinic cell carcinoma** is classified as a low-grade malignancy. Lymphomas and metastatic skin cancer to intra- and periparotid nodes should also be considered in the differential diagnosis.

IV. **Larynx**
   A. **Anatomy and physiology**
      1. The larynx is a critical part of the aerodigestive tract and contributes to airway protection, deglutition, and phonation. It is divided into the **supraglottis, glottis, and subglottis.** The **epiglottis, arytenoid cartilages, aryepiglottic folds, and false vocal folds** compose the supraglottis. The **ventricle** separates the false and true vocal folds. The glottis is 1 cm in height starting rostrally at the horizontal plane running through the apex of the ventricle. The "glottis" includes a portion of the airway immediately below the true vocal folds. The subglottis then extends from this point to the inferior margin of the cricoid cartilage. The rigid support of the larynx consists of the **thyroid and cricoid cartilages** and the **hyoid bone.** The cricoid cartilage is the only complete ring in the airway. Laryngeal elevation, glottic closure, and retroflexion of the epiglottis help prevent aspiration.
      2. The **superior laryngeal nerve** provides sensory innervation to the larynx superior to the glottis, and its external branch provides motor innervation to the cricothyroid muscle. The **recurrent laryngeal nerve** is sensory to the rest of the larynx and is motor to all intrinsic laryngeal muscles. Both are derived from the vagus nerve.
   B. **Congenital laryngeal abnormalities**
      1. **Laryngomalacia** is the most common congenital laryngeal abnormality. An omega-shaped epiglottis and floppy arytenoid towers prolapse into the airway on inspiration. Inspiratory stridor generally worsens for the first 18 months before beginning to improve. If respiratory or feeding difficulties result in failure to thrive, an endoscopic supraglottoplasty is recommended.
      2. The second most common laryngeal abnormality in the newborn is **vocal cord paralysis.** These are often idiopathic but may be related to CNS malformations such as the Arnold-Chiari malformation. Most cases resolve spontaneously, but CNS lesions may require CSF shunts or posterior fossa decompression. Treatment varies based on symptoms and may include tracheostomy.
      3. Other congenital laryngeal abnormalities include laryngeal atresia, stenoses, webs, cysts, laryngeal clefts, and **subglottic stenosis.** Subglottic stenosis is characterized as congenital or acquired and graded by both the residual airway lumen and the craniocaudal length of the stenosis. Surgical laryngotracheal reconstruction or cricotracheal resection are options when dealing with this disease.
   C. **Trauma**
      1. **Blunt or penetrating laryngeal trauma** requires rapid airway assessment and control. This may require intubation or an awake tracheostomy under local anesthesia. Diagnostic modalities include fiberoptic laryngoscopy, high-resolution CT scan, and operative endoscopy. Laryngeal hematomas and small lacerations are managed conservatively with airway observation and humidified air. Displaced fractures and laryngeal instability require urgent tracheostomy followed by open reduction and internal fixation. All mucosal lacerations should be reapproximated, and the larynx may require prolonged stenting.
      2. **Caustic ingestions** can be classified by the type of material ingested. Alkali ingestions result in liquefactive necrosis of the laryngeal suprastructure, pharynx, and esophagus and put the patient at risk for stenosis. Acidic materials cause coagulative necrosis. Endoscopy is recommended 24 to 48 hours after ingestion. Initial therapy includes NG tube placement and high-dose systemic steroids. Strictures occur. These are assessed with barium swallow studies and may require periodic esophageal dilation.
   D. **Inflammation.** Infectious laryngitis is classified as acute or chronic. **Viral laryngitis** is common and generally resolves within 5 days. Treatment is

supportive. **Bacterial laryngitis** (*S. pneumoniae, Streptococcus pyogenes, H. influenzae,* and *M. catarrhalis*) is often associated with pharyngotonsillitis or sinusitis and generally requires antibiotic therapy. Supraglottitis (**epiglottitis**) in children is a medical emergency. Caused primarily by *H. influenzae* type B in the past, the use of HIB vaccine has significantly decreased its incidence. In adults, infection usually involves the entire supraglottis. The severity and time course of the patient's symptoms determines the level of intervention required and the outcome. Those with rapid deterioration within 8 to 12 hours often require intubation or tracheostomy. Other inflammatory lesions within the larynx include sulcus vocalis, contact ulcers, vocal nodules, and granulomas.

E. **Tumors**
   1. Laryngeal growths can cause hoarseness, dyspnea, stridor, dysphagia, odynophagia, and a persistent cough. **Benign tumors** of the larynx are uncommon. **Recurrent respiratory papillomatosis** is the most common benign tumor of the larynx. Human papillomavirus is implicated and is thought to be contracted from the mother during vaginal delivery. Treatment involves repeated débridement with the carbon dioxide laser or laryngeal microdebrider. Tracheostomy is required for severe airway compromise but should be avoided if possible, as it is thought to seed the lower airway with papilloma. Other benign laryngeal tumors include oncocytic papillary cystadenoma, granular cell tumors, lymphangiomas, paragangliomas, and soft-tissue tumors such as fibromas and chondromas.
   2. **Laryngeal cancer** is the second most common head and neck malignancy, and **squamous cell carcinoma** (SCCA) accounts for roughly 90% of all laryngeal cancers. The major risk factors for developing SCCA are tobacco and alcohol abuse. Precancerous lesions include hyperkeratosis, hyperplasia, and various grades of dysplasia. The definitive diagnosis requires a **laryngoscopy and biopsy.** Patients with large, bulky cancers may need a tracheostomy prior to general anesthesia. A CT scan with contrast is important for delineating preepiglottic or paraglottic spread, spread to adjacent structures such as the base of tongue, destruction of laryngeal cartilages, and extension into the neck (cervical adenopathy). Staging is via the American Joint Committee on Cancer system. The treatment of laryngeal cancers depends on the site, stage, and functional status of the patient. Small cancers can be treated with radiotherapy, with endoscopic excision, or via limited open techniques such as laryngofissure with cordectomy. For larger lesions, a vertical hemilaryngectomy, a supraglottic laryngectomy, or a supracricoid laryngectomy may be indicated. The most definitive option is a total laryngectomy with creation of a tracheoesophageal speech fistula. Early-stage lesions may be treated with a single modality (radiation or surgery), but more advanced tumors require multimodality treatment (surgery with postoperative radiation or chemoradiation with surgical salvage). Subglottic cancers are rare. These require a total laryngectomy with thyroidectomy, an ipsilateral neck dissection at a minimum, and postoperative radiation therapy.

F. **Other laryngeal disorders**
   1. A variety of **neuromuscular disorders** affect the larynx. Those discussed here include myasthenia gravis, recurrent laryngeal nerve dysfunction, and focal laryngeal dystonias.
   2. Patients with **myasthenia gravis** develop vocal fatigue and breathiness with prolonged voice use. This is a systemic disease characterized by impaired transmission of impulses at the neuromuscular junction. Concurrent dysfunction of pharyngeal muscles can cause dysphagia and aspiration.
   3. The **recurrent laryngeal nerve** innervates all intrinsic laryngeal muscles. The thyroarytenoid (TA) and lateral cricoarytenoid (LCA) muscles are the primary adductors of the vocal cords, and the posterior cricoarytenoid

(PCA) muscle is the sole abductor. Vocal cord paralysis due to recurrent laryngeal nerve dysfunction can result from pulmonary or other neoplasms along the course of the vagus nerve, iatrogenic nerve injury during surgery, and trauma. Recognized iatrogenic injuries should be repaired by primary epineural anastomosis or cable grafting. Patients presenting with a new diagnosis of vocal cord paralysis require a CT scan of the neck and chest along with an MRI of the head to trace the entire intracranial, neck, and thoracic course of the vagus nerve. Treatment of unilateral vocal cord paralysis starts with observation and speech therapy. Recovery or accommodation may take place. Laryngeal electromyography (LEMG) helps facilitate surgical planning by attempting to predict an individual's likelihood of recovering vocal cord function over time. Surgical options include injection laryngoplasty (with Gelfoam, fat, or Cymetra), medialization of the vocal cord (type I thyroplasty with or without arytenoid adduction), and laryngeal reinnervation. Treatment options for patients with bilateral vocal cord paralysis include endoscopic or open arytenoidectomy, endoscopic cordectomy, and tracheostomy.

   4. **Spasmodic dysphonia** is a type of **focal laryngeal dystonia.** The adductor type produces a strained voice with frequent breaks, and the less common abductor type results in a breathy voice. Both produce vocal fatigue. The pathophysiology of spasmodic dysphonia is unknown. Treatment options include muscle relaxants and recurrent laryngeal nerve sectioning, but the present treatment of choice is selective Botox injection into laryngeal musculature.

V. **The neck**
   A. **Anatomy and physiology.** The neck is divided into **anterior and posterior triangles.** The anterior (viscerovascular) triangle is anterior to the sternocleidomastoid, inferior to the mandible, and superior to the clavicle, while the posterior triangle is posterior to the sternocleidomastoid and anterior to the trapezius. Key fascial layers define various compartments within each triangle. The **superficial fascia** invests the platysma muscle. The **deep fascia** is divided into three layers. The **superficial layer of the deep fascia** is deep to the platysma and invests the strap muscles, sternocleidomastoid, and trapezius. This layer also invests the parotid and submandibular glands. The **middle layer of the deep fascia** surrounds the visceral compartment containing the aerodigestive tract and thyroid gland. The **deep layer of the deep fascia** encloses the vertebral column and its associated musculature. All three layers of the deep fascia contribute to the **carotid sheath.** The carotid sheath contains the carotid artery, the internal jugular vein, the vagus nerve, and the ansa cervicalis.
      There is an extensive network of superficial and deep lymphatics and lymph nodes throughout the head and neck. The neck is divided into six lymphatic levels. The submental and submandibular nodes are in level I, levels II to IV parallel the jugular vein, level V is in the posterior triangle, and level VI is the central compartment medial to the carotid artery. The retropharyngeal nodes also form a distinct nodal group.
   B. **Congenital lesions**
      1. **Thyroglossal duct cysts.** The thyroid forms between the tuberculum impar and the hypobranchial eminence. It descends caudally from the foramen cecum and reaches its normal position anterior to the first three tracheal rings by week 7 of gestation. As the gland descends, the thyroglossal duct behind it is obliterated by week 10. Persistence of the duct may give rise to cystic (essentially midline) masses at any point from the foramen cecum of the tongue to the thyroid gland itself. These sometimes enlarge during upper respiratory tract infections or may get infected. Prior to resection, the surgeon must make sure that the given cyst is not the patient's only functioning thyroid tissue. This can be ascertained by physical exam and a thyroid (nuclear medicine) scan. The cyst is excised surgically using the Sistrunk procedure, which involves

resecting the mass, a central portion of the hyoid bone, and a small block of the tongue base.

2. **Branchial anomalies.** Persistence of any portion of the branchial apparatus results in a cyst (most common), a sinus, or a fistula. A cyst is an epithelium-lined structure with no external or visceral connection, a sinus is a tract that has an internal or external opening, and a fistula is a connection from the upper digestive tract to the skin (two openings). **First branchial anomalies** usually present as painless swellings in the region of the parotid gland, ear, or high sternocleidomastoid muscle. There are type I and type II first branchial anomalies, and these differ in type of tissue present within the anomaly, location and direction of the tract, and its relationship to the facial nerve. **Second branchial anomalies** are the most common. These anomalies course from the tonsillar fossa deep to the stylohyoid ligament, superficial to cranial nerves IX and XII, between the internal and external carotid arteries, and open to the skin anterior to the sternocleidomastoid muscle. **Third branchial fistulas** connect the pyriform sinus to the skin. The tract is deep to both the internal and external carotid arteries, deep to cranial nerve IX, and superficial to cranial nerve XII. The tract pierces the thyrohyoid membrane above the internal branch of the superior laryngeal nerve to open into the pyriform sinus. **Management** of these lesions requires complete excision. Infected branchial anomalies require antibiotics or even incision and drainage to resolve the infection prior to any attempts at resection.

3. **Cystic hygroma** is an older term for a macrocystic lymphatic malformations of the head and neck. These masses are soft, compressible, and usually nontender unless complicated by infection or hemorrhage. MRI is the imaging modality of choice, and surgical resection is the preferred therapy. Care is taken to preserve all vital neural and vascular structures during surgery even if it means performing a subtotal resection.

4. **Teratomas and dermoid cysts.** Teratomas are composed of ectoderm, mesoderm, and endoderm while dermoids contain ectoderm and mesoderm. Tissues within these masses can have varying degrees of differentiation and are sometimes found on preterm ultrasound.

C. **Infections**

1. Facial compartments in the head and neck can develop **deep neck space infections.** While a dental source is most common, these can also result from trauma, tonsillitis, or suppuration of lymph nodes. **Ludwig angina** is inflammation in the sublingual and submandibular spaces. These patient are toxic, presenting with a firm floor of mouth and retrusion of the tongue. Emergency airway control and incision with drainage is required. An abscess is rarely found, and the histology is more consistent with fasciitis. Peritonsillar, parapharyngeal, and retropharyngeal abscesses are discussed in later sections.

2. **Cervical lymphadenopathy** may be caused by viruses, bacteria, or fungi. Viral infections of the upper respiratory tract caused by adenoviruses, rhinoviruses, and enteroviruses are the most common cause of acute infectious cervical lymphadenopathy. **Infectious mononucleosis,** due to the Epstein-Barr virus, causes bilateral cervical lymphadenopathy along with prolonged malaise and myalgia in adolescents and young adults. Cytomegalovirus, herpes viruses, and the human immunodeficiency virus can also cause cervical lymphadenopathy. Group A streptococci and *S. aureus* account for the majority of bacterial lymphadenitis. Oral antibiotics usually suffice, but abscess formation requires incision and drainage. Lymphadenopathy may also be caused by *Mycobacterium tuberculosis* (**scrofula**) or atypical mycobacteria such as *Mycobacterium avium-intracellulare.* **Cat-scratch disease,** due to *Rochalimaea henselae,* also causes prolonged cervical adenopathy, but its course is self-limited. Fungi are a rare cause of lymphadenopathy. **Histoplasmosis, blastomycosis, aspergillosis, and coccidioidomycosis** may occur in

immunocompetent individuals, whereas mucormycosis and cryptococcosis cause severe disease in the immunocompromised.

D. Neoplasms

1. **Benign neoplasms** in the neck include hemangiomas, lymphangiomas, fibromas, lipomas, schwannomas, neurofibromas, and paragangliomas.

   a. **Paragangliomas** arise from the paraganglionic cells of the autonomic nervous system. These are classified as jugulotympanic, vagal, sinonasal, laryngeal, and carotid body tumors. Ten percent are multicentric, and while usually benign, approximately 10% are malignant. Patients with a family history of these lesions tend to have more multicentric and malignant lesions. Histologically, there are clusters of epithelial cells (Zellballen) surrounded by sustentacular cells. Although <3% of these paragangliomas produce catecholamines, all patients should be screened by measuring urine catecholamines. Angiography is the most definitive diagnostic technique and allows for embolization prior to surgical excision (within 24 to 48 hours). Surgery is the preferred treatment modality, but those unable to tolerate the procedure can undergo radiotherapy.

   b. **Schwannomas** are tumors derived from the Schwann cells of peripheral nerves. They can develop in the neck from various cranial nerves, the cervical sensory plexus, the cervical sympathetic chain, or the brachial plexus.

   c. **Neurofibromas** also arise from peripheral nerves and are usually associated with neurofibromatosis type I. These may form massive plexiform accumulations in the neck.

2. **Malignant neck masses.** A persistent neck mass in an adult must be considered malignant until proven otherwise. These neck masses are generally metastatic squamous cell carcinoma from the upper aerodigestive tract. Distant primaries account for <10% of cases, and in <5% of cases no known primary tumor is ever found. Once the patient develops cervical metastasis from an aerodigestive tract primary, overall survival drops by approximately 50%. Primary tumors arising in the neck are less common but include lymphoma, soft-tissue sarcomas, thyroid carcinoma, salivary gland carcinoma, and neuroendocrine malignancies. Each patient deserves a systematic approach to diagnosis and management.

   The patient evaluation begins with a thorough history and physical examination focusing on the head and neck. Symptoms, their duration, a history of tobacco and alcohol use, weight loss, a history of occupational exposures, otalgia (ear pain), and a history of radiation exposure must be ascertained. A thorough office head-and-neck exam includes otoscopy, anterior rhinoscopy, visualization and palpation of the oral cavity, palpation of the base of tongue, fiberoptic nasopharyngoscopy and laryngoscopy, and a thorough palpation of the neck. Suspicious primary lesions should be biopsied, and neck masses should undergo fine-needle aspiration with cytology (and culture if necessary). The initial radiographic test of choice is a CT scan with contrast. Other helpful imaging modalities include ultrasound, nuclear medicine scans, MRI, a positron emission tomography (PET) scan, and angiography as needed. Most surgeons elect to perform a laryngoscopy and esophagoscopy under general anesthesia to both diagnose and describe the lesion in question and look for synchronous tumors. These initial staging procedures also help in planning the definitive management of the patient. Neck masses with no discernable primary tumor on laryngoscopy require a tonsillectomy and directed biopsies of the nasopharynx, base of tongue, and pyriform sinuses. A primary tumor may be found in up to 30% of these biopsies. Treatment options vary by tumor site, stage, and patient comorbidities. Options often include surgery with or without radiation as well as primary chemoradiation with surgical salvage. Tumor resections can be highly disfiguring and compromise speech, respiration, and swallowing to varying degrees. Therefore, treatment must be tailored to the lesion, the individual's overall performance status, and the wishes of the patient.

VI. Oral cavity and pharynx

   A. Anatomy and physiology. The oral cavity extends from the vermilion border of the lips to a ring formed by the circumvallate papillae of the tongue, the anterior tonsillar pillars, and the junction of the hard and soft palates. It includes the lips, buccal mucosa, oral tongue, floor of mouth, hard palate, alveolar ridges, and retromolar trigone. The oropharynx starts at the soft palate and includes the soft palate, tongue posterior to the circumvallate papillae, the tonsils, the posterior tonsillar pillars, the posterior and lateral oropharyngeal walls, and the vallecula. The oral cavity's general sensory innervation is from cranial nerve V, and the chorda tympani and cranial nerve IX provide taste information from the tongue. General sensory information from the oropharynx is transmitted by cranial nerve IX. The blood supply to the oral cavity and oropharynx arises from branches of the external carotid artery, including the ascending pharyngeal artery, lingual artery, and internal maxillary artery. The muscles of mastication are innervated by cranial nerve V. The hypopharynx has three divisions, including the piriform sinuses bilaterally, the postcricoid region, and the posterior hypopharyngeal wall. The hypopharynx is continuous with the cervical esophagus through the upper esophageal sphincter (cricopharyngeus muscle). With the exception of the stylopharyngeus (innervated by cranial nerve IX), the pharyngeal constrictors are innervated by cranial nerve X. Swallowing is a complex task involving soft palate elevation, elevation and retrusion of the tongue, laryngeal elevation, glottic closure, epiglottic retroflexion, and pharyngeal/esophageal peristalsis.

   B. Congenital issues
      1. A variety of congenital abnormalities can affect the **oral cavity and pharynx.** Detailed discussion of these lesions is beyond the scope of this chapter, but a few congenital lesions deserve mention. The Pierre-Robin sequence includes micrognathia, glossoptosis, and a U-shaped cleft. Airway obstruction and feeding difficulties ensue but can be treated with prone positioning, glossopexy, mandibular advancement, closure of the cleft palate, or tracheostomy. A variety of syndromes such as Apert craniosynostosis, Crouzon craniosynostosis, Treacher Collins syndrome, and velocardiofacial syndrome may also create breathing and swallowing problems through midface abnormalities. Treatments vary based on cause.
      2. Cleft lip and palate. Clefts form as a result of developmental fusion abnormalities of the midface skeleton and soft tissues. They are categorized as cleft lip, cleft palate, or combined cleft lip and palate. Clefts may be complete or incomplete, unilateral or bilateral, and can involve the primary or secondary palate (or both). The primary and secondary palates are separated anatomically by the incisive foramen. The cause is multifactorial, and clefts are often associated with named syndromes. Patients with cleft lip and palate deformities should be managed by a multidisciplinary cleft team that addresses feeding, hearing, respiratory, cosmetic, speech, and psychosocial issues. Cleft lips are usually closed during the first year of life, and cleft palate surgery is undertaken between 6 months and 2 years of life. These procedures are staged and may require a variety of cosmetic "touch-ups" as the child ages.

   C. Trauma. Midface fractures were addressed in Section II.I. Patients with **mandible fractures** present with pain, malocclusion, trismus (inability to open the mouth), loose teeth, intraoral lacerations, and varying degrees of sensory loss over the ipsilateral lower lip and chin. Concomitant injuries to the C-spine, intracranial contents, eyes, and midface should be ruled out, and imaging with a Panorex (panoramic plain film), a mandible series, or a CT scan is necessary. Treatment requires stabilization of the fractured segments. Patients may be treated initially in the emergency room with antibiotics and an antiseptic mouthwash (Peridex), but these injuries should be repaired within 7 to 10 days. Closed reduction with maxillary-mandibular wiring is one treatment option. However, such interdental wiring must be maintained for 4 to 8 weeks (depending on age and extent of injury). Open reduction and internal fixation (ORIF) with plates and screws allows for precise anatomic fracture reduction, immediate removal of interdental wires, and early mobilization of the jaw. The patient can resume a soft diet immediately after surgery. ORIF is now the preferred means of fracture repair, and a variety of plating systems are commercially available. Complications of mandible fracture repair include infection, nonunion, malunion, temporomandibular joint ankylosis, and persistent malocclusion.

D. Infections

1. **Ulcers** in the oral cavity are common and usually related to viral infections, nutritional deficiencies, or glandular changes. Treatment is generally supportive, although a variety of oral rinses are available containing antifungals, antihistamines, antibiotics, steroids, and coating agents.

2. **Pharyngotonsillitis** may be caused by a virus or bacteria. Although viral causes are more common, it is important to screen for β-hemolytic streptococci. Fever, a sore throat, and otalgia are common presenting symptoms, and the physical exam reveals swollen, erythematous tonsils with or without exudate. Other infectious diseases to consider in the differential diagnosis are diphtheria, infectious mononucleosis, Vincent angina, candidiasis, syphilis, gonococcal pharyngitis, and tuberculosis. A **peritonsillar abscess** ("quinsy") occurs immediately lateral to the tonsil, most often at its superior pole. These are generally unilateral, and the classic symptoms include a severe sore throat, varying degrees of trismus, difficulty controlling secretions, a muffled "hot potato voice," and a fever. The physical exam reveals a bulging erythematous tonsil and soft palate with uvular deviation. Treatment includes hydration, incision and drainage, antibiotics, and oral care. Young children may require general anesthesia during the draining of these abscesses. The risk of recurrence is 10% to 15%, and some physicians advocate immediate (quinsy) or delayed tonsillectomy as definitive treatment.

3. **Retropharyngeal abscesses** occur primarily in children. The lymph nodes in the retropharyngeal space suppurate as a result of an upper respiratory tract infection. Symptoms include a sore, stiff neck and throat; odynophagia; dysphagia; and systemic signs of infection. Examination shows a posterior pharyngeal bulge, but it can be missed if not specifically sought. Lateral soft-tissue films are helpful, but a CT scan better delineates the lesion. A chest radiograph is mandatory to look for evidence of mediastinitis. Incision and drainage in the operating room and intravenous antibiotics constitute the treatment of choice. Airway management should always be considered during the diagnostic and treatment plan.

4. **Parapharyngeal space abscesses** occur between the skull base and the hyoid immediately lateral to the pharynx. Referred otalgia and trismus can be severe. The infection may initially arise in the tonsils or from poor dentition but spreads quickly. Therefore, extension from another head and neck fascial compartment (retropharyngeal, peritonsillar, masticator, parotid, submandibular, or sublingual) is not uncommon. Timely intervention avoids complications such as cranial neuropathies, thrombosis of the internal jugular vein, airway compromise, and sepsis. Intravenous antibiotics and surgical drainage are indicated.

E. Tumors

1. **Benign tumors** of the oral cavity and pharynx include papillomas, hemangiomas, lymphatic malformations, mucous cysts, benign salivary gland neoplasms, and dental lesions. Premalignant changes include leukoplakia (white hyperkeratotic patches) and erythroplakia (velvet red patches).

2. **Malignancies** of the oral cavity and pharynx are categorized by site of origin and histology of tumor. The oral cavity is divided into subsites, including the lips (vermilion), buccal mucosa, alveolar ridges, retromolar trigone, hard palate, anterior tongue, and floor of mouth. Being that these sites are contiguous, tumors originating in one area spread easily to others and can require complex surgical resections of mucosa, soft tissues, and even bone. Squamous cell carcinoma and its variants account for the majority of oral cavity malignancies. Other cancers include salivary gland malignancies, basal cell carcinomas on the lips, melanomas, and soft-tissue sarcomas. Regional spread can involve perifacial, submental, submandibular, jugular chain, or retropharyngeal nodes depending of the lesion type, site of origin, and depth of invasion. These malignancies usually present as nonhealing painful ulcers and require an incisional biopsy to make the diagnosis. For small lesions, radiation and surgery demonstrate equivalent survival rates, whereas larger tumors require multimodality treatment. Mohs micrographic surgery is popular for the treatment of lip cancers, and a variety of reconstruction techniques exist to repair the residual defects.

3. **Cancers of the oropharynx, tongue base, and hypopharynx** tend to be particularly aggressive. Patients often present with odynophagia, trismus, cervical adenopathy, and weight loss. An adequate physical examination requires laryngoscopy and esophagoscopy. CT scans or an MRI help in staging the lesion and planning multimodality therapy. Surgical options include transoral techniques, a mandibular swing, a lateral pharyngotomy, or a suprahyoid pharyngotomy. Because of the proximity to the larynx, varying degrees of laryngectomy may be required to achieve oncologic margins. New endoscopic CO_2 laser techniques for resection can help decrease the surgical morbidity of these lesions by avoiding external incisions and preserving normal tissue. Reconstruction options for open procedures include healing by secondary intention, skin grafts, pedicled regional flaps, and free tissue transfer.

F. **Sleep apnea**
1. **Pediatric obstructive sleep apnea (OSA)** is characterized by loud snoring and intermittent obstruction to airflow, with continued respiratory effort. It is caused primarily by adenotonsillar hypertrophy, which makes this condition highly treatable with tonsillectomy and adenoidectomy. Consequences of OSA include daytime somnolence, cardiopulmonary dysfunction, bedwetting, night terrors, and behavioral disturbances. Secondary developmental problems of the palate can ensue. The diagnosis is made by history and physical examination but can be confirmed with a formal sleep study.
2. **Adult OSA** is associated with obesity and can result in obstruction to airflow at the palate, oropharynx, or base of tongue. These patients snore loudly and are plagued by daytime hypersomnolence. Long-term cardiopulmonary complications, including pulmonary hypertension and right heart failure, may ensue. The diagnosis is made by sleep study, during which a **respiratory disturbance index (RDI)** is calculated (RDI 5 to 20, mild OSA; 21 to 40, moderate; >40, severe). The location of collapse or obstruction to airflow must be determined clinically during the physical exam. The Müller maneuver involves a flexible fiberoptic examination of the upper airway (looking for the area of collapse) while the patient inspires against a closed mouth and nose. Most patients are treated with CPAP (**continuous positive airway pressure**) during sleep. Those who cannot tolerate CPAP may elect to undergo a variety of surgical procedures, including an uvulopalatopharyngoplasty, tongue base reduction, maxillomandibular advancement, or tracheostomy.

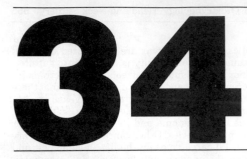

34

Plastic and Hand Surgery

Rodney E. Schmelzer,
Benjamin W. Verdine,
Christopher J. Hussussian,
and Susan E. Mackinnon

Several topics germane to the broad discipline of reconstructive plastic surgery—including wound healing, thermal injury, head and neck surgery, and skin and soft-tissue tumors—are covered in other chapters and so are not reviewed here. Having no specific involvement with a particular organ system or region of the body, plastic surgeons generally concern themselves with the solution of difficult wound healing problems in a way that optimizes form and function. Although specific approaches to select problems are covered, the focus of this chapter is on basic principles that may be applied to a number of surgical issues.

BASIC TECHNIQUES AND PRINCIPLES

I. **The reconstructive ladder.** When considering surgical problems, the simplest approach is often the best approach. This is illustrated by the reconstructive ladder of soft-tissue coverage, in which planning begins with consideration of the least complex alternative (healing by secondary intention) and ends with the most complex (free tissue transfer). The advantage of this approach is that it ensures the existence of alternatives in the case of initial failure.

A. Allowing a wound to heal by **secondary intention** is the simplest approach but is not always feasible. Absolute contraindications include exposed vessels, nerves, tendons, viscera, or bone. Relative contraindications include a large or poorly vascularized wound with a prolonged (>3 weeks) anticipated period of healing and undesirable esthetic consequences.

B. **Primary closure** usually provides the most esthetically pleasing result but can be contraindicated by excessive tension on the skin, which may cause displacement of neighboring structures (e.g., lower eyelid) or necrosis of the skin flaps.

C. **Skin grafting** is the most common method of closure for large wounds. Its use is contraindicated by exposed vessels, nerves, or viscera (except as temporary cover). A healthy bed is required for skin graft take; wound surfaces that do not support skin grafts include bare tendon, bone, or cartilage; radiation-damaged tissue; and any infected wound.

D. **Local tissue transfers** of skin or muscle may be used in regions with convenient tissue nearby. Local flaps become less useful when the wound is in an area without available local tissue (e.g., the distal leg) or when coverage of the wound requires more bulk than is available.

E. **Distant tissue transfers** were the mainstays of difficult wound closure until free flaps were developed. This approach involves the transfer of tissue in staged procedures and has the inherent disadvantages of multiple operations, prolonged wound healing, immobilization for at least 3 weeks, and a limited choice of donor sites.

F. **Free tissue transfer** is the most technically demanding approach to wound closure but has several potential advantages. These include single-stage wound closure, a relatively wide variety of flaps to ensure closure specifically tailored to coverage needs, and, in many cases, a more acceptable esthetic outcome.

II. Types of grafts

A. Skin grafts

1. **Split-thickness grafts** consist of epidermis and a variable thickness of dermis. Skin is composed of two layers, the epidermis and dermis. The epidermis is stratified squamous epithelium consisting primarily of keratinocytes in progressive stages of differentiation. The epidermis has no blood vessels and derives its nutrition by diffusion. The dermis may be further partitioned into a smaller superficial papillary layer and a deeper reticular layer. Thinner grafts (<0.016 inches) have a higher rate of engraftment, whereas thicker grafts, with a greater amount of dermis, are more durable and esthetically acceptable. Common donor sites are the thigh, buttock, and scalp.

2. **Full-thickness grafts** include epidermis and a full layer of dermis. Common donor sites include groin, postauricular, and supraclavicular sites, but the hypothenar eminence and instep of foot can also be used. The donor site is usually closed primarily. These grafts are generally used in areas for which a high priority is placed on the esthetic result (e.g., face and hand). Thinner grafts have greater secondary contraction and do not grow commensurate with the individual. They have less adnexal cells and therefore have variable pigment, less hair, and less sebum, with a proclivity toward dryness and contractures. Full-thickness grafts, with more dermis and the requisite adnexal structures, exhibit less contraction and better cosmesis.

3. Grafts can be meshed in **expansion ratios** from 1.5:1.0 to 6:1. Meshing a graft allows it to cover a wider area and decreases the risk of seroma accumulating under the graft because fluid can escape through the fenestrations. The interstices are covered within 1 week by advancing keratinocytes. However, because the entire area is not covered by dermis, meshed grafts are less durable, and the meshing pattern remains after healing, making them inappropriate for esthetically important areas, such as the face.

4. **Graft healing.** Initial metabolism is supported by imbibition or diffusion of nutrients from the wound bed. Revascularization occurs between days 3 and 5 by ingrowth of recipient vessels into the graft (inosculation). Therefore, for a graft to take, the bed must be well vascularized and free of infection, and the site must be immobilized for a minimum of 3 to 5 days. Prevention of shear forces is particularly important during this period of inosculation. Although bare bone and tendon do not engraft, periosteum and peritenon can support skin grafts, especially if they are first left to form a layer of granulation tissue. Graft failures are most often the result of hematoma, seroma, or shear force prohibiting diffusion and vascular ingrowth.

B. Tendon grafts are used to replace or augment tendons. Preferred donor sites are palmaris longus and plantaris tendons.

C. Bone grafts are used for repair of bony defects. Iliac bone is commonly used for donor cancellous bone, and ribs or outer table of cranium are commonly used for donor cortical bone.

D. Cartilage grafts are used to restore the contour of the ear, nose, and eyelid. Preferred donor sites include costal cartilage, concha of ear, and nasal septum.

E. Nerve grafts are used to repair damaged nerves when primary repair is not feasible. Preferred donor sites include the sural nerve and lateral or medial antebrachial cutaneous nerves. Allogenic nerve grafting has been described using a short course of immunosuppression (*Plast Reconstr Surg* 1992;90:695).

F. Dermal or dermal-fat grafts are used for contour restoration. Preferred donor sites include back, buttock, and groin. The long-term survival of grafted fat is variable but is generally unreliable.

III. Types of flaps. A flap is any tissue that is transferred to another site with an intact blood supply.

A. Classification based on blood supply

    1. Random cutaneous flaps have a blood supply from the dermal and subdermal plexus without a single dominant artery. They generally have a limited length-to-width ratio (usually 3:1), although this varies by anatomic region (e.g., the face has a ratio of up to 5:1). These flaps are usually used locally to cover adjacent tissue defects but can be transferred to a distant site by use of a staged procedure. Depending on the size of the defect to be covered, moving a local tissue flap can create a donor defect, which may require skin grafting. All local flaps are comparatively easier to use with the loose skin of the elderly.

        a. Flaps that rotate around a pivot point include rotation flaps (Fig. 34-1) and transposition flaps (Fig. 34-2). Planning for shortening of the effective length through the arc of rotation is important when designing these flaps. More complex rotation flaps include bilobed flaps (Fig. 34-3) and rhomboid flaps (Fig. 34-4).

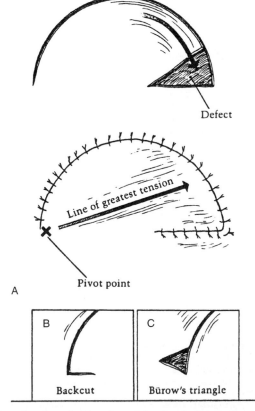

Figure 34-1. Rotation flap. **A:** The edge of the flap is four to five times the length of the base of the defect triangle. **B and C:** A backcut or Bürow triangle can be useful if the flap is under tension.

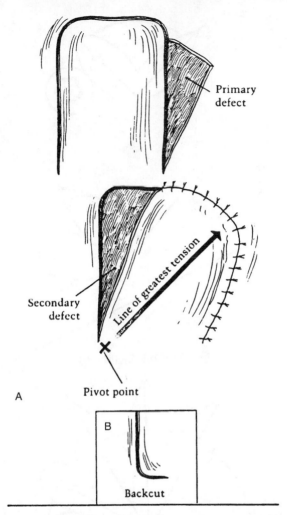

Figure 34-2. A: Transposition flap. The secondary defect is typically covered with a skin graft. **B:** A backcut may be added to reduce tension at the pivot point.

  b. Advancement of skin directly into a defect without rotation can be accomplished with a simple advancement, a V-Y advancement (Fig. 34-5), or a bipedicle advancement flap.
 2. Axial cutaneous flaps contain a single dominant arteriovenous system. This results in a potentially greater length-to-width ratio.
  a. Peninsular flaps are those in which the skin and vessels are moved together as a unit.
  b. Island flaps are those in which the skin is divided from all surrounding tissue but maintained on an isolated, intact vascular pedicle.
  c. Free flaps are those in which the vascular pedicle is isolated and divided. The flap and its pedicle are then moved to a new location and microsurgically anastomosed to vessels at the recipient site, allowing for long-distance transfer of tissue.

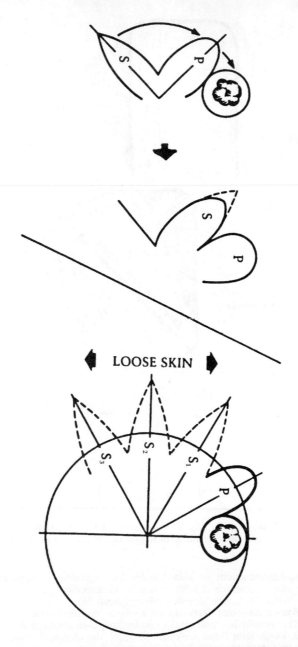

Figure 34-3. Bilobed flap. After the lesion is excised, the primary flap (P) is transposed into the initial defect, and the secondary flap (S) is moved to the site vacated by the primary flap. The bed of the secondary flap is then closed primarily. The primary flap is slightly narrower than the initial defect, whereas the secondary flap is half the width of the primary flap. To be effective, this must be planned in an area where loose skin surrounds the secondary flap site. Three choices for the secondary flap are shown (S_1, S_2, S_3).

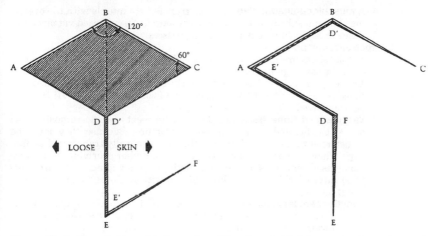

Figure 34-4. Rhomboid or Limberg flap. The rhomboid defect must have 60- and 120-degree angles so that the length of the short diagonal is the same as the length of the sides. The short diagonal is extended by its own length to point E. The line EF is parallel to CD, and they are equal in length. There are four possible Limberg flaps for any rhomboid defect; the flap should be planned in an area where loose skin is available to close the donor defect primarily.

    B. Classification based on tissue type
        1. Cutaneous flaps include the skin and subcutaneous fat. These are generally random flaps because the axial blood supply is deep to the fat.
        2. Fasciocutaneous flaps are axial flaps with a single dominant blood supply contained in the deep fascia along with the overlying fat and skin. A wide variety of fasciocutaneous flaps have been described, but those commonly used include radial forearm, parascapular, lateral arm, and groin flaps. These flaps are often utilized for coverage of mobile structures such as tendons.
        3. Muscle flaps use the specific axial blood supply of a muscle to provide well-vascularized soft-tissue bulk. These flaps can often be transferred with the overlying skin as a myocutaneous flap (see "Basic Techniques and Principles," Section III.B.4). Alternatively, they may be transferred without the overlying skin to fill a cavity or may be covered with a skin graft. Considerations in the transfer of vascularized muscle include the pattern of circulation, arc of rotation, donor-site contour, and donor-site functional defects. Commonly used muscle flaps include the latissimus dorsi, pectoralis major, rectus abdominis, gastrocnemius, soleus, gracilis, tensor fascia lata, trapezius, and gluteus maximus, but any muscle can potentially be transferred as a flap.

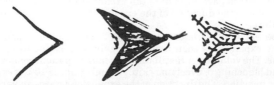

Figure 34-5. V-Y advancement. The skin to the sides of the V is advanced.

4. **A musculocutaneous flap** involves transfer of a muscle with the overlying skin and subcutaneous tissue. The skin is vascularized via myocutaneous or septocutaneous perforating vessels.
   C. **Specialized flaps**
   1. **Fascial flaps** are used when thin, well-vascularized coverage is needed (e.g., for coverage of ear cartilage or the dorsum of the hand or foot). The temporoparietal fascia flap is a classic example, but other fasciocutaneous flaps (see "Basic Techniques and Principles," Section III.B.2) can be transferred without the overlying skin.
   2. **Vascularized bone flaps** are designed to meet specific reconstructive needs, as dictated by loss of bony structure. Because they must be transferred to a specific location, they are generally transferred as free flaps. They may or may not include muscle and/or overlying skin. Commonly used bone flaps include free fibula, scapular spine, iliac (with overlying internal oblique muscle), and rib (with pectoralis major or intercostal muscle).
   3. **Functional muscle** may be transferred with its accompanying dominant nerve. Common functional muscle transfers include transfer of gracilis for restoration of facial movement or latissimus for replacement of biceps function.
   4. **Segmental muscle flaps** can be used when the blood supply to the muscle derives from more than one source. A portion of the muscle is used as a flap, leaving behind a vascularized, innervated, functional muscle, thus minimizing donor-site functional loss. Examples of muscles that can be transferred based on segmental blood supply include the serratus anterior and gluteus maximus.
IV. **Tissue expansion** is a reconstructive technique that uses an inflatable silicone balloon to serially expand surrounding skin. This expansion adjacent to the wound provides donor tissue of similar color, texture, thickness, and sensation, with minimal scar formation and donor-site morbidity. The technique takes advantage of the skin's ability to accommodate a slowly enlarging mass beneath it by increasing its surface area. The idea is to create and develop donor tissue, harvest it, and leave the original donor site preserved.
   A. **The advantages** are that it results in low donor-site morbidity and enables the provision of donor tissue of similar quality to the recipient tissue. It is a versatile technique that is simple and produces robust flaps.
   B. **The disadvantages** are that it is a staged technique, there is a visible deformity during the period of expansion, it requires frequent visits for expansion, and there is a relatively high rate of complications, including infection and extrusion.
   C. **Technique**
   1. **Preoperative planning** involves assessing the defect size, locating matching tissue to be expanded, and deciding where final scars will be.
   2. **Expander placement** is usually performed through an incision at the junction of the lesion and the area of proposed expansion. The length of the incision is controversial, with some proposing one-third the length of the expander (it should be big enough to ensure full pocket creation). The filling port can be incorporated into the expander or placed in a separate pocket. The port may be externalized to minimize anxiety and pain during filling, especially in the pediatric population. There may be advantages to partially filling the expander upon initial placement in that it reduces the duration of the expansion phase and may reduce fold flaw failure.
   3. **The expansion phase** begins 2 to 3 weeks after expander placement. The expander is then inflated weekly with saline using sterile technique. The volume per instillation depends on patient comfort, skin tension, and blanching of overlying skin. A rough guide is 10% of expander volume per injection. The duration of the expansion phase can vary from 6 weeks

to 3 months. Waiting 2 to 3 weeks after the desired volume is achieved allows the expanded skin to soften, decreasing the contraction at the time of flap transposition.
  4. **Removal of expander** is straightforward. However, premature removal may be required secondary to infection, exposure, or rupture.
  5. **The expanded tissue** is usually in the form of a random flap (rotation, advancement, or transposition). If more than one flap is created from expanded tissue, one needs to ensure that all flaps have adequate blood supply.
 D. The **origin of the new tissue** is not completely understood. One potential source is new tissue created in response to the expansion process. Alternatively, tissue may derive from recruitment of adjacent tissues by stretching or creep and by stress relaxation. These possibilities are not mutually exclusive. Studies have shown expansion gives rise to an increase in the thickness of the epidermis, a decrease in the thickness of the dermis, and atrophy of the underlying muscle and fat (*Clin Plast Surg* 1987;14:435).
 E. **Tissue expanders are indicated** in patients in whom flap creation is otherwise not possible. In areas where little suitable tissue is available (e.g., scalp), it can be the esthetically superior option. The patient must be motivated and understand the process. Common indications include burn alopecia, congenital nevi, male pattern baldness, and postmastectomy breast reconstruction.
 F. **Relative contraindications** include malignancy or an open wound, active infection, and unwillingness to comply with multiple procedures. Similarly, tissue expanders cannot be placed under burned tissue, scar, skin graft, or a prior incision. In addition, tissue expanders are less effective in areas that will be irradiated, as the skin in those areas thickens, scars, and contracts, minimizing the degree of expansion possible.
 G. **Complications** include pain, seroma, hematoma (rates widely variable), infection (1% to 5%), exposure or extrusion (5% to 10%) and skin necrosis. Less common complications include striae, resorption of underlying bone, and neurapraxia.

SPECIFIC PROBLEMS IN RECONSTRUCTIVE PLASTIC SURGERY

  I. **Peripheral neuropathy**
  A. **Clinical assessment** of neuropathy requires evaluation of both motor and sensory function as well as electrodiagnostic evaluation of nerve conduction and muscle innervation.
    1. **Standard classification schemes** are available for classification of motor nerve function (Table 34-1). In addition, specific testing of moving or static two-point discrimination, vibration and pressure thresholds, or grip strength may be appropriate.

Table 34-1. Classification of motor function

Grade	Motor function
M0	No contraction
M1	Perceptible contraction in proximal muscles
M2	Perceptible contraction in proximal and distal muscles
M3	All important muscles powerful enough to act against gravity
M4	Muscles act against strong resistance; some independent movement possible
M5	Normal strength and function

Adapted from SE Mackinnon, AL Dellon. *Surgery of the Peripheral Nerve.* New York: Thieme; 1988:118.

Table 34-2. Classification of nerve injuries

Sunderland[a]	Seddon[b]	Structure injured	Prognosis
First degree	Neurapraxia	Schwann cell (demyelination)	Complete recovery within 12 weeks
Second degree	Axonotmesis	Axon (wallerian degeneration)	Complete recovery regeneration 1 mm per day
Third degree		Endoneurium	Incomplete recovery
Fourth degree		Perineurium	No recovery
Fifth degree	Neurotmesis	Epineurium	No recovery
Sixth degree		Mixed injury, neuroma incontinuity[c]	Unpredictable recovery

[a]Sunderland S. A classification of peripheral nerve injuries producing loss of function. *Brain* 1951;74:491.
[b]Seddon HJ. Three types of nerve injury. *Brain* 1943;66:237.
[c]Mackinnon SE. New direction in peripheral nerve surgery *Ann Plast Surg* 1989 Mar;22(3):257–73. [Review]

2. **Diagnostic studies** for quantification of nerve dysfunction include nerve conduction studies (NCSs) and electromyography (EMG). An NCS characterizes the conduction of large-diameter, myelinated nerves, and normal values may be present despite partial nerve injury. NCSs are useful in determining the degree of nerve dysfunction, the presence of segmental demyelination or axonal degeneration, the site of injury, and whether the injury is unifocal, multifocal, or diffuse. EMG samples the action potentials from muscle fibers and can detect individual motor unit potentials, which may indicate early reinnervation, and fibrillations, which represent denervation owing to axonal degeneration.

B. **Acute nerve injury** results from transection, crush, or compression and represents the loss of nerve function distal to the area of injury. Axons are myelinated by Schwann cells and organized into fascicles surrounded by the perineurium. The fascicles are bundled into nerves by the epineurium. The prognosis of injury to a peripheral nerve is dictated by which structures are disrupted. It is important to recognize in the acute setting that an injured nerve may be responsive to stimuli distally for 48 to 72 hours after transection. The severity of nerve injury has been organized into a grading scheme (Table 34-2). Operative repair is indicated for fourth- through sixth-degree injury.

1. **The technique of nerve repair** affects the eventual degree of recovery. Several basic concepts are used to optimize outcome.
   a. **Microsurgical technique** should be used, including magnification and microsurgical instruments and sutures. When conditions allow, a **primary repair** should be performed. The repair should be tension free.
   b. Positioning a limb or digit in extreme flexion or extension to facilitate an end-to-end repair is discouraged because of the joint and ligamentous problems that result. If a tension-free repair cannot be achieved in **neutral position**, transposing the nerve or placing an interposition nerve graft should be used.
   c. An **epineural repair** is typically performed, but a grouped fascicular repair should be performed whenever the internal topography of the nerve is segregated into motor, sensory, or regional components.
   d. **Postoperative motor and sensory reeducation** will help to optimize outcome.
2. **Indications** for peripheral nerve repair include partial or complete transection or in-continuity conduction block. These represent fourth- to sixth-degree nerve injuries and can be difficult to distinguish from

lesser grades of injury based on clinical examination alone. This is
true because all grades of injury can lead to complete loss of function.
Some guidelines for surgical intervention are listed in the following
sections.

a. **Nerves inadvertently divided** during operation are fifth-degree injuries and should be repaired immediately.

b. **Closed-nerve injuries that localize near an anatomically restrictive
site** (e.g., the ulnar nerve at the elbow or the common peroneal nerve at
the knee) can result in neurologic deficit secondary to conduction block
from edema and compression. If no recovery occurs within 3 weeks,
management includes surgical decompression at that site. Iatrogenic
nerve deficit from positioning during long operative procedures is managed similarly.

c. **Closed-nerve injury from blunt trauma or traction** is usually a first-,
second-, or third-degree injury, and full recovery can be expected in
most cases. Patients are closely followed for signs of recovery, including
an advancing Tinel sign, indicating regenerating axons. Baseline NCS
and EMG are obtained at 6 weeks. If there is no evidence of return
of function at 3 months, repeat studies are obtained. If there is no
improvement, the nerve is explored and repaired.

d. **Nerve deficit after sharp trauma** (e.g., a stab wound) usually is the
result of partial or complete transection, and the nerve should be explored and repaired urgently.

e. **Loss of nerve function after gunshot or open blunt trauma** is usually
the result of first- or second-degree injury, and recovery can be expected
in most cases. These cases are usually treated as for closed injuries.
If the nerve is visible or the wound is explored for other reasons (e.g.,
vascular repair), the nerve is explored. If the nerve is in continuity, it
is managed as for a closed injury. If the nerve is not in continuity, it is
usually best to tag the ends of the nerve for ease of identification and
delay definitive repair until the zone of injury to the nerve is clearer
(generally by 3 weeks).

f. **Nerve deficit from compartment syndrome** is treated by emergent
fasciotomy. If decompressed early (within 6 hours), there is usually a
rapid return of function.

g. **Decompression of injured nerves** (e.g., ulnar nerve transposition or
carpal tunnel release) at sites distal to trauma can be useful to avoid
retardation of nerve regeneration across these areas. Multiple sites of
injury or compression can have additive effects, and for first- through
third-degree injuries, decompression can improve outcome.

h. **Division of a sensory nerve** can lead to a painful neuroma as the regenerating axons grow into the surrounding soft tissue. If the resulting
neural deficit results in loss of function or protective sensation, these
nerves can be repaired. If not, the neuroma is excised and the cut
end of the nerve is transposed proximally well away from the wound,
preferably into a nearby muscular environment.

C. **Chronic entrapment neuropathy** due to compression or repetitive trauma
is a common clinical problem. Typically involved nerves include the median
nerve at the wrist (carpal tunnel syndrome), the ulnar nerve at the elbow
or wrist (cubital tunnel syndrome), the anterior or posterior interosseous
nerves in the forearm, the brachial plexus at the thoracic outlet, the common
peroneal nerve at the knee, and the posterior tibial nerve at the ankle (tarsal
tunnel syndrome).

1. **Clinical assessment** of these conditions involves assessment of motor
and sensory function as well as provocative testing (reproducibility of
symptoms with extrinsic nerve compression) and determination whether
Tinel sign is present. EMG and NCS are appropriate if the clinical picture
is unclear.

2. **Initial management** is usually physical therapy, behavior modification, and splinting to avoid repetitive compression. At least 6 weeks of nonsurgical management without improvement is usually recommended before operation, although nerve compression at the cubital tunnel or thoracic outlet typically requires prolonged nonsurgical management. Operations generally involve **decompression** of the affected nerve or transposition to an unrestricted site.

II. **Scalp, calvarial, and forehead reconstruction**
   A. **Anatomy**
      1. The **scalp** consists of five layers: skin, subcutaneous tissue, galea aponeurotica, loose areolar tissue, and pericranium.
      2. **Five major paired vessels** provide the scalp with an ample collateral blood supply: the supraorbital, supratrochlear, superficial temporal, posterior auricular, and occipital arteries.
      3. The **scalp receives sensory innervation** from the supraorbital and supratrochlear, branches of cranial nerve V1, the lesser occipital branch of C2 or C3, the greater auricular nerve, and the auriculotemporal branch of cranial nerve V3. The motor innervation to the frontalis derives from the frontal branch of the facial nerve.
   B. **Scalp lacerations** are common concomitant sequelae of blunt trauma to the head. As such, there may be associated skull, cervical spine, or intracranial injuries. The rich blood supply to the scalp can produce significant blood loss, and hemostasis is important to prevent subgaleal hematoma. Radical débridement is seldom indicated, and primary repair is usually feasible. Repair of the galea generally helps to prevent hematoma formation.
   C. **Partial-thickness scalp loss from avulsion** usually occurs at the subaponeurotic layer. Large avulsions may be skin grafted. One can expect 20% to 40% contraction of the skin graft over the first 6 to 8 months. After this has leveled off, the grafted area can be removed by serial excisions.
   D. **Full-thickness scalp loss** can occur from trauma or tumor extirpation. The optimal treatment varies depending on the size of the defect.
      1. **Small defects** (<3 cm) can often be closed primarily after undermining of flaps. Local flaps, either random or based on blood supply, can be raised. Scoring the galea in a grid pattern of perpendicular lines spaced 1 cm apart can allow for expansion of the flap. Rotation flaps should involve a margin of at least five times the length of the defect. Bipedicled flaps are well-suited for coverage of the poles of the head (forehead, temporal areas, and nape of neck).
      2. **Medium-sized defects** (3 to 10 cm) are usually covered with a scalp flap combined with skin grafting of the donor pericranium. Several specific flaps have been described for medium-sized defects, including the pinwheel flap, three-flap, and four-flap techniques described by Orticochea. All have been used with variable success.
      3. **Large defects** (>10 cm) often require free tissue transfer. If the deficit is due to trauma, replant may be attempted. Because most of these injuries are from industrial accidents involving avulsion, however, the injury to the arterial intima can extend far into the scalp. Latissimus dorsi or omental free flaps with split-thickness skin grafts are described for complete scalp loss.
   E. **Calvarial defects** in the parietal or occipital regions require cranioplasty for protection. Temporal defects are somewhat protected by the temporalis muscle.
      1. **Alloplastic material** can be used to cover these defects, including calcium hydroxyapatite and methylmethacrylate. Polymethylmethacrylate (PMMA) is the most commonly employed, as it is both durable and easy to use. However, it is exothermic upon initial application, has a reported infection rates of approximately 5%, and the rates can be as high as 30% with infection nearby. Newer alloplastic materials are being developed to promote bony ingrowth and decrease the risk of infection. Some can be

custom-made, based on three-dimensional reconstructions of computed tomographic scans.

2. **Autogenous tissue for cranioplasty** includes split-rib grafts, split-table calvarial bone grafts, and bone paste. These are somewhat more difficult to use but have the advantage of a lower complication rate.

III. Trunk

A. Breast

1. **Postmastectomy breast reconstruction** offers restoration of an important symbol of femininity and sexual intimacy. Reconstruction of breast symmetry can lead to a significant improvement in body image and is an important part of cancer rehabilitation for many women (*Scand J Plast Reconstr Surg* 1984;18:221).

   a. **The aims of reconstruction** are to create symmetric breast mounds and, if desired, a new nipple-areola complex. The esthetic goal is defined by the patient and includes a symmetric appearance both clothed and unclothed. Extensive preoperative consultation is required to allow women to explore their options. It should be emphasized that each approach to breast reconstruction usually requires at least two procedures and that the reconstructed breast will never completely replicate the original. Reconstruction can be accomplished with or without the use of an implant, and most procedures can be performed either immediately at the time of the mastectomy or in a delayed fashion.

   b. **Reconstruction of the breast mound** is accomplished with an implant in approximately two-thirds of cases (*Probl Gen Surg* 1996;13:75). In most cases, enough skin is removed with the mastectomy that the desired size of the breast precludes closure of the wound without tension. When this is the case, a tissue expander is placed and serial expansions performed until the desired size is reached (usually after 6 weeks of expansion). At this time, the expander is replaced with a permanent implant filled with silicone gel or saline. The advantages of this approach to reconstruction are that minimal operative time is required, additional scars are minimized, and the recovery period is shorter. The disadvantages include the risks of permanent implants (rupture, infection) and the inability to reproduce certain natural contours.

   c. **Autologous tissue** can be used to recreate a breast mound in the form of pedicled (rectus abdominis, latissimus dorsi) or free (rectus abdominis, gluteus maximus) myocutaneous flaps. The advantages include a more natural appearance for some patients, permanent reconstruction without the potential for future procedures to replace a ruptured implant, and fewer complications with subsequent radiation therapy. Disadvantages include a relatively long procedure, additional scars, and potential donor-site morbidity.

   d. **Reconstruction of the nipple-areola complex** is chosen by approximately 50% of patients undergoing breast reconstruction. A variety of methods are used and include local flaps or nipple-sharing grafts to reconstruct a nipple-like prominence. Split-thickness skin grafting or tattooing can be used to recreate an areola.

   e. **Procedures on the contralateral breast to improve symmetry** may be performed concomitantly or subsequently and include modification of an inframammary fold, removal of dog ears, liposuction of flaps, or reduction mammoplasty or mastopexy of the contralateral side. Symmetry procedures are almost always covered by insurance.

2. **Reduction mammoplasty** is performed for women with a variety of physical complaints and aberrations in body image.

   a. **Common symptoms** are listed below and are considered indications for reduction mammoplasty.

      (1) **Personal embarrassment and psychosocial problems**

      (2) **Shoulder and back pain**

(3) **Grooving of the soft tissue of the shoulders by bra straps**
(4) **Chronic inframammary skin breakdown, rash, or infection (intertrigo)**
(5) **Inability to engage in vigorous exercise**
(6) **Symptoms of brachial plexus compression (rare)**
   b. A variety of procedures are designed to **reduce breast size.** All of them move the nipple-areola complex superiorly on the chest wall. The nipple-areola complex is maintained on a pedicled blood supply when possible, but in certain instances (e.g., pedicle length >15 cm or a patient who smokes), tenuous blood supply to the nipple-areola complex may require a full-thickness graft. There are always scars resulting from the movement of the nipple and resection of excess skin, and the configuration of these scars varies by the procedure chosen.
B. **Chest wall reconstruction**
   1. **Before beginning chest wall reconstruction,** one must ensure complete resection of tumor and radiation-damaged or infected tissue.
   2. **Dead space** in the chest allows for potential empyema and must be obliterated. This space is best filled with pedicled muscle (latissimus dorsi, pectoralis major, serratus anterior, or rectus abdominis) or omental flaps.
   3. **Skeletal stabilization** is required if more than four rib segments or 5 cm of chest wall are missing. This can be achieved using autologous (rib, dermis, or fascial grafts or bulky muscle flaps) or prosthetic (Prolene mesh, Gore-Tex, Marlex-methylmethacrylate sandwich) material.
   4. **Optimal soft-tissue coverage** usually requires pedicled myocutaneous flaps but can be achieved with pedicled muscle or omentum covered with split-thickness skin graft. Rarely, free tissue transfer is required.
   5. **Median sternotomy dehiscence** owing to infection occurs in 1% to 2% of cardiac procedures. Predisposing factors include bilateral internal mammary artery harvest, diabetes mellitus, obesity, and multiple operations. Closure requires removal of wires and débridement of all infected tissue, including bone and cartilage. Closure of the resultant dead space is usually accomplished by advancing or rotating the pectoralis major and/or rectus abdominis muscles. The rectus abdominis muscle cannot be used as a rotational flap if the ipsilateral internal mammary artery has been harvested. Pedicled omental flaps are reserved as alternatives in case of initial failure.
C. **Abdominal wall reconstruction**
   1. **Reconstruction of full-thickness abdominal wall defects** includes recreation of a fascial barrier and skin coverage. Restoration of a functional muscle layer is also helpful in maintaining abdominal wall functionality.
   2. **Complete absence of all layers of the anterior abdominal wall** is usually the result of direct trauma or infection, with or without intra-abdominal catastrophe. The open abdomen can be temporized by skin grafts placed directly on bowel serosa, omentum, or absorbable mesh through which granulation tissue has formed. This allows for resolution of intra-abdominal edema and maturation of adhesions but usually results in a large ventral hernia.
   3. **Primary closure of fascial defects** represents the best approach and can be assisted by sliding myofascial advancement flaps. Lateral release of the external oblique fascia, or "component separation," is ideal for midline musculofascial defects >3 cm in size. Using bilateral relaxing incisions and release, a total of 10 cm, 18 cm, and 6 to 10 cm of advancement may be obtained in the upper, middle, and lower thirds of the abdomen, respectively (*Plast Recon Surg* 1990;86:519). The anterior sheath of one or both rectus muscles can be divided and turned over to provide additional fascia for closure. Synthetic mesh may be used when fascial defects cannot

be primarily closed. AlloDerm®, freeze-dried cadaveric dermis devoid of antigenic cells, may also be utilized for large fascial defects. **Muscle flaps** are required when the existing fascia is insufficient for closure after advancement. The most frequently used flaps are the tensor fascia lata, rectus femoris, and vastus lateralis. These flaps are usually not useful for closing defects of the upper abdomen.
4. **Skin coverage** is accomplished with split-thickness skin grafts, the cutaneous portion of a myocutaneous flap, or local tissue rearrangement (e.g., bipedicled flap, V-Y advancement flap). As skin grafts cannot survive directly on synthetic mesh, a muscle flap may be required to provide an adequate bed for skin grafting.
D. **Pressure sores**
1. The **etiology and staging criteria** are described in Chapter 9.
2. **Principles of nonoperative management** of pressure sores include (1) relief of pressure by positioning changes and appropriate cushioning; (2) bedside débridement of devitalized tissue; (3) optimization of the wound environment with aggressive wound care; (4) avoidance of maceration, trauma, friction, or shearing forces; and (5) reversal of underlying conditions that may predispose to ulcer development. This type of aggressive nonoperative management is often optimally coordinated by specially trained wound care nurses.
3. **Operative management** with soft-tissue flap closure is only indicated for large, deep, or complicated ulcers and then only in patients who are able to care for their wounds. A high degree of cooperation from the patient and caregivers is essential because the recurrence of pressure sores at the same site or new sores at other sites after operation is high. This is especially true for individuals who have spinal cord transection from firearm injuries, whose rate of recurrence is 91%, with a mean time to recurrence of 18 months (*Adv Wound Care* 1994;7:40). This is most likely the result of breakdown in the postoperative support and care systems in this population. Most surgeons, therefore, require demonstration of the patient's ability to care for wounds before embarking on operative closure. Flaps commonly used for closure of pressure ulcers around the pelvic girdle include gluteus maximus, tensor fascia lata, hamstring, or gracilis-based rotation or advancement flaps.
IV. **Lower extremity.** Soft-tissue defects from trauma to the lower extremity are common. A multidisciplinary approach involving orthopedic, vascular, and plastic surgeons provides optimal care.
A. Lower-extremity injuries are first assessed according to **advanced trauma life support guidelines.** The general sequence of priorities is as follows:
1. The first priority is assessment for **concomitant life-threatening injuries and control of active bleeding.** Blood loss from open wounds is often underestimated, and patients must be adequately resuscitated.
2. The **neurovascular status** is determined. If a nerve deficit is progressive during observation in the emergency room, it is likely the result of ischemia from arterial injury or compartment syndrome.
3. **Bony continuity** is assessed by radiographs of all areas of suspected injury.
4. **Operative management** addresses bone stabilization followed by venous and arterial repair. Fasciotomies are indicated for compartment pressures >30 mm Hg and by clinical suspicion from preoperative neurovascular examination. Fasciotomy must be performed within 6 hours to avoid ischemic contracture. Nonviable tissue is débrided, and an assessment is made about delayed or immediate soft-tissue coverage.
B. **Soft-tissue defects of the thigh** are usually closed by primary closure, skin grafts, or local flaps. The thick muscular layers ensure adequate local tissue for coverage of bone and vessels and adequate vascular supply to any fracture sites.

C. **Open tibial fractures** frequently involve degloving of the thin layer of soft tissue covering the anterior tibial surface. The distal tibia is a watershed zone, and fracture with loss of periosteum or soft tissue leads to increased rates of infection and nonunion.

1. Open tibial fractures are classified according to the scheme of **Gustilo** (Tables 34-3 and 34-4).

2. **Gustilo types IIIb and c** frequently require flap coverage of exposed bone.

a. The **proximal third** of the tibia or knee can often be covered by a pedicled hemigastrocnemius flap.

b. The **middle third** of the tibia is often covered by a pedicled hemisoleus flap.

c. **Large defects of the distal third** of the tibia generally require coverage by free muscle transfer.

D. **Limb salvage reconstruction for neoplasm** differs from that for trauma in that large segments of bone, nerve, or vessels may require replacement.

1. **Skeletal replacement** can be accomplished using an endoprosthesis, allogeneic bone transplant, or vascularized free bone (fibula) transfer.

E. **The foot** is divided into regions for purposes of soft-tissue defects caused by trauma or ischemic, diabetic, or infectious ulceration. Optimal coverage of the plantar surface provides a durable, sensate platform.

1. **Small defects of the heel** can be covered using the nonweightbearing skin of the midsole. Larger defects require free muscle transfer and split-thickness skin grafting.

2. **The metatarsal heads** are often successfully covered using plantar V-Y advancement and fillet of toe flaps. Multiple fillet of toe flaps or free muscle transfer may be required for large defects.

3. **For fitting of proper footwear,** coverage of the dorsum of the foot must be thin. If paratenon is present, the dorsum can usually be covered with a skin graft. Small areas of exposed tendon may granulate, but larger

Table 34-3. Gustilo open fracture classification

Classification	Characteristics
I	Clean wound <1 cm long
II	Laceration >1 cm long; no extensive soft-tissue damage, flaps, or avulsions
III	Extensive soft-tissue laceration, damage, or loss; open segmental fracture; or traumatic amputation

Reprinted with permission from RB Gustilo, JT Anderson. Prevention of infection in the treatment of one thousand and twenty-five open fractures of long bones: retrospective and prospective analyses. *J Bone Joint Surg Am* 1976;58A:453.

Table 34-4. Gustilo type III subtypes

Classification	Characteristics
IIIa	Adequate periosteal cover of the bone despite extensive soft-tissue damage; high-energy trauma with small wound
IIIb	Extensive soft-tissue loss with periosteal stripping and bone exposure; usually associated with massive contamination
IIIc	Arterial injury requiring repair

Reprinted with permission from RB Gustilo, JT Anderson. Prevention of infection in the treatment of one thousand and twenty-five open fractures of long bones: retrospective and prospective analyses. *J Bone Joint Surg Am* 1976;58A:453.

areas require thin fascial free flaps (temporoparietal, parascapular, or radial forearm) covered by skin grafts.

HAND SURGERY

I. **Assessment** must be done using a systematic, efficient, and reproducible approach. Underestimating the extent of a hand injury or infection can lead to extended recovery or permanent loss of function.

   A. **History.** The mechanism and timing of the injury, hand position at the time of injury, hand dominance, and patient occupation are all important to diagnosis and treatment.

   B. **Examination**

   1. **Inspect the position of the patient's hand,** paying attention to the resting position of the digits and any swelling or asymmetry as compared with the contralateral hand.

   2. **Vascular assessment** requires observation of color, temperature, capillary refill, and the presence of pulses (palpable or Doppler) and an Allen test to verify the integrity of the palmar arches. Bleeding is controlled by application of direct pressure, not by blindly clamping tissue, as this often results in serious injury to surrounding structures. The use of tourniquets should be reserved for life-threatening exsanguinations, as serious and irreversible damage may result.

   3. **Motor examination,** both active and passive, involves testing for integrity of the tendons.

      a. **Flexor digitorum profundus (FDP)** is tested by stabilizing the proximal interphalangeal (PIP) joint in extension and having the patient flex the distal interphalangeal (DIP) joint.

      b. **Flexor digitorum superficialis (FDS)** is tested by blocking all other fingers in full extension before asking the patient to flex at the PIP joint.

      c. **Extensor tendons** are tested by having the patient extend each finger individually. It should be noted that connections between neighboring tendons (juncturae tendinum) can mask a proximal laceration.

   4. **Sensory testing** includes gross examination of the ulnar, radial, and median nerves, which innervate the muscles in the hand and forearm (Table 34-5). It also involves careful examination of two-point discrimination on the palmar aspect of both the radial and ulnar sides of the digits and comparison with the uninjured hand. Normal two-point discrimination is 3 to 6 mm at the distal tip of the digit.

   5. **Skeletal examination** involves palpating for any tenderness, soft-tissue swelling, or deformity of the bones. Joint integrity is assessed by gently stressing the ligaments and noting any instability, crepitus, or pain. Any suspicion of fracture or dislocation requires radiographic examination.

   C. **Diagnostic radiology.** Plain radiographs of the injured area, including the joint above and below if the physical examination warrants it, are indicated for almost all hand trauma and should be considered in cases of hand

Table 34-5. Unambiguous tests of hand nerve function

Test	Radial nerve	Median nerve	Ulnar nerve
Sensory	Dorsum first web	Index fingertip	Little fingertip
Extrinsic motor	Extend wrist	FDP index	FDP small
Intrinsic motor	None	Abduct thumb perpendicular to palm	Cross long finger over index (interossei)

FDP, flexor digitorum profundus.

infections, particularly in penetrating trauma. Images should include true posteroanterior, lateral, and oblique views. If the injury involves the digits, separate laterals of the involved digits are indicated. The description of the fracture pattern should include the following: the bone(s) involved, simple versus comminuted, displaced versus nondisplaced, transverse versus oblique versus spiral, angulation or rotation of the distal fragment, and intra-articular versus extra-articular. Fractures in children involving the growth plate use the Salter-Harris classification.

II. **Fractures**
  A. **Principles of management**
    1. **Reduction of displaced fractures** can be attempted in the emergency room using local or regional anesthesia. However, early referral to a hand surgeon is essential for all hand fractures.
    2. **Postreduction radiographs** should be done for all fractures after splinting or casting.
    3. **Splinting the fracture** in a position that does not impair function during the healing phase is imperative. A splint made of plaster or fiberglass, appropriately padded and with the hand in the "intrinsic-plus" position, may be used for almost all hand injuries. The intrinsic-plus position places ligamentous structures in their longest position and minimizes stiffness should immobilization be required to treat the fracture. The interphalangeal (IP) joints are in full extension, the metacarpophalangeal (MCP) joints are at 60 to 90 degrees of flexion, and the wrist is at 20 to 30 degrees of extension. Individual digits can be splinted without involving the remainder of the patient's hand and wrist. A thumb spica splint is used for fractures that involve the thumb proximal to the IP joint. The MCP joint is placed in extension, the thumb abducted, and the wrist placed in 20 to 30 degrees of extension. Even if operative management of the fracture is planned, a reduction with splinting in the emergency room is still appropriate for patient comfort and to prevent stiffness.
    4. **Early motion** is used whenever possible to minimize joint stiffness.
    5. **Operative intervention** is considered if closed treatment does not obtain or maintain reduction of the fracture. Contaminated open fractures, associated soft-tissue injuries, malalignment (uncorrected rotated, angulated, or shortened deformities of the digit), and articular incongruity of >1 mm are also indications for operative management.
  B. **Specific fractures**
    1. **Phalangeal fractures** require closed reduction and protective splinting for 4 to 6 weeks. Fractures of the distal phalanx may involve the nail bed apparatus or insertion of either the flexor or extensor mechanisms. Disruption of the extensor mechanism at the distal phalanx results in a mallet finger deformity (see "Hand Surgery," Section IV.B.1) and can be treated by splinting the DIP joint in extension. Other fractures of the distal phalanx can generally be treated with a protective splint. Stable middle and proximal phalanx fractures can be adequately treated by taping the injured finger to its neighbor. Certain fracture patterns are considered unstable and require operative fixation. As always, the goal of early motion is desirable.
    2. **Boxer's fracture** is a common transverse fracture at the distal portion of the ring or small finger metacarpal, with volar angulation of the distal fragment. Volar angulation of the distal fragment of up to 45 degrees is acceptable in the fifth metacarpal because of its mobility, although this may cause prominence of the metacarpal head in the palm. Less angulation is accepted in the fourth metacarpal, and in the second and third metacarpals, angulation >15 degrees is unacceptable. Any rotation or scissoring of the finger must be corrected by reduction as well. It is unnecessary to immobilize the MCP joint, and protection with a volar splint brought to the middle palmar crease is used until the patient sees

a hand surgeon. Buddy taping of the ring and small fingers may also be helpful.

3. **Transverse metacarpal shaft fractures** are caused by axial loading and follow the same guidelines as neck fractures in terms of angulation. Oblique and spiral fractures result from torsional forces and are often best treated with operative fixation, protective splinting, and early range-of-motion exercises.

4. **Bennett's fracture** is an intra-articular fracture at the base of the first metacarpal resulting from an axial load to the thumb. The distal fragment subluxes radially through the pull of the abductor pollicis longus and angulates volarly through the force of the adductor pollicis. The ulnar fragment of the base is held fixed by the volar beak ligament. Closed reduction and splinting often yield a reduction that is anatomic; however, the deforming forces usually move the fragments out of reduction, and these fractures are best treated with open reduction and fixation. Less common is the "baby Bennett's," or "reverse Bennett's," fracture of the fifth metacarpal base; it is similar to the Bennett's fracture, with the extensor carpi ulnaris representing the deforming force on the distal fragment.

5. **Epiphyseal fractures in children** can lead to alterations in the growth of the involved bone. Treatment is similar to that for adults, although healing is often faster and immobilization is more acceptable because joint stiffness is less of a problem in children. Although reduction of the fracture is important, bone remodeling allows for angulation deformities of up to 20 or 30 degrees in the phalanges and metacarpals, provided it is in the anteroposterior plane. Rotatory deformity or deviation in the coronal plane should not be accepted because remodeling does not correct these deformities (*Clin Orthop* 1984;188:12).

6. **Open fractures** require adequate irrigation, reduction, and fixation as necessary, with prophylactic antibiotic coverage.

III. **Dislocations and ligament injuries**
  A. **Principles of management**
    1. **Pre- and postreduction films** to confirm joint alignment and look for associated fractures
    2. **Joint stability assessment** by stressing the periarticular structures and putting the joint through its range of motion. If instability is demonstrated, operative management should be considered. A stable joint is managed with protective splinting and early range-of-motion exercise.
    3. **Distal neurovascular assessment** before and after manipulation.
  B. **Specific dislocations**
    1. **DIP joint and thumb IP joint dislocations** are uncommon injuries treated with closed reduction followed by splinting for 3 weeks, along with early protective range-of-motion exercise, provided tendon function is normal.
    2. **PIP joint injuries** are commonly known as "jammed fingers" and require careful assessment and follow-up to prevent long-term stiffness.
      a. **Dislocations may be dorsal or volar.** Volar dislocations may be difficult to reduce owing to interposition of the extensor apparatus. Volar dislocations may also result in disruption of the extensor tendon central slip, and need close observation to watch for boutonniere deformity. Postreduction care consists of early hand therapy, or operative management if unstable or irreducible.
      b. **Volar plate injuries** are common and result from hyperextension of the PIP joint. The ligament can be strained, ruptured, or avulsed from the base of the middle phalanx with or without a bone fragment. If the injury is to soft tissue only or the avulsion represents <20% of the articular surface with a stable joint, treatment involves buddy taping or extension block splinting with the joint in 30 degrees of extension and immediate range of motion. If the bone fragment represents 20% or more of the articular surface and there is associated

instability, open reduction and internal fixation or volar plate arthroplasty are required.

3. **Finger MCP joint dislocations** are usually caused by forced hyperextension and are most often seen in the index and small fingers. The dislocation is usually dorsal and is usually reducible in the emergency room. If the volar plate is interposed in the joint, however, open reduction may be required. If the joint is stable after reduction, it should be splinted for protection and early motion started. Occasionally, the metacarpal head can be held volarly by the flexor tendons on one side and the intrinsic muscles on the other side such that longitudinal traction tightens the "noose" around the head and prevents reduction. Open reduction is required in these situations.

4. **Thumb MCP joint dislocations** are uncommon. The dislocation is usually dorsal and results from forced abduction. Closed reduction with a thumb spica splint and early range of motion is the usual treatment. The ulnar collateral ligament can be partially or completely torn and may avulse with a bone fragment from the proximal phalanx. If there is joint stability and congruity, the MCP joint is splinted for 4 weeks, leaving the IP joint free. If the joint is unstable or the proximal portion of the torn ulnar collateral ligament is displaced superficial to the adductor pollicis (Stener lesion), open reduction and internal fixation are required. **Of note, a stable lesion may be converted to an unstable (Stener) lesion by inexperienced examiners aggressively stressing the joint.**

5. **Carpometacarpal injuries** are usually dislocations with or without fractures. Ligamentous injuries are less common because the carpometacarpal articulation has less movement than do other joints. Dorsal dislocations with and without fractures result from a direct blow and are more common on the ulnar part of the hand. Closed reduction is frequently possible, but maintaining the reduction often requires percutaneous pinning of the joint.

IV. **Tendon injuries**
   A. **Flexor tendons** are frequently lacerated during everyday activities. Assessment and management of these injuries by a hand surgeon are critical to a satisfactory outcome.
   1. **The assessment** involves a careful history and examination; the examiner should look for a change in the resting tone of the digits (cascade) and assess the profundus and superficialis tendons independently. If flexion against resistance elicits pain, a partial laceration must be suspected. A careful neurovascular examination, including evaluation of two-point discrimination, should be performed to evaluate for concomitant nerve or vessel injury.
   2. **Emergency room management** involves a thorough examination, then irrigation and closure of the wound, dorsal splinting with the patient's wrist in 20 to 30 degrees of flexion, the MCP joint at 90 degrees of flexion, and the IP joints in extension. Operative exploration and repair are appropriate for all lacerations through the tendon sheath, since wrist and digit position at the time of injury can result in significant retraction with respect to skin laceration.
   3. **Anatomy: flexor tendon zones**
      a. **Zone I:** distal to the superficialis (FDS) insertion
      b. **Zone II:** from proximal A1 pulley (distal palmer crease) to FDS insertion
      c. **Zone III:** from distal transverse carpal ligament (carpal tunnel) to A1 pulley
      d. **Zone IV:** within the carpal tunnel
      e. **Zone V:** proximal to the carpal tunnel
   4. **Technique of repair** involves a core, locking suture and an epitendinous repair. For tendon ruptures and lacerations within 1 cm of the FDP

insertion, advancement and reinsertion of the tendon are used. A dorsal splint is applied, and a strict protected motion protocol directed by a hand therapist is started within 24 to 72 hours after repair and continues for 6 to 8 weeks.

B. Extensor tendon injuries result from lacerations and closed axial loading of the digits.

1. **Zone I: over the DIP joint.** Mallet finger is a very common injury that results from forced flexion of the tip of the finger, with rupture of the terminal tendon from the distal phalanx. This leads to inability to extend the DIP. Mallet finger may be associated with an avulsion fracture or joint subluxation. These injuries are treated with splinting of the DIP joint in extension for 6 weeks. Operative management with reduction of the fracture and joint is only occasionally indicated. For open injuries, the tendon should be repaired and the joint pinned or splinted in extension for 6 weeks.

2. **Zone II: over the middle phalanx.** Lacerations in this zone should be repaired using a figure-of-eight or mattress technique. The DIP joint may be transfixed with a pin or splinted for 4 to 6 weeks.

3. **Zone III: over the PIP joint.** A complicated injury, since injury can occur to the central slip or lateral bands. A clue to central slip injury is if the patient is unable to initiate PIP extension from 90 degrees. If the patient is able to fully extend the PIP and DIP, at least one lateral band is intact. If untreated, these injuries can result in a boutonnière deformity (PIP flexion and DIP hyperextension) of the digit. For open injuries, the tendon should be repaired and the joint transfixed with an oblique pin for 3 to 5 weeks. For tendon injuries associated with a fracture that is displaced, reduction and fixation of the fracture are advised. Protective splinting of the joint should be maintained for 6 weeks.

4. **Zone IV: over the proximal phalanx.** The lacerations are often partial because of the width of the tendon at this level. Splinting of the PIP joint in extension for 3 to 4 weeks is often sufficient for these injuries. Repair of the tendon is required if there is any extension lag of the IP joints.

5. **Zone V: over the MCP joint.** These injuries often occur as a result of a punching incident, particularly with a blow to the mouth. Contamination of the wound with oral flora can produce serious infection (see "Hand Surgery," Section VI.B.5). Aggressive wound exploration must be undertaken to rule out joint space involvement, as intra-articular infection can rapidly destroy the delicate cartilaginous surfaces. This often requires elongation of the laceration for adequate visualization and irrigation of the full extent of the wound. Only after the full extent of the wound has been evaluated and the wound aggressively cleansed can the tendon or tendons be repaired and the joint splinted in 20 to 30 degrees of flexion. The wrist is splinted in 30 degrees of extension. Dynamic splinting is useful to avoid adhesions and improve early motion.

6. **Zone VI: over the dorsum of the metacarpals and carpus.** Repair and splint as for zone 5 injuries.

7. **Zone VII: at the level of the extensor retinaculum.** Repair and splint as for zone 5.

8. **Zone VIII: proximal to the extensor retinaculum.** Injury is often at the musculotendinous junction. Repair and splinting for 4 to 6 weeks are required.

V. Amputation

A. Replantation or revascularization

1. **Indications** for replantation include amputation of the thumb; amputation of multiple digits; amputation at the metacarpal, wrist, or forearm level; and amputation at any level in a child. More controversial indications include amputation of the proximal arm and amputation of a single digit distal to the FDS insertion.

2. **Contraindications** for replantation include coexisting serious injuries or diseases that preclude a prolonged operative time, multiple levels of amputation, severe crush or degloving injury to the part, and prolonged ischemia time (12 hours for fingers and 6 hours for proximal limb amputations). Avulsion injury is a relative contraindication to replantation because of the extensive vascular and soft-tissue trauma.

3. **Preparation for transfer** involves a moist dressing on the stump and splinting for comfort. The amputated part should be wrapped in saline-moistened gauze and placed in a clear plastic bag on a mixture of ice and water. The part should never be placed directly on ice or immersed in saline. Radiographs of the stump and the amputated part are essential and can be done at the transferring facility, provided that this does not significantly delay transfer to the microsurgery center. Intravenous fluids, prophylactic antibiotics, and tetanus toxoid, when indicated, should be begun immediately to facilitate prompt transfer to the appropriate facility for replantation. The sequence of repair involves identification of neurovascular structures and tendons and preparation of the bone for fixation. After providing bony stability, the arteries are repaired, followed by repair of the tendons and then veins, nerves, and skin. The postoperative care involves careful monitoring of the splinted part (temperature, color, and turgor) and adequate intravenous hydration in a warm environment.

B. Revision amputation (nonreplantable amputation) management
1. **Principles**
   a. **Complete assessment,** including radiographs
   b. **Antibiotics** when bone is involved or soft tissues are crushed or contaminated
   c. **Preservation of length**
   d. **Maintenance of sensation and motion**
   e. **Esthetics**
   f. **Early motion**
2. **Fingertip injuries** are optimally managed using primary closure without shortening. If this is not possible, lateral V-Y advancement or volar advancement flaps or skin grafts can be used to obtain closure. An alternative for small wounds (with no vital structures exposed) is closure by secondary intention.
3. **More proximal amputations** involve shortening and contouring the bone, shortening the tendons, and identifying digital nerves and allowing them to be transposed away from the skin closure.
4. **A protective dressing** that allows joint motion is recommended, with early referral to a hand therapist for range-of-motion exercises and later desensitization of the tip of the stump.

VI. Infections
A. Management. Infections in the hand can progress rapidly via potential spaces and may risk the viability of tendons, bones, joints, and neurovascular structures by creating increased pressure from pus and edema in closed spaces.
1. **Surgical drainage** is required in most hand infections.
2. **Antibiotic coverage** should be directed against common skin flora such as *Staphylococcus aureus, Staphylococcus epidermidis,* and *Streptococcus* species.
3. **Gram stain and culture of wound.**
4. **Splinting and elevation of the hand.**
5. **Tetanus prophylaxis when appropriate.**
B. Local infections
1. **Paronychia** is a soft-tissue infection of the skin and soft tissue of the lateral nail fold; an **eponychial infection** may extend from this and involves the proximal nail fold. These localized infections often arise from

self-inflicted trauma by nail biting or foreign body penetration, such as a needle-stick. Treatment requires incision and drainage, with removal of the nail when the infection extends deep to the nail plate. Oral antibiotics are used if a cellulitis is present. **Chronic paronychia** is sometimes associated with underlying osteomyelitis or fungal organisms.

2. **Felon** is a localized infection involving the pulp of the volar digit and usually originates with a puncture wound, although a paronychial infection may spread volarly. Purulent fluid is usually under pressure in the fibrous septa of the tip of the digit. Management involves incision and drainage of the abscess (which can be between septa) and systemic antibiotics if there is an associated cellulitis. In general, the incision is located where the felon is "pointing"; however, it should be carefully planned to avoid sensitive scars and destabilization of the pulp of the finger. As with a paronychia, aggressive cleansing with soap and water after incision and drainage promotes drainage and avoids premature closing of the wound.

3. **Cellulitis** in the hand usually occurs secondary to a laceration, abrasion, or other soft-tissue injury. Management involves draining an abscess if present. The fluid should be sent for culture and sensitivity, and oral or intravenous antibiotics should be administered, depending on the severity. When associated with swelling of the digits and hand, splinting in the intrinsic-plus position and elevation prevent stiffness.

4. **After an animal bite,** the wound must be thoroughly irrigated to decrease the bacterial load and to remove any foreign body, such as a tooth. Bite wounds should be treated with oral antibiotics prophylactically and with intravenous antibiotics when an established infection is present. Although a greater percentage of cat bites become infected than do dog bites, the jaws of a dog are significantly more powerful and can inflict other injuries. The organisms most often involved from dog or cat bites include *Pasteurella multocida, S. aureus, Bacteroides* species, and *Streptococcus viridans.* Recommended oral antibiotics are amoxicillin-clavulanate or clindamycin with either ciprofloxacin or trimethoprim-sulfamethoxazole.

5. **Human bites** can involve particularly virulent organisms and frequently present in association with extensor tendon injuries or fractures sustained during physical altercations. An open wound, particularly if it overlies the dorsum of the hand with signs of infection or underlying soft-tissue or bony injuries, should prompt patient questioning about the source of the laceration. Typical organisms cultured from human bite wounds are *S. viridans, S. epidermidis,* and *S. aureus,* as well as anaerobic bacteria, such as *Eikenella corrodens* and *Bacteroides* species. Amoxicillin-clavulanate should be used prophylactically, and when signs of infection are present, treatment with ampicillin-sulbactam, cefoxitin, or clindamycin plus either ciprofloxacin or trimethoprim-sulfamethoxazole is recommended. Wound exploration should be carried out as detailed in Section IV.B.5.

VII. **Surgical emergencies**

A. **Compartment syndrome** is seen in the hand and forearm and results from increased pressure within an osseofascial space, leading to decreased perfusion pressure. If it is left untreated, muscle and nerve ischemia may progress to necrosis and fibrosis, causing Volkmann ischemic contracture.

1. **Etiology.** Fractures that cause bleeding, crush and vascular injuries, circumferential burns, bleeding dyscrasias, reperfusion after ischemia, or tight dressings can lead to the syndrome.

2. **Diagnosis** is based on a high index of suspicion, clinical examination, and symptoms of pain that are exacerbated with passive stretch of the compartment musculature, paresthesias, paralysis, or paresis of ischemic

muscles. Pulselessness may occur and indicates a late finding (and is usually also a sign of irreversible damage) or the presence of major arterial occlusion rather than compartment syndrome. Measurement with a pressure monitor of a compartment pressure of >30 mm Hg confirms diagnosis.

3. **Treatment** for incipient compartment syndrome involves close observation and frequent examinations and should include removal of tight casts and dressings. Elevation of the extremity to, or slightly above, the level of the heart is recommended. Acute or suspected compartment syndrome requires urgent fasciotomies of the involved areas. Decompression within 6 hours of established compartment pressures is necessary to prevent irreversible muscle ischemia. Forearm fasciotomies involve volar, carpal tunnel, and dorsal compartments. Hand fasciotomies include dorsal incisions for interossei and adductor pollicis, thenar, and hypothenar compartments as well as midaxial incisions of the digits (ulnar for the index, long, and ring fingers and radial for the thumb and small finger).

B. **Suppurative tenosynovitis** involves infection of the flexor tendon sheath, which is usually caused by a puncture wound to the volar aspect of the digit or palm.
   1. **Diagnosis: cardinal signs of Kanavel**
      a. **Finger held in flexion**
      b. **Fusiform swelling of the finger**
      c. **Tenderness along the tendon sheath**
      d. **Pain on passive extension**
   2. **Management** involves urgent incision and drainage in the operating room, with placement of an irrigating catheter, such as a pediatric feeding tube, in the sheath for continuous irrigation with saline. Irrigation is maintained for 24 to 48 hours. Intravenous antibiotics are administered. Frequent reassessment to verify resolution is critical to avoiding ischemic injury to the tendon secondary to the contained infection.

C. **Palmar abscess** is usually associated with a puncture wound. The fascia divides the palm into thenar, midpalmar, and hypothenar spaces; each involved space must be incised and drained. As with other infections, splinting, elevation, and intravenous antibiotics are required.

D. **Necrotizing infections** threaten both limb and life. The incidence of invasive group A streptococcal infection is on the rise (*N Engl J Med* 1996;335:547) and can occur after surgery or trauma. Aggressive surgical débridement, high-dose penicillin, and supportive management are the mainstays of treatment. Additional therapy with gentamycin or clindamycin provides antibacterial synergy and blocks production of bacterial toxins. Immune globulin and hyperbaric oxygen are adjuvant therapies.

E. **High-pressure injection injuries** result from grease or paint injected at up to 10,000 pounds per square inch. Although the external wounds are often small and unassuming, deep tissue injury can be severe. Injury to the tissue is the result of both direct physical damage and chemical toxicity, and it leads to edema, thrombosis, and subsequent infection. Management involves urgent, thorough débridement, irrigation, decompression, systemic antibiotics, and splinting, with frequent reassessments and repeat débridement in 24 hours as required. When a digit has sustained significant injection, amputation may be required.

35

Cardiac Surgery

Nahush A. Mokadam, Nader Moazami, and Ralph J. Damiano, Jr.

This chapter focuses on the adult patient undergoing common cardiac operations, particularly coronary artery bypass grafting (CABG) and valve replacement. There also is a dicussion of the surgical treatment of heart failure and arrhythmia.

I. **Anatomy**

   A. **Corornary arteries.** The left and right coronary arteries arise from within the sinuses of Valsalva just distal to the right and left coronary cusps of the aortic valve.

   1. The **left main coronary artery** travels posterior to the pulmonary artery, then divides into its main branches, the **left anterior descending artery (LAD)** and the **left circumflex artery (LCx).** The LAD runs in the interventricular groove and arborizes into **septal and diagonal** branches. The LCx runs in the posterior atrioventricular groove and gives off **obtuse marginal** branches. In 10% to 15% of patients, the LCx gives off the **posterior descending artery (PDA),** termed a **left dominant coronary circulation.**

   2. The **right coronary artery (RCA)** descends in the anterior atrioventricular groove, where in 80% to 85% of cases, it gives off the PDA. This is termed a **right dominant coronary circulation.** In addition, the RCA gives off **acute marginal** branches.

   B. **Coronary veins.** There are three principal venous channels for coronary venous drainage.

   1. The **coronary sinus** is located in the posterior atrioventricular groove and receives venous drainage mainly from the left ventricular system. Its main tributaries are the great, middle, and small cardiac veins.

   2. **Thesbian veins** are small venous channels that drain directly into the cardiac chambers.

   3. The **anterior cardiac veins** drain the right coronary system, ultimately into the right atrium.

   C. **Valves.** The valves of the heart are critical to the pump function of the heart. Their proper functioning is essential for the maintenance of pressure gradients and antegrade flow through the heart chambers.

   1. **Atrioventricular valves.** The function of the AV valves is to prevent atrial regurgitation during ventricular contraction. To this end, these valves are fibrous and continuous with the **anuli fibrosi** at the base of the heart. Furthemore, the leaflets are joined at their commisures and are further secured by **chordae tendineae,** which attach the free leaflets to the interventricular papillary muscles.

      a. The **tricuspid valve** separates the right chambers and consists of a large anterior leaflet, a posterior leaflet on the right, and a septal leaflet attached to the the interventricular septum.

      b. The **mitral (bicuspid) valve** separates the left chambers and consists of a large anterior (aortic) leaflet and a posterior (mural) leaflet.

   2. **Semilunar valves.** The pulmonary and aortic valves are essentially identical, except that the coronary arteries arise just distal to the aortic valve. Each cusp comprises two lunulae, which extend from the commisure and meet at the midpoint, a thickening known as the **nodulus of Arantius.** During diastole, the three nodules coapt, forming a seal. Just distal to the valves are gentle dilations of the ascending aorta, known as **sinuses**

of Valsalva. These structures play an important role in the maintenance of sustained laminar blood flow.

II. Physiology

A. Electrophysiology. Like all neuromuscular tissue, the myocardium is dependent on efficient and predictable electrical activation. The myocardium has specialized tissue responsible for the rapid and orderly dispersal of myocardial electrical activation.

1. The **sinoatrial (SA) node** is located at the junction of the anteromedial aspect of the superior vena cava and the right atrial appendage. The **cardiac pacemaker** is determined by the cells that have the most frequent rate of spontaneous depolarization. In most instances, the pacemaker is at the SA node **(sinus rhythm),** which represents an area in the right atrium with the fastest **automaticity.** In general, all myocardium demonstrates automaticity.

2. The **atrioventricular (AV) node** is located in the interatrial septum, on the ventricular side of the orifice of the coronary sinus. It is designed to protect the ventricle from high atrial rates.

3. The **bundle of His** originates in the AV node and descends through the membranous interventricular septum, just inferior to the septal cusp of the tricuspid valve. Also referred to as **Purkinje fibers,** it separates into the right and left branches at the junction of the membranous and muscular portions of the interventricular septum. In normal anatomy, this is the only electrical connection between the atria and the ventricles. The bundle of His functions to rapidly distribute the depolarization to ventricular myocardium, starting with the ventricular septum; to the apex; then throughout the ventricle (via **gap junctions**).

B. Mechanics. The heart functions to convert electrical stimuli to chemical energy and eventually to mechanical energy. The mechanical forces are governed by the pressure, volume, and contractile state of the cardiac chambers. The determination of **rate, rhythm, preload, afterload,** and **contractility** are critical to understanding effective cardiac mechanical function.

1. The **cardiac cycle** describes the relationship between the electrical status of myocardial membranes and the mechanical condition of the cardiac chambers. As the mitral valve opens, diastolic filling commences. Following atrial depolarization and contraction, the ventricle depolarizes and isovolumetric contraction begins (at **end-diastolic volume,** EDV). Once intraventricular pressure exceeds aortic pressure, the aortic valve opens and **ventricular ejection** occurs. As the aortic pressure overcomes ventricular pressure (at EDV), the aortic valve closes. Isovolumetric relaxation commences until intraventricular pressure is lower than left atrial pressure, and the mitral valve opens.

2. **Preload** is defined as the end-diastolic volume of the ventricle. It is practically measured by central venous or **pulmonary capillary wedge pressure.**

3. **Afterload** is most widely defined as "resistance to ejection." It is more practically described as the **aortic pressure gradient.**

4. **Starling's law** describes the relationship between EDV and contractility. As EDV is increased, ventricular contraction is increased as the **optimal sarcomere length** is reached. However, once the optimal length is exceeded, contractility can decrease, as can be seen in pathologic states.

III. Preoperative evaluation. The preoperative evaluation of patients undergoing cardiac surgery is similar to the evaluation of patients undergoing any major operation. All patients should have a complete history and physical examination. Laboratory studies usually include a complete blood cell count; determination of serum electrolyte, creatinine, and glucose levels; determination of prothrombin (PT) and partial thromboplastin times (PTT); and urinalysis. An arterial blood gas is indicated in patients with chronic obstructive pulmonary disease, heavy tobacco abuse, or other pulmonary pathology. In general,

2 to 4 units of packed red blood cells should be available for use during operation. For elective operations, this may be predonated autologous blood. A chest radiograph (posteroanterior and lateral) should be obtained to evaluate calcification of the aortic arch and to assess the proximity of the cardiac silhouette to the sternum in patients undergoing repeat sternotomy. The chest radiograph is also examined for the presence of other intrathoracic pathology. The height and weight of the patient should be measured, and the body-surface area (in square meters) should be calculated.

A. Organ-specific evaluation

1. **Neurologic complications** after cardiac surgery can be devastating. Perioperative cerebrovascular accidents (CVA) occur in 1% to 2% of low-risk patients but in up to 10% of the elderly. CVA may result from aortic atherosclerotic emboli that are loosened by cannulation, cross-clamping, or construction of proximal anastomoses. Postoperative arrhythmias such as atrial fibrillation are also a common cause of CVA following cardiac surgery. Underlying cerebrovascular disease in conjunction with alterations in cerebral blood flow patterns during cardiopulmonary bypass (CPB) may also play a role. Patients with a history of transient ischemic attack, amaurosis fugax, or CVA should undergo noninvasive evaluation of the carotid arteries with Doppler ultrasonography before operation. Because of the strong association between carotid artery and left main coronary stenoses, patients with left main disease should also undergo carotid Doppler examination. Evaluation of asymptomatic carotid bruits is more controversial. In general, only symptomatic **carotid stenoses** are addressed by carotid endarterectomy before or in combination with the planned cardiac surgical procedure.

2. **Pulmonary disease,** particularly the obstructive form, occurs commonly in patients with cardiac disease because cigarette smoking is a risk factor for both disease processes. A preoperative chest x-ray may demonstrate suspicious pulmonary pathology and can be used in combination with a preoperative arterial blood gas to identify patients who are at high risk for difficulty in being weaned from the ventilator postoperatively. Pulmonary function tests are indicated in high-risk patients. Smoking should be discontinued before operation, when possible.

3. **Peripheral vascular examination.** The presence and quality of arterial pulses in the radial, brachial, femoral, popliteal, dorsalis pedis, and posterior tibial arteries should be documented preoperatively as a baseline for comparison if postoperative arterial complications arise. Blood pressure should be measured in both arms to evaluate for subclavian artery stenosis. Significant subclavian artery stenosis may preclude the use of an internal thoracic (mammary) artery (ITA) as a conduit. A preoperative Allen's test should also be performed to assess the palmar arch and the feasibility of using the radial artery for bypass conduit. For patients with varicosities of the saphenous veins or a history of vein stripping, preoperative vein mapping with ultrasonography can be done to assess the availability and quality of saphenous vein for conduit.

4. **Infection.** Operation should be delayed, if possible, in patients with systemic infection or sepsis and in those with cellulitis or soft-tissue infection at the site of planned incisions. Specific infections should be identified preoperatively, if possible, and treated with appropriate antibiotic therapy. In patients who have fever or leukocytosis but require an immediate operation, cultures should be obtained from all potential sources (including central venous catheters), and broad-spectrum intravenous antibiotics should be administered preoperatively.

5. **Medications.** The cardiac surgery patient may be taking a variety of medications before operation. In general, nitrates and β-adrenergic blocking agents should be continued throughout the entire perioperative period. If possible, antiplatelet agents (e.g., aspirin or ibuprofen) are stopped before surgery to prevent hemorrhagic complications. Digoxin and calcium

channel blockers generally are discontinued at the time of operation and restarted only as needed in the postoperative period. For patients receiving heparin preoperatively for unstable angina, the heparin should not be discontinued before operation because this may precipitate an acute coronary syndrome. For patients receiving warfarin preoperatively (including patients with mechanical valves), the warfarin should be discontinued several days before operation. Once the prothrombin time has normalized, anticoagulation can be accomplished using intravenous heparin until several hours before elective operations.

B. Cardiac testing

1. The **electrocardiogram (ECG)** is an important tool for the evaluation of the heart. It demonstrates the electrical activity of the cardiac cycle. **Stress testing** is used to detect coronary artery disease (CAD) or to assess the functional significance of coronary lesions. The exercise ECG is used to evaluate patients who have symptoms suggestive of angina but no symptoms at rest. A positive test is the development of typical signs or symptoms of angina pectoris associated with ECG changes (ST-segment changes or T-wave inversion).

2. A **pulmonary artery catheter (Swan-Ganz)** is often used in the perioperative setting, and it is placed prior to the start of a cardiac procedure. The PA catheter allows for measurement of intravascular and intracardiac pressures, cardiac output, and mixed-venous oxygen saturation (see Table 35-1).

3. The use of **echocardiography** is essential in modern practice. The real-time assessment of chamber size, wall thickness, ventricular function, and valve appearance and motion are possible. With the addition of Doppler imaging, blood flow characteristics can be easily determined. Both **transthoracic** and **transesophageal** echocardiography are widely available. Transesophageal imaging is particularly helpful intraoperatively.

4. **Thallium imaging** is used to identify ischemic myocardium. The thallium in the blood is taken up by the normal myocytes in proportion to the regional blood flow. Decreased perfusion to a region of the myocardium during exertion with subsequent reperfusion suggests reversible myocardial ischemia, whereas the lack of reperfusion suggests irreversibly scarred, infarcted myocardium. In patients who cannot exercise, thallium imaging can be performed after administration of the coronary vasodilator dipyridamole or **adenosine**.

5. **Coronary arteriography** is used to document the presence and location of coronary artery stenoses. Separate injections are made of the right

Table 35-1. Normal hemodynamic parameters

Parameter	Normal value	Unit
Central venous pressure	2–8	mm Hg
Right ventricular pressure (syst/diast)	15–30/2–8	mm Hg
Pulmonary artery pressure (syst/diast)	15–30/4–12	mm Hg
Pulmonary capillary wedge pressure	2–15	mm Hg
Left ventricular pressure (syst/diast)	100–140/3–12	mm Hg
Cardiac output	3.5–5.5	L/min
Cardiac index	2.0–4.0	L/min/m^2 BSA
Stroke volume index	1	mL/kg
Pulmonary vascular resistance	20–130	dynes · sec/cm^5
Systemic vascular resistance	700–1600	dynes · sec/cm^5
Mixed venous oxygen saturation	65–75	percent

and left main coronary arteries. In general, the atherosclerotic process involves the proximal portions of the major coronary arteries, particularly at or just beyond branch points. A 75% decrease in cross-sectional area (50% decrease in luminal diameter) is considered a significant stenosis. Indications for coronary arteriography include suspected CAD (e.g., positive stress test), preparation for coronary revascularization, typical or atypical clinical presentations with normal or borderline stress testing when a definitive diagnosis of CAD is needed, and planned cardiac surgery (e.g., valve surgery) in patients with risk factors for CAD. Concomitant **ventriculography** can be used for assessing left ventricular function.

IV. **Mechanical cardiopulmonary support**
  A. **Cardiopulmonary bypass (CPB),** first introduced in 1954 by Gibbon, revolutionized modern cardiac surgery. It is intended as a support system during surgery and requires systemic anticoagulation.
    1. A **venous reservoir** stores blood volume and allows for escape of bubbles prior to infusion. There are several varieties of **oxygenators,** but all perform the same gas exchange function. A **heat exchanger** is necessary to maintain hypothermia when needed and to assist with patient rewarming. The **arterial pump** is usually a roller pump and requires frequent calibration to ensure accurate flows. The **cannulae** and pump tubing are constructed of Silastic or latex, which remain supple when cold. A **left atrial vent** can be used to remove any blood that enters the left-side circulation.
    2. **Myocardial protection** strategies are critical to good outcome. Hyperkalemic perfusate (warm or cold) based on blood or crystalloid may be infused into the aortic root and coronary ostia (antegrade) or via the coronary sinus (retrograde).
    3. During CPB, the perfusionist, working with the surgeon, can effectively control perfusion rate, temperature, hematocrit, pulmonary venous pressure, and glucose and arterial oxygen levels.
    4. CPB is generally considered safe, but side effects do exist. Most notably, **postperfusion syndrome** is characterized by a diffuse, whole-body inflammatory reaction that can lead to multisystem organ dysfunction. It is believed that most patients experience some form of inflammatory reaction following CPB, but only a fraction develop this syndrome. Other factors contributing to poor CPB tolerance are length of support (>4 hours) and patient age.
  B. **Extracorporeal membrane oxygenation (ECMO)** is primarily used in infants with severe cardiopulmonary failure but can be used in adults. It is not a treatment modality but rather an intermediate-term (days to weeks) artificial heart and lung support system. Most commonly, it is used to allow patients to recover from reversible severe adult respiratory distress syndrome or pulmonary insufficiency of various etiologies.
V. **Disease states and their treatment**
  A. **Coronary artery disease (CAD)** is the leading cause of death in adults in North America. Risk factors for CAD include cigarette smoking, hypertension, diabetes mellitus, hyperlipidemia, male gender, obesity, advanced age, and a family history of CAD. The clinical presentation of CAD is determined by the distribution of the atherosclerotic lesions, the severity of stenosis, the level of myocardial oxygen demand, and the relative acuity or chronicity of the oxygen supply-demand mismatch. The three most common presentations for patients with CAD are angina pectoris, myocardial infarction (MI), and chronic ischemic cardiomyopathy.
    1. **Angina pectoris** is a symptom complex resulting from reversible myocardial ischemia without cellular necrosis. Patients typically complain of retrosternal chest pain or pressure that often radiates to the left shoulder and down the left arm or into the neck. Stable angina occurs with reproducible increases in myocardial oxygen demand (e.g., exercise) and

resolves with rest or the administration of nitrates. Unstable angina refers to chest pain that occurs at rest or episodes of pain that are increasing in frequency, duration, or severity. Silent myocardial ischemia occurs when there is ECG evidence of myocardial ischemia in the absence of any angina or angina-equivalent symptoms. The extent to which the patient's activity is limited can be graded according to the **New York Heart Association classification:** class I, no symptoms; class II, symptoms with heavy exertion; class III, symptoms with mild exertion; class IV, symptoms at rest.

2. **Acute MI** results from interruption of myocardial oxygen supply with irreversible muscle injury and cell death. The patient typically presents with protracted and severe chest pain, possibly associated with nausea, diaphoresis, or shortness of breath. There are increases in the troponin isoenzyme, creatine kinase–MB isoenzyme, or serum lactate dehydrogenase. ECG changes include ST-segment elevation, T-wave inversions, and the development of new Q waves. Early and late sequelae of acute MI can include atrial or ventricular arrhythmias, heart failure, rupture of the interventricular septum or ventricular free wall, dysfunction or rupture of the papillary muscle(s) and new mitral regurgitation (MR), and the development of a ventricular aneurysm.

   a. **Arrhythmias** are common during the first 24 hours after acute MI. In addition to potentially fatal ventricular arrhythmias, patients can develop supraventricular tachycardia, atrial fibrillation, atrial flutter, heart block of any degree, or junctional rhythms.

   b. **Congestive heart failure** (CHF) may result when a large portion (usually >25%) of the left ventricular myocardium is infarcted. Cardiogenic shock and death often occur with loss of more than 40% of the left ventricular myocardium. There is additional discussion of CHF in Section D.

   c. **Rupture of the interventricular septum** occurs in approximately 2% of patients after MI (anterior wall in 60%, inferior wall in 40%) and leads to a **ventricular septal defect (VSD).** Septal perforation typically occurs when the myocardium is at its weakest, approximately 3 to 5 days after an acute MI, but it may develop 2 or more weeks later. An acute VSD is suggested by a new holosystolic murmur and an oxygen step-up from the right atrium to the pulmonary artery, as evaluated with a pulmonary artery catheter. This is determined by comparing the oxygen saturation of samples drawn simultaneously from the central venous port and the distal pulmonary artery port. A step-up of >9% is generally held to be diagnostic of a left-to-right shunt. The diagnosis can be confirmed with echocardiography. More than 75% of patients survive the initial event and are candidates for urgent surgical repair of the VSD before the they develop the sequelae of low-output syndrome (i.e., multiorgan system failure), which greatly increases the operative risk. An intra-aortic balloon pump (IABP) is indicated to support the failing circulation until surgical correction is possible. Ventricular free-wall rupture results in hemopericardium and cardiac tamponade, which usually is fatal. For those patients who survive, emergent surgical repair is indicated.

   d. **Acute mitral regurgitation** is caused by papillary muscle dysfunction or rupture after an infarction that has extended into the region of the papillary muscles (usually the posteroinferior wall). The failing circulation should be supported with an IABP or percutaneous cardiopulmonary bypass (CPB), if necessary, until emergent operation can be performed.

   e. **Ventricular aneurysm,** a well-defined fibrous scar that replaces the normal myocardium, develops in 5% to 10% of individuals after acute MI. The majority of aneurysms develop at the anteroseptal aspect of the left ventricle after infarction in the distribution of the LAD coronary artery. Large dyskinetic left ventricular aneurysms can reduce the left ventricular ejection fraction substantially, resulting in signs and symptoms of congestive heart failure. These scars can also serve as the substrate for ischemic reentrant ventricular arrhythmias. Additionally, the pooled blood that collects in the aneurysm can clot and shower emboli into the peripheral circulation.

3. **Chronic ischemic cardiomyopathy** can develop after several MIs. Diffuse myocardial injury results in diminishing ventricular function and, eventually, signs and symptoms of heart failure. This presentation is most common in patients with diffuse small-vessel disease (e.g., in patients with diabetes mellitus).

4. **Coronary revascularization** may be accomplished via percutaneous transluminal coronary angioplasty (PTCA) or CABG. Indications depend on the patient but generally include intractable symptoms and proximal coronary stenoses that place a significant portion of myocardium at risk.

   a. **PTCA** is often used for focal symmetric stenoses in proximal coronary vessels. It is generally contraindicated if there is significant left main coronary disease, three-vessel disease, or complex obstructive lesions. PTCA is associated with a high incidence of restenosis, which may be reduced with the concomitant placement of an endoluminal stent. The recently developed **drug-eluting stents**, which prevent neointimal hyperplasia, have demonstrated low 1-year restenosis rates. At Washington University in 2003, 2% of patients required repeat PTCA, and 0.6% of patients required surgical referral at the 6-month follow-up (courtesy M. Taniuchi, Barnes-Jewish Cardiac Catheterization database).

   b. **CABG** is indicated for patients with documented atherosclerotic CAD in several settings: (1) patients with unstable angina for whom maximal medical therapy has failed; (2) patients with severe chronic stable angina who have multivessel disease or left main or proximal LAD stenoses; (3) patients with severe, reversible left ventricular dysfunction (documented by stress thallium scan or dobutamine echocardiography); (4) patients who develop coronary occlusive complications during PTCA or other endovascular interventions; and (5) patients who develop life-threatening complications after acute MI, including VSD, ventricular free-wall rupture, and acute MR.

   c. The rate of emergency surgery for failed percutaneous interventions over the past 3 years at Washington University was 0.04% (courtesy M. Taniuchi, Barnes-Jewish Cardiac Catheterization database). This decrease has been due to improved delivery systems and the development of covered stents for perforation. For patients with hemodynamic instability or refractory angina after failed angioplasty, IABP support or percutaneous CPB may be helpful before an emergent operation can be performed. Given the safety record of percutaneous catheter intervention in recent years, the concept of an operating room "at the ready" is dwindling, and some groups have even proposed angiography suites without cardiac surgery backup.

   d. **CABG** results in initial elimination of angina in more than 90% of patients. Perioperative mortality ranges from 1% to 2% in low-risk patients to more than 10% to 15% in high-risk patients. Graft patency after CABG is related to the bypass conduit used and the outflow vessel. The LITA patency at 5 years was 98%, at 10 years it was 95%, and at 15 years it was 88%. The RITA patency at 5 years was 96%, at 10 years it was 81%, and at 15 years it was 65%. The radial artery patency at 1 year was 96%, and at 4 years it was 89% (*Ann Thor Surg* 2004;77:93–101). Reverse saphenous vein grafts have 10-year patency rates of approximately 80% to the LAD and 50% to the circumflex or right coronary artery. Antiplatelet therapy using aspirin (81 to

325 mg per day) beginning immediately after operation and continued indefinitely is recommended to increase the graft patency rate.

B. Valvular heart disease

1. Aortic valve

a. Aortic stenosis (AS). Left ventricular outflow obstruction can occur at the subvalvular, the supravalvular, or (most commonly) the valvular level. Aortic valvular stenosis is usually the result of senile degeneration and calcification of a normal or a congenitally bicuspid aortic valve. Less frequently, AS develops many years after an episode of acute rheumatic fever. AS places a pressure overload on the left ventricle. Adequate cardiac output is usually maintained until late in the course of AS, but at the expense of **left ventricular hypertrophy.** Physical signs include a systolic ejection murmur, diminished carotid pulses, and a sustained, forceful, nondisplaced apical impulse. Symptoms often develop when the valve area decreases to 1.0 cm^2 or less. **Angina pectoris** develops in approximately 65% of patients with severe AS and results from ventricular hypertrophy (e.g., increased myocardial oxygen demand and reduced coronary perfusion) and the high incidence of concomitant CAD. **Syncope** (25% incidence) probably results from fixed cardiac output and decreased cerebral perfusion during systemic vasodilatation. Congestive heart failure is the presenting symptom in approximately one-third of patients and usually manifests as dyspnea on exertion. The development of symptoms is associated with a 50% 2-year mortality (*Am Heart J* 1980;99:419).

b. Aortic insufficiency (AI) is usually the result of valve leaflet pathology from rheumatic heart disease (often associated with mitral valve disease) or myxomatous degeneration. AI also may result from other causes of leaflet dysfunction or aortic root dilatation, including endocarditis, syphilis, connective tissue diseases (e.g., Marfan syndrome), inflammatory disease (e.g., ankylosing spondylitis), hypertension, and aortic dissection. Chronic AI results in volume overload of the left ventricle, causing chamber enlargement and wall thickening (although a relatively normal ratio of wall thickness to volume is usually maintained). Gradual myocardial decompensation often progresses either without symptoms or with subtle symptoms (e.g., weakness, fatigue, or dyspnea on exertion). Physical signs include a hyperdynamic circulation with markedly increased systemic arterial pulse pressure, known as **Corrigan's water-hammer pulse;** forceful and laterally displaced apical impulse; and a decrescendo diastolic murmur. Acute AI is not well tolerated because of the lack of compensatory chamber enlargement and thus often results in fulminant pulmonary edema, myocardial ischemia, and cardiovascular collapse.

c. Aortic valve replacement is usually indicated for AS in symptomatic patients and in asymptomatic patients with critical AS (e.g., a valve area <1.0 cm^2 or a transvalvular pressure gradient >50 mm Hg). Timing of surgery for AI is critical because irreversible myocardial dysfunction often precedes the development of symptoms. Indications for operation include symptoms or objective evidence of ventricular decompensation (e.g., ejection fraction <50%, increased left ventricular end-diastolic volume and end-systolic left ventricular diameter >55 mm). If there is coexistent CAD documented by coronary arteriography, patients should undergo concomitant CABG.

2. Mitral valve

a. Mitral stenosis (MS) is caused by rheumatic fever in almost all cases. Other less common causes include collagen vascular diseases, amyloidosis, and congenital stenosis. MS places a pressure overload on the left atrium, with relative sparing of ventricular function. Left atrial dilatation to more than 45 mm is associated with a high incidence of atrial fibrillation and subsequent thromboembolism. A transvalvular pressure gradient is present when the valve area is <2 cm^2, and critical MS occurs when the valve area is 1 cm^2 or less. Physical signs include an apical diastolic murmur, an opening snap, and a loud S_1. Symptoms usually develop late and reflect pulmonary congestion (e.g., dyspnea), reduced left ventricular preload (e.g., low–cardiac-output syndrome), or atrial fibrillation (e.g., thromboembolism).

  b. Mitral regurgitation (MR) results from abnormalities of the leaflets (e.g., rheumatic disease, myxomatous degeneration, endocarditis), annulus (e.g., calcification, dilatation, or destruction), chordae tendineae (e.g., rupture from endocarditis or MI, fusion, or elongation), or ischemic papillary muscle dysfunction or rupture. The most common cause of MR in the United States is myxomatous degeneration. MR places a volume overload on the left ventricle and atrium, causing chamber enlargement and wall thickening, although a relatively normal ratio of wall thickness to volume is usually maintained. Systolic unloading into the compliant left atrium allows enhanced emptying of the left ventricle during systole, with only slight increases in oxygen consumption. Atrial fibrillation often develops because of left atrial dilatation. Physical signs include a hyperdynamic circulation and a brisk laterally displaced apical impulse; a holosystolic murmur; and a widely split S_2. Gradual myocardial decompensation often progresses in the absence of symptoms (e.g., dyspnea on exertion, fatigue). In acute MR, adaptation is not possible, and fulminant cardiac decompensation often ensues.

  c. Mitral valve repair or replacement is indicated for patients with symptomatic MR, new-onset atrial fibrillation, or objective evidence of left ventricular dysfunction (same as for AI). Operation is indicated in symptomatic MS or asymptomatic patients with critical MS (valve orifice <1 cm^2). With the advent of mitral valve repair, operation is often undertaken earlier if the valvular anatomy suggests that the valve can be repaired rather than replaced.

3. Tricuspid valve

  a. Tricuspid insufficiency (TI) most often results from a functional dilatation of the valve annulus caused by pulmonary hypertension, which, in turn, may be caused by intrinsic mitral or aortic valve disease. Causes of primary TI include rheumatic heart disease, bacterial endocarditis (usually in intravenous drug users), carcinoid tumors, and blunt trauma. Patients have a systolic murmur, a prominent jugular venous pulse, and a pulsatile liver. Mild to moderate TI usually is well tolerated.

  b. Significant **tricuspid regurgitation** may be repaired at the time of surgery for other cardiac anomalies. Intervention for isolated TI is uncommon. The majority of tricuspid valves can be repaired with simple annuloplasty techniques rather than replacement.

4. Selection of a prosthetic valve must be individualized for each patient. Despite years of research, there still is no ideal prosthetic valve. The general considerations for selecting an appropriate prosthetic valve are summarized in Table 35-2.

  a. Bioprostheses are made from animal tissues, usually the porcine aortic valve or bovine pericardium. Examples include the Carpentier-Edwards, Hancock, and Edwards stented valves and the St. Jude and Medtronic stentless valves. These prostheses are associated with a low rate of thromboembolism, even without long-term anticoagulation. However, they are less durable than mechanical valves. Their rate of deterioration depends on the patient's age, being relatively faster in younger patients and slower in the elderly. Overall, the mean time to failure is approximately 10 years. Bioprostheses are the preferred valves for older patients (over 65) or patients with a contraindication

Table 35-2. Selection of a prosthetic valve

Bioprosthetic valve
Reoperation unlikely
Age >65 years
Previous thrombosed mechanical valve
Limited life expectancy
Anticoagulant-related complication or intolerance
Unreliable anticoagulant risk

Mechanical valve
Reoperation likely
Age <60 years
Long life expectancy
Small aortic annulus
Composite graft
Patient fear of reoperation

---

to lifelong anticoagulation (e.g., young women who desire future pregnancies).
   b. **Mechanical valves** have excellent long-term durability, but the high rate of thromboembolic complications (0.5% to 3.0% per year) necessitates lifelong anticoagulation. All of these valves are manufactured from **pyrolytic carbon,** which was first discovered in 1966 and has the unique quality of thromboresistance. Examples include the St. Jude, Medtronic Hall, CarboMedics, Starr-Edwards, and Björk-Shiley valves. These valves typically are used in young patients who have a long life expectancy.
   c. **Allograft and autograft valves** are useful for replacement of the aortic valve, particularly in the setting of endocarditis (*J Heart Valve Dis* 1994;3:377–387). These prostheses have excellent durability and a low incidence of thromboembolism, but experience with them is limited by the supply of allografts and the relative difficulty of the autograft (Ross) procedure, in which a patient's pulmonic valve is used to replace the diseased aortic valve.
5. **Endocarditis.** The main indications for operation include hemodynamic instability, recurrent septic emboli, and persistent evidence of infection despite appropriate antibiotic therapy. Relative indications include severe acute mitral or aortic valvular insufficiency, heart block, and intracardiac fistulas. The risk for prosthetic valve endocarditis in the first year is higher (approximately 5%) in patients with replacement surgery during active infective endocarditis, especially if the causal organism is unknown or the antibiotic treatment is insufficient. The incidence of prosthetic valve endocarditis is similar or slightly lower for mechanical prostheses than for bioprostheses after 1 year following implantation. Antibiotic therapy alone may be sufficient for some late infections, but expeditious valve replacement usually is required.
6. **Perivalvular leak** occurs when the implanted valve dislodges from the valve annulus. This may lead to clinically significant valvular regurgitation, which can be documented by echocardiography. Hemolytic anemia may be documented by an increased reticulocyte count, increased serum lactate dehydrogenase level, and increased urinary iron excretion. Replacement of the valve is indicated for perivalvular leak associated with moderate to severe valvular regurgitation or severe hemolysis.
7. **Thrombosis and thromboembolism.** Thrombus formation may occur on the surface of the artificial valve and lead to valve thrombosis or

embolism. Embolic complications may include transient ischemic attack, stroke, or embolism to the kidneys or extremities. The use of appropriate anticoagulation [international normalized ratio (INR) = 2.5 to 3.5 times control] with mechanical valves may reduce the risk of thromboembolism to the level (approximately 0.5% per year) associated with bioprosthetic valves.

C. Atrial fibrillation affects over 2.2 million people in the United States, with approximately 160,000 new cases per year. It affects nearly 10% of individuals over the age of 80 years. Morbidity includes patient discomfort, hemodynamic compromise, and thromboembolism.

1. Nonsurgical management of atrial fibrillation includes antiarrhythmic drugs, cardioversion, and percutaneous transcatheter ablation. Although drugs can induce **chemical cardioversion,** their failure rate in some series is as high as 60% at 2 years. (*Cardiology* 2001;95:1–8). When cardioversion fails, the use of chronic anticoagulation for stroke prevention has significant associated morbidity. As the pulmonary veins have been shown to be the source of ectopic foci in many patients with paroxysmal atrial fibrillation, the use of catheter-based ablation and isolation of the pulmonary veins has gained popularity and has demonstrated increasing success.

2. Surgical indications for atrial fibrillation in patients who have failed medical therapy include drug or arrhythmia intolerance, cerebrovascular accident, and concomitant coronary artery or valve disease requiring operative repair. The **Cox maze III procedure,** first performed in 1988, was based on the principle that atrial fibrillation originates from multiple macro-reentrant circuits in the atria. Through a median sternotomy, a series of incisions on both atria, excision of the atrial appendages, and isolation of the pulmonary veins prevent the formation of these macro-reentrant circuits. Long-term results have been outstanding, with a freedom from atrial fibrillation of 97% at a median of 5.4 years and an operative mortality of <2% (*J Thorac Cardiovasc Surg* 2003;126:1822–1827). This "cut and sew" procedure is difficult to perform, and consequently few surgeons have become proficient at it. Recently, less invasive surgical procedures have been developed that have replaced the surgical incisions with linear ablations. These techniques include the use of cryosurgery, radiofrequency or microwave energy, and ultrasound. These new approaches have broadened the use of surgery for atrial fibrillation and have had promising early success (*Ann Thorac Surg* 2002;74:2210–2217).

D. Heart Failure. It is estimated that approximately 300,000 people suffer from advanced heart failure in the United States. The management of heart failure involves medical and surgical care and both acute and chronic interventions. The surgical management of heart failure is herein discussed.

1. The **intra-aortic balloon pump** is used as the first-line device to provide circulatory support in acute heart failure (*Ann Thorac Surg* 1992;54:11).

   a. **Physiology.** The principle effect of the IABP is a dramatic reduction in left ventricular afterload. The resulting effects include improved ventricular ejection and reduction in myocardial oxygen consumption. The IABP inflates during early diastole, increasing diastolic BP and thus also diastolic coronary artery blood flow.

   b. **Indications for the IABP** vary in relation to the timing of operation. In the preoperative period, the IABP is indicated for low–cardiac-output states and for unstable angina refractory to medical therapy (e.g., nitrates, heparin, β-adrenergic blocking agents). Intraoperatively, the IABP is used to permit discontinuation of CPB when inotropic agents alone are not sufficient. In the postoperative period, the IABP is used primarily for low–cardiac-output states. The IABP may be used to support the circulation during periods of refractory arrhythmias and can also be used to provide support to the patient awaiting cardiac transplantation.

   c. Insertion of the IABP generally is accomplished percutaneously via the common femoral artery. Sheathless devices, because of their narrower diameter, may have decreased the incidence of lower-extremity ischemic complications. Correct placement should be confirmed by chest x-ray. The radio-opaque tip of the balloon is positioned just below the aortic knob and just distal to the left subclavian artery. At operation, the IABP may be placed directly into the transverse aortic arch, with the balloon positioned down into the descending aorta. Before **removal of the IABP,** the platelet count, PT, and PTT should be normal. Manual pressure should be applied for 20 to 30 minutes after removal to achieve hemostasis and avoid the formation of a femoral artery pseudoaneurysm or arteriovenous fistula.

   d. Management of the device after placement focuses on ensuring proper diastolic inflation and deflation. The ECG and the femoral (or aortic) pressure waveform are monitored continuously on a bedside console. The device may be triggered using either the ECG or the pressure tracing for every heartbeat (1:1) or less frequently (1:2, 1:3). Anticoagulation during IABP support is optional. If the balloon must be repositioned or removed, the device should be turned off first. IABP support is withdrawn gradually by decreasing the augmentation frequency from 1:1 to 1:3 in steps of several hours each.

   e. Complications of IABP therapy include incorrect placement of the device, resulting in perforation of the aorta; injury to the femoral artery; and reduction in blood flow to the visceral or renal arteries. Ischemia of the lower extremity, evidenced by diminished peripheral pulses or other sequelae, may necessitate removal of the IABP or performance of an inflow arterial bypass procedure (e.g., femoral-to-femoral artery). Rupture of the balloon is an indication for immediate removal because blood may clot within the ruptured balloon, necessitating operative removal.

2. Ventricular remodeling. The progression of heart failure leads to dilatation and structural changes in the ventricle by a process known as remodeling. Initially, these changes are compensatory, but eventually they result in pathologic states, including high wall stress, increased neurohormonal levels, and increased inflammatory mediators, that lead to congestive heart failure.

   a. Partial left ventriculectomy. There are several techniques described to reduce the diameter of the left ventricle. In most series, after an initial improvement, heart failure parameters returned to their preoperative state. For the most part, these procedures have been abandoned in favor of assist devices and transplantation.

   b. Ischemic cardiomyopathy. The repair of ischemic left ventricular aneurysms or akinetic infarctions, either by direct excision or patch repair (**Dor procedure**) may play a role in end-stage heart failure. Based on the concept that ventricular contraction begins in the apex, the direct exclusion or patch ventriculoplasty removes both the stagnant blood as well as the low resistance chamber within the ventricle. The Dor procedure remodels the ventricle from the pathologic spherical shape toward the normal and mechanically more favorable elliptical shape.

3. Mitral valve surgery has gained recent popularity for the therapy of congestive heart failure. Mitral regurgitation secondary to ventricular dilatation is dependent on ventricular geometry and results from mitral annular lengthening, leading to poor leaflet coaptation. The use of a mitral ring annuloplasty has been shown to be safe and effective in a large series for improving NYHA class, left ventricular ejection fraction, cardiac output, and left ventricular end-diastolic volume (*Eur J Heart Fail*

2000;35: 365–371). In fact, it has been estimated that up to 10% of patients undergoing heart transplant evaluation may benefit from mitral valve repair (*J Heart Valve Dis* 2002;11: S26–S31). In cases where papillary muscle dysfunction due to ischemia has changed valvular geometry considerably, mitral valve replacement rather than repair may be more appropriate.

4. **Ventricular assist devices (VADs)** may be used to support the left side of the circulation (LVAD) or the right side of the circulation (RVAD). When both an LVAD and an RVAD are used, the combination is termed a **biventricular assist device (BiVAD)**.

   a. The **physiologic effect** of a VAD is decompression of the left or right ventricle (or both) and restoration of cardiac output, resulting in decreased myocardial oxygen consumption. The goal is either to permit recovery of myocardium that is not irreversibly injured (e.g., "stunned" myocardium) or to support the circulation in patients with a failing heart until a heart transplantation is possible.

   b. **Indications for a VAD** include (1) inability to separate from CPB despite inotropic and IABP support ("bridge to recovery"), (2) intermediate-term cardiac support ("bridge to transplant"), and (3) permanent replacement therapy ("destination therapy").

   c. **VAD subtypes**
      (1) Nonpulsatile devices
         (a) Centrifugal pumps (BioMedicus Bio-pump and 3M Sarns Delphin) have been used most frequently as bridges to recovery in patients with postcardiotomy cardiogenic shock. In the subgroup of patients in whom recovery does not occur, these patients become transplant candidates. Advantages include widespread availability, low cost, and simplicity. Disadvantages include the need for systemic anticoagulation, limited duration of support, and the need for continuous supervision by specially trained personnel.
         (b) ECMO. See Section IV.B.
         (c) Axial flow pumps (Transicoil Jarvik 2000, MicroMed DeBakey VAD, Thoratec HeartMate II) are small pumps, consume less power, and may be completely implantable without the need for external cables to power the device. They are based on the concept that pulsatile flow is not necessary to maintain adequate organ perfusion. All these devices have been approved for clinical trials in the United States.
      (2) Pulsatile devices
         (a) External devices (Abiomed BVS 5000 and Thoratec Ventricular Assist Device) have generally the same indications as centrifugal pumps, although the duration of support may be somewhat longer. Advantages are that the devices are designed to allow sternal closure (centrifugal pumps require an open chest) and that they may have a lower incidence of thromboembolism and generally support higher flow. A disadvantage is that systemic anticoagulation is still required.
         (b) Long-term implantable devices (WorldHeart Novacor and Thoratec HeartMate) are used primarily as bridges to transplantation in patients with chronic heart failure. See "Destination Therapy," Section V.D.4.g.

   d. **Insertion** of VADs. In general, RVADs receive inflow from the right atrium and return outflow to the pulmonary artery using flexible cannulae or grafts. LVADs receive inflow from the left atrium or ventricle and return outflow to the ascending aorta.

   e. **Management** of the VAD after placement focuses on maintaining proper function and adequate anticoagulation. The activated clotting time should be monitored frequently and maintained at approximately

200 seconds. Patients should receive medications to ensure adequate sedation, analgesia, and muscle paralysis. Factors that impact **a low-flow state status post-LVAD** include right ventricular dysfunction, pulmonary hypertension, hypovolemia, and tamponade. It is therefore critical that maximum ventilatory support be provided, including the use of nitrous oxide as necessary.

f. **Complications** of VAD therapy include excessive bleeding, thrombus formation, embolization, and hemolysis. Associated complications not related to the device specifically include respiratory failure (due to infection or fluid overload) and renal failure. Long-term complications include infection, stroke, and device failure.

g. **Destination therapy.** The recent Randomized Evaluation of Mechanical Assistance for the Treatment of Congestive Heart Failure (REMATCH) trial compared assist devices with best medical therapy and demonstrated a decrease in mortality of 48% at 2 years in 129 patients. The most dramatic increase in survival occurred in those who required inotropic support at randomization (104% at 1 year). In addition, there was a significant quality-of-life improvement (*N Engl J Med* 2001;345:1435–1443). The Thoratec Heartmate XVE Left Ventricular Assist System (LVAS) has been approved for destination therapy by the FDA.

5. **Cardiac transplantation** can provide relief from symptoms in patients with end-stage cardiomyopathy who are functionally incapacitated despite medical therapy and who are not candidates for any other cardiac operation. The first successful heart transplant occurred in 1967 in South Africa. There were 2,057 heart transplants performed in the United States in 2003, making this intervention an infrequently used but important modality in the management of heart failure. Currently, the 1-year survival following heart transplant exceeds 86% (UNOS database, 2004).

a. **Accepted indications for heart transplant** include cardiomyopathy that is ischemic, idiopathic, postpartum, or chemotherapy induced. These patients are in Class III or IV NYHA CHF, have a Heart Failure Survival Score of high risk, and have a peak V_{O2} <10 mL/kg per minute after reaching an anaerobic threshhold. Relative indications include instability in fluid balance or renal function despite best medical therapy, recurrent unstable angina not amenable to revascularization, and a peak V_{O2} <14 mL/kg per minute.

b. **Contraindications to transplantation** include age older than 65 years, irreversible pulmonary hypertension (>4 Wood units), active infection, recent pulmonary embolus, renal dysfunction (serum creatinine >2.5 mg/dL or creatinine clearance <25 mL/min), hepatic dysfunction (bilirubin >2.5 or ALT/AST >×2), active or recent malignancy, systemic disease such as amyloidosis, significant carotid or peripheral vascular disease, active or recent peptic ulcer disease, brittle diabetes mellitus, morbid obesity, mental illness, substance abuse, or psychosocial instability.

c. **Donor pool expansion.** Due to the shortage of acceptable donors, the use of an expanded donor pool has been advocated. Some centers have tolerated size mismatch, increased age (>55 years), malignancy, infection, or even donor bypass grafting for carefully selected high-risk recipients.

d. **Immunosuppressive therapy** generally includes a calcineurin inhibitor (cyclosporine or sirolimus), steroids and an antimetabolite (mycofenolate or azathioprine). Cyclosporine usually is started preoperatively. The dosage is adjusted to achieve circulating plasma levels of 250 to 350 ng/mL. Levels significantly above this range may cause nephrotoxicity. Steroid therapy is initiated in the operating room. When rejection episodes occur, the majority can be reversed with bolus doses of intravenous steroids. When rejection episodes are resistant to increased steroid doses, the monoclonal antibody OKT3 or rabbit antithymocyte serum can be added to the treatment regimen. Immunosuppression is covered in more detail in Chapter 28.

  e. Acute allograft rejection is diagnosed by **endomyocardial biopsy.** Biopsy forceps are passed into the right ventricle percutaneously, using fluoroscopic or echocardiographic guidance, usually via the right internal jugular or femoral vein, and several biopsies are taken to document the presence and degree of rejection histologically. During the early postoperative period, biopsies are performed several times each month. After the first 6 months, the frequency of biopsies is decreased to one to two times per year. Whenever a patient develops evidence of a rejection episode, a biopsy is performed. Complications of endomyocardial biopsy are rare but include ventricular perforation, pneumothorax, transient ventricular or supraventricular arrhythmias, hematoma, and infection. **Coronary artery vasculopathy (CAV),** thought to represent **chronic vascular rejection,** occurs in a significant percentage of cardiac transplant recipients and is a major limitation on the long-term success of cardiac transplantation. CAV is usually not amenable to conventional revascularization owing to small-vessel, nonfocal disease and often requires retransplantation.

6. Future therapy for heart failure

  a. Device therapy. There has been a substantial improvement in devices over the last 2 decades. They have become smaller, more durable and less prone to thrombotic complications. Devices will ultimately be totally implantable, and there will eventually be a **totally implantable artificial heart.**

  b. Myocyte regeneration. Several approaches, including those using embryonic stem cells, cardiomyocytes, cryopreserved fetal cardiomyocytes, skeletal myoblasts, bone marrow–derived mesenchymal cells, and dermal fibroblasts, are under investigation.

  c. Xenotransplantation. The primary difficulty in xenotransplantation is the management of rejection and cross-species infection, and to date such management has been unsuccessful. Current data do not yet justify clinical trials.

E. Diseases of the **thoracic aorta** include aortic dissection, traumatic disruption of the aorta, and thoracic aortic aneurysms (see Chapter 22 for details).

  1. Dissection of the aorta occurs when blood dissects within the media of the aorta, creating a false lumen. Aortic dissection may be acute or chronic (arbitrarily >14 days).

  a. Classification. Dissections are classified by a number of schemes according to their location; two of the schemes are presented here.

    (1) In the **DeBakey classification,** type I dissections involve the ascending aorta, the aortic arch, and the descending aorta; type II dissections involve the ascending aorta only; and type III dissections involve only the descending aorta. Type III dissections are subdivided into type IIIa, involving only the descending thoracic aorta, and type IIIb, also involving the abdominal aorta.

    (2) The **Stanford classification** is a simpler scheme, for it categorizes any dissection involving the ascending aorta as type A and those involving only the descending aorta as type B.

  b. Risk factors. Medial degeneration of the aorta (formerly cystic medial necrosis) is present in 20% of patients. Approximately 20% to 40% of patients with Marfan syndrome develop acute aortic dissection. Other common associations include annuloaortic ectasia, bicuspid aortic valve, atherosclerosis, and coarctation of the aorta.

  c. Pathophysiology. The **false lumen** typically occupies one-half to two-thirds of the circumference of the aorta. There may be a small leak from the false lumen, producing a mediastinal hematoma. The false lumen may rupture (1) into the pericardium, producing pericardial tamponade; (2) into the pleural space, producing hemothorax; or (3) into the abdomen, though this rarely occurs. During the dissection process, the major branches of the aorta may be uninvolved, may derive their blood supply from the false lumen, or may occlude.

d. **Clinical presentation.** Patients with rupture of the false lumen or occlusion of one or more coronary arteries may present in extremis. Severe hypovolemic shock may result from hemorrhage. Patients with acute dissection present most commonly with a sudden onset of excruciating back or chest pain. Type A dissections can cause acute aortic insufficiency and malperfusion of the coronary arteries. These complications can lead to congestive heart failure and myocardial infarction, respectively. Other symptoms may be referable to occlusion of major arteries (e.g., splanchnic vessels). The differential diagnosis includes acute MI and pulmonary embolism. Unlike patients with MI or pulmonary embolism, patients with acute aortic dissection often present with hypertension.

e. **Diagnosis.** The **chest x-ray** may demonstrate widening of the mediastinum or cardiomegaly. **Computed tomographic (CT) scan** is probably the most common modality for diagnosing acute aortic dissections and may be used to detect the presence of true and false lumens and to evaluate the extent of the dissection process. Although **MRI scans** may be more sensitive and specific than CT, the time delay in obtaining the scans may prove prohibitive in the acute setting. MRI is an excellent diagnostic modality for chronic dissections. **Transesophageal echocardiography** may demonstrate an intimal flap or wall motion abnormalities due to involvement of the coronary arteries and may be used to evaluate the presence of AI. Although transesophageal echocardiography is sensitive and specific, it is operator dependent. **Aortography** is a sensitive diagnostic study but is performed less commonly today because less invasive diagnostic modalities have been developed. **Selective coronary arteriography** is indicated in stable patients with coronary risk factors or evidence of myocardial ischemia because CABG may be performed together with aortic repair (*Ann Thorac Surg* 1995;59:585).

f. **Treatment**
   (1) **DeBakey types I and II and Stanford type A dissections.** Any patient with dissection of the ascending aorta should undergo urgent operation for replacement of the ascending aorta and resection of the intimal tear. Relative contraindications include advanced age and the presence of an incurable disease. Operation is performed through a median sternotomy. Options for replacement of the ascending aorta include tube grafts, composite grafts (aortic valve with conduit graft), and cryopreserved homografts. The aortic valve commissures can be resuspended if they have become detached from the proximal ascending aorta. When the dissection process involves the proximal coronary arteries, bypass grafts may be required.
   (2) **DeBakey type III and Stanford type B dissections.** The **treatment** generally is medical, with the goal of maintaining normal BP using sodium nitroprusside and a reduction in heart rate (to 60 to 70 beats per minute) and left ventricular work with β-adrenergic receptor antagonists. With medical therapy, the 1-year survival rate is approximately 80%. Operation is indicated for patients with complications of the acute dissection process (e.g., hemothorax, persistent pain, limb or visceral ischemia, acute renal failure, paraplegia) and chronic enlargement of the aneurysm to >6 cm or enlargement of more than 1 cm per year.

g. **Follow-up.** Careful control of postoperative hypertension is associated with increased survival, decreased risk of false lumen aneurysm rupture (10% to 20% versus 50% in patients with poorly controlled hypertension), and decreased risk of recurrent dissection. A chest x-ray and CT scan of the chest should be obtained every 6 months to evaluate for the presence of aneurysm formation. The risk of recurrent dissection is approximately 15%.

2. **Traumatic disruption of the aorta** usually occurs after severe blunt traumatic injuries, such as those characteristic of high-speed motor vehicle accidents. The disruption occurs most commonly just proximal to the ligamentum arteriosum in the upper descending aorta (70%) but may occur less commonly in the ascending aorta (10%) or other sites in the descending aorta (20%).

   a. **Clinical presentation.** Patients with traumatic disruption of the aorta often have other severe injuries. Pain due to aortic disruption is uncommon. Decreased blood flow to the brain or extremities due to occlusion of the major arterial branches of the aorta also is uncommon.

   b. **Radiologic evaluation.** The chest x-ray may demonstrate widening of the mediastinum, hemothorax, tracheal shift to the right, or blurring of the aortic knob. The presence of associated injuries to the first and second ribs or the clavicles should raise the suspicion of injury to the aorta. **Aortography** is used to confirm the presence of aortic disruption and should be obtained in most patients before operation. **Transesophageal echocardiography** may be useful for documenting the presence of aortic disruption, as well as for evaluating the function of the aortic valve, and may obviate the need for aortography in selected patients (*N Engl J Med* 1995;332:356). A chest CT scan may demonstrate mediastinal hematoma associated with aortic disruption but should not delay aortography or transesophageal echocardiography.

   c. **Natural history.** The risk of death is greatest in the period immediately after injury. This risk decreases over time, but there is a finite increased risk of death even 10 years after the injury. Late deaths are typically due to rupture of traumatic false aneurysms.

   d. **Operation** is indicated for any patient in whom aortic disruption is discovered within 5 days of injury and is strongly recommended for patients in whom the diagnosis is made later. For repair of aortic disruptions of the upper descending aorta, the patient is positioned in the right lateral decubitus position, and operation is performed through a left posterolateral thoracotomy. The aorta proximal and distal to the tear generally is replaced with a woven polyethylene terephthalate (Dacron) graft. The mortality rate exceeds 20%, and the paraplegia rate exceeds 15%, both of which are independent of concomitant injuries (*Ann Thorac Surg* 1996;61:875–878). Recently, endoluminal stent grafts have been used in this setting and have the potential to decrease operative morbidity and mortality in selected patients.

VI. **Postoperative management.** Postoperative care of the cardiac surgery patient is provided in three phases: in the intensive care unit (ICU), in the step-down unit, and after discharge from the hospital.

   A. **Intensive care.** ICU care resources generally are required for 1 to 3 days after an operation requiring CPB.

      1. **Initial assessment.** Information on the patient's history, indications for operation, and technical details of operation (e.g., coronary arteries bypassed, conduits used, CPB time, and aortic cross-clamp time) should be related to the ICU staff by the surgeon. The anesthesiologist should relate information about the intraoperative course, including preoperative and intraoperative hemodynamic parameters (especially cardiac filling pressures) and current medications. A thorough physical examination

should be performed, with attention to the cardiovascular system. A baseline chest x-ray and ECG are usually obtained.

2. **Monitoring in the immediate postoperative period** is usually extensive. Continuous recordings are made of arterial, central venous, and pulmonary artery pressures; the ECG; and arterial oxygen saturation using pulse oximetry. The pulmonary artery wedge pressure is measured as indicated by the patient's status, and calculations are made of the cardiac output, cardiac index (cardiac output per unit of body-surface area), stroke volume, pulmonary vascular resistance, and systemic vascular resistance (by thermodilution technique). Normal values for these parameters are listed in Table 35-1. Immediate attention is necessary to determine the etiology and to correct deviations from normal values of any of these parameters. **Body temperature** is monitored continuously using a pulmonary artery thermistor. Because early postoperative hypothermia may increase afterload (systemic vascular resistance) and adversely affect blood clotting, hypothermia is treated aggressively by the application of air-warming blankets. Warming is discontinued when the core temperature reaches 36.0°C. A cooling blanket is applied, and acetaminophen is administered if the body temperature is >38.5°C. For patients with persistent fever, an aggressive search should be made for evidence of infection.

3. **Cardiovascular. Cardiac pump function** is assessed as described earlier. A cardiac index of 2.0 L per minute per m^2 is generally a minimum acceptable value. A mixed venous oxygen saturation of <60% suggests inadequate peripheral tissue perfusion and increased peripheral oxygen extraction. Etiologies include reduced oxygen-carrying capacity (e.g., low hematocrit), reduced cardiac output, and increased oxygen consumption (e.g., shivering). Common causes of low cardiac output in the early postoperative period are hypovolemia, increased systemic vascular resistance due to persistent hypothermia or increased circulating catecholamines, and decreased contractility secondary to myocardial stunning.

   a. **Preload** is increased by administering crystalloid solution (e.g., lactated Ringer solution) or colloid solution (e.g., 6% hetastarch, 5% albumin) as needed to maintain the pulmonary arterial wedge pressure in the target range, as determined by the patient's diastolic compliance and systolic performance. Using blood products in a judicious manner is mandatory.

   b. **Afterload reduction** in the volume-restored patient increases ejection fraction and cardiac output and decreases myocardial oxygen consumption. The body temperature should be returned to the normal range, and hypertension should be controlled. In general, the mean arterial BP should be maintained near the preoperative level. For patients with valve replacement or aortic replacement, the systolic BP should be carefully controlled to prevent postoperative bleeding. Afterload is often initially titrated with parenteral infusions of sodium nitroprusside, nitroglycerin, or nicardipine, followed by a change to longer-acting parenteral or enteral agents.

   c. **Contractility. Inotropic agents** are used only after ensuring an adequate preload and an appropriate afterload. Selection of a particular inotropic agent must be individualized based on the agent's specific effects on the heart rate, BP, cardiac output, systemic vascular resistance, and renal blood flow. All these agents increase the work of the heart and increase myocardial oxygen consumption and thus should be used judiciously. **Mechanical support** in the form of an IABP or a VAD can be considered if other measures are ineffective in restoring adequate ventricular ejection.

   d. **Rate control.** The heart can be paced using temporary epicardial pacing electrodes (placed at the time of operation) at 80 to 100 beats per minute to increase the cardiac output. Pacing can be performed using only the atrial leads (atrial pacing, or AAI mode), only the ventricular leads (ventricular pacing, or VVI mode), or with both sets of leads (atrioventricular sequential pacing or atrial tracking with ventricular pacing). Optimal pacing always involves maintaining atrioventricular synchrony. VVI pacing should only be used in patients with atrial arrhythmias. If epicardial pacing is not necessary, the epicardial pacemaker generator is set in a backup mode to provide ventricular pacing only in the event of marked bradycardia. The pacemaker output threshold (in milliamperes) should be set to approximately twice the minimum threshold required to capture.

  e. **Arrhythmias,** including bradycardia from resolving hypothermia, heart block secondary to persistent cardioplegia effect, and supraventricular tachyarrhythmias (e.g., atrial fibrillation or flutter) can be associated with reduced cardiac output and should be corrected. **Arrhythmias** occur in more than 50% of patients after cardiac surgical procedures and are more common in patients who receive inotropic support. ACLS guidelines should be followed.

  (1) **Supraventricular arrhythmias** (atrial fibrillation, atrial flutter, paroxysmal atrial tachycardia) are most common and are associated with an increased risk of transient or permanent neurologic deficit (*Ann Thorac Surg* 1993;56:539). To reduce the incidence of postoperative arrhythmias, patients receiving β-adrenergic blocking agents preoperatively should continue to be given these medications postoperatively. Patients with supraventricular arrhythmias and hemodynamic compromise should undergo immediate electrical cardioversion (with 50 to 100 J). Because the most frequent etiology is hypoxia or hypokalemia, the new onset of a supraventricular arrhythmia should be evaluated by measurement of the arterial oxygen saturation and the serum potassium. In many patients with hemodynamically stable arrhythmias, prompt correction of the pO_2 (to >70 mm Hg) and the serum potassium level (to >4.5 mg/dL) may terminate the arrhythmia. For patients with **atrial flutter,** overdrive pacing may be used to terminate the arrhythmia. The patient's atrial temporary epicardial pacing wires are connected to a pacemaker generator, and either burst pacing (700 to 800 beats per minute for 3 to 4 seconds) or decremental pacing (stepwise decrease from 300 to 180 beats per minute) is used.

  (2) **Ventricular arrhythmias** in the postoperative period are treated as they are in other patients. Ventricular arrhythmias other than premature ventricular contractions suggest significant underlying ischemic pathology.

  f. **Cardiac tamponade** is a potentially lethal cause of low cardiac output early after operation. Clinical features include narrowed pulse pressure, rising cardiac filling pressures, pulsus paradoxus, widened mediastinal silhouette on chest radiograph, and decreased urine output. Definitive diagnosis is usually made by equalization of diastolic heart pressures or transthoracic or transesophageal echocardiography.

  g. **Perioperative MI** occurs in approximately 1% to 2% of patients and can be diagnosed by ECG changes, biochemical criteria (e.g., elevated troponin-I or creatine kinase–MB), or echocardiography. Survival may be adversely affected if complications such as cardiogenic shock or ventricular arrhythmias develop.

  h. **Postoperative hemorrhage** is common after cardiac surgery and necessitates reexploration in up to 5% of patients. Hematologic parameters (complete blood count, PT, PTT) are measured on admission to the ICU and as needed. CPB requires heparinization, causes platelet dysfunction and destruction, and activates the fibrinolytic system. Initial focus is on adequate BP control, metabolic stability, maintenance of normothermia, and adequate reversal of heparin with protamine. For patients with significant postoperative bleeding (>200 mL per hour), consideration should be given to platelet transfusion to maintain the platelet count at >100,000/μL and transfusion of fresh frozen plasma if the INR is abnormal. Some surgeons advocate stripping the chest tubes every hour to prevent clotting. If clotting becomes apparent, sterile suction tubing can be used to evacuate blood clot. The formation of undrained clot in the mediastinum may result in cardiac tamponade. This diagnosis can be made by an unexplained drop in urine output or cardiac index with adequate filling pressures and can be confirmed by echocardiography. Indications for operative reexploration for bleeding include (1) prolonged bleeding (>200 mL per hour for 4 to 6 hours), (2) excessive bleeding (>1,000 mL), (3) a sudden increase in bleeding, and (4) cardiac tamponade. Pleural and mediastinal chest tubes generally are removed when the drainage is <200 mL in 8 hours.

4. **Pulmonary. Mechanical ventilation** is used in the initial postoperative period with typical settings: intermittent mandatory ventilation, 10 to 16 breaths per minute; inspired oxygen concentration, 1.0; tidal volume, 10 to 15 mL/kg; and positive end-expiratory pressure, 5 cm H_2O. The patient can be extubated when (1) he or she is fully awake and has had a normal neurologic examination; (2) weaning parameters are satisfactory (e.g., respiratory rate <20 breaths per minute; minute ventilation <12 L per minute; negative inspiratory pressure >20 mm H_2O); (3) the arterial blood gas, with only continuous positive airway pressure, is satisfactory (pH approximately 7.40; CO_2 tension <45 mm Hg; oxygen tension >70 mm Hg); (4) there is little mediastinal bleeding (<100 mL per 8 hours); and (5) there is hemodynamic stability. Most patients can be extubated several hours after operation. After extubation, oxygen is administered by high-humidity face mask with an initial inspired oxygen concentration of 0.4. The oxygen can be weaned, as tolerated, to keep the arterial oxygen saturation above 93%.

5. **Renal. Renal dysfunction** in the postoperative period can be due to decreased perfusion pressure during CPB or to inadequate perfusion of the kidneys in the postoperative period. Treatment of acute renal insufficiency in the postoperative period includes ensuring adequate hydration and avoiding nephrotoxic medications. Fluid and electrolyte balance is evaluated immediately after operation and then as needed. Early after operation, intravenous fluids are administered slowly (<30 mL per hour). A useful measure of a patient's intravascular volume status is the body weight, which is measured daily and compared to the preoperative weight. Serum potassium levels are maintained at >4.5 mg/dL to prevent atrial and ventricular arrhythmias. Metabolic acidosis can reflect a low–cardiac-output state.

6. **Neurologic. Neurologic examination** of the patient is performed on admission to the ICU and periodically as needed. In general, the patient awakens from anesthesia several hours after operation. Changes in the neurologic examination warrant immediate investigation. Shivering increases oxygen consumption and should be treated in the early postoperative period by warming the patient or by the administration of meperidine (50 to 100 mg intramuscularly or intravenously every 3 hours) or, for the ventilated patient, pancuronium (0.04 to 0.10 mg/kg intravenously) or vecuronium (0.08 to 0.10 mg/kg slow intravenous bolus, then 1 to 5 mg per hour intravenous continuous infusion). **Pain control** is accomplished using parenteral narcotics or nonsteroidal anti-inflammatory agents, or both, during the early postoperative period.

7. **Nutrition.** The patient is given nothing by mouth until after extubation. A clear liquid diet then is begun and is advanced to a regular diet as tolerated. Patients with prolonged ventilation should receive either enteral feedings or parenteral nutrition.

8. **Infectious disease.** **Infectious complications** are uncommon after cardiac surgical procedures but may lead to substantial morbidity and mortality. Perioperative antibiotics should be administered for 24 hours. **Wound infection** occurs in 1% to 2% of sternotomy incisions and a higher proportion of saphenous vein harvest sites. Risk factors for deep sternal wound infection include diabetes mellitus, male gender, and, possibly, the use of bilateral internal thoracic arteries during CABG procedures in patients older than 74 years (*Ann Thorac Surg* 1998;65:1050–1056). Serous drainage from the skin incision is worrisome and should be treated by application of a sterile dressing twice daily and the administration of intravenous antibiotics. Purulent wound drainage, a sternal click, gross movement of the sternal edges, or substernal air on the chest x-ray may indicate a deep sternal infection. A CT scan of the chest can confirm this diagnosis. In general, deep sternal infections require operative débridement of devitalized sternal and substernal tissues, with cultures of the tissue; administration of broad-spectrum intravenous antibiotics; and vascularized muscle flap closure of the soft-tissue defect.

9. **Gastrointestinal.** **Gastrointestinal (GI) complications** are uncommon after cardiac surgical procedures. Stress gastritis is common after CPB and is thought to be secondary to subclinical ischemia of the gut mucosa. Although overt GI hemorrhage is uncommon, when it does occur, it is associated with a high mortality. Patients should receive sucralfate or H_2-receptor antagonist therapy until a regular diet is begun. GI bleeding may arise from throughout the GI tract. Acute cholecystitis, usually acalculous, is associated with high mortality. Acute pancreatitis, evidenced by hyperamylasemia, occurs in approximately 25% of patients after CPB, but only 5% of patients have abdominal pain.

B. **Step-down unit.** Step-down unit care focuses on convalescence, management of fluid balance, activity level, and diet.

1. **Fluid status.** The patient is weighed daily. Patients receiving diuretics preoperatively resume the same regimen postoperatively. For patients who were not receiving diuretics preoperatively, oral diuretics are administered until the patient's weight falls to the preoperative value. For most patients, no restrictions are placed on the daily oral fluid intake.

2. **Activity.** The patient is encouraged to be out of bed to a chair and to ambulate as early as possible after operation. Patients are instructed not to perform any heavy lifting (>10 lb) for a period of 6 weeks postoperatively.

3. **Diet.** A mild postoperative ileus may be present for several days after operation. A regular diet is begun as early as possible after operation. Some patients require a stool softener. Attention should be paid to maintaining a prudent diet that is low in salt and cholesterol.

C. **Postdischarge care.** Care after hospital discharge focuses on continued risk factor modification and surveillance for late complications. Common difficulties during the first 6 to 8 weeks after operation include decreased motivation, decreased appetite, depression, and insomnia. In general, these conditions are temporary, and the physician can provide reassurance.

1. **Physical rehabilitation** with a daily exercise program begins early after operation and continues after discharge from the hospital. Vigorous walking, with increasing distances and longer periods of activity, is the most useful form of exercise for most patients. Bicycling and swimming are acceptable alternatives after 6 to 8 weeks. Patients who were working before operation should return to work within 2 months after operation.

2. **Risk factor modification** may slow or possibly reverse the progression of atherosclerosis in bypass grafts after CABG.

   a. **Smoking** should be discontinued. Referral to organizations with smoking cessation programs should be made before operation, if possible.

   b. **Obesity.** Patients should reach an ideal body weight through planned exercise and dieting, if necessary.

    c. Hyperlipidemia is a major risk factor for the development of graft atherosclerosis and should be treated aggressively, either with diet modification or by pharmacologic intervention. Current American Heart Association guidelines suggest the following target values: total serum cholesterol <200 mg/dL, serum triglycerides <150 mg/dL, and high-density lipoproteins >35 mg/dL.

    d. Hypertension must be controlled.

    e. Postpericardiotomy (Dressler) syndrome is a delayed pericardial inflammatory reaction characterized by fever, anterior chest pain, and pericardial friction rub, and it may lead to mediastinal fibrosis and premature graft occlusion. Treatment includes nonsteroidal anti-inflammatory drugs for 2 to 4 weeks or corticosteroids for refractory cases.

General Thoracic Surgery

**Nirmal K. Veeramachaneni
and Richard J. Battafarano**

Thoracic surgery encompasses the management of both benign and malignant conditions of the esophagus, lung, pleura, and mediastinum. In this chapter, we focus on the systematic evaluation and treatment of the most common conditions. Diseases processes of the esophagus are discussed in Chapter 11.

I. **Lung cancer.** Cancer of the lung remains the leading cause of cancer death in the United States. Approximately 172,000 cases of lung cancer will be diagnosed in 2005, and over 163,000 people will die from this disease. Most newly diagnosed cases are not amenable to surgical resection and have poor prognosis. Lung cancer carries an overall 15% 5-year survival. **Cigarette smoking** remains the leading risk factor and influences risk stratification in the evaluation of a suspicious lesion. Increasing **age** also increases the probability of malignancy. Although trials conducted over 2 decades ago to screen for lung cancer by either sputum cytology or chest x-ray imaging failed to show benefit, spiral CT scanning is currently being actively investigated for the early detection of lung cancer.

A. **Radiographic presentation**
   1. **Solitary pulmonary nodule (SPN).** Due to the widespread application of CT technology, an estimated 150,000 SPNs are diagnosed each year. By definition, these are circumscribed lung lesions in an asymptomatic individual. Lesions >3 cm are called **masses.**
   2. **Radiographic imaging by CT** is used to both follow these lesions and predict outcome. The first step in the evaluation of an SPN is to evaluate any prior films. **Factors favoring a benign lesion** include absence of growth over a 2-year period, size of the lesion, and pattern of calcification. Calcifications that are diffuse, centrally located, "onion skinned" (laminar), or popcorn-like are generally benign. Eccentric or stippled calcifications may indicate malignancy. Lesion >2 cm, intravenous contrast enhancement, or irregular borders **predict malignancy.**
   3. **Positron emission tomography (PET) scanning** has demonstrated 95% sensitivity and 80% specificity in characterizing solitary pulmonary nodules. PET imaging has a high negative predictive value for most lung cancers; however, bronchoalveolar carcinoma and carcinoid tumor can be negative by PET scan, and inflammatory and infectious processes can be falsely positive. The patient's overall risk factor profile must be considered. In the setting of low risk (e.g., young age, nonsmoker, favorable features on CT), a negative PET scan has a high negative predictive value, but the same result in an elderly smoker is less reassuring and further evaluation is warranted.
   4. **Tissue biopsy** remains the gold standard for diagnosis. Tissue may be obtained by bronchoscopy in patients with central lung lesions or by CT-guided biopsy. This later technique has an 80% sensitivity for a malignant process and requires technical expertise. Surgical biopsy of SPN by either minimally invasive techniques or open technique can provide a definitive diagnosis as well as definitive treatment.

B. **Pathology**
   The **two main classes** of lung tumors are small cell (oat cell) carcinoma and non–small cell carcinoma.

1. **Small cell carcinoma** accounts for approximately 20% of all lung cancers. It is highly malignant, usually occurs centrally near the hilum, occurs almost exclusively in smokers, and rarely is amenable to surgery because of wide dissemination by the time of diagnosis. These cancers initially respond to chemotherapy, but overall 5-year survival remains 10%.

2. **Non–small cell carcinomas** account for 80% of all lung cancers and make up the vast majority of those treated by surgery. The three subtypes are **adenocarcinoma** (30% to 50% of cases), **squamous cell** (20% to 35%), and **large cell** (4% to 15%). Most tumors are histologically heterogeneous, possibly indicating common origin. **Bronchioloalveolar carcinoma** is a variant of adenocarcinoma and is known for its ability to produce mucin and its multifocal nature. Over the last decade, it has been appreciated that carcinoid tumors (grade I), atypical carcinoid tumors (grade II), large cell carcinoma, and small cell tumors represent important subgroups of bronchogenic neuroendocrine carcinoma. This may explain the more aggressive behavior of large cell carcinoma relative to other non–small cell cancers.

C. **Symptomatic presentation** of lung cancer implies a worsening stage and is associated with an overall lower rate of survival.

1. **Bronchopulmonary features** include cough or a change in a previously stable smoker's cough, increased sputum production, dyspnea, and new wheezing. Minor hemoptysis causing blood-tinged sputum, even as an isolated episode, should be investigated with flexible bronchoscopy, especially in patients with a history of smoking who are 40 years of age or older. Lung cancer may also present with postobstructive pneumonia.

2. **Extrapulmonary thoracic symptoms** include chest wall pain secondary to local tumor invasion, hoarseness from invasion of the left recurrent laryngeal nerve near the aorta and left main pulmonary artery, shortness of breath secondary to malignant pleural effusion, and superior vena cava syndrome causing facial, neck, and upper-extremity swelling. Pancoast tumor (superior sulcus tumor) can lead to brachial plexus invasion as well as invasion of the cervical sympathetic ganglia, which causes an ipsilateral Horner syndrome (ptosis, miosis, and anhidrosis). Rarely, lung cancer can present as dysphagia secondary to compression or invasion of the esophagus by mediastinal nodes or by the primary tumor.

   The most frequent **sites of distant metastases** include the liver, bone, brain, and adrenal glands. Symptoms may include pathologic fractures and arthritis from bony involvement. Brain metastasis may cause headache, vision changes, or changes in mental status. Adrenal involvement infrequently presents with Addison disease. Lung cancer is the most common tumor causing adrenal dysfunction.

3. **Paraneoplastic syndromes** are frequent and occur secondary to the release of hormone-like substances by tumor cells. They include Cushing syndrome (adrenocorticotropic hormone secretion in small cell carcinoma), syndrome of inappropriate antidiuretic hormone (SIADH), hypercalcemia (parathyroid hormone–related protein secreted by squamous cell carcinomas), hypertrophic pulmonary osteoarthropathy (clubbing of the fingers, stiffness of joints, and periosteal thickening on X-ray), and various myopathies.

D. **Accurate clinical and pathologic staging is critical** in the management of patients with non–small cell carcinoma because surgery is the primary mode of therapy for all stage I and II patients and selected stage IIIa patients who have enough physiologic reserve to tolerate resection. It is critical to exclude metastatic disease prior to resection. The essential elements of staging include evaluation for lymph node involvement and evaluation for adrenal, brain, and bone metastasis. An anatomic staging system using

Table 36-1. American Joint Committee on Cancer staging system of lung cancer

Tumor status (T)

T1	<3 cm without invasion of visceral pleura proximal to lobar bronchus
T2	>3 cm or any size with associated atelectasis or obstructive pneumonitis that does not involve the entire lung; may invade visceral pleura; proximal extent must be >2 cm from carina
T3	Any size with direct extension into chest wall, diaphragm, mediastinal pleura, or pericardium without involvement of great vessels or vital mediastinal structures; cannot involve carina; atelectasis or obstructive pneumonitis of the entire lung
T4	Any size with invasion of heart or mediastinal vital structures or carina, malignant pleural effusion, satellite lesions

Nodal involvement (N)

N0	None
N1	Peribronchial or ipsilateral hilar lymph nodes
N2	Ipsilateral mediastinal lymph nodes, including subcarinal
N3	Contralateral mediastinal or hilar lymph nodes, ipsilateral or contralateral scalene or supraclavicular lymph nodes

Distant metastases (M)

M0	None
M1	Distant metastases present

STAGE

Ia	T1 N0 M0
Ib	T2 N0 M0
IIa	T1 N1 M0
IIb	T2 N1 M0; T3 N0 M0
IIIa	T3 N1 M0; T1,2,3 N2 M0
IIIb	Any T N3 M0; T4, any N, M0
IV	Any T, any N, M1

Reprinted with permission from ID Fleming, JS Cooper, DF Henson, et al., eds. *AJCC Cancer Staging Manual.* 5th ed. Philadelphia: Lippincott Williams & Wilkins; 1998.

the classification for tumor, nodal, and metastatic status was most recently modified in 1997 (Table 36-1).

1. **Chest CT to include the upper abdomen** provides useful information on location, size, and local involvement of tumor and also allows evaluation for liver and adrenal metastasis. CT scanning alone does not accurately determine the resectability of tumor adherent to vital structures. Patients with localized disease may require intraoperative staging to determine resectability. CT also can identify mediastinal lymphadenopathy. However, the sensitivity for identifying metastatic lymph nodes by CT is only 65% to 80% and the specificity is only 65%. With nodes larger than 1 cm, the sensitivity decreases but the specificity increases.

2. **PET imaging** is often used in the staging of patients with non–small cell carcinoma, but its accuracy for detecting primary tumors and metastatic disease may be limited by the presence of inflammation and ongoing infection. In regions endemic for inflammatory processes such as histoplasmosis, the usefulness of PET imaging for investigating mediastinal lymph nodes is limited. However, it can be useful for identifying occult distant metastatic disease to the liver, adrenals, and bone.

3. **Mediastinoscopy** is the most accurate method for staging mediastinal lymph nodes, and it provides access to the pretracheal, subcarinal, and

paratracheal node stations. Although invasive, it is safe, with less than a 1% complication rate. We favor the routine use of this technique in the staging of patients with non–small cell carcinoma. The timing of mediastinoscopy, whether at the time of thoracotomy or before a planned resection, is controversial and depends on the surgeon's preference and the availability of expert pathologic evaluation of mediastinal lymph node frozen sections.

4. **CT or MR imaging of the brain** to identify brain metastases is mandatory in the patient with neurologic symptoms but is controversial as a routine part of the workup of symptomatic patients. Given the reported, albeit low, incidence of CNS metastasis in the setting of even small primary tumors, we advocate the routine use of brain imaging.

5. **Bone scan** is obtained in all patients with specific symptoms of skeletal pain and selectively as part of the preoperative metastatic workup. The routine use of PET imaging in many centers has eliminated the need for this modality.

6. **Fiberoptic bronchoscopy** is important in diagnosing and assessing the extent of the endobronchial lesion. Although peripheral cancers rarely can be seen with bronchoscopy, preoperative bronchoscopy is important for excluding synchronous lung cancers (found in approximately 1% of patients) prior to resection. Bronchial washings with culture can be taken at the time of bronchoscopy in patients with significant secretion.

E. **Preoperative assessment of pulmonary** function and estimation of postoperative pulmonary assessment is the most critical factor in planning lung resection for cancer.

1. **Pulmonary function tests** and **arterial blood gas analysis** are the standard by which the risk of developing postoperative pulmonary failure is determined. In general, pulmonary resection can be tolerated if the preoperative FEV_1 (forced expiratory volume in 1 second) is >60% of predicted. If the FEV_1 is <60% of predicted, measurement of **diffusion capacity, quantitative ventilation perfusion scan, and exercise testing** are indicated. These tests allow the surgeon to determine how much of the area of resection contributes to the overall pulmonary function. In general, an **estimated postresection FEV_1** of 800 cc or greater suggests the patient will tolerate a pneumonectomy. Preoperative hypercapnia (arterial carbon dioxide tension >45 mm Hg) precludes resection.

2. **Evaluation of cardiac disease** is critical for minimizing perioperative complications. Patients with lung cancer are often at high risk for coronary disease because of extensive smoking histories. A detailed history and physical examination to elicit signs and symptoms of ischemia and a baseline ECG are the initial steps. Any abnormal findings should be aggressively pursued with stress tests or coronary catheterization.

3. **Smoking cessation** preoperatively for as little as 2 weeks can aid in the regeneration of the mucociliary function and pulmonary toilet.

F. **In summary,** all patients should have a posteroanterior and lateral chest x-ray and a chest CT scan to evaluate the primary tumor and the mediastinum and to check for metastatic disease to the brain and adrenals. PET imaging or bone scan is required to exclude bone metastasis. Cervical mediastinoscopy with biopsy of the lymph nodes in the paratracheal and subcarinal space should be performed to exclude mediastinal lymph node metastasis prior to resection. All patients should undergo a fiberoptic bronchoscopy by the surgeon before thoracotomy; this is usually done at the same setting as mediastinoscopy.

G. **Operative principles.** In the patient able to tolerate resection, the minimal extent of resection should be an anatomic lobectomy. Even in Stage I disease, a more limited resection, such as a wedge resection, results in a threefold higher incidence of local recurrence and a decreased overall and disease-free survival. Patients with limited pulmonary reserve may be treated by segmental or wedge resection. Most centers report an operative mortality of 2% to 3% with lobectomy and of 6% to 8% with pneumonectomy. Minimally invasive techniques for anatomic resection are in clinical trial.

H. **Five-year survival rates** are 67% for stage Ia (T1N0) disease and 57% for stage Ib (T2N0). Stage I disease is generally treated with surgical resection alone. The presence of ipsilateral intrapulmonary lymph nodes decreases the overall survival to 55% for stage IIa (T1N1) and 39% for stage IIb (T2N1). Stage II cancers are also treated with surgical resection. However, adjuvant chemoradiation is considered in patients with close surgical margins or central N1 lymph node metastasis.

Certain patients with stage IIIa disease appear to benefit form surgical resection alone (T3N1M0). However, selected patients with mediastinal lymph node metastasis (N2 disease) may be candidates for surgical resection in combination with chemotherapy or chemoradiation therapy. Patients with stage IIIa and more advanced disease are treated using multiple modalities. The optimal regimen of chemotherapy, radiation, or a combination of both is currently being investigated in clinical trials. Stage IIIb tumors involve the contralateral mediastinal or hilar lymph nodes, the ipsilateral scalene or supraclavicular lymph nodes, extensive mediastinal invasion, intrapulmonary metastasis, or malignant pleural effusions. These tumors are considered unresectable. Stage IV tumors have distant metastases and are also considered unresectable. However, selected patients with node-negative lung cancer and a solitary brain metastasis have achieved long-term survival with combined resection.

II. **Tumors of the pleura.** The most common tumor of the pleura is the rare but deadly **mesothelioma.** Less common tumors include lipomas, angiomas, soft-tissue sarcomas, and fibrous histiocytomas.

A. **Asbestos** exposure is associated with mesothelioma 70% of the time. Mesotheliomas arise from mesothelial cells but differentiate into a variety of histologic patterns. It is often difficult to differentiate mesothelioma from other tumors without the benefit of special stains or immunohistochemistry.

B. **Epidemiologically,** mesothelioma is primarily a disease of men in the 5th through 7th decades of life. Patients may have been exposed to asbestos decades before (latency >30 years). Patient presentation may be variable. While benign mesothelioma variants are not associated with asbestos exposure and are asymptomatic, patients with the more common malignant form often report chest pain, malaise, cough, weakness, weight loss, and shortness of breath with pleural effusion. One-third of patients report paraneoplastic symptoms of osteoarthropathy, hypoglycemia, and fever.

C. **CT scan** is useful in differentiating pleural from parenchymal disease. Malignant mesothelioma usually appears as a markedly thickened, irregular pleural-based mass or nodular pleura with a pleural effusion. Occasionally, only a pleural effusion is seen. Routine use of MR imaging has not been shown to have significant advantages over use of CT. However, it has been useful for identify transdiaphragmatic extension of tumor into the abdomen.

D. **Diagnosis** based purely on cytology of thoracentesis sample is difficult. Thoracoscopic or open pleural biopsy is usually necessary to confirm the diagnosis.

E. **Classification** is based on histological evaluation: epithelial, sarcomatous, and mixed forms have been identified.

F. **Median survival** in untreated patients with malignant mesothelioma is 4 to 12 months. Patients with mixed or sarcomatous mesothelioma have a poor prognosis and do not appear to benefit from surgical resection. Current aggressive multimodality therapy consists of pleurectomy and decortication or extrapleural pneumonectomy to decrease tumor mass, followed by chemotherapy and radiotherapy. Adjuvant therapy is not beneficial in the setting of incomplete resection. However, patients with epithelial histology,

Table 36-2. Differential diagnosis of tumors located in the mediastinum

Anterior	Middle	Posterior
Thymoma	Congenital cyst	Neurogenic
Germ cell	Lymphoma	Lymphoma
Teratoma	Primary cardiac	Mesenchymal
Seminoma	Neural crest	
Nonseminoma		
Lymphoma		
Parathyroid		
Lipoma		
Fibroma		
Lymphangioma		
Aberrant thyroid		

Modified from Young RM, Kernstine KH, Corson JD. Miscellaneous cardiopulmonary conditions. In: Corson JD, Williamson RCN, eds. *Surgery*. Philadelphia: Mosby; 2001.

no evidence of lymph node metastasis, and complete resection appear to benefit from an aggressive combined modality approach. The most encouraging studies report a 5-year survival of 39%.

III. **Tumors of the mediastinum.** The location of a mass in relation to the heart helps the surgeon form a differential diagnosis (Table 36-2). On the lateral chest x-ray, the mediastinum is divided into thirds, with the heart comprising the middle segment.

   A. **Epidemiology.** In the totality of all age groups, lymphoma is the most common mediastinal tumor. Neurogenic tumors are more likely in children. The likelihood of malignancy is greatest in the 2nd to 4th decades of life. The presence of symptoms is more suggestive of a malignant lesion. Symptoms are often nonspecific and include dyspnea, cough, hoarseness, vague chest pain, and fever.

   B. **Evaluation.** Chest x-ray is often used as a screening tool and can lead to the diagnosis of a mass. This should be followed by a CT scan to further delineate the anatomy.

   C. **Tumors.** Due to the prevalence of germ cell tumors, all anterior mediastinal masses should be evaluated with biochemical markers β-HCG and α-fetoprotein (AFP).

   1. **Teratomas** are usually benign and often contain ectodermal components such as hair, teeth, and bone. Elevation of both β-HCG and AFP suggests a malignant teratoma. Treatment is surgical resection.

   2. **Seminomas** do not present with an elevation in AFP, and <10% present with an elevation in β-HCG. Their treatment is primarily nonsurgical (radiation and chemotherapy), except in the case of localized disease.

   3. **Nonseminomatous germ cell** tumors present with an elevation of both tumor markers. Again, the treatment is primarily nonsurgical, with the exception of obtaining tissue for diagnosis.

   4. Tissue diagnosis is often crucial for the diagnosis and treatment of **lymphoma.** Treatment is primarily nonsurgical. Cervical lymph node biopsy, CT-guided biopsy, or mediastinoscopy with biopsy may be required. These lesions often present as irregular masses on CT scan.

   5. Patients with paravertebral or posterior mediastinal masses should have their catecholamine levels measured to rule out **pheochromocytomas.**

IV. **Thymectomy/thymoma**

   A. The role of the **thymus gland in myasthenia gravis** is poorly understood. However, it appears to be important in the generation of autoreactive antibodies directed against the acetylcholine receptor. Antiacetylcholine receptor antibodies may be used to evaluate for thymoma. Over 80% of cases demonstrate complete or partial response to thymectomy. Chances of improvement are increased if thymectomy is performed early in the course of disease (first signs of muscle weakness) and if the myasthenia is not associated with a thymoma.

B. A **thymoma** is a focal mass in the thymus gland composed primarily of thymic epithelial cells. Most are benign, but the presence of invasion of its fibrous capsule defines malignancy. While 15% of myasthenia gravis patients have a thymoma, ~50% of patients with a thymoma have paraneoplastic syndromes, including myasthenia gravis, hypogammaglobulinemia, and red cell aplasia.

C. **Preoperative preparation** of the patient with myasthenia gravis involves reduction of corticosteroid dosage, if appropriate, and the weaning of anticholinesterases. Plasmapheresis can be performed preoperatively to aid in discontinuation of anticholinesterase agents. Muscle relaxants and atropine should be avoided during anesthetic induction.

D. The **operative approach** for thymectomy for myasthenia in cases in which noninvasive imaging **does not indicate the presence of a thymoma** or a mass lesion is controversial. The options range from median sternotomy to a transcervical thymectomy. The **transcervical approach** involves a low collar incision and is facilitated by using a table-mounted retractor to elevate the manubrium and expose the thymic tissue for resection.

E. **In instances of bulky thymic disease,** a median sternotomy approach is preferred to **provide maximal exposure for complete resection.**

V. **Pneumothorax**
A. Pneumothorax is the presence of air in the pleural cavity, leading to separation of the visceral and parietal pleura. This disruption of the potential space disrupts pulmonary mechanics, and if left untreated, it may progress to tension physiology. In tension pneumothorax, cardiac compromise occurs and presents a true emergency. The etiology may be spontaneous, iatrogenic, or due to trauma. The etiology will determine the most appropriate short- and long-term management strategies.

B. **Physical examination** may demonstrate decreased breath sounds on the involved side if the lung is more than 25% collapsed. Hyperresonance on the affected side is possible. Common symptoms include dyspnea and chest pain. Careful examination for signs of tension pneumothorax (including deviation of the trachea to the opposite side, respiratory distress, and hypotension) must be performed. If there is no clinical evidence of tension pneumothorax, an upright chest x-ray will be required to establish the diagnosis. Smaller pneumothoraces may only be evident on expiration chest x-rays or CT scan. The clinical setting will influence their management.

C. **Management options** include observation, aspiration, chest tube placement with or without pleurodesis, and surgery. The etiology of the pneumothorax will influence management strategy.
  1. **Observation** is an option in a healthy, asymptomatic patient. This should be reserved for small pneumothoraces, unlikely to recur, as failure to fully resolve may lead to fibrous entrapment of the lung. Supplemental oxygen may help reabsorb the pneumothorax by affecting the gradient of nitrogen in the body and in the pneumothorax.
  2. **Aspiration** of the pneumothorax may be done using a small catheter attached to a three-way stopcock. This should be reserved for situations with low suspicion of an ongoing air leak.
  3. **Percutaneous catheters** may be placed using Seldinger technique. Multiple commercial kits exist and allow for the catheter to be placed to a Heimlich valve or to suction. The catheters in these kits are generally of small caliber, and their use is limited to situations of simple pneumothorax.

4. **Tube thoracostomy** remains the gold standard, especially for larger pneumothoraces, for persistent air leaks, when there is an expected need for pleurodesis, or for associated effusion.
   a. Chest tubes may be connected either to a **Heimlich flutter valve,** to a **simple underwater-seal system,** or to **vacuum suction.** The two most commonly used systems are the Pleurovac and Emerson systems. Both systems may be placed to a water seal (providing -3-cm to -5-cm H_2O suction) or to vacuum suction (typically -20-cm).
   b. **If the water-seal chamber bubbles with expiration or with coughing,** this is evidence that an air leak persists. Newer Pleurovac systems allow as much as -40-cm H_2O suction to be applied to the pleural space.
5. **Bedside pleurodesis.** Sclerosing agents may be administered through the chest tube to induce fusion of the parietal and visceral pleural surfaces. Doxycycline, bleomycin, and talc have all been described.
   a. Bedside pleurodesis **can be associated with an inflammatory pneumonitis** in the lung, on the treated side. In patients with limited pulmonary reserve, this may present as clinically significant hypoxia. Pleurodesis can be quite uncomfortable for the patient, and adequate analgesia is mandatory. Patient-controlled analgesic pump and bolus administration of ketorolac (if tolerated) are effective.
   b. **Doxycycline** is used as the sclerosing agent for benign processes.
      (1) It is administered as 500 mg in 100 mL normal saline. Doxycycline is extremely irritating to the pleural surfaces; therefore, 30 mL 1% lidocaine can be administered via the chest tube before the doxycycline is given and used to flush the drug again. The total dose of lidocaine should not exceed the toxic dose, which is usually 5 mg/kg.
      (2) In patients with large air leaks, the chest tube should not be clamped to prevent the development of a tension pneumothorax. Instead, the drainage bottle or suction device should be elevated to maintain the effective water-seal pressure at -20-cm H_2O.
      (3) The patient (with assistance) is instructed to roll from supine to right lateral decubitus to left lateral decubitus every 15 minutes for 2 hours. Prone, Trendelenburg, and reverse Trendelenburg positions should also be part of the sequence if the patient is able to tolerate it.
      (4) The chest tube may be unclamped (if done for the procedure) and returned to suction after the procedure.
   c. **Talc** is a less painful sclerosing agent. Due to concern about introducing a potentially carcinogenic agent and permanent foreign body, it is generally limited to patients with underlying malignant conditions (see "Effusions," Section VIII).
      (1) Talc, 5 g in 180-mL sterile saline, split into 360-mL catheter syringes, is administered via the chest tube and then flushed with an additional 60-mL saline.
      (2) The patient is instructed to change positions as described above.
6. **Surgery** is performed using a video-assisted approach or by thoracotomy. Patients who have a persistent air leak secondary to a ruptured bleb but are otherwise well should be considered for surgery. Patients by this point have already undergone stabilization by chest tube placement (see Section V.D.3 for specific indications for surgery).
D. **Etiology**
   1. **Iatrogenic** pneumothoraces usually are the result of pleural injury during central venous access attempts, pacemaker placement, or transthoracic or transbronchial lung biopsy. A postprocedure chest x-ray is mandatory. Often the injury to the lung is small and self-limited. The extent of pneumothorax and associated injury should determine the need for invasive procedures. Observation or percutaneous placement

of a chest tube may be appropriate in a patient who is not mechanically ventilated.

2. **Spontaneous** pneumothorax is nearly always caused by rupture of an apical bleb. Up to 80% of patients are tall, young adults, and men outnumber women by 6 to 1; it is more common in smokers than in nonsmokers. The typical patient presents with acute onset of shortness of breath and chest pain on the side of the collapsed lung. Patients older than 40 years usually have significant parenchymal disease, such as emphysema. These patients present with a ruptured bulla and often have a more dramatic presentation, including tachypnea, cyanosis, and hypoxia. There is a significant risk of recurrence, and pleurodesis or surgical intervention may be indicated even after the first occurrence. Other etiologies of spontaneous pneumothorax include cystic fibrosis and, rarely, lung cancer.

3. **Indications for operation** for spontaneous pneumothorax include (1) recurrent ipsilateral pneumothoraces, (2) bilateral pneumothoraces, (3) persistent air leaks on chest tube suction (usually >5 days), and (4) first episodes occurring in patients with high-risk occupations (e.g., pilots, divers) or those who live a great distance from medical care facilities. The risk of ipsilateral recurrence of a spontaneous pneumothorax is 50%, 62%, and 80% after the first, second, and third episodes, respectively. Some authors recommend chemical pleurodesis as the minimal therapy for the first occurrence.

   a. **Operative management** consists of stapled wedge resection of blebs or bullae, usually found in the apex of the upper lobe or superior segment of the lower lobe. Pleural abrasion (pleurodesis) should be done to promote formation of adhesions between visceral and parietal pleurae. Video-assisted thoracoscopic techniques have allowed procedures to be less morbid in most cases. Using three small port incisions on the affected side, thoracoscopic stapling of the involved apical bulla and pleurodesis can be done. Alternatively, a transaxillary thoracotomy incision gives excellent exposure of the upper lung through a limited incision.

4. **Traumatic** pneumothoraces may be caused by either blunt or penetrating thoracic trauma and often result in lung contusion and multiple rib injury.

   a. **Evaluation and treatment** begin with the initial stabilization of airway and circulation. A chest x-ray should be obtained.

   b. **Prompt chest tube insertion** is performed to evacuate air and blood. In 80% of patients with penetrating trauma to the hemithorax, exploratory thoracotomy is unnecessary, and chest tube decompression with observation is sufficient. Indications for operation include immediate drainage of >1,500 mL blood after tube insertion or persistent bleeding >200 mL per hour. Patients who have with multiple injuries and proven pneumothoraces or significant chest injuries should have prophylactic chest tubes placed before general anesthesia because of the risk of tension pneumothorax with positive-pressure ventilation.

   c. **Pulmonary contusion** is associated with traumatic pneumothorax. The contusion usually is evident on the initial chest x-ray (as opposed to aspiration, in which several hours may elapse before an infiltrative pattern appears on serial radiographs), and it appears as a fluffy infiltrate that progresses in extent and density over 24 to 48 hours.

   d. The contusion may be associated with multiple rib fractures, leading to a **flail chest**. This occurs when several ribs are broken segmentally, allowing for a portion of the chest wall to be "floating" and to move paradoxically with breathing (inward on inspiration). The paradoxical movement and splinting secondary to pain and the associated pain lead to a reduction in vital capacity and to ineffective ventilation.

e. All patients with suspected contusions and rib fractures should have **aggressive pain control** measures, including patient-controlled analgesia pumps, epidural catheters, and intercostal nerve blocks.

f. **Intravenous fluid should be minimized** to the extent allowed by the patient's clinical status because of associated increased capillary endothelial permeability. Serial arterial blood gas measurements are important for close monitoring of respiratory status. Close monitoring and a high index of suspicion for respiratory decompensation are necessary. Intubation, positive-pressure ventilation, and even tracheostomy are often necessary.

g. **A traumatic bronchopleural fistula** can occur after penetrating or blunt chest trauma. If mechanical ventilation is ineffective secondary to the large air leak, emergent thoracotomy and repair are usually necessary. On occasion, selective intubation of the uninvolved bronchus can provide short-term stability in the minutes before definitive operative treatment.

h. The unusual circumstance known as a **sucking chest wound** consists of a full-thickness hole in the chest wall greater than two-thirds the diameter of the trachea. With inspiration, air preferentially flows through the wound because of the low resistance to flow. This requires immediate coverage of the hole with an occlusive dressing and chest tube insertion to reexpand the lung. If tube thoracostomy cannot be immediately performed, coverage with an occlusive dressing taped on three sides functions as a one-way valve to prevent the accumulation of air within the chest, although tube thoracostomy should be performed as soon as possible.

VI. **Hemoptysis** can originate from a number of causes, including infectious, malignant, and cardiac disorders (e.g., bronchitis or tuberculosis, bronchogenic carcinoma, and mitral stenosis, respectively).

A. **Massive hemoptysis** requires emergent thoracic surgical intervention, often with little time for formal studies before entering the operating room. The surgeon is called primarily for significant hemoptysis, which is defined as more than 600 mL of blood expelled over 48 hours or, more often, a volume of blood that is impairing gas exchange. Because the volume of the main airways is approximately 200 cc, even smaller amounts of blood can cause severe respiratory compromise. Prompt treatment is required to ensure survival. As baseline lung function decreases, a lower volume and rate of hemoptysis is capable of severely compromising gas exchange.

1. A **brief focused history** can often elucidate the etiology of the bleed, such as a history of tuberculosis or aspergillosis. A recent chest x-ray may reveal the diagnosis in up to half of cases. Chest CT is rarely helpful in the acute setting and is contraindicated in patients who are unstable. Trace amounts of hemoptysis can be evaluated by radiologic examinations in conjunction with bronchoscopy.

2. **Bronchoscopy** is the mainstay of diagnosis and initial treatment. Although it may not eliminate later episodes of bleeding, it can allow for temporizing measures, such as placement of balloon-tipped catheters and topical or injected vasoconstrictors. In a setting of massive hemoptysis, the patient should be prepared for a rigid bronchoscopy, which is best performed in the operating room under general anesthesia. Asphyxiation is the primary cause of death in patients with massive hemoptysis. Rigid bronchoscopy allows for rapid and effective clearance of blood and clot from the airway, rapid identification of the bleeding side, and prompt protection of the remaining lung parenchyma (with cautery, by packing with epinephrine-soaked gauze, or by placement of a balloon-tipped catheter in the lobar orifice).

3. In cases in which the **etiology** and the precise bleeding source are not identified by bronchoscopy, ongoing bleeding requires protection of the contralateral lung. Selective ventilation, either with a double-lumen tube or by direct intubation of the contralateral main-stem bronchus, may be critical to avoid asphyxiation.

4. **After isolation of the bleeding site, angiographic embolization** of a bronchial arterial source may allow for lung salvage without the need for resection. The bronchial circulation is almost always the source of hemoptysis. Bleeding from the pulmonary circulation is seen only in patients with pulmonary hypertension.

5. **Definitive therapy** may require thoracotomy with lobar resection or, rarely, pneumonectomy. Infrequently, emergent surgical resection is necessary to control the hemoptysis. The etiology of the bleeding and the pulmonary reserve of the patient are important, because many patients are not candidates for surgical resection.

VII. **Pleural effusion**

A. Pleural effusion may result from a wide spectrum of benign, malignant, and inflammatory conditions. By history, it is often possible to deduce the etiology, but diagnosis is often dependent on the analysis of the pleural fluid. The presentation of symptoms will be dependent on the underlying etiology, and **treatment is based on the underlying disease process.**

1. **Chest x-ray** is often the first diagnostic test. Depending on radiographic technique, an effusion may remain hidden. While decubitus films are the most sensitive for detecting small free-flowing effusions, the same volume may remain hidden in a standard anteroposterior film. A concave meniscus in the costophrenic angle on an upright chest x-ray suggests at least 250 mL pleural fluid. **CT scan** and **ultrasound** can be particularly helpful if the fluid is not free flowing or if history suggests a more chronic organizing process such as empyema.

2. **Thoracentesis**
   a. **The technique** of thoracentesis is described in Chapter 42.
   b. **The fluid should be sent for culture and Gram stain, biochemical analyses [pH, glucose, amylase, lactate dehydrogenase (LDH), and protein levels], and a differential cell count and cytology to rule out malignancy.**
   c. In general, thin, yellowish, clear fluid is common with transudative effusions; cloudy and foul-smelling fluid usually signals infection or early empyema; bloody effusions often denote malignancy; milky white fluid suggests chylothorax; and pH <7.2 suggests bacterial infection or connective tissue disease.
   d. Larger volumes (several hundred milliliters) can often aid the cytopathologists in making a diagnosis. White blood cell count >10,000/mm^3 suggests pyogenic etiology. A predominance of lymphocytes is noted with tuberculosis. Glucose is decreased in infectious processes as well as in malignancy.
   e. Pleural effusions are broadly categorized as either **transudative** (protein-poor fluid not involving primary pulmonary pathology) or **exudative** (resulting from increased vascular permeability as a result of diseased pleura or pleural lymphatics). Protein and LDH levels measured simultaneously in the pleural fluid and serum provide the diagnosis in nearly all settings.
   f. Exudative pleural effusions satisfy at least one of the following criteria: (1) ratio of pleural fluid protein to serum protein >0.5, (2) ratio of pleural fluid LDH to serum LDH >0.6, or (3) pleural fluid LDH greater than two-thirds the upper normal limit for serum.

3. **Transudative pleural effusion** can usually be considered a secondary diagnosis; therefore, therapy should be directed at the underlying problem (e.g., congestive heart failure, cirrhosis, or nephrotic syndrome). Therapeutic drainage is rarely indicated because fluid rapidly reaccumulates unless the underlying cause improves.

4. **Exudative pleural effusion** may be broadly classified based on whether its cause is benign or malignant.
   a. **Malignant** effusions are most often associated with cancers of the breast, lung, and ovary and with lymphoma. Diagnosis is often made by cytology, but in the event that this process is not diagnostic, pleural biopsy may be indicated. Given the overall poor prognosis in these patients, **therapy offered by the thoracic surgeon is generally palliative.**
      (1) **Drainage** of effusion to alleviate dyspnea and improve pulmonary mechanics by reexpanding the lung may be done with chest tube placement.
      (2) **Pleurodesis** with talc or doxycycline may prevent reaccumulation of the effusion.
   b. **Benign exudative effusions** are most often a result of pneumonia (**parapneumonic**). The process begins with a sterile parapneumonic exudative effusion and leads to a suppurative infection of the pleural space, **empyema,** if the effusion becomes infected. The initially free-flowing fluid becomes infected and begins to deposit fibrin and cellular debris (5 to 7 days). Eventually, this fluid becomes organized, and a thick fibrous peel entraps the lung (10 to 14 days).
      (1) **Empyema.** Fifty percent of empyemas are complications of pneumonia; 25% are complications of esophageal, pulmonary, or mediastinal surgery; and 10% are extensions from subphrenic abscesses. Thoracentesis is diagnostic but is sufficient treatment in only the earliest cases.
      (2) The **clinical presentation** of empyema ranges from systemic sepsis requiring emergent care to chronic loculated effusion in a patient who complains of fatigue. Other symptoms include pleuritic chest pain, fever, cough, and dyspnea.
      (3) The **most common offending organisms** are Gram-positive cocci (*Staphylococcus aureus* and streptococci) and Gram-negative organisms (*Escherichia coli* and *Pseudomonas* and *Klebsiella* species). *Bacteroides* species are also common.
      (4) **Management** includes control of the infection by appropriate antibiotics, drainage of the pleural space, and obliteration of the empyema space. Once the diagnosis is made, treatment should not be delayed. Specific management depends on the phase of the empyema, which depends on the character of the fluid. **If the fluid does not layer on posteroanterior and lateral and decubitus chest x-ray, a CT scan should be done.**
         (a) Early or **exudative empyema** is usually adequately treated with simple tube drainage.
         (b) **Fibropurulent empyema** may be amenable to tube drainage alone, but the fluid may be loculated. The loculations of empyema cavities are composed of fibrin.
         (c) In advanced or **organizing empyema,** the fluid is thicker, and a fibrous peel encases the lung. Thoracotomy may be necessary to free the entrapped lung.
         (d) If a patient has a **persistent fluid collection with an adequately placed tube** as evidenced by chest CT, intrapleural fibrinolytic therapy may be indicated. Intrapleural streptokinase, 250,000 units, is divided into three doses, each in 60 mL normal saline. A dose is administered and flushed with 30 mL normal saline. The tube is clamped and the patient rolled as described for pleurodesis; then the tube is returned to suction. The procedure is repeated every 8 hours. Alternatively, 250,000 units can be administered daily for 3 days. The adequacy of treatment is determined by resolution of the fluid collection and complete reexpansion of the lung.

(e) A **postpneumonectomy empyema** is one of the most difficult complications to manage in thoracic surgery. Typically, there is a dehiscence of the bronchial stump and contamination of the pneumonectomy space with bronchial flora. The finding of air in the pneumonectomy space on chest x-ray is often diagnostic. The incidence of major bronchopleural fistula after pulmonary resection varies from 2% to 10% and has a high mortality (16% to 70%). Initial management includes thorough drainage (either open or closed) of the infected pleural space, antibiotics, and pulmonary toilet.

(f) Definitive surgical repair of the fistula may include primary closure of a long bronchial stump or closure of the fistula using vascularized muscle or omental flaps. The residual pleural cavity can be obliterated by a muscle transposition, thoracoplasty, or delayed Clagett procedure.

    (i) **Initially,** a chest tube is inserted to evacuate the empyema. Great caution should be taken in inserting chest tubes into postpneumonectomy empyemas. A communicating bronchial stump–pleural fistula can contaminate the contralateral lung rapidly when decompression of the empyema is attempted. The patient should be positioned with the affected side down so that the remaining lung is not contaminated with empyema fluid. This procedure might best be handled in the operating room.

    (ii) **After the patient is stabilized,** the next step usually is the creation of a **Clagett window** to provide a venue for daily packing and to maintain external drainage of the infected pleural space. This typically involves reopening the thoracotomy incision at its anterolateral end and resecting a short segment of two or three ribs to create generous access to the pleural space. The pleura is then treated with irrigation and debridement. After a suitable interval (weeks to months), the wound edges can be excised and the pneumonectomy space is closed either primarily or with a muscle flap after it has been filled with 0.25% neomycin solution. Alternatively, the space can be filled with vascularized muscle flap.

VIII. COPD, lung volume reduction, and transplantation

  A. The long-term consequences of smoking lead not only to lung cancer but also to **chronic obstructive pulmonary disease (COPD).**

    1. Destruction of lung parenchyma occurs in a nonuniform manner. As lung tissue loses its elastic recoil, the areas of destruction expand. This expansion of diseased areas, in combination with inflammation, leads to poor ventilation of relatively normal lung.

    2. This leads to the **typical findings of hyperexpanded lungs** on chest x-ray: flattened diaphragms, widened intercostal spaces, and horizontal ribs. On pulmonary function testing, patients present with increased residual volumes and decreased FEV_1.

    3. Despite maximal medical and surgical treatment, the **disease is progressive.** Surgical treatment is generally reserved for the symptomatic (dyspnea) patient who has failed maximal medical treatment, with the goal of improving symptoms.

    4. The **goals of surgery** are to remove diseased areas of lung and allow improved function of the remaining lung tissue.

  B. The mainstays of surgical treatment have been bullectomy, lung volume reduction, and transplantation. Prior to any surgical intervention, **patients must be carefully selected. Smoking cessation for at least 6 months is mandatory, as is enrollment in a supervised pulmonary rehabilitation program.**

1. **Bullectomy.** Patients with emphysema may have large bullous disease. Emphysematous bullae are giant air sacs and may become secondarily infected.

2. **Lung volume reduction** may be indicated in patients who have predominantly apical disease, with $FEV_1 > 20\%$ of predicted, and patients who may be too old for transplantation. Through a sternotomy incision, one or both lungs have areas of heavily diseased lung resected. Patients with diffuse emphysema are not candidates for this procedure.

3. Emphysema and α_1-antitrypsin deficiency have become the leading indications for lung transplantation. Other common indications include cystic fibrosis, pulmonary fibrosis, and pulmonary hypertension.

   a. Patients selected for lung transplantation generally are younger, have diffuse involvement of emphysema, and have $FEV_1 < 20\%$.

   b. Both single lung and bilateral lung transplantation have been performed for emphysema, although bilateral transplant patients have improved long-term survival.

   c. The only absolute indication for bilateral lung transplantation is cystic fibrosis, because single lung transplantation would leave a chronically infected native lung in an immunocompromised patient.

   d. Long-term, chronic allograft dysfunction in the form of bronchiolitis obliterans occurs in 50% of patients.

IX. **Issues in the care of the thoracic patient**

A. **Postoperative care of the thoracic surgery patient** focuses on three factors: **control of incisional pain, maintenance of pulmonary function, and monitoring of cardiovascular status.**

1. The **thoracotomy incision is one of the most painful and debilitating** in surgery. Inadequate pain control contributes heavily to nearly all postoperative complications. Chest wall splinting contributes to atelectasis and poor pulmonary toilet. Pain increases sympathetic tone and myocardial oxygen demand, provoking arrhythmias and cardiac ischemic episodes. The routine use of epidural catheter anesthesia perioperatively and during the early recovery period has improved pain management significantly. Other effective analgesic maneuvers include intercostal blocks with long-acting local anesthetic before closure of the chest and intrapleural administration or local anesthetic via catheters placed at the time of thoracotomy.

2. **Maintenance of good bronchial hygiene** is often the most difficult challenge facing the postthoracotomy patient. A lengthy smoking history, decreased ciliary function, chronic bronchitis, and significant postoperative pain all contribute to the ineffective clearance of pulmonary secretions. Even aggressive pulmonary toilet with incentive spirometry and chest physiotherapy delivered by the respiratory therapist, along with adequate analgesia, are insufficient on occasion. **Diligent attention must be paid,** including frequent physical examination and daily chest x-ray and arterial blood gas evaluation to detect any changes in gas exchange. **Atelectasis** and **mucus plugging** can lead to ventilation-perfusion mismatch and ensuing respiratory failure. The clinician should make liberal use of nasotracheal suctioning, bedside flexible bronchoscopy, and mechanical ventilatory support if needed.

3. All physicians caring for the postthoracotomy patient should be familiar with **chest tube placement, maintenance, and removal.** The purpose of chest tube placement after thoracotomy and lung resection is to allow drainage of air and fluid from the pleural space and to ensure reexpansion of the remaining lung parenchyma.

   a. **Chest-tube drainage** is not used routinely with pneumonectomy unless bleeding or infection is present. Some surgeons place a chest tube on the operative side and remove it on postoperative day 1. Balanced pneumonectomy Pleurovacs have been advocated to balance the mediastinum during the first 24 to 48 hours. A chest tube in the patient with a pneumonectomy space should not be placed to conventional suction because of the risk of cardiac herniation.

b. **Chest tubes are removed after the air leak has resolved and fluid drainage decreased** (usually <100 mL over 8 hours). Chest tubes usually are removed one at a time. The patient is instructed to take a large inspiratory breath and hold it while the tube is removed swiftly and the site is simultaneously covered with an occlusive dressing. The technique of chest tube removal is critical to preventing air entry through the removal site.

4. **Cardiovascular complications** in the postoperative period are second in frequency only to pulmonary complications, because the population that develops lung cancer is at high risk for heart disease. The three most common sources of cardiac morbidity are **arrhythmias, myocardial infarctions, and congestive heart failure.** A negative preoperative cardiac evaluation does not preclude the development of postoperative complications.

a. **Cardiac arrhythmias** occur in up to 30% of patients undergoing pulmonary surgery. The highest incidence occurs in elderly patients undergoing pneumonectomy or intrapericardial pulmonary artery ligation. All patients should have cardiac rhythm monitoring after thoracotomy for at least 72 hours.

b. A number of trials have failed to reach consensus on optimal regimen for prophylaxis.

c. **Treatment** of any rhythm disturbance begins with an assessment of the patient's hemodynamic status. Manifestations of these arrhythmias vary in acuity from hemodynamic collapse to palpitations. If the patient is hemodynamically unstable, the advanced cardiac life support protocol should be followed (see Chapter 3). After the patient has been examined and hemodynamic stability confirmed, an electrocardiogram, arterial blood gas sample, and serum electrolyte panel should be obtained. Frequently, supplementary oxygen and aggressive potassium and magnesium replenishment are the only treatment necessary. Premature ventricular contractions often are signs of myocardial ischemia. They should be treated expediently with electrolyte correction, optimization of oxygenation, and evaluation for ischemia.

d. **Chest pain associated with myocardial infarction** often goes unnoticed by caretakers and patients due to thoracotomy incisional pain and narcotic administration.

e. **Perioperative fluid management** of thoracic surgery patients differs from that of patients after abdominal surgery. **Pulmonary surgery does not induce large fluid shifts.** In addition, collapse and reexpansion of lungs during surgery can lead to pulmonary edema. Pulmonary edema should be treated with aggressive diuresis. This is largely due to the limited pulmonary reserve, most graphically demonstrated in the pneumonectomy patient in whom 100% of the cardiac output perfuses the remaining lung. Judicious fluid management, including avoiding fluid overload and pulmonary edema, is critical in patients with limited pulmonary reserve. Discussions regarding intraoperative fluid management should be held with the anesthesiologist before surgery. Physicians may need to accept transiently decreased urine output and increased serum creatinine. Mild hypotension may be treated with intravenous α-agonists such as phenylephrine. Cardiac dysfunction may also be the source of postoperative oliguria, pulmonary edema, and hypotension and should always be considered in patients who are not responding normally. Echocardiography or placement of a Swan-Ganz catheter may guide treatment.

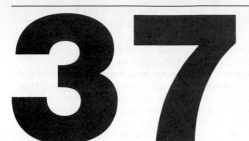

Pediatric Surgery

**Sean E. McLean and
Patrick A. Dillon**

Pediatric surgery involves the care of fetuses, neonates, children, and adolescents with surgical disorders. Although many diseases managed by the pediatric surgeon are unique to this age group, others, such as gastroesophageal reflux or inflammatory bowel disease, are managed similarly in adults. Aside from the obvious difference in the size of the pediatric surgeon's patient, the physiology of children, especially neonates, provides many unique challenges. The scope of this chapter is limited to the diagnosis and treatment of selected problems common to pediatric surgical practice.

CARE OF THE PEDIATRIC SURGICAL PATIENT

I. **Fluid, electrolytes, and nutrition** are essential components in the overall care of the pediatric surgical patient.
    A. **Fluid requirements**
        1. **Normal daily fluid requirements for children,** especially premature infants, must account for insensible losses as a result of the high body-surface area to volume ratio and the immature kidneys in the neonate, which have a limited ability to concentrate urine. Fluid replacement can be calculated based on body weight, as shown:

Weight (kg)	24-hour fluid requirements
<2 (premature)	150 mL/kg
1–10	100 mL/kg
11–20	1,000 mL + 50 mL/kg >10 kg
>20	1,500 mL + 20 mL/kg >20 kg

   A simple method for calculating a child's hourly maintenance fluid requirements is to use 4 mL/kg per hour for each kilogram of the first 10 kg weight, plus 2 mL/kg per hour for each kilogram from 10 to 20 kg, plus 1 mL/kg per hour for each kilogram over 20 kg.
        2. **Postoperative fluid replacement** is determined from the normal daily requirements and losses incurred from any disease process and surgical procedures. Such third-space losses should be replaced with a balanced salt solution such as lactated Ringer solution.
            a. As a **first estimate,** an additional 25% of the calculated daily maintenance volume should be given for each quadrant of the peritoneal cavity involved or entered (*Ann Surg* 1982;196:76).
            b. **Output from tubes and drains** should be matched by replacement fluid with similar electrolyte composition.
            c. The **total fluid administered** ultimately should be adjusted to support urine output between 1 and 2 mL/kg per hour.
            d. **Central venous pressure monitoring** can be used to estimate intravascular volume more accurately.
            e. In **full-term newborns,** total body water is a higher percentage of body weight than in adults (75% in infants versus 60% in adults).
            f. **Total blood volume in the newborn** is approximately 8% of body weight, which decreases to 5% in older infants.

B. **Electrolyte requirements** generally are met in pediatric patients when the normal daily fluid requirements are given according to the following guidelines.
 1. **Children younger than 6 months** should be given 10% dextrose in 0.25% saline with potassium chloride, 20 mEq/dL, as a maintenance fluid.
 2. **Children older than 6 months** should be given 5% dextrose in 0.45% saline with potassium chloride, 20 mEq/dL, for maintenance fluid replacement.
 3. **Daily sodium requirements** are 2 to 3 mEq/kg, and daily potassium requirements are 1 to 2 mEq/kg.
C. **Nutritional requirements** are increased in infants and children compared with adults.
 1. The **minimum daily caloric needs for children** can be calculated using the table shown in Section I.Λ.1 (for daily fluid requirements), substituting kcal/kg for mL/kg.
 2. **Additional nutritional demands** are made on infants and children affected by stresses such as sepsis, burns, trauma, and fever. These excess caloric needs must be met to prevent the development of a catabolic state.
 3. **Carbohydrates** should supply 40% to 45%, **lipids** 35%, and **protein** 15% of total calories in the diet.
 4. **Enteral nutrition** is the preferred method of delivering calories to a patient if the gastrointestinal (GI) tract is functioning. In patients where enteral nutrition in contraindicated, parenteral nutrition should be used.
 5. Most **infant formulas** contain 20 kcal/oz; therefore, caloric needs can be calculated by the following formula:

Weight (kg) × 6 oz = volume of formula necessary to deliver 120 kcal/kg

 6. A **newborn weight gain** of 15 to 30 g per day is expected.
II. **Preoperative preparation**
A. A thorough and succinct **history and physical examination** are always required. Occasionally, patients have **signs and symptoms** of an upper respiratory infection, which may require postponement of an elective operation. The acuteness of the illness and the urgency of the procedure planned must be considered. Other signs, such as fever, leukocytosis, decreased appetite, or lethargy, may necessitate a delay of the procedure. Severe diaper rash with a planned groin surgery and signs of child abuse are other reasons to postpone surgery.
B. **Laboratory tests** are not indicated routinely. The decision to obtain any preoperative laboratory tests should be made jointly by the surgical and anesthesiology teams on an individual basis. Typically, only a hematocrit is required for elective procedures.
C. **Abstinence from food and drink** for a prolonged preoperative period is not required in children. Studies have indicated that clear liquids ingested 2 to 3 hours before induction of anesthesia do not increase the risk of aspiration (*Anesthesiology* 1990;72:593). **Aspiration risks** can also be reduced by administering H_2-receptor antagonists, metoclopramide, and buffering agents such as sodium citrate.
   Standard **nothing-by-mouth (n.p.o.) guidelines** according to age are as follows (Preoperative evaluation. In: Rasch DK, Webster DE, eds. *Clinical Manual of Pediatric Anesthesia*. New York: McGraw-Hill; 1994).
 1. **Newborn to 1-year-old children** may receive regular formula feedings until 5 hours preoperatively. Clear liquids may be given until 2 hours before surgery.
 2. **One- to 14-year-old children** may eat solid food until midnight the night before surgery. Clear liquids may be taken up to 3 hours before the procedure.

3. Fourteen- to 19-year-old children should have nothing to eat or drink after midnight the night before surgery.

D. Preoperative antibiotic prophylaxis is required for patients with cardiac anomalies who are undergoing noncardiac surgery, patients with ventriculoperitoneal shunts, and those who have other prosthetic material. The most commonly recommended antibiotics are ampicillin (50 mg/kg), erythromycin (10 mg/kg), and clindamycin (10 mg/kg). Although specific recommendations may vary, usually one dose is given 1 hour before the procedure, and the final dose is given 6 hours after the procedure.

III. Vascular access

A. Peripheral venous access often is challenging in pediatric patients, especially neonates. However, cannulation of a vein can usually be accomplished in one of the following sites: dorsal vein of the hand, antecubital vein of the arm, saphenous vein at the ankle, dorsal vein in the foot, median tributary at the wrist, external jugular vein, and scalp veins.

B. Percutaneous central venous catheter insertion is the method of choice when peripheral access is not available. The sites most often chosen are the subclavian vein, internal jugular vein, and femoral vein. Central venous catheter insertion often requires sedation before the procedure, but it can be done safely in newborns. Complications of central venous catheters include air embolus, pneumothorax, infection, and thrombosis. Strict adherence to sterile technique and regular dressing care are the best prevention against infection. If thrombosis of the catheter occurs, thrombolytic therapy may be effective at dissolving the clot.

C. Saphenous vein cutdown has been used for the pediatric patient in whom vascular access is not obtainable by a percutaneous approach. Even in experienced hands, however, a venous cutdown can be time consuming, and, therefore, during an emergency situation, alternative routes for the administration of fluids and medications must be sought. When performing a **venous cutdown in an elective situation**, it is helpful to use a peripherally inserted central catheter, or PCVC catheter. The saphenous vein at the saphenofemoral junction or the vena comitantes of the brachial artery are the usual sites chosen.

D. Intraosseous infusion should be used in an emergency setting when other attempts at obtaining vascular access have failed. A location 1 to 3 cm distal to the tibial tuberosity is the recommended site. The needle should be directed inferiorly during insertion. Alternatively, the femur may be reached by inserting the needle in a cephalad direction 3 cm proximal to the condyles. Either a bone marrow aspiration needle or a 16- to 19-gauge butterfly needle is adequate.

E. Arterial catheters are needed in some neonates and infants. The potential sites for placement of an arterial catheter include the umbilical, radial, femoral, posterior tibial, and temporal arteries; however, the radial artery is used most frequently. The typical catheters are 22- to 24-gauge and can be placed percutaneously or by cutdown. In a neonate who is within the first 2 to 4 days of life, the umbilical artery can often be cannulated through the umbilical stump.

IV. Common neonatal surgical problems

A. Congenital diaphragmatic hernia (CDH) occurs when the diaphragm fails to form completely, allowing the abdominal organs to herniate into the chest. This anomaly occurs on the left in 90% of cases and on the right in 10%. The herniated viscera act as a space-occupying lesion, preventing normal lung development, primarily on the affected side. Thus, cardiorespiratory compromise is the hallmark of this disease.

1. Diagnosis of CDH often is made prenatally by routine ultrasonography. Polyhydramnios is present in up to 80% of pregnancies with CDH; thus, the presence of polyhydramnios may prompt a diagnostic prenatal ultrasound that reveals CDH in the fetus. Children that are not diagnosed prenatally will present with cardiorespiratory compromise.

Findings on physical examination will demonstrate an asymmetric "funnel" chest, reduced breath sounds on the affected side, and a scaphoid abdomen. Plain chest x-ray is a good diagnostic modality because it reveals the presence of herniated abdominal viscera within the chest. Once the diagnosis is established, renal ultrasound, cranial ultrasound, and echocardiography must be performed to evaluate for other congenital abnormalities.

2. **Mortality** is directly related to the degree of pulmonary hypoplasia, the degree of pulmonary hypertension, and the presence of associated congenital anomalies.

3. **Management**

   a. **Immediate postnatal care** of an infant who has CDH includes several supportive measures.

      (1) **Supplemental oxygen** is needed to maximize hemoglobin saturation.

      (2) **Adequate ventilation** is critical for maintaining gas exchange. If signs and symptoms of respiratory distress are present, endotracheal intubation is indicated. Avoid bag-mask ventilation, which exacerbates GI distention and further impedes lung ventilation.

      (3) **Intravenous access** is necessary for the administration of fluids to maintain organ perfusion.

      (4) **GI decompression** by orogastric or nasogastric intubation reduces distention of the stomach and intestines if they are encroaching on the lung.

      (5) **Transport of the child** can be done safely once the preceding measures are complete. The patient should be positioned to avoid compression of his or her lung on the unaffected side. In addition, GI decompression should be continued throughout travel.

   b. **Intensive care** delivered once the infant is at an appropriate referral center is aimed at controlling pulmonary hypertension and minimizing the right-to-left cardiac shunt.

      (1) **Mechanical ventilation** is the primary means for respiratory support, with the goal of providing oxygenation while limiting barotrauma to a hypoplastic lung. The important aspects of management include maintaining a preductal oxygen saturation level of >90%, limiting mean and peak airway pressures, and tolerating moderate hypercarbia. **Permissive hypercapnia** is a strategy designed to minimize barotrauma to the hypoplastic lungs. Ventilator settings are adjusted to accept a pH >7.20, an arterial carbon dioxide tension of 60 to 70 mm Hg, and a preductal oxygen saturation >90%. When peak airway pressures exceed 30 cm H_2O and mean airway pressures exceed 20 cm H_2O, consideration is given to placing the child on extracorporeal membrane oxygenation. The high-frequency oscillating ventilator (HFOV) and inhaled nitric oxide are other useful adjuncts that may be used in children that fail conventional modes of ventilation. In some centers, the HFOV is the primary mode of ventilation in children with CDH.

      (2) **Extracorporeal membrane oxygenation (ECMO)** should be considered for patients that decompensate with severe preductal hypoxemia or right to left shunting due to high pulmonary vascular resistance. Patients with overwhelming pulmonary hypoplasia not compatible with life are not candidates for ECMO.

      (3) **Definitive surgical repair** usually is deferred until the patient's pulmonary status is stable. A subcostal incision on the affected side allows the herniated abdominal contents to be replaced in the peritoneal cavity. The defect is either repaired primarily or repaired with a synthetic patch, depending on the size of the defect.

B. Tracheoesophageal malformations represent a spectrum of anomalies, including esophageal atresia (EA) and tracheoesophageal fistula (TEF), separately or in combination (Fig. 37-1). These are believed to arise from an interruption in the normal budding of the trachea from the foregut during embryonic development.

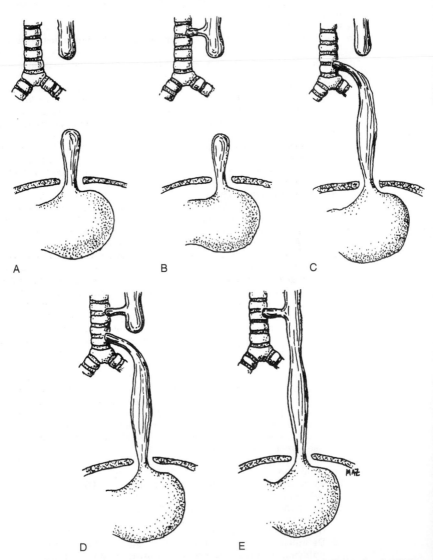

Figure 37-1. Variants of tracheoesophageal fistula. **A.** Atresia without fistula (5% to 7% of cases). **B.** Proximal fistula and distal pouch (<1% occurrence). **C.** Proximal pouch with distal fistula (85% to 90% of cases). **D.** Atresia with proximal and distal fistulas (<1% of cases). **E.** Fistula without atresia (H-type) (2% to 6% occurrence).

1. The **diagnosis** of a tracheoesophageal malformation varies, depending on the type of anomaly present.
   a. **EA,** with or without TEF, should be recognized in the immediate newborn period by the following symptoms and signs.
      (1) **Excessive drooling**
      (2) **Regurgitation** of feedings
      (3) **Choking, coughing, or cyanosis** during feeding
      (4) **Coiled orogastric tube** in the esophageal pouch on plain radiography
      (5) **Gas in the GI tract** on plain radiograph implies the presence of a distal TEF.
   b. **TEF usually is associated with EA.** Isolated TEF ("H-type" fistula; Fig. 37-1E) may present later in childhood and can be identified by the following signs and symptoms.
      (1) **Choking or coughing** during ingestion of **liquids**
      (2) **Recurrent pneumonia**
      (3) **Abdominal distention**
      (4) **Excessive flatulence**
      (5) **Contrast in the trachea** on upper GI study
      (6) A **fistula** visualized at bronchoscopy
2. **Management** of a suspected TEF/EA in a newborn must be carried out expeditiously.
   a. **Prevent aspiration.**
      (1) Place the infant in the **supine position** with the **head elevated 30 to 45 degrees.**
      (2) Insert an **orogastric or nasogastric tube** into the proximal esophageal pouch for decompression and to prevent aspiration.
   b. Administer **ampicillin (50 mg/kg) and gentamicin (2.5 mg/kg)** intravenously.
   c. **Transport** the patient rapidly, accompanied by personnel experienced in neonatal airway management.
   d. Once the child is at a tertiary care facility, an experienced surgeon should urgently gain **control of the TEF.** Performing surgical **ligation of the fistula** and **repair of the EA** at one anesthetic is the preferred management, and the procedures are done through a right extrapleural thoracotomy. In **neonates** too ill to withstand an operation, bronchoscopic placement of a **balloon-tipped catheter** to occlude the fistula is required.
   e. Integral to the **perioperative management** is an investigation for other anomalies that may occur in association with tracheoesophageal malformations. These anomalies are known as **VACTERL** (*v*ertebral defects, imperforate *a*nus, *c*ardiac defects, *t*rache*o*esophageal malformations, *r*enal dysplasia, and *l*imb anomalies). Echocardiography and renal ultrasonography are necessary to screen for associated life-threatening anomalies.
   f. Robotic-assisted minimally invasive surgical techniques have been used in animal models to simulate repair of TEF and EA. This research may produce a new modality of treatment in the near future.
C. **Gastroschisis** is an abdominal wall defect that is believed to arise from an isolated vascular insult in the developing mesenchyme. The defect usually occurs to the right of a normal umbilical cord. Typically, the midgut and stomach herniate through this defect. Unlike omphalocele, there is no membranous sac covering the eviscerated abdominal organs; furthermore, the incidence of associated anomalies in gastroschisis is infrequent.
   1. **Diagnosis.** Gastroschisis is most often discovered during prenatal ultrasound. **Ultrasound examination** of a fetus after 13 weeks may reveal extra-abdominal intestine free within the amniotic fluid. The intestine is located apart from the umbilical cord. Once gastroschisis is detected,

other anomalies should be noted. When an unsuspected abdominal wall defect is not recognized until birth, accurate pathologic description is key to the proper diagnosis. In gastroschisis, the exposed bowel may develop a **serositis,** and it is at risk for strangulation and vascular compromise in the presence of a small abdominal wall defect.

2. **Management**
   a. In **prenatal management,** serial ultrasonography helps to monitor the course of the fetus with gastroschisis. If bowel dilatation and mural thickening of the eviscerated intestine are detected, delivery at the time of lung maturity may be indicated (*Surg Obstet Gynecol* 1993;81:53).
   b. Pregnancies complicated by gastroschisis should be managed at a tertiary care center with both a high-risk obstetrics service and pediatric surgical expertise.
   c. The initial steps for **postnatal management** include fluid resuscitation, electrolyte replacement, antibiotic therapy, close monitoring of urine output, prevention of heat loss, and placement of a nasogastric tube for intestinal decompression.
      (1) **Intravenous fluids** should be started, with an initial bolus of normal saline at 20 mL/kg body weight. Subsequently, 5% dextrose in lactated Ringer solution should be infused at a rate that is three to four times the maintenance requirements until the urine output reaches 1.5 to 2.0 mL/kg per hour.
      (2) **Exposed bowel** should be covered with moistened gauze and placed in a "bowel bag" or wrapped in cellophane to prevent heat loss.
      (3) **Heat and fluid losses** can be decreased by placing the neonate in a plastic bag up to the neck.
      (4) **Position** the neonate in a lateral position to prevent kinking of the bowel and vascular compromise.
      (5) **Extension of the fascial defect** in the midline for 1 to 2 cm can be done if the bowel mesentery appears to be compressed by a narrow opening.
      (6) **Expeditious transport is crucial.** Delays should not occur owing to difficulty in obtaining intravenous access.
      (7) **Definitive treatment.** At our center, we routinely use a transparent spring-loaded silo to aid in the reduction of abdominal viscera. The placement of the silo is performed in the NICU or delivery room under sterile conditions. The abdominal viscera are reduced gradually over time. The abdominal wall defect is then repaired in a primary fashion on an elective basis. Fewer complications arise with this method of management than with immediate reduction of viscera and early primary closure (*J Pediatr Surg* 2000;35:843–846).
D. **Omphalocele** is an abdominal wall defect of the umbilical ring in which the intestines protrude through the base of the umbilical cord and herniate into a sac. The sac consists of an outer layer of amnion and an inner layer of peritoneum, and the umbilical cord inserts into the sac. Associated with the abdominal wall defect is a high incidence (50%) of related anomalies.
   1. **Diagnosis** is made during prenatal ultrasound.
      a. **Ultrasound examination** beyond 13 weeks of fetal development may reveal intestine herniating through the base of the umbilical cord. This intestine is covered by a smooth, echogenic sac. Because of the high incidence of related anomalies, the presence of an omphalocele should direct a thorough search for other birth defects by ultrasonography and amniocentesis.
      b. Amniotic fluid α-fetoprotein levels are elevated.
      c. **Postnatal diagnosis** is unusual, as in gastroschisis, and is made readily on physical examination.

d. Important physical findings include the following:

(1) The presence of the abdominal wall defect at the base of the umbilical cord.

(2) The presence of a sac covering the herniated viscera. The **size of the defect** varies from a few centimeters to absence of most of the abdominal wall.

(3) Rupture of the sac is infrequent, but it is distinguished from gastroschisis by the presence of residual sac in continuity with the umbilical cord.

2. Postnatal management. The care of a patient with an omphalocele should be conducted according to the same principles as for gastroschisis (see Section IV.C.2). Rupture of the sac requires that the defect be treated as a gastroschisis.

3. Due to the presence of other anomalies associated with omphalocele, **the overall prognosis** for infants with omphalocele is significantly worse than that for gastroschisis.

E. Necrotizing enterocolitis (NEC) is a syndrome characterized by discontinuous areas of bowel injury, which range from mucosal ulceration to gangrenous bowel with intestinal perforation. The inciting cause is unknown; however, the pathogenesis is thought to be multifactorial, involving an immature gut barrier defense and virulent bacteria. The incidence of NEC is 1 to 3 cases per 1,000 live births. The disease primarily affects premature infants, for NEC occurs in 10% of all babies born weighing <1,500 g.

1. Diagnosis of NEC begins with clinical suspicion. Radiographic studies and laboratory tests are used to support the diagnosis after a careful history and physical examination.

a. Signs and symptoms that characterize NEC include the following:

(1) Abdominal distention. The abdomen may initially be soft and progress to a firm state. Bowel loops may be palpable.

(2) High gastric residuals

(3) Vomiting or bilious nasogastric tube drainage

(4) Hematochezia

(5) Diarrhea, which can be bloody

(6) Temperature instability

(7) Apnea

(8) Lethargy

(9) Skin pallor or mottling

(10) Edema, erythematic, cellulites, or repentance of the abdominal wall may indicate peritonitis, local response to inflamed bowel, or perforation of bowel.

b. Plain radiographs may reveal any of several findings that are consistent with NEC.

(1) Pneumatosis intestinalis is the most characteristic radiographic sign of NEC, occurring in 98% of patients with the syndrome.

(2) Dilated loops of intestine often are present.

(3) An intestinal loop that is static on serial films may be recognized; it represents a lack of peristalsis due to full-thickness necrosis.

(4) Ascites may appear acutely on serial radiographs.

(5) Intrahepatic portal vein gas is associated with poor prognosis.

(6) Pneumoperitoneum may be apparent if intestinal perforation has occurred.

(7) Gastric distention may be pronounced as a result of a paralytic ileus.

c. Contrast imaging is often avoided due to the risk of perforation.

d. Plain radiographs are most often sufficient. **Ultrasonography** may reveal portal venous gas, pneumatosis, and the presence of free peritoneal fluid, which may aid in the decision for exploratory laparotomy.

e. Laboratory tests also are not specific for NEC, but the following suggest the onset of sepsis:

(1) **Metabolic acidosis**
(2) **Thrombocytopenia**
(3) **Leukocytosis or leukopenia**
2. **Management.** If there is no evidence of bowel perforation or intestinal necrosis, the management of NEC is supportive.
   a. **Nonoperative treatment** for NEC consists of bowel rest, nasogastric decompression, removal of umbilical catheters (if possible), maintenance of proper fluid balance, parenteral nutrition, and broad-spectrum antibiotics. A good response to this therapy is indicated by decreased gastric residuals, diminished abdominal distention, and clearing of blood from the stool. The neonate with NEC should be monitored with serial abdominal examinations, radiographs, and laboratory studies. Enteral nutrition should be withheld until there is evidence of the resolution of NEC and return of peristalsis. Enteral nutrition starts with dilute formula, and it is advanced as tolerated.
   b. **Absolute indications for operative treatment** of NEC are as follows:
      (1) **Intestinal perforation.** This is most often indicated by pneumoperitoneum on plain radiograph.
      (2) **Intestinal obstruction**
      (3) **Intra-abdominal abscess**
      (4) **Intestinal necrosis.** The best indicators of intestinal gangrene are pneumoperitoneum, portal venous gas, and paracentesis fluid positive for organisms.
   c. **Relative indications for surgery** include the following:
      (1) **Sepsis unresponsive to medical treatment**
      (2) **Inflammatory changes in the abdominal wall**
      (3) **Radiographic signs** such as a static intestinal loop, asymmetrically dilated loops, and ascites, all of which suggest intestinal gangrene
      (4) **Laboratory tests** that reveal thrombocytopenia, coagulopathy, severe hyponatremia, or intractable acidosis, all of which suggest bowel necrosis
      (5) **Paracentesis fluid** that is brown and cloudy, contains bacteria (as revealed by Gram stain), or contains a high leukocyte count, with neutrophils predominating
   d. **The operation performed depends on the pathology found.** Most often, resection of the involved intestine is done, with the creation of stomas. When intestinal viability is questionable, reexploration within 24 hours is essential.
   e. **Open peritoneal drainage** in critically ill neonates may be used as a temporizing measure or as primary therapy for extremely low birth weight infants (<1,000 g). This procedure is performed at the isolette by inserting a Penrose drain through a right lower quadrant abdominal incision. If not definitive treatment, this drainage technique may stabilize the infant's condition until he or she is better able to tolerate a laparotomy (*J Pediatr Surg* 1990;25:1034).
V. **Alimentary tract obstruction** in a child may present with nausea, vomiting, GI bleeding, and abdominal pain and distention. Often, within this presentation are clues that can direct an evaluation toward the site of obstruction or signal the presence of a life-threatening illness. For example, nonbilious emesis is the distinguishing feature of obstruction proximal to the ampulla of Vater, particularly pyloric stenosis. As another example, the more distal an obstruction is, the more distended the abdomen can become. Alternatively, bilious emesis in an infant or child may signal intestinal malrotation with midgut volvulus, which can be lethal if not detected early in its course. The etiologies of intestinal obstruction include congenital and acquired diseases. **Congenital causes of alimentary tract obstruction** (topics A through H) typically present in the newborn period. **Acquired causes of alimentary tract**

obstruction (topics I through K) in children can present at any time postnatally but typically present after the newborn period.
A. Intestinal malrotation occurs when the intestine fails to undergo its normal rotation and fixation during embryologic development. The incidence of intestinal malrotation has been reported to be 1 in 500 to 1 in 6,000. Associated anomalies are present in 30% to 59% of patients. Symptoms most often present in the neonatal period but may present as late as adulthood. Once recognized, malrotation must be corrected due to the risk of volvulus.

  1. **Diagnosis** of malrotation is made from the clinical presentation and contrast radiographs.

     a. **Signs and symptoms** may include the following:

        (1) **Bilious emesis** (the most common symptom)

        (2) **Abdominal distention and pain**

        (3) **Hematochezia or hematemesis**

        (4) **Physical examination** findings may range from benign to an acute abdomen.

     b. Radiologic studies are critical in establishing the diagnosis of malrotation with or without midgut volvulus.

        (1) **Plain radiographs** may be nondiagnostic, but certain signs may be helpful.

           (a) **"Double-bubble"** is indicative of duodenal obstruction.

           (b) **"Gasless" abdomen** characterizes volvulus.

        (2) **Contrast imaging** is necessary to establish the diagnosis. Upper GI with a small-bowel follow-through is the study of choice. Major signs of malrotation include evidence of failure of the ligament of Treitz to cross to the right of the spine (midline) and a right-sided jejunum. Hallmark signs for volvulus include the "bird's beak" sign and a corkscrew appearance of the small intestine.

  2. **Management** of malrotation involves surgical correction. Exploratory laparotomy and the Ladd procedure is the standard for treating malrotation with or without volvulus. If the intestine is not necrotic, the volvulus should be reduced by counterclockwise rotation and the peritoneal bands (Ladd bands) divided. Infarcted bowel should be removed and a primary anastomosis performed. The bowel is placed in a state of nonrotation, in which the colon is positioned on the left side of the abdomen and the small bowel on the right to restore a long distance between the duodenojejunal junction and the ileocecal junction. To complete the procedure, an appendectomy is performed. If there is a possibility that the child will develop short-gut syndrome, questionably viable intestine should not be resected. A repeat laparotomy 24 hours later is necessary to assess the viability of the intestine.

  3. **Laparoscopic surgical management** can be performed in patients with malrotation with or without volvulus. The major steps of laparoscopic management are (1) inspection of the mesenteric base and detorsion of bowel, (2) lysis of peritoneal bands, (3) placement of bowel in a state of nonrotation with broadening of the mesenteric base, and (4) appendectomy (*J Am Coll Surg* 1997;185:172–176).

B. Intestinal atresia or stenosis can occur anywhere from the duodenum to the colon. The distal ileum, proximal jejunum, and duodenum are the most common sites for atresias. Atresias are thought to be caused by intrauterine vascular insults.

  1. **Diagnosis** of intestinal atresia may be suspected antenatally if polyhydramnios is present on ultrasonography. In the newborn period, babies typically present with bilious vomiting, abdominal distention, and failure to pass meconium. Infants with intestinal stenosis may **present** at a few weeks to months of age with vomiting, failure to thrive, and poor feeding. A **plain abdominal radiograph** should be obtained to delineate the level of obstruction. A "double-bubble" sign is diagnostic of duodenal

obstruction. Contrast enema may be used to rule out a functional obstruction, such as meconium ileus or meconium plug syndrome.

2. **Management** of intestinal atresia should begin with nasogastric decompression and intravenous fluid administration to maintain a urine output of 2 mL/kg per hour. Ampicillin (50 mg/kg) and gentamicin (2.5 mg/kg) should be started immediately. Surgical repair consists of resection of the dilated proximal segment and primary anastomosis. In contrast, for duodenal atresia, a duodenoduodenostomy is created to bypass the obstruction. Finally, during the operation, saline should be infused into the distal bowel to rule out synchronous intestinal atresias.

C. **Hirschsprung disease** is a congenital disorder characterized by a variable length of intestinal aganglionosis of the hindgut. Hirschsprung disease may show a familial pattern of inheritance, or it may be sporadic in nature. Up to 7.8% of cases occur in patients where more than one family member is affected. Many genetic mutations have been linked to intestinal aganglionosis. Mutations in the *RET* proto-oncogene have been found to be present in both familial and sporadic cases of Hirschsprung disease.

1. **Diagnosis** of Hirschsprung disease is suggested by the history and confirmed by histological proof of the absence of ganglion cells within the bowel wall.

   a. Neonates classically **present** with abdominal distention, infrequent defecation, or failure to pass meconium within the first 48 hours of life. In some patients, the first manifestation of Hirschsprung disease is enterocolitis with sepsis. Older infants and children present with chronic constipation or failure to thrive.

   b. **Plain abdominal radiographs** of patients with Hirschsprung disease commonly show a pattern of distal obstruction.

   c. **Barium enema** usually demonstrates a transition zone between distal nondilated bowel and proximal dilated bowel. This transition zone is found most commonly in the rectosigmoid, but it may be seen anywhere in the colon. In neonates, a transition zone may not be identifiable. Patients with total colonic aganglionosis do not have a transition zone.

   d. **Rectal biopsy** is essential for making the diagnosis of Hirschsprung disease. Full-thickness specimens are the ideal tissue samples to allow identification of the absence of ganglion cells in the Auerbach myenteric and Meissner submucosal plexus. In neonates, rectal suction biopsy often is sufficient to make the definitive diagnosis of Hirschsprung disease.

2. **Preoperative management** of patients with Hirschsprung disease initially should include **colonic decompression** to prevent enterocolitis. Saline enemas may be used to evacuate impacted stool. A **nasogastric tube** should be placed if the child is vomiting.

3. **Operative treatment** in patients who are unstable or who have massively dilated bowel involves placing a **diverting colostomy** proximal to the aganglionic segment until definitive reconstruction is performed. Daily rectal irrigations may obviate the need for a colostomy. **Reconstruction of intestinal continuity** involves bringing ganglionated bowel to within 1 cm of the anal verge. The three classic methods for this reconstruction are the procedures developed by Swenson, Duhamel, and Soave. Each of these operations has been modified to improve functional results and usually is reserved until the patient reaches 6 to 12 months of age. Recent advances in the surgical management of Hirschsprung disease have led to earlier surgical intervention, as early as the first week of life, and to alterations in technique. Operative techniques that have shown great promise include the laparoscopic endorectal pull-through advocated by Georgeson and the transanal one-stage endorectal pull-through advocated by Langer. The advocates of these two approaches cite decreased recovery time, decreased hospital stay,

decreased complications, a potential for decreased adhesions, and decreased cost as some of the advantages of these two minimal access approaches in comparison with open transabdominal procedures (*Ann Surg* 1999;229:678–682; *J Pediatr Surg* 2000;35:820–822).

D. Anorectal anomalies are a constellation of congenital defects associated with fecal and urinary incontinence and sexual inadequacy. The classification proposed by Pena and colleagues is linked to the sex of the affected neonate (*Am J Surg* 2000;180:370): **Males:** perineal fistula, rectourethral bulbar fistula, rectourethral prostatic fistula, rectovesical (bladder neck) fistula, imperforate anus without fistula, rectal atresia and stenosis; **Females:** perineal fistula, vestibular fistula, imperforate anus with no fistula, rectal atresia and stenosis, persistent cloaca. The lesions may also be classified as high, intermediate, or low depending on whether the atresia is below, at the level, or above the puborectalis sling.

1. **Diagnosis.** Diagnosis of anorectal anomalies is typically made upon physical examination of the affected infant. Plain radiographs, contrast studies, and MR may aid in the definition of the anatomical defect of the affected infant.

2. **Management.** When the diagnosis of an anorectal anomaly is discovered, it is important to define associated defects that may have life-threatening consequences. Cardiovascular (12% to 22%) and anomalies in the VACTERL complex are frequently associated with anorectal anomalies.

   The decision to create a protective colostomy is the next major decision in the management of infants with anorectal anomalies. Protective colostomy is not necessary if primary repair can be performed safely.

   Inspection of the perineum is usually sufficient to establish the need for a colostomy. It is important to wait 24 hours for the passage of meconium prior to the creation of a stoma. This will allow confirmation of the presence of a perineal fistula. Earlier determinations concerning the anatomy may lead to errors in treatment. If the anatomy is in doubt after 24 hours, lateral radiographs of the pelvis with the infant in a prone position should be obtained.

3. **Definitive operative repair.** The main goal of caring for a baby with an anorectal malformation is bowel and urinary continence. For perineal fistulas, primary repair may be performed without a protective colostomy. For other anorectal anomalies, a three-step methodology is advocated with a diverting colostomy after birth, definitive repair, and colostomy closure. Recently, in some centers pediatric surgeons are advocating primary repair for malformations other than perineal fistulas. Of note, laparoscopic management of anorectal anomalies has been performed.

E. Omphalomesenteric duct abnormalities result from incomplete involution of the vitelline duct, which connects the primitive gut to the yolk sac. The omphalomesenteric duct remnant may persist as any of the following (which occur within 60 cm proximal to the ileocecal valve): (1) a simple ileal outpouching found on the antimesenteric side of the intestine, known as **Meckel's diverticulum** (a true diverticulum); (2) a **patent duct** between the ileum and the umbilicus; (3) an **umbilical cyst** lined by intestinal mucosa; or (4) a **fibrous cord** between an ileal diverticulum and the umbilicus or mesentery.

1. **Diagnosis** of omphalomesenteric duct abnormalities depends on the type of remnant that persists. A **patent duct** is recognized by spillage of ileal contents through the child's umbilicus. **Umbilical cysts** of vitelline duct origin secrete a mucoid discharge at the umbilicus. A **fibrous band** remnant between the ileum and the abdominal wall usually presents as an internal hernia or intestinal volvulus around this cord of tissue, with the accompanying signs of intestinal obstruction. A **Meckel's diverticulum** frequently contains ectopic gastric mucosa, resulting in peptic

ulceration and hemorrhage in 22% of cases. This is recognized as painless rectal bleeding, which is often substantial and can be life-threatening but usually is self-limited. Other complications of a Meckel's diverticulum include bowel obstruction caused by internal hernia around a vitelline duct band (13%), diverticulitis with abdominal pain (2%), and intussusception, with the Meckel's diverticulum acting as a lead point (<1%) (*Arch Surg* 1987;122:542). More than one-half of the children with a symptomatic Meckel's diverticulum present before 2 years of age. Diagnostic evaluation of a patient suspected of having a Meckel's diverticulum should begin with a technetium-99m pertechnetate scintiscan. This isotope is taken up by the ectopic gastric mucosa of the Meckel's diverticulum.

2. **Management** of omphalomesenteric duct abnormalities involves **surgical resection** of the remnant. When GI bleeding is the indication for the operation, a diverticulectomy plus either oversewing or resection of the bleeding site is recommended. **Laparoscopic resection** of the diverticulum using a stapling device can be performed. Occasionally, a large feeding vessel crosses onto the surface of the diverticulum from the mesentery, and this may require separate dissection and clipping or ligation. When radiographic reduction of an intussusception is unsuccessful, surgical reduction of the invaginated intestine and diverticulectomy should be attempted. If gangrenous bowel is present, bowel resection with primary anastomosis should be done. In infants or young children who have a Meckel's diverticulum discovered incidentally at laparotomy, diverticulectomy should be performed, particularly when a palpable mass is present within this enteric outpouching, because it may contain gastric mucosa, with the potential for ileal mucosal ulceration.

F. **Meconium ileus** is an intestinal obstruction that occurs in neonates with cystic fibrosis and is caused by inspissated meconium.

1. **Diagnosis** of meconium ileus can be suspected prenatally by the detection of polyhydramnios on prenatal ultrasound. However, the typical **presentation** is abdominal distention, bilious vomiting, and failure to pass meconium within 24 to 48 hours of life. Complicated meconium ileus has an acute onset within 24 hours of birth and is characterized by progressive abdominal distention, pneumoperitoneum, peritonitis, and abdominal wall inflammation. Hypovolemia and sepsis may ensue. **Plain abdominal radiographic findings** are variable. Dilated loops of small bowel are common. A mixture of air bubbles and meconium produces a **ground-glass, coarse, granular, or soap bubble–like** appearance. Air-fluid levels are infrequent. Intra-abdominal calcifications suggest prenatal perforation and subsequent meconium peritonitis. Ascites or pneumoperitoneum suggests perforation after birth. Alternatively, up to 35% of infants with complicated meconium ileus show no plain radiographic abnormalities. A **water-soluble contrast enema** can confirm the diagnosis by demonstrating a microcolon and pellets of inspissated meconium in the ileum.

2. **Management** of meconium ileus depends on the severity of the illness. **Nonsurgical treatment** for uncomplicated cases consists of the administration of a hyperosmolar, water-soluble contrast enema, which is both diagnostic and therapeutic. This solution draws fluid into the bowel lumen and causes an osmotic diarrhea. The patient should be well hydrated and given broad-spectrum antibiotics before this therapy. **Operative intervention** is indicated for complicated meconium ileus or when enema therapy fails. Initially, an ileotomy is performed, and irrigation with an acetylcysteine solution is attempted. If gentle irrigation does not flush out the meconium, a 14 French ileostomy T tube may be placed, and routine irrigations are done beginning on postoperative day 1. This operation generally has good results. If intestinal volvulus, atresia,

perforation, or gangrene complicates the illness, nonviable bowel must be resected, and an ileostomy with mucous fistula is made. Irrigation can then be accomplished through the stoma until primary anastomosis is performed 2 to 3 weeks later. When oral feedings are advanced postoperatively, pancreatic enzyme supplementation is started.

G. **Meconium plug syndrome** has classically been described in patients without cystic fibrosis to distinguish it from meconium ileus. Altered colonic motility or a viscous meconium mass is believed to cause impaired transit of bowel contents and obstruction of the intestinal lumen.

1. **Diagnosis** (see Section V.F.)
2. **Management** (see Section V.F.). Rarely, surgery is needed to relieve the obstruction. Further evaluation includes a suction biopsy to rule out Hirschsprung disease and a sweat chloride test to ensure that cystic fibrosis is not the etiology of the disease.

H. **Intestinal duplications** are cystic or tubular structures lined by various types of normal GI mucosa, which usually are located dorsal to the true alimentary tract. These lesions frequently share a common muscular wall and blood supply with the normal GI tract and may occur anywhere from the mouth to the anus. In 20% of cases, enteric duplications communicate with the true GI tract.

1. **Diagnosis** of alimentary tract duplication can occasionally be made by prenatal ultrasonography. Postnatally, obstructive symptoms, such as vomiting, abdominal pain, and distention, may occur if the duplication compresses the lumen of the adjacent hollow viscus. Additionally, on physical examination, the neonate may have a palpable abdominal mass. **Ultrasonography or GI contrast studies** most commonly confirm the diagnosis by demonstrating external compression or displacement of the normal alimentary tract. In cysts that contain ectopic gastric mucosa, technetium radioisotope scans may aid in the diagnosis.

2. **Management** of alimentary tract duplications involves **surgical resection** or **internal drainage** of the cyst. When the cyst is within the bowel mesentery, resection of the adjacent bowel often is necessary because of a shared blood supply. Duodenal duplications usually are managed by marsupialization of the cyst into the lumen of the duodenum, which minimizes the risk of damage to the biliary system. If the duplication cyst is tubular, a common channel between the cyst and the adjacent hollow viscus can be made. When gastric mucosa is found in a cyst distant from the stomach, either the cyst is excised or the gastric mucosa is stripped and the cyst lumen joined to the adjacent intestine.

I. **Pyloric stenosis** is the most common surgical cause of nonbilious vomiting in infants. It occurs in 1 of 400 live births. It affects male infants four times more frequently than female infants.

1. **Diagnosis** of pyloric stenosis can be made clinically and confirmed by imaging studies. **Vomiting** is characteristically forceful or projectile and occurs 30 to 60 minutes after feeding in neonates who are 2 to 5 weeks of age. Undigested formula in the vomitus may lead to switching formulas in an attempt to improve feeding tolerance, but this maneuver typically is unsuccessful. Dehydration may occur and is manifested by lethargy, absence of tears, a sunken anterior fontanelle, dry mucous membranes, and decreased urine output (measured by a reduction in the weight of diapers and the frequency of diaper changes). The physical examination is most reliable if the infant is calm and the abdomen is relaxed. This task may be accomplished with the infant suckling in the mother's arms. **Palpation of the abdomen to the right and above the umbilicus may reveal the hypertrophied pylorus. This "olive" is approximately 2 cm in diameter, firm, and mobile.** To relax a hungry, agitated child, sugar water may be given by mouth. This technique consists of placing a nasogastric tube to decompress the stomach and providing a means of removing the fluid. An **upper GI contrast study** is helpful

when physical examination is nondiagnostic. An enlarged stomach, poor gastric emptying, and an elongated, **narrow pyloric channel or "string sign"** are consistent with pyloric stenosis. **Abdominal ultrasonography** may be useful when the history and physical examination are equivocal. Identification of a pyloric diameter >14 mm, muscular thickness >4 mm, and pyloric length >16 mm is diagnostic of pyloric stenosis with 91% to 100% sensitivity and 100% specificity (*J Pediatr Surg* 1987; 22:950).

   2. **Management** of a patient with pyloric stenosis should begin once evidence of dehydration is found. Preoperative fluid resuscitation and correction of the hypochloremic metabolic alkalosis that results from long-standing vomiting are paramount. Initially, a 20 mL/kg intravenous bolus of normal saline is given, followed by 5% dextrose in normal saline at a rate needed to achieve a urine output of 2 mL/kg per hour. When urine output is adequate, 20 mEq/L potassium chloride can be added to the solution. As the serum Na^+ and Cl^- concentrations return toward normal, the intravenous solution can be switched to 0.45% saline. Surgery should be undertaken only after the patient has received adequate resuscitation, which is determined by the following: (1) normal skin turgor, (2) normal fontanelle pressure, (3) moist mucous membranes, (4) a urine output of 2 mL/kg per hour, and (5) electrolyte values within normal limits, especially a total carbon dioxide of <30 mEq/L. **Operative treatment** is a pyloromyotomy, which divides the hypertrophied pyloric muscle, leaving the mucosa intact. This may be performed with either an **open technique** or **laparoscopic technique** (see Section X.C.3). Postoperative feedings can begin 8 hours after pyloromyotomy, with small volumes of sugar water given frequently. Over the next 12 hours, formula or pumped breast milk can be started. The volume of feedings should increase, with a concomitant decrease in the feeding frequency. Full oral nutrition should be under way 24 to 36 hours after operation. Parents should be advised that vomiting may occur postoperatively as a result of swelling at the pyloromyotomy, but this problem is self-limited. If the pyloric mucosa is perforated and repaired during surgery, nasogastric drainage is recommended for 24 hours before feeding is started.

J. **Intussusception** is an invagination of proximal intestine into adjacent distal bowel, with resultant obstruction of the lumen. If prolonged, this obstruction may compromise the mesenteric venous return and arterial supply. It is a frequent cause of bowel obstruction in infants, toddlers, and young children, but the highest incidence is at 5 to 10 months of age. In 30% of cases, an antecedent viral gastroenteritis or upper respiratory infection may exist. Ileocolic intussusceptions are the most common. A lead point of the intussusception is identified in only 5% of patients and is most commonly a Meckel's diverticulum (see Section V.E).

   1. **Diagnosis** of intussusception should be considered in a previously healthy infant who **presents** with a history of periods of abrupt crying and retraction of the legs up to the abdomen. These attacks usually subside over a few minutes but recur every 10 to 15 minutes. Some children become lethargic between attacks. Normal stool is passed early on, but eventually dark red mucoid stool, referred to as **"currant jelly,"** may be passed. Vomiting is common. On **physical examination,** hyperperistaltic rushes may be heard on auscultation of the abdomen during an attack. A **sausage-shaped abdominal mass** may be palpated, or the tip of the intussusception may be felt on rectal examination. If the presentation is early, the vital signs usually are within normal limits. However, a delay in obtaining medical attention can lead to dehydration, sepsis, or shock. A **barium or air-contrast enema** confirms the diagnosis by demonstrating a **"coiled spring" sign.**

2. **Management** of a patient with intussusception should involve surgical consultation before an attempt at nonoperative reduction. Before obtaining a barium or air-contrast enema, a nasogastric tube should be placed, intravenous fluid resuscitation started, and broad-spectrum antibiotics given. **Pneumatic or hydrostatic reduction** of the intussusception by air insufflation under radiographic guidance should be attempted if no evidence of peritonitis exists and the patient is stable. This technique has a 90% success rate. The maximum safe intraluminal air pressure for young infants is 80 mm Hg, and that for older children is 110 to 120 mm Hg. After successful pneumatic or hydrostatic reduction, the child should be admitted for 24 hours of observation. A liquid diet can be started once the child is awake and alert, and the diet is advanced as tolerated. Recurrent intussusception occurs in 8% to 12% of patients treated nonoperatively, and most of these patients should be managed the same as for an initial presentation. If a recurrence happens in an older child, however, surgery is advised because small-bowel tumors, which can serve as the lead point for the intussusception, occur more frequently in this age group. **Surgery** is required when nonoperative reduction fails or the child presents with peritonitis, sepsis, or shock. A transverse incision can be made to deliver the bowel. Gentle retrograde pressure is applied to the telescoped portion of the intestine in an attempt at manual reduction. Proximal and distal segments should not be pulled apart because of the risk of injury to the bowel. If manual reduction is not possible, resection of the involved segment and primary anastomosis should be done. An incidental appendectomy should also be performed. Recurrence of intussusception after operative treatment is approximately 1%.

K. **Distal intestinal obstruction syndrome (DIOS)**, formerly known as *meconium ileus equivalent*, is an intestinal obstruction caused by impaction of inspissated intestinal contents in older patients with cystic fibrosis. This problem occurs in 10% to 40% of patients with cystic fibrosis who are followed long term.

1. **Diagnosis** of DIOS should be suspected in a child with cystic fibrosis who presents with chronic or recurrent abdominal pain and distention, vomiting, and constipation. An inciting cause, such as abrupt cessation of pancreatic enzyme supplementation, dehydration, dietary change, or exacerbation of respiratory symptoms, may precipitate an acute presentation. **Plain abdominal radiographs** show the typical **ground-glass appearance** of the intestine. Dilated small-bowel and air-fluid levels may be present. Diagnosis may be confirmed by water-soluble contrast enemas, which demonstrate the inspissated intestinal contents.

2. **Management** of a patient with DIOS most often is accomplished at the time of diagnostic enema, which induces an osmotic diarrhea to flush the intestine and relieve the obstruction. Only rarely, when intussusception or volvulus complicates DIOS, is surgery required.

VI. **Jaundice** is a physical sign that reflects the presence of hyperbilirubinemia. In infants, when jaundice is present, the total serum bilirubin usually exceeds 7 mg/dL. This elevated bilirubin may reflect a rise in either the conjugated (direct) or unconjugated (indirect) bilirubin, or both. This distinction is key for establishing a differential diagnosis for jaundice.

A. **Unconjugated hyperbilirubinemia** results when bilirubin that has not been metabolized in the liver rises above normal serum values. The most common causes of this condition are hemolytic disorders, breast-feeding, and physiologic jaundice of the newborn. Treatment with phototherapy or exchange transfusions for severe hyperbilirubinemia should be considered in infants with these conditions. Less common causes of unconjugated hyperbilirubinemia include meconium ileus, Hirschsprung disease, and pyloric stenosis, which indirectly cause an increase in the enterohepatic circulation of bilirubin. Surgical treatment of the underlying disorder corrects the jaundice in these patients.

B. Conjugated hyperbilirubinemia is an elevation of the serum bilirubin, which has been linked to monoglucuronides and diglucuronides in the liver. This abnormality can be caused by biliary obstruction, hepatitis of infectious, toxic, or metabolic etiology, and conditions of chronic bilirubin overload. Because of these various causes, serologic titers for the TORCH (*to*xoplasmosis, *r*ubella, *c*ytomegalovirus, and *h*erpes simplex virus) infections and screening tests for inherited etiologies of elevated direct bilirubin should be part of the initial evaluation. However, only the obstructive causes are amenable to surgical therapy and are discussed here.

1. **Biliary atresia** is the most common cause of infantile jaundice that requires surgical correction. The etiology is unknown, but the disease is characterized by a dynamic and progressive obliteration and sclerosis of the biliary tree. As the infant gets older, obliteration of the extrahepatic bile ducts, proliferation of the intrahepatic bile ducts, and fibrosis or cirrhosis of the liver progress at an unpredictable rate.

    a. **Diagnosis** of biliary atresia often is difficult to make because clinical and laboratory information is nonspecific. Typically, these infants are well nourished and appear otherwise healthy but present with jaundice, acholic stools, dark urine, and hepatomegaly. **Percutaneous liver biopsy** usually is the first test obtained. Some biopsy specimens demonstrate unequivocally the pattern of biliary atresia. More often, however, the histology cannot be differentiated from that in α_1-antitrypsin deficiency or neonatal hepatitis. An α_1-antitrypsin level can rule out this disorder. Subsequently, the distinction between liver parenchymal disease and biliary obstructive disease can be made using **hepatobiliary imaging** with technetium-99m iminodiacetic acid. In biliary atresia, the liver readily takes up this tracer molecule, but no excretion into the duodenum is seen. **Ultrasonography** of the biliary tree can provide some structural information. Patients with biliary atresia characteristically show shrunken extrahepatic ducts and a noncontractile gallbladder on ultrasonography.

    b. **Management** of biliary atresia begins with repeat liver biopsy by open technique and an intraoperative cholangiogram. The common bile duct is visualized by cholangiography in only 25% of patients with biliary atresia. Cholangiography in the remaining 75% of patients demonstrates an atretic biliary tree. After diagnosis has been confirmed, operative correction is undertaken by performing a Kasai procedure (hepatoportoenterostomy). In this operation, the obliterated extrahepatic ducts are excised, and a hepaticojejunostomy is performed. When the distal common bile duct is patent, a choledochojejunostomy is constructed. Postoperatively, patients require supplementation with medium-chain triglycerides and the fat-soluble vitamins A, D, E, and K until normal bile flow is restored. In large series, the overall results for children treated with a Kasai procedure are that one-third show long-term improvement, one-third obtain temporary benefit, and one-third experience treatment failure. Survival for infants treated before 2.5 months of age with a Kasai procedure is 50% at 5 years (*Ann Surg* 1989;210:289). Approximately one-fourth of these same patients survive until adolescence. When liver failure results or the Kasai procedure fails, liver transplantation is the only option available.

2. **Choledochal cysts** make up a spectrum of diseases characterized by cystic dilatation of the extrahepatic and intrahepatic biliary tree. Types I to V, plus a forme fruste variant, are recognized. However, type I (fusiform cystic dilatation of the common bile duct) and type IV (cystic disease of the intrahepatic and extrahepatic bile ducts) are the most common forms. Although the pathogenesis of choledochal cysts is

unclear, an embryologic malformation of the pancreaticobiliary system is believed to be the origin of this disease.

   a. Diagnosis of more than 50% of choledochal cysts is made during the first 10 years of life. Infants most commonly present with unremitting, asymptomatic jaundice, whereas older children and adults manifest mild intermittent but long-standing jaundice. Approximately one-third of older patients present with the symptom triad of abdominal pain, jaundice, and an abdominal mass. Cholangitis and pancreatitis also are possible presentations for this disease. Previously unrecognized, choledochal cysts may even present as cholelithiasis, cirrhosis, portal hypertension, hepatic abscess, biliary carcinoma, or cyst rupture. **Ultrasonography** is the common initial test to identify a suspected choledochal cyst. **Hepatobiliary scintigraphy** can reveal intrahepatic cystic dilatation as well as biliary obstruction. **Transhepatic cholangiography and endoscopic retrograde cholangiopancreatography** are each superior to ultrasound and to scintigraphy for delineating intrahepatic and extrahepatic ductal disease.

   b. Management of a choledochal cyst is most commonly accomplished by cyst excision. This operation involves removing the entire cyst or shelling out the inner wall and its contents. It is important to identify the entrance of the pancreatic duct into the biliary tree before the excision is complete. After the cyst is removed, a choledochojejunostomy is constructed for biliary drainage. In rare cases, hepatic resection may be necessary when the disease is intrahepatic and is limited to a lobe or segment of the liver. If the intrahepatic component of the disease is diffuse or extensive, liver transplantation may be required.

VII. Groin masses in the pediatric population are most often hernias or hydroceles, but the examiner must exclude less common causes, such as acute testicular torsion, an undescended or retractile testicle, idiopathic scrotal edema, epididymitis, and inguinal lymphadenitis.

   A. The **indirect inguinal hernia** is more common in children than are **direct** or **femoral hernias.** This inguinal defect occurs in 1% to 5% of children, and boys outnumber girls 8:1. Prematurity may increase the incidence of inguinal hernia to between 7% and 30%. The true incidence of bilateral hernias is difficult to quantitate exactly, but it probably ranges from 10% to 40%. Bilateral hernias occur more frequently in premature infants and in girls.

   1. Diagnosis of an inguinal hernia is made most often on physical examination by identification of a groin bulge extending toward the scrotum or vulva. Frequently, a child is referred with a history of a hernia, but no mass can be found on examination. If the patient can be induced to laugh, cry, or stand, the hernia may be reproduced. If these maneuvers prove ineffective, the presence of a thickened spermatic cord with a clear history from a reliable observer is sufficient to proceed with hernia repair.

   2. Management of an inguinal hernia begins with assessment for incarceration. Most hernias reduce spontaneously with relaxation. Some hernias require manual reduction, however, which may be accomplished with gentle direct pressure on the hernia. Simultaneously applying caudal traction on the testicle in addition to direct pressure on the hernia may be necessary in some cases. If the hernia cannot be reduced, emergent operative repair is indicated. A child referred with an incarcerated hernia that is then reduced should be admitted to the hospital and scheduled for herniorrhaphy the next day. Premature infants in the nursery should have the hernia repair a few days before discharge from the hospital. Repair of a hernia is accomplished by high surgical ligation of the processus vaginalis through an inguinal incision. The hernia sac is found lying anterior and medial to the spermatic cord in boys. Sac contents can include small bowel, omentum, or ovary. In these cases, the viability of the sac contents must be ensured before repair.

B. Hydroceles are fluid collections within the processus vaginalis that envelop the testicle. This fluid may communicate freely with the peritoneal cavity if the processus is patent and can thus be regarded as a hernia. Alternatively, after the portion of the processus that traverses the inguinal canal obliterates normally, any fluid accumulation remains confined to the scrotum as a noncommunicating hydrocele. Hydroceles occur in approximately 6% of full-term male newborns. A newly discovered hydrocele, a history of a change in size of this mass, or persistence of the hydrocele for longer than 12 months suggests the presence of a patent processus vaginalis. In these cases, elective repair of the hydrocele should be scheduled to prevent subsequent incarceration. Noncommunicating hydroceles are self-limiting and usually resolve in 6 to 12 months.

VIII. Abdominal pain is a very common complaint in the pediatric age group. There are multiple causes of abdominal pain, some of which are unrelated to an intra-abdominal process. In constructing a differential diagnosis for acute abdominal pain, one must consider the age, gender, duration, circumstances at onset, and modifying factors. The following is a list of causes of abdominal pain in children, according to prevalence. Many of these entities are discussed in depth in other sections of this chapter or in other chapters of this book.

A. Differential diagnosis of acute abdominal pain
  1. **Very common**
     a. **Acute appendicitis**
     b. **Viral infection, nonspecific**
     c. **Gastroenteritis**
     d. **Constipation**
     e. **Urinary tract infection**
  2. **Less common**
     a. **Intussusception**
     b. **Lower-lobe pneumonia**
     c. **Intestinal obstruction**
     d. **Urinary tract obstruction**
     e. **Inguinal hernia**
     f. **Meckel diverticulum**
     g. **Cholecystitis**
     h. **Intra-abdominal tumors or masses**
  3. **Rare**
     a. **Henoch-Schönlein purpura**
     b. **Primary peritonitis** (nephrotic syndromes)
     c. **Pancreatitis**
     d. **Hepatitis**
     e. **Diabetic ketoacidosis**
     f. **Lead poisoning**
     g. **Acute porphyria**
     h. **Herpes zoster**
     i. **Sickle cell anemia**
     j. **Hemophilia** (retroperitoneal hematoma)

B. A **history** of the present illness can often be difficult to obtain from a child, and consequently the examiner must rely on the parents for accurate information. Several characteristics of the pain can be helpful in guiding the investigation of the symptom(s). Assess the quality of the pain, such as whether it is sharp or dull, episodic or constant. Determine the onset, location, duration, and presence of exacerbating or relieving factors for the pain. Associated symptoms, such as vomiting (bilious versus nonbilious), diarrhea, changes in bowel habits, hematemesis, melena, or hematochezia help to elucidate the cause of the abdominal pain.

C. The **physical examination** should be performed with the child in a comfortable position and with full access to his or her abdomen and groin. Early in the examination, it is imperative to determine whether the child has peritonitis. Palpation of the abdomen may reveal guarding or rebound tenderness when the peritoneum is involved in the disease process. Guarding is best assessed by palpating lateral to the rectus abdominis muscles bilaterally. In a child who does not relax for examination, percussion of the abdomen also should produce guarding and rebound tenderness if peritonitis is present. Tenderness usually is most impressive in the region of underlying pathology. Abdominal pain either on manipulation of the hip or with deep respiratory movements suggests peritoneal irritation. In addition, on rectal examination, movement of the peritoneal reflection causes severe pain if peritonitis is present. One technique for performing a rectal examination in a child includes positioning the patient supine with the knees and hips maximally flexed and the legs spread apart. Younger children may pose a challenge to the examiner who attempts to perform a rectal examination. In these cases, diverting the child's attention or examining the child while asleep or cuddling with the mother may facilitate the task. Whereas in adults auscultation of the abdomen is important, this technique is of limited value in infants and young children.

IX. Tumors and neoplasms

A. Neuroblastoma is a neoplasm of the sympathochromaffin system. It has an incidence of approximately eight new cases per million children per year. This tumor is the most common extracranial tumor of childhood and accounts for 10% of all pediatric malignancies. The median age at diagnosis is 2 years, with 85% of the tumors being diagnosed before age 5.

  1. Diagnosis of neuroblastoma usually is made during radiographic studies performed for other reasons or after the finding of an abdominal mass by the parents or pediatrician. Occasionally, children present with symptoms of fever, malaise, or abdominal pain. At the time of discovery, up to 75% of neuroblastomas are metastatic. The most common sites of spread are regional lymph nodes, liver, skin, and bone. Metastasis to the orbits may produce the raccoon's-eye appearance.

  2. Management of neuroblastoma includes initial staging of the disease because age and tumor stage at the time of diagnosis are the most significant predictors of outcome. Several staging systems are available; however, the proposed **International Neuroblastoma Staging System** incorporates clinical, radiographic, and surgical information to define tumor stage (Table 37-1). **Plain radiographs** of the chest and skull, along with a **bone scan** and **bone marrow aspirate**, should be performed. **Computed tomographic (CT)** scanning or **MR** scanning studies are useful in delineating tumor surrounding the spinal canal. Operative evaluation may also be necessary for accurate staging. Children younger than 12 months at the time of diagnosis have a better prognosis for cure, whereas in older patients with disseminated disease, the prognosis remains poor.

  3. Surgical treatment for local disease is complete excision of the tumor with lymph node sampling. A liver biopsy should also be performed if the tumor is intra-abdominal. When bulky or metastatic disease is present, a tumor biopsy is performed, followed by chemotherapy, radiotherapy, or both. N-*myc* amplification in the tumor is associated with a worse prognosis. A good response to chemotherapy is indicated by shrinkage of the tumor. Delayed resection then is undertaken.

B. Wilms tumor is the most common renal malignancy in children. The annual incidence is approximately 5.0 to 7.8 per million children younger than 15 years. It is bilateral in 5% of cases and accounts for 6% of all malignancies in children. The gender distribution is equal, and most Wilms tumors are diagnosed between 1 and 3 years of age.

Table 37-1. International Neuroblastoma Staging System

Stage	Characteristics
1	Localized tumor confined to the area of origin; complete gross excision with or without microscopic residual disease; identifiable ipsilateral and contralateral lymph nodes negative microscopically
2A	Unilateral tumor with incomplete gross excision; identifiable ipsilateral and contralateral lymph nodes negative microscopically
2B	Unilateral tumor with complete or incomplete gross excision; with positive ipsilateral regional lymph nodes; identifiable contralateral lymph nodes negative microscopically
3	Tumor infiltrating across the midline with or without regional lymph node involvement; or unilateral tumor with contralateral regional lymph node involvement; or midline tumor with bilateral tumor involvement
4	Dissemination of tumor to distant lymph nodes, bone, bone marrow, liver, or other organs (except as defined in stage 4S)
4S	Localized primary tumor as defined for stage 1 or 2 with dissemination limited to liver, skin, or bone marrow

1. **Diagnosis** of Wilms tumor is made from a combination of clinical, radiographic, and pathologic information. The **history** reveals abdominal pain in almost one-half of patients with Wilms tumor; one-fourth of patients have fever, hematuria, or a urinary tract infection.

   On **physical examination,** 85% of these children have a palpable flank or abdominal mass. Anomalies associated with Wilms tumor include hemihypertrophy (2%), aniridia (1%), and genitourinary anomalies (5%). **Abdominal ultrasonography** usually can distinguish an intrarenal mass, more consistent with Wilms tumor, from an extrarenal mass, more characteristic of a neuroblastoma. This test also is useful in ruling out tumor extension into the renal vein or vena cava. **Abdominal and chest CT scans** are necessary for staging, particularly to evaluate the contralateral kidney and to screen for pulmonary metastases. **Histological examination** of tissue obtained at surgery confirms the diagnosis.

2. **Management** of patients with a Wilms tumor combines surgery and chemotherapy, which together result in a better than 90% chance of cure. A radical nephrectomy with sampling of the para-aortic lymph nodes is performed through a transabdominal approach. Isolation of the hilar vessels and examination of the contralateral kidney also are required. If the Wilms tumor is found initially to be unresectable because of size or bilaterality, a second-look operation can be done after chemotherapy. Vincristine, doxorubicin, and dactinomycin are the most effective chemotherapeutic agents. Radiotherapy is used for advanced stages of Wilms tumor.

C. **Hepatic tumors** in children are malignant in 70% of cases, but they make up fewer than 5% of all intra-abdominal malignancies. **Hepatoblastoma** accounts for 39% of liver tumors. Ninety percent occur before the age of 3 years, and 60% are diagnosed by 1 year of age. **Hepatocellular carcinoma** usually presents in older children. Approximately one-third of these patients have cirrhosis secondary to an inherited metabolic abnormality.

   1. **Diagnosis** of a hepatic tumor often begins with a child who presents with an enlarging abdominal mass that may be painful. The mass is best imaged by a **CT** or **MR scan. Angiography** can be useful in distinguishing benign from malignant tumors. Most patients with hepatoblastoma have an **elevated serum AFP** levels; this is a useful parameter to monitor for recurrence after resection.

   2. **Management** of hepatic malignancies involves resecting the primary tumor. If the tumor is deemed unresectable at the initial operation,

however, chemotherapy is administered, followed by surgical reexploration at 4 months. Lymph node sampling and frozen-section analysis of the liver margins is necessary to confirm complete removal of the tumor. Survival is dismal for patients in whom the tumor cannot be completely resected.

  D. **Teratomas** are composed of tissues from all germ layers (endoderm, ectoderm, and mesoderm). In neonates, sacrococcygeal teratomas are the most common. These tumors are much more common in girls (4:1). A family history of twinning is observed in 10% of cases.

 1. **Diagnosis** is usually made on prenatal ultrasound. If the tumor is large, delivery by cesarean section may be needed. The tumor presents as a mass extending from the sacrum. **Ultrasound** of the tumor may show extension of the tumor into the pelvis and abdomen.

 2. **Management** includes elective resection through a chevron-shaped buttocks incision during the first week of life. Occasionally, arteriovenous shunting in the tumor produces a shocklike syndrome with metabolic acidosis. This situation requires emergency resection. Principles important in resection of the tumor include preservation of the rectal sphincter muscles, resection of the coccyx with the tumor, and early control of the midsacral vessels that supply the tumor. The latter helps to control hemorrhage, the most common complication of this operation. Failure to resect the coccyx results in a high recurrence rate. **Malignancy** is rarely seen in neonates but increases with the age of the child. If the tumor is malignant, a thorough search for metastases is in order, and combination chemotherapy is given, which may shrink the tumor and allow for resection.

  E. **Soft-tissue sarcomas** account for 6% of childhood malignancies, more than one-half of which are rhabdomyosarcomas.

 1. **Diagnosis** of a soft-tissue sarcoma is best accomplished with a multidisciplinary approach. The mass should be imaged by **CT scan** or **MR scan**. An **incisional biopsy** usually is required to determine the histologic type preoperatively. Consultation with a radiotherapist and oncologist before initiating therapy is advised.

 2. **Management** of nonrhabdomyosarcomas includes wide surgical excision. If the tumor is a rhabdomyosarcoma, however, treatment is determined by the location of the tumor. Complete resection of head and neck tumors is rarely possible, and they usually are treated with biopsy followed by chemotherapy. Trunk and retroperitoneal tumors are treated with wide excision whenever possible. Rhabdomyosarcomas of the extremity also are treated with wide excision, but resection of muscle groups and the use of radiotherapy or brachytherapy should also be considered (*Surg Clin North Am* 1992;72:1417). A biopsy of the regional lymph nodes should be included in the procedure.

X. **Minimal access surgery for children.** With the development of new instruments designed for pediatrics, laparoscopy is now safe and effective treatment for a wide variety of surgical diseases in children and infants. The instruments used in pediatric laparoscopy are predominantly 3 to 5 mm in diameter but may be as small as 1.7 mm. Endoscopic robotics will aid in broadening the applications of minimal access surgery. Presently robotics are being used at certain institutions for difficult minimal access anastomoses (such as for esophageal atresia).

  A. **General technique.** All patients should receive **general anesthesia.** The patient should be positioned according to the procedure to be performed. The **stomach and bladder** should be **decompressed** with an **orogastric tube** and **Foley catheter,** respectively. CO_2 insufflation should be performed with **warmed gas in small children or infants.** A pressure of 15 Torr is well tolerated in most patients, but infants with poor pulmonary function may encounter ventilatory compromise. A multitude of interventions can be performed with minimal access surgery, including interventions for general and thoracic surgical diseases treated by pediatric surgeons (see Section X.C.4). With present-day instrumentation, minimal access surgeons may perform biopsies, excise tissue, perform anastomoses, and suture.

B. Potential complications

1. **Injuries associated with port placement** include vascular injury, intestinal perforation, and solid organ injury.

2. **Herniation** may occur at port sites as small as 3 mm.

C. Common minimal access procedures in pediatric surgery

1. **Laparoscopic appendectomy.** The procedure may be performed in any patient with the presumptive diagnosis of appendicitis. It is particularly useful in patients with an atypical presentation where diagnostic tests are equivocal. The appendix and the mesoappendix may be amputated and ligated with the use of clips and endoscopic stapling instruments. The technical advantage of laparoscopic technique is that it provides access to a most of the abdominal cavity and pelvis. Other advantages include the shorter hospital stay and earlier return to normal activities that it makes possible.

2. **Laparoscopic antireflux procedures.** For the treatment of gastroesophageal reflux disease, Nissen fundoplication and alternate antireflux procedures may be performed with laparoscopic technique. Advanced laparoscopic skills are necessary for dissection and mobilization of the esophagus, mobilization and wrapping of the fundus of the stomach, and suturing of the fundus. The advantages of laparoscopic antireflux procedures are that it decreases the time to feeding, lowers the analgesic requirements, and shortens the length of hospitalization.

3. **Laparoscopic treatment of pyloric stenosis.** Pyloromyotomy may be performed laparoscopically through three 2-mm incisions. The advantages over open technique include that it allows earlier resumption of feeds and earlier discharge.

4. **Other minimal access procedures performed in children** include cholecystectomy, repair of diaphragmatic hernia, Ladd's procedure, small-bowel and colon resections, Kasai procedure, herniorrhaphy, undescended testes excision or orchiopexy, ventriculoperitoneal shunt placement/manipulation, patent ductus arteriosus ligation, resection of mediastinal mass, lobectomy, and ligation of tracheoesophageal fistula.

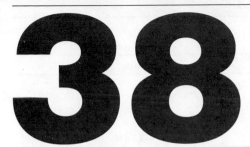

Neurosurgical Emergencies

Dennis J. Rivet and Michael R. Chicoine

Neurosurgical emergencies involve a broad spectrum of illness, including traumatic injury to the head and spine. Several nontraumatic settings also require emergent intervention, among these intracranial hemorrhage, elevated intracranial pressure (ICP), spinal cord compression, and infections. In many cases, rapid assessment and immediate neurosurgical consultation and intervention can prevent significant neurologic injury and can even be lifesaving.

NEUROSURGICAL TRAUMA

I. Intracranial trauma
- **A. Evaluation.** Initial management of head injury focuses on hemodynamic stabilization through establishment of an adequate airway, ventilation, and support of circulation, followed by rapid diagnosis and treatment of intracranial injuries.
  - **1. Airway and ventilation.** Severe head injury frequently leads to failure of oxygenation, ventilation, or airway protection; therefore, intubation in these cases is essential. A rapid neurologic assessment performed before sedation and paralysis are induced is critical. A low threshold for intubation must be present for agitated patients requiring sedation. Even with adequate oxygenation (e.g., by pulse oximetry), inadequate ventilation can occur.

    When possible, cervical spine films should be assessed before intubation. In situations of acute compromise, intubation should proceed even before complete evaluation of the cervical spine. Two-person in-line intubation is performed, with the second individual securing the patient's neck with axial traction to avoid extension of the neck during intubation. Nasal intubation can be performed if craniofacial injuries do not otherwise contraindicate this procedure. Associated cervical spine injuries should be assumed in the patient with a head injury until they are ruled out.
  - **2. Circulatory support** requires aggressive fluid resuscitation for treatment of arterial hypotension, followed by blood products, if necessary, and identification of the etiology of the hypotension. Head injury with intracranial hemorrhage is almost never the sole cause of systemic hypotension (in the absence of profuse scalp bleeding). When clinical signs of adequate oxygen perfusion are present, patients with head injuries should not be overresuscitated with fluids. Impairment in mental status cannot be adequately assessed until mean arterial pressure (MAP) and thus cerebral perfusion pressure (cerebral perfusion pressure = MAP – intracranial pressure) are corrected.
- **B. Neurologic evaluation**
  - **1. A rapid but systematic** neurologic examination is performed on the scene and is repeated frequently during transport and on initial presentation to the emergency room. Examination focuses on the three components of the **Glasgow Coma Scale** (GCS) (Table 38-1): eye opening, verbal response, and motor response (*Lancet* 1974;2:81). This score indicates injury severity and measures changes in the impairment of consciousness. Pupillary response, extraocular movements, facial movements should be

Table 38-1. Glasgow Coma Scale*

Components	Points
Eye opening	
Spontaneous	4
To voice	3
To stimulation	2
None	1
Motor response	
To command	6
Localizes	5
Withdraws	4
Abnormal flexion	3
Extension	2
None	1
Verbal response	
Oriented	5
Confused but comprehensible	4
Inappropriate or incoherent	3
Incomprehensible (no words)	2
None	1

*Glasgow Coma Score = best eye opening + best motor response + best verbal response. If patient is intubated, the verbal score is omitted and an addendum of "T" is given to the best eye opening + best motor response score.

examined, and the remainder of the cranial nerve examination should be performed. The **pupils** of a head-injured patient should never be pharmacologically dilated in the acute setting because changes in pupillary reaction can be early signs of herniation. Strength and symmetry of the extremities should be noted as part of the search for evidence of cerebral or spinal cord damage. The sensory examination should be performed as thoroughly as the level of consciousness permits. Useful landmarks for sensory dermatomes include the nipple (T4 level) and the umbilicus (T10 level). Reflexes and sphincter tone should also be assessed. Finally, the head-injured patient has a high incidence of associated injuries. Cervical spine evaluation is obligatory (see Sections IV.A.3 and IV.A.4). Thorough examination is essential, even in patients thought to have an isolated closed head injury. Unnecessary sedation and prolonged pharmacologic paralysis in head-injured patients can make neurologic assessment difficult and should be avoided.

2. **Systemic causes** of mental status impairment must be ruled out. Metabolic (electrolyte or acid-base abnormalities, hypo- and hyperglycemia), toxic (drugs, uremia), hypothermic, or respiratory (hypoxia, hypercapnia) derangements can underlie mental status changes, even if closed head injury is present. Recent seizures or cardiac arrest can also impair neurologic function severely. Corrective measures, such as dextrose for hypoglycemia, thiamine (100 mg intramuscularly) in the setting of alcohol abuse, naloxone for suspected opioid overdose, and oxygenation or ventilatory support, should be initiated as immediately indicated.

C. **Radiographic evaluation** begins with cervical spine plain x-rays, including anteroposterior, lateral, and open-mouth (odontoid) views. The initial emergency room evaluation should proceed rapidly to head computed tomographic (CT) scanning. Mass lesions are not diagnosed or excluded reliably by clinical examination. Delay caused by evaluation of non-life-threatening injuries should be avoided until the patient's head is imaged. Centers without this capability should stabilize the vital signs, secure the airway, and arrange for rapid transfer of the patient to a facility with head CT scanning and neurosurgical facilities.

D. **Initial therapies**
  1. **If elevated intracranial pressure (ICP)** is suspected, such as with signs of herniation or acute neurologic deterioration, therapy should be initiated until the ICP can be measured. **Mannitol** (0.25 to 1.0 g/kg intravenous bolus) is effective in controlling raised ICP acutely. A Foley catheter should be placed to follow the osmotic diuresis closely after mannitol administration. Fluid replacement may be necessary to avoid hypotension as a euvolemic, hyperosmolar situation is desirable. Systemic causes of neurologic deterioration must also be ruled out. Ventilatory support to maintain a mildly hypocapnic partial pressure of carbon dioxide (PCO_2; $\sim$35 mm Hg) should be instituted. For refractory elevated ICP, **hyperventilation** (PCO_2; $\sim$30 mm Hg) may be used only in the acute setting for **brief** periods. Prolonged use of hyperventilation should not be used to control elevated ICP and may worsen ischemia by compromising cerebral blood flow. No proven role for steroids in the management of acute head injury exists.
  2. **Seizures** should be controlled rapidly in patients with head injury. Intravenous lorazepam can be administered in 1-mg boluses and repeated until seizures are controlled. Airway protection must be available if significant doses of benzodiazepines are to be given. Phenytoin (Dilantin) should also be administered for seizures and is indicated for seizure prophylaxis in patients at high risk for early posttraumatic seizures (GCS = 10 or less, intracranial hematoma, depressed skull fracture, cortical contusion visible on CT, penetrating or open injuries) for a duration of no more than 7 days if the patient remains seizure free (*N Engl J Med* 1990;323:497). A loading dose of phenytoin or fosphenytoin (Cerebyx) in patients with poor intravenous access or status epilepticus may be given. With either phenytoin or fosphenytoin, the rate of intravenous infusion should be slow (no greater than 50 mg/minute for phenytoin) to avoid hypotension, and close monitoring of the ECG, blood pressure, and respiratory function should be performed during administration. Maintenance doses of phenytoin should then be started and drug levels followed to guide dosing.

II. **Types of head injury**
  A. **Focal (mass) lesions** are best diagnosed by emergent CT scan of the head without contrast. Hemiparesis, unilateral pupillary dysfunction (the fixed and dilated pupil), or both, can herald brainstem herniation from mass lesions, but these are imperfect localizing signs (*Neurosurgery* 1994;34:840); therefore, CT scan is imperative. Relative indications for surgical evacuation include neurologic symptoms referable to the mass lesion, midline shift >5 mm, and elevated ICP that is refractory to medical management. Posterior fossa mass lesions can be particularly dangerous because brainstem herniation may have very few specific warning signs before death occurs (see Section V.A.2.b).
    1. **Epidural and subdural hematomas (SDHs)** can cause rapid deterioration and usually require surgical evacuation. Classically, epidural hematomas present with a "lucid interval" after injury, which precedes rapid deterioration. This sign is inconsistent and nonspecific and may also be seen with SDHs. Epidural hematomas appear on head CT scan as biconvex hyperdensities that typically respect the suture lines, and they are operated on emergently if they are causing significant mass effect, symptoms, or both. A frequent association with simultaneous SDH exists.
    2. **Acute SDHs** typically appear on head CT scan as hyperdense crescents as the blood spreads around the surface of the brain. Often, SDHs are associated with severe intracranial injury. If surgical evacuation is indicated

and delayed for more than 4 hours, these lesions have a high mortality (*J Neurosurg* 1991;74:212; *N Engl J Med* 1981;304:1511).

3. **SDHs** also can present, especially in the elderly, days to weeks after head injury. These **chronic SDHs** can cause focal neurologic deficit, mental status changes, and seizures. A symptomatic chronic SDH large enough to be drained can be treated with burr-hole drainage or twist-drill craniostomy with subdural drain placement (*J Neurosurg* 1986;65:183). Prophylactic anticonvulsants are considered, and steroids may be beneficial. Diagnosis is best made with CT scan because MR scan can give an inconsistent picture of lesion size.

B. **Nonfocal** sequelae of head injury include **cerebral edema** and **diffuse axonal injury (DAI).** Hallmarks of cerebral edema on head CT scan include obliteration of the basal cisterns and coronal sulci and loss of differentiation of the gray and white matter. In DAI, severe head injury is associated with minimal changes on head CT scan (*J Neurosurg* 1982;56:26). DAI represents the pathologic result of shearing forces on the brain. Often, small hemorrhages are seen in corpus callosum, midbrain, deep white matter, or other deep cerebral structures. Microscopic injury to axons may result in severe neurologic dysfunction. Radiographic evidence of diffuse edema or a severely impaired neurologic condition may be an indication for monitoring and treatment of elevated ICP.

C. **Open injuries and fractures**
1. **Open skull fractures** require operative irrigation, débridement of nonviable tissues, and dural closure. Evaluation of scalp lacerations should include attention to the presence of underlying skull fractures. Prophylactic antibiotics may reduce the risk of infection. Surgical treatment of **depressed skull fractures** usually is required for depressions greater than the thickness of the skull table. Open, depressed skull fractures require elevation and débridement of depressed skull fragments as well as devitalized tissue, followed by a course of antibiotics. Fractures through the paranasal air **sinuses,** especially with associated pneumocephalus and dural tears, may require repair. Often, repair is performed in combination with repair of associated facial fractures. The prophylactic use of broad-spectrum antibiotics to prevent meningitis in these cases is controversial.

D. **Basilar skull fractures** can be complicated by **cerebrospinal fluid (CSF)** leaks, and are managed nonoperatively. The use of prophylactic antibiotics is controversial. If drainage continues or recurs, a lumbar drain or surgical repair may be required because persistent leakage can lead to meningitis. Temporal bone fractures can be associated with damage to the seventh and eighth cranial nerves, the middle ear apparatus, or both.

E. **Missile injuries** require débridement, closure, and prophylactic antibiotics similar to those used for other open head injuries. However, injuries from gunshot wounds present several associated problems. Shock waves can result in widespread destruction of brain tissue and vasculature. Operative management must address removal of accessible foreign bodies and bone fragments, evacuation of intracranial hematomas, débridement of entrance and exit wounds, and closure of dura and scalp. Overaggressive débridement near large vessels should be avoided to prevent further damage to vascular structures.

III. **Management of elevated ICP**
A. **Monitoring**
1. **Indications.** ICP monitoring generally is recommended in head injury if serial neurologic examinations cannot be used as a reliable indicator of progressive intracranial pathology. This usually corresponds to a GCS score of <9. Head CT scans demonstrating mass lesions, diffuse cerebral edema, or other pathology associated with elevated ICP are also indications for monitoring or for empiric treatment until monitoring is available.

2. **ICP pressure monitors** are of several types. The **parenchymal bolt** consists of a fiberoptic or strain gauge catheter tip that measures ICP at the brain surface. **Intraventricular catheters** (ventriculostomy) are placed in the lateral ventricle with the tip at the foramen of Monro. Additionally, intraventricular catheters allow for the drainage of CSF in the treatment of elevated ICP (see Section I.D.1). Other monitors include subdural catheters, usually placed intraoperatively.

B. **Treatment**

1. In addition to initial treatment of elevated ICP (e.g., mannitol, mechanical ventilation), **simple measures** are taken, such as head elevation to 30 degrees, a neutral head position to enhance venous drainage, avoidance of circumferential taping around the patient's neck when securing the endotracheal tube, appropriate fitting of cervical spine collars if indicated, and adequate sedation before any stimulation, such as intubation. Elevated intrathoracic pressures (as with coughing, straining, or high positive end-expiratory pressure) can elevate ICP. Fever can also exacerbate ICP, and aggressive treatment with antipyretics and cooling blankets should be instituted to prevent hyperthermia.

2. Further treatment is aimed at keeping ICP <20 mm Hg (*J Neurosurg* 1991;75:S59), usually with **osmotic and loop diuretics** (mannitol, 25- to 50-g intravenous boluses every 6 hours, or furosemide). Fluid balance, serum electrolytes, and serum osmolarity should be carefully monitored; euvolemia must be maintained. Diuretics generally are held if serum osmolarity exceeds 320 mOsm/L. In addition, hypotension should be avoided in these patients, and there are some data that suggest better outcomes occur with maintenance of cerebral perfusion pressure (MAP − ICP) of 70 mm Hg or greater (see Section III.C.1).

3. **Sedation** can also be used to control ICP. Benzodiazepine or narcotic (e.g., fentanyl) infusions can be given and titrated to effect, with a goal of Ramsay 3 (*Br Med J* 1974;11:659). Intubation and mechanical ventilation usually are needed. Refractory elevation of ICP may require neuromuscular paralysis or even barbiturate coma with invasive hemodynamic monitoring.

4. **Surgical interventions** are directed primarily at removal of **mass lesions,** if present. In the absence of a mass lesion, uncontrollable ICP and a deteriorating neurologic examination may require **craniectomy,** with removal of a large bone flap to relieve pressure on the intracranial contents (*Neurosurgery* 1991;29:62). Removal of CSF by **ventriculostomy** can reduce ICP; however, the small intracranial volume occupied by the CSF limits this effect.

C. **Frequently associated complications**

1. **Cardiac considerations.** Adequate blood pressure should be maintained in the setting of elevated ICP, with care taken to avoid hypotension (systolic blood pressure <90 mm Hg), which has been associated with worse outcome in severely head injured patients (*Br J Neurosurg* 1993;7:267). Maintenance of cerebral perfusion pressure >70 mm Hg (or MAP >90 mm Hg) can be used as a treatment guideline. Administration of isotonic crystalloid, colloid, and/or easily titratable vasopressors, such as phenylephrine or dobutamine, can be used to maintain an adequate perfusion pressure.

2. **Respiratory considerations.** Early airway control is essential in the head-injured patient. Severe head injury is also associated with ventilation-perfusion mismatch and development of pulmonary edema or adult respiratory distress syndrome. Delayed complications of pneumonia and pulmonary embolism are common, as are associated injuries, such as pneumothorax or pulmonary contusions.

3. **Gastrointestinal (GI) considerations.** Patients with severe head injury and increased ICP are at risk of developing Cushing (stress) ulcers and GI

bleeding. These patients should undergo prophylaxis with H_2 antagonists or sucralfate.

4. **Fluid and electrolytes.** Head-injured patients are at risk for development of either diabetes insipidus or the syndrome of inappropriate antidiuretic hormone. Initially, the use of isotonic saline (with glucose and, if necessary, potassium) avoids exacerbating cerebral edema. Close monitoring of electrolytes is essential because alterations in sodium and water balance are common. **Diabetes insipidus** can develop rapidly and must be treated aggressively. Fluid hydration should match output. Often, the process is self-limiting, but persistent output of large amounts (>300 mL per hour) of urine with a low specific gravity may necessitate vasopressin treatment [desmopressin (DDAVP), 1 μg intravenously every 12 hours]. If the syndrome of inappropriate antidiuretic hormone with hyponatremia develops, treatment with restriction of free water intake usually is sufficient, although infusion of hypertonic (1.5% NaCl) saline may be necessary. As mentioned previously, treatment with osmotic diuretics may require large-volume fluid replacement. In this case, electrolytes (including potassium, magnesium, and phosphorus) should be monitored closely.

5. **Hematologic considerations.** Disseminated intravascular coagulopathy can occur with severe head injury, such as missile injuries, often developing several hours after the disruption of brain tissue. Coagulopathies should be aggressively treated with fresh frozen plasma and vitamin K (10 mg per day intramuscularly), especially if intracranial hemorrhage is present.

6. **Nutrition.** Nutritional demands are increased in head injury (*Neurosurg Clin North Am* 1991;2:301). High-osmolarity tube feedings can reduce the risk of cerebral edema and provide adequate caloric intake. If tube feedings are not tolerated, parenteral nutrition may be necessary. Replacement of 140% of the expected resting metabolism expenditure in nonparalyzed patients and 100% of the expenditure in paralyzed patients by the 7th day after injury can be used as a guideline.

7. **Associated injuries.** A thorough assessment for other systemic and orthopedic injuries is essential. The unconscious patient should always be assumed to have a cervical spine injury until this is ruled out with appropriate radiographic tests.

8. **Mild head injury.** Management of the patient with a mild head injury (presenting GCS score of 13 to 15) focuses on detecting and rapidly treating those at risk for subsequent deterioration (*J Neurosurg* 1986;65:203). Selection of those at higher risk for delayed mass lesion, associated fracture, elevated ICP, and CSF leaks is needed. A normal CT scan without altered level of consciousness, neurologic deficit, or open injuries may allow the patient to be discharged to home with reliable supervision. Any exceptions may indicate a more severe injury with a higher risk of associated or delayed lesions and may require the patient to be admitted for observation.

IV. **Spinal trauma. Evaluation** for spinal injury is indicated if focal pain, neurologic examination, or mechanism of injury warrants. Neurologic deficit involving the lower extremities after trauma may require evaluation of the entire spine to find an injury.

A. **Initial support**
   1. **Airway and breathing.** Intubation should be performed early in patients demonstrating respiratory fatigue or otherwise requiring airway protection or ventilatory support. In the presence of cervical spine injury, fiberoptic intubation requires less manipulation and reduces the risk of further neurologic injury. When this is not available, two-person intubation with in-line stabilization of the neck can be performed safely.
   2. **Circulation.** Nonneurologic sources of hypotension must be pursued thoroughly. In patients with obvious external hemorrhage or suspected

hypovolemic shock, standard fluid resuscitation should be initiated. In the paraplegic or quadriplegic patient, if no blood loss is suspected and fluid challenges do not improve perfusion, diagnosis of **spinal shock** should be considered. Hypotension associated with the loss of sympathetic tone seen in some high thoracic and cervical spine injuries does not respond to fluids alone. Pressors (e.g., dopamine) reduce peripheral vasodilatation and improve cardiac output. Excessive fluid administration can worsen respiratory difficulty and spinal cord edema.
3. **Neurologic examination.** This includes a careful assessment of motor and sensory function and deep tendon reflexes. Multiple sensory modalities (light touch, pinprick, temperature sensation, and joint position sense) should be assessed, especially in the patient with an incomplete lesion. Deep tendon reflexes, sphincter tone, and cremasteric and bulbocavernosus reflexes should be documented. Incomplete lesions are common and, as with sacral sparing of sensory function, carry prognostic significance (*Neurosurgery* 1987;20:742).
4. **Radiographic evaluation**
   a. Standard radiographic evaluation of the cervical spine includes **anteroposterior, lateral, and open-mouth (odontoid)** views. A **swimmer's** view may be necessary to visualize C7 and the C7-T1 interspace, which is essential in complete evaluation of the cervical spine. CT scanning is necessary if adequate plain films cannot be obtained, although plain films remain the best means of surveying for fractures or subluxations that may suggest occult ligamentous instability. Anteroposterior and lateral views of the thoracic and lumbar spine are obtained as indicated. If a spinal fracture is found, the entire spine should be imaged with plain radiographs, owing to the high rate of coincident injuries (*J Spinal Disord* 1992;5:320).
   b. Other imaging modalities include **CT scans** to further evaluate known or suspected fractures. **MR scan** are sensitive for ligamentous injuries, intraspinal hemorrhage, and protruded intervertebral discs (*J Neurosurg* 1993;79:341), which can cause deficit with or without bony abnormalities seen on plain films. Damage to the vertebral artery can occur with cervical injuries, especially if fracture of the foramen transversarium occurs. CT angiography or conventional angiography usually is pursued if neurologic damage is referable to vertebral artery injury.
B. **Instability.** Spinal instability must be suspected until ruled out. Ligamentous injury can occur in the absence of fracture, and instability can occur with normal plain films. Severe pain or apprehension of neck movement also warrants careful assessment. In the minimally symptomatic, alert patient, cervical flexion-extension films can aid in the assessment of spinal stability. Flexion and extension must be done under the patient's own power, and motion should be stopped if pain or other symptoms arise.
C. **Treatment**
   1. **Steroids** have been reported to improve outcome from spinal cord injury if given within 8 hours (*N Engl J Med* 1990;322:1405). Patients seen between 3 to 8 hours after injury should be treated emergently with **methylprednisolone, 30 mg/kg intravenous bolus** over 15 minutes, followed 45 minutes later by a **5.4-mg/kg per hour intravenous infusion** continued over the next 48 hours (*JAMA* 1997;277:1597). If steroids are administered within 3 hours of injury, intravenous infusion is given for only 24 hours. If patients are seen more than 8 hours after injury, this protocol is not of proven benefit and is contraindicated. Steroids are also contraindicated in cases of spinal gunshot wounds (*Neurosurgery* 1997; 41:576).
   2. **Immobilization and reduction.** Suspected or known spine injuries require immobilization, initially with a rigid cervical collar and long backboard. Cervical spine subluxations and dislocations must be reduced under

neurosurgical supervision. Fractures may be treated by external immobilization (e.g., halo external fixation) or by operative fusion, depending on the nature of the fracture and degree of instability.

Thoracic and lumbar spine fractures are managed with operative stabilization or immobilization with an orthosis. Injuries with associated neurologic deficit, with excessive displacement or angulation of the spinal column, or with loss of vertebral body height are more likely to require operative stabilization. Before stabilization, patients are managed with bedrest with frequent logrolling. Although early surgical decompression and stabilization promote mobilization of the patient, the timing of surgery and the role of emergency surgery in the patient with acute neurologic deficit remain somewhat controversial (*Neurosurgery* 1994; 35:240).

3. **Cervical spine injuries are associated** with the development of adult respiratory distress syndrome, hyponatremia, hypotension, bradyarrhythmias, ileus, and urinary retention. Patients with cervical spine injuries may require cardiorespiratory monitoring, isotonic fluid support, nasogastric decompression, urinary catheter placement, laxatives, and stool softeners to address these issues. Bladder and bowel dysfunctions also are seen with lower spine injuries, although autonomic problems are rare in injuries below the upper thoracic spine.

4. **Penetrating injuries** to the neck and torso may result in fractures of the spine or penetration of the spinal canal, along with other injuries.

V. Other emergencies

A. Nontraumatic intracranial hypertension and herniation syndromes

1. **Etiology.** Elevation of the ICP may lead to compression of neurologic structures and irreversible neurologic damage. Nontraumatic causes include hemorrhagic and nonhemorrhagic mass lesions.

   a. Spontaneous **intraparenchymal hemorrhages** may occur owing to hypertension, vascular malformations (arteriovenous malformations or aneurysms), tumor, angiopathy, vasculitis, or secondary hemorrhage into a large infarction.

   b. **Nonhemorrhagic lesions** include tumor, infection, and mass effect from edema after cerebral infarction.

2. Clinical **herniation syndromes** exist with presentations referable to the location of the lesion.

   a. **Supratentorial** sites of herniation include uncal, central transtentorial, and subfalcine herniation. Progressive lethargy, unilateral pupillary dysfunction, and/or hemiparesis suggest uncal herniation. Compression of vascular and brain structures requires immediate intervention. **Uncal** herniation often is the result of temporal lobe lesions. **Central transtentorial** herniation results from downward compression of brainstem structures. Unresponsiveness, deep coma, and cranial nerve dysfunction are observed. Central transtentorial herniation suggests a bilateral process or an interhemispheric lesion. **Subfalcine** herniation results from lesions causing a shift across the inferior aspect of the falx and can present with only lethargy or lower-extremity weakness. Both falcine and uncal herniation can progress to a central transtentorial picture as further structures are compressed.

   b. **Infratentorial** herniation results from posterior fossa masses compressing the brainstem or from herniation of the cerebellar tonsils through the foramen magnum. Signs of infratentorial herniation include lower cranial nerve dysfunction and the rapid onset of respiratory or cardiac arrest with little warning.

3. **Treatment** of herniation requires control of the ICP. The obtunded patient must have his or her airway controlled. Mannitol can be used, often with ICP monitoring (see Section III.A) to guide medical treatment. Mass lesions may need to be evacuated. The underlying cause of a hemorrhagic lesion should be determined if time permits.

B. Nonhemorrhagic lesions. Diffuse cerebral edema also can produce ICP elevations that require treatment. **Metabolic derangements,** such as those seen in hepatic encephalopathy, can elevate the ICP.

Edema can also develop secondary to large **infarctions** in the cerebral hemispheres, leading to delayed deterioration. Management of elevated ICP may be indicated in large cerebral infarctions, whether hemorrhagic or nonhemorrhagic.

1. **Brain tumors** rarely are surgical emergencies. Presenting symptoms include progressive headache, seizures, and localizing neurologic deficit. Uncommonly, acute neurologic deterioration is seen, usually suggestive of hemorrhage into the tumor. Evaluation and treatment are similar to those for any other acute intracranial mass lesion. High-dose **steroids** may have a potent effect on the brain edema associated with tumors. Urgent **surgical evacuation** of the mass lesion occasionally is required.
2. **Hydrocephalus** may result from a variety of causes and can lead to rapid neurologic deterioration.
   a. **Cerebellar tumors** or other mass lesions may cause fourth ventricle obstruction without preceding symptoms. Tuberculosis and bacterial meningitis also can cause hydrocephalus. Patients classically present with lethargy, headache, papilledema, sixth nerve palsy, or abnormalities of upward gaze ("setting-sun" sign). **Treatment** involves urgent placement of a catheter for external **ventricular drainage** (see Section III.A.2) to relieve the buildup of CSF.
   b. **Shunt malfunction.** Internal ventricular drainage systems (shunts) require special attention. Malfunction can present with warning symptoms, such as headache or nausea, or with rapid deterioration of mental status. Imaging, such as an emergency CT scan, can help in the diagnosis, but emergent operative revision may be indicated if mental status deterioration is present and shunt malfunction is suspected. A shunt series (plain films of the head, neck, chest, and abdomen) can visualize the entire course of the shunt and its connections, possibly leading to identification of a malfunction.

C. Intracranial hemorrhage. Spontaneous intracranial hemorrhage requires emergent intervention, and the sequelae of the associated mass effect also need to be addressed.

1. **Subarachnoid hemorrhage (SAH)** secondary to aneurysmal hemorrhage is a common neurosurgical emergency.
   a. The clinical **presentation** usually includes a history of severe sudden headache, nuchal rigidity, photophobia, lethargy, agitation, or a comatose state. Acute blood from an SAH appears bright on CT scan. Blood usually is seen in the cisterns or sylvian fissure. Lumbar puncture can make the diagnosis if the history is suggestive, even with a normal CT scan, but is not required when the scan is diagnostic. The principal goal of treatment is the prevention of rebleeding by surgical clipping or endovascular techniques. Without treatment, rebleeding occurs in 50% of patients with a ruptured aneurysm in the first 6 months (*J Neurosurg* 1985;62:321).
2. **Spontaneous intraventricular hemorrhage** may result from vascular malformations, hypertensive hemorrhage, or extension of intraparenchymal hemorrhage. Angiography can be used in determining the etiology. Patients are observed for the development of hydrocephalus, which requires external CSF drainage (ventriculostomy).
3. **Pituitary apoplexy** occurs after hemorrhage into the pituitary gland, usually related to an underlying pituitary adenoma. Patients typically present with acute headache and visual symptoms, such as decreased acuity, visual field cut, ptosis, or diplopia, which result from compression of nearby cranial nerves. Life-threatening panhypopituitarism can occur. Treatment involves hormonal replacement, correction of any electrolyte abnormalities, and emergent CT or MR scan to evaluate for

hemorrhagic pituitary lesions. Emergent evacuation of hematoma may preserve vision.

D. Infections

1. **Cerebral abscesses** can result from hematogenous or local traumatic spread of a septic process. Infections may also involve the epidural or subdural spaces. Underlying abnormalities are common, such as an immunocompromised state or systemic arteriovenous shunting. Presenting symptoms include those of increased ICP, focal deficits, and seizures. A head CT scan with intravenous contrast shows an enhancing lesion. Early-stage cerebral abscess may respond to medical management alone. Abscesses larger than 3 cm, failure of medical management, and need for tissue diagnosis are common indications for surgical drainage by open craniotomy or stereotactic drainage. Prolonged intravenous antibiotics are indicated.

2. **Spinal epidural abscesses** can become a surgical emergency. Severe neck or back pain in the setting of fever should raise concern. Although neurologic deficit may not occur initially, often progressive evidence of cord compression exists. MR scan or myelography demonstrates the lesion. Surgical evacuation is most often necessary, although antibiotics alone can be attempted if neither neurologic compromise nor a large collection is present. Even with surgical drainage, an extended course of antibiotics is required. Disc space infection and spinal osteomyelitis can occur in association with or separately from spinal epidural abscesses. Antibiotic therapy usually is effective. An elevated erythrocyte sedimentation rate generally is present and falls with effective treatment.

E. Spinal cord compression

1. **Diagnosis.** Nontraumatic spinal cord compression can result from metastatic tumor or another adjacent mass lesion. Patients present initially with pain, followed by progressive or sudden neurologic symptoms. Lung, breast, and prostate are the most common sources of metastases (*Neurosurgery* 1987;21:676). Examination usually reveals weakness, long-tract signs (spasticity, hyperactive reflexes, upgoing toes), or sphincter dysfunction. It is important to distinguish myelopathy from radiculopathy. The latter presents with pain, sensory changes, and weakness in a dermatomal pattern. Emergent MR scan or myelography to demonstrate the presence and level of the lesion confirms diagnosis of cord compression. Imaging should extend to higher spinal levels if no lesion is found because, for example, a cervical lesion can present with only lower-extremity symptoms; alternatively, multilevel involvement can be present.

2. **Treatment** begins with **steroids** (dexamethasone, 10 mg intravenously, followed by 4 to 10 mg orally or intravenously every 6 hours; higher doses frequently are given for severe deficits); these are administered immediately if spinal cord compression is suspected. The neurosurgical priorities include **decompression** if a deficit is present and spinal **stabilization and fusion** if bony destruction is prominent (*Neurosurgery* 1985;17:424). Emergent **radiation therapy** to the area of compression may be preferable to surgical intervention in some cases.

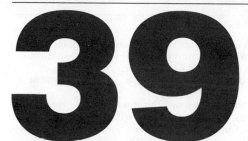

Orthopedic Injuries

J. R. Rudzki and
Joseph Borrelli, Jr.

TREATMENT OF ORTHOPEDIC INJURIES

I. **Initial assessment**
   A. **Priorities of management. ABCs** (airway, breathing, and circulation) take precedence over extremity injuries, but multisystem-injured patients benefit from aggressive treatment of extremity and pelvic trauma.
   B. **History.** Understanding the mechanism of injury, along with details of the accident, helps to direct assessment and management of patients with musculoskeletal injuries. Knowledge of patient age, associated medical conditions, and preinjury functional status are important.
   C. **Examination**
      1. **Remove all of the patient's clothing.** Observe the extremities for deformity and asymmetry. **Palpate** all extremities, noting tenderness, crepitus, deformity, or instability. Assess joint **range of motion.** In suspected cervical spine injury, maintain immobilization in a cervical collar until radiographs are obtained and the patient is able to comply with a physical examination. Logroll the patient to examine the back.
      2. **Assess vascular status** by checking pulses, body temperature, and color, with comparison to the opposite side. **Note:** normal pulses do not rule out compartment syndrome.
      3. **Sensorimotor evaluation.** Little value exists in grading muscle strength in the acute setting, except for spinal cord injury in which the neurologic status is evolving. If an abnormality is detected, a more detailed examination is needed. Sensory examination should be performed with light touch and pinprick, along with two-point discrimination in upper-extremity or cervical spine trauma.
      4. **Associated injuries.** Relate the location of the trauma to structures present at that level. If the patient is unconscious, spinal and pelvic injuries must be ruled out.
II. **Radiologic examination.** All trauma patients and unconscious patients must have screening chest, pelvis, and cervical spine radiographs. The lateral cervical spine radiograph must include all cervical vertebrae down through the C7-T1 junction. Assessment of extremity fractures and dislocations should include two views, 90 degrees to each other, of the affected area and should include the joints above and below the injured area. Dislocations of the knee and any other joint (e.g., ankle) that involve neurovascular or soft-tissue compromise should be reduced as soon as possible.
III. **Fractures and dislocations**
   A. **Terminology and classification**
      1. **Anatomic location** refers usually to the proximal, middle, or distal portion of the bone. *Epiphyseal, metaphyseal,* and *diaphyseal* as well as *head, base,* and *shaft* are also acceptable descriptive terms. **A fracture is considered to be transverse when it is oriented** perpendicular to the long axis of the bone and **oblique** if angled 45 to 60 degrees to the bone. **Spiral** fractures are intuitively spiral in appearance and caused by a torsional mechanism. **Comminuted** injuries have more than two fragments.
      2. **Alignment** refers to the amount of angulation between the proximal (closest to the trunk) fragment and distal (closest to the end of the extremity)

fragment. **Apposition** denotes the amount of cortical contact between fragments. **Displacement** denotes the distance between cortical surfaces. Intra-articular fractures involve the joint surface.
3. **Stable** fractures do not displace after reduction, whereas **unstable** injuries do displace.
4. **Soft-tissue injury. Closed** fractures are those with the overlying skin intact. **Open (compound)** fractures are those with a disruption of the overlying skin so that the fracture communicates with the external environment. **Complicated** fractures are those with associated neurovascular, ligamentous, or muscular injury.
5. **Subluxation** refers to joint disruption, with partial contact between joint surfaces. **Dislocation** refers to complete loss of contact between joint surfaces. Both are described by the position of the distal bone in relation to its proximal articulation.
B. **General management principles**
   1. **Dislocation**
      a. All dislocated joints, especially in the setting of **neurovascular compromise,** should be reduced in the emergency room if adequate and safe anesthesia can be administered (see Section VI. B). Successful reduction reduces the risk of soft-tissue (e.g., pressure necrosis) and neurovascular compromise.
      b. **Hip and knee** dislocations require immediate reduction in an attempt to avoid secondary complications, including avascular necrosis (hip) and neurovascular compromise (knee). Postreduction angiography is performed after knee dislocations when pulses are asymmetric before or after reduction, or both. Serial physical examinations are critical. **Note:** the incidence of concomitant vascular injury with knee dislocation is ~ 30%, and pedal pulse examination has a low sensitivity (79%) for detecting a significant vascular injury.
      c. **Wrist, ankle, and foot** dislocations often are associated with a fracture, thus creating an unstable joint. In this setting, reduction may not be maintained in a splint or cast, necessitating definitive surgical intervention.
   2. **Fracture** is diagnosed by history of the injury and symptoms of pain, loss of motion, and swelling. Physical examination findings include crepitus, tenderness, swelling, and/or deformity. Because any of these signs may be absent, a high index of suspicion is needed. Confirmation of fracture is obtained via radiographs.
      a. **Treatment** is directed toward reduction, if indicated, and immobilization. Uncontrolled movement is avoided to prevent further injury. In open fractures, the wound is irrigated thoroughly and covered with a sterile dressing soaked with normal saline (see Section IV.C.). Direct pressure over pulsatile bleeding or clamping of obvious bleeding vessels is usually effective. Tourniquets may be utilized in extreme cases of near or complete traumatic amputation. Gentle realignment of the limb before radiographic assessment is beneficial and mandatory when the overlying skin or distal blood flow is compromised.
         (1) **Stable fractures** do not displace without additional trauma but are immobilized to decrease pain and allow healing.
         (2) **Unstable fractures** require immobilization and, often, surgical stabilization. Intra-articular fractures with more than 2 mm of articular displacement are treated similarly. **Closed reduction** is performed as described in Section VI.C. In the case of skin, soft-tissue, or neurovascular compromise, immediate reduction to improve alignment is performed. Reduction may not be attainable because of the fracture pattern or soft-tissue interposition. In these cases, the fracture may be immobilized in the best attainable position

until early surgical stabilization, especially when neurovascular, soft-tissue, or skin compromise is present.
b. **Open fractures** (see Section IV.D).
c. **Pediatric musculoskeletal fractures**
(1) **Younger patients have a greater potential for bony remodeling,** and therefore a greater amount of angulation is acceptable. However, limited reduction of deformity may be beneficial to decrease the risk of permanent deformity.
(2) **Physeal plate injuries** are common because this is the weakest part of the bone. The physeal plate is the cartilage region responsible for longitudinal growth. The Salter-Harris classification categorizes these fractures into five types. Type I injuries involve a fracture through the growth plate without any bony involvement. Type II injury occurs when disruption of the growth plate is associated with a metaphyseal fracture. Type III involves growth-plate disruption and an epiphyseal fracture. Fracture through the metaphysis and across the growth plate and epiphysis define a type IV injury. Type V occurs with a crush injury to the growth plate.
(3) **Only qualified personnel should perform reductions,** unless skin or neurovascular compromise mandates immediate improvement of position. Adequate immobilization of the injured area and the joints above and below is necessary.
d. **Hazards in fracture management.** Observe patients closely for possible compartment syndrome, especially in leg and forearm injuries. Neurovascular compromise after plaster immobilization usually is secondary to swelling, and splints and bandages should be loosened to accommodate anticipated swelling. Circumferential casting in the acute setting should generally be avoided. If the patient is to return home, he or she should be instructed on the warning signs of early compartment syndrome and told to return to the hospital immediately if these symptoms develop (see Section IV.C).
C. **Upper extremity**
1. **Clavicle.** Injury usually occurs after a fall on an outstretched hand or shoulder and, less commonly, secondary to a direct blow. Deformity may be clinically apparent, and pain occurs with motion. Close attention to neurovascular status is needed because subclavian structures may be damaged. These fractures may be treated with a sling to counter the weight of the arm or a figure-of-eight splint. Most clavicle fractures heal with nonoperative treatment.
2. **Sternoclavicular joint.** Injury ranges from simple sprains to subluxations and dislocations. Computed tomographic (CT) scan is often necessary to determine the direction of dislocation. Anterior dislocations are treated with a sling or shoulder immobilizer if the skin is not compromised. Posterior dislocations can compress the mediastinal structures, causing hoarseness, dyspnea, dysphagia, and engorged neck veins, and they require emergent reduction. To facilitate reduction, a rolled towel is placed between the scapulae, posterior pressure is applied to both shoulders, and the clavicle is pulled from the retrosternal area. A towel clip can be used to grasp the proximal clavicle to facilitate reduction under general anesthesia. This should be performed with a general or thoracic surgeon available in case of injury to the lung or great vessels. A figure-of-eight bandage or sling is subsequently applied.
3. **Acromioclavicular joint.** Injury occurs after a direct blow to the acromion or a fall on the extremity, with injury ranging from sprain to complete dislocation. Pain, swelling, tenderness to palpation, and limited motion are present. Stress views are obtained with 5 to 10 lb of weight tied to each hand. Sprains and subluxations are treated with a sling and early motion, but dislocations may require reduction and fixation, especially if the skin is compromised.

4. Shoulder
a. Dislocations. Anterior dislocations (most common) occur after forced abduction or external rotation (or both). Posterior dislocations result from a direct blow or seizure and often are missed on initial examination. Inferior dislocations occur after hyperabduction injuries. Pain with motion and shoulder asymmetry are present, with the humeral head often palpable anteriorly, posteriorly, or inferiorly. Neurovascular status, especially deltoid function and sensation about the lateral proximal arm to assess axillary nerve function, must be adequately documented before reduction. Anteroposterior, scapular lateral, and axillary radiographs are needed to look for humeral head defects and associated fractures. Reduction is performed as described in Section VI.C. Reduction is confirmed with radiographs, and neurovascular status is documented. A sling or shoulder immobilizer is applied, and motion is initiated early (3 to 5 days). Anterior dislocations are stable in internal rotation, whereas posterior dislocations are stable in external rotation and may require prolonged immobilization. Dislocations in older patients are associated with acute tears of the rotator cuff, causing weakness or pain with abduction and rotation. The redislocation rate is inversely proportional to the patient's age.
b. Soft-tissue injury (see Section V).
5. Humerus
a. Proximal fractures commonly occur in older patients after a fall on the extremity. Examination reveals swelling, tenderness, pain with motion, and ecchymosis of the shoulder and lateral chest wall. When the fracture is nondisplaced, treatment involves a sling and early circumduction exercises. Displaced fractures require reduction and can be associated with neurovascular injury. Fracture-dislocations of the glenohumeral joint are often irreducible by closed means, requiring emergent surgical intervention. Attempts at closed reduction can result in further displacement and neurovascular injury.
b. Diaphyseal fractures usually are in the middle third of the humerus. Neurovascular status is checked closely. The radial nerve is especially vulnerable and should be evaluated by checking for active wrist and thumb extension and intact sensation in the dorsal first web space. Transverse fractures of the middle third are most commonly associated with radial neuropraxia, whereas spiral fractures of the distal third present a higher risk of laceration or entrapment of the radial nerve. Treatment involves immobilization in a coaptation splint or hanging arm cast and eventual stabilization in a fracture brace. In the acute setting, operative fixation is indicated in cases of polytrauma, inadequate closed reduction, radial nerve palsy after reduction, open fracture, segmental fracture, bilateral humerus fracture, and ipsilateral forearm fracture.
c. Distal (supracondylar) fractures are most common in children and older individuals and occur after a fall on the elbow. Careful examination for neurovascular compromise should be performed because these injuries may constitute a surgical emergency. In adults, closed reduction and repositioning in the emergency room are performed to improve or protect neurovascular status. Definitive treatment in the operating room is required for displaced fractures in children and comminuted fractures with intra-articular extension in adults.
6. Elbow
a. Olecranon fractures are usually evident by lack of active elbow extension and by a palpable defect, if displaced. Nondisplaced fractures are treated with a posterior splint and with the elbow flexed to 90 degrees, and displaced fractures are reduced and stabilized surgically.
b. Elbow dislocations usually occur posteriorly, after a fall on an outstretched arm, but can also occur anteriorly, medially, or laterally.

Examination reveals asymmetry, and neurovascular status should be checked closely. Radiographs confirm the diagnosis and reveal the direction and any associated fracture. Treatment involves immediate reduction (see Section VI.C). After reduction, the elbow is assessed for stability, and neurovascular status is documented. The joint is splinted in a stable position. When immobilized, the elbow has the propensity to become stiff, and thus for stable reductions, early motion exercises are mandatory.

7. Forearm

    a. Radial head fractures commonly occur after a fall on an outstretched hand; the patient presents with tenderness over the proximal radius and pain with forearm rotation. Elbow motion should then be documented. Motion block, articular fractures involving more than 25% to 30% of the joint surface, and fractures with severe comminution or displacement require surgical intervention. Otherwise, treatment involves sling immobilization for 3 to 5 days and early motion exercises.

    b. Fracture of the proximal ulna can be associated with dislocation of the radial head (Monteggia fracture). This fracture commonly occurs in children, and closed reduction and splinting usually are successful. When reduction is unsuccessful or when Monteggia fracture occurs in adults, it is treated operatively, with open reduction and internal fixation of the ulna.

    c. Diaphyseal (radial and ulnar) fractures may be associated with compartment syndrome, and careful examination is needed (see Section IV.C). In children, closed reduction and casting usually are effective, but in adults, open reduction and surgical fixation are required. For either group, nondisplaced fractures are placed in a posterior long-arm splint. Fractures of the distal half of the radius can be associated with disruption of the distal radioulnar joint (Galeazzi fracture). If the distal radioulnar joint cannot be reduced or if the reduction is unstable, open reduction and internal fixation is indicated.

    d. Distal fractures occur usually after a fall on an outstretched hand. Volar or dorsal displacement of the distal fragment may occur. These fractures can be severely comminuted or have intra-articular extension. Children should be assessed for possible physeal involvement. Closed reduction and splinting above the elbow are indicated. Operative reduction and fixation are necessary in cases of unstable fractures, inadequate closed reduction, or displaced intra-articular fragments.

8. Wrist fractures

    a. Scaphoid fractures present with painful wrist motion and anatomic "snuffbox" tenderness. Even if a fracture is not evident on x-ray, a thumb spica splint is applied until repeat radiographic examination is performed. Nondisplaced fractures are treated similarly. Fractures with >1 mm of displacement require surgical intervention.

    b. Lunate and perilunate injuries usually occur after wrist hyperextension and present with pain, tenderness, limitation of motion, and possible fullness on the volar wrist. Median neuropathy may also be present. Reduction is performed by applying longitudinal traction, hyperextending the wrist, and then applying pressure over the lunate. Surgical stabilization is often needed to maintain reduction and reestablish normal ligamentous anatomy.

    c. Carpometacarpal dislocations are rare and are difficult to diagnose clinically because of considerable swelling. Radiographic evaluation usually is diagnostic. Closed or open reduction, if needed, and splinting are performed to prevent further injury or displacement.

9. Hand. Although the position of immobilization ultimately depends on the particular injury treated, the "safe position" can always be used (see Section VI.A.2.d).

a. **Extra-articular fractures** are treated with reduction, if needed, and immobilization in a splint. Radial or ulnar gutter or thumb spica splints are used for metacarpal fractures, depending on their location. Prefabricated aluminum splint material usually is adequate for phalangeal fractures. Intra-articular and unstable fractures often require surgical intervention.

b. **Dislocations** are treated with closed reduction and immobilization. Dorsal metacarpophalangeal joint dislocations irreducible by closed technique require immediate open reduction in the operating room. Fracture dislocations can occur at any joint, especially the base of the first or fifth metacarpal. These injuries are often unstable and treated surgically.

c. **Fingertip injuries.** Painful **subungual hematomas** are decompressed by burning a hole in the nail with a hand-held portable electrocautery or by penetrating the nail with a large-bore needle after a digital block. When concurrent fracture of the distal phalanx is present, nail plate removal and nail bed repair may be needed. Small areas of skin loss require dressing changes and possible skin graft. Larger, full-thickness loss without nail involvement may require a graft or local coverage. **Amputations** through bone are treated with skeletal shortening and closure.

D. **Pelvic fractures**

1. **History.** Pelvic fractures are typically high-energy injuries and are a common cause of death when associated with significant soft-tissue injury and bleeding. With patients in hypovolemic shock, it is often difficult to distinguish intra-abdominal bleeding from pelvic hemorrhage. Pelvic bleeding may result in a loss of 2 to 3 L of blood or more, and replacement must be handled aggressively.

2. **Examination**

a. **A high index of suspicion is needed,** especially when tenderness, crepitus, or instability with compression or distraction of the iliac wings is present. A screening anteroposterior pelvic radiograph is essential in the initial examination. Minimizing manipulation of the pelvis when radiographs demonstrate significant fracture or dislocation decreases the risk of bleeding, dislodging clots, or causing further soft-tissue damage.

b. **Pelvic and rectal examinations** are performed to check for blood, masses, a high-riding prostate, and open communication with fracture. Open pelvic fractures are associated with a high morbidity and mortality. Although placement of an indwelling urinary catheter helps monitor volume status, genitourinary tract injury is common and suspected when blood is present at the urethral meatus, when a high-riding prostate is found, or when pubic symphysis diastasis is present. In these cases, a retrograde urethrogram and cystogram should be performed before placing a Foley catheter. Once stabilized, the patient should undergo further x-rays, including **pelvic inlet and outlet views,** to better assess the pelvic injury. CT is extremely helpful in assessing sacroiliac joint and sacral injuries.

3. **Treatment**

a. **Maintenance of blood volume, fracture fragment reduction, and immobilization** are essential first steps to decrease further hemorrhage. If the patient is hemodynamically stable, surgical intervention can be performed electively to allow complete assessment of associated injuries and resuscitation of the patient. If, however, the patient is hemodynamically unstable after fluid resuscitation and has an unstable pelvic injury, he or she should undergo temporary reduction of the pelvis (i.e., tying a sheet around the pelvis, laying the patient on his or her side, or applying a pelvic C-clamp) to reduce pelvic volume until an anterior pelvic external fixation can be applied. An intra-abdominal source of bleeding must then be ruled out before pelvic angiography and embolization are performed.

   b. Fractures not involving weightbearing regions (i.e., pubic rami) or without associated pelvic ring disruption are treated symptomatically, with increased weightbearing as pain resolves. Pelvic ring disruptions or fractures involving weightbearing areas require restricted weightbearing, traction, and, possibly, surgical intervention.

E. Lower-extremity fractures and dislocations
   1. Hip dislocation
      a. Hip dislocation usually occurs secondary to severe trauma in association with considerable soft-tissue damage. Examination reveals pain with attempted range of motion. Anterior dislocations occur with forced abduction, leaving the extremity abducted, externally rotated, and flexed. Posterior dislocations occur when a force is applied to a flexed knee, such as occurs with striking the dashboard, leaving the extremity internally rotated, shortened, and adducted. Dislocations may be associated with a fracture of the femoral head or acetabulum. Central fracture-dislocation results from a blow to the greater trochanter, by which the extremity is shortened. In all cases, radiographs are essential to confirm the direction of dislocation and assess for associated femoral or acetabular fracture.
      b. Treatment. Immediate closed reduction, and open reduction if necessary, is performed after careful assessment and documentation of the patient's neurovascular status (see Section VI.C). Skeletal traction through the distal femur should then be applied when femoral head or acetabular fractures are identified. Postreduction x-rays (including anteroposterior and Judet views) are mandatory to assess joint congruity and rule out the presence of intra-articular fragments. CT scans are obtained to determine the presence of incarcerated fragments and to assess femoral head fractures or acetabular fractures, particularly when incongruence is noted on radiographs.
      c. Complications. Hip dislocations are associated with neurovascular compromise (peroneal division of the sciatic nerve), avascular necrosis, and posttraumatic osteoarthritis. Immediate congruent reduction is imperative.
   2. Femur
      a. Femoral neck fractures usually occur after low-energy injuries, such as a stumble or fall in older patients, but are generally the result of high-energy injuries in younger individuals. A high index of suspicion is needed because patients often present with minimal groin or medial knee pain. If routine radiographs do not reveal any abnormality in the older patient, MR or bone scan may be needed. Displaced fractures cause shortening and external rotation of the extremity. In younger patients, stress fractures and nondisplaced fractures are treated with nonweightbearing ambulation and, possibly, surgical stabilization. Displaced fractures require immediate anatomic reduction and internal fixation to minimize the risk of avascular necrosis. Older patients generally require surgical intervention, with reduction and percutaneous screw fixation for nondisplaced fractures and hemireplacement for displaced fractures.
      b. Peritrochanteric fractures. Older patients usually present after a fall or a direct blow to the hip. The extremity is shortened and externally rotated, and there is pain on attempted motion. Treatment consists of gentle skin traction to decrease pain until surgery is performed. Younger patients sustain subtrochanteric fractures secondary to direct high-energy trauma. Surgical stabilization is needed. The patient is maintained in skeletal traction until operation, with careful monitoring of hemodynamic status and the limb's neurovascular status.

Methods of stabilization include plate and screw fixation and use of a reconstruction intramedullary nail.

c. **Femoral shaft fractures** occur with significant trauma and are associated with considerable bleeding, soft-tissue damage, and other extremity injuries. The injury is obvious, but adequate examination of the remainder of the extremity is necessary. Ipsilateral injuries of the hip and knee are common. x-ray evaluation must include the hip and knee joint to detect the presence of other fractures. Hare traction splints should be removed promptly after orthopedic evaluation in the emergency room, and skeletal traction or surgical stabilization are needed for further management. The gold standard of treatment is an antegrade, reamed, statically locked intramedullary nail. **Note:** a high index of suspicion for ipsilateral femoral neck fractures is critical.

d. **Supracondylar femur fractures.** Careful assessment of neurovascular status is essential. Nondisplaced fractures can be treated with splint and cast immobilization, but displaced fractures are typically treated with surgical intervention.

3. **Knee**

a. **Patellar fracture or dislocation.** Nondisplaced fractures in association with an intact extensor mechanism are treated with an immobilizer or a cylinder cast. Displaced fractures require surgical intervention to restore the integrity of the extensor mechanism. A patellar dislocation is evident clinically and reduced with sedation, extension of the knee, and pressure to push the patella toward the midline. Radiographs confirm reduction, and a knee immobilizer should be applied.

b. **Knee dislocations** are rare but require immediate reduction and careful assessment of the neurovascular status. When pulses are diminished before or after reduction, immediate arteriography is needed to rule out vascular injury. If vascular repair is required, a spanning external fixator can be applied to stabilize the knee. After repair of vascular injury, prophylactic fasciotomy should be performed. Often, ligamentous reconstruction is necessary to restore knee stability.

4. **Tibia**

a. **Plateau fractures** can be displaced, nondisplaced, or comminuted. The knee must be examined for stability. If the fracture is nondisplaced, early mobilization but limited weightbearing should be instituted. Displaced fractures of >2 mm require surgical intervention to restore articular congruity and joint stability.

b. **Diaphyseal fractures** may occur with either torsional, low-energy, or high-energy mechanisms. Given that the anteromedial tibia is subcutaneous, open fractures are common, and soft-tissue compromise is a frequent clinically relevant issue (see Section V). Soft tissues should be thoroughly assessed, and neurovascular status must be checked frequently to rule out the development of a compartment syndrome. Skin compromise secondary to severe fracture angulation requires immediate reduction and splint immobilization. Treatment by either splint/cast immobilization or intramedullary nailing depends on the fracture pattern and the amount of comminution, shortening, rotation, and angulation.

c. **Distal tibia articular fractures (pilon fractures)** are typically associated with severe soft-tissue injury and involve the joint surface. In the case of displaced and shortened fractures, initial management includes closed reduction and application of a temporary ankle-spanning external fixator, which acts as a form of portable traction. External fixation is maintained until soft tissues can tolerate formal open reduction and internal fixation.

5. **Ankle fracture.** The precise location of pain, swelling, and tenderness must be assessed. Radiographs, including anteroposterior, lateral, and mortise views, are obtained when history and physical examination suggest fracture. Bimalleolar (medial and lateral) fractures represent unstable ankle injuries and require surgical intervention. Isolated lateral malleolar fractures without medial tenderness are stable; they are treated with splint immobilization and early weightbearing. When lateral malleolar fractures occur together with medial tenderness on examination, a mortise stress x-ray (stabilizing the distal tibia and externally rotating the patient's foot) is obtained to assess joint stability. Widening of more than 2 mm of the medial joint space represents an unstable ankle. Initial management of ankle fractures includes closed reduction, splinting, and strict elevation to help avoid soft-tissue complications or swelling.

6. **Foot**
   a. **Calcaneus fractures** usually occur from a fall or motor vehicle crash. These injuries are often bilateral and can be associated with lumbosacral spine injuries as well. Examination of these areas is necessary, as is radiologic assessment. CT scans help to further delineate these fractures and direct treatment. These injuries are associated with considerable swelling and blister formation, and therefore a well-padded splint should be applied and the limb elevated and the patient observed. Fractures with severe subtalar joint depression and comminution may require open reduction and internal fixation. Surgery is typically delayed for 10 to 14 days to allow recovery of the soft tissues.
   b. **Talus**
      (1) **Peritalar dislocation** occurs after varying degrees of forced foot inversion. **Skin disruption or fracture of the talar neck** may occur. Examination often reveals deformity, with the patient's foot medial to his or her leg, the lateral skin tented, and the talus palpable under the skin. Emergent reduction is performed to decrease the chance of avascular necrosis and eliminate skin compromise. Soft-tissue interposition can prevent closed reduction, in which case immediate open reduction is required. Associated fractures must be anatomically reduced and stabilized.
      (2) **Fractures of the talar neck** occur with forced ankle flexion or extension. A high index of suspicion is needed because these fractures may not be apparent on examination or radiographs. Displaced fractures of >2 mm require anatomic reduction and fixation to minimize the risk of complications. Nondisplaced fractures can be treated with strict weightbearing avoidance, immobilization, and close follow-up.
   c. **Fracture dislocations of the tarsometatarsal joints** (Lisfranc fracture-dislocation) are complex and difficult to treat. These injuries are diagnosed radiographically by incongruity of the tarsometatarsal joints, most commonly between the medial base of the second metatarsal and the medial edge of the middle cuneiform, which normally are collinear. Treatment consists of splinting, elevation, avoidance of weightbearing, and eventually operative reduction and fixation.
   d. **Lesser metatarsal fractures** are treated with a pressure dressing and elevation until pain and swelling subside. First metatarsal fractures, if displaced, may require surgical intervention. Transverse fractures of the diaphysis of the fifth metatarsal ("Jones" fracture) requires a strict nonweightbearing cast, immobilization, and possible surgery, whereas avulsion fractures of the proximal fifth metatarsal metaphysis ("pseudo-Jones") can be treated with early weightbearing.
   e. **Toe injuries** are best treated by "buddy" taping to the adjacent digit. The patient may then ambulate in a hard-soled shoe.

IV. Orthopedic emergencies

A. Infection must be considered in any patient with localized findings (pain, redness, swelling, warmth) or systemic findings (malaise, fever, tachycardia).

   1. Acute infections often respond to prompt assessment, medical treatment with appropriate antibiotic therapy (cellulitis), and surgical decompression (abscess, septic bursitis).

      a. Septic arthritis usually occurs secondary to immunosuppression, systemic infection, preexisting joint disease, previous arthrotomy, or intravenous drug abuse.

         (1) Examination reveals tenderness, effusion, increased warmth, and **pain with motion.** The patient may have an elevated erythrocyte sedimentation rate, C-reactive protein, and/or white blood cell (WBC) count. Diagnosis is confirmed by needle aspiration and laboratory analysis of synovial fluid. Inflammatory and noninflammatory processes (e.g., gout) are ruled out by analyzing the synovial fluid for cell count and differential, Gram stain, routine aerobic and anaerobic cultures, and crystals.

         (2) Baseline radiographs (significant changes occur late, in 7 to 10 days) should be obtained and broad-spectrum intravenous antibiotics (first-generation cephalosporin and gentamicin) initiated after adequate specimens are obtained and the limb is immobilized. If septic arthritis is diagnosed, some means of cleansing the joint should be performed (serial aspirations, arthroscopic débridement, or arthrotomy) to prevent cartilage degradation and further systemic illness.

   2. Osteomyelitis. Childhood osteomyelitis most commonly results from hematogenous spread of bacteria to the metaphysis. Adult osteomyelitis typically occurs from direct inoculation via surgery, an open fracture, or chronic soft-tissue ulcers. Hematogenous spread may occur in cases of intravenous drug abuse, sickle cell disease, and immunosuppression.

      a. Physical examination findings are similar to those in septic arthritis but also may reveal bony tenderness and drainage.

      b. Imaging studies, including bone scan, MR scan, or both, may confirm the diagnosis, along with needle aspiration, bone biopsy, elevated erythrocyte sedimentation rate, elevated C-reactive protein, elevated WBC count, and culture.

      c. Treatment typically involves débridement and assessment of soft-tissue coverage, followed by an extended course of intravenous antibiotics.

   3. Suppurative flexor tenosynovitis. Patients present with tenderness along the flexor sheath, a semiflexed finger position, pain on extension, and fusiform swelling of the entire finger (Kanavel signs). Skin wounds may appear innocuous. The patient's entire hand must be examined because infection may extend into other spaces. Immediate surgical decompression, irrigation, and débridement are indicated.

   4. Abscess

      a. Hand. Numerous potential spaces exist that can be infected. All present with pain, tense swelling, induration, and tenderness to palpation. Systemic signs of infection may or may not be present. Immediate surgical drainage is mandatory.

      b. Others. Infection in the soft tissue may occur anywhere and presents with pain, tenderness, swelling, possible fluctuation, and induration. Fluid collections are readily localized with large-bore needle aspiration. Surgical drainage is performed on a semielective basis unless systemic involvement compromises patient health or management.

B. Fat embolism

   1. Fat embolism occurs within 3 days of a long-bone fracture and is characterized by mental status changes, tachycardia, dyspnea, and petechiae.

2. **Laboratory data** reveal a decrease in platelet count (<15,000 μL), an arterial oxygen tension of <60 mm Hg, increased serum lipase, and, possibly, fat in the urine. Patchy infiltrates appear on the chest x-ray. Electrocardiography can reveal tachycardia, inverted T waves, right bundle-branch block, and depressed ST segments.

3. **Treatment** involves respiratory support to keep the arterial oxygen tension at 50 to 100 mm Hg; intubation may be necessary. Positive end-expiratory pressure and corticosteroid administration have been used to treat this complication.

C. **Compartment syndrome** is characterized by an increase in tissue pressure within a closed osteofascial space, which may compromise microcirculation, leading to irreversible muscle injury and eventual rhabdomyolysis. Acute renal failure may then ensue.

1. **Location.** Most frequently, compartment syndrome occurs in the anterior, lateral, or posterior compartments of the leg or the volar or dorsal compartments of the forearm.

2. **Causes.** Bleeding after fracture, crush, or vascular injury is a likely cause. Increased capillary permeability secondary to postischemic swelling, trauma, or burns may also contribute to compartment syndrome. Muscle hypertrophy, tight dressings, and pneumatic antishock garments (e.g., military antishock trousers) are less common causes.

3. **Examination.** Patients at risk for compartment syndrome should be identified early and examined frequently. Signs to watch for are as follows:
   a. **Pain** out of proportion to the injury and not controlled with appropriate narcotics
   b. **Pain with passive motion** of involved muscles or tendons traversing the suspicious compartment
   c. **Paresthesias** in the distribution of the peripheral nerves traversing the suspicious compartment
   d. **Paralysis, pallor, and pulselessness** are very late signs and likely indicate irreparable soft-tissue injury; if pulses are altered or absent, major arterial occlusion rather than compartment syndrome should be considered in the diagnosis.
   e. **Elevated compartment pressures** should be measured in high-risk patients when the clinical examination is suspicious. Infusion, wick, or injection techniques are used to measure the pressure of all compartments in the involved extremity. Several measurements should be taken in different locations, and comparison with pressures in uninvolved compartments can be helpful.

4. **Treatment.** Circumferential bandages, splints, or casts should be removed. For pressures of <30 mm Hg or for pressures of 30 to 40 mm Hg without clear evidence of the syndrome clinically, observation with hourly examination and pressure measurements is appropriate. If examination is equivocal or worrisome, fasciotomy should be performed. For pressures within 20 to 30 mm Hg of the diastolic blood pressure with equivocal clinical examination or for pressures exceeding 40 mm Hg regardless of examination, fasciotomy is in order.

D. **Open fractures and joints.** Lacerations or wounds near fractures or joints often communicate. If exposed bone is not evident, wounds should be probed to determine if communication to fracture is present. Joints may be distended with sterile saline to check for extravasation from adjacent wounds, which would indicate open communication. Air in the joint on x-ray and fat droplets in blood from the wound also confirm communication with a joint or fracture.

1. **Treatment**
   a. **Assess wounds.**
   b. **Irrigate grossly contaminated wounds with normal saline.**
   c. **Apply moist saline-soaked dressing, reduce the fracture or joint, and splint the extremity.**

> **d. Administer tetanus prophylaxis and intravenous antibiotics.** Type
> I injuries with a skin opening <1 cm require a first-generation
> cephalosporin. With type II and III injuries (skin opening >1 cm and
> significant soft-tissue stripping), an aminoglycoside should be added.
> Farm injuries require administration of penicillin to cover for *Clostridium perfringens*.
> **e. Check neurovascular status closely and frequently.**
> 2. **Gunshot injuries**
>   a. The **weapon caliber and type** must be identified. High-energy injuries (shotgun, rifle, or high-caliber handguns) require operative débridement secondary to severe soft-tissue or bony damage. With low-energy injuries (low-caliber handguns), débridement is not always needed because less damage occurs.
>   b. **Neurovascular status** should be checked closely and frequently, especially if the wound is near major neurovascular structures, and radiographs to assess bony damage should be obtained. If the wound is near a joint without evident intra-articular involvement, aspirate for hemarthrosis, sterilely distend the joint capsule with saline, and look for extravasation from the wound.
>   c. **Treatment.** Clean the skin, débride the wound edges, and irrigate thoroughly. Apply a dressing and splint the extremity if a fracture is found. If no neurovascular compromise or compartment syndrome exists, isolated soft-tissue injury is treated with local wound care and oral antibiotics.
> 3. **Traumatic amputation**
>   a. **A team approach is needed** to evaluate for possible replantation, and all necessary consultants should be contacted early.
>   b. **The proximal stump is cleaned,** and a compressive dressing is applied. Tourniquets are not used. Amputated parts are wrapped in moist gauze, placed in a bag, and cooled by placing on ice (freezing should be avoided).

V. Soft-tissue injury
A. Principles of management
  1. **In general,** isolated soft-tissue injuries, such as ligament sprains and muscle strains, are treated with *r*est, *i*ce, *c*ompression bandage, and *e*levation (RICE therapy) with or without immobilization.
  2. **Skin.** All devitalized tissue should be débrided. If the wound cannot be closed due to excessive tension, it should be covered with a moist saline dressing, and a delayed primary closure or skin grafting should be planned.
  3. **Muscle**
    a. **Trauma to the musculotendinous unit** usually is secondary to violent contraction or excessive stretch, and it ranges from stretch of the fibers to a complete tear and loss of function.
    b. **Swelling, tenderness, and pain with movement occur.** A defect may be palpable. Immobilization of the extremity and any associated joints on which the muscle acts is adequate for less severe injuries.
  4. **Tendon.** Lacerated, ruptured, or avulsed tendons, especially of the upper extremity, should be surgically repaired because failure to do so results in loss of function. Examination reveals loss of motion or weakness. If associated with a tendon laceration, the wound is irrigated thoroughly, débrided, and closed primarily. In grossly contaminated wounds, incision and débridement in the operating room are needed. Splints are applied with the extremity in a functional position.
  5. **Ligament.** Injury ranges from mild stretch to complete tear. Pain, localized tenderness, abnormal joint motion or position, or instability may be present on examination. Radiographs may reveal joint incongruence. If the joint is clinically or radiographically unstable, treatment involves immobilization in a reduced position. If no evidence of instability is present,

treatment based on the RICE principle is used, and early range of motion is encouraged.
- **B. Common injuries**
  1. **Rotator cuff tear.** Acute rupture is most commonly associated with traumatic dislocation of the glenohumeral joint in patients over 40 years old or with the acute onset of pain while lifting with the humerus in abduction and forward elevation. Avulsion fractures of the greater tuberosity may be seen as well. Weakness and pain with attempted shoulder forward elevation, abduction, or external rotation is present.
  2. **Rupture** of the **pectoralis major** and **biceps brachii** tendon often occurs with heavy lifting or exertion and is diagnosed by pain, weakness, and a visible, palpable defect. Initial treatment consists of placement of the extremity in a sling and initiation of early motion.
  3. A **ruptured heel cord** (Achilles tendon) usually occurs during running, jumping, or vigorous activity, with sudden pain and difficulty in walking. Examination reveals a palpable defect, weak plantar flexion, and no passive ankle plantar flexion on squeezing the patient's calf (positive "Thompson sign"). Older patients often can be treated in a splint, with the ankle plantar flexed. Serial casting with progressive dorsiflexion of the foot is then initiated. In younger patients, rerupture rates are less with surgical repair of the tendon.
  4. **Ankle sprains** commonly occur with inversion or external rotation of the ankle. Patients present with swelling, ecchymosis, and maximal tenderness along all injured ligaments. Radiographs are normal or reveal clinically insignificant, small cortical avulsions. Initial treatment based on the RICE principle is adequate, followed by physical therapy for proprioceptive training.
  5. **Knee ligament disruption.** Dislocation must be considered. Stability is assessed. An effusion may be aspirated to examine for lipohemarthrosis and thus confirm the presence of a fracture. If no fracture or dislocation exists, an immobilizer is applied for comfort with weightbearing, and early range of motion is emphasized. Common knee injuries include anterior cruciate ligament tears, medial collateral ligament tears, and meniscal tears.
- **VI. Practical procedures**
  - **A. Common splints.** Splints limit further soft-tissue injury and swelling and help to minimize pain. They also facilitate further clinical and radiographic evaluation. Air splints are used only in the emergency setting because they increase pressure in the extremity and compromise blood flow.
    1. **Preparation and application.** Prefabricated splints and immobilizers can be used, if available. Plaster splints consist of plaster and cast padding. The required length, to include a joint above and below the injury, is measured from the uninjured side. Two layers of soft roll are applied against the skin, and extra padding is placed over bony prominences. A 10-layer-thick stack of plaster splint material is wetted in cold to lukewarm water and squeezed until damp. The splint is applied over the soft-roll padding and wrapped lightly with an elastic bandage. The extremity is held in the appropriate position until the plaster is firm.
    2. **Upper-extremity splints.** Remove all of the patient's jewelry!
       a. **Commercial shoulder immobilizers, Velpeau dressing, and sling and swathe** are used for shoulder dislocations, humerus fractures, and some elbow fractures. A pad is placed in the axilla to prevent skin maceration.
       b. **Figure-of-eight slings** can be used for clavicle fracture stabilization but are often poorly tolerated by adults.
       c. **Posterior and sugar tong splints** are used in elbow, forearm, and wrist injuries. They are applied with the patient's elbow flexed to 90 degrees, wrist extended 20 to 30 degrees, and forearm in neutral rotation.

    d. Thumb spica, ulnar/radial gutter, and volar/dorsal forearm splints are used for forearm, hand, and wrist injuries. Finger injuries may be treated with prefabricated aluminum splint material. For wrist and hand injuries, immobilization is performed with the patient's hand and wrist in a so-called **safe position:** the wrist in 20 to 30 degrees of extension, the metacarpophalangeal joints in 70 to 80 degrees of flexion, and the interphalangeal joints extended.

3. Lower-extremity splints

    a. Thomas/Hare traction splints are used by primary responders for femur fractures. Traction is applied by an ankle hitch, with countertraction across the ischial tuberosity. The splint should not be left in place for longer than 2 hours because sloughing of the skin can occur about the ankle and groin.

    b. A **Jones dressing** with or without plaster reinforcements is used in acute knee, ankle, calcaneus, and some tibial fractures, where considerable swelling is expected. The injured extremity is wrapped with cotton, followed by a lightly wrapped elastic bandage. Plaster splints can be applied to the posterior, medial, and lateral aspects for added stability. Circumferential plaster should be avoided.

    c. Short leg splints are used in acute leg or foot trauma. They extend from below the knee to the toes and incorporate posterior, medial, and lateral plaster slabs. The ankle should be immobilized in the neutral position.

4. Precautions. Bony prominences should be padded. Casts or circumferential splints are avoided in acute trauma when swelling is anticipated, unless they are bivalved or split (including padding) to allow swelling. To split the cast, cut a 1-inch strip of plaster from the full length of the cast, split the padding, and spread the cast edges.

B. Anesthesia for fracture and joint reduction

1. Local anesthesia. Appropriate sterile technique must be used.

    a. Peripheral nerve block. The peripheral nerves of the hands and feet can be easily blocked using 1% lidocaine without epinephrine (sometimes mixed with 0.25% to 0.50% bupivacaine for longer-lasting analgesia). The digital nerves of the fingers or toes can be blocked by infiltrating 2 to 5 mL into the web spaces adjacent to the injured digit. An ankle block may be performed by infiltrating (often with 0.5% bupivacaine) (1) 10 mL posterior to the medial malleolus to block the posterior tibial nerve, (2) 5 mL subcutaneously from the medial malleolus to the lateral malleolus dorsally to block the saphenous and superficial peroneal nerves, (3) 2.5 mL posterior to the lateral malleolus to block the sural nerve, and, finally, (4) 2.5 mL posterior to the extensor hallucis longus tendon anteriorly to block the deep peroneal nerve. At the wrist, the median nerve and ulnar nerves may be blocked by infiltrating 5 mL local anesthetic into the carpal tunnel and the space dorsal to the flexor carpi ulnaris tendon, respectively.

    b. Hematoma block is especially effective with fractures of the distal radius. A 21-gauge needle is inserted into the fracture site through the dorsal forearm. Aspiration of blood confirms appropriate position of the needle in the fracture site. Approximately 8 to 10 mL 1% lidocaine without epinephrine is then infiltrated. A hematoma block in conjunction with light sedation often provides excellent analgesia and relaxation for reduction.

    c. Intra-articular injection is used to provide analgesia for reduction of fractures and joints and to position joints for splinting. Some joints may be easily injected with local anesthetic. Aspiration of blood in the case of fracture and easy flow of the anesthetic confirm entry into the joint. The ankle may be infiltrated anteriorly adjacent to either malleolus. The elbow may be entered laterally in the triangle formed by the lateral epicondyle, radial head, and olecranon. Finally, the shoulder is infiltrated either anteriorly lateral to the coracoid process or posteriorly 2 cm distal and 1 cm medial to the posterolateral edge of the acromion.

2. **Sedation.** Midazolam (Versed) and fentanyl are administered intravenously slowly over 2 to 5 minutes to achieve easily arousable sedation and pain control (usually a total of 2 to 5 mg midazolam is needed). Close observation of respiratory status and monitoring with a pulse oximeter are required. Midazolam sedation is readily reversed with flumazenil (Romazicon) and fentanyl with naloxone hydrochloride (Narcan). Patients are monitored for 60 minutes after manipulation.

C. **Technique for reduction of fracture or dislocation**

1. **Dislocation.** After adequate analgesia and sedation as noted, longitudinal traction of the affected extremity (avoiding sudden, forceful movements) is applied, initially gently and progressively with increasing force until reduction is achieved. The dislocated fragment is manipulated by applying pressure in the direction of reduction. Gentle rotation may help but is performed cautiously because long-bone fracture may occur.

2. **Fracture.** Traction is applied first in the direction of the angulation (recreating the injury to release the impaction of the bony ends) and then in line with the long axis of the limb to correct the alignment, rotation, and length. Pressure is applied to the distal fragment in the direction of the reduced position. Postreduction x-rays are obtained in all cases, and the joint or extremity is immobilized.

Urologic Surgery

**Jay S. Belani and
Arnold D. Bullock**

EVALUATION OF HEMATURIA

I. **Hematuria** is the hallmark of disease in the genitourinary tract and warrants a thorough investigation. Pain associated with hematuria may suggest a benign etiology such as cystitis or urinary calculi. However, painless hematuria should be regarded as secondary to a tumor until proven otherwise.

   A. All of the following warrant a hematuria workup:
   1. One or more episodes of gross hematuria
   2. At least 3 red blood cells (RBCs) per high-power field on 2 of 3 urine specimens.

   B. **Evaluation of hematuria**
   1. **Freshly voided** urine is evaluated with a dipstick and microscopic analysis for the following:
      a. **Specific gravity** is noted because RBC rupture occurs in hypotonic urine (specific gravity <1.008).
      b. **Urinary pH** can aid in the diagnosis of disease.
      c. **Microscopic analysis** evaluates RBC morphology, casts, crystals, white blood cell (WBC) count, and bacteria.
      d. The presence and character of **clots** can be revealing; upper tract bleeding may cause vermiform clots, whereas bladder clots may be amorphous.
   2. **Complete blood cell (CBC) count, coagulation parameters, and serum creatinine** are essential.
   3. **Radiologic evaluation** of the upper urinary tract with an intravenous pyelogram (IVP) or retrograde pyelogram is mandatory. Renal parenchymal imaging with an ultrasound may be used as an adjunct. Computed tomographic (CT) urography may be performed instead of IVP and ultrasound.
   4. The lower urinary tract is visualized with **cystoscopy.**
   5. **Urine is sent for culture and cytology.**
   6. If a diagnosis still is not made, a repeat urinalysis in 6 months is necessary, with another complete workup if the hematuria persists. Evaluation of microscopic hematuria can be performed on an outpatient basis. Anticoagulation at therapeutic levels does not predispose patients to hematuria; these patients require complete evaluation.

   C. **Treatment.** Gross hematuria requires urgent evaluation.
   1. **Patients passing blood clots** may require irrigation and initiation of continuous bladder irrigation with normal saline via a three-way Foley catheter [22 to 26 French (Fr.)]. Prostatic bleeding may be controlled with gentle catheter traction.
   2. **Bladder irrigation** with 1% alum or 1% silver nitrate can alleviate persistent bleeding. It is imperative that the bladder be free of clots before initiating alum or silver nitrate irrigation. Silver nitrate and alum are astringents that act by protein precipitation over the bleeding surfaces. Initiation of intravenous ε-aminocaproic acid (Amicar; 5 g in 250 mL D5W infused over 1 hour, then 1 g per hour continuous infusion) can also be used to help control bleeding. ε-Aminocaproic acid is an inhibitor of fibrinolysis and can be associated with thromboembolic complications. It should

be used judiciously and should not be used in any patient suspected of disseminated intravascular coagulopathy. It may also be given orally or administered intravesically.
3. **Persistent bleeding** on continuous bladder irrigation or significant gross hematuria in the unstable patient requires immediate cystoscopic evaluation to localize and control bleeding.

DISEASES OF THE KIDNEY

I. **Evaluation of renal masses**
   A. Increased use of abdominal CT scanning and ultrasonography has resulted in detection of more asymptomatic **renal masses.** These masses must be characterized as benign or malignant.
   B. **The vast majority of masses are benign cysts** (*Radiology* 1991;179:307).
   C. **Renal cysts** occur in one-half of persons older than 50 years. Other **benign lesions** include infarction, abscess, hemangioma, angiomyolipoma, and adenoma. **Most solid renal masses** (85% to 90%) are renal cell carcinomas (RCCs). Up to 25% of these cancers measure <3 cm in diameter and are diagnosed incidentally by imaging obtained for other reasons (*Radiology* 1989;170:699). Over the last 20 years, the incidence of RCC has been increasing. Improved imaging and early diagnosis have dramatically increased the number of patients who present with curable disease. **Other malignant lesions** include transitional cell carcinoma, oncocytoma (benign in the vast majority of cases), sarcoma, lymphoma, leukemia, and metastatic tumor (lung, breast, gastrointestinal, prostate, and pancreatic tumors and melanoma).
   D. **Presentation.** The historical triad of flank pain, hematuria, and flank mass occurs <10% of the time.
   E. Ten percent to 40% of renal cell carcinomas are associated with **paraneoplastic syndromes.**
      1. Hypertension from **renin overproduction** is common.
      2. **Stauffer syndrome** (nonmetastatic hepatic dysfunction) is seen in some patients and resolves after tumor removal.
      3. **Hypercalcemia** from parathyroid hormone–like protein produced by the tumor also may occur.
      4. **Erythrocytosis** can occur as a result of production of erythropoietin by the tumor.
   F. **Staging.** Adequate staging of renal cell carcinoma is imperative to properly guide therapy. In addition to complete history, thorough physical examination, and blood work [CBC, electrolytes (including calcium), creatinine, and liver function tests], a chest radiograph and cross-sectional abdominal imaging (CT or MR scan with contrast) should be obtained. Radionuclide bone scan is not necessary in patients who have normal alkaline phosphatase and serum calcium and do not have symptoms of skeletal involvement. Symptoms and results of these basic tests should guide additional radiographic staging. The TNM (tumor, node, metastasis) staging system is outlined in Table 40-1.
   G. **Imaging modalities**
      1. **CT scan** with and without intravenous contrast is the preferred diagnostic study for evaluating a renal mass. Precontrast images may be hypodense, isodense, or hyperdense compared with normal renal parenchyma; renal cell carcinomas generally enhance, but to a lesser degree than surrounding parenchyma. CT also provides staging information, including local extent of the tumor, presence of regional lymphadenopathy, or presence of distant metastatic lesions (lung, liver, adrenal gland).
      2. **Ultrasonography** is the modality of choice in determining whether a lesion is solid or cystic.
         a. **Bosniak** classification (*Radiology* 1991;179:307).

Table 40-1. American Joint Committee on Cancer staging for kidney cancer

Stage	Tumor (T)[a]	Node (N)[b]	Metastasis (M)[c]
I	T1	N0	M0
II	T2	N0	M0
III	T1	N1	M0
	T2	N1	M0
	T3	N0, N1	M0
IV	T4	N0, N1	M0
	Any T	N2, N3	M0
	Any T	Any N	M1

[a]T1, tumor ≤7 cm in greatest dimension, limited to the kidney; T2, tumor >7 cm in greatest dimension, limited to the kidney; T3, tumor extends into major veins or invades adrenal gland or perinephric tissues, but not beyond the Gerota fascia; T3a, tumor invades adrenal gland or perinephric tissues but not beyond the Gerota fascia; T3b, tumor grossly extends into renal vein or vena cava below diaphragm; T3c, tumor grossly extends into vena cava above the diaphragm; T4, tumor grossly extends beyond the Gerota fascia.
[b]N0, no regional lymph node metastasis; N1, metastasis in a single regional lymph node, 2 cm in greatest dimension; N2, metastasis in a single regional lymph node, >2 cm but not >5 cm in greatest dimension, or multiple lymph nodes, none >5 cm in greatest dimension; N3, metastasis in a lymph node >5 cm in greatest dimension.
[c]M0, no distant metastasis; M1, distant metastasis.

    (1) **Category I:** simple cyst.
    (2) **Category II:** high-density cyst; thin, smooth septa; or linear calcification.
    (3) **Category III:** indeterminate lesions; numerous or thick septa, or both; thick calcification. These lesions require surgical management.
    (4) **Category IV:** high probability of malignancy with cystic component, irregular margins, and solid vascular elements. These lesions require surgical management.
  3. Doppler ultrasonography may be useful for evaluating the extent of vena caval involvement.
  4. MR scan is useful for staging renal tumors (especially in patients with renal insufficiency or allergies to contrast dye) and for detecting tumor thrombus in the renal vein and inferior vena cava.
  5. Angiography rarely is used in evaluating an indeterminate renal mass, but it may be helpful in planning nephron-sparing surgery (partial nephrectomy). Renal cell carcinoma is characteristically hypervascular on arteriography.
  6. IVP remains the standard diagnostic modality for evaluating the upper urinary tract of patients presenting with hematuria (38% of renal cell cancers). Renal masses may distort the collecting system. Tomograms may detect 85% of lesions >3 cm.
 II. Management of renal masses
  A. Radical nephrectomy remains the most effective treatment modality. Radical nephrectomy involves removing the kidney outside of the Gerota fascia. Ten-year survival after nephrectomy for Robson stage I and II lesions was >78% in one modern series (*J Urol* 1998;159:192). Nephron-sparing surgery (partial nephrectomy) has been proven to have results similar to those of radical nephrectomy for small (<4 cm) lesions (*Urology* 1995;46:149). Laparoscopic nephrectomy and partial nephrectomy increasingly is being performed for renal cell cancer and has been shown to have efficacy comparable to that of open nephrectomy (*J Urol* 2002;167:1257; *Curr Opin Urol* 2003;13:439). For smaller tumors, renal cryoablation and radiofrequency ablation are being studied.
  B. Renal cell carcinoma is resistant to radiation and chemotherapy. Immunotherapy protocols using interferon and interleukin-2 have

demonstrated increased survival after nephrectomy for metastatic renal cell carcinoma (*J Urol* 2000;163:154S).

DISEASES OF THE URETER

III. Ureteropelvic junction obstruction (UPJO)

A. UPJO is often a **congenital anomaly** that results from a stenotic segment of ureter. Acquired lesions may include tortuous or kinked ureters as a result of vesicoureteral reflux; benign tumors such as fibroepithelial polyps; or scarring as a result of stone disease, ischemia, or previous surgical manipulation of the urinary system. The role of crossing vessels (present in one-third of cases) has not been firmly established, although their presence may be associated with treatment failures.

B. **Presentation.** Although UPJO can be a congenital problem, patients may present at any age. Common symptoms are flank pain, which may be intermittent; hematuria; infection; and, rarely, hypertension.

C. **Radiographic studies** should determine the site and functional significance of the obstruction. Useful studies include IVP, diuretic renal scintigraphy, and retrograde pyelography. Ultrasound may demonstrate a hydronephrosis, but this is not diagnostic of functional obstruction.

D. **Open pyeloplasty** is the gold standard treatment, with success rates >90%. Recently, a variety of minimally invasive procedures have been developed to avoid the morbidity of open surgery. Options include laparoscopic pyeloplasty, percutaneous endopyelotomy, and ureteroscopic or retrograde endopyelotomy with a balloon-cutting device.

IV. Urolithiasis

A. **Epidemiology.** The peak incidence of urinary calculi is in the 3rd to 5th decade. Stones are more prevalent in men than in women. Stone incidence is increased during the late summer months. Dietary factors leading to stone formation include low water intake and high protein or oxalate (leafy green vegetable) consumption. Calcium restriction is not recommended as a means of preventing stone formation; however, a low-sodium diet may decrease calciuria. Citrus juices, particularly lemonade, may increase urinary levels of citrate, an inhibitor of stone formation. Various drugs, including high-dose vitamin C and D, acetazolamide, triamterene, and some protease inhibitors (indinavir) [*Lancet* 349(9061):1294, 1997], have been associated with stone formation. Disease states, such as inflammatory bowel disease, and metabolic disorders, such as type I renal tubular acidosis or cystinuria, can also contribute to stone formation.

B. **Clinical features.** Acute onset of severe flank pain or renal colic, often associated with nausea and vomiting, results from urinary obstruction by the stone. Common locations for stones to become impacted include the renal infundibulum, the ureteropelvic junction, the crossing of the iliac vessels, and the ureterovesical junction, which is the most constricted area through which the stone must pass. Patients may present with microscopic or gross hematuria. Up to 15% of patients may have no hematuria.

C. **Types of calculi**

1. **Calcium stones** make up approximately 70% of all stones. Disorders of calcium metabolism, such as increased intestinal absorption or increased renal excretion of calcium or oxalate, can cause calcium stones. Systemic disorders, such as hyperparathyroidism, sarcoidosis, immobilization (causing calcium resorption from bone), and type I renal tubular acidosis, can lead to these derangements of calcium metabolism.

2. **Uric acid stones** make up approximately 10% of all stones. They occur as a result of hyperuricosuria, persistently acidic pH, and low urine volumes.

3. **Cysteine stones** account for 4% of stones. They are caused by a defect in tubular reabsorption of cysteine that is inherited in an autosomal recessive manner. Hexagonal crystals in the urine are highly suggestive of cysteine stones.

4. **Magnesium ammonium phosphate or struvite stones** account for 15% of stones and are associated with urinary tract infection, commonly with urea-splitting organisms, and a chronically alkaline urinary pH (>7.2). Urinalysis may demonstrate rectangular "coffin lid" crystals.

D. **Evaluation of urinary calculi**

1. **Urinalysis,** including microscopic examination and urine culture, should be performed on all patients suspected of having calculi.

2. **Serum electrolytes,** including calcium, and creatinine levels are also part of the standard workup. Additionally, uric acid levels and parathyroid hormone levels may be helpful. A CBC with differential can be obtained in patients with signs of concurrent infection.

3. **KUB (kidneys, ureters, bladder)** should be the initial radiographic study. Calcium phosphate and calcium oxalate stones are the most radiopaque, whereas uric acid stones are radiolucent.

4. **Noncontrast spiral CT** has replaced IVP as the diagnostic study of choice in the acute setting (*J Urol* 1998;160:679). Spiral CT is quick and easy to obtain, and it does not require the use of contrast. For patients with suspected nephrolithiasis but atypical symptoms, CT may elucidate other causes of abdominal pain. Signs of obstruction include hydroureteronephrosis and perinephric fat stranding.

E. **Management of urinary calculi**

1. **Hydration.** Intravenous fluids are required if the patient is nauseated and cannot take oral fluids. Normal saline usually is initiated at 150 mL per hour in appropriate patients.

2. **Pain management.** Patients whose pain is not adequately managed with oral analgesics require hospitalization for administration of parenteral narcotics. Parenteral nonsteroidal compounds, such as ketorolac, can be effective in reducing the pain of renal colic but should not be used in patients who may undergo lithotripsy. Shock-wave lithotripsy is contraindicated within 72 hours of administration of any nonsteroidal analgesics to minimize the risk of renal hematoma.

3. **Urine should be collected and strained** to retrieve the stone. The stone should be analyzed for composition.

4. **Any patient found to have an obstructing stone in the presence of infection or fever needs emergent decompression** with percutaneous nephrostomy tube or stent placement. This situation can deteriorate quickly into a life-threatening crisis, particularly in the diabetic or immunosuppressed patient.

5. **Ninety-five percent of stones 4 mm or smaller in size pass spontaneously** (*J Urol* 1997;158:1915). Patients may be given up to 4 weeks to pass a partially obstructing stone without permanent renal damage. Patients with stones larger than 4 mm or with intractable symptoms of pain, nausea, or vomiting may need early surgical treatment to relieve obstruction with a ureteral stent, shock-wave lithotripsy, or ureteroscopy with stone ablation or retrieval.

6. Patients who have had one episode of nephrolithiasis do not require further workup. Those who have recurrent episodes require a 24-hour urine collection for volume, creatinine, pH, sodium, calcium, magnesium, phosphorous, oxalate, citrate, uric acid, and protein.

7. Potassium citrate may help prevent stone recurrence by increasing urinary citrate levels and alkalizing the urine. Uric acid stones may dissolve by increasing urinary pH, and calcium stones may be prevented with thiazide diuretics.

DISEASES OF THE URINARY BLADDER

I. **Bladder cancer.** Bladder cancer is found in up to 10% of patients with microscopic hematuria.

Table 40-2. American Joint Committee on Cancer staging for bladder cancer

Stage	Tumor (T)[a]	Node (N)[b]	Metastasis (M)[c]
0_a	Ta	N0	M0
0_{is}	Tis	N0	M0
I	T1	N0	M0
II	T2a	N0	M0
	T2b	N0	M0
III	T3a	N0	M0
	T3b	N0	M0
IV	T4a	N0	M0
	T4b	N0	M0
	Any T	N1–3	M0
	Any T	Any N	M1

[a] Ta, noninvasive papillary carcinoma; Tis, carcinoma *in situ*; T1, tumor invades subepithelial connective tissue; T2, tumor invades muscle; T2a, tumor invades superficial muscle (inner half); T2b, tumor invades deep muscle (outer half); T3, tumor invades perivesical tissue; T3a, microscopically; T3b, macroscopically (extravesical mass); T4, tumor invades any of the following: prostate, uterus, vagina, pelvic wall, or abdominal wall; T4a, tumor invades prostate, uterus, or vagina; T4b, tumor invades pelvic wall or abdominal wall.
[b] N0, no regional lymph node metastasis; N1, metastasis in a single lymph node d2 cm or less in largest dimension; N2, metastasis in a single lymph node >2 cm but not >5 cm in greatest dimension, or multiple lymph nodes, none >5 cm in greatest dimension.
[c] M0, no distant metastasis; M1, distant metastasis.

A. **Transitional cell carcinoma** accounts for up to 90% of bladder tumors in the United States; squamous cell carcinoma and adenocarcinoma are correspondingly less common. Transitional cell carcinoma has been linked directly to cigarette smoking, aniline dyes, aromatic amines, and chronic phenacetin use. Patients who have received cyclophosphamide are at increased risk for developing transitional cell carcinoma; use of the uroprotectant mesna may reduce this risk as well as reduce the risk of hemorrhagic cystitis.

B. **Transitional cell cancer is categorized as superficial or invasive.** Staging is outlined in Table 40-2.

C. **Superficial tumors** are exophytic papillary lesions that do not invade the muscular bladder wall. These tumors can be treated with transurethral resection. Sixty-five percent to 85% of superficial tumors recur; therefore, diligent follow-up is necessary. Recurrent tumors are treated with transurethral resection and intravesical therapy (bacillus Calmette-Guérin, mitomycin C, or thiotepa). In 10% to 15% of patients with superficial bladder tumors, the tumors progress to muscle-invasive disease; their tendency to progress is dependent on stage and grade.

D. **Muscle-invasive transitional cell carcinoma** is treated with radical cystectomy and urinary diversion. Radical cystectomy involves radical cystoprostatectomy (removal of bladder, prostate, and possibly urethra) in the male and anterior exenteration (removal of bladder, urethra, uterus, cervix, and anterior wall of vagina) in the female. Appropriate metastatic evaluation for patients with invasive bladder cancer includes chest radiograph, IVP, CT scan of the abdomen and pelvis, bone scan, and liver function tests. Bladder-sparing protocols combining external-beam radiation therapy and chemotherapy can be used for patients who desire to keep their native bladder or for those who are not operative candidates. Despite this aggressive management, only 50% of patients with invasive bladder cancer are rendered completely free of tumor because many have occult metastases at the time of surgery.

E. **Chemotherapy** [methotrexate, vinblastine, doxorubicin (Adriamycin), and *cis*-platinum (MVAC)] and radiotherapy are used for the treatment of advanced or residual disease. Gemcitabine is a new agent that appears to be effective against transitional cell carcinoma and has less renal toxicity than platinum-based chemotherapy (*J Clin Oncol* 2000;17:3068).

DISEASES OF THE PROSTATE

I. **Prostate cancer**

   A. **Prostate examination. Digital rectal examination (DRE)** of the prostate is an important part of the physical examination. The **normal prostate** is chestnut-sized and measures 3.5 cm wide at the base, 2.5 cm long, and 2.5 cm deep; it weighs approximately 20 g. The prostate should feel smooth, having the consistency of the contracted thenar eminence of the thumb. The prostate is best examined when the patient is standing with the knees slightly flexed and elbows resting on a table or in the lateral decubitus position with the hips flexed.

   B. **Prostate nodules** usually are small (pea-sized) or larger firm areas within the peripheral zone of the prostate. They can represent prostate cancer and must be evaluated with transrectal ultrasonography (TRUS) and prostate biopsy. In men older than 50 years, 15% have a suspicious rectal examination, and 21% of those men have cancer. Serum prostate-specific antigen (PSA) is a more sensitive test than DRE for detection of prostate cancer, but the tests should be used together to maximize cancer detection (*J Urol* 1994;151:1283).

   C. **Prostate cancer** is the most common noncutaneous malignancy in American men and the second leading cause of cancer death. Twenty percent of men with prostate cancer die of the disease. Prostate cancer rarely causes symptoms until it becomes locally advanced or metastatic and is no longer curable.

   D. **Current American Urological Association and American Cancer Society guidelines** recommend that men age 50 and older begin prostate cancer screening with a yearly DRE and PSA measurement. African American men and men with a family history should begin screening at age 45 (*Oncology* 2000;14:267). Abnormalities in either the DRE (manifest as indurated nodules) or the PSA (>4.0 ng/mL) should be evaluated by TRUS and needle biopsy of the prostate.

   E. **New assays for measuring the percentage of free PSA** have the potential to categorize men with intermediate levels of total PSA (4 to 10 ng/mL) into low and high cancer risk groups. Prostate cancer is more likely to be found on biopsy in men with a low percentage of free PSA (<25%). This could result in a reduction of unnecessary prostate biopsies in men with a high percentage of free PSA (*JAMA* 1998;279:1542).

   F. **Appropriate staging workup includes DRE and PSA.** Table 40-3 outlines current staging for prostate cancer. Bone scan is not necessary for patients with well-differentiated or moderately differentiated tumors and a PSA <10. CT is of limited value for patients with well-differentiated or moderately differentiated tumors and a PSA <20.

   G. Prostate cancer is graded by the **Gleason scoring system.** A grade from 1 to 5 is given for the primary and secondary grade, and the total score is added together. The primary score is the first number, and the secondary score is the second number. Well-differentiated tumors have a Gleason sum of 2 to 4, moderately differentiated tumors have a sum of 5 or 6, and poorly differentiated tumors have a sum of 8 to 10. For Gleason sum 7, patients with 3 + 4 are considered moderately differentiated, while those with a 4 + 3 are considered poorly differentiated.

   H. **Treatment options** for men with organ-confined prostate cancer include radical prostatectomy, external-beam radiation therapy, and interstitial radiotherapy (brachytherapy).

      1. For **radical prostatectomy,** the overall 5-year freedom from PSA progression was reported as being 61% to 87% in several published series (*Urol Clin North Am* 1993;20:713). Overall, 10-year disease-specific survival following radical prostatectomy for clinically localized prostate cancer is 85% (81% to 87%, 95% confidence interval) (*JAMA* 1996;276:615).

Table 40-3. American Joint Committee on Cancer staging for prostate cancer

Stage	Tumor (T)[a]	Node (N)[b]	Metastasis (M)[c]
I	T1a	N0	M0[d]
II	T1a	N0	M0
	T1b	N0	M0
	T1c	N0	M0
	T2a, T2b	N0	M0
III	T3	N0	M0
IV	T4	N0	M0
	Any T	N1	M0
	Any T	Any N	M1

[a]T1, clinically inapparent tumor neither palpable nor visible by imaging; T1a, tumor incidental histologic finding in ≤5% of tissue resected; T1b, tumor incidental histologic finding in >5% of tissue resected; T1c, tumor identified by needle biopsy (e.g., because of elevated PSA levels); T2, tumor confined within the prostate; T2a, tumor involves one lobe; T2b, tumor involves both lobes; T3, tumor extends through the prostatic capsule; T3a, extracapsular extension (unilateral or bilateral); T3b, tumor invades seminal vesicles; T4, tumor is fixed or invades adjacent structures other than the seminal vesicle(s) structures, bladder neck, external sphincter, rectum, levator muscles, and/or pelvic wall.
[b]N0, no regional lymph node metastasis; N1, metastasis in regional lymph node(s).
[c]M0, no distant metastasis; M1, distant metastasis; M1a, nonregional lymph node(s); M1b, bone(s); M1c, other site(s).
[d]Includes only well-differentiated (Gleason grade 24) tumors.

2. **External-beam radiotherapy** with delivery of 6,500 to 7,500 cGy achieves disease-free rates of 45% to 85% for localized disease (*N Engl J Med* 1994;331:996). Certain patients may also benefit from adjuvant hormonal therapy in addition to radiotherapy (*Lancet* 2002;360:103).

3. **Technical improvements in dosimetry and implantation** combined with reports of low morbidity have led to a renewed interest in brachytherapy. Some authors have suggested that brachytherapy alone may have a higher rate of PSA progression than other treatment modalities (*Urology* 1998;51:884). The optimal form of treatment for clinically localized prostate cancer has not been conclusively determined.

4. **Hormonal therapy** with either bilateral orchiectomy or luteinizing hormone–releasing hormone agonists usually is reserved for men with locally advanced or metastatic disease.

5. **Watchful waiting** is appropriate for men with a life expectancy of <10 years and low-stage, low-grade prostate cancer (*J Urol* 1998;159:1431).

II. **Prostatitis** is a diagnosis that spans a spectrum of disease entities. The classification and diagnostic criteria for the different forms of prostatitis recently have been changed in an effort to standardize diagnosis to improve research and clinical treatment.

A. **Signs and symptoms of urinary tract infection** mark acute bacterial prostatitis; many patients have significant voiding complaints, fevers, and malaise. DRE reveals a tender, boggy prostate. Repeat exams should be minimized to avoid spread of infection. Antibiotics are the mainstays of treatment. Those patients with high fevers may require admission for intravenous antibiotics. Drainage of the urinary bladder via a suprapubic tube or a small urethral catheter may be required for those patients in urinary retention.

B. **Chronic bacterial prostatitis** is differentiated from other categories by the presence of documented recurrent bacterial infection of expressed prostatic secretions, postprostatic massage urine, or semen. Treatment is with antibiotics; fluoroquinolones have excellent prostatic penetration.

III. **Prostatic abscess** can be difficult to diagnose.

A. **Patients typically have acute urinary retention, fever, dysuria, urinary frequency, and perineal pain.**

B. Prostatic enlargement is the most common finding on examination; other findings, such as tenderness and fluctuance, are more variable (*Rev Infect Dis* 1988;10:239).

C. CT scan or TRUS confirms the diagnosis.

D. Treatment is with percutaneous or transurethral drainage and appropriate parenteral antibiotics.

IV. Urinary retention may result from BPH, prostate cancer, or urethral stricture disease. Retention also can be associated with pelvic trauma, neurologic conditions, or various medications or the postoperative setting.

A. Evaluation. A history usually elicits the cause of retention. Common signs and symptoms of BPH include hesitancy, decreased force of stream, frequency, urgency, postvoid dribbling, double voiding, incomplete bladder emptying, and nocturia. Patients with BPH who are treated with decongestants containing an α-agonist may develop urinary retention from increased smooth-muscle tone at the bladder neck and the prostate. Anticholinergic medications can cause urinary retention through relaxation of the detrusor muscle.

B. Physical examination reveals a distended lower abdomen. Prostatic enlargement is common on DRE. Serum electrolytes and creatinine levels, urinalysis, and urine culture should be obtained. Serum PSA concentration obtained during acute urinary retention often is spuriously elevated and is best measured at least 4 to 6 weeks after the acute event.

C. Treatment

1. Sterile technique is used. The proper technique of urethral catheter placement involves passing the catheter to the hub and inflating the balloon *only* after the return of urine.

2. When a standard Foley catheter cannot be passed easily, sterile 2% viscous lidocaine can be injected through the urethra. This anesthetizes and relaxes the sphincter, allowing gentle passage of a 16 to 22 Fr. Coudé tip catheter. The viscous lidocaine is given 5 to 10 minutes before passing the catheter. The catheter is passed gently with the tip directed upward. If the Coudé tip catheter does not pass easily, a urology consultation is required.

3. Catheterization should not be attempted when a urethral injury is suspected. Urethral stricture requires calibration and dilation or placement of a suprapubic tube by a urologist. Urinary clot retention usually requires bladder irrigation.

4. Patients should be monitored for postobstructive diuresis, especially if the patient is azotemic. This is a physiologic response to a hypervolemic state. Occasionally, it can become a pathologic diuresis and may warrant hospital observation, with fluid and electrolyte replacement. Five-percent dextrose in 0.45% saline should be used for hydration. Urine output >200 mL per hour for more than 2 hours should be replaced with 0.5 mL intravenous 0.45% saline for each 1 mL urine. Electrolytes should be checked every 6 hours initially and replaced as needed.

V. BPH is most commonly treated medically with alpha-blockers, such as doxazosin, terazosin, and tamsulosin. Another class of medications, 5-α-reductase inhibitors, such as finasteride, may help improve voiding symptoms. If medications are ineffective, surgical intervention with transurethral resection is warranted.

DISEASES OF THE PENIS

I. Priapism is a persistent erection that is not associated with sexual stimulation or that continues after orgasm. The corpora cavernosa are affected, but the corpus spongiosum usually is spared. Priapism can be classified as low flow or high flow.

A. Low-flow priapism is an ischemic state in the corpora, secondary to prolonged erection and resultant edema of the cavernosal trabeculae. Symptoms include pain and tenderness. Stasis, thrombosis, fibrosis, and scarring of the corpora cavernosa eventually can result in erectile dysfunction (ED). The diagnosis is made by penile corporal aspiration, which demonstrates dark, crankcase oil–like blood with an acidic pH. Ischemia and acidosis appear after approximately 6 hours.

B. Priapism may occur in association with sickle cell anemia and has a 6% incidence among sickle cell patients. Patients may have a history of stuttering priapism lasting 2 to 6 hours, usually at night. Initial treatment should include aggressive hydration with intravenous fluid supplemented with 1 ampule of $NaHCO_3/L$ and oxygen to prevent further sickling. If these measures are unsuccessful, corporal aspiration injection as described below may be necessary.

C. Iatrogenic priapism can occur secondary to intracavernous injection of vasoactive substances (prostaglandin E_1, phentolamine, papaverine) used to treat ED. Oral α-agonists, such as terbutaline or pseudoephedrine, may be effective up to one-third of the time in iatrogenic priapism. If oral treatment fails, aspiration and irrigation of the corpora (see below) should be performed. Psychotropic agents, antihypertensive agents (hydralazine, guanethidine, prazosin), and alcohol account for 20% of priapism. The antidepressant trazodone has been shown to induce priapism (*Med Lett Drugs Ther* 1984; 26:35).

D. Neoplasm (especially leukemia), with venous occlusion, stasis, and emboli, can result in priapism. Treatment is with chemotherapy and radiotherapy.

E. Treatment
 1. For patients with sickle cell disease, primary treatment involves aggressive hydration, supplemental oxygen, and blood transfusion if the hematocrit is low.
 2. **First-line treatment** involves aspiration of old blood from the corpora via a 21-gauge needle.
 3. An **α-adrenergic agent** (phenylephrine, 250 to 500 μg) can then be injected. The solution is prepared by mixing 1 mL of phenylephrine (10 mg/mL) in 19 mL sterile normal saline. Each mL contains 500 μg phenylephrine. Doses can be repeated every 5 to 10 minutes. Patients should be monitored for the possible hemodynamic effects of phenylephrine. Topical or subcutaneous injection of lidocaine before therapeutic injection or irrigation can be helpful for patient comfort. Injections and aspiration should be performed laterally at the 3 o'clock and 9 o'clock positions to avoid the dorsal blood supply of the penis.
 4. If evacuation of old blood and injection of α-adrenergic agents fails, **surgical shunting** should be considered.
    a. The **Winter shunt** involves creation of a fistula between the glans penis (corpus spongiosum) and corpus cavernosum. This is done with a core (Tru-Cut) needle after a penile block.
    b. The **Al-Ghorab procedure** is a more aggressive open surgical modification of the Winter shunt. It involves a glandular incision, exposing the tips of the corpora; a 5-mm ellipse of the tunica albuginea is removed to create a cavernosospongiosal shunt.
    c. Finally, the more proximal **side-to-side cavernosospongiosal shunt (Quackels shunt) or the cavernosaphenous shunt** may be necessary when distal shunting procedures fail. Circumferential compressive dressings should never be used after shunting because they can obstruct venous drainage, resulting in further tissue ischemia.

F. High-flow priapism is a nonischemic state usually brought about by perineal or genital trauma. A traumatic pudendal arterial fistula or cavernosal artery laceration may give rise to a high-flow state. Diagnosis is confirmed by aspiration of bright-red, well-oxygenated blood. Blood gas analysis can be helpful in differentiating low-flow priapism from high-flow priapism. Treatment is accomplished by embolization of the ipsilateral branch of the pudendal artery.

II. Erectile dysfunction (ED) recently has received increasing attention from the public and lay media as a result of new treatment modalities. Minimal, moderate, or complete ED may affect up to 50% of men aged 40 to 70 years; incidence increases with age.

A. Initial evaluation includes complete history and physical examination, with a focus on eliciting possible underlying causes of ED, including heart disease, hypertension, diabetes, renal insufficiency, and endocrine abnormalities (hypogonadism, hyperprolactinemia). Smoking alone or in combination with any of these risk factors can increase the incidence of ED.

B. Attention should be paid to medications, such as antihypertensives [central-acting agents (clonidine), α-adrenergic blocking agents (prazosin), beta-blocking agents], antipsychotics, tricyclic antidepressants, and histamine H_2 blockers (cimetidine), that may be associated with ED. Cigarette smoking and heavy use of alcohol can also lead to ED. Previous pelvic or penile surgery may be associated with ED. The timing of onset of ED (sudden versus gradual) should be noted, as should the presence of nocturnal or morning erections. Loss of libido may signal hormonal disturbances.

C. Physical examination should focus on genital development and signs of endocrinologic or neurologic abnormalities.

D. Appropriate laboratory testing includes serum chemistries, including creatinine, CBC count, urinalysis, and, when indicated, a limited hormonal evaluation (testosterone and prolactin). Additionally, screening for diabetes and hypercholesterolemia should be done.

E. For the majority of patients, ED is multifactorial, and no single cause is identified. In these cases, it is appropriate to counsel patients about available nonsurgical options for treatment and to allow them a trial of one or more of these methods until a satisfactory solution is found. Available medical options include the following:

1. **Hormone replacement.** Exogenous testosterone is available in a variety of delivery methods, including parenteral preparations and transdermal therapy. Liver function tests should be monitored. This treatment is best suited for patients with a low libido and documented hypogonadism. The effect of testosterone on erectile function is variable.

2. **Oral therapies.** Sildenafil citrate (Viagra) is a selective type 5 phosphodiesterase inhibitor that inhibits the breakdown of cyclic guanosine monophosphate, allowing smooth-muscle relaxation in the corpus cavernosum. Typical doses are 50 to 100 mg taken 1 hour before sexual activity. Sildenafil is effective in 60% of men, regardless of etiology. Side effects include headache, facial flushing, and dyspepsia. Sildenafil citrate is contraindicated in patients who are taking nitrates because of a synergistic effect, which results in excessive reduction in blood pressure. Also, sildenafil should not be used within 6 hours of taking an alpha-blocker. Other oral therapies, tadalafil and vardenafil, have recently been introduced. Tadalafil has the advantage of having a prolonged half-life.

3. **Intracavernosal therapy.** Injection of vasoactive medications, such as alprostadil (prostaglandin E_1), directly into the corpus cavernosum is effective in 70% to 80% of patients. Side effects are pain with injection, hematoma or ecchymosis, and priapism. An intraurethral alprostadil suppository is also available and is effective in some men.

4. **Medical devices.** For men who do not desire or are not candidates for medical therapy, there are several devices that may aid in getting and maintaining an erection. A vacuum pump is efficacious, but many couples find it cumbersome and uncomfortable. Patients with difficulty in maintaining an erection due to cavernosal venous insufficiency may benefit from a constriction band.

5. **Surgical options.** For patients who are refractory to noninvasive therapy, consideration may be given to a surgically placed penile implant. These devices have a high degree of success but have the disadvantage of being

irreversible, and there are potential complications, such as infection (2%) and mechanical malfunction (2%).

DISEASES OF THE SCROTUM AND TESTICLES

I. **Management of scrotal emergencies.** Acute scrotal pathology can result in significant morbidity, testicular loss, and infertility. The diagnosis can be difficult to make and may require scrotal exploration.

  A. **Testicular torsion** develops most often in the peripubertal (12 to 18 years old) age group, although it can occur at any age.

   1. The **clinical picture** is one of acute onset of testicular pain and swelling, commonly associated with nausea and vomiting. Some patients give a history of a prior episode that spontaneously resolved (intermittent torsion). There usually is no history of voiding complaints, dysuria, fever, or exposure to sexually transmitted diseases.

   2. **Physical examination** reveals an extremely tender, swollen testicle high in the scrotum with a transverse lie. The cremasteric reflex (elicited by stroking the inner thigh) is absent on the affected side. In contrast to epididymitis, elevation of the scrotum does not provide relief of pain (Prehn sign) in torsion. Normal urinalysis and the absence of leukocytosis help to rule out epididymitis.

   3. When the **clinical diagnosis** is equivocal, radiographic studies may be helpful. Depending on availability, nuclear scintigraphy and color Doppler ultrasound have similar sensitivity in evaluating testicular torsion (*Radiol Clin North Am* 1997;35:959).

   4. **Treatment** should not be delayed to obtain imaging. If testicular torsion is suspected, urgent scrotal exploration is indicated. Manual detorsion of the testicle may be attempted in the emergency room, but orchiopexy is still indicated. Typically, the testicle is detorsed by rotating from a medial to lateral direction. Testicular viability is a function of the reestablishment of perfusion (Table 40-4). Contralateral testicular fixation should be performed at the time of surgery.

  B. **Torsion of testicular appendage (appendix testis)** can present with symptoms similar to those of torsion of the testicle, usually in a prepubertal boy. The onset commonly is over 12 to 24 hours.

   1. **Extreme tenderness over the appendage** exists, usually on the superior aspect of the testicle. The "blue dot" sign may be present when the ischemic appendage can be seen through the scrotal skin. The testicle has a normal position and lie. Careful examination reveals that the testicle and the epididymis are not diffusely tender or swollen. The cremasteric reflex usually is present. Imaging studies may be necessary if the clinical diagnosis is unclear (see above).

   2. **Torsion of the testicular appendage** usually is managed expectantly. Pain is best controlled with anti-inflammatory agents and gradually resolves over 7 to 14 days.

Table 40-4. Rate of salvage in testicular torsion

Duration of ischemia (hr)	Salvage rate (%)
0–6	85–97
6–12	55–85
12–24	20–80
>24	<10

Adapted from American Urological Association. *Torsion of the Testis: Changing Concepts.* AUA Update Series IX. American Urological Association; 1990.

C. Mild epididymitis usually presents with a 1- to 2-day onset of unilateral testicular pain and swelling associated with dysuria or urethral discharge.
  1. Typically, the **findings** include a painful, indurated epididymis and pyuria. Urinalysis, urine culture, and CBC count are obtained. When clinically indicated, urethral swabs for gonococci and chlamydiae are sent for culture.
  2. With **appropriate antibiotic coverage,** these patients can be managed as outpatients. For patients in whom the etiology is gonococcal or chlamydial, ceftriaxone (125 to 250 mg intramuscularly) is given in the emergency room, followed by doxycycline (100 mg orally two times a day for 7 days). Azithromycin, 1 g orally as a one-time dose, is as effective as doxycycline in the treatment of chlamydial infections [*MMWR* 1998;47(RR-1):51]. In older men (>35 years of age), enterobacteria are more common, and a fluoroquinolone, such as ciprofloxacin (500 mg orally two times a day), provides broad coverage until culture sensitivities can be obtained. Nonsteroidal analgesics and scrotal elevation can reduce inflammation and provide symptomatic relief.
  3. Moderate to severe cases of epididymitis may require hospital admission. Symptoms usually have been present for several days. Fever and leukocytosis are present. Broad-spectrum antibiotics and supportive measures of bedrest with scrotal elevation should be instituted. Ultrasonography can be useful to rule out abscess formation and assess testicular perfusion.
D. Fournier gangrene is a severe polymicrobial soft-tissue infection involving the genitals and perineum. Although the term *Fournier gangrene* usually is applied to men, necrotizing fasciitis of this area can occur in women. Prompt diagnosis and institution of treatment may be lifesaving. Roughly 25% of the patients have a genitourinary source, 25% have an anorectal source, up to 10% have an intra-abdominal source, and nearly 40% have an unidentified source. Diabetic, alcoholic, and other immunocompromised patients appear more susceptible. The clinical course is one of abrupt onset with pruritus, rapidly progressing to edema, erythema, and necrosis, often within a few hours. Fever, chills, and malaise are accompanying signs.
  1. **Physical examination** reveals edema and erythema of the skin of the scrotum, phallus, and perineal area. This may progress rapidly to frank necrosis of the skin and subcutaneous tissues, with extension to the skin of the abdomen and back, reaching as high as the clavicles and down the thighs. Crepitus in the tissues suggests the presence of gas-forming organisms.
  2. **Laboratory evaluation** should include a CBC count, serum electrolytes, creatinine, arterial blood gas, coagulation parameters, urinalysis, urine, and blood cultures. A KUB plain film may reveal subcutaneous gas.
  3. **The patient should be stabilized and prepared emergently for the operating room.** Broad-spectrum antibiotics that are active against both aerobes (including *Staphylococcus aureus*, β-hemolytic *Streptococcus* species, *Pseudomonas* species, *Escherichia coli*, and *Klebsiella* species) and anaerobes (including *Bacteroides* and *Clostridium* species) should be started immediately. Aerobic and anaerobic wound cultures are usually polymicrobial.
  4. **Wide débridement** is required, with aggressive postoperative support. The testicles are often spared, as they have a blood supply discrete from the scrotum; orchiectomy is rarely indicated. Wound closure and dermal coverage often is an extensive process, and recovery requires intense physical therapy and wound care. Despite improvements in critical care, antibiotics, and surgical technology, **mortality** still exceeds 30% in some recent series (*Urology* 1996;47:935).
II. Nonacute scrotal masses
  A. Hydroceles generally are asymptomatic fluid collections around the testicle that transilluminate. Ultrasound evaluation is recommended to rule out serious underlying causes such as testicular malignancies. If hydroceles

do enlarge and become symptomatic, they can be repaired by a variety of transscrotal techniques. Hydroceles in infants may be associated with a patent processus vaginalis; parents give a history of intermittent scrotal swelling. These hydroceles usually resolve by 1 year of age. Those that persist can be repaired by an inguinal approach.

B. Spermatoceles are benign cystic dilations involving the tail of the epididymis or proximal vas deferens.

C. Varicoceles are abnormal tortuosities and dilations of the testicular veins within the spermatic cord. On physical examination, they feel like a "bag of worms." A varicocele may diminish in size when the patient is supine. Because the left gonadal vein drains directly into the renal vein, varicoceles are much more common on the left side. Right-sided varicoceles may be associated with obstruction of the inferior vena cava. Varicoceles are the most common surgically correctable cause of male infertility; however, most men with varicoceles remain fertile. Varicocele repair results in improved semen quality in approximately 70% of patients. Treatment of varicoceles is indicated for diminished testicular growth in adolescents, infertility, or significant symptoms. Varicoceles may be treated by spermatic vein embolization or spermatic vein ligation via a laparoscopic, open, or microvascular approach. Any patient who presents with a new-onset varicocele later in life warrants retroperitoneal imaging to rule out a malignancy causing venous obstruction.

III. Testicular tumors are the most common solid tumors in 15- to 35-year-old men. The estimated lifetime risk for testicular malignancy is 1 in 500. Owing to improved multimodality therapy, overall 5-year survival for testis cancer is now 95%.

A. The typical clinical finding is a painless testicular mass, although one-third of patients may present with pain. Pulmonary or gastrointestinal complaints or the presence of an abdominal mass may reflect advanced disease. Scrotal sonography is mandatory; seminomas appear as a hypoechoic lesion, and nonseminomatous tumors appear inhomogeneous. α-Fetoprotein, β-human chorionic gonadotropin, and lactic acid dehydrogenase are serum tumor markers that help to identify the tumor type and completely stage the tumor. The markers are used to monitor the effectiveness of therapy and to screen for recurrence.

B. Staging of testicular tumors is outlined in Table 40-5. Serum tumor markers have recently been added to the staging system.

C. Initial therapy for all testicular tumors is radical inguinal orchiectomy. The type of tumor and the stage of the disease determine further therapy.

   1. Seminomas constitute 60% to 65% of germ cell tumors. Low-stage seminomas are treated with adjuvant radiation therapy to the retroperitoneum. Advanced disease is usually treated with a platinum-based chemotherapy regimen.

   2. Nonseminomatous tumors include the histologic types of embryonal carcinoma, teratoma, choriocarcinoma, and yolk sac elements, alone or in combination. Nonseminomatous tumors are more likely to present with advanced disease. Patients with clinically negative retroperitoneal nodes with normal tumor markers are treated with retroperitoneal lymph node dissection, prophylactic chemotherapy, or close observation. Patients with high-stage disease with elevated markers receive platinum-based chemotherapy followed by retroperitoneal node dissection if there is residual disease.

GENITOURINARY TRAUMA

Genitourinary injuries should be identified during the secondary survey after life-threatening injuries have been addressed and initial resuscitation has been undertaken.

   I. Renal injury is a component of approximately 10% of abdominal traumas. Blunt trauma accounts for 80% to 90% of renal injuries. Penetrating trauma occurs

Table 40-5. American Joint Committee on Cancer staging of testicular cancer

Stage	Tumor (T)[a]	Node (N)[b]	Metastasis (M)[c]	Serum tumor markers (S)
0	Tis	N0	M0	S0
IA	T1	N0	M0	S0
IB	T2–4	N0	M0	S0
IS	Any T	N0	M0	S1–3
IIA	Any T	N1	M0	S0
	Any T	N1	M0	S1
IIB	Any T	N2	M0	S0
	Any T	N2	M0	S1
IIC	Any T	N3	M0	S0
	Any T	N3	M0	S1
IIIA	Any T	Any N	M1a	S0
	Any T	Any N	M1a	S1
IIIB	Any T	Any N	M0	S2
	Any T	Any N	M1a	S2
IIIC	Any T	Any N	M0	S3
	Any T	Any N	M1a	S3
	Any T	Any N	M1b	Any S

	Serum tumor markers		
	Lactate dehydrogenase	Human chorionic gonadotropin (mIU/mL)	Alpha-fetoprotein (ng/mL)
S0	≤Normal	≤Normal	≤Normal
S1	<1.5 × N	<5,000	<1,000
S2	1.5–10 × N	5,000–50,000	1,000–10,000
S3	>10 × N	>50,000	>10,000

[a]Tis, intratubular germ cell neoplasia; T1, limited to testis; T2, beyond tunica albuginea or into epididymis; T3, invades spermatic cord; T4, invades scrotum.
[b]N0, no node metastasis; N1, one node metastasis, <2 cm; N2, one node metastasis, 25 cm, or multiple nodal metastases, each <5 cm; N3, node metastasis >5 cm.
[c]M0, no metastasis; M1, nonregional nodal or pulmonary metastasis; M2, nonpulmonary visceral metastasis.

as a result of gunshot wounds or stab wounds and accounts for 10% to 20% of renal injuries. The grading system for renal injuries is shown in Table 40-6.

A. Blunt renal trauma should be suspected in patients with abdominal tenderness, lower rib fractures, vertebral fractures, or flank contusions.

B. Microscopic hematuria (>3 RBCs per high-power field) or gross hematuria is present in more than 95% of patients with a renal injury. A voided specimen is best for urinalysis, but if the patient cannot void or is unconscious and no blood is at the meatus, a well-lubricated urethral catheter should gently be passed.

C. All patients with **gross hematuria and blunt trauma** should be evaluated with a CT scan using intravenous contrast. Patients with microscopic hematuria and shock (systolic blood pressure <90 mm Hg) should be imaged with a CT scan after they are stabilized. Patients with microscopic hematuria, no shock, and no evidence of significant deceleration or renal injury do not need radiographic evaluation of their urinary system (*J Urol* 1989;141:1095).

D. The **degree of hematuria** does not correlate with the severity of the injury (*J Urol* 1978;120:455), and any patient with a suspected renal injury due to rapid deceleration requires radiographic evaluation. Disruption of the

Table 40-6. Renal injury scale of the American Association for the Surgery of Trauma

Renal injury scale	Injury	Description
I	Contusion	Microscopic or gross hematuria; urologic studies normal
	Hematoma	Nonexpanding perirenal hematoma confined to the renal retroperitoneum
II	Hematoma	Subcapsular, nonexpanding without parenchymal laceration
	Laceration	<1 cm parenchymal depth of renal cortex without urinary extravasation
III	Laceration	>1 cm parenchymal depth of renal cortex without collecting system rupture or urinary extravasation
IV	Laceration	Parenchymal laceration extending through the renal cortex, medulla, and collecting system
	Vascular	Main renal artery or vein injury with contained hemorrhage
V	Laceration	Completely shattered kidney
	Vascular	Avulsion of renal hilum that devascularizes the kidney

ureteropelvic junction should be considered in children with deceleration or hyperextension injuries.

- **E.** The majority of **blunt renal injuries** can be managed conservatively; fewer than 10% of blunt renal injuries require surgery (*World J Urol* 1999;17:71).
- **F.** **Penetrating renal trauma** with microscopic hematuria (>3 RBCs per high-power field) or gross hematuria requires radiographic assessment with CT scan or an IVP. Preferably, this is done before exploration to evaluate the injured kidney and to confirm function of the contralateral kidney. The presence of a normal contralateral kidney may influence the surgeon's decision (repair versus nephrectomy) on management of the injured kidney. Intraoperative palpation of a contralateral kidney may be misleading.
- **G.** A **high-dose, single-shot IVP** with a 2-mL/kg bolus injection of contrast followed by a single film at 10 minutes can be performed in the trauma suite or in the operating room without interfering with other critical elements of the trauma evaluation and resuscitation.
- **H.** **Indications for intraoperative renal exploration** include an expanding, pulsatile, or unconfined retroperitoneal hematoma; all grade V renal injuries; and renal injuries that have not been completely staged.
- **II. Ureteral injuries** account for approximately 3% of all urologic traumas. A high index of suspicion often is necessary to make the diagnosis, and many ureteral injuries have a delayed presentation.
  - **A.** The most common scenario is **penetrating trauma with multiple associated injuries.** The absence of gross or microscopic hematuria has been documented in 30% of patients.
  - **B.** **Radiographic findings** include extravasation and, more commonly, delayed function; proximal dilation; and deviation of the ureter. A CT may demonstrate medial extravasation; delayed images are necessary to assess ureteral patency. Retrograde pyelography is the most sensitive diagnostic tool but may be difficult to obtain in the setting of acute trauma.
  - **C.** **Adequately visualizing the ureter during laparotomy** is important for diagnosing ureteral injury; intravenous or intraureteral injection of indigo carmine or methylene blue may help to assess the integrity of the urothelium.
  - **D.** For purposes of determining the **type of repair,** the ureter is divided into thirds.
    - **1.** Injuries to the distal one-third of the ureter are best managed by **ureteral reimplantation.** Additional length to provide a tension-free anastomosis

may be gained by using a Psoas hitch and, if necessary, a Boari bladder flap.

  2. Injuries of the middle or upper third of the ureter are best managed by **ureteroureterostomy.** An omental wrap may be used to protect the repair. Stents and drains are recommended for all ureteral repairs (*World J Urol* 1999;17:78).

III. Bladder injuries result from blunt trauma, penetrating trauma, and iatrogenic injury during surgical procedures.

  A. Ninety-five percent of bladder injuries present with **gross hematuria.** Anyone with a history of blunt or penetrating trauma, gross hematuria, and difficulty in urinating should be evaluated with a cystogram.

  B. A **Foley catheter** is placed if a urethral injury is not suspected (see Section IV below). A scout film is obtained. Standard radiographic contrast is diluted to a 50:50 mix with saline and is infused under gravity. When 100 mL have been instilled, an anteroposterior radiograph is taken. If no extravasation is seen, the bladder is filled to 350 mL under gravity, and an anteroposterior and oblique radiograph is obtained. A postdrainage film is mandatory.

  C. **Upper tract imaging** can then be done. If a CT scan is obtained, a CT cystogram may be substituted for a plain radiographic or fluoroscopic cystogram. The bladder should be filled retrograde by gravity via an indwelling Foley catheter with 350 mL dilute (3% to 5%) contrast. Postdrainage films are not necessary; merely clamping the Foley to allow bladder filling with excreted contrast does not constitute an adequate study. An IVP or CT scan alone is not adequate to evaluate bladder trauma.

  D. **Management**
    1. All patients with penetrating trauma to the bladder and intraperitoneal extravasation of contrast require **surgical exploration and repair** of the bladder (*World J Urol* 1999;17:84).
    2. Often, patients with blunt trauma and extraperitoneal extravasation of contrast can be managed nonoperatively with **catheter drainage** for 10 days.

IV. Genital and urethral injuries

  A. **Urethral injuries** occur in 5% of patients with pelvic fractures. Posterior urethral injuries involve the prostatic and membranous urethra to the level of the urogenital diaphragm. These injuries are caused mainly by blunt trauma.

  B. **Urethral injury** should be suspected when blood is at the meatus or the mechanism of injury is such that urethral injury might have occurred. Physical examination in patients with urethral injury may reveal penile and scrotal edema and ecchymosis. Rectal examination can reveal a high-riding prostate or boggy hematoma in the expected position of the prostate.

  C. A **retrograde urethrogram** is performed by placing a 14 or 16 Fr. Foley catheter into the urethra so that the balloon is 2 to 3 cm beyond the meatus. The balloon is inflated with 1 to 2 cc to seat it in the fossa navicularis. With the patient in a 30-degree oblique position, 25 to 30 mL half-strength contrast medium is injected through the catheter. The radiograph is exposed when the contrast is nearly completely injected. If the urethra is normal, the balloon can be deflated, the catheter advanced into the bladder, and a cystogram performed.

  D. **Anterior urethral injuries** include injuries to the bulbous and penile urethra distal to the urogenital diaphragm. Straddle injuries and penetrating trauma are the most common causes of these types of injuries. Injuries contained by the Buck fascia often have a characteristic "sleeve of penis" pattern, whereas urethral or penile injuries in which the Buck fascia is disrupted are contained by the Colles fascia and have a "butterfly" appearance on the perineum.

  E. **Complete disruptions** of the posterior urethra can be managed by primary endoscopic realignment or by suprapubic diversion and delayed repair. **Partial disruptions** may be managed with catheter drainage for 14 to 21 days

(*World J Urol* 1998;16:69). These injuries are often associated with formation of urethral strictures and with impotence.

F. **Minor penile lacerations and contusions** can be managed in the emergency room. **Serious blunt or penetrating trauma** with injury to the corpus cavernosum is best managed with surgical exploration, débridement, and repair of the corporal injury. A retrograde urethrogram is necessary to rule out urethral injury. Broad-spectrum antibiotics should be given, particularly in human bite injuries.

G. **Testicular injury** may occur as a result of blunt or penetrating trauma. History and physical examination are the keys to diagnosis of testicular rupture. The presentation is marked by acute and severe pain, often with associated nausea and vomiting. Physical examination may reveal a hematoma or ecchymosis of overlying skin. All penetrating scrotal gunshot wounds deep to the dartos fascia require surgical exploration. Ultrasonography only has a specificity of 75% and a sensitivity of 64% in identifying testicular injury. The orchiectomy rate is below 10% for ruptured testicles explored within 72 hours after injury. Repair consists of hematoma evacuation, débridement of the necrotic tubules, and closure of the tunica albuginea (*World J Urol* 1999;17:101).

H. **Scrotal avulsion and skin loss** are most often a result of motor vehicle accidents. Because of the redundancy and vascularity of scrotal skin, a variety of options are available for local flaps and coverage of the testicles. Wounds should be copiously irrigated and débrided; clean wounds may be closed in layers, whereas grossly contaminated wounds should be cleaned and packed with sterile gauze dressings.

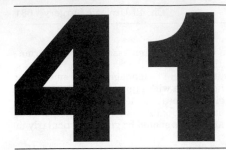

Obstetric and Gynecologic Surgery

Mary E. Abusief,
Barbara M. Buttin,
David E. Cohn, and
Thomas J. Herzog

OBSTETRIC AND GYNECOLOGIC DISORDERS

I. **Vaginal bleeding** to an abnormal degree may result from a variety of causes. A thorough history, including pattern and intensity of bleeding, and physical examination is sufficient to determine the etiology. A pregnancy test must be performed in all women of reproductive age. Hemoglobin (Hgb) and hematocrit (Hct) should be determined if the abnormal bleeding is chronic or heavy. Endometrial biopsy should be performed in all postmenopausal women to rule out endometrial carcinoma or if hormonal intervention is planned. Evaluation and treatment depend on the presentation and etiology.

   A. **Obstetric etiologies.** Approximately 30% to 40% of all pregnancies are associated with some vaginal bleeding, and approximately half of these are spontaneously aborted.

   1. **Terminology**
      a. **Threatened abortion:** any vaginal bleeding during the first half of pregnancy, cervix closed
      b. **Missed abortion:** fetal death with retention of products of conception, cervix closed
      c. **Inevitable abortion:** cervical dilatation with or without ruptured membranes
      d. **Incomplete abortion:** partial passage of products of conception, cervix open
      e. **Complete abortion:** expulsion of all products of conception from the uterine cavity, cervix closed

   2. **Presentation and clinical features.** Patients classically present with vaginal bleeding and crampy midline lower abdominal pain. Bleeding from the urethra or rectum or from lacerations of the cervix or vagina should be excluded. Complaints of passage of tissue may represent a complete or incomplete abortion.

   3. **Physical examination.** Vital signs are within normal ranges unless extensive vaginal bleeding or septic abortion occurs, with resultant tachycardia and hypotension. Septic abortions can cause elevated temperatures, marked suprapubic tenderness, or purulent discharge through the cervical os.

   4. **Laboratory investigation**
      a. **Hgb and Hct.** Plasma volume expansion in pregnancy may result in a lower mean Hgb during the second trimester. With acute blood loss, the Hgb and Hct can be normal until compensatory mechanisms restore normal plasma volume.
      b. **White blood cell (WBC) count with differential** is useful to evaluate elevated temperatures. Septic abortion is associated with a left shift and an elevated WBC count.
      c. **Blood type and screen** are useful to identify Rh-negative patients at risk for isoimmunization (see Section I.A.6.g).
      d. **Quantitative beta subunit of human chorionic gonadotropin (hCG).** The sensitivity of a pregnancy test (urine or serum) can vary greatly depending on the type of test performed (i.e., latex agglutination, enzyme-linked immunosorbent assays, radioimmunoassay). Most institutions

use very sensitive serum pregnancy tests; however, the sensitivity of the urine pregnancy test may be more variable. A urine pregnancy test has the advantage of requiring only a few drops of urine and gives a rapid result. Unlike the serum pregnancy test, however, the urine pregnancy test is unable to be quantified, which is helpful when evaluating the status of a pregnancy. Serial quantitative (serum) hCG values may be used along with ultrasonography to distinguish an early viable pregnancy from an abnormal pregnancy. In most normal intrauterine pregnancies near 6 weeks' gestation, hCG increases by at least 66% every 48 hours (*ACOG Pract Bull 3*, December 1998). Patients with stable clinical examinations can be followed with serial hCG values until reaching the sonographic threshold values at which ultrasound visualization of an intrauterine pregnancy is possible (see Section I.A.5).

- **e. Progesterone levels** in excess of 15 ng/mL usually are associated with a normal intrauterine pregnancy. Below this range, pregnancy is likely abnormal, but location may be intrauterine or extrauterine.

5. Imaging studies. Ultrasonography may be useful in demonstrating a viable pregnancy. The sonographic threshold value of hCG for vaginal probe ultrasonography is generally >2,000 mIU/mL, international reference preparation, although you should be able to see a gestational sac at 1,500 mIU/mL. For abdominal ultrasonography, the threshold is >6,000 mIU/mL. Cardiac activity can be seen at 10,000 mIU/mL.

6. Treatment

- **a. Threatened abortion.** Patients with a pregnancy that is viable or of indeterminate viability, vaginal bleeding, and a closed internal cervical os are followed expectantly with repeat ultrasound in 7 days or repeat hCG in 48 hours, or both.
- **b. Missed abortion.** Patients may be followed expectantly or undergo evacuation. If they are followed expectantly for more than 3 to 4 weeks, coagulation studies [i.e., complete blood cell (CBC) count, prothrombin time, partial thromboplastin time, fibrinogen, and fibrin degradation products] should be monitored because of the risk of disseminated intravascular coagulopathy. Counsel patients to bring any tissue passed back to the hospital for pathologic verification. Generally, after 3 weeks evacuation is suggested, and the individual should be scheduled as an outpatient.
- **c. For inevitable abortion,** the uterus usually begins to contract, resulting in expulsion of products before infection develops. Patients occasionally are followed expectantly with monitoring for infection but typically undergo uterine evacuation. If fever develops, intravenous antibiotics with polymicrobial coverage are administered, followed by evacuation of the uterus. These patients require admission and careful monitoring of coagulation factors.
- **d. For incomplete abortion,** bleeding, cramping, and an open internal os usually are found. Uterine evacuation is indicated. If products of conception are not recovered, ectopic pregnancy should be considered.
- **e. For complete abortion,** all products of conception have been expelled, and the cervix is closed. Bleeding and cramping are minimal. Only short-term observation for stability is necessary.
- **f. Evacuation of the uterus.** Suction curettage is done safely in the first trimester and can be performed in the emergency room if significant cervical dilatation exists. A stable patient with a first-trimester missed abortion that requires dilation of the cervix undergoes dilation and curettage (D & C) as an outpatient. In the second trimester, a dilation and evacuation or medical induction of labor under gynecologic consultation is performed. After curettage, prophylactic antibiotics (doxycycline, 100 mg orally two times a day for 7 days), ergot alkaloids (methylergonovine maleate, 0.2 mg orally three times a day for 2 to 3 days), and antiprostaglandins (ibuprofen, 800 mg orally every

8 hours as needed for pain) commonly are prescribed. If heavy vaginal bleeding, abdominal pain, or fever occurs after evacuation, investigation for retained products, uterine perforation, and endometritis is warranted.

g. **Rho immune globulin (RhoGAM)** is given to any pregnant patient with vaginal bleeding who is Rh negative and has a negative antibody screen. The recommended dose of RhoGAM is 300 μg intramuscularly after the first trimester. For first-trimester events, 50 μg intramuscularly is sufficient (*ACOG Pract Bull 4*, May 1999).

h. **Pathology.** Any tissue passed or obtained on uterine evacuation must be evaluated for chorionic villi. If villi are not identified, further investigation is necessary to exclude ectopic pregnancy or incomplete abortion.

B. **Nonobstetric etiologies of vaginal bleeding** (Table 41-1)

II. **Abdominal pain.** The differential diagnosis for nongynecologic causes includes appendicitis, gastroenteritis, ischemic bowel, ureteral colic, urinary tract infection, and cholecystitis. Pregnancy should be excluded in all women of reproductive age.

A. **Ectopic pregnancy** occurs when the blastocyst implants outside the uterine cavity; 97% of cases occur in a fallopian tube (tubal pregnancy).

1. **Presentation and clinical features.** Although more than 90% of patients with tubal pregnancies have abdominal or pelvic pain, some may be asymptomatic. Early (unruptured) pregnancies often present with amenorrhea, vaginal spotting, and colicky, vague lower abdominal pain, whereas ruptured ectopics often present with severe pain, syncope, dizziness, and lightheadedness. Pleuritic chest pain and shoulder pain from diaphragmatic irritation can also occur.

2. **Physical examination.** Vital signs vary greatly, from normal blood pressure and pulse to hypotension and tachycardia from cardiovascular collapse secondary to hemorrhage. Whereas patients with unruptured ectopic pregnancy may demonstrate only mild tenderness, peritoneal signs, including marked tenderness, rigidity, guarding, and rebound, may be found. Pelvic masses sometimes are palpable, but lack of a mass does not exclude ectopic pregnancy. The uterus may appear small for dates.

3. **Laboratory investigation**

a. **CBC.** Hgb and Hct may indicate the degree of hemorrhage except in acute cases. The WBC count typically is normal or slightly elevated and **lacks a left shift.**

b. **Blood type and screen** should be obtained to identify Rh-negative patients and to cross-match blood for possible transfusion (see Section I.A.6.g).

c. **hCG.** Although ectopic pregnancy can occur with any quantitative serum hCG value, these data can be useful for ultrasound interpretation. Serial hCG values that do not increase appropriately are suspicious for an ectopic pregnancy (see Section I.A.4.d).

d. **Progesterone** values rarely aid in the diagnosis of ectopic pregnancy (see Section I.A.4.e).

4. **Imaging studies.** Ultrasonography is most useful in excluding a tubal pregnancy by demonstrating an intrauterine gestational sac or fetus. With a quantitative hCG <1,500 mIU/mL, this may not be possible, and stable patients should be followed with serial hCG titers. However, with an hCG <2,500 mIU/mL, absence of a gestational sac in the uterus indicates either nonviable intrauterine or ectopic pregnancy. Ultrasound findings consistent with ectopic pregnancy include a uterus without a well-formed gestational sac, possibly free intraperitoneal fluid, and, sometimes, an adnexal mass representing the tubal pregnancy.

5. **Diagnostic studies**

a. **Culdocentesis** is useful for detecting hemoperitoneum but is painful and contraindicated in the presence of a cul-de-sac mass or bleeding

Table 41-1. Nonobstetric causes of vaginal bleeding

Differential diagnosis	Laboratory data	Signs and symptoms	Treatment
Menses	CBC count, urine hCG	Cyclic bleeding every 21–35 days	Iron therapy if indicated
Dysfunctional uterine bleeding	CBC count, urine hCG, endometrial biopsy if >35 yr, duration >6 mo	Noncyclic bleeding; may have associated dysmenorrhea, fatigue, or dizziness	Hormonal therapy if patient is hemodynamically stable; if hemodynamically unstable, transfuse as needed, i.v. estrogen or high-dose oral contraceptive pills
Infection: gonorrhea/chlamydia cervicitis	Cervical culture, wet prep	Purulent vaginal discharge, possible spotting	Ceftriaxone, 125 mg i.m. × 1; azithromycin, 1 g p.o. × 1
Trichomonas vaginitis	Wet prep	Yellow-green frothy vaginal discharge, possible spotting	Metronidazole, 500 mg p.o. b.i.d. × 7 days or 2 g p.o. × 1 (if pregnant, defer treatment to second trimester)
Sexual trauma	Rape kit	Vaginal bleeding and/or discharge	Emergency contraception, prophylactic treatment for sexually transmitted diseases; if laceration, pack vagina, possible surgical repair
Malignancy	Endometrial biopsy, Pap smear, cervical biopsy	Postmenopausal bleeding, postcoital bleeding, intermenstrual bleeding	Refer to gynecologic oncologist

CBC, complete blood cell; hCG, human chorionic gonadotropin.

diathesis. It is used infrequently because sonographic evaluation for free intraperitoneal fluid often is sufficient. A culdocentesis is performed with a speculum in the vagina and a single-toothed tenaculum on the posterior cervical lip to lift the cervix anteriorly and expose the uterosacral ligaments. An 18-gauge spinal needle with a 10-mL syringe is placed aseptically in the midline of the posterior vaginal fornix. Aspiration of clear yellow fluid is normal. If no fluid is obtained, the test is nondiagnostic. If clotting blood is obtained, an intravascular source is likely, and no conclusions can be drawn. If nonclotting blood is obtained, especially with an Hct above 15%, there is a hemoperitoneum, consistent with (but not diagnostic of) ruptured ectopic pregnancy.

b. D & C can be performed to differentiate between ectopic pregnancy and incomplete abortion after excluding a normal early intrauterine pregnancy. Chorionic villi are suggested if curettage products float in saline. If villi are not identified, laparoscopy to exclude ectopic pregnancy is indicated.

6. Treatment

a. Surgical therapy. The majority of ectopic pregnancies are treated surgically.

(1) **Laparoscopy** is preferred for diagnosis and treatment of tubal pregnancy; however, laparotomy is indicated if the patient is hemodynamically unstable.

(2) **Conservative surgical therapy** is recommended in patients who wish to preserve reproductive potential. **Linear salpingotomy** in the antimesosalpinx portion of the tube performed with fine-tip electrocautery is preferable when the ectopic pregnancy is unruptured and is located in the ampulla of the tube. After removal of the pregnancy from the tube, the base is irrigated, and hemostasis is achieved with cautery. The tube is left to heal by secondary intention. **Segmental resection** often is performed when the tube is ruptured and the ectopic pregnancy is in the isthmic (proximal) portion of the tube; interval reanastomosis can be performed.

(3) **Nonconservative surgical therapy** includes **salpingectomy** (removal of tube) for tubal rupture or severe hemorrhage and **cornual resection** for interstitial pregnancies. Pregnancy rates after salpingectomy have been shown to be equivalent to those following linear salpingotomy, although the incidence of recurrent ectopic pregnancy may be slightly higher with salpingostomy.

(4) **Follow-up.** Patients treated with conservative surgical management, or after rupture or spillage of trophoblastic tissue, have a 5% incidence of persistent viable trophoblastic tissue. Weekly quantitative hCG values should be followed until negative. If the levels plateau or increase, reevaluation is indicated.

b. Medical therapy with methotrexate, a folic acid antagonist, can be used in compliant outpatients who are hemodynamically stable. Indications for ectopic pregnancy treatable with methotrexate include size of ectopic ≤3.5 cm in diameter, an intact tube, no fetal heart motion or evidence of hemoperitoneum, and an hCG <10,000 mIU/mL. Prior to treatment, patients should be extensively counseled about risks, benefits, and need for follow-up. Baseline labs, including hCG, Rh factor, CBC, and hepatic enzymes, should be obtained. The most common side effects of therapy are bloating and flatulence. Transient rise in hepatic enzymes may be observed. Less frequent side effects include stomatitis, hair loss, and anemia. Repeat quantitative hCG levels should be drawn on day 4 and day 7. If hCG levels fail to decline <15% between days 4 and 7, a second dose of methotrexate should be administered and a new day 1 assigned. Methotrexate quantitative hCG values are followed until negative. Approximately 20% of patients have an inappropriate fall in hCG levels and require surgical intervention. *Separation pain* refers to the increase in abdominopelvic discomfort that is commonly experienced by patients undergoing treatment and is thought to be caused by tubal stretching during resolution of the pregnancy. Patients are counseled to rest and take oral analgesics but warned to seek immediate reevaluation to rule out rupture if pain does not resolve within 1 hour (Copeland LJ, *Textbook of Gynecology.* 2nd ed. Philadelphia: W.B. Saunders; 2000).

B. Pelvic inflammatory disease (PID) is a polymicrobial infection of the upper genital tract. The majority of cases occur in sexually active young women between the ages of 15 and 30 years. It rarely occurs in nonmenstruating women and is extremely rare during pregnancy. Factors promoting progression of infection from the lower to upper genital tract can result from events that cause breakdown of the cervical mucus barrier, including douching, IUD insertion, hysteroscopy, D & C, endometrial biopsy, and hysterosalpingography. Risk factors include a history of sexually transmitted diseases or PID, multiple sexual partners, and age <25 years.

1. **Presentation and clinical features.** Patients with PID typically have lower abdominal and pelvic pain, which may be constant, dull, sharp, or crampy. PID is aggravated by movement and often occurs around or during menses. Approximately 75% of patients have purulent vaginal discharge, fewer than 50% have abnormal vaginal bleeding, and only 33% manifest fever. Nausea and vomiting with associated ileus may occur but are usually late symptoms.

2. **Physical examination** reveals lower abdominal tenderness, including peritoneal signs of guarding and rebound, adnexal tenderness, and cervical motion tenderness; an adnexal fullness or a mass may be found. PID is often accompanied by a mucopurulent vaginal discharge. Cervical motion tenderness is a nonspecific sign of peritoneal irritation that can be elicited in any female patient with peritonitis from any cause, and therefore it is not pathognomonic of PID.

3. **Laboratory investigation.** Pregnancy must be excluded. Elevated WBC count and elevated erythrocyte sedimentation rate suggest a severe infection. A wet-smear examination of a drop of vaginal discharge in a few drops of isotonic saline under high magnification usually reveals numerous WBCs. A cervical swab for DNA probe analysis of *Neisseria gonorrhoeae* and *Chlamydia trachomatis* should be obtained. Bloody samples may give false-negative results. Alternatively, cultures for *N. gonorrhoeae* and *C. trachomatis* can be obtained by using a urine assay (uriprobe).

4. **Imaging studies.** Ultrasonography is used to detect tubo-ovarian abscess if a mass is palpated on examination or if no improvement is noted after 48 hours of antibiotic treatment. In general, the management of patients with PID is rarely modified by ultrasound results. Abdominal plain films, ultrasonography, or computed tomographic (CT) scan also may be used to investigate other etiologies of a patient's pain if the diagnosis is uncertain.

5. **Diagnostic studies**
   a. The Centers for Disease Control and Prevention (CDC) has issued guidelines for diagnosis of acute PID that are intended to serve as clinical criteria for initiating treatment. **Minimum criteria** include low abdominal tenderness, adnexal tenderness, and cervical motion tenderness. **Additional criteria** include temperature $>101°F$ (38.3°C), abnormal cervical/vaginal discharge, elevated erythrocyte sedimentation rate, elevated C-reactive protein, and documented infection with *N. gonorrhoeae* or *C. trachomatis*. **Definitive criteria** include histopathologic evidence of endometritis on endometrial biopsy, transvaginal ultrasound showing fluid-filled tubes or tubo-ovarian abscesses (TOAs), and laparoscopic abnormalities consistent with PID.
   b. **Culdocentesis** seldom is necessary to make the diagnosis of PID. However, aspiration of purulent material confirms an infectious process (see Section II.A.5.a).
   c. **Laparoscopy** revealing erythema and edema of the fallopian tubes and purulent material confirms the diagnosis and provides the opportunity to collect direct cultures of infected organs. Laparoscopy should not be considered a routine means of establishing a diagnosis.

6. **Treatment** of PID depends on the severity of the infection.
   a. **Inpatient therapy** is indicated for patients with nausea and vomiting, possible surgical emergencies, pregnancy, suspicion for TOA, immunodeficiency, or failed outpatient therapy or for patients in whom preservation of reproductive potential is very important. According to CDC guidelines from 2000, inpatient treatment is provided by cefotetan, 2 g intravenously every 12 hours, or cefoxitin, 2 g intravenously every

6 hours, and doxycycline, 100 mg orally or intravenously every 12 hours (alternatively, clindamycin, 900 mg intravenously every 8 hours, and gentamicin, 2 mg/kg intravenous load followed by 1.5 mg/kg intravenously every 8 hours, can be used). Other alternative regimens include ofloxacillin, 400 mg intravenously every 12 hours, and metronidazole, 500 mg intravenously every 8 hours; ampicillin/sulbactam, 3 g intravenously every 6 hours, and doxycycline, 100 mg intravenously or orally every 12 hours; and ciprofloxacin, 200 mg intravenously every 12 hours, doxycycline, 100 mg intravenously or orally every 12 hours, and metronidazole, 500 mg every 8 hours. Inpatient treatment is continued until the patient is afebrile for 48 hours and has decreased pain on pelvic examination. Patients then are treated with oral doxycycline for a total of 14 days. Patients with discrete pelvic fluid collections and TOAs may be candidates for drainage by interventional radiologists; concurrent antibiotics should be administered.

   b. **Outpatient therapy** includes one dose of ceftriaxone, 250 mg intramuscularly, followed by doxycycline, 100 mg orally two times a day for 14 days (alternatively, ofloxacin, 400 mg orally two times a day, and metronidazole, 500 mg orally two times a day for 14 days, can be used) [*MMWR* 2002;51(RR06):1–80]. Patients should be followed up within 48 to 72 hours to ensure adequate progress.

   c. In patients with TOAs who are not responding to intravenous antibiotics after 48 hours, **surgery** should be considered. Generally, surgery should be reserved for patients with symptomatic pelvic masses or ruptured TOAs and for draining TOAs in patients failing intravenous antibiotics. Ultrasound-guided transvaginal aspiration of TOAs is another option that may benefit patients who are not responding to intravenous antibiotics.

C. **Corpus luteal cysts** develop from mature follicles in the ovary. Intrafollicular bleeding can occur 2 to 4 days after ovulation, creating a hemorrhagic cyst. Corpus luteal cysts usually are ≤4 cm in diameter but can be >12 cm. These can occur in the pregnant or nonpregnant state. Diagnosis can be difficult in pregnancy, as a cyst may be confused with ectopic pregnancy.

   1. **Presentation and clinical features.** Patients can be asymptomatic or may present with unilateral dull lower abdominal and pelvic pain. If the cyst has ruptured, the patient may complain of sudden, severe lower abdominal pain.

   2. **Physical examination** reveals adnexal enlargement or tenderness, or both; if the cyst has ruptured, signs of peritoneal irritation can be present. Hemodynamic stability must be ensured, as some patients can bleed significantly from a hemorrhagic cyst.

   3. **Laboratory investigation.** A CBC count and an hCG should always be obtained. Ultrasound can aid in visualizing a cyst or free fluid in the pelvis, indicative of recent cyst rupture. Culdocentesis may be performed to search for blood in the cul-de-sac in cases of suspected cyst rupture.

   4. **Treatment** usually is conservative, allowing for spontaneous resolution. Oral contraceptive pills (OCPs) to suppress ovulation and future cyst formation, as well as analgesia with nonsteroidal anti-inflammatory drugs or short courses of narcotics, can be prescribed. Surgical treatment with laparoscopic cystectomy is rarely indicated unless significant intraperitoneal hemorrhage is present.

D. **Adnexal torsion** accounts for an estimated 3% of gynecological emergencies requiring immediate operative intervention. Torsion occurs when the ovary or tube, or both, twist on the infundibulopelvic ligament. Incomplete torsion results in occlusion of the venous and lymphatic channels, causing cyanotic and edematous adnexa. With complete torsion, the arterial supply is interrupted, with subsequent ischemia and necrosis of the adnexa. Adnexal torsion occurs most commonly in the reproductive age group, more frequently on the right side, and typically with large ovaries or ovarian masses. In 20%

of cases, concurrent pregnancy is present, in 50% to 60% of cases a benign ovarian tumor may be present (Copeland LJ, *Textbook of Gynecology.* 2nd ed. Philadelphia: W.B. Saunders; 2000).

1. **Presentation and clinical features.** Patients with torsion present with acute, severe, sharp, intermittent unilateral lower abdominal or pelvic pain. The pain is proportional to the degree of vascular obstruction. Intermittent torsion may present with periodic pain for days to weeks from twisting and untwisting of the adnexa. The pain often is related to a sudden change in position. Approximately two-thirds of patients experience nausea, whereas few have fever.

2. **Physical examination** can reveal tachycardia or bradycardia (from vagal stimulation) and fever if there is necrosis. Unilateral abdominal tenderness or a tender adnexal mass often is found on pelvic examination.

3. **Diagnostic studies.** Ultrasonography may visualize an adnexal mass. Doppler ultrasound has moderate sensitivity and specificity in diagnosing torsion. Blood flow around the adnexa is reassuring but does not exclude the diagnosis of torsion. Laparoscopy confirms the diagnosis.

4. **Treatment** involves immediate surgical intervention. If only partial torsion or no evidence of tissue necrosis exists and the patient desires future fertility, preservation of adnexa with untwisting and stabilization is possible. Cyst resection and exclusion of underlying malignancy (rare) should be performed. If necrosis of the adnexa is present or the ovary is felt to be definitively nonviable, salpingo-oophorectomy should be undertaken.

E. **Fibroids or leiomyomas** are benign tumors of uterine smooth muscle that vary in size from <1 cm to >20 cm.

1. **Presentation and clinical features.** Although most fibroids are asymptomatic, one-third of patients have dysmenorrhea or abnormal menstrual bleeding, including menorrhagia (heavy menses) or metrorrhagia (intermenstrual bleeding). Symptoms also can result from local compression of the bladder or rectum. Fever and acute pain responsive to high-dose NSAID therapy may be associated with fibroid degeneration.

2. **Physical examination** reveals an enlarged, irregular uterus.

3. **Diagnostic studies.** Ultrasonography confirms uterine size and the presence of myomas. In patients older than 35 years with abnormal bleeding, an endometrial biopsy should be performed to rule out endometrial pathology, including hyperplasia and carcinoma.

4. **Treatment** is determined by symptoms and the patient's desire for future fertility. Prostaglandin synthetase inhibitors, including ibuprofen (200 to 800 mg every 6 to 8 hours) or naproxen sodium (220 to 550 mg every 6 hours); hormonal therapy, including OCPs and medroxyprogesterone acetate to regulate bleeding; and gonadotropin-releasing hormone agonist to shrink the tumor can be used. Surgery (myomectomy or hysterectomy) is reserved for patients with failed medical management.

F. **Dysmenorrhea** is painful lower abdominal cramping that occurs just before and during menses. It affects 40% of women of reproductive age and often is accompanied by other symptoms, including diaphoresis, tachycardia, headache, nausea, vomiting, and diarrhea.

1. The **etiology** of dysmenorrhea is thought to be related to increased prostaglandin levels.

2. **Treatment** includes prostaglandin synthetase inhibitors, such as ibuprofen (400 to 800 mg) or naproxen sodium (220 to 550 mg orally every 6 hours) beginning before the onset of menses, or OCPs to suppress ovulation.

G. **Adnexal masses** are often found incidentally either on pelvic examination or intraoperatively. To guide the surgeon in their management, criteria have been developed that aid in assessing the malignant potential of adnexal masses.

1. **Presentation and clinical features.** Most adnexal masses are asymptomatic unless they are associated with torsion or large enough to

compress surrounding structures. Less than 2% of adnexal masses are malignant.
2. **Physical examination** reveals adnexal fullness or a discrete mass. Attention should be paid to the mobility of the mass and to the solid versus cystic components.
3. **Diagnostic studies.** Ultrasound can reveal the size and characteristics of adnexal masses. CT is less useful for visualizing the pelvis.
4. **Treatment.** A very large (>10 cm) adnexal mass warrants laparotomy. Smaller masses in premenopausal women may be observed for 6 to 8 weeks unless certain factors make it likely to be malignant. If it grows or persists on repeat ultrasound, surgery is indicated. Controversy exists regarding the management of small, asymptomatic adnexal masses in postmenopausal women. Small, unilocular cysts may be observed for some time, although most practitioners have a lower threshold for surgery in this age group. Laparoscopy has been shown to be as effective and safe as laparotomy for the removal of masses <10 cm, with decreased associated morbidity and shorter hospital stays. Fixed and solid masses or those associated with ascites require laparotomy and a gynecologic oncologist on standby. Benign adnexal masses frequently encountered include benign cystic teratomas (dermoid cysts), endometriomas, and serous and mucinous cystadenomas. Dermoids and serous cystadenomas are frequently bilateral and warrant close inspection of the contralateral ovary. Mucinous cystadenomas can be associated with pseudomyxoma peritonei. In those cases, inspection of the appendix is important, as appendiceal mucoceles and carcinomas can also result in pseudomyxoma. Other benign, solid ovarian tumors include Brenner tumors, fibromas, and thecomas.
III. **Nonobstetric surgery in the pregnant patient.** Common indications for major surgery in the pregnant patient are appendicitis, adnexal mass, and cholecystitis. It is preferable to treat pregnant patients conservatively, if possible, deferring surgery to the postpartum period; however, delay of an indicated surgical procedure can be devastating. If nonemergent surgery is required, it is safest to proceed in the second trimester. Surgery in the first trimester carries a risk of fetal loss and malformation because organogenesis occurs during this period. Surgery in the third trimester carries a risk of inducing preterm labor.
A. **Preoperative considerations.** Patients are at increased risk for aspiration because of upward displacement of the stomach and the inhibitory effects of progesterone on gastrointestinal motility. A nonparticulate antacid should be given shortly before induction of anesthesia. In the second half of pregnancy, the left lateral position should be used to decrease venacaval and aortic compression. Fetal heart tones should always be documented pre- and postoperatively.
B. Trocar placement for **laparoscopy in pregnancy** is best accomplished by an open technique, with the additional trocars inserted under direct visualization. Laparoscopy in pregnancy has primarily been used for cholecystectomy. The second trimester is the maximum gestational age for safe laparoscopy in pregnancy because the uterus is not large enough to obstruct visualization and room for manipulation exists. Intra-abdominal carbon dioxide insufflation appears safe up to 14 mm Hg and is unlikely to alter the acid-base balance in the fetus. Preliminary data suggest that laparoscopic surgical procedures may result in decreased morbidity and mortality, a lower overall cost with shorter hospitalizations, and a decreased risk of thromboembolic disease compared with laparotomy.
C. **Anesthetic** selection is based on the maternal condition and the planned surgical procedure. For general anesthesia, all patients should be intubated using cricoid pressure to minimize the risk of aspiration. Anesthetic inhalation agents and narcotic analgesia commonly are used. Regional anesthesia may be complicated by episodes of hypotension, which is potentially poorly tolerated by patient and fetus. Most commonly administered anesthetics are acceptable for use in pregnancy.

D. Postoperatively, fetal-uterine monitoring and tocolytic agents are used, depending on gestational age and degree of maternal symptoms.

IV. Trauma in pregnancy

A. Presentation and clinical features. Trauma is a frequent event during pregnancy; it is the leading cause of morbidity and mortality in the United States in women younger than 40 years of age. Initial interventions are aimed at stabilization of the mother according to advanced cardiac trauma life support protocols. After initial survey of the mechanism and extent of injury, establishment of fetal age and monitoring of fetal heart tone (if feasible) are undertaken.

B. Types of abdominal trauma

1. **Penetrating trauma** places the uterus and fetus at great risk during the later stages of pregnancy. Evaluation and treatment are similar to those in the nonpregnant patient, with the usual necessity of surgical exploration. Amniocentesis to establish fetal lung maturity or to detect bacteria or blood may be helpful if time permits.

2. **Blunt trauma** in pregnancy is associated most often with motor vehicle accidents. Despite the concern for abdominal seat-belt injuries, restrained pregnant patients fare better than those who are unrestrained. Intrauterine or retroplacental hemorrhage must be considered because 20% of the cardiac output in pregnancy is delivered to the uteroplacental unit.

3. **Abruptio placentae** occurs in 1% to 5% of minor and 40% to 50% of major blunt traumas. Focal uterine tenderness, vaginal bleeding, hypertonic contractions, and fetal compromise frequently occur. Disseminated intravascular coagulopathy may occur in almost one-third of abruptions, and a disseminated intravascular coagulation panel, including fibrinogen and a Kleihauer-Betke screen to assess for fetal-maternal hemorrhage in Rh-negative patients, should be ordered.

   a. **Management of abruptio placentae** depends on fetal age and degree of placental separation and blood loss as estimated on ultrasonography. At viability, continuous fetal heart monitoring is done, and route of delivery is dictated by both fetal and maternal cardiovascular stability, with immediate cesarean section undertaken if evidence of severe compromise exists.

C. Special considerations of trauma in pregnancy

1. **Fetal-uterine monitoring** is effective in determining fetal distress, abruptio placentae, and preterm labor caused by trauma. These measures are instituted for gestations >20 weeks. Doptones are sufficient for previable pregnancies after 12 weeks of gestation.

2. **Ultrasonography** is an effective tool for establishing gestational age, fetal viability, placental state, and placental location.

3. In **positioning** the pregnant patient, avoid placing her supine to optimize venous return. During cardiopulmonary resuscitation, a 10- to 15-degree wedge into the left lateral decubitus position should be used, if possible.

4. **Tetanus prophylaxis** should be administered in the same manner and for the same indications as in the nonpregnant patient.

5. **Peritoneal lavage,** usually by the open, supraumbilical technique, can be used to detect intraperitoneal hemorrhage while avoiding the uterus, which is localized by examination and ultrasonography (*J Trauma* 1989;29:1628).

6. **Radiation** in the form of diagnostic studies places the fetus at potential risk for spontaneous abortion (first several weeks of pregnancy), teratogenesis (weeks 3 to 12), and growth retardation (>12 weeks of gestation). These effects and secondary childhood cancers are unlikely at doses of <10 rads (chest film, <1 rad; CT scan of abdomen and pelvis, 5 to 8 rads). Uterine shielding should be used when possible. Studies should be ordered judiciously, but x-rays that are deemed important for evaluation should not be omitted (*ACOG Educ Bull* 236, April 1997).

7. **Perimortem or postmortem cesarean section** should be accomplished within 10 minutes of maternal cardiopulmonary arrest to optimize neonatal prognosis and maternal response to resuscitation.

8. **Isoimmunization** must be considered in the Rh-negative patient, and RhoGAM is administered when fetal maternal hemorrhage is suspected (see Section I.A.6.g).

9. All blood product **transfusions should be screened** and negative for cytomegalovirus.

10. **Prophylactic cephalosporins** are safe in all trimesters of pregnancy.

V. **Gynecologic malignancies.** The female genital tract accounts for more than 80,000 new cases of invasive carcinoma annually in the United States, resulting in approximately 27,000 deaths in 2001. Mortality would be reduced by earlier detection because 5-year survival rates approach 90% with proper treatment when these cancers are diagnosed at stage I (confined to primary organ) but fall to 30% to 50% when diagnosed at advanced stages. A brief overview of vulvar, cervical, endometrial, and ovarian cancers is presented, with emphasis on diagnosis and initial management. A complete discussion of gynecologic malignancies, including less common cancers (vaginal, fallopian tube, and gestational trophoblastic disease), is beyond the scope of this manual. Patients should be referred to a gynecologic oncologist for specialized care and comprehensive management.

A. **Vulvar carcinoma.** Vulvar cancer is primarily a disease of postmenopausal women, and the average age at diagnosis is 68 years. The etiology has been linked to human papillomavirus infection in younger patients, and vulvar cancer is associated with chronic vulvar conditions, including dystrophies, lichen sclerosis, and condylomata. Squamous cell histology predominates (90%), followed by melanoma and adenocarcinoma.

1. **Presentation and clinical features.** Vulvar cancer often presents as a hyper- or hypopigmented lesion. It may be ulcerating, pruritic, painful, or asymptomatic and may have been treated with a variety of antibiotics and ointments before diagnosis.

2. **Diagnosis.** Accurate diagnosis requires biopsy and histopathologic evaluation of suspicious areas.

3. **Treatment** of vulvar cancer depends on the stage. Surgery ranging from local excision to radical vulvectomy with bilateral groin lymph node dissection generally is the primary treatment. Local, groin, and pelvic adjuvant radiation is administered, depending on the surgical pathologic findings. In cases of basal cell carcinoma, wide local excision is sufficient.

4. **Prognosis** depends on the extent of disease. Patients with stage I tumors have a 5-year survival of ≥90%, whereas those with positive lymph nodes have a 5-year survival of <40%, depending on the number and location of positive lymph nodes.

B. **Cervical carcinoma.** The incidence of invasive cervical cancer has dramatically decreased (but preinvasive disease has markedly increased) in the United States, owing largely to widespread institution screening by cervical cytology (Papanicolaou smears). This success in cervical screening has not been duplicated worldwide; cervical cancer remains by far the leading cause of mortality among gynecologic malignancies in less developed countries. Approximately 12,000 new cases were diagnosed in 2003, with an estimated 4,000 deaths. The goal is to diagnose and treat disease of the cervix in the preinvasive state. This is accomplished by aggressive evaluation of abnormal Papanicolaou smears with colposcopy-guided biopsies for appropriate patients (see ALTS trial, 2001). Risk factors for cervical cancer include a history of sexually transmitted diseases, HIV infection, human papillomavirus, multiple sex partners, engaging in sexual intercourse at an early age, lower socioeconomic status, and smoking.

1. **Presentation and clinical features.** Patients may be asymptomatic or present with irregular or postcoital vaginal bleeding. A foul-smelling or watery discharge may also be present. Advanced stages may present with

leg pain (sciatic nerve involvement), flank pain (ureteral obstruction), or renal failure.

2. **Diagnosis** is by biopsy via speculum examination of a visible or palpable nodule, or both. Staging remains clinical and is based on a thorough bimanual and rectovaginal examination, cystoscopy, and proctoscopy. Appropriate adjuvant radiographs include chest x-ray, intravenous pyelogram, and barium enema. PET scan is a useful diagnostic modality for assessing distant disease activity. Stage is never changed by intraoperative findings and remains the most important prognostic factor, with an 88% 5-year survival for stage I disease and a 38% 5-year survival for stage III disease (Table 41-2).

3. **Treatment** depends on stage and lymph node status.

   a. **Microinvasive disease** (stage IA1, depth of invasion <3 mm, diameter <7 mm, negative lymph vascular space invasion) can be treated with cervical conization alone or with extrafascial hysterectomy. Lesions with greater depth of invasion, multifocal disease, or upper-vaginal involvement (stages IA2 to IIA) require a radical hysterectomy, which removes the parametria and upper vagina and includes a complete pelvic and sometimes para-aortic lymphadenectomy. Although radical hysterectomy is only appropriate for a subset of patients, radiotherapy is applicable to any patient with early-stage cervical cancer. The most common complication after radical hysterectomy is bladder dysfunction. Ureteral fistulas, infection, hemorrhage, and lymphocyst formation are more rare.

   b. **Radiotherapy** is the appropriate treatment for advanced-stage disease. Combined surgery and radiotherapy for advanced stages does not increase survival but dramatically increases the rate of complications

Table 41-2. Cervical cancer staging

TNM	FIGO	Definition
T1	I	Cervical carcinoma confined to the uterus (extension to the corpus should be disregarded)
T1a	IA	Preclinical invasive carcinoma, diagnosed by microscopy only
T1a1	IA1	Microscopic stromal invasion no greater than 3 mm in depth and no wider than 7 mm
T1a2	IA2	Tumor with stromal invasion between 3 and 5 mm in depth and no wider than 7 mm
T1b	IB	Tumor confined to the cervix but larger than IA2
T1b1	IB1	Clinical lesions no greater than 4 cm in size
T1b2	IB2	Clinical lesions greater than 4 cm in size
T2	II	Tumor invades beyond the cervix but not to the pelvic side wall or the lower third of the vagina
T2a	IIA	Tumor without parametrial involvement
T2b	IIB	Tumor with parametrial involvement
T3	III	Tumor extends to the pelvic side wall and/or involves the lower one-third of the vagina and/or causes hydronephrosis or nonfunctioning kidney
T3a	IIIA	Tumor invades lower third of the vagina with no extension to the pelvic side wall
T3b	IIIB	Tumor extends to the pelvic side wall and/or causes hydronephrosis or a nonfunctioning kidney
T4	IVA	Tumor invades mucosa of the bladder or rectum and/or extends beyond the true pelvis
M1	IVB	Distant metastasis

FIGO, International Federation of Gynecology and Obstetrics; TNM, tumor, node, metastasis.

in the form of obstruction, strictures, and fistula formation. The prescription of radiation is based on stage, lesion size, and lymph node status. Both external-beam (teletherapy) and intracavitary (brachytherapy) radiation are used in various combinations. Complications from radiotherapy depend on dose, volume, and tissue tolerance. Acute complications include transient nausea and diarrhea. Early complications occur within the first 6 months after treatment and include skin ulceration, cystitis, and proctitis. Late complications may occur any time thereafter and include bowel obstruction secondary to strictures, fistulas, and chronic proctosigmoiditis. Recent studies indicate that adding cisplatin to radiation in locally advanced (stages IIB to IVA) and early-stage high-risk disease (stages IB to IIA with pelvic node involvement, parametrial involvement, or positive surgical margins) decreases the risk of dying from cervical cancer by 30% to 50% over radiation alone.

   c. Patients with **pelvic recurrence** after radical hysterectomy are often treated with radiation. Following primary radiation treatment, patients with central recurrence may be candidates for pelvic exenteration. Five-year survival ranges from 20% to 62% after exenteration, with an operative mortality of 10%. Response to chemotherapy in recurrent cervical cancer is generally poor.

 4. **Uncontrolled bleeding** from cervical cancer per vagina occasionally is encountered in the emergency department. In most cases, bleeding can be stabilized with tight vaginal packing, after which a transurethral Foley catheter should be placed. Acetone-soaked gauze is the most effective packing for vessel sclerosis and control of hemorrhage from necrotic tumor. Emergent radiotherapy may be necessary.

C. Endometrial carcinoma. Endometrial carcinoma is the most common gynecologic malignancy in the United States. Approximately 40,000 new cases were diagnosed in 2003. Most (approximately 90%) of these tumors are adenocarcinomas arising from the lining of the uterus. African American women have mortality rates nearly twice as high as Caucasian women. Risk factors for endometrial cancer include Caucasian race, obesity, early menarche and late menopause, nulliparity, tamoxifen therapy, estrogen replacement therapy, infertility, hereditary nonpolyposis colon cancer (HNPCC), and factors leading to unopposed estrogen exposure. Pregnancy and oral contraceptive use appear to be protective. Atypical endometrial hyperplasia is a precursor lesion and progresses to carcinoma in 23% of cases if left untreated. Only 1% to 3% of hyperplasia without atypia progresses to carcinoma. Hyperplasia can be treated conservatively with progestins and close observation. Extrafascial hysterectomy is suggested for persistent hyperplasia in patients who have completed their childbearing.

 1. **Presentation and clinical features.** The most common symptom is abnormal vaginal bleeding, often in the form of postmenopausal bleeding. Approximately three-fourths of patients present with stage I disease. Endometrial sampling should be considered mandatory in all postmenopausal patients with vaginal bleeding and any patient over 35 years of age with anovulatory uterine bleeding. Although endometrial carcinoma is rare in women younger than 35 years, patients in this age group who have persistent noncyclic vaginal bleeding or are nonresponsive to medical management should undergo endometrial assessment (*ACOG Pract Bull* 14, March 2000).

 2. **Physical examination** should include an assessment for obesity, hirsutism, and other signs of hyperestrogenism. The uterus may be enlarged or of normal size.

 3. **Diagnosis** is by transcervical aspiration (e.g., Pipelle), which usually is performed as an office procedure, or by hysteroscopy/D & C, which is performed in the operating room. Ultrasound can help suggest an intrauterine abnormality. Staging is done surgically.

4. **Treatment** generally consists of extrafascial total hysterectomy and bilateral salpingo-oophorectomy; pelvic and para-aortic lymphadenectomy is considered therapeutic and should be performed in all patients. Intraoperative evaluation of the uterus should be performed by bivalving the uterus and obtaining a frozen section as needed. Pelvic fluid should be obtained for cytology; omentectomy is sometimes performed. Adjuvant radiotherapy and/or chemotherapy is used postoperatively in patients with poor prognostic factors who are at high risk for recurrence. Hormonal therapy or chemotherapy is used for advanced disease, but response to chemotherapy has been poor.

5. **Prognosis** generally is favorable, with 5-year survival >90% for patients with surgical stage I tumors (Table 41-3). Prognosis depends on the grade of tumor as well as the depth of myometrial invasion, adnexal involvement, pelvic fluid cytology, and lymph node spread. Less common histologies, such as clear-cell or papillary serous cancers, and the sarcomas arising from the wall of the uterus do not enjoy the overall good prognosis of early-stage adenocarcinomas.

D. **Ovarian carcinoma.** Ovarian cancer is the deadliest of all the gynecologic malignancies. There were approximately 25,000 new cases diagnosed in 2003. More than two-thirds of patients in whom epithelial ovarian cancer is diagnosed eventually die from this disease (14,300 per year in the United States) (*CA* 2003;51:23). Besides tumors arising from the ovarian coelomic surface, which are the most common, germ cell (often in younger patients) and stromal primary tumors can occur. Two-thirds of epithelial ovarian cancers are diagnosed at advanced stages, with extraovarian metastasis. Incidence increases steadily with advancing age to a total lifetime incidence of 1 in 57. Risk factors include nulliparity, late menopause, early menarche, use of infertility drugs, and personal or family history of breast or ovarian cancer. Genetic cancer syndromes including the presence of *BRAC1* or *BRAC2* mutations, and hereditary nonpolyposis colon cancer (HNPCC) also has been associated with an increased risk of ovarian cancer. Prophylactic removal of ovaries and fallopian tubes has been suggested as a way to decrease the risk of gynecological cancer in these patients. Use of oral contraceptives, pregnancy, and tubal ligation appear to be protective.

Table 41-3. Endometrial cancer staging

TNM	FIGO	Definition
T1	I	Tumor confined to the corpus uteri
T1a	IA	Tumor limited to the endometrium
T1b	IB	Tumor invades less than or up to half of the myometrium
T1c	IC	Tumor invades more than half of the myometrium
T2	II	Tumor invades the cervix but does not extend beyond the uterus
T2a	IIA	Endocervical glandular involvement only
T2b	IIB	Cervical stromal invasion
T3	III	Local and/or regional spread as specified
T3a	IIIA	Tumor involves the serosa and/or adnexa and/or positive washings
T3b	IIIB	Vaginal involvement
N1	IIIC	Metastasis to the pelvic and/or para-aortic lymph nodes
T4	IVA	Tumor invades the bladder mucosa or the rectum and/or bowel mucosa
M1	IVB	Distant metastasis including intra-abdominal and/or inguinal lymph nodes

FIGO, International Federation of Gynecology and Obstetrics; TNM, tumor, node, metastasis.

Table 41-4. Ovarian cancer staging

TNM	FIGO	Definition
T1	I	Tumor limited to one or both ovaries
T1a	IA	Tumor limited to one ovary; capsule intact, no tumor on ovarian surface, no malignant cells in ascites or peritoneal washings
T1b	IB	Tumor limited to both ovaries; capsule intact, no tumor on ovarian surface, no malignant cells in ascites or peritoneal washings
T1c	IC	Tumor limited to one or both ovaries with any of the following: capsule ruptured, tumor on ovarian surface, malignant cells in ascites or peritoneal washings
T2	II	Tumor involves one or both ovaries with pelvic extension
T2a	IIA	Extension and/or implants on uterus and/or tubes; no malignant cells in ascites or peritoneal washings
T2b	IIB	Extension to other pelvic tissues; no malignant cells in ascites or peritoneal washings
T2c	IIC	Pelvic extension with malignant cells in ascites or peritoneal washings
T3	III	Tumor involves one or both ovaries with microscopically confirmed peritoneal metastasis outside the pelvis and/or regional lymph node metastasis
T3a	IIIA	Microscopic peritoneal metastasis beyond the pelvis
T3b	IIIB	Macroscopic peritoneal metastasis beyond the pelvis 2 cm or less in greatest dimension
T3c	IIIC	Peritoneal metastasis beyond the pelvis more than 2 cm in greatest dimension and/or regional lymph node involvement
M1	IV	Distant metastasis (excludes peritoneal metastasis)

FIGO, International Federation of Gynecology and Obstetrics; TNM, tumor, node, metastasis.

1. **Presentation and clinical features.** Women with early-stage disease are generally asymptomatic. In later stages, patients may present with vague abdominal pain or pressure, nausea, early satiety, weight loss, or swelling.
2. **Diagnosis** of ovarian cancer at early stages has proved clinically difficult (Table 41-4). No cost-effective screening test has yet been proved reliable in detecting stage I disease (confined to the ovaries). Bimanual examination remains the most effective means of screening, followed by surgery for histologic diagnosis. Ultrasonography of the pelvis (preferably transvaginal) and CT scan are effective adjuncts. CA 125 antigen is not effective for mass screening but serves as an effective tumor marker once diagnosis has been established and treatment is initiated.
3. **Treatment** is primarily surgical, with aggressive debulking and complete staging, even if inspection intraoperatively suggests that disease may be confined to one ovary. Complete staging is performed surgically and includes pelvic washings on entering the peritoneum, total abdominal hysterectomy, bilateral salpingo-oophorectomy, omentectomy, pelvic and para-aortic lymph node dissection, and peritoneal biopsies. Optimal cytoreduction (residual disease <1 cm) improves response to adjuvant chemotherapy and overall survival. In young women with early-stage disease, fertility-sparing surgery can often be performed, with removal of the uterus and contralateral ovary after childbearing is completed. However, complete staging at initial surgery is still necessary. Patients with disease outside the ovary are treated with six cycles of paclitaxel and platinum–based chemotherapy.

4. **Prognosis** correlates directly with stage and with the residual disease remaining after debulking. Median survival depends on optimal cytoreduction, with removal of all possible tumor at initial laparotomy. Median survival for optimally debulked advanced-stage tumors is nearly 80% at 1 year; the 5-year relative survival rate for all stages is 53% (*CA* 2003;51:23).

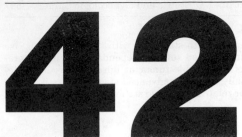

Common Surgical Procedures

Sunil M. Prasad and
Matthew G. Mutch

CATHETERIZATION, DRAINAGE, AND EMERGENCY AIRWAY PROCEDURES

I. **Central venous catheterization.** The ability to gain access to the central venous circulation rapidly and safely is essential for the management of surgical patients. Central venous catheterization is an important diagnostic tool for the measurement of central venous pressure, pulmonary wedge pressure, cardiac output, and mixed venous blood gases, as well as an important therapeutic tool in the delivery of intravenous fluids, blood products, medications, and total parenteral nutrition. Hemodialysis, plasmapheresis, chemotherapy, and the placement of inferior vena cava filters are also indications for central venous access. Several approaches to the central venous system exist, and depending on the indication, each has its advantages and disadvantages.

Absolute and relative contraindications for central venous catheterization exist. Venous thrombosis is an absolute contraindication to catheter placement in that vein. This may not become evident until the vein has already been cannulated, but once noted, an alternative approach should be used. Relative contraindications include coagulopathies (international normalized ratio >2 or partial prothrombin time >55 seconds), thrombocytopenia (platelet count <50,000/μL), ongoing sepsis, or the restless, combative patient in whom safe placement of a central venous catheter is difficult. The needle used to cannulate the venous system has the potential to cause significant damage to blood vessels, lung parenchyma, nerves, and soft tissue. Therefore, it is very important for the surgeon to set a limit on the number of unsuccessful passes to be made with the needle before abandoning the procedure and obtaining assistance.

A. **Internal jugular approach**
   1. **Indications.** The internal jugular vein is easily and rapidly accessible in most surgical patients. Several advantages of obtaining central venous access through the internal jugular vein exist: decreased risk of pneumothorax compared with the subclavian approach, direct access to the vessels in the case of bleeding, and the fact that the right internal jugular offers the most direct route to the right atrium. Therefore, it is the preferred route of access for short-term catheters; for thin, frail patients; and for the coagulopathic or thrombocytopenic patient. The right internal jugular vein is the preferred site for the placement of Swan-Ganz catheters because it offers the most direct path to the right atrium and pulmonary vasculature. In contrast, the left internal jugular vein has an indirect route to the pulmonary vasculature; therefore, Swan-Ganz catheters should be placed here only if the other approaches have been exhausted. For the unsedated or ambulatory patient, this is a difficult site to maintain. An internal jugular catheter is an uncomfortable site and may hinder the patient's neck movement. Keeping the insertion site dressed and sterile can be difficult. It is a site that should not be used for long-term access.
   2. **Technique.** The pulse of the common carotid artery is palpated at the medial border of the sternocleidomastoid (SCM) at midneck. The internal jugular vein is located lateral to the common carotid artery and courses slightly anterior to the artery as it joins the subclavian vein (Fig. 42-1). Two equally effective approaches to the internal jugular vein are

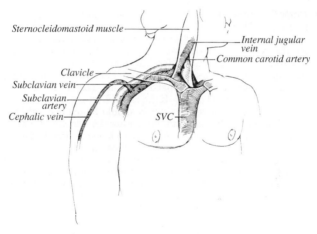

Sternocleidomastoid muscle

Internal jugular
vein
Common carotid artery

Clavicle
Subclavian vein
Subclavian
artery
Cephalic vein

SVC

Figure 42-1. Anatomy of the upper chest and neck, including the vasculature and important landmarks. SVC, superior vena cava.

advocated: the central and posterior approaches. The patient is placed in the Trendelenburg position at an angle of 10 to 15 degrees with his or her head flat on the bed and turned contralateral to the side of the line placement. The skin is prepared with povidone-iodine, and 1% lidocaine is infiltrated subcutaneously over the belly and lateral border of the SCM. The physician stands at the head of the bed for either approach. For the central approach, a 21-gauge "seeker" needle is introduced approximately 1 cm lateral to the carotid pulse into the belly of the SCM. At a 45-degree angle to the floor, the needle is slowly advanced toward the ipsilateral nipple. For the posterior approach, the seeker needle is introduced at the lateral edge of the SCM and directed toward the sternal notch at a 45-degree angle to the floor. The vein should be entered within 5 to 7 cm with both approaches. If the vein is not entered, the needle should be withdrawn and redirected for another pass. Redirection of the needle should be done just below the surface of the skin because the tip of the needle is capable of lacerating the vessels in the area. As previously mentioned, a limit on the number of passes should be set. Constant negative pressure is exerted on the syringe at all times, and entry into the vein is confirmed by the return of venous blood. A 14-gauge needle is then introduced just inferior to the seeker needle and is advanced along the same path until dark venous blood is aspirated. The **Seldinger technique** is carried out, whereby a flexible guidewire is passed into the vein through the 14-gauge needle, the needle is removed over the wire, and a nick is made in the skin at the puncture site to allow passage of the dilator. It is very important to maintain control of the guidewire at all times. The dilator creates a tract for the passage of the less rigid central venous catheter. The catheter is introduced over the wire and advanced to 15 to 20 cm so that its tip is at the junction of the superior vena cava (SVC) and the right atrium. In patients with difficult anatomy or vena cava filters fluoroscopy may be used to assess the position of the wire tip immediately. Aspiration of blood from all ports and subsequent flushing with saline confirm that the catheter is positioned in the vein and that all its ports are functional. The catheter is then secured to the patient's neck at a minimum of two sites, and a sterile dressing is applied. A chest x-ray is obtained to confirm the location of the catheter tip and to rule out the presence of a pneumothorax.

3. **Complications.** All percutaneously placed neck lines carry a risk of pneumothorax. This should be evaluated immediately after placement of the catheter with an anteroposterior chest x-ray. Every attempt at placement of a central venous catheter, successful or unsuccessful, should be followed by a chest x-ray before the catheter is used or line placement is attempted at another site. Inadvertent carotid artery puncture is usually tolerated in the noncoagulopathic patient. This is treated by direct pressure over the carotid artery. If the carotid artery is punctured, no further attempts at central venous access should be made on either side of the patient's neck. The patient's neck must be watched for the next 10 to 15 minutes for the development of a neck hematoma. In the hemodynamically unstable or poorly oxygenating patient, it is not always possible to distinguish venous blood from arterial blood by appearance. This can lead to inadvertent cannulation of the carotid artery. When this complication is recognized, the dilator or catheter should not be removed because this can lead to life-threatening hemorrhage, and help should be sought. The dilator is a rigid, large-bore device that is capable of injuring the subclavian or brachiocephalic vein during its advancement; therefore, great care must be taken when it is introduced and advanced. Advancement of guidewire into the right atrium can cause an arrhythmia, which usually resolves once the wire is withdrawn from the right atrium. Venous stenosis can occur at the site where the catheter enters the vein, which can lead to thrombosis of the vessel. Because the upper extremities and neck have extensive venous collaterals, stenosis or thrombosis is usually well tolerated. If the patient develops symptoms from a stenosis, the lesion can either be stented or undergo venoplasty. Air embolus, perforation of the right atrium or ventricle with resultant hemopericardium, and cardiac tamponade injury to the trachea, esophagus, thoracic duct, vagus nerve, phrenic nerve, or brachial plexus can all complicate the placement of neck catheters.

4. Treatment of **catheter-associated infections and sepsis** comprises removal of the catheter and institution of appropriate antibiotic therapy. Some advocate the routine replacement of indwelling central venous catheters every 3 to 7 days to prevent line sepsis (*Ann Surg* 1988;208:651). Other studies have failed to show significant reduction of catheter-associated infections with the prophylactic exchange of catheters versus replacing them as needed (*Crit Care Med* 1997;25:257). One study demonstrated that catheters made of polyurethane and impregnated with chlorhexidine and silver sulfadiazine reduced the incidence of catheter-related infections and increased the time that they could be left in place (*Ann Intern Med* 1997;127:257). Cuffs impregnated with antibiotics are advocated in some centers to prevent the migration of skin flora along the catheter tract in long-term catheters (*Am J Infect Control* 1988;16:79).

B. **Subclavian vein approach**

1. **Indications.** The subclavian approach to the central venous system is the least cumbersome to the patient and easiest to maintain. Therefore, it is the preferred site for long-term indwelling catheters. Because the left subclavian vein offers a direct route to the right atrium and the pulmonary vasculature, it is the second best site for the placement of a Swan-Ganz catheter. The clavicle overlies the subclavian vessels and does not allow direct access to the vessels; therefore, this approach should not be used in the coagulopathic or thrombocytopenic patient. Because of the significant risk of pneumothorax and lack of ability to control the vessels, the subclavian approach should be discouraged in emergency situations.

2. **Technique.** The subclavian vein courses posterior to the clavicle, where it joins the internal jugular vein and the contralateral veins to form the SVC (Fig. 42-1). The subclavian artery and the apical pleura lie just posterior to the subclavian vein. The patient is placed in the Trendelenburg

position with a rolled towel between the scapulas, which allows the shoulders to fall posterior. The skin is prepared with povidone-iodine, and 1% lidocaine is infiltrated subcutaneously in the infraclavicular space near the middle and lateral third of the clavicle. The infusion is carried into the deep soft tissue and to the periosteum of the clavicle. A 14-gauge needle is introduced at the middle third of the clavicle in the deltopectoral groove. Keeping the needle parallel to the plane of the floor, the needle is slowly advanced toward the sternal notch, deep to the clavicle. Constant negative pressure is applied to the syringe. Once the needle enters the subclavian vein, the guidewire, dilator, and catheter are introduced using the **Seldinger technique**, as previously described. As with the other approaches, all catheter ports are aspirated and flushed to ensure that they are functional. A chest x-ray is obtained to confirm the location of the catheter tip and to evaluate for pneumothorax. A supraclavicular approach to the subclavian vein has also been described (*South Med J* 1990;83:1178).

3. **Complications.** The complications of subclavian venous catheterization include those described in the previous section. Puncture of the subclavian artery can be troublesome because the clavicle prevents the application of direct pressure to achieve homeostasis. Therefore, this approach should be avoided in the patient with coagulopathy. If the artery is punctured, the patient should be monitored for the next 30 to 45 minutes to ensure that bleeding is not ongoing. Inadvertent cannulation of the subclavian artery with the dilator or catheter is a potentially fatal complication. The dilator or catheter should be left in place, and removal of the catheter and repair of the arteriotomy are to be done in the operating room. Particular attention must be paid to the placement of left subclavian catheters to avoid injuring the thoracic duct, brachiocephalic vein, and SVC with the needle or dilator because of the course of these vessels. Attention must be paid to the final position of the catheter tip when placed on the left side to avoid abutting the SVC wall, which poses the immediate or delayed risk of SVC perforation (*Chest* 1992;101:1633).

C. **Femoral vein approach**
1. **Indications.** The femoral vein is the easiest site for obtaining central access and is therefore the preferred approach for central venous access during cardiopulmonary resuscitation. This approach does not interfere with the other procedures of cardiopulmonary resuscitation. It should be remembered that a femoral vein catheter does not actually reach the central circulation and may not be ideal for the administration of vasoactive drugs. This may be the only site available in patients with upper-body burns. The femoral vein catheter inhibits patient mobility, and the groin is a difficult area in which to maintain sterility. Therefore, it should not be used in elective situations, except when upper-extremity and neck sites are not available.

2. **Technique.** The femoral artery crosses the inguinal ligament approximately midway between the anterosuperior iliac spine and the pubic tubercle. The femoral vein runs medial to the artery as they cross the inguinal ligament (Fig. 42-2). If possible, placing the patient in the reverse Trendelenburg position may help with venous cannulation. The skin is prepared with povidone-iodine, and 1% lidocaine is infiltrated in the subcutaneous tissue medial to the femoral artery and inferior to the inguinal ligament. The pulse of the femoral artery is palpated below the inguinal ligament, and a 14-gauge needle is introduced medial to the pulse at a 30-degree angle to the floor. It is directed cephalad with constant negative pressure until the vein is entered. The catheter is placed using the **Seldinger technique** previously described. When a femoral pulse cannot be palpated, as in cardiopulmonary arrest, the position of the femoral artery can be estimated to be at the midpoint between the anterosuperior iliac spine and the pubic tubercle, and the vein then lies 1 to 2 cm

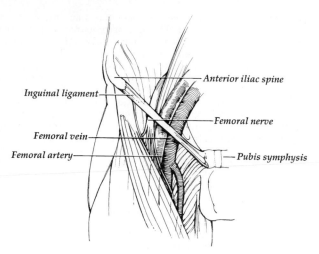

Figure 42-2. Anatomy of the femoral vessels.

medial to this point. Once the catheter is successfully placed, all three ports are aspirated and flushed to ensure that they are functional.

3. **Complications.** Injury to the common femoral artery or its branches during cannulation of the femoral vein can result in an inguinal or retroperitoneal hematoma, a pseudoaneurysm, or an arteriovenous fistula. The femoral nerve can be also be damaged. Injury to the inguinal lymphatic system can result in a lymphocele. The possibility of injuring peritoneal structures also exists, particularly if an inguinal hernia is present. Errant passages of the guidewire and the rigid dilator run the risk of perforating the pelvic venous complex and causing retroperitoneal hemorrhage. Late complications include infection and thrombosis of the femoral vein.

D. **Cephalic vein cutdown**

1. **Indications.** Cannulation of the cephalic vein under direct visualization has several advantages over the percutaneous approach to the central venous system. A decreased risk of pneumothorax exists, and bleeding complications are easily controlled. It is indicated in the patient with coagulopathy, the patient who cannot tolerate the Trendelenburg position, and the patient who would tolerate pneumothorax poorly. When repeated percutaneous attempts at vascular access have failed, cephalic vein cutdown should be considered. Some consider this the preferred approach for the placement of long-term vascular access devices. This approach should be attempted under strict sterile conditions, such as the operating room; bedside cephalic vein cutdown is discouraged.

2. **Technique.** The cephalic vein courses anterior along the deltoid muscle. It is reached most easily where it passes through the deltopectoral groove before turning posterior to enter the axillary vein (Fig. 42-1). Once the area over the lateral third of the clavicle has been prepared with povidone-iodine, 1% lidocaine is infiltrated subcutaneously over the deltopectoral groove, just medial to the coracoid process. A 3- to 4-cm incision is made in the skin parallel to the deltopectoral groove. The incision is carried down to the level of the clavicopectoral fascia. This fascia is incised, and the cephalic vein should then be easily identified. The vein is mobilized and ligated distally. A transverse venotomy is made, and the catheter is passed into the vein under direct visualization, with or without the assistance of a vein pick. The catheter position is confirmed via radiography or fluoroscopy.

3. **Complications.** Compared with the percutaneous approach, no significant difference in the complications of cephalic vein cutdown exists. Risk of pneumothorax, bleeding, air embolus, damage to the vessels, thrombosis, and infection remains, but the risk of pneumothorax and arterial injuries is significantly lower. Inadequate vein size and difficulty in cannulating the vein do lead to prolonged operative times and increase the need for additional cutdown sites (*Am Surg* 1984;208:651). Because the vein is ligated, its future use is compromised.

II. **Thoracic drainage procedures**
   A. **Thoracentesis**
      1. **Indications.** A diagnostic thoracentesis is indicated for any pleural effusion of unknown etiology. Pleural effusions are generally categorized as transudative or exudative. This differentiation of pleural fluid is based on its microscopic, gross, and biochemical characteristics. A wide variety of laboratory studies are available for studying pleural fluid. The patient's clinical presentation should guide the studies obtained. A pleural fluid–serum lactate dehydrogenase (LDH) ratio >0.6 and a fluid–serum protein ratio >0.5 indicate an exudative effusion, whereas a fluid–serum LDH ratio <0.6 and a fluid–serum protein ratio <0.5 indicate a transudative effusion. Fluid glucose level, amylase level, lipid level, and pH should also be measured when analyzing pleural fluid. Cytologic examination for malignant cells should be obtained when a malignant effusion is considered. If an infectious etiology is suspected, Gram stain and culture for bacteria and fungi are necessary (*Chest* 1997;111:970). Therapeutic thoracentesis is indicated to relieve shortness of breath or discomfort from large pleural effusions. When repeated therapeutic thoracentesis is needed to treat recurrent pleural effusions, chest tube drainage and pleurosclerosis should be considered (*Am Rev Respir Dis* 1989;140:257).
      2. **Technique.** The site for thoracentesis depends on the location of the effusion, which can be determined by physical and radiographic examination. For free-flowing effusions, the patient is seated upright and slightly forward. The thorax should be entered posteriorly, 4 to 6 cm lateral to the spinal column and one to two interspaces below the cessation of tactile fremitus and where percussion is dull. Loculated effusions can be localized by ultrasonography, and the site for thoracentesis is marked on the skin. The site is prepared with povidone-iodine and draped with sterile towels. Lidocaine 1% is infiltrated into the subcutaneous tissue covering the rib below the interspace to be entered. The infiltration is carried deep to the periosteum of the rib. Next, placing negative pressure on the syringe, the needle is advanced slowly over the top of the rib, with care taken to avoid injury to the neurovascular bundle. The needle is advanced until pleural fluid is returned; then it is withdrawn a fraction, and lidocaine is injected to anesthetize the pleura. Lidocaine is then infiltrated into the intercostal muscles as the needle is withdrawn.

      Most thoracentesis kits contain a long 14-gauge needle inserted into a plastic catheter with an attached syringe and stopcock. The needle-catheter apparatus is introduced at the level of the rib below the interspace to be entered. With negative pressure applied to the syringe, the needle is slowly advanced over the top of the rib and into the pleural cavity until fluid is returned. Aspiration of air bubbles indicates puncture of the lung parenchyma; the needle should be promptly removed under negative pressure. Once the needle is in the pleural space, the catheter is advanced over the needle toward the diaphragm. Special attention is taken not to advance the needle as the catheter is being directed into the pleural space. A drainage bag is attached to the stopcock to remove the pleural fluid. The amount of fluid removed depends on the indication for the thoracentesis. A diagnostic tap requires 20 to 30 mL fluid for the appropriate tests, and a therapeutic tap can drain 1 to 2 L fluid. A chest x-ray should be obtained after the procedure to evaluate for pneumothorax and resolution of the effusion.

   3. Complications. Pneumothorax is the most common complication of thoracentesis. It must be treated with a tube thoracostomy and negative suction until the air leak seals. Reexpansion pulmonary edema is common
   after therapeutic thoracentesis when a large amount of fluid is removed
   at one time. To minimize the occurrence of this complication, no more
   than 1.5 to 2.0 L should be removed at a time. Hemothorax, infection, injury to the neurovascular bundle, and subcutaneous hematoma are other
   complications that can follow this procedure.
B. Tube thoracostomy
   1. Indications. Tube thoracostomy is indicated for a pneumothorax, hemothorax, recurrent pleural effusion, chylothorax, and empyema. The need for
   a chest tube may be emergent (e.g., a trauma situation) or elective (e.g.,
   the drainage of a recurrent malignant effusion). Under either circumstance, a good understanding of thoracic anatomy is needed to prevent
   injuries to the lung parenchyma, diaphragm, intercostal neurovascular
   bundles, and mediastinum. The lung may have adhesions to the chest wall
   that make insertion and advancement of the thoracostomy tube difficult.
   The intercostal neurovascular bundle runs in a groove on the inferior aspect of each rib; therefore, the tube should be passed over the top of the
   rib to avoid injury. Because, during normal respiration, the diaphragm
   can rise to the level of the fourth intercostal space, insertion of the chest
   tube lower than the sixth interspace is to be discouraged. Profound coagulopathy is a relative contraindication to the placement of a chest tube,
   and all efforts should be made to correct the coagulopathy before the tube
   is placed.
   2. Technique. The size of thoracostomy tube needed depends on the material
   to be drained. Generally, a 24 to 28 French tube directed apically is used
   for a pneumothorax, and a 28 to 32 French tube directed basally is used
   for the evacuation of a hemothorax and a dependent pleural effusion. The
   patient is placed in the lateral position with the unaffected side down,
   and the head of the bed is inclined 10 to 15 degrees. The patient's arm
   on the affected side is extended forward or above the head. With the
   skin prepared, 1% lidocaine is infiltrated over the fifth or sixth rib in
   the middle or anterior axillary line by the technique described in the
   previous section. A 2- to 3-cm transverse incision is made through the
   skin and subcutaneous tissue. A curved clamp is used to bluntly dissect
   an oblique tract to the rib (Fig. 42-3A). With careful spreading, the clamp
   is advanced over the top of the rib. The parietal pleura is punctured with
   the clamp, and an efflux of air or fluid is usually encountered. A finger is
   introduced into the tract to ensure passage into the pleural space and to
   lyse any adhesions at the point of entry (Fig. 42-3B). With the clamp as
   a guide, the chest tube is introduced into the pleural space (Fig. 42-3C).
   It is directed apically for pneumothorax and basally and posteriorly for
   dependent effusions. A clamp placed at the free end of the chest tube
   prevents drainage from the chest until the tube can be connected to a
   closed suction or water-seal system. The chest tube is advanced until the
   last hole of the tube is clearly inside the thoracic cavity. When the tube is
   positioned properly and functioning adequately, it is secured to the skin
   with two heavy silk sutures and covered with an occlusive dressing to
   prevent air leaks. Some surgeons place a U-stitch around the chest tube
   to be used as a purse-string suture when the tube is removed. A chest x-
   ray is obtained after the procedure to assess reexpansion of the lung and
   the tube position. The trocar insertion technique has been discouraged
   because of a high incidence of complications, but safe modifications of the
   technique have been described (*J Am Coll Surg* 1994;179:230).
   3. Complications. The majority of complications are due to improper insertion technique and tube placement. Low placement of a chest tube can
   result in injury to the diaphragm, with associated injury to the liver or
   spleen. Management of a punctured diaphragm or intraperitoneal chest

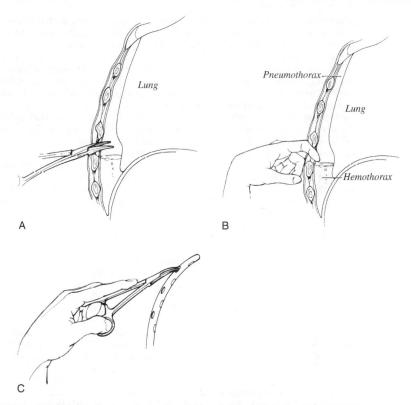

Figure 42-3. Tube thoracostomy placement. **A:** Pleural space entered by blunt spreading of the clamp over the top of the adjacent rib. **B:** A finger is introduced to ensure position within the pleural space and to lyse adhesions. **C:** The chest tube is placed into the tunnel and directed with the help of a Kelly clamp. The tube is directed caudal for an effusion or hemothorax and cephalad for a pneumothorax.

tube must be tailored to the particular situation. Some tubes may be removed without significant consequence, and others may require operative management. Failure to guide the tube into the pleural space can result in dissection of the extrapleural plane. This can be a difficult diagnosis, but anteroposterior and lateral chest radiographs should reveal a lung that has failed to reexpand and suggest a chest tube placed outside the thorax. The tube should be removed and placed within the thoracic cavity to reexpand the lung. Parenchymal or hilar injuries or cardiac contusions can occur with overzealous advancement of the tube or dissection of pleural adhesions. Other complications include subcutaneous emphysema, reexpansion pulmonary edema, phrenic nerve injury, esophageal perforation, contralateral pneumothorax, and neurovascular bundle injury. Late complications include empyema, infection along the chest tube tract, and abscess.

III. Peritoneal drainage procedure
    A. Paracentesis
        1. Indications. Bedside paracentesis is a useful diagnostic and therapeutic tool. A diagnostic paracentesis is indicated in the case of ascites with an unknown etiology. Measurement of the fluid protein, LDH, amylase,

specific gravity, red blood cell count, white blood cell count with differential, and fibrinogen can help establish a diagnosis. Cytology, Gram stain, and culture are other useful laboratory tests. A therapeutic paracentesis is indicated for patients with respiratory compromise or discomfort caused by tense ascites and in patients with ascites refractory to medical management. Relative contraindications include previous abdominal surgery, pregnancy, coagulopathy, and progressive liver failure with encephalopathy or hepatorenal syndrome.

2. **Technique.** The patient's bladder is emptied, either by the patient or by the placement of a Foley catheter. With the patient lying supine, the level of the ascites can be determined by locating the transition from dullness to tympany with percussion. Depending on the height of the ascites, a midline or lateral approach can be used. Care must be taken with the midline approach because the air-filled bowel tends to float on top of the ascites. The skin at the site of entry should be prepared and draped. One-percent lidocaine is infiltrated subcutaneously and is carried to the level of the peritoneum. For the midline approach, a needle is introduced at a point midway between the umbilicus and the pubis symphysis. For the lateral approach, the point of entry can be in the right or left lower quadrant in the area bound by the lateral border of the rectus abdominis muscle, the line between the umbilicus and the anterior iliac spine, and the line between the anterior iliac spine and the pubis symphysis. A simple diagnostic tap can be achieved by inserting a 22-gauge needle into the peritoneal cavity and aspirating 20 to 30 mL fluid. Constant negative pressure should be applied to the syringe, and care is taken not to advance the needle beyond the point where ascites is encountered. For a therapeutic paracentesis, a 14-gauge needle fit with a catheter allows for efficient drainage of larger volumes of ascites. With either the midline or the lateral approach, once ascites is returned, the catheter is advanced over the needle and directed toward the pelvis. A drainage bag is attached to the catheter to collect and measure the fluid removed. Intravenous volume replacement with 10 g 25% albumin for each liter of ascites removed helps prevent hypovolemia and hypotension with large-volume taps.

3. **Complications.** Injuries to the bowel or bladder can occur with percutaneous paracentesis. Emptying the bladder, avoiding the insertion of the needle near surgical scars, and maintaining control of the needle once inside the peritoneum help to minimize these injuries. Intraperitoneal hemorrhage from injury to a mesenteric vessel can occur. Laceration of the inferior epigastric vessels can lead to a hematoma of the rectus sheath or the abdominal wall. In patients with large, recurrent ascites, a persistent leakage of ascites from the site of entry can result. These fistulas usually close spontaneously, but they can persist and develop into difficult management issues. Late complications include peritonitis and abdominal wall abscess.

IV. **Emergency airways**

A. **Endotracheal (ET) intubation**

1. **Indications.** Establishment of a secure airway is the first priority in the management of an acutely ill patient. The airway can be secured either mechanically, with an ET tube, or surgically, with a tracheostomy or cricothyroidotomy. ET intubation is indicated when a patient is unable to adequately oxygenate and ventilate. Cardiac arrest, pneumonia, adult respiratory distress syndrome, pulmonary edema, inhalation injury, multisystem trauma, sepsis, postoperative hemodynamic instability, and altered mental status owing to trauma, anesthesia, or coma are reasons for failure to oxygenate or ventilate. The oral approach under direct vision is the most common method of intubating the trachea. Other approaches include nasotracheal and endoscopic intubation; however, only orotracheal intubation is described here. Relative contraindications to orotracheal

intubation include maxillofacial trauma, laryngeal injury, and cervical spine injury.

2. **Technique.** Whether orotracheal intubation is emergent or elective, the principles are the same. Preoxygenation with a bag-valve-mask apparatus and 100% oxygen suction, adequate sedation, and muscle relaxation; an appropriately sized ET tube; and a functional laryngoscope are required. Two types of laryngeal scope blades are available: a straight blade (Miller) and a curved blade (Macintosh). The straight blade may provide better visualization in children, and the curved blade may be better for patients with short, thick necks. The physician should be comfortable using either blade. With the physician at the patient's head, the head is positioned so that the pharyngeal and laryngeal axes are in alignment (Fig. 42-4A). The patient's head and neck are fully extended into the "sniffing" position. With the nondominant hand, the physician opens the patient's mouth with the thumb and index finger on the patient's lower and upper teeth, respectively. Using the middle finger, the physician sweeps the patient's tongue to the side. The oropharynx is inspected, and foreign bodies or secretions are removed. The blade of the laryngoscope

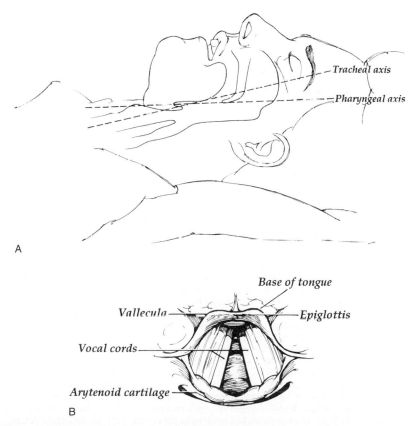

Figure 42-4. Orotracheal intubation. **A:** Fully extending the patient's head into the "sniffing" position aligns the pharyngeal and laryngeal axes. This allows for the best visualization of the airway. **B:** View of the larynx and airway during oral intubation of the trachea.

is introduced and advanced with gentle traction upward and toward the patient's feet. Once the epiglottis is visualized, the tip of the blade is positioned in the vallecula. Great care must be taken not to use the handle as a lever against the patient's teeth and lips. The glottic opening and vocal cords should come into view (Fig. 42-4B). If not, gently increase the upward and caudal traction or have an assistant place external pressure on the cricoid and thyroid cartilage. If still unable to visualize the glottic opening, remove the blade, oxygenate and reposition the patient, and try again. Once the glottic opening is adequately visualized, the ET tube is advanced under direct vision until the cuff passes through the vocal cords. The cuff is inserted roughly 2 cm past the vocal cords, and the patient's incisors should rest at the 19- to 23-cm markings on the tube. The stylet and laryngoscope are carefully removed while maintaining control and the position of the ET tube. The cuff is inflated, and proper position is confirmed by osculating bilateral breath sounds or monitoring end-tidal carbon dioxide. Once position is confirmed, the ET tube is secured to the patient. An anteroposterior chest x-ray is obtained to confirm position. When in the ideal position, the tip of the ET tube is 2 to 4 cm above the carina.

   3. **Complications.** Unsuccessful attempts to intubate the trachea must be followed by face-mask ventilation and oxygenation with 100% oxygen. Do not allow the patient to go for more than 30 seconds without ventilation and oxygen when attempting to intubate the trachea. If the patient cannot be manually ventilated or the most experienced person is unable to intubate the trachea, an emergent surgical airway must be secured (discussed in the following section). Intubation of the esophagus or right main-stem bronchus can readily be diagnosed by absent breath sounds associated with epigastric gargling on manual ventilation and right-sided breath sounds with absent left-sided breath sounds, respectively. Chipped teeth, emesis, vocal cord injury, laryngospasm, and soft-tissue injury to lips, tongue, and gums may all complicate ET intubation.

B. **Cricothyroidotomy**
   1. **Indications.** Cricothyroidotomy is indicated when attempts at oral or nasal intubation have failed or when maxillofacial injury prohibits oral or nasal intubation. In cases of trauma, blood or maxillofacial injuries may prevent direct visualization of the larynx. In this instance, cricothyroidotomy is the procedure of choice. Other indications for a surgical airway include cervical spine injuries and difficulty intubating the patient because of his or her location. In extreme cases, a large-bore needle can be placed through the cricothyroid membrane as a temporary mode of ventilation until a more secure airway can be obtained. Laryngeal tracheal separation and laryngeal trauma are contraindications to this procedure. Percutaneous dilational cricothyroidotomy is a safe and effective method of emergently obtaining an airway, and it is gaining widespread use (*Intensive Care Med* 1996;22:937).
   2. **Technique.** Because the vast majority of cricothyroidotomies are done in emergent situations, an excellent understanding of the anatomy in the region of the trachea is necessary to minimize complications. The thyroid cartilage is easily identified in the midline of the neck (Fig. 42-5). The cricoid, the only complete cartilaginous ring, is the first ring inferior to the thyroid cartilage. The cricothyroid membrane joins these two cartilages and is an avascular membrane. Inferior to the cricoid and straddling the trachea is the isthmus of the thyroid gland. The thyroid lobes lie lateral to the trachea, and the superior poles can extend to the level of the thyroid cartilage. If time permits, the area is prepared, draped, and anesthetized with 1% lidocaine. The cricoid cartilage is identified and held firmly and circumferentially in the physician's nondominant hand until the end of the procedure. Using a No. 11 or 15 blade, a small 3- to 5-cm transverse incision is made over the cricothyroid membrane. The incision is carried

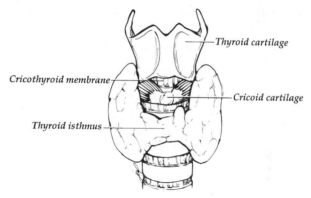

Figure 42-5. Anatomy of the larynx.

deep until the airway is entered through the cricothyroid membrane. The index finger of the physician's nondominant hand can be used to identify landmarks as the dissection proceeds. Using a clamp, a tracheal dilator, or the end of the scalpel handle, widen the tract. Insert the tracheostomy tube along its curve into the trachea, inflate the cuff, and check for bilateral breath sounds. If breath sounds are present, secure the tracheostomy to the skin by suturing the tabs to the skin with heavy, nonabsorbable, monofilament suture.

3. **Complications.** Creation of a false passage when inserting the tracheostomy tube is the most common complication. This should become evident by the absence of breath sounds and the development of subcutaneous emphysema. Pneumothorax can also occur. Injury to surrounding structures, such as the thyroid, parathyroids, esophagus, anterior jugular veins, and recurrent laryngeal nerves, can occur in situations of extreme urgency. Subglottic stenosis and granuloma formation are potential long-term complications.

C. **Percutenous tracheostomy**

1. **Indications.** The theoretical advantages of percutenous tracheostomy (PDT) over standard operative tracheostomy are primarily related to reduced tissue trauma and ease of use at the bedside, allowing it to be done in conjunction with other bedside procedures, such as percutaneous endoscopic gastrostomy. Following the skin incision, the remainder of the PDT procedure is dilational. Less tissue devitalization should result in less bleeding, fewer infections, a low risk of subglottic stenosis, and a better cosmetic result. The ability to perform PDT at the bedside ensures that patients who could benefit from tracheostomy have the procedure performed as soon as possible and at the same time helps avoid the transportation of critically ill patients to the operating room.

2. **Technique.** Although the technique may be performed blind, whenever possible the trachea should be visualized via an intubating fiberoptic bronchoscope passed down the tracheal tube. Two operators are required for the procedure, one performing the tracheostomy, and one at the head of the patient looking after the airway, anaesthesia, and bronchoscopy. The bronchoscope is passed through a tracheal tube and the anatomy of the airway visualized. The aim of the fiberoptic scope is to ensure correct initial placement of the introducer needle, in the midline and through the second or third tracheal rings. Subsequent to this, it will be used to monitor dilation of the trachea and ensure the introducer does not remain in the trachea. After an initial 1.5-cm skin incision over the first

tracheal ring, blunt dissection is performed down to the level of the pre-tracheal fascia using a mosquito hemostat, and the existing endotracheal tube is withdrawn into the proximal larynx, permitting a needle to be introduced between the first and second or second and third tracheal rings. Placement of a guidewire is followed by progressive dilation of the tracheostoma using beveled plastic dilators. Once the tracheostoma has been adequately dilated, the tracheostomy tube is introduced into the trachea over the same guidewire utilizing a dilator as an obturator.

3. **Complications.** In many studies, there was no significant difference in the rate of intraprocedural complications; however, postprocedural complications (accidental decannulation, bleeding, stomal infection) occurred significantly more frequently in patients randomized to open tracheostomy (12% for PDT versus 41% for open tracheostomy).

Commonly Used Formulas*

Cardiovascular formulas

Formula	Normal range
Arterial carbon dioxide tension (Pa_{CO_2})	35–45 mm Hg
Arterial carbon dioxide content (Ca_{CO_2})	48–50 mL/dL
Arterial oxygen content (Ca_{O_2})	20 vol%
$\quad Ca_{O_2} = 1.36$ [hemoglobin (Hgb)] $(Sa_{O_2}) + 0.003 (Pa_{O_2})$	
Arterial oxygen saturation (Sa_{O_2})	93–98%
Arterial oxygen tension (Pa_{O_2})	70–100 mm Hg
Body-surface area (BSA)	1.73 m^2 for 70-kg adult
Carbon dioxide production (V_{CO_2})	2.3 mL/kg per min
Heart rate (HR)	60–100 beats per min
$\quad$ Maximum age-adjusted HR $= 220 -$ age in yr	
Cardiac output (CO)	4–8 L per min
$\quad$ Fick equation: $V_{O_2}/8.5 (Ca_{O_2} - C\bar{v}_{O_2})$	
Physiologic: CO $=$ HR $\times$ SV	
Cardiac index (CI)	2.5–4.0 L per min
$\quad$ CI $=$ CO/BSA	
Central venous pressure (CVP)	0–8 mm Hg
Fraction of inspired oxygen (F_{IO_2})	0.21–1.0
Left atrial pressure (LAP)	3–12 mm Hg
Left ventricular ejection fraction (LVEF)	55–70%
Left ventricular end-diastolic volume (LVEDV)	70 mL/m^2
Left ventricular systolic pressure (LVS)	100–140 mm Hg
Mean arterial pressure (MAP)	70–105 mm Hg
$\quad$ MAP $= [(SBP - DBP)/3] + DBP$	
$\quad$ SBP $=$ systolic blood pressure	
$\quad$ DBP $=$ diastolic blood pressure	
Mixed venous carbon dioxide tension ($P\bar{v}_{CO_2}$)	41–51 mm Hg
Mixed venous oxygen content ($C\bar{v}_{O_2}$)	15 vol%
$\quad C\bar{v}_{O_2} = 1.36$ (Hgb) $(S\bar{v}_{O_2}) + 0.003 (M\bar{v}_{O_2})$	
$\quad$ Mixed venous oxygen saturation ($S\bar{v}_{O_2}$)	75%
$\quad$ Mixed venous oxygen tension ($M\bar{v}_{O_2}$)	35–40 mm Hg
Oxygen consumption (V_{O_2})	250 mL per min
Oxygen delivery (O_2 del)	640–1,000 mL per min at rest
$\quad O_2$ del $=$ CO $\times$ Ca$_{CO_2}$	
Pulmonary artery pressure, mean (PAP)	5–10 mm Hg
Pulmonary artery diastolic pressure (PAD)	5–12 mm Hg
Pulmonary artery systolic pressure (PAS)	15–30 mm Hg
Pulmonary capillary wedge pressure (PCWP)	5–12 mm Hg
Pulmonary vascular resistance (PVR)	<3 dynes $\times$ sec/cm^3
$\quad$ PVR $=$ (PAP $-$ PCWP)/CO	
Pulse pressure (PP)	40 mm Hg
PP $=$ SBP $-$ DBP	
Right atrial pressure (RAP)	0–8 mm Hg
Right ventricular diastolic pressure (RVD)	0–8 mm Hg
Right ventricular systolic pressure (RVS)	15–28 mm Hg

*Compiled by Sunil M. Prasad.

Formula	**Normal range**
Stroke volume (SV)	60–100 mL/beat
$SV = CO/HR$	
Stroke volume index (SVI)	33–47 mL/beat/m^2
$SVI = 1,000\ (CO)/(HR)\ (BSA)$	
Systemic vascular resistance (SVR)	<20 dynes $\times$ sec/cm^3
$SVR = (MAP - RAP)/CO$	

Pulmonary formulas

Formula	**Normal range**
Alveolar arterial oxygen gradient (P[A-a] O_2)	3–16 mm Hg
Age correction: A-a gradient = $2.5 + age/4$	
Alveolar oxygen tension (PaO$_2$)	Room air: 100 mm Hg
$PaO_2 = 713\ (FIO_2) - (PaCO_2/0.8)$ at sea level	100%: 673 mm Hg
Alveolar carbon dioxide tension (PaCO$_2$)	40 mm Hg
$PaCO_2 = \dot{V}\ CO_2 \times 0.863/VA$	
Alveolar ventilation (VA)	4 L per min
$VA = 0.863\ (\dot{V}\ CO_2)/PaCO_2$	
Arterial blood gas format	
pH/PaCO$_2$/PaO$_2$/HCO$_3{}^-$, FIO$_2$	
pH	7.35–7.45
PaCO$_2$	35–45 mm Hg
PaO$_2$	70–100 mm Hg
HCO$_3{}^-$	24–30 mmol/L
FIO$_2$	21% room air
Expiratory reserve volume (ERV)	25% VC
$ERV = FRC - RV$	
Forced expiratory volume in 1 sec (FEV$_1$)	$FEV_1 = 83\%$
Forced expiratory volume in 2 sec (FEV$_2$)	$FEV_2 = 94\%$
Functional residual capacity (FRC)	1.8–3.4 L
$FRC = ERV + RV$	
Henderson-Hasselbalch equation	pH 7.4
$pH = pK + log\ (base/acid)$	
$H_2O + CO_2 \leftrightarrow H_2CO_3 \leftrightarrow HCO_3{}^- + H^+$	
$pH = 6.1 + log\ (HCO_3{}^-/CO_2)$	
Inspiratory capacity (IC)	1.0–2.4 L
$IC = $ inspiratory reserve volume (IRV) $ + V_T$	
Minute ventilation (V$_E$)	90 mL/kg per min
$V_E = V_T \times RR$ (respiratory rate)	
Negative inspiratory force (NIF)	60–100 cm H$_2$O
Pulmonary blood flow (QT)	5 L per min
Pulmonary shunt blood volume (QS)	150 mL per min
Pulmonary shunt fraction (QS/QT)	2–3%
Residual volume (RV)	1.0–2.4 L
Tidal volume (V$_T$)	6–7 mL/kg
Total lung capacity (TLC)	4–6 L
$TLC = VC + RV$	
Vital capacity (VC)	3–5 L
$VC = IRV + ERV + V_T$	

Renal formulas

Degree of renal impairment indicated by creatinine clearance (Cl$_{Cr}$)

Cl$_{Cr}$ (mL per min)	**Degree of renal impairment**
>100	Normal
40–60	Mild
10–40	Moderate
<10	Severe

Fractional excretion of sodium (FeNa⁺)

$FeNa^+ = $ (urine $Na^+ \times$ serum Cr)/(urine Cr $\times$ serum Na^+) $\times$ 100%

Fractional excretion of X [X = K^+, blood urea nitrogen (BUN), amylase, and so forth] can be calculated by replacing Na^+ with X in preceding formula.

Free water clearance (Cl_{H_2O})

Normal value = −20

$Cl_{H_2O} = V - (U_{osm} \times V)/P_{osm}$

where V = urine volume $\times$ (mL/min), U_{osm} = measured urine osmolality, and P_{osm} = plasma osmolality.

Glomerular filtration rate (GFR)

GFR = ultrafiltrate/time
Normal GFR = 80 L per day

Daily renal solute and water exchange for a normal adult man

	Filtered	Excreted	Percentage reabsorbed
Na^+ (mEq)	26,000	100–250	>99
Cl^- (mEq)	21,000	100–250	>99
K^+ (mEq)	800	40–120	85–95
HCO_3^- (mEq)	4,800	0	100
Glucose (mmol/L)	900	0	100
Urea (mmol/L)	900	400	44
Creatinine (mmol/L)	15	15	0
H_2O (L)	180	0.5–3.0	98–99

Urine output (UO)

UO = 0.5–1.0 mL/kg per hr
Oliguria = <500 mL/day

Metabolic and fluid formulas

Anion gap (AG)
$\quad$ AG = $Na^+ - (Cl^- + HCO_{3-})$
Plasma osmolality (calculated)
Sodium deficit = total body water $\times$
$\quad$ [140 − Na^+ (mmol)]
Total body water (TBW)

Extracellular fluid (ECF)
Interstitial fluid (ISF)
Plasma
Whole blood
Intracellular fluid (ICF)

Normal range
8–12 mEq/L

270–300 mOsm/L

Male, 0.6 $\times$ lean body wt (kg)
Female, 0.5 $\times$ lean body wt (kg)
$^1/_3$ TBW
$^3/_4$ ECF
$^1/_4$ ECF
75 mL/kg
$^2/_3$ TBW

Bodily fluid composition (mEq/L)

Fluid	Na^+	Cl^-	K^+	HCO_3^-	H^+	Volume (L/day)
Saliva	30–60	15–40	20	15–50	—	0.5–1.5
Gastric	60–100	90–140	10	—	30–100	1.0–4.0
Duodenum	140	80	5	50	—	1.0–3.0
Bile	140	100	5	50	—	0.5–1.5

Fluid	Na$^+$	Cl$^-$	K$^+$	HCO$_3$$^-$	H$^+$	Volume (L/day)
Pancreas	140	75	5	90	—	1.0
Jejunum	100	100	5	10	—	1.0–2.0
Ileum	130	110	10	30	—	1.0–2.0
Colon	60	40	30	20	—	—

Composition of commonly used intravenous fluids (mEq/L)

Fluid	Na$^+$	Cl	K$^+$	Ca^{2+}	Base	Glucose	pH	mOsm/L
0.9% normal saline	154	154	—	—	—	—	5.0	292
5% dextrose 0.9% NS	154	154	—	—	—	50	5.0	565
Lactated Ringer solution	130	109	4	4	28	—	6.5	277
D5W	—	—	—	—	—	50	4.0	274
5% albumin	154	154	—	—	—	—	7.0	~300
Hetastarch	154	154	—	—	—	60	5.5	310

Nutrition formulas

Actual energy expenditure (AAE)

AAE = basal energy expenditure (BEE) × [metabolic activity factor (MAF) + 1.0]

Basal energy expenditure in kcal/day (Harris-Benedict equation)

Men: kcal/24 hr = 66 + [13.7 × wt (kg)] + [5 × ht (cm)] − (6.8 × age)
Women: kcal/24 hr = 655 + [9.6 × wt (kg)] + [1.8 × ht (cm)] − (4.7 × age)
Estimate: 25–30 kcal/kg/day

Body mass index

BMI = (weight in kilograms/(height in meters) × (height in meters))

Calorie conversion

Substrate	Kcal
Carbohydrate	1 g = 3.4
Fat, long chain	1 g = 9.0
Fat, medium chain	1 g = 7.1
Protein	1 g = 4.0

Ideal body weight (estimate)

Men: 50 kg for 5 ft + 2.3 kg for every 1 in. thereafter
Women: 45.5 kg for 5 ft + 2.3 kg every 1 in. thereafter
Ideal calorie-nitrogen ratio = 135–200:1

Metabolic activity factor

Activity factor + injury factor + fever factor + growth factor

Condition	Activity factor
Bedrest	0.2
Moderately active	0.35
Active	0.5

Condition	Injury factor
Minor surgery	0.2
Major surgery	0.35
Major burn	1.0

Condition	Growth factor
Moderate weight loss	0.05
Severe weight loss	0.13

Fever factor: $0.13°C$ above $37°C$

Protein requirement and nitrogen balance

Must be adjusted for renal insufficiency.

Nitrogen (N_2): 0.8–2.0 g/kg per 24 hr
6.25 g protein = 1 g
N_2 balance = protein uptake (g)/6.25 − [UUN + 4 g (insensible loss)]
Urinary urea nitrogen (UUN) = collected urinary N_2 in 24 hr

Respiratory quotient

$\dot{V}CO_2/\dot{V}O_2$

Oxidized substrate	Value
Pure fat	0.7
Pure protein	0.8
Pure carbohydrate	1.0
Fat synthesis	1.3

Unit conversions

Length
1 in. = 2.54 cm
1 cm = 0.3973 in.

Pressure
1 mm Hg = 0.735 cm H_2O
1 cm H_2O = 1.36 mm Hg

Temperature
$°F = 9/5 \ °C + 32$
$°C = 5/9 \ (°F − 32)$

Weight
1 lb = 0.454 kg
1 kg = 2.204 lb

Volume
1 qt = 0.943 L
1 L = 1.06 qt

Index

anticoagulants in, endogenous, 89
evaluation of, 90–91
fibrinolytic system in, 89–90
mechanisms of, 88, 89f
in wounds, acute, 156
Hemostatic agents, 109. *See also* specific agents
Hemothorax, 430, 443
Heparin
for arterial occlusion of extremity, 347, 348
for deep venous thrombosis
perioperative prophylaxis against, 14, 14t
postoperative, 28
in ICU, 195t
perioperative, 13, 13t
Heparin, low-molecular-weight, 14, 99, 392
Heparin, unfractionated, 14, 98–99, 392
Heparin-induced thrombocytopenia (HIT), 92–93, 92t
Hepatic. *See also* Liver entries
Hepatic abscess, 300–301
Hepatic adenoma, 295
Hepatic artery aneurysms, 372–373
Hepatic artery thrombosis, after liver transplantation, 480
Hepatic cysts, 301–302
Hepatic encephalopathy, 306
Hepatic failure, nutrition in, 51
Hepatic injuries, 446–447
Hepatic resection, 293–294. *See also* Liver cancer
Hepatic transplantation, 476–482. *See also* Liver transplantation
Hepatic tumors, pediatric, 636–637
Hepatoblastoma, pediatric, 636–637
Hepatocellular carcinoma (HCC), 296–298
pediatric, 636–637
Hepatoma, 296–298
Hereditary elliptocytosis, splenectomy for, 328
Hereditary hemolytic anemias, 103–104, 103t, 328
Hereditary nonpolyposis colorectal cancer syndrome (HNPCC), 398
Hereditary renal carcinoma (HRC), 402
Hereditary spherocytosis, 328
Hereditary tumor syndromes, 395–403
ataxia-telangiectasia, 396
breast cancer, 395–396
colorectal cancer, 396–399 (*See also* Colorectal cancer, hereditary)
Cowden disease, 396
endocrine tumors, 399–401
multiple endocrine neoplasia type 1 (MEN-1), 399–400
multiple endocrine neoplasia type 2 (MEN-2), 400–401
genetic testing and counseling for, 403
introduction to, 395
Li-Fraumeni syndrome, 396
melanoma, 402–403
neurofibromatosis type 1 (NF1), 401
renal carcinoma, 402
retinoblastoma, 401
sarcomas, 401
Von Hippel-Lindau syndrome, 402
Wilm tumor (nephroblastoma), 402
Hernias, 510–520
abdominal wall, 519–520
combined, 510
congenital diaphragmatic, 618–619
direct, 510

epigastric, 519
femoral, 517–518
pediatric, 633–634
hiatal, 197–198
incarcerated, 226, 510
incisional, 519
indirect sacs, 510
inguinal, 510–517 (*See also* Inguinal hernias)
pediatric, 633–634
internal, 518–519
lumbar, 519
obturator, 519
pantaloon, 510
sliding, 510
Spigelian, 519
umbilical, 519
Herniation, 432, 646
Herniation syndromes, 646
Herpes simplex virus (HSV) infection, in immunocompromised, 464t, 465
Hetastarch, in fluid therapy, 80t, 81
Heterotopic pancreas, 289
Hiatal hernia, 197–198
Hickman catheter, 127–128
Hidradenitis suppurativa, 268
High-frequency oscillatory ventilation (HFOV), 184
High-humidity mask, 181, 181t
High-pressure injection injuries, of hand, 578
Hilar tumor, 319–321
Hill posterior gastropexy, 201
Hip dislocation, 650, 655
Hirschsprung disease, 626–627
Hirudin, 99
Histocompatibility, of transplant organ, 462
Hodgkin lymphoma, 330
Hohn catheter, 127
Hormone replacement therapy, venous thromboembolism from, 390
Hospital notes, 32–33, 33t, 34t
Hospital orders, 31–32
Howship-Romberg sign, 519
Human bite, 169, 577
Humerus fractures, 652
Hutchinson freckle, 502
Hydatid cysts, 292, 301–302, 330
Hydralazine, 190t
Hydroceles, 634, 676–677
Hydrocephalus, 647
Hydrocolloids, in wound care, 166, 172t
Hydrofibers, in wound care, 167
Hydrogels, in wound care, 166, 172t–173t
Hydrogen peroxide, in wound care, 174t
Hydromorphone, 124, 180
Hydroxyethyl starch, in fluid therapy, 80t, 81
Hygroma, cystic, 551
Hyoid bone, 548
Hyperbilirubinemia, 631–632
Hypercalcemia, 75–76, 412
Hypercoagulable states, 96–98
Hypercortisolism, 420–421, 425
Hyperglycemia, 46, 49
Hyperhomocysteinemia, 97
Hyperlipidemia, after cardiac surgery, 600
Hypermagnesemia, 79
Hypernatremia, 46, 49, 70–72, 71f
Hyperosmolarity, 46, 49
Hyperoxaluria, in short-bowel syndrome, 339
Hyperparathyroid crisis, 415

Mucoepidermoid carcinoma, 547
Mucosa, intestinal, 223
Mucus plugging, after thoracic surgery, 614
Muir-Torre syndrome (MTS), 398–399
Multinodular goiter, 407
Multiple endocrine neoplasia type 1 (MEN-1), 399–400
Multiple endocrine neoplasia type 2 (MEN-2), 400–401
Multiple hamartoma syndrome, 396
Multiple polyposis coli, 272
Mumps, 547
Murph's sign, 244, 309
Muscle flaps, 561, 562
Muscle infections, postoperative, 27
Muscle relaxants, nondepolarizing, 119–120, 119t
Muscularis mucosae, intestinal wall, 223
Muscularis propria, intestinal wall, 223
Musculocutaneous flaps, 562
Myasthenia gravis, 549, 606–607
Mycophenolate mofetil, 463
Mycosis fungoides, wound healing in, 159
Myelodysplastic disorders, splenectomy for, 329
Myeloid metaplasia, splenectomy for, 329
Myeloproliferative disorders, splenectomy for, 329
Myocardial infarction (MI)
  acute, 584–585
  after thoracic surgery, 614
  perioperative, 597
  postoperative, 20–22
  preoperative evaluation and management after, 3
Myocardial ischemia, postoperative, 20–22
Myocyte regeneration, 593

N
N-acetylcysteine, for renal dysfunction, 193
Narcotics. *See also* specific drugs
  as anesthetics, 120
  in critical care, 180
  for postoperative analgesia, 123–124
Nasal cannula, 181, 181t
Nasal choanae, 542
Nasal choanal atresia, posterior, 543
Nasal disorders, 543–545
  adenoid hypertrophy, 544
  congenital, 543
  diagnostic tests for, 543
  foreign bodies, 544
  inflammatory, 543–544
    nasal polyps, 544
  neoplasms, 544–545
  septal deviation, 544
  trauma, 545–546
Nasal endotracheal intubation, 181. *See also* Endotracheal (ET) intubation
Nasal fractures, 439, 545
Nasal polyps, inflammatory, 544
Nasal septal deviation, 544
Nasal valve, 542
Nasobiliary (NB) tubes, 143
Nasoenteric (NET) feeding tubes, 141–142
Nasogastric (NG) tubes, 139–140
Nasojejunal feeding tubes, 141–142
Nasopharyngeal angiofibroma, juvenile, 545
Nasopharyngeal neoplasms, 544–545
Native vein fistulas, 135–137
Nausea, after anesthesia, 121

Neck
  anatomy of, 550, 699f
  physiology of, 550
  trauma survey of, 436–437
Neck disorders, 550–553
  branchial anomalies, 551
  congenital lesions, 550–551
  cystic hygroma, 551
  infections, 551–552
  neoplasms
    benign, 552
    malignant, 552–553
  teratomas and dermoid cysts, 551
  thyroglossal duct cysts, 550–551
Neck injuries, 440–441
Necrotizing enterocolitis (NEC), 623–624
Necrotizing infections
  anorectal, 267
  clostridial, severe postoperative, 26
  enterocolitis, 623–624
  hand, 578
  pancreatitis, 282
Needle localization biopsy, for breast cancer, 524
Neointimal hyperplasia, in synthetic graft, 137
Neoplasms. *See also* specific neoplasms
  colorectal, 271–279 (*See also* Colorectal neoplasia; specific cancers)
  esophageal, benign, 210–211
  nasal and nasopharyngeal, 544–545
  small intestine, 226, 235–239
  thyroid, 409–411 (*See also* Thyroid cancer)
Nephrectomy. *See also* specific indications
  pretransplant native, 470
  radical, 666
  for renovascular disease, 361
Nephroblastoma (Wilms tumor), 402
  pediatric, 635–636
Nephrogenic diabetes insipidus, 72
Nephrolithiasis, in short-bowel syndrome, 339
Nephrotoxins, perioperative, 8. *See also* specific nephrotoxins
Nerve block
  brachial plexus, 116–117
  cervical plexus, 117
  digital, 118
  intercostal, 117–118, 117f
  peripheral, for fracture/joint reductions, 662
Nerve graft, 557
Nerve injury, classification of, 564, 564t
Nerve palsies, after anesthesia, 122
Nerve repair, 564–565
Neurapraxia, 564t
Neuritis, vestibular, 542
Neuroblastoma, pediatric, 635, 636t
Neurofibromas, 236, 500–501, 552
Neurofibromatosis type 1 (NF1), 401
Neurogenic shock, 187t, 188, 191
Neurologic complications
  of cardiac surgery, 598
  perioperative, 18 (*See also* specific complications)
  postoperative, 18–20
Neurologic deficit, ischemic reversible, 356
Neuromuscular blockade, 119–120, 119t
Neuromuscular paralysis, in mechanical ventilation, 185
Neuropathy, 161
  peripheral (*See* Peripheral neuropathy)